Gorbach's
5-Minute Infectious Diseases Consult

2ND EDITION

Gorbach's
5-Minute
Infectious
Diseases
Consult

2ND EDITION

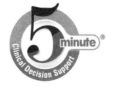

Editors

Matthew E. Falagas, MD, MSc, DSc
Director, Alfa Institute of Biomedical Sciences (AIBS)
Athens, Greece
Adjunct Associate Professor of Medicine
Tufts University School of Medicine
Boston, Massachusetts
Director, Infectious Diseases Clinic
Henry Dunant Hospital
Athens, Greece

Eleftherios Mylonakis, MD, PhD, FIDSA
Associate Professor of Medicine
Harvard Medical School
Massachusetts General Hospital
Division of Infectious Diseases
Boston, Massachusetts

Wolters Kluwer | Lippincott Williams & Wilkins
Health
Philadelphia · Baltimore · New York · London
Buenos Aires · Hong Kong · Sydney · Tokyo

Acquisitions Editor: Frances DeStefano
Product Manager: Leanne Vandetty
Production Manager: Bridgett Dougherty
Senior Manufacturing Manager: Benjamin Rivera
Marketing Manager: Kimberly Schonberger
Design Coordinator: Teresa Mallon
Production Service: Aptara, Inc.

© **2012 by LIPPINCOTT WILLIAMS & WILKINS, a WOLTERS KLUWER business**
Two Commerce Square
2001 Market Street
Philadelphia, PA 19103 USA
LWW.com

First Edition © 2001 by LIPPINCOTT WILLIAMS & WILKINS

Printed in the United States of America

Library of Congress Cataloging-in-Publication Data
Gorbach's 5-minute infectious diseases consult / [edited by] Matthew E. Falagas, Eleftherios Mylonakis ; associate editors, Isaac I. Bogoch . . . [et al.]. − 2nd ed.
 p. ; cm. − (5-minute consult series)
 5-minute infectious diseases consult
 Rev. ed. of: 5-minute infectious diseases consult / cditors, Sherwood L. Gorbach, Matthew Falagas ; associate editors, Eleftherios Mylonakis, David R. Stone. c2001.
 Includes bibliographical references and index.
 Summary: "Using the two-page, templated organization of the 5-Minute Consult series, Gorbach's 5-Minute Infectious Diseases Consult, Second Edition provides comprehensive coverage for clinicians dealing with infectious diseases. The two major sections of the book cover chief complaints and individual diseases and disorders. Additional materials include summary information about individual microorganisms as well as numerous elements related to drugs for infectious disorders. A team of international authorities provides actionable information, supported by current research and practice guidelines. Features Include: Comprehensive coverage of infectious diseases, important symptoms, microorganisms, and anti-infective drugs Coverage of emerging infectious diseases such as H1N1 flu Increased coverage of tropical diseases Two-page, tightly written chapters Updated information about management of HIV/AIDS" —Provided by publisher.
 ISBN 13: 978-1-60913-386-3 (hardback : alk. paper)
 ISBN 10: 1-60913-386-2 (hardback : alk. paper)
 I. Falagas, Matthew E.   II. Mylonakis, Eleftherios.   III. Gorbach, Sherwood L., 1934-   IV. 5-minute infectious diseases consult.   V. Title: 5-minute infectious diseases consult.   VI. Series: 5-minute consult.
 [DNLM: 1. Communicable Diseases−Handbooks. WC 39]
 616.9−dc23   2011035305

To purchase additional copies of this book, call our customer service department at (800) 638-3030 or fax orders to (301) 223-2320. International customers should call (301) 223-2300.

Visit Lippincott Williams & Wilkins on the Internet: at LWW.com. Lippincott Williams & Wilkins customer service representatives are available from 8:30 am to 6:00 pm, EST.

10 9 8 7 6 5 4 3 2 1

CONTRIBUTORS

Murat Akova, MD
Professor of Medicine
Department of Medicine
Hacettepe University
Attending Physician
Section of Infectious Diseases
Hacettepe University School of
    Medicine
Ankara, Turkey

Stavros S. Athanasiou, MD
First Department of Obstetrics and
    Gynecology
Athens University School of Medicine
Alexandra Hospital
Athens, Greece

Isaac I. Bogoch, MD, FRCP(C)
Division of Infectious Diseases
Massachusetts General Hospital
    Harvard Medical School
Boston, Massachusetts

**Herman A. Carneiro, MBBS, MSc,
DLSHTM**
Harvard Medical School
Division of Infectious Diseases
Massachusetts General Hospital
Boston, Massachusetts

West London Renal and Transplant
    Centre
Hammersmith Hospital
Imperial College Healthcare NHS Trust
London, United Kingdom

Girish Chinnaswamy, MD, MBBS
Pediatric Oncologist
Christian Medical College
Vellore, South India

Matthew E. Falagas, MD, MSc, DSc
Director, Alfa Institute of Biomedical
    Sciences (AIBS)
Athens, Greece
Adjunct Associate Professor of
    Medicine
Tufts University School of Medicine
Boston, Massachusetts
Director, Infectious Diseases Clinic
Henry Dunant Hospital
Athens, Greece

Theodoros Filippopoulos, MD
Clinical Lecturer
Department of Ophthalmology
University of Athens Medical School
Attikon Hospital
Head of Glaucoma
Department of Ophthalmology Athens
Vision Eye Institute
Athens, Greece

Renato Finkelstein, MD
Clinical Professor
Department of Medicine
Bruce Rapport Faculty of Medicine
Technion Israel Institute of Technology
Director
Department of Infectious Disease
Rambam Health Care Campus
Haifa, Israel

Georgia G. Georgantzi, MD
Research Fellow
Alfa Institute of Biomedical Sciences
    (AIBS)
Paediatrician in Training
Department of Pediatrics
University General Hospital Attikon
Athens, Greece

Abdul Ghafur, MBBS
Consultant in Infectious Diseases and
    Clinical Mycology
Apollo Hospital
Chennai, India

Jason B. Harris, MD
Assistant Professor of Pediatrics
Division of Infectious Diseases
Massachusetts General Hospital
Boston, Massachusetts

Emily P. Hyle, MD
Instructor
Department of Medicine
Harvard Medical School
Assistant in Medicine
Department of Medicine
Massachusetts General Hospital
Boston, Massachusetts

Cameron J. Jeremiah, MBBS
Infectious Diseases Registrar
Infectious Diseases Unit and Department
    of Microbiology
Alfred Hospital
Melbourne, Australia

Hong-ni Jiang, MD, PhD
Department of Pulmonary Medicine
Shanghai Medical College of Fudan
    University
Attending Physician
Department of Pulmonary Medicine
Zhongshan Hospital
Shanghai, China

Jennifer A. Johnson, MD
Instructor in Medicine
Department of Medicine
Harvard Medical School
Associate Physician
Department of Medicine, Division of
    Infectious Diseases
Brigham and Women's Hospital
Boston, Massachusetts

Souha S. Kanj, MD, FACP, FIDSA
Professor of Medicine
Department of Internal Medicine
Head, Division of Infectious Diseases
Department of Internal Medicine
American University of Beirut Medical
    Center
Beirut, Lebanon

Anastasios M. Kapaskelis, MD
Alfa Institute of Biomedical Sciences
    (AIBS)
Athens, Greece

Drosos E. Karageorgopoulos, MD
Researcher
Alfa Institute of Biomedical Sciences
Athens, Greece
Attending Physician
Department of Medicine
Tzaneio General Hospital
Piraeus, Greece

Petros M. Karsaliakos, MD
Internal Medicine Specialist
Director of Internal Medicine Sector
Hygeia Hospital
Tirana, Albania

Bettina M. Knoll, MD, PhD
Infectious Diseases Fellow, Transplant
Department of Internal Medicine
Massachusetts General Hospital
Boston, Massachusetts

Irene S. Kourbeti, MD
Doctorate Fellow
Graduate Program
University of Crete Medical School
Heraklion, Crete, Greece
Attending Physician
Department of Medicine, Infectious
 Disease
General Hospital of Chalkida
Chalkida, Greece

Katherine M. Langan, MD
Department of Infectious Diseases
Alfred Hospital
Melbourne, Victoria, Australia

Wei Lu, MD
Department of Infectious Diseases
Peking Union Medical College Hospital
No. 1, Shuanfuyuan, Wangfujing
Beijing, China

Michael K. Mansour, MD, PhD
Clinical Fellow
Department of Medicine
Harvard Medical School
Clinical and Research Fellow
Department of Medicine
Massachusetts General Hospital
Boston, Massachusetts

Catherine Marshall

Michael N. Mavros, MD
Research Fellow
Department of Surgery
Alfa Institute of Biomedical Sciences
Marousi, Athens, Greece

Maged Muhammed, MD
Research Fellow
Department of Medicine
Harvard Medical School
Postdoctoral Fellow
Department of Infectious
Disease/Medicine
Massachusetts General Hospital
Boston, Massachusetts

Eleftherios Mylonakis, MD, PhD, FIDSA
Associate Professor of Medicine
Harvard Medical School
Massachusetts General Hospital
Division of Infectious Diseases
Boston, Massachusetts

Francisco M. Nacinovich, MD
Chief
Department of Infectious Diseases and
 Infection Control
Instituto Cardiovascular de Buenos Aires
Buenos Aires, Argentina

Vasant Nagvekar
Internal Medicine Physician
Lilavati Hospital and Research Centre
Mumbai, India

Eleni Patrozou, MD
Clinical Instructor
Department of Medicine
Brown University
Providence, Rhode Island, United States
 of America
Hygeia Hospital
Athens, Greece

Anton Y. Peleg
Senior Lecturer
Department of Microbiology
Monash University
Infectious Diseases Physician
Department of Infectious Diseases
Alfred Hospital
Melbourne, Victoria, Australia

Georgios Peppas, MD, PhD
Alfa Institute of Biomedical Sciences
 (AIBS)
Athens, Greece

Mary L. Pisculli, MD, MPH
Division of Infectious Disease
Brigham and Women's Hospital
Boston, Massachusetts

Jie-ming Qu, MD, PhD
Professor
Department of Pulmonary Medicine
Shanghai Medical College of Fudan
 University
Chief Physician
Department of Pulmonary Medicine
Huadong Hospital
Shanghai, China

Petros I. Rafailidis, MD, MRCP(UK), MSc
Researcher
Department of Medicine
Alfa Institute of Biomedical Sciences
Attending Physician
Infectious Diseases Clinic
Henry Dunant Hospital
Athens, Greece

Alejandro Restrepo, MD
Assistant Professor
Department of Medicine
University of Arkansas for Medical
 Sciences
Infectious Diseases/Hospitalist
Department of Medicine
University of Arkansas for Medical
 Sciences—MIRT
Little Rock, Arkansas

Abiola C. Senok, MBBS, PhD
Assistant Professor, Microbiology &
 Immunology
College of Medicine
Alfaisal University
Riyadh, Saudi Arabia

Konstantinos S. Sgouros, MD
Internist
2nd Department of Internal Medicine
Asclepion Voulas General Hospital
Voula, Greece
Internist, ICU Subspecialization
Intensive Care Unit
Metaxa Hospital
Piraeus, Greece

Erica S. Shenoy, MD, PhD
Division of Infectious Diseases
Massachusetts General Hospital
Boston, Massachusetts

Atef M. Shibl, MD, PhD
Professor of Microbiology
Departement of Pharmaceutics
College of Pharmacy
King Saud University
Riyadh, Saudi Arabia

Rachel P. Simmons, MD
Instructor
Department of Medicine
Harvard University
Assistant in Medicine
Department of Medicine
Massachusetts General Hospital
Boston, Massachusetts

Padma Srikanth, MD
Professor
Department of Microbiology
Sri Ramachandra Medical College &
 Research Institute
Senior Consultant
Sri Ramachandra Medical Centre
Sri Ramachandra University
Porur, Chennai, India

Luisa M. Stamm, MD, PhD
Clinical Fellow
Division of Infectious Diseases
Massachusetts General Hospital
Boston, Massachusetts

Martin E. Stryjewski, MD, MHS
Associate Professor
Department of Medicine, Division of
 Infectious Diseases
Instituto Universitario CEMIC
Attending
Department of Medicine, Division of
 Infectious Diseases
Centro de Educación Médica e
 Investigaciones Clínicas (CEMIC)
Buenos Aires, Argentina

Hanssa Summah
Department of Pulmonary Medicine
Shanghai Medical College of Fudan
 University
Physician
Department of Pulmonary Medicine
Huadong Hospital
Shanghai, China

Sarah Taimur, MD
Clinical Fellow
Transplant Infectious Diseases
The Cleveland Clinic Foundation
Cleveland, Ohio

Li-li Tao, MMed
PhD Candidate
Department of Pulmonary Medicine
Shanghai Medical College of Fudan
 University
Physician
Department of Pulmonary Medicine
Huadong Hospital
Shanghai, China

Balaji Veeraraghavan, MD
Professor
Department of Microbiology &
Antimicrobial Resistance Surveillance
Christian Medical College
Vellore, South India

Paschalis Vergidis, MD
Post-Doctoral Fellow
Division of Clinical Microbiology
Mayo Clinic College of Medicine
Rochester, Minnesota

Evridiki K. Vouloumanou
Alfa Institute of Biomedical Sciences
 (AIBS)
Athens, Greece

Jatin M. Vyas, MD, PhD
Assistant Professor
Department of Medicine
Harvard Medical School
Assistant in Medicine
Department of Medicine, Division of
 Infectious Disease
Massachusetts General Hospital
Boston, Massachusetts

Jia-yi Xu
Department of Pulmonary Medicine
Shanghai Medical College of Fudan
 University
Physician
Department of Pulmonary Medicine
Huadong Hospital
Shanghai, China

Ata Nevzat Yalçin, MD
Professor
Department of Infectious Diseases and
 Clinical Microbiology
Akdeniz University
Antalya, Turkey

Ioanna M. Zarkada, MD
Alfa Institute of Biomedical Sciences
 (AIBS)
Athens, Greece

Jing Zhang, MD, PhD
Department of Pulmonary Medicine
Shanghai Medical College of Fudan
 University
Attending Physician
Department of Pulmonary
 Medicine
Zhongshan Hospital
Shanghai, China

Ying-gang Zhu, MD
Candidate
Department of Pulmonary Medicine
Shanghai Medical College of Fudan
 University
Physician
Department of Pulmonary Medicine
Huadong Hospital
Shanghai, China

FOREWORD

There are times when brevity can capture the essence of wisdom. This is the challenge that the authors accepted in the first edition of this book by providing brief and authoritative vignettes of the full range of infectious diseases. Matthew Falagas and Eleftherios Mylonakis have readdressed as authors of this second edition.

It has been said that "Knowledge comes, but wisdom lingers." So, these clinical descriptions include not only the basic information about specific clinical conditions but also, more importantly, the distilled recommendations of experienced clinicians who know how to diagnose and treat infection and also how to guide others in the practice of the possible. In many instances, a clinician could consult an entire treatise on the topic. Yet, such detail does not serve the busy practitioner who needs to know the essentials about a specific condition in a practical and comprehensive manner—all within 5 minutes. And it must be right because a sick patient is at the other end of the thought process. When the illness is contagious, others are impacted by the decision, adding to the need for accuracy in diagnosis and infection control.

Most disciplines of Medicine are confined to a single species—Homo sapiens—or a single organ, the heart, the kidney, or the lungs. When confronting infection, however, the health care provider must know about diverse microorganisms, from prions to parasites, about vectors and foods, and about winged creatures and stalking insects—what Major General Stanley takes pride in pronouncing: "I know the scientific names of beings animalculous." Every organ in the human can be attacked by these silent, usually microscopic life forms. The authors of this book have seen virtually all of them and can lead by acumen and experience to the best possible outcome.

Francis Bacon opined "Some books are to be tasted, others to be swallowed, and some few to be chewed and digested" (1605). This book is intended for consumption in the latter category as a guide to best practice by the clinician who needs to know practical information without compromise.

SHERWOOD L. GORBACH, MD

PREFACE

Since the first edition of the book, the field of infectious diseases has gone through significant changes. The implementation of new diagnostic assays, the development of antimicrobial stewardship programs, the greater recognition of polymicrobial infections and pathogen-pathogen interactions, and the new directions in antimicrobial discovery that include immunomodulatory and antivirulence compounds and probiotics are a few of the most recent developments that are expected to transform our field. However, emerging infections, drug-resistant pathogens, and the discrepancies in healthcare are quickly becoming major threats.

In addition to these changes, the second edition of the book gives us an opportunity to reflect to our personal developments. Importantly, the book is now named in honor of Dr. Sherry Gorbach. Sherry is a pioneer in our field and a prominent physician-scientist who has shaped our field over decades. His extensive contributions in research, clinical practice, and education are only paralleled by his mentoring that has shaped the professional lives of many members of the infectious disease community around the world. It is a great honor for us to edit a book that caries the name of such a legend in our field.

In its core, managing infectious diseases continues to be practicing "Medicine of the Possible," as we noted on the first edition. Most of the common infections are treatable by anti-infective drugs or have a self-limited course that can be ameliorated by symptomatic therapy. Upon making a diagnosis and starting treatment, both the patient and the physician are generally assured a favorable outcome. While this homily is widely accepted, the "problem is in the details." The correct diagnosis must be established, usually on clinical grounds by a careful history and physical examination.

If indicated, the proper laboratory tests must be obtained. And last, but certainly not least, effective treatment must be applied. What this book provides is a quick and ready reference for most of the infections seen in medical practice, with expert guidance on these critical issues—clinical diagnosis, laboratory tests, and appropriate therapy. While key articles are provided for more detailed study, the main need that is served by this book is for a brief, easily digested source of critical information that can be applied instantly in managing infection.

"Medicine of the Possible" means that physicians and healthcare workers can make a substantial difference in improving the outcome of a patient with an infectious disease by applying the principles of correct diagnosis and judicious treatment. Many illnesses in medicine are chronic and unrelenting conditions which can be improved but not necessarily cured by treatment. On the other hand, most infections are transient interruptions in the course of life which, if managed properly, can pass without significant damage to the fabric of one's existence.

Despite advances in antimicrobial agents, vaccines, and preventive medicine, infection continues to cause significant morbidity and mortality on all strata of our population, with its greatest impact on the young, the old, and the infirm. The authors of this book have tried to provide guidance to manage infectious diseases, thereby relieving the patient's misery and giving physicians the satisfaction of performing their sacred calling of curing disease and relieving suffering.

MATTHEW E. FALAGAS, MD, MSc, DSc
ELEFTHERIOS MYLONAKIS, MD, PhD, FIDSA

CONTENTS

Section I
Chief Complaints

Eleftherios Mylonakis, Editor

ABDOMINAL PAIN AND FEVER

Isaac I. Bogoch

 BASICS

DESCRIPTION
Definition
- This chapter examines diseases associated with fever and abdominal pain.

Approach to the Patient
- The first major decision in examining a patient with fever and abdominal pain is to determine if this is an emergency requiring surgical attention.
- Be mindful to exclude potentially critical conditions when examining the patient, and consider pain "referred" from other areas which masquerade as abdominal pain.
- Patients with catastrophic abdominal infections may present with subtle signs or symptoms. This is more common among neonates, elderly, and immunocompromised patients.
- The physician needs to quickly clarify the severity, onset, and characteristics of the symptoms; check vital signs; and perform a thorough physical examination.
- In addition to a detailed abdominal exam, a full physical exam should be performed with particular attention to the pulmonary and cardiovascular systems.
- Rectal examination should be performed, unless the patient is severely neutropenic (in which case, clinicians should perform careful inspection).

EPIDEMIOLOGY
- Patients with appendicitis frequently present to emergency departments with abdominal pain and fever.
- Most cases of typhoid fever in the US are acquired abroad, usually in Mexico, India, and Pakistan.
- Travel to tropical areas: Consider malaria as a cause of fever and abdominal pain.
- Travel to areas where louse-borne relapsing fever is endemic (Ethiopia, South America, the East Asia) raises the possibility of *Borrelia recurrentis* infection.
- HIV can cause fever and abdominal pain from many mechanisms. Consider HIV risk factors and those from areas of high endemicity (e.g., Sub-Saharan Africa and Southeast Asia, intravenous drug exposure).
- Ingestion of unpasteurized milk and milk products, malnutrition, and HIV infection are associated with intestinal tuberculosis.
- Animal contact may suggest leptospirosis, toxoplasmosis, brucellosis, or Q fever.
- Other vector exposure: Dengue fever (mosquito), typhus (flea, mite, louse), and psittacosis (parrots and related birds).
- Patients with sickle cell disease or splenectomy are more prone to salmonellosis.
- Consider solid tumors or lymphomas in patients with melena or guaiac-positive stools and weight loss.
- Cardiovascular disease is the most common cause of death in Western societies and frequently presents as abdominal pain.

ETIOLOGY
- Generalized abdominal pain and fever; consider peritonitis, ileus/obstruction, enteric vascular disease, ruptured aneurysm, or metabolic disorder.
- Infectious causes of abdominal pain per anatomic region:
  - Right upper quadrant pain: Acute cholecystitis (including perforation), hepatitis, Fitz-Hugh–Curtis syndrome, pyelonephritis, pneumonia, liver abscess.
  - Left upper quadrant pain: Pyelonephritis, pneumonia, and splenic abscess
  - Epigastric pain: Diverticulitis, appendicitis (early phase), peritonitis (primary, secondary, tuberculous), acute gastroenteritis, pancreatitis, cholangitis, Crohn's disease, ulcerative colitis, and colitis due to *Clostridium difficile*, mediastinitis
  - Right lower quadrant pain: Appendicitis, salpingitis, psoas muscle abscess, mesenteric adenitis, pelvic inflammatory disease, and bowel perforation
  - Left lower quadrant pain: Diverticulitis, salpingitis, psoas muscle abscess, mesenteric adenitis, pelvic infection, and bowel perforation
- Selected noninfectious causes of abdominal pain include:
  - Acute porphyria
  - Addisonian crisis
  - Collagen and granulomatous diseases (polyarteritis nodosa or other vasculitis, sarcoidosis, Crohn's disease, Still's disease, granulomatous hepatitis, etc.)
  - Diabetic ketoacidosis
  - Esophageal disease
  - Familial Mediterranean fever
  - Lead intoxication
  - Malignancy (intraabdominal or hematologic)
  - Mediastinal tumors
  - Mesenteric artery embolus
  - Mesenteric vessel thrombus
  - Myocardial infarction
  - Pancreatitis
  - Pneumothorax complicating pneumonia (e.g., due to *Pneumocystis carinii*)
  - Pulmonary embolism
  - Ruptured ovarian follicle
  - Sickle cell anemia crisis
- Enteric fever is characterized by fever and abdominal pain, but may also be associated with headache, hepatomegaly, splenomegaly, and a macular rash ('rose spots').
- Typhoid fever (caused by *Salmonella typhi*) is the prototype of enteric fever, but several bacteria can cause enteric fever including *Salmonella paratyphi*, and a range of systemic bacterial, rickettsial, viral, fungal, and parasitic infections can cause enteric fever-like syndrome (e.g., *Yersinia enterocolitica*, *Yersinia pestis*, *Leptospira*, *Mycobacterium tuberculosis*, Chlamydia, viral hepatitis, Epstein–Barr virus, etc.).

- Mesenteric adenitis, a syndrome that may mimic acute appendicitis, most frequently is due to a viral infection or *Y. enterocolitica*.
- Eosinophilia associated with abdominal cramps or diarrhea is often accompanied by fever and may be associated with parasitic infection (usually helminths) or intestinal lymphoma.
- Patients infected with enterohemorrhagic *Escherichia coli* (e.g., *E. coli* O157:H7) often present with abdominal cramps before developing bloody diarrhea, many are afebrile.
- Abdominal pain and fever in patients with HIV: Consider infectious and noninfectious etiologies. These patients develop typical causes as seen in immunocompetent hosts, and other causes including typhlitis, small bowel or colonic perforation with associated abscess, HIV-related cholangiopathy, hepatic abscesses, hepatic bacillary angiomatosis, pancreatitis, splenic infarction or abscess. Intestinal manifestations from gastrointestinal tuberculosis, cytomegalovirus colitis or esophagitis, Candida esophagitis, histoplasmosis, *Mycobacterium avium complex*, enteritis with cryptosporidium, *Isospora*, microsporidia. Also consider *Giardia*, *Strongyloides*, Kaposi's sarcoma, lymphoma.

Dx **DIAGNOSIS**

HISTORY
The location of pain, intensity, quality, and radiation of pain, palliating and provoking factors, relation to eating, presence of diarrhea (see relevant chapter) or constipation, recent travel, food, and animal exposures, cardiovascular risk factors.

PHYSICAL EXAM
- The physical examination should include auscultating for bowel sounds and bruits, the location and degree of tenderness (if any), palpation for splenomegaly and hepatomegaly.
- Stigmata of acute and chronic liver disease such as jaundice, scleral icterus, spider angiomata, clubbing, ascites.
- Evaluation of the oropharynx and anus for lesions (e.g., herpes, adenovirus, aphthous ulcerations).
- Relative bradycardia suggests enteric fever. Conjunctivitis, pharyngitis, or abnormal lung examination may also be present in enteric fever.
- Acute diarrhea and nonsuppurative arthritis are often prominent features of infection with *Y. enterocolitica*.
- Pain and rebound tenderness localized in the lower right quadrant, mimicking acute appendicitis may be associated with mesenteric adenitis.
- Only half of patients with acute appendicitis present with classic peri-umbilical pain migrating to the right lower quadrant.

DIAGNOSTIC TESTS & INTERPRETATION
Lab
- CBC with differential, Lytes, BUN, Cr, Liver enzymes, liver function tests, calcium profile
- Blood cultures prior to the initiation of empiric antibiotics
- Urine culture
- ECG
- Blood, stool, and urine specimens should be obtained for cultures from every patient with a syndrome compatible with enteric fever before initiating antimicrobial therapy. Consider bone marrow cultures if typhoid fever is suspected in the context of negative blood cultures.
- Widal's reaction (a serology test) is not helpful in the diagnosis of enteric fever caused by organisms other than *S. typhi*.
- Leukopenia is common in typhoid fever.
- With eosinophilia present, stool should be sent for ova and parasites.
- Fever with *Giardia* infections is only present in 10–15% of individuals. Stool ova and parasite examination, small bowel biopsy, and immunoassays (e.g., ELISA) can aid in diagnosis.
- Malaria: Thick and thin blood smear q24h × 3. Rapid tests are also available.
- Stool evaluation: In the correct clinical context examine for *C. difficile*, ova, and parasites. Culture for *E. coli* O157:H7, *Shigella*, *Yersinia*, *Campylobacter*, *Salmonella*.
- Most cases of appendicitis present with leukocytosis.

Imaging
- Flat and upright abdominal radiographs can provide clues for the diagnosis of abdominal pain (free air, loss of psoas muscle shadow, radiopaque stones, etc.). Further testing with ultrasonography or computed tomography (CT) is often necessary.
- Ultrasound remains the initial investigation of choice in patients with suspected biliary or renal infection; however, it is of limited value particularly in imaging deep structures like the pancreas and in postoperative patients.
- CT scans are often diagnostically superior and accuracy rises with contrast agents. Caution over nephrotoxicity with contrast use.
- Ultrasonography is generally used for the initial evaluation of patients presenting with symptoms consistent with biliary disease (cholecystitis, cholangitis, choledocholithiasis).
- Diagnostic accuracy of endoscopic ultrasonography for biliary tract stone disease is >95%.
- Magnetic resonance cholangiography is a noninvasive and accurate method of imaging the biliary tract.

- Acute acalculous cholecystitis accounts for 2–15% of all cases of acute cholecystitis. Hydroxyindole diaminoacetic acid scanning is costly and rarely used as a first-line study to evaluate biliary tract disease, but it is occasionally useful in evaluating acalculous cholecystitis.
- Endoscopic retrograde cholangiography, percutaneous transhepatic cholangiography, and intraoperative cholangiography are considered the best diagnostic methods for common bile duct stones; however, these procedures are invasive and associated with complications such as pancreatitis.

TREATMENT
MEDICATION
- For many patients with fever and abdominal pain, antimicrobial therapy must be initiated before a diagnosis can be confirmed.
- It is vital to tailor antibiotics to a suspected clinical infectious syndrome.
- The patient's travel history should be considered before initial empiric antimicrobial therapy.
- Mesenteric adenitis is usually a self-limited illness, and specific antimicrobial therapy often is not required. Therapeutic agents to be considered include trimethoprim–sulfamethoxazole, a third-generation cephalosporin, or a fluoroquinolone.
- Mild-to-moderate community-acquired intraabdominal infections like acute cholecystitis could be treated with a fluoroquinolone plus metronidazole OR with a beta-lactam/beta-lactamase inhibitor (e.g., ampicillin/sulbactam, piperacillin/tazobactam).
- Vancomycin is frequently added if there is suspected methicillin-resistant *S. aureus*.
- Ampicillin is preferred over vancomycin for *Enterococcus* coverage if it is susceptible to both agents.
- For high-severity community-acquired infections and health-care intraabdominal (complication after surgery) associated infection, early treatment with complex multidrug regimens, appropriate for the nosocomial flora, is recommended and often involves antipseudomonal cephalosporins (e.g., ceftazidime, cefepime) or carbapenems.

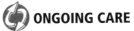

ONGOING CARE
FOLLOW-UP RECOMMENDATIONS
- Beware of subtle or atypical symptoms in the elderly and the neonates and infants.
- Watch patients closely until fever resolves.
- Consider CT imaging of the abdomen for persistent fevers and abdominal pain that evades diagnosis on history, physical exam, and ultrasound.

ADDITIONAL READING
- Solomkin JS, Mazuski JE, Baron EJ, et al. Guidelines for the selection of anti-infective agents for complicated intra-abdominal infections. IDSA guidelines. *Clin Infect Dis* 2003;37:997–1005.
- Grant TH, Rosen MP, Fidler JL, et al. *ACR Appropriateness Criteria: Acute abdominal pain and fever or suspected abdominal abscess.* Reston, VA: American College of Radiology, 2006.
- Samuels J, Aksentijevich I, Torosyan Y, et al. Familial Mediterranean fever at the millennium: Clinical spectrum, ancient mutations, and a survey of 100 American referrals to the National Institutes of Health. *Medicine* 1998;77:268–297.
- Wagner JM, McKinney WP, Carpenter JL. Does this patient have appendicitis? *JAMA* 1996;276: 1589–1594.
- Kaltenthaler EC, Walters SJ, Chilcott J, et al. MRCP compared to diagnostic ERCP for diagnosis when biliary obstruction is suspected: A systematic review. *BMC Med Imaging* 2006;6:9.

CODES

ICD9
- 541 Appendicitis, unqualified
- 780.60 Fever, unspecified
- 789.00 Abdominal pain, unspecified site

CLINICAL PEARLS
- Fever and abdominal pain may indicate abdominal pathology or referred pathology from nearby anatomic structures.
- Immunocompromised patients (e.g., chemotherapy, steroids, AIDS) and the elderly may have severe abdominal infections with mild symptoms.

ANIMAL BITE AND CLENCHED-FIST INJURY RELATED INFECTIONS

Isaac I. Bogoch

 BASICS

DESCRIPTION

Definition

- Animal bites may cause puncture wounds, scratches, or open lacerations, with variable tissue damage. Clenched fist injuries or bites occur as a result of an individual's tooth penetration to another individual's skin and the inoculation of mouth flora.

Approach to the Patient

- Initial rapid investigation for life or limb-threatening tissue damage and bleeding. Perform a detailed neurologic and vascular exam of the affected limb.
- If patients present with symptoms of shock, initial hemodynamic support, empiric antibiotics, and possible surgical evaluation are warranted.
- Important to discriminate if animal bite or puncture wound is from a potentially poisonous species.
- Essential to carefully explore the wound for possible detection of deeper tissue damage (tendons, vessels, nerves, joints, organs).
- Also essential to evaluate for evidence of foreign bodies (e.g., teeth).
- Irrigation with ample sterile water or normal saline, and careful debridement of necrotic tissue and foreign material. Often will require local anesthesia to facilitate irrigation and debridement.
- The area of trauma should be kept moist with topical antibacterial cream and should be covered with the aim to reduce the microbial burden.
- Generally after extensive debridement and high-pressure irrigation, some carefully selected traumas – even in hands and feet – can undergo primary closure; however, most animal and human bite wounds and scratches should be healed by secondary intention.
- Very close follow-up of the wound is required due to high risk of infection.
- An X-ray or further imaging with CT or MRI may be needed for the detection of foreign bodies and to determine if deeper trauma exists.
- Bites and punctures to the hands and feet frequently require surgical consultation as deep tendon infections can spread quickly and cause sepsis and irreparable damage.
- Tetanus and rabies immunizations should be considered.
- Suspicious human bites may reflect child and domestic abuse.

EPIDEMIOLOGY

- In the US, roughly 40% of households own a dog, and 33% own a cat.
- Children are the most frequent victims of animal bites, and often have trauma to the head and neck.
- Up to 2.5% of dog bites have clinical evidence of infection by the time patients present to medical attention.

RISK FACTORS

Morbidity from animal bites raises with the following factors:

- Age: Children are more prone to expose themselves to hazardous bites including the upper thorax, neck, and head.
- Occupation: Veterinarians and animal breeders are more vulnerable.
- Immune status: Immunocompromised hosts at higher risk for sepsis. HIV, active malignancy or chemotherapy, steroid use, asplenia, liver disease.
- Diabetes mellitus: Difficult wound healing on extremities with peripheral vascular disease and neuropathy.

ETIOLOGY

- Most infections are polymicrobial with aerobic and anaerobic pathogens. Infections represent mouth flora of the perpetrator and skin flora of the victim. Note that *methicillin-resistant Staphylococcus aureus* (MRSA) is now a very frequent colonizer of human skin and may be introduced to the wound at time of injury.
- Common infections from dog bites include *Capnocytophaga* spp. and *Pasteurella canis*. *Pasteurella multocida* is a common isolate from cat bites.
- Other pathogens associated with animal exposure include the following:
  – *Bartonella henselae*
  – *Francisella tularensis*
  – *Leptospira* spp.

- Less common aerobes include *Streptococcus* spp., *Staphylococcus* spp., *Moraxella* spp., and *Neisseria* spp. Anaerobes are usually involved in polymicrobial infections and include *Fusobacterium* spp., *Bacteroides* spp., *Porphyromonas* spp., and *Prevotella* spp.
- In human bites, common aerobic isolates include *Streptococcus* spp., *Staphylococcus aureus*, *Eikenella corrodens*, and *Haemophilus influenzae*. Anaerobic species include *Fusobacterium nucleatum*, *Prevotella* spp., *Porphyromonas* spp., *Peptococcus* spp., and *Peptostreptococcus* spp.
- Bite wounds from aquatic animals may be exposed to waterborne infections such as *Aeromonas*, *Vibrio* spp., *Erysipelothrix*, and *Mycobacterium marinum*.
- Small rodents, including rats, mice, and gerbils, as well as animals that prey on rodents, may transmit *Streptobacillus moniliformis* or *Sarracenia minor* causing rat-bite fever.

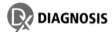 DIAGNOSIS

HISTORY

- Have the patient describe the events before, during, and after trauma.
- Ask about biting animal: Is it poisonous, domestic, wild? Has it received the appropriate shots? Is it available for rabies evaluation?
- Assess the immune history (e.g., Hepatitis B) and vaccination status (e.g., Tetanus) of the victim.
- Ask about allergies to antibiotics.
- Inquire about potential liver disease and immunocompromised status of the victim, such as malignancy, HIV, steroids, asplenia, as these are risk factors for more severe infection.

PHYSICAL EXAM
- Vital signs
- Complete physical examination
- Complete exposure of bitten area
- Secondary dermatologic exam to assess for other less obvious areas of trauma
- Careful evaluation as to the depth of puncture. Assess if bone, joint, or tendon involved. Look for pain along tendon sheath. Also look for spreading erythema, enlarged lymph nodes, exudates, purulence, fluctuance under skin
- Detailed neurologic and vascular exam of affected region
- Clinical manifestations:
  – A patient may present with a single or multiple bites with variable severity.
  – Symptoms and signs of systemic toxicity and hemodynamic instability due septic shock or hemorrhage are the most emergent issues.
  – Osteomyelitis may result from deep penetrating wounds and may present remotely from time of injury.
  – Meningitis, peritonitis, and endocarditis are rare but serious complications of disseminated infection.
  – Ecchymosis or hematoma without finding superficial wound may reflect tissue reaction to a venom.

DIAGNOSTIC TESTS & INTERPRETATION
Lab
- CBC, Lytes, BUN, Cr, liver enzymes, and liver function tests.
- At least 2 sets of blood cultures (aerobic and anaerobic) prior to initiating antibiotics.
- Some oral flora may take longer to culture from blood, so samples should be held for >14 days.
- Gram stain and culture of trauma swab might be helpful but frequently not specific.

- *Pasteurella* spp. are the most commonly isolated microbes from dog and cat bites, they are Gram-negative bacilli and grow on blood and chocolate agar.
- MRSA is extremely common on host skin and may be inoculated into wound around the time of injury.

Imaging
- X-rays to assess for foreign body (e.g., tooth fragment).
- CT and MRI will better elucidate hemorrhage, abscess, tendon sheath involvement, osteomyelitis.

 TREATMENT

MEDICATION
- Always remember tetanus and rabies prophylaxis when indicated.
- Strongly consider prophylactic antibiotic treatment for all bites except those which are very superficial.
- The prophylactic treatment should be determined by the respective mouth flora of the animal.
- Empiric coverage for human, cat, or dog bites should include a beta-lactam/beta-lactamase inhibitor such as amoxicillin/clavulanate.
- Alternative regimens include combining trimethoprim-sulfamethoxazole (TMP-SMX), penicillin, fluoroquinolone, or doxycycline with either metronidazole or clindamycin.
- Note that clindamycin, TMP-SMX, and clindamycin potentially have MRSA coverage.
- Intravenous formulations are necessary for systemic toxicity.
- Venomous serpent: Antivenom and ceftriaxone.

 ONGOING CARE

FOLLOW-UP RECOMMENDATIONS
- Daily wound inspection and dressing changes.
- Low threshold for expedited surgical care if deep penetrating wound, presence of foreign body, or tendon sheath involvement.
- Patients should be informed of infectious signs and symptoms prior to discharge.
- Immunization for tetanus or rabies might be life-saving.

ADDITIONAL READING
- Oehler RL, Velez AP, Mizrachi M, et al. Bite-related and septic syndromes caused by cats and dogs. *Lancet Infect Dis* 2009;9(7):439–447.
- Singer AJ, Dagum AB. Current management of acute cutaneous wounds. *N Engl J Med* 2008;359(10): 1037–1046.

 CODES

ICD9
- 879.9 Open wound(s) (multiple) of unspecified site(s), complicated
- 882.1 Open wound of hand except fingers alone, complicated
- 958.3 Posttraumatic wound infection, not elsewhere classified

CLINICAL PEARLS
- Early and aggressive treatment of the wound is key to successful and uncomplicated healing.
- Most bite wounds are polymicrobial.
- Do not forget tetanus booster and rabies vaccination if indicated.

BACK PAIN (LOW) AND FEVER

Anton Peleg

 BASICS

DESCRIPTION

- The term back pain is usually used to describe acute or chronic spinal or paraspinal pain.
- Patients who present with back pain and fever should have a thorough evaluation to detect possible sources of nonmechanical pain.
- Clinicians should obtain a careful history and inquire for symptoms of weight loss, recumbency pain, morning stiffness, and acute severe or colicky pain.
- Repeated spinal and neurological examinations are essential, and when there is spinal pain or tenderness, full investigation is warranted.
- Back pain exacerbated by motion and unrelieved by rest, spine tenderness over the involved spine segment, and an elevated erythrocyte sedimentation rate (ESR) are the most common findings in vertebral osteomyelitis.
- Pain due to neoplastic infiltration of nerves is typically continuous, progressive in severity, and unrelieved by rest at night. In contrast, mechanical low back pain is usually improved with rest.
- Patients will generally require a plain roentgenographic examination with subsequent scintography, magnetic resonance imaging (MRI), computed tomography (CT), laboratory work, and biopsy as indicated by any positive findings during the diagnostic work-up.

EPIDEMIOLOGY

- The exact origin of pain is of difficult approach and may be exactly determined in less than 25% of cases.
- Mechanical low back pain comprise the great majority of cases—about 97%. Of them, degenerative disk disease and lumbar sprain or strain comprise the 80%.
- Spine is 1 of the commonest sites of bone metastasis.
- Vertebral osteomyelitis is a rare disease with nearly 1 case per 100.000 people per year. An increasing incidence during last years might be attributed to vascular devices and intravenous drug users.
- Vertebral osteomyelitis predilects early childhood and patients after 50 years.
- 1 per 10.000 hospital admissions per year is the incidence of spinal epidural abscess.
- *Methicillin-resistant Staphylococcus aureus* (MRSA) vertebral osteomyelitis and epidural abscesses are of increasing frequency.
- Although tuberculosis cases are globally augmented, extrapulmonary manifestations as Pott's disease remain constant.
- Pott's disease (usually affecting lower thoracic vertebrae) is the commonest extrapulmonary musculoskeletal tuberculosis manifestation.
- With the survival of sickle cell patients having increased, Salmonella vertebral osteomyelitis became more prevalent.

RISK FACTORS

- Infections have been attributed to bites from many animal species, often as a consequence of occupational exposure (farmers, laboratory workers, veterinarians) or recreational exposure (hunters, campers, owners of exotic pets).
- Systemic infections after animal or human bites are particularly likely in hosts with edema or compromised lymphatic drainage in the involved extremity and in patients who are immunocompromised by medication or disease.
- When fever occurs in immunosuppressed patients after a dog bite, the possibility of an infection with *Capnocytophaga canimorsus*, an invasive organism, should be considered.

ETIOLOGY

- Infectious causes of back pain and fever:
  - Biliary tract infection
  - Chronic prostatitis
  - Herpes zoster
  - Pyelonephritis
  - Retroperitoneal abscess
  - Spinal epidural abscess
  - Vertebral osteomyelitis
- Noninfectious causes of back pain and fever:
  - Colonic neoplasms
  - Diseases of the pancreas
  - Histiocytosis X
  - Metastatic carcinoma (breast, lung, prostate, thyroid, kidney, gastrointestinal tract)
  - Multiple myeloma
  - Neoplastic invasion of pelvic nerves
  - Lymphoma
  - Pregnancy
  - Vertebral fracture
  - Renal artery or vein thrombosis
  - Renal stones
  - Retroperitoneal hemorrhage and tumors
  - Tumor of the posterior wall of the stomach or duodenum
- *Staphylococcus aureus* is the most commonly recognized causative organism of spinal epidural abscess and accounts for 57–73% of reported abscesses. Other pathogens include the following:
  - *Actinomyces israelii*
  - *Aspergillus* spp.
  - *Blastomyces* spp.
  - *Brucella* spp.
  - *Cryptococcus* spp.
  - *Haemophilus parainfluenzae*
  - *Mycobacterium tuberculosis*
  - *Streptococcus milleri*
- Vertebral osteomyelitis is usually caused by staphylococci, but other bacteria or *M. tuberculosis* (Pott's disease) may be the responsible organisms. However, this is variable. In a retrospective multicenter study conducted in the south of Spain, 48% of patients had vertebral osteomyelitis due to *Brucella* spp., 33% had pyogenic vertebral osteomyelitis, and 19% had tuberculous vertebral osteomyelitis.

COMMONLY ASSOCIATED CONDITIONS

- Conditions commonly associated with vertebral osteomyelitis and spinal epidural abscess include the following:
  - Diabetes mellitus (in up to 25–33% of cases)
  - Injecting drug use
  - Chronic renal failure
  - Ethanol abuse
  - Focal infections and bacteremia
  - Malignancy
- Most spinal epidural abscesses are thought to result from the hematogenous spread of bacteria, usually from a cutaneous or mucosal source. The direct spread of infection into the epidural space from a source adjacent to the spine is also well described. Postoperative abscesses account for 16% of all spinal epidural abscesses, and epidural catheter insertion is another recognized predisposing factor.
- Blunt trauma is reported to precede the symptoms of spinal epidural abscess in 15–35% of cases, and it is postulated that trauma may result in the formation of an epidural hematoma that subsequently becomes infected.

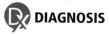 **DIAGNOSIS**

- The typical features of spinal epidural abscess include fever, spinal pain and tenderness, and radiating root pain followed by limb weakness. Pain is the most consistent symptom and occurs in virtually all patients at some time during their illness. However, spinal pain and fever can be the only features before a precipitous neurological deterioration occurs.
- When septicemia dominates the clinical picture, the neurological symptoms may go unnoticed. This also may be the case in patients confined to bed.
- Fever can be absent in up to 30% of patients with pyogenic vertebral osteomyelitis. The absence of fever is more frequent in the group of tuberculous vertebral osteomyelitis.

HISTORY

- Age, constitutional symptoms (fever, weakness, weight loss, perspiration), previous history of trauma infection or cancer, character of pain, immune status, and glycemic status in diabetic patients and history of IVDU are of great importance.
- Ask for neurological symptoms (motor weakness, paresthesia, numbness, bowel, bladder, or sexual dysfunction).
- Consider if your patient appears with any of the following risk factors:
  - Older than 50 years
  - User of steroid
  - Having HIV
  - On immunosuppressive drugs
  - History of previous surgery

PHYSICAL EXAM

- General appearance of the patient, vital signs, peripheral pulses, rapid cardiopulmonary, and abdominal clinical examination in case of the patient being in a critical condition.
- Exclude referral cause of pain by thoroughly examining any potential primary site for sensitivity.
- Is there a neurological disability? Is there a possibility of spinal cord compression or damage? A complete neurological examination may indicate the level of spinal cord damage.
- Spinal cord compression below T12 presents with low motor neuron syndrome. Cauda equina syndrome additionally may present with fecal or bladder incontinence.
- Fever in the elderly might be of low grade. Its height and pattern does not represent the gravity of the disease.
- Spinous processes percussion may detect a sensitive vertebra with trauma, cancer, or infection.
- Search for endocarditis signs or signs of remote septic emboli.

DIAGNOSTIC TESTS & INTERPRETATION
Lab

- The usual hematological and biochemical parameters are of little value in the diagnosis of vertebral osteomyelitis. However, when leukocytosis, neutrophilia, and very high values of ESR and C-reactive protein are present, they suggest pyogenic vertebral osteomyelitis.
- CT and MRI have significantly improved the sensitivity and specificity of simple radiography in the diagnosis of vertebral osteomyelitis.
- Blood culture is the most useful routine test, resulting in the isolation of the responsible microorganism in about half the cases of vertebral osteomyelitis due to pyogenic and *Brucella* spp.
- Bone biopsy is necessary to establish the diagnosis in 50% of pyogenic vertebral osteomyelitis and in almost 75% of tuberculous vertebral osteomyelitis.

Imaging

- Plain x-ray films of the spine may be normal early in vertebral osteomyelitis.
- The extent and location of a spinal epidural abscess are best visualized using MRI.
- MRI or CT-myelography are the studies of choice in the setting of suspected spinal metastasis.

Diagnostic Procedures/Other

- CT-guided needle biopsy is a reliable procedure for diagnosing carcinoma but not lymphoma. The reliability of needle biopsy for the diagnosis of lymphoma has improved with the advent of CT guidance, the addition of immunophenotyping, and the use of larger bore needles, but the failure rate is still high.
- Etiologic diagnosis of vertebral osteomyelitis is frequently difficult, requiring in 30–70% of cases the performance of percutaneous or surgical vertebral bone biopsies.

DIFFERENTIAL DIAGNOSIS

- Tuberculosis tends to be 1 of the early opportunistic infections occurring in AIDS patients, often an AIDS-defining illness, whereas MAC infection tends to occur in the late stage of HIV infection when the CD4 count is usually 50–75 cells per milliliter or less.
- Pertussis should be considered in anyone who has a pure or predominant complaint of cough, especially if there is a history of paroxysmal coughing, inspiratory whoop, posttussive vomiting, cough resulting in sleep disturbance, or close contact with others who have similar symptoms.

TREATMENT
MEDICATION

- In case of vertebral osteomyelitis or epidural abscess, start empiric therapy with vancomycin (1 g b.i.d.) to treat possible MRSA infection. Add a third- or fourth-generation cephalosporin if a gram-negative bacteremia is suspected (especially if pyelonephritis co-exists).
- Adapt therapy after the identification of the causal therapy. If methicillin-sensitive *Staphylococcus aureus* is isolated, consider nafcillin, oxacillin, or cefazolin.
- Duration of therapy at least 6 weeks.
- Treatment of tuberculosis, brucellosis, and salmonellosis bone involvement is described in the respective chapters.
- Corticosteroids might be useful in acute cord compression.
- NSAIDS with their analgesic effect as a symptomatic treatment.
- Biphosphates in fractures due to breast cancer.

ADDITIONAL TREATMENT
General Measures

- Prompt diagnosis and selective treatment related to the specific disease is needed.
- Surgical treatment with early decompression and antibiotic coverage are essential for epidural abscess.
- Spinal cord compression is a neurosurgery emergency. Decompression with surgery or radiotherapy in the first 24 hours of the symptoms is required to avoid permanent neurological complications.
- In spinal or paraspinal infections, empirical antibiotic treatment with bactericidal drugs should be immediately initiated.

 ## ONGOING CARE
FOLLOW-UP RECOMMENDATIONS

- If back pain remains more than 6 weeks, repeat laboratory and imaging tests.
- After 6 weeks of antibiotic treatment due to osteomyelitis or epidural abscess, reevaluation is needed to continue therapy.
- Screening for drug toxicity is essential. Remember that the elderly are more vulnerable as far as undesirable drug reactions are concerned.

ADDITIONAL READING

- Darouiche R. Spinal epidural abscess. Review article. *N Engl J Med* 2006;355:2012–2020.
- Deyo R, WeinsteinJ. Low back pain. *N Engl J Med* 2001;344(5):363–370.
- NICE guideline. Management of acute low back pain. 2008.

 ## CODES

ICD9
- 724.2 Lumbago
- 780.60 Fever, unspecified

CLINICAL PEARLS

- Imaging techniques may detect vertebral osteomyelitis after 4–8 weeks of the infection onset.
- In epidural abscesses, early decompression surgery is mandatory due to unpredicted neurological complications.
- Remember: If there is altered mental status, neurological evaluation is frequently inadequate.

COUGH AND FEVER

Mary L. Pisculli

BASICS

DESCRIPTION
- Cough is an explosive expiration that provides a protective mechanism for clearing the tracheobronchial tree of secretions and foreign material.
- Fever is generally defined as a rise in body temperature 2°F above normal or >100.4°F. The rise in temperature set-point is often part of an immune response.
- Acute cough lasts less than 3 weeks, subacute persists 3–8 weeks, and chronic cough is defined as cough persisting for 8 weeks or longer.
- In areas of high TB prevalence, chronic cough is defined as >2–3 weeks duration.

EPIDEMIOLOGY
- Cough is among the most common complaints in outpatient care.
- Cough and fever are common symptoms of respiratory illnesses, but may occur with other disorders as well.

RISK FACTORS
- Immunodeficiency
- Smoking
- Asthma, COPD
- The elderly and young children are at most risk for the development of pneumonia.
- Swallowing disorders (neurologic including stroke, Parkinson's disease; postsurgical/radiation treatment of oral, throat, or esophageal cancers) increase the risk of aspiration.
- Environmental or occupational exposures including unpasteurized dairy (brucellosis), birds (*Chlamydia psittaci*, psittacosis), residence/travel to Southwest US (coccidiomycosis), rodents (hantavirus), bat droppings (histoplasmosis), aerosolized water (legionellosis), or water contaminated with animal urine (leptospirosis).
- Inhalational anthrax, tularemia, plague, and other unusually severe pneumonia in a previously healthy host or clusters warrant consideration of bioterrorism.
- Pandemic influenza and SARS may also present in clusters.

GENERAL PREVENTION
- Up-to-date immunization against influenza and *Streptococcus pneumoniae*.
- Immunization against pertussis and *Haemophilus influenzae* type b especially important in pediatric patients.
- Smoking cessation

PATHOPHYSIOLOGY
Cough can be initiated as a protective mechanism by a variety of airway irritants that enter the tracheobronchial tree by inhalation (smoke, dust, fumes) or aspiration (upper airway secretions, gastric contents, foreign bodies).

ETIOLOGY
- Acute cough and fever is most frequently associated with viral nasopharyngitis with the usual causes including influenza virus, parainfluenza virus, respiratory syncytial virus, rhinovirus, coronavirus, and adenovirus.
  - In adults with "common cold," a slight fever (elevation of 1°F) is not uncommon, but an elevation greater than this is atypical.
- Other illnesses that may present with acute cough and fever include:
  - Upper respiratory tract infection (URI): Acute sinusitis, bronchitis. Both are often caused by viruses. Cough is the predominant symptom of acute bronchitis.
  - Lower respiratory tract infection (LRI): Pneumonia (bacterial, viral, fungal, and aspiration), exacerbation of bronchiectasis, lung abscess
  - Mediastinitis
  - Endocarditis
  - Malaria
  - Pulmonary embolism
  - Note: Some of the above disorders may also present with chronic cough and recurrent fever.
- Subacute cough may be due to bacterial sinusitis.
  - Although fever is generally absent or minimal, subacute cough is concerning in case of pertussis. Infection may be mild or atypical in previously immunized persons; however, pertussis is highly contagious and may be life-threatening to infants.
- Chronic cough and fever may represent TB in persons with risk factors (homelessness, HIV/AIDS) or from endemic areas. Other causes of chronic cough and fever include:
  - Chronic sinusitis
  - Chronic melioidosis (*Burkholderia pseudomallei*, endemic in Southeast Asia)
  - Endobronchial sarcoidosis
  - Kaposi's sarcoma
  - Lymphoma
  - Neoplasms infiltrating the airway wall, such as bronchogenic carcinoma or carcinoid tumor
  - Pulmonary embolism
  - Pulmonary inflammatory pseudotumor
- Cough and fever may be unrelated symptoms, especially if the onset is not simultaneous.
  - Chronic cough has many causes not limited to gastroesophageal reflux, postnasal drip, ACE inhibitor side effect, or asthma.
  - Subacute cough may also be postinfectious.

COMMONLY ASSOCIATED CONDITIONS
- HIV/AIDS
- Other immunodeficiency

DIAGNOSIS

HISTORY
- As severe febrile respiratory illnesses can rapidly progress to acute respiratory failure (bacterial pneumonia, influenza, SARS, agents of bioterrorism, pulmonary emboli), the initial approach is to determine if the illness is life-threatening or associated with signs of significant systemic disease.
- Assess for the following:
  - Dyspnea
  - Hemoptysis
  - Production of sputum
  - Symptoms suggestive of respiratory infection
  - Immunodeficiency
- Obtain a detailed history to assess for environmental or occupational exposures and travel history.
- Careful history may also suggest noninfectious causes (i.e., prolonged immobility and pulmonary emboli; smoking, weight loss, and hemoptysis in the absence of TB risk factors suggest malignancy).

PHYSICAL EXAM
- In addition to examination of the lungs, upper airway (mouth, throat, nose, sinuses), and ears, pay careful attention to overall appearance to assess severity of illness and possible respiratory compromise or fatigue.
  - Assess for tachycardia (heart rate >100 beats/min), tachypnea (>24 respirations/min), and difficulty oxygenating
- Physical findings supportive of LRI include focal rales and egophony. Physical examination is often insufficient to diagnose pneumonia.

DIAGNOSTIC TESTS & INTERPRETATION
Lab

Initial lab tests
- Purulent sputum suggests chronic bronchitis, bronchiectasis, pneumonia, or lung abscess. Blood in the sputum may be seen in the same disorders, but may also indicate an endobronchial tumor.
- Sputum microscopic examination and Gram stain may identify causative infectious organisms while culture results may guide antibiotic therapy. The diagnostic yield for both studies is low due to operator variability and lack of sputum production in many patients with pneumonia.

Follow-Up & Special Considerations
Chest X-ray as well as sputum smears and cultures for acid fast bacilli should be obtained for patients with chronic cough from areas with high TB prevalence.

Imaging
Initial approach
- Chest radiography is useful to distinguish upper versus lower respiratory disease or infection, as well as to identify the presence of an intrathoracic mass lesion.
- Patients with a clinical syndrome suggestive of acute bronchitis, with normal vital signs and normal pulmonary exam do not need CXR imaging as probability of pneumonia is low.
- While some features may aid in the diagnosis of pneumonia, infiltrate pattern does not confirm a specific infectious etiology. See chapter "Pneumonia."
  - Lobar consolidation, cavitation, and large pleural effusions suggest a bacterial infection.
  - Bilateral diffuse pulmonary involvement can be seen in patients with *Pneumocystis carinii*, *Legionella* spp., viral or *M. pneumoniae* infection.
  - Necrotizing pneumonia with cavitation and empyema suggests aspiration, Gram-negative or staphylococcal infection.
  - A nodular or cavitary pattern may be observed with bacterial lung abscess or infection with *Nocardia* spp., actinomycosis, atypical mycobacteria, cryptococcosis, or aspergillosis.
  - Focal infiltrates are common with bacteria (including *Nocardia* spp.), mycobacteria, *Cryptococcus* spp., or *Aspergillus* spp.
- HRCT is the procedure of choice for demonstrating dilated airways and confirming the diagnosis of bronchiectasis. Chest CT also aids in the evaluation of infections unresponsive to therapy and to define lung abscesses and postobstructive pneumonia due to tumor or other mass lesion.

Follow-Up & Special Considerations
- Consider sinus imaging and otolaryngology consultation if diagnosis unclear.
- Assess for extrapulmonary spread (especially brain abscess) in all patients with pulmonary infection who have neurologic or other extrapulmonary symptoms.

Diagnostic Procedures/Other
- Fiberoptic bronchoscopy is useful to collect specimens for histopathological analysis in the evaluation of an endobronchial tumor. Bronchoscopy with a protected specimen brush can assist in determining organism sensitivities in a patient with pneumonia not responding to therapy.
- Pleural biopsy and analysis of pleural fluid may assist in the diagnosis of TB or malignancy.

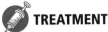 TREATMENT
MEDICATION
- Definitive treatment of cough depends on determining the underlying cause and then initiating specific therapy.
- Antimicrobials are generally not indicated for acute URI.
  - At presentation it is difficult to distinguish a diagnosis of bacterial sinusitis from a viral URI; antibiotic prescription should be delayed for 7 days.
- Antibiotics are indicated for pneumonia, TB, and pertussis.
- An irritative, nonproductive cough may be suppressed by an antitussive agent which increases the latency or threshold of the cough: Codeine (15 mg q.i.d.) or dextromethorphan (15 mg q.i.d.).
- Other pharmacologic agents that may decrease cough include:
  - NSAIDs such as naproxen
  - Sedating antihistamines may decrease cough due to "common colds"; newer generation nonsedating antihistamines are ineffective.
  - Ipratropium bromide (2–4 puffs q.i.d.) in patients with chronic bronchitis
- Cough productive of significant quantities of sputum should usually not be suppressed, as retention of sputum in the tracheobronchial tree may interfere with the distribution of ventilation, alveolar aeration, and the ability of the lung to resist infection.
- Hydration and expectorants such as guaifenesin may thin mucus and aid in expectoration.
- Although usually resected, inflammatory pseudotumors have been treated successfully with antibiotics, radiation, and corticosteroids. Spontaneous regression may also occur.

ADDITIONAL TREATMENT
General Measures
- Maintain hydration
- Smoking cessation

IN-PATIENT CONSIDERATIONS
Initial Stabilization
- Intubation and positive pressure ventilation should be considered in patients with respiratory fatigue or severe alterations of oxygenation and ventilation determined by arterial blood gas measurement.
  - Infection control measures (e.g., isolation and airborne precautions) should be implemented for patients with severe febrile respiratory illness and epidemiologic risk factors concerning for possible widespread transmission including appropriate travel history, exposure to an animal vector or laboratory pathogen, and bioterrorism event.

Admission Criteria
Although developed for pneumonia, the Pneumonia Severity Index may be applied to any patient with a febrile respiratory illness to help determine whether hospitalization is appropriate. Advanced age and significant medical comorbidities along with altered vital signs including tachypnea, tachycardia, and hypotension are markers for increased morbidity and mortality.

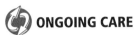 ONGOING CARE
FOLLOW-UP RECOMMENDATIONS
Encourage smoking cessation

PROGNOSIS
The mortality rate for community-acquired pneumonia is 13%.

COMPLICATIONS
- Paroxysms of coughing may precipitate syncope.
- Patients with TB and cough are considered infectious and can spread the infection.

ADDITIONAL READING
- Donowitz GR, Mandell GL. Acute pneumonia. In: Mandell GL, Bennett JE, Dolin R, eds. *Mandell, Douglas, and Bennett's principles and practice of infectious diseases*, 6th ed. Philadelphia: Elsevier, 2005:819–845.
- Gwaltney JM. The common cold. In: Mandell GL, Bennett JE, Dolin R, eds. *Mandell, Douglas, and Bennett's principles and practice of infectious diseases*, 6th ed. Philadelphia: Elsevier, 2005: 747–752.
- Irwin RS, Baumann MH, Bolser DC, et al. Diagnosis and management of cough executive summary: ACCP evidence-based clinical practice guidelines. *CHEST* 2006;129:1S–23S.
- Stanton MW. *Improving treatment decisions for patients with community-acquired pneumonia.* Research in Action, Issue 7. AHRQ Pub. No. 02-0033. Rockville, MD: Agency for Healthcare Research and Quality, 2002.

 CODES
ICD9
- 460 Acute nasopharyngitis (common cold)
- 780.60 Fever, unspecified
- 786.2 Cough

CLINICAL PEARLS
- Most causes of acute cough and fever are viral and self-limited.
- Consider infection control measures in cases of severe febrile respiratory illness until a cause can be determined to lessen spread to other patients and protect healthcare workers.
- Encourage smoking cessation.

DIARRHEA AND FEVER
Rachel P. Simmons

 BASICS

DESCRIPTION
- Diarrhea is formally defined as an increase in daily stool weight above 200 g and more generally defined as 3 or more loose stools per day.
- Diarrhea is considered acute when lasting <14 days and chronic when lasting >4 weeks.
- An inflammatory diarrheal syndrome is characterized by frequent, small-volume, mucoid or bloody stools (or both). It may be accompanied by tenesmus, fever, or severe abdominal pain. The hallmark of inflammatory diarrheas is the presence of leukocytes in the stool.
- A noninflammatory diarrheal syndrome is characterized by watery stools that may be of large volume (>1 L/d), without blood, pus, severe abdominal pain, or fever.

EPIDEMIOLOGY
Incidence
- 200–375 million episodes of acute diarrhea occur in the US each year.
- Approximately 38 million of these episodes are attributable to a known pathogen (bacteria, parasite, or virus). Food borne transmission accounts for approximately 36% of diarrheal illnesses due to known pathogens.
- Of the 9 bacterial enteropathogens tracked by FoodNet, the most common causes in 2007 were non-typhoid salmonella (14.86 cases/100,000 population), campylobacter (12.78), *shigella* (6.24), cryptosporidium (2.67), and Shiga toxin-producing *E. coli* (STEC) O157 (1.19).
- The incidence of bacterial diarrhea caused by salmonella, campylobacter, and yersinia is highest in infants <1 year of age.
- The incidence of post-diarrheal hemolytic uremic syndrome (HUS) in the US is 0.65 cases per 100,000 population and is highest in children under the age of 5.
- Traveler's diarrhea affects 20–60% of international travelers.

RISK FACTORS
- Consuming undercooked eggs, meat, seafood, poultry, or unpasteurized dairy products.
- Drinking untreated stream or river water.
- Conditions associated with increased severity of illness or increased risk for specific pathogens include HIV infection, immunosuppressing medications (glucocorticoids, TNF inhibitors, chemotherapy, etc), recent antibiotic use, liver disease, neutropenia, malnutrition, zinc deficiency, IgA deficiency
- Oral–anal sexual contact
- Exposure to antibiotics is a risk factor for *C. difficile* associated diarrhea.

GENERAL PREVENTION
- Wash hands with soap before eating or preparing food
- Avoid raw or undercooked eggs or poultry, meat, fish, and seafood
- Avoid unpasteurized dairy products
- Avoid consuming untreated stream or river water
- When traveling, avoid tap water and ice in areas with potentially contaminated water.
- Vaccines are available to prevent *Salmonella typhi* associated with international travel. Please see CDC website for recommended vaccinations based on destination (http://www.cdc.gov/).
- Rotavirus vaccine is recommended by The Advisory Committee on Immunization Practices for infants in the US.

ETIOLOGY
- Bacteria (Campylobacter, *Salmonella* species, *E. coli* [a. Enterotoxigenic (ETEC), b. Enteropathogenic (EPEC), c. Enteroinvasive (EIEC), d. Shiga toxin-producing *E. coli* (STEC) including E. coli O157:H7 and e. Enteroaggregative E. coli (EAEC)], *Shigella* species, *Yersinia enterocolitica*, *Clostridium difficile*, *Vibrio cholera*, *Vibrio parahaemolyticus*, *Aeromonas species*, *Plesiomonas shigelloides*
- Viruses (Rotavirus, human caliciviruses including noroviruses, Adenovirus, and Cytomegalovirus)
- Parasites (*Giardia intestinalis*, *Cryptosporidium parvum*, *Entamoeba histolytica*, *Cyclospora cayetanensis*, *Isospora belli*, and *Strongyloides stercoralis*)
- Toxin-mediated diarrhea (*Staphylococcus aureus*, *Bacillus cereus*, and *Clostridium perfringens*)

DIAGNOSIS

HISTORY
- A detailed medical history and a physical examination are essential in determining the possible etiology, degree of severity, and presence of complications.
- Enquire about recent travel, diet, antibiotic use, sexual activity, day-care attendance, other illnesses, outbreaks, and season.
- Determine the frequency, duration, and character of diarrhea (watery, bloody, etc)
- Infectious diarrhea can be associated with fever and chills, vomiting, nausea, abdominal pain, tenesmus.
- A history of dizziness, syncope, or presyncope indicates volume depletion.
- Bloody stools (dysentery) suggests an invasive pathogen such as shigella, salmonella, campylobacter, Shiga toxin-producing *E. coli* (especially if no fever), or yersinia.
- Shiga toxin-producing *E. coli*, including O157:H7 causes watery progressing to bloody diarrhea and is associated with consuming contaminated beef or produce in about half. Fever is often absent.

- Yersinia and salmonella can infect the terminal ileum and cecum and present with right lower quadrant pain and tenderness suggestive of acute appendicitis.
- Watery diarrhea is clinically nonspecific.
- Gastroenteritis caused by an enterotoxin (food poisoning) can be due to S. *aureus*, B. *cereus*, or C. *perfringens*. Such cases can present with vomiting alone (S. *aureus* or C. *perfringens*) or watery diarrhea (B. *Cereus* or C. *perfringens*). Fever is generally absent. The incubation period is short (2–7 h for S. *aureus*; 8–14 hours for C. *perfringens*; C. *perfringens* can have either) and duration is short.
- Extraintestinal manifestations such as arthritis, skin lesions, or ocular symptoms suggest inflammatory bowel disease.
- If recent international travel, the cause depends on destination, setting, and season. The most common pathogens include enterotoxigenic E. coli, enteroaggregative E. coli, campylobacter, salmonella, and norovirus. The CDC Travelers' Heath website or other travel medicine resource can aid in diagnostic workup.

PHYSICAL EXAM
- Assess blood pressure, heart rate, respiratory rate, temperature, and mental status to ascertain the severity.
- Check for signs of dehydration including dry mucous membranes, poor skin turgor, sunken eyes, diminished capillary refill, low jugular venous pressure, or postural hypotension.
- Evaluate for abdominal tenderness, signs of peritonitis (guarding, rebound tenderness), hepatomegaly, and splenomegaly.

DIAGNOSTIC TESTS & INTERPRETATION
Lab
Initial lab tests
- Indications for diagnostic testing include the following: Fever, systemic illness, bloody diarrhea, dehydration, a known or suspected outbreak of food-borne infection, recent overseas travel, immunosuppression, or recent antibiotic use.
- Send stool for culture. In most microbiology laboratories, stool sent for culture of enteric pathogens will be processed for shigella, salmonella, and campylobacter. Therefore, if the clinical suspicion for *E. coli* (STEC, ETEC, EPEC, EIEC), yersinia, vibrio, and so on is high, notify the microbiology lab. The diagnostic yield of stool cultures ranges from 1.5–5.6%.
- If bloody diarrhea, culture stool for salmonella, shigella, campylobacter, and Shiga toxin-producing *E. Coli* and send immunoassay for Shiga toxin. If *E. coli* is isolated, send to a reference lab for serotyping.
- If recent antibiotic exposure, recent hospitalization, day care exposure, or recent chemotherapy, stool should be tested for *C. difficile* toxins A and B.

- For persistent diarrhea for more than 7 days, send multiple stool specimens for ova and parasite testing specifically for Giardia, cryptosporidium, Isospora belli, and Cyclospora. Consider noninfectious cause. In patients with AIDS or immunosuppression, also test for microsporidia, *Mycobacterium avium* complex, and cytomegalovirus.
- Positive fecal testing for polymorphonuclear cells suggests an inflammatory diarrhea.

Follow-Up & Special Considerations
If evidence of dehydration or severe illness, check serum electrolytes, kidney function, liver function, complete blood count, and blood cultures.

Imaging
If diagnosis remains uncertain, critical illness, prominent abdominal pain, or evidence of peritonitis, consider a CT scan with oral and intravenous contrast.

Diagnostic Procedures/Other
For further evaluation, consider upper gastrointestinal endoscopy or colonoscopy with diagnostic biopsies.

DIFFERENTIAL DIAGNOSIS
- Acute inflammatory diarrheal syndrome can also be of noninfectious etiology (ulcerative colitis, Crohn's disease, radiation or ischemic colitis, partial bowel obstruction, or diverticulitis, laxative abuse, rectosigmoid abscess, Whipple's disease, pernicious anemia, diabetes, malabsorption, scleroderma, or celiac sprue).
- Diarrhea and fever also may result from infection outside the gastrointestinal tract, as in malaria or sepsis.

 TREATMENT

MEDICATION
- The key components of treatment include **rehydration** and **antibiotics**.
- Oral rehydration is the most appropriate cost-effective management for both developing and developed countries. Intravenous repletion of volume is indicated in severe dehydration or severe electrolyte disturbance. Rice-based oral solution is superior in adults and children with cholera.
- Antimicrobial therapy is indicated in severe infection and recommended for persistent gastroenteritis, in adults >65 years, in immunocompromised persons, in patients with prostheses, and in invasive infections with the exception of Shiga toxin-producing *E. coli*.

Empiric therapy:
- For febrile community-acquired invasive diarrhea or moderate to severe traveler's diarrhea, treat with ciprofloxacin 500 mg twice daily or levofloxacin 500 mg daily pending stool studies unless Shiga toxin-producing *E. coli* is suspected. If recent travel to Southeast Asia, consider fluoroquinolone resistant campylobacter.

- If recent antibiotic use or nosocomial diarrhea, treat with metronidazole or vancomycin pending assay for *C. difficile* toxin.

Selected pathogens and their therapy:
- Salmonella (non-typhi species) – Bacteremia occurs in 2–8%. Treat if severe disease, age <12 months, age >50 years, valve disease, severe atherosclerosis, prosthesis, cancer, HIV, uremia, sickle cell disease, and other immunocompromised diseases. Ciprofloxacin 500 mg PO twice daily or levofloxacin 500 mg daily for 5–7 days. If susceptible, TMP-SMX DS twice daily for 5–7 days, ceftriaxone 2 g IV/IM daily for 5–7 days. Treat for 14 days if immunocompromised. Antibiotics may increase shedding.
- Shigellosis – ciprofloxacin 500 mg PO twice daily or levofloxacin 500 mg once daily for 3 days or if susceptible, TMP-SMX DS twice daily for 3 days. Treat 7–10 days in severe disease or if immunocompromised.
- Campylobacter – erythromycin 500 mg twice daily for 5 days. High fluoroquinolone resistance, especially in Southeast Asia.
- *E. coli*, Shiga toxin-producing (STEC) – **NO** antibiotics as may increase risk of HUS. Supportive care.
- *E. coli* (ETEC, EPEC, EIEC) – ciprofloxacin 500 mg PO twice daily or levofloxacin 500 mg daily for 3 days. If susceptible, TMP-SMX DS twice daily for 3 days.
- *Yersinia* – antibiotics not usually required. For severe infections or immunocompromise, doxycycline plus aminoglycoside, fluoroquinolones, or TMP-SMX.
- *C. difficile* – stop unnecessary antibiotics and metronidazole 500 mg 3 times daily for milder cases or vancomycin 125 mg 4 times daily for 10–14 days. Please see relevant topic.
- Cholera: Fluid replacement is the key. Check local susceptibilities. Can be treated with doxycycline, tetracycline, TMP-SMX, or fluoroquinolone.
- Amebiasis: Metronidazole 750 mg 3 times daily for 5 days (10 days in severe infection), followed by paromomycin 500 mg 3 times daily for 7 days, or iodoquinol 650 mg 3 times daily for 20 days.
- Giardiasis: Metronidazole 250–750 mg 3 times daily for 7–10 days or tinidazole 2 g for 1 dose
- Cyclospora & Isospora – TMP-SMX 1 DS twice daily for 7–10 days. If immunocompromised, extend treatment and consider suppression.

ADDITIONAL TREATMENT
General Measures
- Most mild cases are self-limited. Symptomatic treatment includes hydration and anti-motility agents such as loperamide.
- Loperamide is the antidiarrheal agent of choice in adults with mild to moderate diarrhea without bloody stools. It is contraindicated in cases of severe, inflammatory, or bloody diarrheas, *C. difficile infection*, and children <2 years.
- Bismuth salicylate is an antisecretory agent; can reduce stool output in children and adults.

Issues for Referral
- For cases of severe or persistent diarrhea of unknown etiology, consider gastroenterology and/or infectious diseases consultation.
- Report cases of *Salmonella* species, *Shigella*, *Campylobacter*, *E. coli*, *Cholera*, cryptosporidiosis, cyclosporiasis, *Vibrio* species, and suspected or confirmed outbreaks.

IN-PATIENT CONSIDERATIONS
Initial Stabilization
Prompt rehydration and empiric antibiotics in inflammatory diarrhea are warranted in severe acute diarrhea with systemic toxicity.

Admission Criteria
Hospitalize patients with severe dehydration or inability to maintain fluid intake.

IV Fluids
Intravenous repletion of volume is indicated in severe dehydration or if the patient has altered mental status.

Discharge Criteria
Patients may be discharged when fevers abate for >24 h, vital signs normalize, and patient can maintain adequate fluid and food intake.

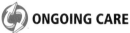 ONGOING CARE

FOLLOW-UP RECOMMENDATIONS
Test and treat family with similar symptoms.

DIET
- Food can be started 4 hours after initiation of oral or intravenous hydration.
- Give frequent, small meals of easily digestible food.
- Avoid fruit juices which are hyperosmolar and can exacerbate diarrhea.

PATIENT EDUCATION
Educate patients about general food safety and how to avoid food-borne illnesses, especially while traveling.

PROGNOSIS
Gastrointestinal illness is responsible for more than 900,000 hospitalizations and 6,000 deaths in the US annually.

COMPLICATIONS
Complications include dehydration, electrolyte abnormalities, bacteremia and sepsis, malnutrition and vitamin loss, HUS, and systemic amebiasis.

ADDITIONAL READING
- DuPont HL. Clinical practice. Bacterial diarrhea. *N Engl J Med* 2009;361:1560–1569.
- Theilman NM, Guerrant RL. Clinical practice. Acute infectious diarrhea. *N Engl J Med* 2004;350:38–47.

 CODES

ICD9
- 009.2 Infectious diarrhea
- 558.9 Other and unspecified noninfectious gastroenteritis and colitis

CLINICAL PEARLS
- Avoid raw or undercooked eggs or poultry, meat, fish, and seafood and unpasteurized dairy products, especially when traveling.
- Stool culture for enteric pathogens is the test of choice.
- Do not give antibiotics if Shiga toxin-producing *E. coli* is suspected.
- Avoid antimotility drugs in invasive, inflammatory, bloody diarrheas.

DYSURIA AND FEVER

Anton Y. Peleg

 BASICS

DESCRIPTION
- The term dysuria is used to describe painful urination.
- Acute urethral syndrome can also be used to describe symptoms of dysuria, urgency, and frequency that is not associated with significant bacteriuria.

Approach to the Patient
- Irritation of the urethral and vesical mucosa causes frequent and painful urination of small amounts of urine.
- Many physicians equate dysuria with urinary tract infection (UTI) and treat with antibiotics. This therapeutic trial represents undertreatment for some and inappropriate treatment for others.
- A careful history and examination (including rectal and pelvic examination where appropriate) can lead to a diagnosis and allow directed therapy.
- Sexually-transmitted infections such as *Chlamydia trachomatis, Neisseria gonorrhoeae,* or herpes simplex virus (HSV) can cause dysuria in men and women.
- Prostatitis is an important diagnosis to make in men due to the difficulty with treatment and risk of recurrent infection.
- Fever is rare in lower-urinary tract infection (cystitis) but may be present in acute prostatitis.
- If dysuria is accompanied by fever, consider an upper-tract infectious etiology such as pyelonephritis. Primary genital herpes can also produce dysuria with fever. Chlamydia, gonorrhea, and nonspecific urethritis are uncommonly associated with fever unless pelvic inflammatory disease or Fitz-Hugh-Curtis syndrome (perihepatitis) are present.
- If dysuria is accompanied by hematuria, consider infectious or noninfectious cystitis, including tuberculous cystitis, bladder carcinoma, trauma, renal calculus, and schistosomiasis.

- If dysuria is accompanied by urethral or vaginal discharge, consider a sexually-transmitted infection such as gonorrhea or Chlamydia, as well as nonspecific urethritis (with or without joint involvement and conjunctivitis, known as Reiter's syndrome), and prostatitis.
- Urinalysis and urine culture are the most common initial diagnostic tests. However, for young women with characteristic symptoms of UTI and no risk factors for complicated or recurrent infection, empiric antibiotic treatment may be warranted.

EPIDEMIOLOGY
Incidence
- UTIs are among the most prevalent infectious syndromes and they are responsible for a huge financial burden.
- The annual cost of the prescribed antibiotics for UTIs in the US is estimated over 1 billion dollars.
- 80% of patients with primary symptomatic genital herpes will have dysuria; however, dysuria is usually not present if the infection recurs.
- Sexual intercourse is associated with several causes of dysuria. Women with postcoital cystitis typically develop symptoms within a few days of intercourse, whereas women with urethritis develop symptoms 1–2 weeks later, and women with vaginitis develop symptoms weeks to months later.
- Pyelonephritis is one of the commonest reasons for hospital admission.
- UTIs in the US account for more than 100,000 admissions per year.
- About 40% of healthcare-associated infections are UTIs and the majority of them catheter-related.
- Up to 25% of patients with a urinary catheter in for more than 7 days develop bacteriuria, with a 5% daily risk of UTI.
- A single bladder catheterization may lead to UTI in 1–2%.
- *E. coli* is the causative organism in 50–75% of uncomplicated UTIs.
- 20–40% of those with asymptomatic bacteriuria during pregnancy will develop pyelonephritis, with subsequent risks of premature labor.

ETIOLOGY
- In addition to the causes noted above, dysuria can be due to the following:
  - Atrophic vaginitis, Vaginitis secondary to *Candida* spp.
  - Bladder irritation from a distal urethral stone
  - Chemical exposure
  - Compression from an adnexal mass
  - Radiation
  - Vaginal and urethral trauma, including sexual abuse and the insertion of a foreign body
- Among women presenting with acute dysuria and frequency, most have significant bacteriuria, but most of those without significant bacteriuria also have infections of the kidneys, bladder, or urethra.
- *Ureaplasma urealyticum* has frequently been isolated from the urethra and urine of patients with dysuria, but it is also found in specimens from patients without urinary symptoms.
- *U. urealyticum* and *Mycoplasma hominis* have been isolated from prostatic and renal tissues of patients with dysuria.
- Adenoviruses cause acute hemorrhagic cystitis in children and in some young adults, often in epidemics.
- Although many other viruses can be isolated from urine, they are thought not to cause urinary infection in immunocompetent patients.

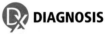 **DIAGNOSIS**

HISTORY
- Dysuria, frequency, urgency, and suprapubic tenderness are common symptoms of bladder and urethral inflammation.
- Prostatitis leads to frequency, dysuria, and urgency, and the prostate may be boggy and tender on rectal examination.
- Symptoms of acute pyelonephritis generally develop rapidly over a few hours or a day and include a fever, shaking chills, nausea, vomiting, and diarrhea. Symptoms of cystitis may or may not develop. In addition to fever, tachycardia, and generalized muscle tenderness, physical examination reveals marked tenderness on deep pressure in one or both costovertebral angles.

- Assess for predisposing factors for UTI or pyelonephritis, including atrophic vaginitis, which is associated with decreased vaginal discharge, vaginal tenderness, bloody vaginal spotting (especially after intercourse), and dyspareunia.

PHYSICAL EXAM
- Assess vital signs and hydration status, especially if pyelonephritis suspected.
- Suprapubic sensitivity and positive flank sensitivity may reflect the presence of lower or upper urinary tract infection respectively.
- Genital exam may be necessary if symptoms are suggestive of a sexually-transmitted infection.
- Prostate exam is always necessary in men.

DIAGNOSTIC TESTS & INTERPRETATION
Lab
- The most sensitive laboratory indicator for UTI is pyuria. A positive leukocyte esterase dipstick test is 75–95% sensitive in detecting pyuria secondary to infection.
- Bacterial colony counts of 10^5 organisms per milliliter or greater in urine generally indicate urinary tract infection. Levels above 10^2 colonies per milliliter are sufficient to indicate infection in symptomatic patients and in urine samples obtained by suprapubic aspiration or bladder catheter.
- Most bacterial pathogens (with the exception of *Staphylococcus saprophyticus* and *Enterococcus* spp.) can convert urinary nitrate to nitrite. Positive nitrite is >90% specific for urinary tract infections, but sensitivity is only about 30%.
- Rapid methods of detection of bacteriuria have been developed as alternatives to standard culture methods. These methods detect bacterial growth by photometry, bioluminescence, or other means and provide results rapidly, usually in 1–2 hours. However, the sensitivity of these tests falls less than 80% when 10^2–10^4 colony-forming units per milliliter is the standard of comparison.
- Pyuria in the absence of bacteriuria (sterile pyuria) may indicate infection with unusual bacterial agents, such as *C. trachomatis*, *U. urealyticum*, and *Mycobacterium tuberculosis*, or with fungi.
- Sterile pyuria may also indicate prostatitis and noninfectious urologic conditions such as calculi, anatomic abnormality, nephrocalcinosis, vesicoureteral reflux, interstitial nephritis, or polycystic disease.

 TREATMENT
- The choice of treatment for patients with acute urethritis depends on the etiology.
- Short course antibiotic therapy (3–5 days) is indicated for lower tract urinary infection in women. This should be extended to 10–14 days in men or those with upper tract involvement.
- If prostatitis is suspected or confirmed, longer periods of antibiotic therapy are required (at least 4 weeks).
- See other chapters for more detail: Section I, "Urethritis and Urethral Discharge" and Section II, "Prostatitis" and "Vaginal Discharge/Vaginitis."
- Women with acute dysuria and frequency, negative urine cultures, and no pyuria usually do not respond to antimicrobial agents.

 ONGOING CARE
FOLLOW-UP RECOMMENDATIONS
- >30% of women will experience at least one episode of cystitis in their lifetime, 20% will have recurrent cystitis.
- Recurrent urinary tract infections are usually reinfections separated by an asymptomatic interval of at least 1 month's duration. They are usually caused by vaginal and rectal colonization with uropathogens. Anatomic abnormalities in young women with recurrent cystitis are rare.

COMPLICATIONS
Cystitis may result in upper tract infection.

ADDITIONAL READING
- Grabe M, Bjerklund-Johansen TE, Botto H, et al. Guidelines on urological infections. European association of Urology, March 2011.
- Hooton TM, Bradley SF, Cardenas DD, et al. Diagnosis prevention and treatment of catheter-associated urinary tract infection in adults: 2009 International Clinical Practice Guidelines from the Infectious Diseases Society of America. *Clin Infect Dis* 2010;50(5):625–63.

 CODES

ICD9
- 597.81 Urethral syndrome nos
- 788.1 Dysuria

CLINICAL PEARLS
- Classic symptoms of dysuria, frequency and urgency in a young female, warrants empiric treatment for UTI. Further testing is required if recurrent UTI occurs.
- Always consider sexually-transmitted infections, including HIV.
- Always consider prostatitis in male patients with dysuria, especially if >50 yrs of age.
- Renal tract imaging is indicated in those with recurrent infections, first infection in males and urinary infections in children.
- Think TB with sterile pyuria.

EAR PAIN
Isaac I. Bogoch

BASICS

DESCRIPTION
- Otalgia refers to pain involving the ear.
- Approach to the patient:
  - The age of the patient and the presence of other associated symptoms such as sore throat, fever, headache, visual changes, and the duration of these symptoms should be investigated.
  - A careful exam of all aspects of the ear is crucial for patients presenting with ear pain. The auricle and external auditory meatus should be examined first, followed by the auditory canal and the tympanic membrane. This will help generate a differential diagnosis.
  - A complete physical examination of the head and neck may also reveal lymphadenopathy, posterior nasal or pharyngeal inflammation, thyroiditis, or oral/dental pathology.
  - Otoscopic examination of the tympanic membrane may be obscured by cerumen (ear wax). This should be carefully removed to ensure proper visualization of auditory structures.
  - Exudate in the auditory canal should be sent for culture and sensitivity testing.
  - Pain on moving the ear suggests otitis externa, foreign body, and sometimes impacted wax.
  - Perichondritis, an infection of the outer ear, must be distinguished from relapsing polychondritis, a rheumatologic condition.

EPIDEMIOLOGY
- It is estimated that 50% of ear pain is referred from non-otologic sites.
- Acute otitis externa (or "swimmer's ear") occurs mostly in the summer.
- About 20% of children have multiple, recurrent episodes of acute otitis media.

- Most head and neck cancers occur after age 50, although these cancers can appear in younger patients, including those without known risk factors. Many forms of nasopharyngeal carcinoma have been linked to Epstein-Barr virus (EBV) infection.
- In auricular cellulitis, there may be a history of minor trauma to the ear.
- Perichondritis (infection of the perichondrium of the ear) usually follows burns or trauma to the ear and are occasionally associated with piercings of the upper ear. *Pseudomonas aeruginosa* and *Staphylococcus aureus* are the most common pathogens.
- Chronic otitis externa is often due to irritation from either repeated minor trauma to the canal such as scratching or the use of cotton swabs. Drainage of a chronic middle ear infection may be mistaken for chronic otitis externa.
- Malignant otitis externa is an erosive disease of the auditory canal and skull base.

ETIOLOGY
- Otalgia is often referred pain from other head and neck structures. Pain may be experienced in the ear as it is richly innervation from cranial nerves V, VII, VIII, IX, and X.
- Otalgia can be referred from the following:
  - Diseases of the teeth and gingiva (abscess, impacted teeth, etc.)
  - Inflammatory, neoplastic, and other diseases of the larynx and nasopharynx.
  - Sinus pathology such as sinusitis
  - Temporomandibular joint disorders
  - Tonsillitis
  - Tongue pathology
  - Diseases of the cervical spine like degenerative disc disease
  - Damage or irritation to nerves (e.g. acoustic neuroma, trigeminal neuralgia)
  - Gastroesophageal reflux (in infants and children)
  - Thyroiditis
  - Inflammation and thrombosis of the lateral sinus
  - Inflammatory or infectious processes of the posterior fossa
  - Medications (such as mesalazine and sulfasalazine)

- Otalgia secondary to ear pathology has a broad differential diagnosis that includes the following:
  - Acute otitis media
  - Chronic otitis media
  - Traumatic rupture of the tympanic membrane
  - Fracture of the anterior wall of the body canal
  - Mastoiditis
  - Ménière's disease
  - Eustachian tube dysfunction
- Malignant otitis externa is almost always caused by *P. aeruginosa*.
- Ear pain is also associated with migraine headaches, atypical facial pain, and herpes simplex of the fifth and seventh cranial nerves and the glossopharyngeal nerve.
- Herpes zoster in the external canal is often accompanied by ipsilateral facial paralysis (Ramsay Hunt syndrome) due to the involvement of the geniculate ganglion of cranial nerve VII.
- Cranial nerve seven palsy may be caused by herpes zoster and Lyme disease.
- The infratemporal fossa is a relatively protected region that may be the site of neoplasms presenting as otalgia.
- The most common pathogens of acute otitis externa are *P. aeruginosa*, *S. aureus*, and streptococcal species. Risk factors include swimming or trauma to the auditory canal.

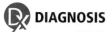

DIAGNOSIS

CLINICAL-MANIFESTATIONS
- Auricular cellulitis usually presents as a swollen, erythematous, hot, mildly tender ear.
- Perichondritis is associated with infection of the skin and tissue surrounding the cartilage of the outer ear. Patients present with a swollen, hot, red, and exquisitely tender pinna, usually with sparing of the lobule.
- Chronic otitis externa typically causes pruritus rather than ear pain.
- Nasopharyngeal carcinoma may be asymptomatic until it is locally or regionally advanced. It often causes unilateral serous otitis media due to obstruction of the eustachian tube, unilateral or bilateral nasal obstruction, or epistaxis.
- Advanced nasopharyngeal carcinoma can present with cranial nerve palsies typically affecting nerves III, IV, VI, and VII.

- Patients with malignant otitis externa are usually elderly patients with diabetes or HIV positive individuals. Presentation typically involves severe ear pain and otorrhea. Cranial nerve VII is most commonly involved, and palsies of other cranial nerves may be seen as well. There may be a loss of hearing, the pinna is typically tender, and trismus indicates temporomandibular involvement. Constitutional symptoms such as fever and weight loss are relatively uncommon. Physical examination usually reveals abnormalities of the external auditory canal, including swelling, erythema, purulent discharge, debris, and granulation tissue in the canal wall.
- A vesicular rash of the external auditory canal may indicate herpes zoster. Also look for ipsilateral cranial nerve VII palsy suggestive of the Ramsay Hunt syndrome.
- Hearing loss with an abnormal tympanic membrane (e.g. loss of cone of light) suggests serous or bacterial otitis media or cholesteatoma.
- Polyposis, severe deviation of the nasal septum, or a nasopharyngeal tumor may be associated with otitis media.

PHYSICAL EXAM
- Erythematous ear canal with discharge, swollen preauricular lymph nodes, and sensitive tragus or pinna may suggest otitis externa.
- Fever, irritation in children, and otoscopic findings such as an erythematous or bulging tympanic membrane associated with an absent cone of light indicates otitis media. In addition, you may see pus in the canal if the tympanic membrane is ruptured.
- Altered mental status and signs of meningeal irritation such as headache and neck stiffness are indicative of CNS involvement and should be treated emergently.

DIAGNOSTIC TESTS & INTERPRETATION
Lab
Peripheral leukocytosis is relatively infrequent in malignant external otitis, while the erythrocyte sedimentation rate is typically elevated. Cerebrospinal fluid occasionally exhibits pleocytosis and an elevation in the protein level.

Imaging
- Dental disease can be evaluated by radiographic examination (Panorex films).
- In malignant external otitis, computed tomography (CT) of the mastoid or temporal bone typically reveals bony erosions and new bone formation, while the floor of the skull may have soft-tissue densities associated with areas of cellulitis. Magnetic resonance imaging (MRI) will delineate soft-tissue involvement with greater sensitivity and accuracy.

 TREATMENT

MEDICATION
- Treatment of acute otitis externa involves careful cleaning of the ear and canal, along with the administration of topical antiseptic agents, or topical antibiotics such as polymyxin–neomycin (4 drops 4 times daily for 5 days). In addition, patients should be counseled on proper ear hygiene and avoiding water exposure during infection.
- Malignant otitis externa should be promptly evaluated by an otolaryngologist. It is usually treated with antipseudomonal agents such as cefepime or ceftazidime, carbapenems, or with fluoroquinolones like ciprofloxacin. Treatment should be extended for 3–4 weeks and even longer if bone is involved.
- Treatment of auricular cellulitis consists of warm compresses and intravenous administration of antibiotics active against *S. aureus* and streptococci.
- Severe perichondritis should be treated with antibiotics, such as piperacillin/tazobactam or nafcillin plus ciprofloxacin for at least 4 weeks. Incision and drainage may be helpful for culture and for resolution of infection, which is often slow.
- Ramsay Hunt is commonly treated with acyclovir and corticosteroids. Early initiation of therapy may prevent permanent cranial nerve VII palsy. Ophthalmology should examine for eye involvement of zoster.

 ONGOING CARE

FOLLOW-UP RECOMMENDATIONS
Referral to an otolaryngologist is usually indicated if otalgia does not resolve after initial diagnosis and management.

COMPLICATIONS
- Complications of otitis media include mastoiditis, epidural abscess, dural venous thrombophlebitis (usually sigmoid sinus), meningitis, and brain abscess.
- The cavernous sinus can become involved in malignant external otitis, as can the contralateral petrous apex; meningitis and brain abscess are relatively rare but serious complications.

ADDITIONAL READING
- Lieberthal AS. Acute otitis media guidelines: Review and update. *Curr Allergy Asthma Rep* 2006;6(4): 334–341.
- Osguthorpe JD, Nielsen DR. Otitis externa: Review and clinical update. *Am Fam Physician* 2006;74(9): 1510–1516.

 CODES

ICD9
- 380.00 Perichondritis of pinna, unspecified
- 380.10 Infective otitis externa, unspecified
- 388.70 Otalgia, unspecified

CLINICAL PEARLS
- Otalgia may arise from ear pathology but is also commonly referred from nearby structures.
- Serious infections of the ear may involve adjacent regions of the CNS.

E

FEVER OF UNKNOWN ORIGIN

Cameron J. Jeremiah
Anton Y. Peleg

 BASICS

DESCRIPTION

- Fever of unknown origin (FUO) is a term applied to a clinical syndrome characterized by persistence of fever beyond the time expected for resolution of an acute febrile illness.
- The term is intended to exclude self-limiting infections, conditions diagnosed on basic baseline investigations, and patients with benign fevers (i.e., <38.3°C).
- Current accepted criteria for FUO are a revised version of those originally proposed by Petersdorf and Beeson in 1961 (1):
  - An illness of at least 3 weeks duration
  - A fever above 38.3°C on several occasions
  - And no diagnosis after thorough investigation
- Durack and Street have defined subtypes of FUO to reflect differences in etiology and diagnostic approach in a variety of clinical scenarios (2):
  - Classical FUO (as defined above)
  - Immune-deficient FUO
  - Healthcare-associated FUO
  - HIV-related FUO
  - Based on this approach, immune-deficient patients, hospitalized individuals afebrile prior to their admission, and those with HIV can be considered as having FUO after 3–5 days of evaluation in hospital, with 48 hours of negative cultures.

Approach to the Patient

- FUO is one of the most challenging and frustrating clinical problems for both patient and physician. Bearing this in mind, the key management goals of FUO must be considered:
  - Identify an etiology.
  - Reach a diagnosis with efficient and safe use of appropriate investigations. Some patients will require periods of observation, while others will need rapid and extensive investigation.
  - Institute appropriate treatment once a diagnosis is made or, if necessary, commence a therapeutic trial.
- Evaluation of an FUO must be tailored to the patient in order to avoid over-investigating unlikely causes and under-investigating likely causes. Therefore strict diagnostic algorithms are discouraged.
- When evaluating an FUO, the clinician should aim to assess the following five points:
  - Confirm the fever and characterize its pattern. Fever >41°C is rarely due to infection.
  - Assess the tempo and severity of the illness.
  - Attempt to identify localizing symptoms.
  - Explore the context including past medical history and medications.
  - Identify any disease risk factors or exposures, e.g., travel, occupational and sexual histories, animal exposure, vaccination, and intravenous drug use.
- In order to qualify for the diagnosis of FUO, a minimum diagnostic evaluation should include at least the following:
  - Detailed history
  - Repeat physical examination
  - Complete blood count with blood film, differential and platelet count
  - Routine blood chemistry, including liver enzymes, lactate dehydrogenase, and bilirubin
  - Urinalysis (including microscopy and culture)

- Chest radiograph
- Erythrocyte sedimentation rate and C-reactive protein
- Antinuclear antibodies
- Rheumatoid factor and anti-cyclic citrullinated peptide
- Three sets of routine blood cultures (while not on antibiotics)
- Tuberculin skin test (TST) or interferon gamma release assay (IGRA)
- CT of abdomen and pelvis
- Serological evaluation for infectious diseases (described in etiology) should be based on the clinical scenario

Geriatric Considerations (3)

- Polymyalgia rheumatica
- Less undiagnosed causes of FUO

Pediatric Considerations

- HHV6/7/8 common in children/infants
- Ultrasound is preferable over CT in children due to lower radiation and greater resolution in children
- Connective tissue diseases and neoplasms are rare in those <12 months
- Kawasaki disease is common in those <5 years
- Still's disease is often seen in children and young adults
- Arthritis in children generally signals serious pathology
- Hyper-IgD, cyclic neutropenia, and nephroma all need to be considered in pediatric patients

Pregnancy Considerations

- Pregnant women are at increased risk of venous thromboembolism
- Consider septic pelvic thrombophlebitis post obstetric surgery
- Consider sexually transmitted infections – HIV and syphilis
- Pyometra

EPIDEMIOLOGY

- True FUO is an uncommon presentation.
- Patient series have demonstrated that the relative frequencies of specific etiologies of FUO vary with population, geographic location, institution, age, local disease prevalence, and medical practice.
- Over time, the proportion of infectious and neoplastic causes of FUO have reduced, while undiagnosed patients have increased.

DIAGNOSIS

The diagnostic approach in FUO includes a thorough history, careful physical examination, laboratory tests, and radiographic studies.

HISTORY

- A thorough history is important, and this should include information about alcohol intake, medications, occupational and sexual exposures, pets, travel, familial diseases, and previous illnesses.
- Specific fever patterns have been described for many infectious and noninfectious causes of FUO. However, entities that usually have a distinctive fever pattern (e.g., malaria) are rare, and fever patterns thought to be distinctive for other diseases, such as Pel-Ebstein fever in lymphoma, are uncommon.

PHYSICAL EXAM

- The specific findings that have led to a diagnosis in FUO are diverse, and thorough repeated clinical assessment is the cornerstone for diagnosis. This should include evaluation of the following:
  - Oropharynx (dental abscess)
  - Thyroid (thyroiditis)
  - Temporal area (temporal arteritis)
  - Heart murmurs (endocarditis or atrial myxoma)
  - Skin (vasculitis, Whipple's disease)
  - Any wounds or lines, including removal of occlusive dressings for thorough inspection
  - Regional lymph node groups
  - Genitals and perineum
  - May require vaginal or rectal exam
- Relative bradycardia may be useful, but it is associated with a substantial differential diagnosis, including brucellosis, drug fever, factitious fever, hepatitis A, Legionnaires' disease, leptospirosis, neoplasms, psittacosis, subacute necrotizing lymphadenitis, and typhoid fever.
- Fever due to solid tumors and many collagen diseases may subsides with the use of nonsteroidal anti-inflammatory drugs, while fever due to other causes may persist (4).
- Other features, such as sweats, chills, or weight loss, have not discriminated among causes of FUO.
- Clues for factitious fever include: Absence of tachycardia and tachypnea, temperature >41°C, lack of diurnal variation, and absence of sweating post-fever.

DIAGNOSTIC TESTS & INTERPRETATION

Lab

- Noninvasive laboratory tests have provided a diagnosis in perhaps one-fourth of FUO cases. These include serologic tests for microbial pathogens or rheumatologic diseases, biochemical markers (e.g., ferritin in Still's disease), and genetic markers (e.g., Familial Mediterranean fever).
- Imaging has been used primarily to localize abnormalities for subsequent evaluation. Abdominal CT, in particular, has increased the rate of positive results when subsequent invasive diagnostic procedures are done.
- False-negative CT results have occasionally been reported, even with abscesses in solid organs.
- MRI is preferred if a spinal or paraspinal lesion is suspected.
- When infection or malignancy is the cause of FUO, scanning with gallium-67- or indium-111-labeled autologous leucocytes has occasionally been helpful. Limitations include false-negative gallium results with secondary infected lesions (e.g., hematomas or pseudocysts), difficulty detecting splenic abscesses due to a high level of background uptake in the spleen, and a low-positive predictive value with indium.
- FDG PET/CT has been found to be helpful in establishing neoplastic, inflammatory, or infective diagnoses in at least a third of patients (5).
- If imaging and serologic studies are unrevealing, invasive studies (including liver and bone marrow biopsy) should be considered.
- Diagnosis in fewer than half the cases of FUO has resulted from excisional or needle biopsy or laparotomy.
- Temporal artery biopsy in elderly patients with a very high Erythrocyte Sedimentation rate may often be

rewarding, even in the absence of prior localizing inflammation.

- Disseminated tuberculosis is probably the most treatable cause of death in patients with FUO and warrants vigorous diagnostic efforts when the disease is suspected. TST and IGRA may be negative in up to one-half of patients, and sputum smears may be positive for acid-fast bacilli in only one-fourth to one-half of cases. Biopsies of lymph nodes, bone marrow, or liver are often required for confirmation.
- Excisional lymph node biopsy may be helpful if nodes are enlarged. Inguinal nodes are often palpable but are seldom diagnostically useful.

DIFFERENTIAL DIAGNOSIS

- The five main etiologic categories of FUO and their relative frequencies are: Infections (33%), neoplasms (25%), connective tissue or inflammatory conditions (13%), miscellaneous (20%), undiagnosed (8%) (6)
- Although rare causes of FUO are often sought, unusual presentations of common conditions and conditions difficult to diagnose account for far more FUOs than rare diseases.
- It is useful to think in terms of FUO subtype to provide an insight into likely etiology.
- Etiology of classical FUO
  - Infections:
    ○ Tuberculosis, bacterial endocarditis, and abdominal collections remain the most common infectious cause of FUO
    ○ Systemic bacterial infections: Bartonellosis, brucellosis, *Campylobacter* infection, cat-scratch disease/bacillary angiomatosis, ehrlichiosis, gonococcemia, HACEK organisms, legionellosis, leptospirosis, listeriosis, Lyme disease, meningococcemia, rat-bite fever, relapsing fever (*Borrelia recurrentis*), salmonellosis (including typhoid fever), syphilis, tularemia, and yersiniosis
    ○ Chlamydial infections
    ○ Fungal infections
    ○ Parasitic infections
    ○ Viral infections
  - Also, FUO can be caused by localized infections such as:
    ○ Intravascular infections: Endocarditis, aortitis, intravenous catheter infection, septic jugular phlebitis, vascular graft infection
    ○ Intra-abdominal infections: Appendicitis, cholangitis, cholecystitis, diverticulitis, abscess (such as subphrenic, liver, splenic, pancreatic, perinephric, and pelvic), mesenteric lymphadenitis, pelvic inflammatory disease, and pyometra
    ○ Prosthesis-related infections: Bone and joint prostheses, pacemakers, implantable defibrillators, shunts, and vascular access devices
    ○ Others: Dental abscess, intracranial abscess, lung abscess, mastoiditis, otitis media, sinusitis, prostatic abscess, and wound infection
  - The most common noninfectious causes of FUO are the following:
    ○ Malignant neoplasms (renal cell carcinoma, hepatomas, Hodgkin's and non-Hodgkin's lymphomas, colon cancer, leukemia, malignant histiocytosis, pancreatic cancer, and sarcoma)
    ○ Benign neoplasms (atrial myxoma)
    ○ Connective tissue and inflammatory conditions (adult Still's disease, Behçet's syndrome, cryoglobulinemia, etc.)

- Miscellaneous conditions: Neuroleptic malignant syndrome, hematoma, recurrent pulmonary embolism, aortic dissection, after myocardial infarction (Dressler's syndrome), subacute thyroiditis, hyperthyroidism, Addison's, drug fever, factitious fever, gout, pseudogout, hypersensitivity pneumonitis, cerebrovascular accident, Familial Mediterranean fever, and pheochromocytoma
- Healthcare-associated FUO
  - Infections:
    ○ Intravascular catheter infections, septic thrombophlebitis, and prosthetic device related infections
    ○ Surgical wound infections, particularly deep abdominal collections
    ○ *Clostridium difficile* associated colitis. In a minority of patients, ileus rather than diarrhea is present, and is a marker of severe disease
    ○ Septic pelvic thrombophlebitis, usually in post-operative obstetric or gynecology patients
    ○ Acalculous cholecystitis
    ○ Sinus infections are common in the ICU associated with nasogastric feeding and endotracheal intubation
  - Miscellaneous:
    ○ Venous thromboembolism
    ○ Drug fever. Although eosinophilia and rash are helpful when present, their absence is the rule rather than the exception. Typical drugs include antimicrobials (beta-lactams, sulfonamides, vancomycin), diuretics, anti-seizure medications, neuroleptics, anti-hypertensives, and anti-arrhythmics
    ○ Factitious fever
  - Undiagnosed:
    ○ Fever is a common component of the post-operative inflammatory response to major surgery
- Immune-deficient FUO
  - Majority are due to infection, with a pathogen identified in 40–60% of patients
  - Type of infection is dependent on duration and nature of immunodeficiency
  - Neoplastic: Progressive or recurrent disease is a common cause of persistent fever in hematology–oncology patients
  - Inflammatory conditions: Graft versus host disease
  - Miscellaneous: Venous thromboembolism, drug fever, adrenal insufficiency
- HIV-related
  - Greater than 80% of FUOs in this subtype are due to infections
  - The incidence of HIV-related FUO has decreased in the anti-retroviral therapy era correlating with fewer opportunistic infections (7)
  - Etiology is primarily dictated by CD4 count
  - Common scenarios
    ○ HIV seroconversion illness as a cause of FUO
    ○ Opportunistic infections: Mycobacterial, *Pneumocystis jiroveci*, cytomegalovirus, toxoplasmosis, histoplasmosis, leishmaniasis
  - Inflammatory and connective tissue conditions: Immune reconstitution syndrome, Castleman's disease, and hemophagocytic lymphohistiocytosis
  - Malignancy: Lymphoma and Kaposi's sarcoma
  - Miscellaneous: Drug fever

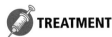 TREATMENT

MEDICATION
Therapy varies based on the underlying condition.

- If the TST or IGRA is positive, or if granulomatous disease (with possible anergy) is present, then a therapeutic trial for tuberculosis should be undertaken, with treatment continued for up to 6 weeks. Failure of the fever to respond over this period suggests an alternative diagnosis.
- Glucocorticoids and nonsteroidal anti-inflammatories could mask fever, while permitting the spread of infection, so their use should be avoided unless infection has been largely excluded.
- In severely immune-deficient patients with FUO, an empirical trial antimicrobial therapy is often required because of the high prevalence of infections and associated mortality.

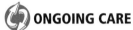 ONGOING CARE

FOLLOW-UP RECOMMENDATIONS
- All inpatients with FUO should be followed closely for new clinical symptoms or signs.

REFERENCES

1. Petersdorf RG, Beeson PB. Fever of unexplained origin: report on 100 cases. *Medicine* 1961;40: 1–30.
2. Durack DT, Street AC. Fever of unknown origin–reexamined and redefined. *Curr Clin Top Infect Dis* 1991;11:35–51.
3. Norman DC, Wong MB, Yoshikawa TT. Fever of unknown origin in older persons. *Infect Dis Clin North Am* 2007;21(4):937–945.
4. Cunha BA, Fever of unknown origin: Focused diagnostic approach based on clinical clues from the history, physical examination, and laboratory tests. *Infect Dis Clin N Am* 2007;21:1137–1187.
5. Ballink H, Collins J, Bruyn GA, Gemmel F. F-18 FDG PET/CT in the Diagnosis of Fever of Unknown Origin. *Clin Nucl Med* 2009;43:862–868.
6. Mackowiak PA, Durak DT. Fever of Unknown Origin. In: Mandell GL, Bennett JE, Dolin R, eds. *Principles and Practice of Infectious Diseases*, 7th Ed. Philadelphia: Churchill Livingstone Elsevier, 2010:779–789.
7. Abellan-Martinez J, Guerra-Vales JM, Fernandez-Cotarello MJ, et al. Evolution of the Incidence and Aetiology of Fever of Unknown Origin (FUO), and survival in HIV-infected Patients after HAART (Highly Active Antiretroviral Therapy). *Eur J Intern Med* 2009;20:474–477.

 CODES

ICD9
- 672 Pyrexia of unknown origin during the puerperium
- 780.60 Fever, unspecified

CLINICAL PEARLS

- In half of cases of FUO, the abnormalities are detected only by repeat history and examinations.
- As the duration of fever increases, the likelihood of an infectious cause decreases.
- FUO patients who remain undiagnosed after extensive evaluation generally have a favorable outcome.
- The elderly are more likely to have sinister, non-infectious causes for their FUO, and thus have a poorer prognosis.

GENITAL LESIONS AND ULCERS
Mary L. Pisculli

 BASICS

DESCRIPTION
- Lesions involving the reproductive organs
- Several infectious and noninfectious conditions cause genital lesions.

EPIDEMIOLOGY
- Genital ulcers are the most common type of genital lesion caused by sexually transmitted diseases.
- In North America and Europe, sexually transmitted diseases most likely to cause genital ulcers are genital herpes and syphilis.
- About 1 of 6 people aged 14–49 years in the US have genital HSV-2 infection. HSV I is the causal agent in up to 30% of genital infection cases.
- Chancroid is more prevalent in Africa, Asia, and Latin America, although sporadic outbreaks occur in the US.
- Lymphogranuloma venereum (LGV) is rare in industrialized nations; however, outbreaks have been reported among men who have sex with men (MSM).

RISK FACTORS
- 50% of sexual partners will acquire genital warts (HPV) following sexual contact with an infected partner.
- Syphilis transmission rate through sexual contact may be as high as 30%.

GENERAL PREVENTION
- Abstinence, condom use, limiting the number of sex partners, practicing safer sex, and HPV vaccination reduce the risk of sexually transmitted infections.
- Prophylaxis
  - 2 HPV vaccines are available for females aged 9–26 years and protect against serotypes 6 and 11 (the cause of 90% of genital warts), and 16 and 18 (70% of cervical cancers): a quadrivalent (Gardasil), and a bivalent (Cervarix) vaccine.
  - Administration of the quadrivalent vaccine to males aged 9–26 years may prevent genital warts

ETIOLOGY
- Infectious ulcers: Genital herpes, syphilis (*Treponema pallidum*), chancroid (*Haemophilus ducreyi*), lymphogranuloma venereum (LGV, Chlamydia trachomatis serovars L1, L2, or L3), donovanosis or granuloma inguinale (Klebsiella granulomatis), tuberculosis, and tularemia
  - Other less common causes include: Candidiasis, histoplasmosis, amebiasis, gonorrhea, and trichomoniasis
  - Acute or primary HIV infection may present with genital ulcerations
  - Up to 10% of patients with genital ulcers have more than one pathogen.

- Noninfectious ulcers: Trauma, fixed drug eruption, malignancy (skin cancer, leukemia, etc.), systemic lupus erythematosus, and Behçet's disease
- Less common genital lesions include:
  - Papules: Candidiasis, molluscum contagiosum, scabies (Sarcoptes scabiei), syphilis, venereal warts or condylomata acuminata (human papillomavirus; types 6 and 11 most common, types 16, 18, 31, 33, and 35 associated with cervical dysplasia)
  - Vesicles and bullae: Herpes genitalis, impetigo, scabies
  - Diffuse erythema: Candidiasis, erysipelas (usually associated with trauma or surgery), contact dermatitis, drug eruption, psoriasis, trauma
  - Benign cysts
  - Nodules: Hidradenitis, furunculosis
  - Crusts: Herpes genitalis, scabies

COMMONLY ASSOCIATED CONDITIONS
- HIV
- Other STDs

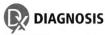 **DIAGNOSIS**

HISTORY
- Obtain a detailed history. When did the genital lesion(s) first appear? Any possible accompanying symptoms? Underlying immunodeficiency? Previous sexually transmitted diseases? History of similar genital lesions? Any travel history?
- Usual incubation period:
  - Herpes genitalis: 2–7 days (can be up to 4 weeks)
  - Genital warts: 4–12 weeks (occasionally longer)
  - Syphilis: 1–3 weeks (can be up to 3 months)
  - Chancroid: 5–7 days (can be from 1 day to 3 weeks)
  - Donovanosis: 2–3 weeks
  - Molluscum contagiosum: Up to 8 months
  - Pubic lice and scabies: 4–6 weeks
- Genital lesions that develop within hours of sexual exposure suggest trauma, chemical irritation, or hypersensitivity.
- Pruritus is present in patients with herpes genitalis (especially early), scabies, and pubic lice.
- Mild itching can be present in secondary syphilis.

PHYSICAL EXAM
- Identify the type and extent of the lesions; whether confined to the genitalia or spread to other skin areas; evaluate for associated tenderness, inguinal or generalized lymphadenopathy, or any vaginal or urethral discharge; and perform a careful examination of the buccal mucosa and the perianal area.
- Pelvic examination or evaluation of the prostate is often indicated.

- The classic initial lesion of genital herpes is grouped vesicles on an erythematous base. Umbilications are sometimes observed. The lesion is extremely painful, and the vesicles have often ruptured by the time the patient seeks medical attention.
- Tenderness characterizes herpes genitalis, chancroid, and tularemia.
- Ulcerated lesions of donovanosis are non-tender.
- Ulcer base
  - Behçet's disease: Yellow and necrotic
  - Chancroid: Necrotic
  - Donovanosis: Beefy red with hypertrophy
  - Syphilitic and herpetic ulcers: Clean
- Ulcer edge
  - Chancroid: Non-indurated ("soft chancre"), erythematous, irregular
  - Donovanosis: White
  - Herpetic ulcers: Erythematous
  - Syphilitic: Indurated
- Primary syphilis usually causes a single lesion, while chancroid usually presents as multiple ulcerations of variable size.
- Behçet's disease can present with recurrent, multiple genital ulcerations involving the scrotum or vulva. Other symptoms of Behçet's include recurrent oral ulcerations and lesions of the skin or the eyes. Diagnosis may be difficult as symptoms often do not present simultaneously.
- Linear tracks suggest scabies, while reddish flecks can be due to crab louse excreta.
- Urethral discharge suggests gonorrhea or Reiter's syndrome.
- Inguinal lymphadenopathy is not always associated with acute or local disease; however, its presence in an adult with a genital lesion suggests the following:
  - Chancroid
  - Lymphogranuloma venereum
  - Syphilis
  - Genital herpes
  - Lymphoma
  - Tuberculosis
- The genital ulcer caused by LGV can go unnoticed by the patient. The ulcer spontaneously heals, and 2–4 weeks later, painful inguinal lymphadenopathy develops, often associated with systemic symptoms (headache, arthralgia, leukocytosis, and hypergammaglobulinemia).
  - LGV can lead to elephantiasis distortion of the genitalia.
- Inguinal lymphadenopathy is usually unilateral in chancroid and LGV, and bilateral in genital herpes.
- The finding of painful perianal ulcers or mucosal ulcers on anoscopy should be treated presumptively for HSV and LGV.

- Molluscum contagiosum is mildly infectious. Lesions are usually umbilicated and vary in size up to 1 cm. Patients with advanced HIV infection may have generalized molluscum contagiosum or large lesions.
- Tuberculous lesions can manifest as chronic, minimally painful "sores" that are red, moderately firm, and nodular.
- For details on the diagnosis and treatment of syphilis, please see the chapter, "Syphilis" (Section II). Gonorrhea is discussed in the Section I chapter, "Urethral Discharge/Urethritis."
- Frequently, an accurate diagnosis cannot be made on the basis of history and/or morphology alone.

DIAGNOSTIC TESTS & INTERPRETATION
Lab
Initial lab tests
- All patients with genital, anal, or perianal ulcer(s) should undergo:
  - A serologic test for syphilis and dark-field examination (if available)
  - Diagnostic evaluation for HSV – either culture or PCR test for HSV or serologic testing for type specific HSV antibody
  - HIV testing
- If there is clinical or epidemiologic suspicion, and culture is available, obtain a culture specimen for *H. ducreyi*.
- Donovanosis: Intracellular "Donovan bodies," using Giemsa or Wright stain, may be seen in lesion scrapings or biopsies (do a biopsy when malignancy is also a possibility.)
- Chancroid: Culture is >80% sensitive, but selective culture media are not readily available.
- A probable diagnosis of chancroid is based on the presence of one or more painful ulcers, clinical presentation typical for chancroid, no evidence of *T. pallidum* on dark field or by serologic testing for syphilis performed >7 days after ulcer onset, and no evidence of HSV on the ulcer exudate.
- Diagnosis of LGV is based on serology or by isolating *C. trachomatis* and confirming serovars L1, 2, or 3 (definitive diagnosis).
- Diagnosis of molluscum contagiosum can be confirmed by histology and electron microscopy.

Follow-Up & Special Considerations
- Chancres may remain unnoticed in up to 30% of patients.
- Nontreponemal tests may be negative in up to 40% of patients with primary syphilis.
- When the diagnosis is unclear or the lesion could be due to skin cancer, biopsies should be obtained.

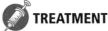 **TREATMENT**
MEDICATION
- Chancroid
  - Azithromycin (1 g orally) or
  - Ceftriaxone (250 mg intramuscular injection) given once
- Condylomata acumulata
  - No optimal treatment established.
  - Imiquimod 5% cream 3 times per week for 16 weeks or
  - Podophyllotoxin (podofilox 0.5% solution or gel) twice daily for 3 days, followed by 1 day off; repeat 4 times
- Donovanosis
  - Trimethoprim-sulfamethoxazole (1 double-strength tablet orally b.i.d) or
  - Tetracycline (500 mg orally q.i.d) or
  - Doxycycline (100 mg orally bid) – all for >3 weeks
- Herpes simplex virus infection
  - Acyclovir (400 mg orally t.i.d or 200 mg 5 times a day) for 7–10 days
  - Famciclovir (250 mg orally t.i.d) for 7–10 days
  - Valacyclovir (1 g orally b.i.d) for 7–10 days
  - For severe disease, Acyclovir 5–10 mg/kg every 8 hours may be necessary
  - See also Section II chapter, "Herpes Simplex Virus Infections."
- Tuberculous lesions: Systemic antituberculosis treatment
- LGV: Doxycycline (100 mg b.i.d orally) for 21 days
- Molluscum contagiosum: Desiccation, freezing, or curettage of lesions

COMPLEMENTARY & ALTERNATIVE THERAPIES
- Chancroid
  - Erythromycin (500 mg orally q.i.d) for 7 days or
  - Ciprofloxacin (500 mg orally b.i.d) for 3 days
- Condylomata acuminata: Cryosurgery, excision, electrosurgical destruction, and laser evaporation
- Donovanosis: Ciprofloxacin (750 mg orally b.i.d) for >3 weeks, erythromycin, chloramphenicol
- LGV: erythromycin (500 mg q.i.d orally) for 21 days

 ONGOING CARE
FOLLOW-UP RECOMMENDATIONS
- Encourage patients to refer their sexual partners for evaluation and treatment.
- At the time of diagnosis of a genital lesion, patients should be tested for HIV. If negative, serologic testing for HIV and syphilis should be performed 3 months after diagnosis.
- Consider Pap smears for all patients evaluated for sexually transmitted diseases that did not have a documented Pap smear within the preceding 12 months.
- Counsel women with human papilloma virus infection of the need for regular cytologic screening.

Pediatric Considerations
The presence of sexually transmitted lesions in a child should prompt evaluation for sexual abuse.

COMPLICATIONS
- Primary syphilis progresses to secondary syphilis in 2–8 weeks after the appearance of chancre by disseminating hematogenously.
- Chancroid, genital herpes, and syphilis are risk factors for HIV transmission.

ADDITIONAL READING
- CDC. *Sexually transmitted disease surveillance 2009*. Atlanta: U.S. Department of Health and Human Services, 2010.
- CDC. Sexually transmitted diseases treatment guidelines, 2010. *MMWR Morb Mortal Wkly Rep* 2010;59(RR-12):1–116.
- *Mandell Douglas, and Bennett's Principles and Practice of Infectious Diseases*, 7th ed. 2009.

 CODES

ICD9
- 054.10 Genital herpes, unspecified
- 099.0 Chancroid
- 099.1 Lymphogranuloma venereum

CLINICAL PEARLS
- All patients with genital ulcers should undergo testing for syphilis and HSV.
- Perform a comprehensive screening for other sexually transmitted infections.
- Counsel patients to abstain from sexual intercourse until the entire course of treatment is completed.

G

GONORRHEA

Eleni Patrozou

 BASICS

DESCRIPTION
- Gonorrhea results from infection with the gram-negative intracellular diplococcus *Neisseria gonorrhoeae*, an obligate human pathogen.
- Transmission results from direct inoculation of gonococci from one mucous membrane to another, during sexual contact or labor. Gonorrhea is transmitted from males to females more efficiently than in the opposite direction. The transmission rate to females after one sexual encounter is up to 50%.

EPIDEMIOLOGY
- Gonorrhea remains a major public health problem worldwide and is a significant cause of morbidity in developing countries.
- Worldwide new gonococcal infections are estimated to reach 62 million cases each year, with the highest rates occurring in sub-Saharan Africa, south and Southeast Asia, the Caribbean, and Latin America.
- In 2008, 336,742 cases of gonorrhea were reported by state health departments in the US (111.6 cases per 100,000). The incidence of gonorrhea was highest in females 15–19 years of age and in males 20–24 years of age. Gonorrhea was more common in African Americans and Hispanics populations than in Whites.

RISK FACTORS
Female sex, age <25 years, a previous diagnosis of gonorrhea or other sexually transmitted disease, new or multiple sex partners, inconsistent condom use, commercial sex work, drug use, and overseas travel to countries of high prevalence are risk factors for gonococcal infection.

GENERAL PREVENTION
- Early detection of disease, treatment at the time of diagnosis and treatment of sexual partners are the cornerstones of gonorrhea control.
- Any partner within 60 days of the onset of symptoms should be screened and treated.
- Behavioral modifications, such as delaying sexual debut and limiting the number of sexual partners, decrease the transmission of gonorrhea.
- Consistent condom use reduces the risk of infection.

ETIOLOGY
Gonorrhea is caused by *N. gonorrhoeae*, a nonmotile, nonspore-forming gram-negative diplococcus.

COMMONLY ASSOCIATED CONDITIONS
Gonococcal infections frequently coexist with other sexually transmitted diseases. Coinfection with *Chlamydia* can occur in one-third of cases. Furthermore, gonorrhea has been shown to facilitate acquisition of HIV.

DIAGNOSIS

- The spectrum of clinical symptoms is influenced by a number of factors, such as, the initial site of infection, the type of strain of *N. gonorrhoeae*, host factors including sex and the presence of other coinfections.
- Asymptomatic infection is common in both men and women.
- The incubation period is 2–7 days after exposure.
- Urethritis in men presents with dysuric symptoms that is followed by purulent discharge. The most common complication is acute epididymitis.
- Women with urethritis may complain of dysuria, urinary frequency, and urgency.
- Women may also develop cervicitis. Cervicitis is a clinical syndrome that includes purulent vaginal discharge, abdominal cramps, dyspareunia, and postcoital or intermenstrual bleeding. Infection commonly becomes symptomatic during menstruation. If left untreated, the infection may progress to pelvic inflammatory disease with ultimate sterility and chronic pelvic pain.
- Conjunctivitis is usually a result of autoinoculation from another infected site and may present with profuse purulent discharge and can rapidly progress to panophthalmitis and loss of the eye unless treated promptly.
- In neonates, gonococcal infection most commonly manifests as ophthalmia neonatorum and is acquired during passage from the birth canal. Ocular installation of prophylactic agents (1% silver nitrate eyedrops or tetracycline ointment) is used for prevention.

- Disseminated gonococcal disease may present with fever, rash, tenosynovitis, and septic arthritis. Frequently, the illness is characterized as influenza-like with low grade temperature and mucosal symptoms may not be present. Therefore, all mucosal sites (urethra or cervix, rectum, and pharynx) should be sampled.

DIAGNOSTIC TESTS & INTERPRETATION
Lab
- Gram stain of the urethral discharge of symptomatic males may reveal polynuclear cells and gram-negative intracellular diplococci. However, Gram stain is less sensitive in endocervical, rectal, and pharyngeal specimens.
- Cultures have the additional benefit of providing antimicrobial susceptibility data. Cultures should be performed in modified Thayer-Martin or other gonococcal selective medium (Martin Lewis, New York City medium etc.). Gonococci require aerobic conditions with increased carbon dioxide for growth. Immediate processing is crucial, since gonococcus cannot tolerate drying.
- Gonococcal strains that tend to cause disseminated gonococcal infection are more fastidious and difficult to culture.
- Nucleic acid probe tests can be used for the direct detection of *N. gonorrhoeae* in cervical and urethral swab specimens and in urine samples. Sensitivity and specificity are comparable or superior to culture of swab specimens. Limitations are the increased cost, and cross reaction with nongonococcal *Neisseria* sp.

DIFFERENTIAL DIAGNOSIS
- Nongonococcal urethritis (*Chlamydia*, *Ureaplasma urealyticum*, *Mycoplasma genitalium*, *Haemophilus vaginalis*, Herpes Simplex Virus, Adenovirus etc.)
- Vaginitis due to candidiasis, bacterial vaginosis, and trichomoniasis as well as noninfectious causes such as chemical irritation, allergic reactions, vesicovaginal or rectovaginal fistula, and leukorrhea of pregnancy.
- The differential diagnosis for disseminated gonococcal infection is extensive and includes meningococcemia, Ecthyma gangrenosum, and other causes of bacteremia. The arthritis of disseminated gonococcal infection should be differentiated from septic arthritis of other bacterial cause and reactive arthritis.

TREATMENT

MEDICATION

- Current CDC guidelines for treatment of gonorrhea are confined in a single antibiotic class: Cephalosporins.
- For uncomplicated gonococcal infections of the urethra, cervix, and rectum, the recommended regimens are the following: Ceftriaxone 125 mg intramuscularly in a single dose or cefixime 400 mg orally in a single dose, or spectinomycin 2 gm intramuscularly in a single dose.
- For gonococcal infection of the pharynx, the treatment recommendations differ as it is a more difficult infection to eradicate and the recommended agent is only ceftriaxone 125 mg intramuscularly in a single dose.
- Gonococcal conjunctivitis should be treated with a single dose of ceftriaxone 125 mg intramuscularly. Saline lavage of the infected eye may also be considered.
- For disseminated gonococcal infection, a cephalosporin-based regimen (such as ceftriaxone 1 gm intravenously/intramuscularly daily or cefotaxime 1 gm intravenously 3 times daily or ceftizoxime 1 gm intravenously 3 times daily or spectinomycin 2 gm intramuscularly twice daily) is recommended. Parenteral antibiotics should be continued for 24–48 hours after improvement begins. At that time switching to an oral regimen is reasonable, such as cefixime 400 mg orally twice daily to complete 1 week of treatment.
- In all the above cases, treatment for *Chlamydia* should also be given if chlamydial infection is not excluded.
- Quinolones are no longer recommended in the US as first-line treatment because of widespread chromosomally mediated resistance.

ADDITIONAL TREATMENT
General Measures
Coinfection with *C. trachomatis* occurs frequently. Initial treatment regimens should be effective against chlamydial infections (e.g., azithromycin or doxycycline).

 ONGOING CARE

FOLLOW-UP RECOMMENDATIONS
Patient Monitoring
- Patients with uncomplicated infections do not routinely need a test of cure, after treatment is concluded.
- Cultures for *N. gonorrhoeae* along with antimicrobial susceptibility testing should be performed if symptoms persist after therapy.
- The most common cause for treatment failure is repeated exposure to untreated sexual partners.

PATIENT EDUCATION
- Patients should be advised to use condoms consistently to reduce the risk of infection.
- Patients should be instructed about the proper use of condoms.

COMPLICATIONS
- Pelvic inflammatory disease is the most important complication of gonorrhea. It results from the migration of *N. gonorrhoeae* from the site of primary infection into the upper genital tract.
- Pelvic inflammatory disease can produce tubo-ovarian abscess and extend to pelvic peritonitis and Fitz-Hugh-Curtis syndrome (perihepatitis). Sterility and chronic pelvic pain are long term complications.
- Epididymitis, periurethritis, balanitis, acute and chronic prostatitis, orchitis, seminal vasculitis, and infection of the Tyson and Cowper glands are complications of gonococcal infections in male patients.
- Disseminated gonococcemia is more common in women and follows the dissemination of gonococci from the primary site by the bloodstream. Menstruation is a risk factor for dissemination. Tenosynovitis, migratory arthritis, and peripheral skin lesions ranging from maculopapular to pustular are typical findings.
- Blood cultures are positive in only 20–30% of cases.
- Gonococcal endocarditis and meningitis are rarely encountered in the antibiotic era.

ADDITIONAL READING
- Centers for Disease Control and Prevention (CDC). Update to CDC's sexually transmitted diseases treatment guidelines, 2006. Fluoroquinolones no longer recommended for treatment of gonococcal infections. *MMWR Morb Mortal Wkly Rep* 2007; 56(14):332–336.
- Golden MR, Whittington WL, Handsfield HH, et al. Effect of expedited treatment of sex partners on recurrent or persistent gonorrhea or chlamydial infection. *N Engl J Med* 2005;352:676–685.
- Greer L, Wendel GD Jr. Rapid diagnostic methods in sexually transmitted infections. *Infect Dis Clin North Am* 2008;22:601–617.
- Workowski KA, Berman SM. Centers for Disease Control and Prevention. Sexually transmitted diseases treatment guidelines, 2006. *MMWR Recomm Rep* 2006;55(RR-11):1–94.

 CODES

ICD9
- 098.0 Gonococcal infection (acute) of lower genitourinary tract
- 098.10 Gonococcal infection (acute) of upper genitourinary tract, site unspecified
- 098.2 Gonococcal infection, chronic, of lower genitourinary tract

CLINICAL PEARLS
- Patients being tested for gonorrhea should also be offered testing for all other sexually transmitted infections.
- Terminal complement complex (C5–9) deficiency predisposes to systemic infection with both *N. gonorrhoeae* and *Neisseria meningitides*.

G

HEPATOSPLENOMEGALY AND FEVER

Cameron J. Jeremiah
Anton Y. Peleg

 BASICS

DESCRIPTION
- Liver span (midclavicular line) equal to or greater than 12.5 cm suggests hepatomegaly (1).
- Any spleen greater than 250 g or that is palpable is deemed enlarged. The ultrasound criterion of enlargement is a cephalocaudal diameter of 13 cm or more (2).

Approach to the patient
- Evaluation for hepatosplenomegaly
  - Palpate to locate the lower liver border in the midclavicular line.
  - With a palpable lower edge, the midclavicular line span can be ascertained by light percussion of the upper border. Liver span should be measured and if ≥12.5 cm, then defined clinically as hepatomegaly. Given that lung hyperexpansion can displace the liver inferiorly, the upper border of the liver must be assessed.
  - The bedside examination of the spleen should consist of both palpation and percussion.
  - Palpation is best performed by bimanual palpation in both supine and right lateral positions.
  - Percussion techniques described by Castell and Nixon have the best diagnostic value (1).
  - Nixon's technique: The patient is positioned on their right side and percussion is commenced in the posterior axillary line at the lower level of pulmonary resonance and progresses in an oblique line toward the lower mid-anterior costal margin. A dull percussion span >8 cm suggests splenomegaly, with 59% sensitivity and 94% specificity.
  - Castell's technique: With the patient supine, percussion in the left anterior axillary line in the lowest intercostals space will be resonant with a normal sized spleen and remains resonant throughout respiration. Sensitivity and specificity are 82% and 83%, respectively
  - If the possibility of missing splenic enlargement remains an important clinical concern, ultrasonography or scintigraphy is indicated.
- Approach to the patient with liver and/or spleen enlargement and fever
  - A thorough history is required including history of travel, immigration, occupation, sexual and intravenous drug use history, animal exposure, and family history of malignancies, connective tissue diseases, and other heritable conditions.
  - Evaluate for associated features:
    o The presence of jaundice
    o The duration and characteristics of fever
    o The presence of lymphadenopathy
    o Cutaneous manifestations and bites
    o Consistency, nodularity, and tenderness of a palpable liver edge
    o The presence of enlarged gallbladder or another abdominal mass
    o The size and the consistency of the spleen
  - Diagnostic tests include general laboratory evaluation, monospot test, hepatitis profile, imaging studies, and, in certain cases, bone marrow examination, endoscopy, and/or liver biopsy.

EPIDEMIOLOGY
- The epidemiology of a palpable liver or spleen in young adults has been defined by several studies. One study reported data on a palpable liver among 1000 healthy military personnel. In 57% of subjects, the liver either was not palpable in the right upper quadrant or was felt just at the costal margin. An additional 28% descended only 1–2 cm below the costal margin (3).
- In 2 other studies, about 3% of otherwise healthy students entering a US college had unexplained palpable spleens, and 12% of otherwise normal postpartum women at a Canadian hospital had palpable spleens (4–5).

ETIOLOGY
Hepatomegaly and Fever
- Infectious causes
  - Abscess – either pyogenic or amoebic
  - Ascending cholangitis
  - Chronic granulomatous disease of childhood
  - Chronic Q fever
  - Ehrlichiosis
  - Histoplasmosis
  - HIV
  - Infectious hepatitis
  - Infectious mononucleosis
  - Leptospirosis
  - Syphilis
  - Tuberculosis
  - Parasitosis (see below)
- Malignant
  - Diffuse hepatic carcinoma
  - Diffuse metastases
  - Myeloproliferative disorder
  - Lymphoma
  - Angiosarcoma
- Inflammatory
  - Sarcoidosis
  - Autoimmune hepatitis
  - Familial Mediterranean fever
  - Still's disease

Splenomegaly and Fever
- Infectious causes
  - Viral
    o Infectious hepatitis
    o Infectious mononucleosis
    o HIV
  - Bacterial
    o Endocarditis
    o Pyogenic abscess
    o Salmonellosis
    o Leptospirosis
    o Brucellosis
    o Bartonella
  - Fungal
    o Histoplasmosis
  - Mycobacterial
    o Miliary tuberculosis
    o Non-tuberculous mycobacteria
  - Parasitic

  o Malaria
  o Toxoplasmosis
  o Amoebic liver abscess
  o Schistosomiasis (Katayama fever)
  o Visceral leishmaniasis
  o Babesiosis
  o Ehrlichiosis
- Inflammatory
  - Rheumatoid arthritis
  - Sarcoidosis
  - Systemic lupus erythematosus
  - Hemophagocytic lymphohistiocytosis
- Malignant
  - Lymphomas
  - Acute and chronic leukemias
  - Myelodysplastic and myeloproliferative syndromes
- Numerous parasitic diseases can lead to liver and spleen enlargement. The causes vary based on epidemiologic data and include the following:
  - Malaria
  - Schistosomiasis
  - Hydatidosis
  - Leishmaniasis
  - Toxocariasis
  - Toxoplasmosis
  - Liver flukes including fascioliasis (*Fasciola hepatica*)
  - Echinococcal cysts can cause liver and spleen enlargement but rarely associated with fever
- Fever is found in nearly 50% of cases with either *Toxoplasma* or *Toxocara* infections.

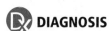 **DIAGNOSIS**

HISTORY
Clinical Manifestations
- In a young adult, fatigue, sore throat, fever, lymphadenopathy, and hepatosplenomegaly are almost always due to infectious mononucleosis.
- A constellation of fever, abdominal pain (whether or not localized in the right upper abdomen), vomiting or anorexia, hepatomegaly, elevated white blood cell count and sedimentation rate, and an unexplained anemia should prompt the clinician to include liver abscess in the differential diagnosis.
- Biliary disease remains the most common cause of pyogenic liver abscess, with enteric pathogens being the most common causative organisms, including *Eshcherichia coli*, *Klebsiella*, enterococci, anginosis group streptococci and anaerobes. Most commonly seen in adults in 5th and 6th decades of life.
- Pyogenic liver abscess associated with metastatic infection (endophthalmitis, meningitis, or other focal abscess) is likely due to *Klebsiella pneumoniae* and is primarily found in those with diabetes and from East Asia (6).

- Nowadays, amebic liver abscess is almost always found in travelers and migrants. Men have a 10 times greater risk of invasive *Entamoeba histolytica* infection, which includes liver abscess. Nausea, vomiting, and diarrhea are not that common (15–35% of patients), and symptoms can occur years after exposure to endemic area.
- In patients with HIV and low CD4 counts, fever with associated lymphadenopathy and splenomegaly is usually due to mycobacterial infection, but lymphoma must be excluded.
- Leptospirosis has a variable presentation but needs to be considered in those with an appropriate exposure history associated with fever, rigors, headache, and myalgias. Severe forms may have associated pulmonary, liver and renal dysfunction, aseptic meningitis, and bleeding diathesis.
- In the tropics, a finding of splenomegaly can be due to tropical splenomegaly syndrome (also known as hyper-reactive malarial splenomegaly). This syndrome is characterized by fever, anemia, weight loss, abdominal discomfort, and lassitude. Laboratory hallmarks include abnormal results of liver function tests, elevated IgM levels, and hepatic sinusoidal lymphocytosis.

PHYSICAL EXAM

- Apart from fever, and hepatosplenomegaly, which has been discussed, associated clinical signs should be looked for and will give clues to diagnosis
- Associated lymphadenopathy (lymphoma, infectious mononucleosis, brucellosis, schistosomiasis, HIV, mycobacterial infection)
- Cutaneous eruptions (schistosomiasis, rickettsia, leishmaniasis, infectious mononucleosis, Still's disease, syphilis)
- Throat (infectious mononucleosis)
- Embolic phenomenon and cardiac murmur (endocarditis, *Bartonella*, and brucellosis)
- Jaundice (viral hepatitis, cholangitis, leptospirosis)
- Conjunctival suffusion (leptospirosis)
- Joints (rheumatoid arthritis, systemic lupus erythematosus, Still's disease)

DIAGNOSTIC TESTS & INTERPRETATION
Lab

- An elevated WBC with a shift to the left is suggestive of a bacterial infection.
- Lymphocytosis (>50% of differential) with >10% atypia on a blood film is suggestive of infectious mononucleosis. This may be confirmed with a monospot test in the 1st few weeks of illness. Alternatively, IgM to viral capsid antigen may be tested.
- Eosinophilia may be found in cases of liver or spleen enlargement caused by certain parasitic diseases but is not found in amebic infection.
- 3 sets of blood cultures taken while off antibiotics exclude most cases of endocarditis. *Bartonella*, *Brucella* and Q fever are best excluded by serology.
- Depending on travel, sexual, and occupational history:
  – HIV, syphilis, and viral hepatitis serology
  – Rickettsial, amoebic, toxoplasma, *Schistosoma*, Q fever, *Fasciola*, leptospirosis and *Ehrlichia* serology
  – Blood film for malaria and babesiosis
- Biochemistry, autoimmune markers, and ferritin
- If abscess is seen on imaging, imaging-guided aspirate can be diagnostic.

- An excisional lymph node biopsy or liver biopsy has the highest diagnostic yield for lymphoma
- Bone marrow biopsy or splenic aspirate for leishmaniasis. Alternatives include tissue PCR and serology.

Imaging

- Ultrasonography enables confirmation of examination findings and may identify an underlying cause, e.g., abscess, hepatocellular carcinoma, cholangitis.
- Contrast-enhanced computerized tomography is useful where ultrasound is non-diagnostic and clinical suspicion remains high for a focal lesion or lymphoma.
- MRI is rarely required but may be useful in distinguishing between abscess and neoplasia.

 TREATMENT

MEDICATION

- Treatment is obviously guided by the final diagnosis.
- If liver abscess is confirmed, antibiotics targeting the causative organisms are indicated.
- Unlike amebic liver abscess, for pyogenic liver abscess, percutaneous aspiration in combination with antibiotics is the preferred therapy (7). If percutaneous aspiration fails or multiple complex abscesses are present, then surgery may be indicated (8).
- Praziquantel is an effective and well-tolerated drug for treatment of *Schistosoma mansoni* infection in patients with advanced hepatosplenic schistosomiasis, and it is the drug of choice for patients with coexisting *Schistosoma haematobium* infection.
- Fascioliasis is usually managed with triclabendazole, at a dose of 10 mg/kg for 1–2 days (9). Bithionol 40 mg/kg in 3 divided doses on alternate days for 10–15 doses is an alternative, but the efficacy of praziquantel is controversial.

 ONGOING CARE

FOLLOW-UP RECOMMENDATIONS
Patients with splenomegaly should be advised to avoid contact sports and should be monitored for the development of signs and symptoms suggestive of spontaneous splenic rupture. Severe upper abdominal pain is the presenting complaint in virtually all patients with spontaneous splenic rupture. The pain usually begins in the left upper quadrant and spreads throughout the abdomen, frequently radiating to the left shoulder.

COMPLICATIONS
In the US, nearly all cases of spontaneous splenic rupture are associated with infectious mononucleosis. Splenic rupture is a rare complication that is estimated to occur in 0.1–0.5% of the patients with infectious mononucleosis. However, this complication is the most frequent cause of death associated with infectious mononucleosis

REFERENCES

1. Naylor CD. Physical examination of the liver. *JAMA* 1994;271:1859–1865.
2. Yang JC, Rickman LS. The Clinical Diagnosis of Splenomegaly. *West J Med* 1991;155:47–52.
3. Palmer ED. Palpability of the liver edge in healthy adults. *U S Armed Forces Med J* 1958;9: 1685–1690.
4. McIntyre OR, Ebaugh FG. Palpable spleens in college freshmen. *Ann Intern Med* 1967;66: 301–306.
5. Berris B. The incidence of palpable liver and spleen in the postpartum period. *Can Med Assoc J* 1966;95:1318–1319.
6. Fang CT, Lai SY, Yi WC, et al. Klebsiella pneumoniae genotype K1: an emerging pathogen that causes septic ocular or central nervous system complications from pyogenic liver abscess. *Clin Infect Dis* 2007;45(3):284–293.
7. Liu CH, Gervais DA, Hahn PF, et al. Percutaneous hepatic abscess drainage: do multiple abscesses or multiloculated abscesses preclude drainage or affect outcome? *J Vasc Interv Radiol* 2009;20: 1059–1065.
8. Hope WW, Vrochides DV, Newcomb WL, et al. Optimal treatment of hepatic abscess. *Am Surg* 2008;74:178–182.
9. Keiser J, Utzinger J. Chemotherapy for major food-borne trematodes: a review. *Expert Opin Pharmacother* 2004;5:1711–1726.

ADDITIONAL READING

- Abramson JS, Digumarthy S, Ferry JA. Case 27–2009: A 56-year old woman with fever, rash, and lymphadenopathy. *N Engl J Med* 2009;361: 900–911.
- Hunt DP, Thabet A, Rosenberg ES. Case 29–2010: A 29-year-old woman with fever and abdominal pain. *N Engl J Med* 2010;363:1266–1274.
- O'Reilly RA. Splenomegaly in 2,505 patients at a large university medical center from 1913 to 1995. 1963 to 1995: 449 patients. *West J Med* 1998;169:88–97.

CODES

ICD9
- 780.60 Fever, unspecified
- 789.1 Hepatomegaly
- 789.2 Splenomegaly

CLINICAL PEARLS

- All returned travelers from a malaria endemic region with fever +/– splenomegaly must have an urgent blood film
- An accurate and extensive history of travel and animal exposure combined with relevant infectious disease prevalence data is essential in evaluating infectious causes of hepatosplenomegaly
- Massive splenomegaly with associated fever has a limited number of causes: Lymphoma, infections associated with either myelofibrosis or CML, leishmaniasis, malaria, and mycobacterial avium infections in HIV patients

INSECT BITES AND STINGS

Isaac I. Bogoch

 BASICS

DESCRIPTION
- Zoonosis refers to any infection transmitted to humans by other nonhuman animals.
- A vector refers to the nonhuman animal transmitting infections.

Approach to the Patient
- Insect bites and stings can cause an array of infectious illnesses which can present with acute, subacute, and sometimes protean manifestations. Awareness of the geographic distribution, life cycle, and clinical manifestations of these infections is crucial.
- In addition to infectious complications, patients may present with anaphylaxis or other inflammatory responses to insect bites and stings.
- A history of mosquito or tick bites and the timing of exposure can be helpful in ruling in or ruling out certain infections.
- A thorough travel history, with dates of departure, return, and intermediate stops, is very important. A history of pretravel medical care should be obtained, as well as adherence to any recommended therapy such as pretravel vaccinations, malaria prophylaxis, mosquito net use, or insect repellant use.
- In many cases, diagnostic laboratory tests will confirm the clinical diagnosis of insect-borne illness, but may not be available at the time of acute illness (e.g. dengue serology).
- Patients may have multiple infections from a single insect exposure. For example, *Borrelia burgdorferi*, *Ehrlichia* spp, and *Babesia microti* are transmitted to humans by *Ixodes scapularis*, and patients can have infection with more than one of these pathogens.
- Malaria should be considered in febrile patients returning from endemic regions, and should be treated as a medical emergency. Because of the substantial morbidity and mortality associated with a delay in diagnosing and treating these infections, empiric administration of appropriate antimicrobial therapy is often justified.

EPIDEMIOLOGY
- Close to 250,000 cases of Lyme disease were reported in the US between 1992 and 2006, with 19,931 cases reported in 2006. Most cases were in the Northeast US, Minnesota, and Wisconsin. Rocky Mountain spotted fever occurs in North and South America, and primarily in the south and southeastern parts of the US. It is more common in the spring and summer months. Infection rates are 0.5–16 cases per one million people, depending on race and geography.
- West Nile virus was first detected in the US in 1999. Between 1999 and 2008 there were 28,961 cases reported to the Centers for Disease Control and Prevention (CDC). An estimated 80% of infections are asymptomatic, and the number of people with exposure is very likely to be significantly higher.
- Eastern equine encephalitis is a life-threatening, mosquito-borne arboviral infection found principally along the East and Gulf coasts of the US. Cases have occurred sporadically and in small epidemics: 223 cases were reported to the CDC between 1955 and 1993.
- In 2008 there were 1298 cases of malaria reported in the US.

GENERAL PREVENTION
- In regions where tick exposure is likely, preventive measures are recommended and should include wearing long-sleeved shirts, pants, and closed-toed shoes. To remove an embedded tick, use tweezers to grasp the tick as close as possible to the skin, then pull slowly and steadily, perpendicular to the skin – it will often back out of the skin. Care should be taken not to crush the tick, or pull too briskly as parts of the tick may be left under the skin.
- N, N-diethyl-3-methylbenzamide (DEET) is the most effective and best studied insect repellent currently on the market. DEET-based repellents combined with permethrin-treated clothing offers excellent protection against mosquito bites. Products with 10–30% DEET have excellent efficacy, and higher concentrations do not seem to offer more protection. Lower concentrations may still be effective; however, the duration of efficacy may be shorter and will require more frequent re-application of the product. Other topical products include plant-based repellents such as picaridin, PMD (P-menthane-3, 8-diol), or citronella. These have some efficacy; however, DEET is the "gold standard." The US Environmental Protection Agency has a comprehensive web page on repellents and insecticides at http://www.epa.gov/pesticides/

ETIOLOGY
Physicians in the US may encounter the following local or imported vector-borne illnesses:
- Mosquitoes
  - Malaria
  - West Nile virus
  - Dengue
  - Eastern equine encephalitis and other viral encephalitides
  - Yellow fever
  - Chikungunya virus
- Ticks
  - Lyme disease
  - Babesiosis
  - Human ehrlichiosis and anaplasmosis
  - Rocky Mountain spotted fever
  - Tularemia
  - Southern tick-associated rash illness
  - *Bartonella henselae*
  - Tick paralysis
  - Other rickettsial illnesses

- Flies
  - *Bartonella bacilliformis*
  - African trypanosomiasis
  - Filariasis
  - Onchocerciasis
  - Leishmaniasis
  - Fly larvae embedded in skin ("myiasis")
- Fleas
  - Plague
  - Tungiasis
  - Murine typhus

Please see the appropriate chapters for details of abovementioned infections.

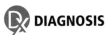 DIAGNOSIS

- Please see relevant chapters for specific conditions. The incubation period for Falciparum malaria is 12–14 days. Patients may present with fever, chills, headache, neck or abdominal pains, nausea, and vomiting. Patients may appear jaundiced as well.
- Incubation of West Nile virus is between 2 and 14 days, and most infected patients are asymptomatic. Symptomatic patients typically have fever, myalgias, and headache lasting less than 1 week, with a diffuse maculopapular rash in about half of these patients. West Nile virus can affect the central nervous system and cause symptoms of meningitis or encephalitis as well.
- Patients with Colorado tick fever, after an incubation period of 3–6 days, develop the primary phase of illness that begins with fever, chills, severe headache, photophobia, and myalgias. These symptoms persist for 5–8 days, then, after resolution, recur within 3 days in approximately 50% of patients. This secondary phase of illness usually lasts 2–4 days. A transient petechial or macular rash may develop.
- Dengue infection has a 3–14 day incubation period, and classically presents with fever, headache (especially behind the eyes), rash, and often severe muscle and joint pains.

DIAGNOSTIC TESTS & INTERPRETATION
Lab
- Please see relevant chapters for specific conditions.
- Blood film should be performed on all patients presenting with fever returning from malaria-endemic regions.
- Lyme infection can be diagnosed by sending blood for enzyme-linked immunosorbent assay, and confirmed with a Western Blot test in patients with compatible symptoms.
- *Babesia* requires a blood film for diagnosis. Parasites can be visualized inside red blood cells. Parasites may be outside of red blood cells in cases of severe infection. PCR and serologic tests are also available.
- West Nile virus can be diagnosed with IgM studies on the blood or cerebral spinal fluid.

Imaging
Eastern equine encephalitis has characteristic MRI brain findings in the thalamus and basal ganglia.

 TREATMENT

Please see relevant chapters for specific conditions.

 ONGOING CARE

COMPLICATIONS
- The mortality rate in eastern equine encephalitis is 35%, and one third of the survivors are moderately or severely disabled.
- A delay in diagnosing and treating Falciparum malaria may result in permanent neurologic injury and elevated mortality rates.
- Lyme disease may affect the central and peripheral nervous systems (e.g., meningitis, encephalitis, cranial nerve palsies), and cardiac conduction systems resulting in arrhythmias.

- Epistaxis and scattered petechiae are often noted in uncomplicated dengue, and preexisting gastrointestinal lesions may bleed during the acute illness.
- Rare complications, such as encephalitis, aseptic meningitis, hemorrhage, pericarditis, orchitis, atypical pneumonitis, and hepatitis, have been described among patients with Colorado tick fever.

ADDITIONAL READING

- Bacon RM, Kugeler KJ, Mead PS, et al. Surveillance for Lyme disease – United States, 1992–2006. *MMWR Surveill Summ* 2008;57(10):1–9.
- Cutler SJ, Fooks AR, van der Poel WH. Public health treat of new, reemerging and neglected zoonoses in the industrialized world. *Emerg Infect Dis* 2010;16:1–7.
- Lindsey NP, Staples JE, Lehman JA, et al. Surveillance for human West Nile virus disease – United States, 1999–2008. *MMWR Surveill Summ* 2010;59(2):1–17.
- Mali S, Steels S, Slutsker L, et al. Malaria surveillance – United States, 2008. *MMWR Surveill Summ* 2010;59(7):1.
- Pollack RJ, Marcus LC. A travel medicine guide to arthropods of medical importance. *Infect Dis Clin N Am* 2005;19:169–183.

 CODES

ICD9
- 919.5 Insect bite, nonvenomous, of other, multiple, and unspecified sites, infected
- 989.5 Toxic effect of venom

I

JAUNDICE AND FEVER

Katherine M. Langan
Anton Y. Peleg

 BASICS

DESCRIPTION

- Jaundice (or icterus): Hyperbilirubinemia and deposition of bile pigment in the skin, mucous membranes, and the sclera.
- For further discussion on this topic, please see also the Section I chapters, "Abdominal Pain and Fever" and "Hepatosplenomegaly and Fever," and the Section II chapters, "Cholecystitis/Cholangitis" and "Hepatitis."

Approach to the Patient

- Historic evaluation should include the following:
  - Determination of the length of symptoms before the jaundice
  - Duration of fever
  - Presence and character of abdominal pain
  - Presence of pruritus, myalgias, constitutional symptoms, and changes in appetite, weight, and bowel habits
  - History of medication (including over-the-counter drugs)
  - History of blood product transfusions or injecting drug use
  - History of travel to developing countries
- Once jaundice is recognized clinically or chemically, it is important to clarify whether hyperbilirubinemia is predominantly unconjugated or conjugated. Absence of bilirubin in the urine suggests unconjugated hyperbilirubinemia

EPIDEMIOLOGY

- Please refer to Section II chapter, "Hepatitis."
- The National Notifiable Disease Surveillance System (NNDSS) in 2007 reported rates of acute hepatitis A infection to be 1.0 per 100,000, acute hepatitis B infection to be 1.5 per 100,000, and acute hepatitis C to be 0.5 per 100,000 population. This is falling. These figures are underestimates, and for every reported acute case, there are probably 2–5 unreported cases.

ETIOLOGY

- The most common causes of unconjugated hyperbilirubinemia and fever include the following:
  - Sepsis that can cause decreased hepatic uptake and bilirubin conjugation.
  - Hepatitis that can cause hepatocellular disease. Acute viral infection with either hepatitis A, B, C, D, or E is the most common cause. Other viral infections such as Epstein–Barr virus (infectious mononucleosis), cytomegalovirus, herpes simplex, mumps, rubella, rubeola, varicella zoster virus, adenovirus, coxsackievirus, and yellow fever may also cause a hepatitis-like illness. Other infectious organisms which can cause hepatic inflammation include *Toxoplasma*, *Leptospira*, *Brucella*, *Coxiella*, *Treponema*, *Plasmodium*, *Candida*, *Mycobacteria*, *Babesia* spp., and *Pneumocystis*. Right ventricular failure with passive hepatic congestion or hypoperfusion syndromes can cause hepatic injury that can be confused with viral hepatitis.
  - Patients with Gilbert's syndrome (who have an impairment in the bilirubin conjugation process) often develop jaundice with febrile illnesses. They have normal liver function tests.
- Chronic hepatitis can present with a history of unexplained episodes of acute hepatitis.
- Patients with chronic hepatitis B can develop acute hepatitis with concomitant hepatitis D infection and during hepatitis B eAg to eAb seroconversion.

Pregnancy Considerations

- In pregnant women, acute fatty liver of pregnancy and HELLP syndrome should be considered.
- The most common causes of conjugated hyperbilirubinemia and fever include the following:
  - Sepsis that can impair hepatic excretion
  - Extrahepatic biliary obstruction due to malignancy, inflammation (pancreatitis), parasitic infection (*Ascaris*, *Clonorchis*, schistosomiasis, etc.), and gallstones (that may lead to cholecystitis/cholangitis)
  - Hemolytic anemia
- Hepatic metastases can mimic acute or even fulminant viral hepatitis.

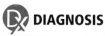 **DIAGNOSIS**

HISTORY

- Jaundice is usually visible in the sclera or skin when the serum bilirubin value exceeds 50 μmol/L (3 mg/dL).
- The diagnosis of anicteric hepatitis is difficult and requires a high index of suspicion, and it is based on clinical features and on aminotransferase elevations.

PHYSICAL EXAM

- Epigastric or right upper quadrant tenderness is frequently associated with choledocholithiasis and cholangitis or cholecystitis.
- The presence of splenomegaly may provide a clue to the presence of portal hypertension, from chronic active hepatitis, severe alcoholic, or acute viral hepatitis or from cirrhosis.

DIAGNOSTIC TESTS & INTERPRETATION
Lab
- A blood film should be performed to exclude hemolytic anemia.
- In viral hepatitis, serum alkaline phosphatase is often not particularly raised compared with obstructive jaundice, where it is often raised more than 3 times the upper level of normal.
- In the appropriate clinical setting, serologic studies are extremely helpful for establishing or excluding the diagnosis of hepatitis A; acute and chronic hepatitis B; hepatitis C, D, and E; and cytomegalovirus or Epstein–Barr virus.
- When acute viral hepatitis is considered, the patient should undergo 4 serologic tests:
  - HBsAg
  - IgM anti-HAV
  - IgM anti-HBc
  - Anti-HCV
- Tests such as the differential heterophile and serologic tests for other viral agents may be helpful in the differential diagnosis. The heterophile test is a specific but not sensitive test. In acute EBV, it may be negative, especially in children.

Imaging
- For patients whose clinical evaluation and liver chemistries suggest cholestasis or extrahepatic biliary obstruction, biliary imaging is an important early diagnostic tool to differentiate intrahepatic causes from extrahepatic obstruction. Both ultrasonography and computed tomography detect dilated extrahepatic biliary ducts with great sensitivity.
- Further definition and relief of extrahepatic biliary obstruction can frequently be accomplished by percutaneous or endoscopic cholangiography.

Diagnostic Procedures/Other
- Endoscopic retrograde cholangiopancreatography (ERCP) is frequently the preferred technique for diagnosing and treating distal biliary obstructions.
- In some cases, identification of focal lesions by computed tomography, transabdominal ultrasonography, or magnetic resonance imaging can increase the diagnostic accuracy of liver biopsy.
- The results of percutaneous, transjugular, or laparoscopic biopsy may also provide important information for optimal therapy.

 TREATMENT

- See the Section II chapter, "Hepatitis."
- Symptomatic management and supportive care if due to viral hepatitis.
- Cholecystectomy is the definitive treatment for acute cholecystitis and is usually performed acutely. The IDSA recommends that antibiotics be given in acute calculous cholecystitis if there is radiological and clinical suspicion of infection. Gram negative, but not enterococcal, cover is recommended.

ADDITIONAL READING
- Julka K, Ko CW. Infectious diseases and the gallbladder. *Infect Dis Clin North Am* 2010; 24:885–898.
- Fingeroth JD. Herpesvirus infection of the liver. *Infect Dis Clin North Am* 2000;14(3):689–719.
- Hanau LH, Steigbigel NH. Acute (ascending) cholangitis. *Infect Dis Clin North Am*. 2000;14(3): 521–546.
- Solomkin JS, Mazuski JE, Baron EJ, et al. Guidelines for the selection of anti-infective agents for complicated intra-abdominal infections. *Clin Infect Dis* 2003;37:997–1005.
- Daniels D, Grytdal S, Wasley A; Centers for Disease Control and Prevention (CDC). Surveillance for acute viral hepatitis – United States, 2007. *MMWR Surveill Summ* 2009;58(3):1–27.
- Hunt DP, Thabet A, Rosenberg ES. Case records of the Massachusetts General Hospital. Case 29–2010. A 29-year-old woman with fever and abdominal pain. *N Engl J Med* 2010;363(13):1266–1274.
- Bonilla MF, Kaul DR, Saint S, et al. Clinical problem-solving. Ring around the diagnosis. *N Engl J Med* 2006;354(18):1937–1942.

CLINICAL PEARLS
- Patients over 40 years most often have cholangitis or other surgical diagnoses.
- Those aged less than 40 years are more likely to have viral hepatitis or another infection such as EBV.
- Fever with rigors in the presence of jaundice is unlikely to be due to viral hepatitis.
- If abdominal pain and tenderness are present, imaging of the liver and biliary tree and a surgical opinion is warranted.
- Absence of bilirubin in the urine suggests unconjugated hyperbilirubinemia.
- Hepatitis A, B, and C (+/− D, E) serology should be performed when acute viral hepatitis is suspected.
- Gilbert's syndrome may be present if there an isolated hyperbilirubinemia.

J

JOINT PAIN AND FEVER

Catherine Marshall
Anton Y. Peleg

 BASICS

DESCRIPTION
- Joint disorders are classified as monarticular (1 joint involved), oligoarticular (2-to-3 joints involved), or polyarticular (more than 3 joints involved).
- Joint disorders may be symmetrical (affecting the same joints on both sides of the body) or asymmetrical.
- Arthritis describes inflammatory process that involves the joint(s). It is not a diagnosis.
- Arthralgia refers to pain that involves the joint(s).

Approach to the Patient
- Musculoskeletal disorders can be classified as inflammatory (infectious, crystal-induced, immune-related, reactive, idiopathic) or noninflammatory and are called acute if they last less than 6 weeks and chronic if they last longer. Acute arthropathies tend to be infectious, crystal-induced, or reactive.
- Noninflammatory disorders may be related to trauma, osteoarthritis, or fibromyalgia and usually are not associated with fever.
- History is important, including family history, recent travel and illnesses, prior trauma, and sexual history. The chronology of the complaint (onset, evolution, and duration) is an important diagnostic feature. The onset of certain disorders, such as septic arthritis and gout, tends to be abrupt.
- Septic arthritis should be considered in a child who suddenly develops a limp or refuses to use a limb.
- The goal of the physical examination is to determine the structures involved, the nature of the underlying pathology, the extent and functional consequences of the process, and the presence of systemic or extraarticular manifestations.
- Examination of joints involves assessing for the presence of warmth, erythema, swelling, tenderness, or limitation of movement. This can help determine the presence of arthritis as opposed to arthralgia.

- Aspiration and analysis of synovial fluid are always indicated in acute monoarthritis or when an infectious or crystal-induced arthropathy is suspected.
- If examination and cultures of the synovial fluid are nondiagnostic, the likelihood of viral arthritis, reactive arthritis, or systemic rheumatic illness increases. Serologic studies should be obtained, particularly assays for antinuclear and antistreptococcal antibodies and for antibodies to *Borrelia burgdorferi* in the case of patients who live in or have visited areas where Lyme disease is endemic.

EPIDEMIOLOGY
- In bacterial arthritis, only 10–20% of adults have polyarticular involvement, with simultaneous onset in several large joints or serial onset over 1 or 2 days.
- Risk factors for bacterial arthritis include underlying joint disease, chronic diseases such as diabetes mellitus, malignancy and chronic renal failure, immunosuppression, trauma, intravenous drug use, and prosthetic joints.
- Musculoskeletal symptoms are frequent in endocarditis, occurring in 45% of patients in 1 large series.
- Since 2004, there have been large outbreaks of chikungunya virus in the Indian Ocean region, India, and parts of Asia. Many cases have occurred in travelers returning from these areas.
- A large-joint oligoarthritis occurs in 10–20% of patients with inflammatory bowel disease, usually during periods of active disease. In these patients, it can be a reflection of the intraabdominal process.
- Familial Mediterranean fever appears during childhood, with brief episodes of fever, arthritis, and abdominal and pleuritic pain.
- The post-Q-fever fatigue syndrome (inappropriate fatigue, myalgia and arthralgia, night sweats, changes in mood and sleep patterns) has been reported in up to 20% of laboratory-proven, acute primary Q-fever cases.

ETIOLOGY
- Septic arthritis is the most important diagnosis to consider. *Staphylococcus aureus* is the most common pathogen found.
- Fever and arthritis have also been reported in a number of other local and systemic infections, including the following:
  - Bacterial infections
    - Chronic meningococcemia caused by *Neisseria meningitidis*
    - Disseminated gonococcal infection
    - Endocarditis
    - Lyme disease
    - Rickettsial diseases
    - Secondary syphilis
    - Whipple's disease
    - Rat bite fever caused by *Streptobacillus moniliformis*
  - Viral infections
    - Rubella
    - Acute HIV conversion
    - Dengue virus
    - Alphavirus: Chikungunya and Ross River virus
    - Epstein–Barr virus
    - Parvovirus B19 infection
    - Viral hepatitis
    - Mumps
    - Enterovirus
- Rheumatic fever remains common in developing countries and some Indigenous groups.
- Mycobacterium including mycobacterium tuberculosis and nontuberculous mycobacterium can cause a chronic monoarthritis.
- The systemic form of juvenile rheumatoid arthritis (Still's disease) is characterized by high fever and polyarthritis. It may appear in young adults and occasionally in older adults, either as a new illness or as a recrudescence of a dormant childhood disease.
- Fever and polyarthritis can be early features of systemic lupus erythematosus and vasculitis.
- Fever is frequent in polyarticular gout. In pseudogout, high fever has been reported, even with monoarthritis.
- Lymphoma and other neoplasias can rarely present with arthritis and fever.

DIAGNOSIS

HISTORY

- An asymmetric, additive polyarthritis predominantly involving large joints in a lower extremity may be a sequel to enteritis (usually caused by *Salmonella*, *Shigella*, *Campylobacter*, or *Yersinia*) or urogenital infection with certain organisms (principally *Chlamydia trachomatis*).
- The clinical manifestations of Whipple's disease are many and diverse. Almost all organ systems can be involved. In approximately two-thirds of patients, the disease begins insidiously with either arthralgia or a migratory, nonerosive, nondeforming seronegative arthritis. This may precede any other features by up to 24 years.
- Dissemination of *B. burgdorferi*, the causative agent of Lyme disease in the US, is often accompanied by fever and migratory arthralgia, with little or no joint swelling, but frank arthritis may appear weeks or months later (mean interval, 6 months).
- Neisseria arthritis may present as a migratory arthritis with chills, fever, and tenosynovitis, especially in the wrist and ankle extensor-tendon sheaths.
- In mycobacterial and fungal arthritis, an indolent monoarthritis is usual, but occasionally 2 or 3 large joints may be involved. Because fever is either absent or mild, an infectious process may not be considered.
- Systemic candidiasis may present with polyarthritis, particularly in immunosuppressed patients and intravenous drug users.
- Among patients with hepatitis B virus infection, the arthritis precedes the symptoms of hepatitis and resolves when jaundice appears.
- In children with rheumatic fever, cardiac involvement is a dominant feature, but adults generally present with abrupt onset of polyarthritis and fever. The arthritis is usually migratory and typically very responsive to nonsteroidal anti-inflammatory agents (NSAIDs). Monoarthritis can be a presenting feature in high-risk groups.
- Chikungunya virus usually presents with an acute febrile illness with polyarthritis. Forty to seventy-five percent have skin manifestations, usually a maculopapular rash. The acute illness usually lasts 7—10 days but >65% have persistent arthralgia for >2 months.

PHYSICAL EXAM

- Assess for signs of joint inflammation including warmth, erythema, swelling, and restriction of movement.
- Assess for extraarticular manifestations that may suggest an etiology such as rash, enthesitis, cardiac murmurs, stigmata or endocarditis, gouty tophi or rheumatoid nodules

DIAGNOSTIC TESTS & INTERPRETATION
Lab

- Examination of the synovial fluid may identify bacterial and crystal-induced arthritis and is often helpful in reducing the number of conditions warranting continued consideration.
- Synovial fluid leukocyte counts over 50,000/mL suggest a bacterial infection but are occasionally seen in rheumatoid, crystal-induced, and reactive arthritis.
- Infectious synovial fluid is turbid and opaque, with a predominance of polymorphonuclear leukocytes (>75%) and low viscosity. Whenever infection is suspected, synovial fluid should be Gram stained and cultured appropriately.
- Culture synovial aspirates for mycobacterium and fungus in clinically compatible cases.
- Blood cultures should be taken in acute arthritis.
- Blood and synovial cultures are often negative in disseminated gonococcal infection. It is important to culture swabs from potential mucosal portals of entry.
- Serological markers are useful for diagnosis of rheumatological conditions. Anti-nuclear antibodies are sensitive for systemic lupus erythematosus.
- Elevations of peripheral white blood cell count, CRP, and ESR are more suggestive of bacterial than viral infection.
- Transiently positive rheumatoid factors have been reported early in the course of Lyme disease.
- Patients with adult Still's disease often have markedly elevated ferritin >3000 ng/mL, in some patients >10,000 ng/mL.

 TREATMENT

- For patients with septic arthritis, therapy should be initiated promptly after the samples for cultures have been obtained (see Section II chapter, "Septic Arthritis").
- Surgical intervention with joint aspiration and drainage or washout is required in most cases of nongonococcal bacterial septic arthritis.
- Gonococcal arthritis usually does not require surgical management and is best treated with ceftriaxone or oral ciprofloxacin or levofloxacin in regions without significant fluoroquinolone resistance.
- Analgesia and early joint immobilization provide symptom control. Non-steroidal anti-inflammatory agents can be beneficial in viral and reactive arthritis.
- Gentle mobilization is necessary after infection is controlled.

 ONGOING CARE

COMPLICATIONS
For septic arthritis, spread to bone or frank bacteremia

 CODES

ICD9
- 719.40 Pain in joint, site unspecified
- 719.49 Pain in joint involving multiple sites

CLINICAL PEARLS

- Septic arthritis should always be considered in acute monoarthritis with limitation of joint movement; early diagnosis and prompt treatment are critical to preserve joint function
- Patients with underlying rheumatological conditions such as rheumatoid arthritis are at greater risk for septic arthritis; don't assume a single pathology
- If in doubt aspirate at joint
- Always consider gonococcal arthritis in a sexually active person with polyarthritis and fever

J

LUNG NODULES

Isaac I. Bogoch

 BASICS

DESCRIPTION

- Pulmonary nodules by definition are surrounded by lung tissue and are typically defined as being smaller than 3–4 cm. Larger sized structures are referred to as lung masses.
- There are both pathologic and radiologic definitions of pulmonary nodules; the pathologic definition is "a small, approximately spherical, circumscribed focus of abnormal tissue." The radiologic definition is "a round opacity, at least moderately well marginated and no more than 3 cm in maximum diameter."
- Opacities with linear characteristics or two dimensions are not considered nodules.
- Radiography may reveal a solitary lung nodule (also referred to as a "coin lesion"), or multiple lung nodules.

Approach to the Patient

- One of the primary goals is to differentiate whether the patient has a benign or malignant nodule.
- The physician should begin with the patient's history.
- The probability of malignancy rises with age. It is rare for a lung nodule to be malignant under the age of 35 years.
- Evaluate for malignancy risk factors: Previous lung cancer, lung cancer in first degree relatives, smoking history, exposure to other smoke (e.g., second-hand smoke, burning wood), occupational exposures to carcinogens (e.g., asbestos and radon), fibrosis, chronic obstructive pulmonary disease, and alpha-1 antitrypsin deficiency.
- Greater smoking burden is associated with greater cancer risk.
- If malignancy is suspected or confirmed, it is important to determine if the nodule is primary or metastatic.
- History of fevers may indicate an infectious process.
- The immunologic status of the patient is very important as opportunistic infections may present as solitary or multiple lung nodules.
- Clinical examination may reveal additional signs of malignancy as cachexia, anemia, icterus, clubbing, bone pain due to fracture, abdominal mass, and superior vena cava syndrome.
- The radiologic appearance often offers helpful diagnostic clues. The size, distribution (upper or lower lungs, central or peripheral), shape, pattern of calcification, presence of cavitation, coexistence of lymphadenopathy or pleural effusion, and the clustering of multiple nodules should be noted.
- Some nodules deemed low risk for malignancy can be monitored with serial CT scans.
- Transthoracic needle biopsy should be considered in larger nodules with the suspicion of cancer.
- Positron emission tomography (PET) scan and video-assisted thoracoscopic surgery (VATS) may aid in diagnosis and therapy in cases of malignancy.
- Initiate empiric antibiotic treatment in immunocompromised hosts or those who are at risk of rapid clinical deterioration.

EPIDEMIOLOGY

- Up to 51% of smokers aged 50 years or older have pulmonary nodules on CT scans.
- Fewer than 1% of very small nodules (<5 mm) in patients without a history of cancer are malignant.
- The likelihood of malignancy is 0.2% for nodules smaller than 3 mm, 0.9% for those between 4–7 mm, 18% for 8–20 mm, and greater than 50% for those larger than 20 mm.
- The relative risk for developing lung carcinoma in male smokers is about 10 times than that in nonsmokers. The risk is 15–35 times higher for heavy smokers.
- *Paragonimus westermani* is a fluke endemic in parts of China, Korea, Japan, the Philippines, and Taiwan which may present as a lung nodule.
- The most common radiologic finding in patients with tuberculosis is hilar lymphadenopathy (65%).
- Histoplasmosis is the most common cause of hospitalization from endemic mycoses in the US.

GENERAL PREVENTION

Speech–language pathology, occupational and physical therapists can help reduce the risk of aspiration in high-risk patients with special diets, support, and training.

ETIOLOGY

- The following etiologies may present as solitary lung nodules:
  - Bronchogenic carcinoma:
    - Adenocarcinoma
    - Squamous cell carcinoma
    - Large cell carcinoma
    - Small cell carcinoma
  - Metastases from the following sites:
    - Breast
    - Head and neck
    - Thyroid
    - Melanoma
    - Colon
    - Kidney
    - Sarcoma
    - Germ cell tumor
    - Other
  - Carcinoid
  - Infectious disease:
    - Bacterial abscess
    - Histoplasmosis
    - Blastomycosis
    - Coccidioidomycosis
    - Cryptococcal infection
    - Aspergilloma
    - Tuberculosis
    - Atypical mycobacteria
    - Nocardia
    - *Dirofilaria immitis*
    - Echinococcus cyst
    - Ascariasis
    - Pneumocystis
    - *Paragonimus westermani*

- Benign neoplasm's:
  - Hamartoma
  - Lipoma
  - Fibroma
- Other:
  - Arteriovenous malformation
  - Bronchogenic cyst
  - Wegener's granulomatosis
  - Sarcoidosis
  - Rheumatoid nodule
  - Amyloidoma
  - Rounded atelectasis
  - Intrapulmonary lymph node
  - Hematoma
  - Pulmonary infarct
  - Mucoid impaction
- Multiple lung nodules are more frequently benign if less than 1 cm. In those with known malignancy, pulmonary nodules >0.5 cm are more likely to be metastatic.
- Infections which may present as multiple pulmonary nodules include:
  - Abscesses
  - Septic emboli (e.g., tricuspid valve endocarditis, Lemierre's syndrome)
  - Fungal infections (e.g., Cryptococcus, Aspergillosis, Histoplasmosis, Coccidioidomycosis)
  - Tuberculosis
  - Atypical mycobacterium
  - Paragonimiasis.
- Other causes of multiple pulmonary nodules include inflammatory conditions like Wegener's granulomatosis, rheumatoid arthritis, and sarcoidosis. Pneumoconiosis and pulmonary arteriovenous malformations may also have this appearance.

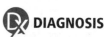 **DIAGNOSIS**

PHYSICAL EXAM

- Careful history to see if patients have TB risk factors, immunocompromised state, and exposure to areas that put them at risk for endemic fungal infection.
- Patients with recurrent aspiration, tricuspid valve endocarditis, septic thrombophlebitis from jugular veins (e.g., Lemierre's syndrome) or with bacteremia may present single or multiple lung abscesses.
- Patients who form lung abscesses from aspiration often have poor dentition as a source of infection or have long periods in a recumbent position (e.g., decreased level of consciousness from drugs, seizure, and debilitation).
- Evaluate for cough, sputum production, and shortness of breath.
- Patients with chronic infection or malignancy may present with nonspecific symptoms and signs such as fevers, night sweats, unintentional weight loss, and anorexia. Look for muscle wasting and clubbing on physical exam.

DIAGNOSTIC TESTS & INTERPRETATION
Lab
- Blood cultures in the case of sepsis. In the right clinical setting, blood cultures with fungal isolator should be obtained.
- Sputum gram stain and culture may aid in diagnosis.
- Blood for cryptococcal antigen.
- Blood for galactomannan and beta-D-glucan may provide clues for invasive fungal infection.
- Sputum staining for acid-fast bacilli (e.g., Ziehl-Nielsen stain) and mycobacterium culture for TB or non-tuberculous mycobacterial infections. Sputum should also be sent for fungal cultures and stains.
- Serologic tests for Histoplasma, Blastomycosis, Coccidioides, if history of travel to endemic location.
- Urine Histoplasma antigen.

Imaging
- High resolution CT scanning can detect nodules as small as 1–2 mm.
- Calcification patterns typically associated with benign nodules include homogeneous, "popcorn," concentric, and central.
- Calcification patterns more suggestive of malignant nodules include amorphous, eccentric, and nodules with spiculated borders.
- Ghon complex: a tuberculous lesion in the lung with an associated lymph node. Perifocal ground-glass opacity is useful in differentiating fungal infiltrates from older scars. Look for a "halo" of ground glass opacity around a nodule. This is classic for invasive pulmonary Aspergillosis.
- PET scan may indicate a metabolically active cancerous lesion and its primary focus.
- Transthoracic echocardiography is recommended if pulmonary abscesses are thought to be secondary to tricuspid valve endocarditis.
- CT neck looking for jugular vein thrombosis if *Fusobacterium* species identified in blood cultures (Lemierre's syndrome).

Diagnostic Procedures/Other
Percutaneous needle biopsy and VATS should be considered in cases where there is a high risk of malignancy.

DIFFERENTIAL DIAGNOSIS
- The upper lung fields are typically involved in the following disorders:
  - Sarcoidosis
  - Tuberculosis
  - Hypersensitivity pneumonitis
  - Langerhans cell histiocytosis
  - Silicosis
  - Ankylosing spondylitis
- The lower fields are involved in:
  - Aspiration abscesses
  - Bronchiectasis
  - bronchiolitis obliterans with organizing pneumonia (BOOP)
  - Rheumatoid disease
  - Scleroderma
  - Asbestosis
  - Acute Interstitial Pneumonia (Hamman-Rich Syndrome)

 TREATMENT
MEDICATION
- Early empiric antibiotic treatment should be initiated in cases where fever or systemic toxicity is present. Blood cultures should be drawn prior to antibiotic therapy.
- If tuberculosis is suspected, it is crucial to differentiate between latent and active infection with a thorough history, physical exam, chest radiography, and induced sputum for acid-fast bacilli and mycobacterial growth.
- Pulmonary Histoplasmosis does not have to be treated in many mild cases with focal lung findings; however itraconazole is recommended if symptoms persist. Acute cases that are moderate-to-severe are treated initially with lipid formulations of amphotericin B followed by itraconazole.
- Lung abscesses are commonly polymicrobial and involve oral anaerobic bacteria. Treat with a beta lactam/beta lactamase inhibitor (e.g., piperacillin/tazobactam) or clindamycin.
- Voriconazole is the drug of choice for invasive Aspergillosis. Surgical debridement is indicated in many patients although many are too unstable for surgery due to neutropenia or thrombocytopenia.
- Paragonimiasis is treated with praziquantel or triclabendazole.

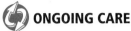 ONGOING CARE
FOLLOW-UP RECOMMENDATIONS
- Malignant solitary pulmonary nodules will typically double in volume between 20–400 days.
- Solitary nodules that are low probability for malignancy or <1 cm can be followed by serial CT scans. Solitary nodules that are high probability for malignancy should be excised.
- PET scanning is helpful in intermediate-risk solitary nodules that are >1 cm. Active nodules can be excised and non-active nodules can be followed with serial CT scans.

COMPLICATIONS
- Lung abscesses that go untreated may cause progressive pulmonary symptoms and respiratory arrest requiring mechanical ventilation.
- Many infectious, malignant, and inflammatory lung nodules will undergo cavitation.
- Cavitary lung lesions are commonly superinfected with Aspergillus spp.

ADDITIONAL READING

- MacMahon H, Austin JHR, et al. Guidelines for management of small pulmonary nodules detected on CT scans: A statement from Fleischner society. *Radiology* 2005;237:395–400.
- Van Klavern RJ, Oudkerk M, Prokop M, et al. Management of lung nodules detected by volume CT scanning. *N Engl J Med* 2009;361:2221–2229.

 CODES

ICD9
- 162.9 Malignant neoplasm of bronchus and lung, unspecified
- 212.3 Benign neoplasm of bronchus and lung
- 518.89 Other diseases of lung, not elsewhere classified

CLINICAL PEARLS
- The presence of a solitary lung nodule in the upper lung fields increases the likelihood of malignancy.
- Solitary pulmonary nodules in smokers, >2 cm, growing in size or with irregular borders are more likely to be malignant.

L

LYMPHADENOPATHY AND FEVER

Isaac I. Bogoch

 BASICS

DESCRIPTION

- Lymphadenitis is the inflammation of one or more lymph nodes, lymphangitis refers to inflammation of the lymphatic channels – both may be seen in acute or chronic conditions.
- Mesenteric lymphadenitis is caused by inflammation of the mesenteric lymph nodes and clinically resembles acute appendicitis and.
- Lymph nodes >1 cm in diameter are considered significantly enlarged in most parts of the body. Epitrochlear nodes >0.5 cm, and inguinal nodes >1.5–2.0 cm should be regarded as abnormal.
- It is common for healthy adults to present with palpable inguinal lymph nodes.
- Generalized lymphadenopathy refers to abnormalities in two or more noncontiguous lymph node regions.

Approach to the Patient

- Most causes of lymph node enlargement can be associated with fever. Infection is a leading cause of fever and lymphadenopathy.
- Lymphadenopathy may either be an incidental finding or a presenting sign or symptom. The clinician must decide whether observation or further investigations are necessary based on the clinical information available.
- A detailed history and physical exam should be performed.
- The duration of lymphadenopathy may be helpful. Most suppurative infections produce a short (<1 week) history of symptoms. Long-standing lymphadenopathy may be caused by a variety of diseases, including infections (e.g., HIV, tuberculosis), malignancy, inflammation, and autoimmune diseases.
- Focus on possible epidemiologic clues such as travel, sick contacts, and exposure to animals (e.g., cats).

- Investigate for symptoms such as weight loss, fever, night sweats, sore throat, cough, pruritus, fatigue, lymph node pain, and myalgia/arthralgia.
- A full examination of all nodal sites should be performed to determine whether the disease process is localized or generalized. Abdominal examination should determine the presence of liver and splenic enlargement.
- Anemia, petechiae, or bleeding may be seen in infiltrative disease of the bone marrow.
- Many infectious agents cause fever and lymphadenopathy, but only a few, including *Francisella tularensis*, *Bartonella henselae*, and various mycobacterium, typically present with a single prominent lymph node and fever.

EPIDEMIOLOGY

- More than two-thirds of patients who present in the primary care setting with lymphadenopathy have nonspecific causes or upper respiratory illnesses.
- The frequency of malignant lymphadenopathy rises in those over 50 years of age.
- In the primary care setting, up to 1% of patients presenting with lymphadenopathy have an underlying malignancy as the cause.
- Acute mesenteric lymphadenitis is more common among children.
- In developed countries, lymphadenopathy due to mycobacterium is more likely to be nontuberculous.

ETIOLOGY

- Infectious diseases
  - Viral etiologies include Epstein-Barr virus (EBV), cytomegalovirus, herpes simplex viruses, dengue fever, rubella, measles, HIV, and West Nile virus.
  - Bacterial etiologies include: Streptococcal species, *Staphylococcus aureus*, cat-scratch disease (*Bartonella henselae*), brucellosis, tularemia, plague, melioidosis, tuberculosis and nontuberculous mycobacterium, listeriosis, leptospirosis, syphilis (secondary), diphtheria, typhoid fever, and lymphogranuloma venereum (Chlamydia).
  - Fungal infections include: Histoplasmosis, coccidioidomycosis, paracoccidioidomycosis, and cryptococcosis.
  - Parasitic infections include: Toxoplasmosis, leishmaniasis, trypanosomiasis, and filariasis.
  - Rickettsial infections.

- Immunologic diseases, such as lupus, rheumatoid arthritis, Churg-Strauss vasculitis, Still's disease, dermatomyositis, graft—versus—host disease, juvenile rheumatoid arthritis, mixed connective-tissue disease, serum sickness, and Sjögren's syndrome.
- Malignant diseases (hematologic)
  - Hodgkin's disease, non-Hodgkin's lymphomas, acute or chronic lymphocytic leukemia, hairy-cell leukemia, and amyloidosis.
- Malignant diseases (non-hematologic)
- Sarcomas and metastasis
- Lipid storage diseases: Gaucher's, Niemann-Pick disease, and Fabry disease
- Endocrine disease
  - Hyperthyroidism, Addison's disease
- Others: Disorders such as Castleman's disease, Kikuchi's disease, drugs (particularly phenytoin, carbamazepine, hydralazine, and allopurinol), familial Mediterranean fever, and Kawasaki disease
- Lymphadenopathy is a common finding in patients with HIV infection ranging from generalized follicular hyperplasia seen early in disease to opportunistic infections and neoplasms. In this population, non-Hodgkin's lymphoma, mycobacterial infection, toxoplasmosis, systemic fungal infection, and bacillary angiomatosis are potential causes of lymphadenopathy.

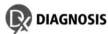 **DIAGNOSIS**

- When examining a patient, note the size, shape, texture/consistency, and mobility of lymph nodes. Also note whether or not they are tender. Hard lymph nodes may be associated with carcinoma, rubbery firm nodes that are non-tender are often associated with lymphoma, and tender nodes that are mobile are frequently reactive to an underlying infection.
- Some malignant diseases, such as acute leukemia, produce rapid lymph node enlargement and pain.

DIAGNOSTIC TESTS & INTERPRETATION
Lab
- Initial laboratory evaluation of fever and lymphadenopathy should be reflective of the patient's risk factors. This may include blood cultures, HIV screen, Rapid Plasma Reagin (RPR), heterophile test, Toxoplasma IgG/IgM, CMV IgG/IgM, EBV IgG/IgM, Bartonella serology, urine histoplasma antigen, ANA, rheumatoid factor, or other tests based on the differential diagnosis listed above.
- Fine-needle aspiration has an important role in evaluating lymphadenopathy, however an excisional biopsy is far better for making a diagnosis of several conditions, most notably non-Hodgkin lymphoma.
- The lymph node can be sent for routine culture and sensitivity, stains for mycobacterial infection (acid fast stains), mycobacterial culture, fungal stains and culture, cytology, and molecular diagnostic assays.

Imaging
- The chest x-ray may indicate pulmonary infiltrates and mediastinal or hilar lymphadenopathy.
- Ultrasonography is often helpful in determining lymphadenopathy in superficial locations like the head and neck. This is a poor test to evaluate deeper nodes like those around the pancreas and retroperitoneum.
- CT and MRI are helpful for distinguishing lymph nodes from other surrounding tissues and may aide in guiding biopsies. They are superior for assessing deeper nodes like those in the retroperitoneum.
- PET-scan will indicate lymph nodes with high metabolic activity.

Diagnostic Procedures/Other
In cases where there are no worrisome features to suggest malignancy or severe infection and initial investigations do not reveal a diagnosis, it is usually safe to watch the enlarged lymph nodes clinically for 2–4 weeks to see if they ultimately return to a normal size. A biopsy is recommended should lymphadenopathy not resolve in this time frame.

DIFFERENTIAL DIAGNOSIS
- The most frequent site of regional adenopathy is the neck, commonly from upper respiratory tract infections, oral and dental infections, and infectious mononucleosis.
- Occipital adenopathy often reflects an infection of the scalp, while preauricular adenopathy accompanies conjunctival infections and cat-scratch disease. Preauricular lymphadenopathy is a finding in tularemia, tuberculosis, sporotrichosis, and syphilis.
- Enlargement of supraclavicular and scalene nodes is always abnormal. Tuberculosis, sarcoidosis, and toxoplasmosis are nonmalignant causes of supraclavicular adenopathy. Assess for metastases from distant sites (e.g., lung, breast, gastrointestinal tract, gonads) especially with a left enlarged supraclavicular node (Virchow's node). Axillary adenopathy is usually due to injuries or localized infections of the ipsilateral upper extremity, or regional malignancies such as breast cancer.
- Mediastinal adenopathy is often associated with infectious mononucleosis, lymphoma, or sarcoidosis. Consider TB or fungal infections in endemic regions. Enlarged intra-abdominal or retroperitoneal nodes are frequently malignant.

 TREATMENT

Treatment of lymphadenitis depends on the underlying etiology. Please refer to relevant chapters in Section II.

 ONGOING CARE

FOLLOW-UP RECOMMENDATIONS
After an initial history, physical examination, and routine investigations, a period of clinical observation for 2–4 weeks is appropriate prior to pursuing lymph node biopsy in the absence of symptoms suggestive of malignancy or serious infection.

COMPLICATIONS
Failure to promptly diagnose and treat many infectious causes of lymphadenopathy can result in disseminated or severe infection.

ADDITIONAL READING
- Abramson J, Digumarthy S, Ferry JA. Case records of the Massachusetts General Hospital. Case 27-2009. A 56-year-old woman with fever, rash and lymphadenopathy. *N Engl J Med* 2009;361: 900–911.
- Ferrer R. Lymphadenopathy: Differential diagnosis and evaluation. *Am Fam Physician* 1998;15;58(6): 1313–1320.
- Hurt C, Tammaro D. Diagnostic evaluation of mononucleosis-like illnesses. *Am J Med* 2007; 120(10):911.
- Leggett J. Approach to Fever and Suspected Infection in the Normal Host. Chapter 302. Cecil's Medicine, 23rd Edition, Saunders, 2008:2112–2118.
- Vassilakopoulos TP, Pangalis GA. Application of a prediction rule to select which patients presenting with lymphadenopathy should undergo a lymph node biopsy. *Medicine (Baltimore)* 2000;79(5): 338–347.

 CODES

ICD9
- 017.2 Tuberculosis of peripheral lymph nodes
- 135 Sarcoidosis
- 785.6 Enlargement of lymph nodes

CLINICAL PEARLS
- The most common infectious cause of fever and generalized lymphadenopathy is infectious mononucleosis due to EBV.

L

LYMPHOCYTOSIS

Isaac I. Bogoch

 BASICS

DESCRIPTION

Definition

- Lymphocytosis can be divided into either reactive or neoplastic causes.
- Reactive lymphocytosis can be caused by infectious or noninfectious etiologies.
- Infectious causes of reactive lymphocytosis include viral, bacterial, protozoal, and parasitic (discussed below) diseases. Noninfectious causes include drugs, autoimmune disorders, and a few endocrinopathies.
- The atypical lymphocyte is a non-neoplastic cell that presents in the blood in response to various immunogenic stimuli.
- Lymphocytosis is defined as >4000 lymphocytes per cubic millimeter in peripheral blood.
- Atypical lymphocytes are typically larger than normal lymphocytes and have nucleoli in the nuclei, unevenly stained cytoplasm, and often have surrounding red blood cells close enough to impinge on the periphery of the cell.

Approach to the Patient

- Use the history and physical exam to help differentiate lymphocytosis between neoplastic and non-neoplastic disorders.
- Certain conditions are more common at different ages: Acute Epstein-Barr virus (EBV) is common in the first 2 decades of life, and Chronic Lymphocytic Leukemia after the fifth decade.
- Enquire about the chronicity of symptoms, vaccination history (e.g., measles, mumps, rubella), and preexisting medical conditions.
- Evaluate for HIV risk factors: Unprotected heterosexual or homosexual sex, intravenous drug use, occupational exposures.
- Evaluate for TB risk factors: Close contacts, travel to an endemic area, and homeless, institutionalization.
- Detailed travel history: Ensure appropriate prophylactic measures against water-borne, food-borne, and arthropod-borne infections.
- Clinical examination to determine if lymphadenopathy or organ involvement (e.g., hepatomegaly, splenomegaly) is present.
- Many patients with chronic symptoms and without systemic toxicity can be evaluated in an outpatient setting.
- Experienced lab personnel should examine the blood smear as atypical lymphocytes may be difficult to recognize.

EPIDEMIOLOGY

- Lymphocytosis is a frequent finding in many common and uncommon conditions.
- Immunologic evidence of prior EBV infection can be found in over 90% of adults.
- Primary EBV infection is very common and mostly asymptomatic in infants and children.

- Cytomegalovirus (CMV) seroprevalence increases with age and may differ among ethnic groups. In the US, about 35% of 6–11 year olds are seropositive, compared to over 90% of people over the age of 80 years.
- About 33 million people are living with HIV/AIDS worldwide, and there are about 56000 new cases per year in the US. Patients with acute HIV infection may present with a flu-like illness with the presence of atypical lymphocytosis.
- The World Health Organization estimates that there are 2 billion individuals infected with tuberculosis, with over 14 million active infections.

ETIOLOGY

- Atypical lymphocytes are activated T-lymphocytes that polyclonally proliferate due to activation of B-lymphocytes by any of the following stimuli
- The most common infections which present with lymphocytosis are:
  - EBV
  - Cytomegalovirus
  - Coxsackie virus
  - Rubella
  - Roseola
  - Herpes simplex
  - Herpes Zoster or Varicella
  - Dengue fever
  - Rickettsial pox
  - Measles
  - Pertussis
  - Rubella
  - Mumps
  - Adenovirus
  - Influenza
  - HIV (1+2)
  - Hepatitis A
  - Hepatitis B
  - Listeria monocytogenes
  - Tuberculosis
  - Q fever
  - Bartonella
  - Mycoplasma pneumonia
  - Syphilis
  - Brucellosis
  - Toxoplasma
  - Malaria
  - Babesiosis
- Noninfectious causes of lymphocytosis include the following:
  - Drug and Toxic reactions:
    - Phenothiazine
    - Lead
    - Dapsone
  - Post-perfusion syndrome
  - Immunizations/Vaccinations
  - Radiation

- Endocrine disorders:
  - Catecholamine secretion (stress)
  - Addison's disease
  - Glucocorticoids deficiency
  - Panhypopituitarism
  - Thyrotoxicosis
- Autoimmune diseases:
  - Rheumatoid arthritis
  - Systemic lupus erythematosus
  - Idiopathic thrombocytopenic purpura
  - Autoimmune hemolytic anemia
- Agammaglobulinemia
- Malignant disease:
  - Acute Lymphocytic leukemia
  - Chronic lymphocytic leukemia
  - Hodgkin's disease and Non Hodgkin lymphomas-Burkitt's lymphoma
  - Hairy cell leukemia
  - Solid tumors
  - Cancer
  - Paraneoplastic neuropathies
- Miscellaneous disorders:
  - Sarcoidosis
  - Thymoma
  - Myasthenia Gravis
  - Guillain-Barré syndrome
  - Serum sickness
- Graft rejection
- Smoking

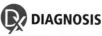 **DIAGNOSIS**

HISTORY

Exposure to an infectious agent, sick contacts, epidemiologic risk factors, country of origin, travel history, local epidemics, immune status, history of vaccinations, history of past infectious diseases, and current and recent medication should also be noted. Ask about acute versus chronic symptoms to help distinguish between the various etiologies.

PHYSICAL EXAM

- Acute infection with EBV, CMV, HIV can include a syndrome of fever, lymphadenopathy.
- Pharyngitis (classically exudative in EBV and non-exudative in CMV or HIV), weakness, anorexia, and sometimes hepatomegaly/splenomegaly. CMV is less likely to present with hepatosplenomegaly and more likely to present with fevers.
- *Bartonella henselae* (Cat-scratch fever) presents as lymphadenopathy near the site of inoculation.
- Fevers may be a prominent feature in infectious and noninfectious etiologies of lymphocytosis. Watch for Pel-Ebstein fevers (cycling fevers that last for days or weeks) classically associated with Hodgkin's lymphoma.
- Rash is a prominent aspect of many viral syndromes.

- Generalized lymphadenopathy can be seen in many infections including EBV, CMV, HIV, toxoplasmosis, tuberculosis, or in noninfectious etiologies like chronic or acute leukemias and lymphomas or sarcoidosis.
- Massive splenomegaly may be seen in myeloproliferative disorders, lymphomas, visceral Leishmaniasis, malaria, or glycogen storage diseases like Gaucher's.
- Viral hepatitis may present with jaundice, right upper quadrant abdominal tenderness, and hepatomegaly.

DIAGNOSTIC TESTS & INTERPRETATION
Lab
- The blood smear should be evaluated by experienced laboratory personnel.
- Review old blood work to determine chronicity of lymphocytosis.
- Patients with acute EBV present with an absolute increase of mononuclear cells, heterophile antibodies, and often with elevated aminotransferases.
- Monospot test, which evaluates the existence of heterophile antibodies, is 100% specific and about 85% sensitive. No further testing is necessary on most individuals if this is positive in the context of a compatible syndrome.
- Antibodies toward EBV viral capsid antigen (VCA) include IgM in acute infection, whereas IgG to VCA appear later and typically persist for life. Antibodies to EBV nuclear antigen ("EBNA") are suggestive of past infection. Note that antibodies to VCA can cross react with toxoplasma, or other herpes viruses (like CMV).
- CMV IgM represents acute infection, and IgG denotes past infection, appearing roughly 4 weeks after exposure and typically lasting for life. Other diagnostic tests are available but are usually reserved for hospitalized or immunocompromised individuals. These include PCR for CMV DNA, or detecting intranuclear inclusions on biopsy samples from tissue where there is active CMV infection (e.g., esophagus, colon)
- HIV diagnosis involves an initial ELISA based test with sensitivity and specificity greater than 99%, followed by confirmation with Western blot. IgG antibodies take about 6 weeks to be present in sufficient quantity for a positive test, and are positive in 95% of individuals 6 months after infection. In the setting of acute infection, PCR for HIV viral load is warranted, as no antibodies will be present.
- Antibodies (IgG and IgM) are the tests of choice for the detection of toxoplasma. IgM will be positive 1 week after infection.

- Influenza A (including H1N1) and B are routinely diagnosed with a nasopharyngeal swab. Rapid antigen tests have poor sensitivity (40–50%), immunofluorescence antibody staining is often higher yield, and PCR is used in some institutions with the highest sensitivity and specificity. Samples should also be concurrently tested for other respiratory illnesses like parainfluenza and respiratory syncytial virus.
- Further tests to examine whether lymphocytosis is secondary to malignancy or infiltrative granulomatous disease may include bone marrow biopsy, flow cytometry, and cytogenetics.

Imaging
- Images should only be obtained if clinically indicated. Many benign causes of lymphocytosis are self-limited and require no radiography.
- Chest x-ray to be taken if there are symptoms of pneumonia. Note that CT Chest is of higher yield in detecting consolidations and is of higher diagnostic yield in immunocompromised patients.
- Abdominal ultrasound to evaluate for hepatomegaly or splenomegaly if there is a high pre-test probability or detected on clinical exam.
- Disseminated toxoplasmosis in immunocompromised patients may manifest as multiple brain lesions, and can be visualized on CT or MRI.

 ## TREATMENT
- Treatment should be tailored to the specific etiology.
- Uncomplicated EBV infection requires only supportive care. Monitor for rare complications such as hemolytic anemia, aplastic anemia, splenic rupture, respiratory obstruction from tonsillar enlargement, Guillain Barré syndrome, encephalitis, myocarditis, and bacterial superinfection such as pneumonia.
- Counsel patients with infectious mononucleosis and hepatomegaly/splenomegaly to refrain from contact sports until this resolves (usually up to 2 months) given the risk of splenic rupture.
- Ampicillin (and less frequently penicillin) given to those with EBV infection will commonly cause a diffuse maculopapular rash.
- Treatment or prophylaxis for CMV infection is typically reserved for immunocompromised patients.

MEDICATION
- Acetaminophen or NSAIDs are helpful in symptomatic uncomplicated EBV infections. Corticosteroids can be used in respiratory distress and impending airway obstruction.
- CMV treatment includes Valganciclovir, Ganciclovir, Foscarnet, or Cidofovir and is typically reserved for immunocompromised hosts.
- HIV/AIDS is treated with highly active antiretroviral therapy, initiated and closely supervised by an HIV specialist.
- Many herpes virus 1 and 2 infections are treated with acyclovir or valacyclovir.
- Oseltamivir or zanamivir are both used for the treatment of influenza A (including H1N1) and B.

 ## ONGOING CARE
FOLLOW-UP RECOMMENDATIONS
- Inform patients of EBV complications and have them return to the clinic should these appear.
- Follow liver function tests to ensure resolution of hepatitis in mononucleosis.
- Consultation with a hematologist if blood abnormalities are excessive or persistent.

ADDITIONAL READING
- van der Meer W, van Gelder W, de Keijzer R, et al. The divergent morphological classification of variant lymphocytes in blood smears. *J Clin Pathol* 2007;60: 838–839.
- Luzuriaga K, Sullivan JL. Infectious mononucleosis. *N Engl J Med* 2010;362(21):1993–2000.

 ## CODES

ICD9
- 078.89 Other specified diseases due to viruses
- 288.61 Lymphocytosis (symptomatic)

CLINICAL PEARLS
- Detection of lymphocytes in the blood smear warrants further clinical evaluation and correlation with a patient's history, physical exam, and investigations to determine the etiology.
- EBV is the most frequent infective agent causing atypical lymphocytosis.

L

NEUROLOGIC SYMPTOMS/SIGNS AND FEVER

Isaac I. Bogoch

 BASICS

DESCRIPTION
- Clouding of consciousness refers to very mild changes in consciousness, inattentiveness, and slightly reduced wakefulness.
- Obtunded patients have slowed responses to external stimuli, decreased alertness, and increased sleepiness.
- Coma indicates a state from which the patient cannot be aroused by stimulation, and no purposeful attempt is made to avoid painful stimuli.
- Encephalitis refers to inflammation of the brain associated with neurologic or mental status changes.
- Meningitis refers to inflammation of the meninges surrounding the central nervous system (CNS), and can be acute (presenting in hours) or chronic (lasting >4 weeks).

Approach to the Patient
- Patients with fever and neurologic symptoms should be evaluated for localized infections of the CNS, systemic infections, and for noninfectious pathology.
- Obtain details of any preceding neurologic symptoms, the use of medications, illicit drugs or alcohol, trauma, travel, animal exposures, past medical history, and family medical history. Try to corroborate the history with someone accompanying the patient.
- A complete physical examination from head to toe, with particular focus on dermatologic, head and neck, and cardiopulmonary exams.
- A detailed neurologic exam should be performed and should include mental status, cranial nerves, funduscopy, gait, tone, power, reflexes, sensation, and cerebellar signs.
- Level of consciousness should be assessed and documented with the Glasgow Coma Scale.
- Physical examination for meningitis includes assessing for neck stiffness, testing for Kernig and Brudzinski signs, and assessing jolt accentuation of headache.
- The funduscopic examination is used to detect subarachnoid hemorrhage, hypertensive encephalopathy, and increased intracranial pressure.

EPIDEMIOLOGY
- Herpes simplex virus type 1 accounts for approximately 10% of all cases of encephalitis.
- In countries where tuberculosis is highly endemic, tuberculomas account for a significant proportion of intracranial masses.
- The annual incidence of bacterial meningitis ranges from approximately 1.5 per 100,000 population in the US.
- A study looking at the etiology of bacterial meningitis showed that 51% were from *Streptococcus pneumoniae*, 37% *Neisseria meningitidis*, and 4% *Listeria monocytogenes* in adults. Other cases were due to *Staphylococcus aureus*, *Haemophilus influenzae*, and Gram-negative organisms. It should be noted that *S. aureus* is an increasingly common infection, including methicillin-resistant *S. aureus*.

GENERAL PREVENTION
- Headache accompanied by fever and meningismus is a medical emergency.
- Vaccination against *S. pneumoniae*, *H. influenzae*, and *N. meningitidis*

ETIOLOGY
- Fever in a patient with acute neurologic signs and symptoms suggests systemic infection, bacterial meningitis, encephalitis, or possibly an infectious brain lesion. These are potentially rapidly fatal conditions, and should be treated as medical emergencies.
- Granulomas involving the CNS can be due to syphilis, cysticercosis, tuberculoma, fungal infections, or rarely sarcoid. Although more frequently associated with chronic meningitis, *Cryptococcus neoformans* infections can cause solitary lesions as well.
- Enterovirus (for example coxsackievirus and echovirus) is most often implicated in aseptic meningitis. In addition, several opportunistic infections with advanced HIV infection can cause fever with neurologic signs and symptoms.
- *Listeria* rhombencephalitis is associated with signs of cranial nerve or brainstem involvement and can often be detected on MRI scan.

- *Echinococcus granulosus* is a major cause of cerebral infection worldwide.
- Schistosomiasis may affect the spinal canal, producing myelopathy. In rare cases, it may cause intracranial lesions.
- Amebiasis (*Entamoeba histolytica*) can be complicated by meningoencephalitis and suppurative brain abscesses in a small percentage of individuals. Patients will typically have hepatic abscesses and are acutely ill.
- Paragonimiasis is a frequent cause of solitary brain masses in East Asia.
- Cryptococcal infections are the most common fungal etiology of meningitis. Coccidioidomycosis and histoplasmosis can disseminate to the nervous system as well. Blastomycosis generally infects the brain and meninges late in the course of advanced disease. *Aspergillus* spp., mucormycosis, and *Pseudallescheria boydii* can cause widespread disease in immunocompromised persons.
- Cerebellar encephalitis has occurred in patients with measles, varicella, Lyme disease, rabies, and legionellosis.
- Amoebas like *Naegleria fowleri*, found in fresh water, can cause acute fulminant meningitis in immunocompetent hosts, whereas *Acanthamoeba* and *Balamuthia* are associated with a chronic form of meningitis/encephalitis, usually in immunocompromised hosts.
- Some noninfectious etiologies include:
  - Drug intoxication or withdrawal, including anticholinergic agents
  - Malignancies such as lymphoma
  - Subarachnoid hemorrhage

DIAGNOSIS

- Bacterial meningitis typically presents with an acute onset of fever, headache, neck stiffness, and may be associated with photophobia, phonophobia, nausea, and vomiting.
- Absence of headache and jolt accentuation effectively eliminates bacterial meningitis. However, individual items of the clinical history have low accuracy for the diagnosis of meningitis in adults (for headache, 50%, and for nausea/vomiting, 30%).
- 80% of individuals with tuberculosis affecting their CNS will have fever
- *Brucella* can cause chronic granulomatous meningitis, but it is typically associated with fever, constitutional symptoms, and a history of exposure to infected animal tissues or products.

DIAGNOSTIC TESTS & INTERPRETATION
Lab
- CBC, electrolytes, creatinine, liver function tests
- Blood cultures
- Lumbar puncture is important, and may include tests for opening pressure, white blood cell (WBC) count (and differential), red blood cell count, protein, glucose, Gram stain, culture and sensitivity, mycobacterial cultures, fungal culture and stains, cryptococcal antigen, syphilis screening, and PCR for herpes simplex virus or varicella zoster virus. Caution should be taken in individuals with suspected raised intracranial pressure or bleeding disorders.

Imaging
- Blood cultures
- CT or MRI scans of the head are important for ruling out space-occupying lesions.
- In some cases, infectious meningitis presents as leptomeningeal enhancement, and carcinomatous meningitis presents as dural enhancement.

Diagnostic Procedures/Other
Cerebrospinal Fluid
In bacterial meningitis, opening pressures are typically above normal (>200 mm H_2O). WBC counts can be >1000 cells/μL, but may be less if early in the course of infection, and these will be mostly neutrophils. Protein levels are usually >250 mg/dL, and glucose may be low to normal. Viral meningitis typically has lower WBC counts compared to bacterial infections, and more lymphocytes will be seen. Protein levels should be in the 50–250 mg/dL range, and glucose tends to be in the 10–45 mg/dL range.

DIFFERENTIAL DIAGNOSIS
Consider infectious etiologies (bacterial, mycobacterial, viral, protozoal, amoebic) and noninfectious etiologies such as neoplasms, drugs, and metabolic abnormalities.

TREATMENT

- Empiric therapy for bacterial meningitis in adults includes a third- or fourth-generation cephalosporin (such as ceftriaxone or cefepime) plus vancomycin. In patients over the age of 50 or with immunocompromised states, ampicillin should be added to cover *Listeria* infections. Steroids (usually dexamethasone) are also an important empiric treatment that is beneficial in *S. pneumonia* meningitis, and should be continued if this is suspected or cultured.
- Therapy with acyclovir should be instituted if the diagnosis of herpes virus is suspected.
- Treatment with antibiotics should not be delayed by imaging or lumbar puncture studies in suspected cases of meningitis.

ADDITIONAL TREATMENT
Patients should be cared for by a multidisciplinary team, and may require support from physiotherapists, occupational therapists, and speech language pathologists after an acute illness.

ONGOING CARE

FOLLOW-UP RECOMMENDATIONS
Early clinical recognition of meningitis is imperative to allow clinicians to efficiently complete further tests and initiate appropriate therapy.

COMPLICATIONS
- Meningitis
- Death
- Deafness, visual impairment, seizures, stroke, cognitive impairment
- Increased intracranial pressure

ADDITIONAL READING

- Tunkel AR. Approach to the patient with central nervous system infection. In: Mandell GL, Bennett JE, Dolin R (eds.) *Principles and Practice of Infectious Diseases* (Chapter 83). New York: Elsevier, 2010.
- Tunkel AR, Hartman BJ, Kaplan SL, et al. Practice guidelines for the management of bacterial meningitis. *Clin Infect Dis* 2004;39(9):1267–1268.
- Tunkel AR, Glaser CA, Bloch KC, et al. The management of encephalitis: Clinical practice guidelines by the Infectious Diseases Society of America. *Clin Infect Dis* 2008;47(3):303–327.
- van de Beek D, de Gans J, Spanjaard L, et al. Clinical features and prognostic factors in adults with bacterial meningitis. *N Engl J Med* 2004 351(18): 1849–1859.

CODES

ICD9
- 323.9 Unspecified cause of encephalitis, myelitis, and encephalomyelitis
- 780.60 Fever, unspecified
- 781.99 Other symptoms involving nervous and musculoskeletal systems

N

PANCYTOPENIA AND FEVER

Bettina M. Knoll

 BASICS

DESCRIPTION
- Pancytopenia is the deficiency of all formed elements of the blood.
- Anemia is defined by a hemoglobin <13.5 g/dL (male) or <12 g/dL (female).
- Absolute neutropenia is defined by an absolute neutrophil count of $1.5 \times 10^3/\mu L$.
- Thrombocytopenia is defined by a platelet count $<150 \times 10^9/L$.

Approach to the Patient
- Cytopenias in the settings of infections can be due to cytokine/chemokine effects, cytopathic effects, and/or bone marrow infiltration.
- Fever in neutropenic patients is a medical emergency. The first step is to determine whether the patient is suffering from a febrile illness that is associated with cytopenias or whether the fever is caused by a secondary infection during absolute neutropenia in the setting of a hematologic malignancy or chemo-/radiation therapy.
- History should include:
  Complete medication list inclusive of over-the-counter medication, herbal remedies (i.e., leukopenia due to Echinacea).
- Travel, sexual, and work-related exposures, imprisonment, drug use (i.e., agranulocytosis due to levamisole adulterated cocaine).
- Patients should be questioned about the presence of concurrent symptoms (such as weight loss, night sweats, etc.).
- Review of previous complete blood counts results is helpful.
- In evaluating anemia without reticulocytosis, especially in the setting of pancytopenia, one must consider infiltrative diseases of the marrow.
- Patients with cytopenia(s) and fever should undergo blood cultures and serologic evaluation and be considered for an evaluation of the bone marrow that includes histology and cultures for bacteria, parasites, mycobacteria, and fungi.

EPIDEMIOLOGY
- The lower limit of the normal neutrophils count differs among different ethnicities. Yemenite Jews present very low normal neutrophils counts.
- Aplastic anemia prognosis worsens as the age increases.

Bacterial Diseases
- Tuberculosis:
  - Thrombocytopenia, a shift to the left in the neutrophil count, and pancytopenia have been described in patients with tuberculosis. In a study of miliary tuberculosis, thrombocytopenia was recorded in 83% of the patients, leukopenia in 15%, lymphopenia in 87%, and pancytopenia in 5%; in 3 of the 6 patients with pancytopenia, it was reversed by antituberculosis treatment.
- Brucellosis:
  - Anemia is very common in patients with brucellosis, neutropenia presents in up to 30% and pancytopenia in up to 20% of cases.
- Typhoid fever:
  - Associated with leukopenia and increased percentage of band forms in 25–50% of cases and with pancytopenia in <10% of cases.

Viral Diseases
- Hepatitis:
  - 2–5% of patients have aplastic anemia.
- Human immunodeficiency virus:
  - Thrombocytopenia is more common in drug users with HIV (36.9%) than in non-HIV IVDU (8.7%).
  - About 30% of patients with end-stage AIDS present with marrow hypoplasia.

Vector Born
- Rickettsialpox
- 75% of patients have leukopenia.
- Human granulocytic ehrlichiosis.
- 50–90% of patients have lymphopenia or neutropenia.
- Dengue fever
- Thrombocytopenia in dengue fever is characteristic for the disease with up to 55% with platelets below 100,000 cells/mm^3.

ETIOLOGY
- Reactive hemophagocytic syndrome:
  - Benign histiocytic disorder is characterized by hemophagocytosis by stimulated histiocytes in the bone marrow and reticuloendothelial system, resulting in pancytopenia, liver dysfunction, and disseminated coagulopathy.
  - Associated with viral (particularly herpes viruses) or bacterial infection, lymphoma, and other malignancies.

- Human ehrlichiosis should be considered in the differential diagnosis in patients with fever and cytopenia associated with hemophagocytosis. Pancytopenia associated with ehrlichiosis is usually transient; however, it may be severe when it is associated with destruction of normal blood elements.
  - The underlying disease sometimes remains unclear.
- Bone marrow necrosis:
  - Destruction of hematopoietic tissue, including the stroma, with preservation of the bone.
  - Rare condition associated with sickle cell diseases, AIDS, leukemia, lymphoma, metastatic carcinoma, anemia, parvovirus infections, enterovirus infection, sepsis, Kaposi's sarcoma, mucormycosis, disseminated tuberculosis, and other systemic diseases.
- Bone marrow invasion:
  - Associated with leishmaniasis, histoplasmosis, tuberculosis, malignancy, and myelodysplastic syndromes.
  - Kala Azar can present with fever, hepatosplenomegaly, and pancytopenia.
  - In AIDS patients, Mycobacterium tuberculosis, histoplasmosis, and cryptococcosis, can cause massive bone marrow infiltration in the setting of widely disseminated disease; the patients typically have fever, chills, sweats, and lymphadenopathy and/or hepatosplenomegaly.
  - Disseminated Mycobacterium avium complex infection can cause pancytopenia as a result of massive bone marrow infiltration, but unlike other systemic infections, this disorder is often associated with a profound anemia disproportionate to the degree of leukopenia and thrombocytopenia.
- Bone marrow suppression:
  - Of the disseminated viral opportunistic infections, cytomegalovirus (CMV) infection is most commonly associated with bone marrow suppression in patients with AIDS and transplant recipients, but the pancytopenia that results usually does not include a disproportionately pronounced anemia.
  - In transplant recipients, human herpes virus 6 and Epstein-Barr viru (EBV) can cause leukopenia in addition to CMV.
  - Neutropenia can occur during dengue fever, yellow fever, Colorado tick bite fever, phlebotomus fever.

- Hyperreactive malarial splenomegaly syndrome:
  - Malaria can present with mild neutropenia and/or thrombocytopenia. Massive splenomegaly and pancytopenia are characteristic of the hyperreactive malarial splenomegaly syndrome.
- Aplastic anemia:
  - Infectious causes include EBV, hepatitis viruses, and HIV.
- Pure red cell aplasia:
  - The infectious agent most often associated is parvovirus B19.
- Life-threatening thrombocytopenia:
  - Can be seen in acute infectious mononucleosis.

Noninfectious
- Systemic lupus erythematosus:
  - Can present with lymphadenopathy, fever, anemia, and leukopenia.
- Familial erythrophagocytic lymphocytosis:
  - Rare, nonmalignant class II histiocytosis characterized by fever, irritability, hepatosplenomegaly, pancytopenia, and hemophagocytosis.

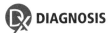 **DIAGNOSIS**

Patients with virus-associated hemophagocytic syndrome have high fever, skin rash, hepatosplenomegaly, pancytopenia, and coagulopathy. Morphologic examination of lymph node and bone marrow demonstrates prominent phagocytosis of erythrocytes and nucleated blood cells.

DIAGNOSTIC TESTS & INTERPRETATION
Diagnostic Procedures/Other
Bone Marrow Biopsy
- Indicated for work-up/diagnosis of:
  - Lymphoma.
  - Infections such as toxoplasmosis, leishmaniasis, and disseminated fungal infections, including those caused by *Histoplasma capsulatum* and *Penicillium mameffei*.
  - HIV-infected patients with pyrexia without localizing signs.
  - Pancytopenia.
- However, bone marrow biopsy is of little diagnostic utility in the investigation of afebrile patients with isolated thrombocytopenia, anemia, or leukopenia.

 TREATMENT

ADDITIONAL TREATMENT
General Measures
- Neutropenic fevers must be treated timely with parenteral, broad-spectrum antibiotics. Empiric antifungal therapy should be added when patients are persistently febrile despite broad spectrum antibiotic therapy.
- For the treatment of aplastic anemia, bone marrow or peripheral blood stem-cell transplantation from a histocompatible sibling usually cures the underlying bone marrow failure. Survival rates have been reported to be as high as 90% from a single experienced institution and 77% for registry data, which reflect the more general experience.
- Treatment of infectious mononucleosis-induced thrombocytopenia with steroids is variably successful. Intravenous immunoglobulin and, in selected cases, splenectomy are also used.
- Aggressive antiretroviral treatment may effectively diminish transfusion requirements among HIV-infected individuals with pure red blood cell aplasia resulting from parvovirus B19 infection.
- Anemia and thrombocytopenia can be corrected by transfusion.

 ONGOING CARE

FOLLOW-UP RECOMMENDATIONS
Limited numbers of blood transfusions probably do not affect the outcome of stem-cell transplantation; to avoid alloimmunization, family donors should not be used.

COMPLICATIONS
The prognosis in aplastic anemia is directly related to the quantitative reduction in peripheral blood cell counts, particularly the neutrophil number. Prior to the introduction of practical blood transfusions, patients died of congestive heart failure caused by anemia or of hemorrhaging due to thrombocytopenia. Historically, mortality figures at 1–2 years were

80–90% in patients who were treated only with blood transfusions and antibiotics. Today, the most serious complication of aplastic anemia is the high risk of infection secondary to the absence of neutrophils; overwhelming bacterial sepsis and, especially, fungal infections are the most frequent causes of death. Patients who satisfy the criteria for severe disease, but who are refractory to treatment, have a <20% chance of long-term survival.

ADDITIONAL READING

- Abdool Gaffar MS, Seedat YK, Coovadia YM, et al. The white cell count in typhoid fever. *Trop Geogr Med* 1992;44:23.
- Hughes WT, Armstrong D, Bodey GP, et al. 2002 guidelines for the use of antimicrobial agents in neutropenic patients with cancer. *CID* 2002;34:730.
- Lichtman MA, Beutler E, Kaushansky K, et al. *Williams Hematology*. 7th ed. McGraw-Hill Medical. New York: 2005.
- Stefos A, Georgiadou SP, Gioti C, et al. Leptospirosis and pancytopenia: Two case reports and review of the literature. *J Infect* 2005;51:e277–280.

 CODES

ICD9
284.1 Pancytopenia

CLINICAL PEARLS

- Bone marrow infiltrative disorders need bone marrow biopsy.
- In difficult diagnostic cases, the sensitivity may be increased from bone marrow biopsy of different sites.

P

PLEURAL EFFUSION AND FEVER

Eleni Patrozou

 BASICS

DESCRIPTION

- A pleural effusion is defined as the presence of fluid in the pleural space, due to increased production or decreased absorption.
- Light's criteria are used to discern transudates and exudates, with a sensitivity of 98% and a specificity of 83%.
- Exudative pleural effusions meet at least one of the following criteria:
  – Pleural fluid protein/serum protein >0.5
  – Pleural fluid lactate dehydrogenase (LDH)/serum LDH >0.6
  – Pleural fluid LDH more than two-thirds normal upper limit for serum
- The term parapneumonic effusion is used when the pleural effusion is secondary to a bacterial process in the thoracic cavity:
  – A patient has a simple (uncomplicated) parapneumonic effusion if the pleural fluid is free-flowing and sterile. A simple parapneumonic effusion usually resolves with antibiotic treatment and does not require drainage.
  – Complicated parapneumonic effusions are usually larger than simple effusions and exhibit low pH, low glucose, and loculation.
  – Empyema is grossly purulent fluid in the pleural space. The most common organism associated with empyema is *Streptococcus pneumoniae*. A patient has a simple empyema if the pleural fluid is frank pus and if the fluid is free-flowing or is in a single loculus. A patient has a complex empyema if the pleural fluid is frank pus and if the fluid is multiloculated.

Approach to the Patient

- When the patient is first evaluated, a thorough history should be obtained. Symptoms associated with pleural effusions depend on the underlying disease process and can include dyspnea, chest pain, lower extremity edema, fever, weight loss, hemoptysis and so on.
- A careful physical exam and a diagnostic thoracentesis should be performed. Initial laboratory studies include measurement of the levels of protein, glucose, amylase, and LDH and pleural fluid cytology. If the patient has an acute febrile illness or if the pleural fluid smells putrid or is turbid, the fluid should be analyzed for cell count, and Gram stain and aerobic and anaerobic cultures should be obtained. Also, consider evaluation of pH, acid-fast bacillus smear, tuberculosis culture, fungal smear, and fungal culture.
- If pleural tuberculosis or malignancy is strongly suspected, needle biopsy of the parietal pleura should follow. Bronchoscopy is also recommended in this case.
- If indicated, the patient should be subjected to thoracoscopy or open pleural biopsy.

EPIDEMIOLOGY

- The incidence of pleural effusion in the US is estimated to be at least 1.5 million cases annually.
- In many parts of the world, the most common cause of exudative pleural effusions is tuberculosis, but this is relatively uncommon in the US.
- In the medical intensive care unit, about 10% of the pleural effusions are parapneumonic.

ETIOLOGY

- Transudative pleural effusions are caused by systemic factors that alter the capillary hydrostatic pressure, the colloid osmotic pressure, or both. Usually fever does not accompany transudative effusions. The most common causes include the following:
  – Congestive heart failure
  – Nephrotic syndrome
  – Cirrhosis (hepatic hydrothorax)
  – Constrictive pericarditis
  – Malignancy (through lymphatic obstruction)
  – Myxedema
  – Pulmonary emboli
  – Peritoneal dialysis
  – Superior vena cava obstruction
  – Urinothorax
- Exudative effusions are a result of local factors, like a change in pleural surface permeability, obstruction of lymphatic drainage of the pleural cavity, and so on. All leading causes of exudative pleural effusions can be accompanied by fever and include the following:
  – Infections (bacterial, fungal, mycobacterial, viral, or parasitic)
  – Malignancies (usually lung carcinoma, mesothelioma, and lung metastases from breast carcinoma, and lymphoma)
  – Pulmonary embolism
  – Collagen-vascular diseases (rheumatoid pleuritis, systemic lupus erythematosus, Wegener's, Churg-Strauss, etc.)
- Other causes of exudative pleural effusions include the following:
  – Gastrointestinal disease (esophageal perforation, pancreatitis, intra-abdominal abscesses, etc.)
  – Asbestos related pleural disease
  – Chylothorax
  – Hemothorax
  – Drug-induced pleural disease (nitrofurantoin, amiodarone, etc.)
  – Electrical burns
  – Iatrogenic injury
  – Meigs' syndrome
  – Pericardial disease
  – Post-lung transplant
  – Post-cardiac injury syndrome
  – Dressler's syndrome
  – Radiation therapy
  – Sarcoidosis
  – Uremia
  – Yellow nail syndrome

- Among hospitalized patients with AIDS, most causes of pleural effusion are noninfectious and include hypoalbuminemia, cardiac failure, atelectasis, Kaposi's sarcoma, uremic pleurisy, and adult respiratory distress syndrome. Most common infectious causes include bacterial pneumonia, *Pneumocystis carinii* pneumonia, Mycobacterium tuberculosis, septic embolism, *Nocardia asteroides*, *Cryptococcus neoformans*, and *Mycobacterium avium-intracellulare*.
- Tuberculous pleurisy usually occurs 3–7 months after infection. The fluid is straw colored and at times hemorrhagic; it is an exudate with a protein concentration >50% of that in serum, a normal to low glucose concentration, a pH that is generally <7.2, and, usually, 500–2,500 WBC/mL. Neutrophils may predominate in the early stage, while mononuclear cells are the typical finding later.
- Vertebral osteomyelitis should be considered in the differential diagnosis of pleural effusion, especially if there is associated back pain.
- Hantavirus pulmonary syndrome often is associated with pleural effusion. The fluid is initially transudative but may take on characteristics of an exudate.
- Consider testing for antibodies to *Toxocara larvae* in patients with eosinophilic pleurisy, particularly when associated with blood eosinophilia.
- Chagas' disease can cause a transudative effusion due to congestive heart failure.

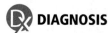 **DIAGNOSIS**

- Patients with aerobic bacterial pneumonia and pleural effusion present with an acute febrile illness consisting of chest pain, sputum production, and leukocytosis. Patients with anaerobic infections commonly present with a subacute illness, associated with weight loss, leukocytosis, mild anemia, and a history of some factor that predisposes them to aspiration.
- Tuberculous pleuritis is associated with primary TB and represents a hypersensitivity reaction to the presence of tuberculous protein in the pleural space. Patients with tuberculous pleuritis present with fever, weight loss, dyspnea, and/or pleuritic chest pain. Pleural pain is absent in about one-fourth of the cases.

DIAGNOSTIC TESTS & INTERPRETATION

Lab

- Neutrophilic predominance in the pleural fluid is characteristic for parapneumonic effusions, pulmonary embolism, and pancreatitis. A predominance of lymphocytes (>50%) is typical for cancer, tuberculous pleurisy, and rheumatologic disease.
- A high pleural fluid eosinophil count is noted in hemothorax, asbestos exposure, parasitic diseases (i.e., paragonimiasis), Churg-Strauss, and pulmonary embolism.
- Pleural fluid glucose concentration levels below 60 mg/dL suggest pleuritis due to bacterial infection, malignancy, or rheumatoid arthritis.
- A low PH (<7.3) can be seen in the following conditions: Empyema, malignancy, collagen vascular disease, tuberculous pleurisy, urinothorax, and esophageal rupture.
- In cases of tuberculous pleurisy, acid-fast stains and cultures of the pleural effusion have a low sensitivity. Pleural biopsy has a higher yield: A specimen from a single, closed pleural biopsy can show granulomas in about 60%, while 3 biopsies can demonstrate granulomas in about 80%. Mycobacterial culture of the biopsy specimen increases the diagnostic yield to about 90%. Thoracoscopic biopsy probably has an even higher sensitivity. The use of polymerase chain reaction has not been found to be clinically useful.
- An ADA level of pleural fluid >70 U/L has significant sensitivity and specificity for the diagnosis of tuberculosis. However, in countries with low prevalence of tuberculosis, the diagnostic yield of ADA is lower.
- Pleural fluid interferon-γ (IFN-γ) levels are increased in patients with tuberculous pleurisy. INF-γ levels >140 pg/mL are highly sensitive (98% sensitivity). INF-γ levels are also increased in emphysemas and rheumatoid pleurisy.
- Elevated pleural effusion amylase is seen in pancreatic disease (pancreatitis or pancreatic pseudocyst), lung adenocarcinoma, and esophageal rupture.
- By Light's criteria, an exudate may be diagnosed in cases of heart or renal failure after diuretic therapy.
- Routine diagnostic bronchoscopy should not be performed for undiagnosed pleuritic effusion.

Imaging

- In tuberculous pleuritis, only about one-third of the cases have parenchymal disease visible radiographically.
- In tuberculosis and other lung processes, computed tomography of the chest can reveal parenchymal disease that is not evident on simple radiographs.

- Parapneumonic pleural effusion >1 cm height on lateral decubitus radiograph is indicative for paracentesis.
- In ICU patients, pleural effusion may manifest as hazy opacities in plain x-ray, due to the gravity effects on lying position.
- Fibrinous pleural septations are better visualized on ultrasound than on CT scans.
- Helical CT is the test of choice in case of suspected pulmonary embolism.
- Recent studies have shown that PET scan may aid to differentiate benign from malignant pleural diseases.

 TREATMENT

ADDITIONAL TREATMENT

General Measures

- Antibiotic therapy alone is adequate for the treatment of a simple (uncomplicated) parapneumonic effusion.
- The appropriate management of patients with complicated parapneumonic pleural effusion is tube thoracostomy (usually relatively small chest tubes inserted percutaneously).
- Streptokinase or urokinase administered through the chest tube can facilitate the drainage of loculated effusions. If drainage is still inadequate, thoracoscopy with the breakdown of adhesions and the optimal positioning of the chest tube or decortication is indicated.
- Patients with a simple empyema should be treated with a relatively large chest tube. If a sizable empyema cavity persists after 7 days of chest tube drainage, consideration should be given to perform more extensive drainage and a decortication.
- Patients with complex empyemas should initially be managed with large chest tubes and intrapleural thrombolytic therapy. However, most patients will require decortication.

ONGOING CARE

FOLLOW-UP RECOMMENDATIONS

In persistently undiagnosed effusions, the possibility of pulmonary embolism and tuberculosis should be reconsidered.

COMPLICATIONS

- Even though the pleural reaction itself abates without treatment, active tuberculosis develops in approximately 65% of patients with tuberculous pleurisy within 5–7 years. Treatment for active tuberculosis, therefore, is mandatory.
- Tuberculous empyema is usually the result of the rupture of a tuberculous cavity and may result in severe pleural fibrosis and restrictive lung disease.

ADDITIONAL READING

- Sahn SA. The value of pleural fluid analysis. *Am J Med Sci* 2008;335(1):7–15.
- Maskell N, Butland RJA. BTS guidelines for the investigation of a unilateral pleural effusion in adults. *Thorax* 2003;58:8–17.
- Porcel J, Light RW. Diagnostic approach to pleural effusion in adults. *Am Fam Physician* 2006;73;1211–1220.
- Gopi A, Madhavan SM, Sharma SK, et al. Diagnosis and treatment of tuberculous pleural effusion in 2006. *Chest* 2007;131(3):880–889.
- Krenke R, Safianowska A, Paplinska M, et al. Pleural fluid adenosine deaminase and interferon gamma as diagnostic tools in tuberculosis pleurisy. *J Physiol Pharmacol* 2008;59(Suppl 6):349–360.

 CODES

ICD9

- 012.00 Tuberculous pleurisy, confirmation unspecified
- 510.9 Empyema without mention of fistula
- 511.9 Unspecified pleural effusion

CLINICAL PEARLS

- Early in the process of a parapneumonic effusion, the effusion may appear transudative.
- HIV transmission has been reported from needles contaminated with pleural fluid.
- In cases of symmetric bilateral effusions, without fever or chest pain, in which congestive heart failure is suspected, diuresis can be performed prior to thoracentesis.
- To increase the sensitivity of pleural fluid cultures, immediate inoculation in blood – culture bottles can be performed.

P

PLEURITIC CHEST PAIN AND FEVER

Eleni Patrozou

 BASICS

DESCRIPTION

Definition
- The term pleuritic chest pain is used to describe pain that is located in the chest, is related to respiratory movements and, is aggravated by cough and/or deep inspiration.
- Because the pleuritic component is not always apparent, chest pain in general is discussed.

Approach to the Patient
- Chest discomfort is one of the most frequent complaints for which patients seek medical attention.
- Failure to recognize a serious disorder, such as ischemic heart disease, may result in the dangerous delay of the much-needed treatment.
- Clinicians should determine whether the syndrome represents new, acute, recurrent, episodic pain; or pain that is persistent, perhaps for days.
- A thorough history and a physical examination are needed to diagnose potentially life-threatening conditions, such as coronary artery disease, aortic dissection, or pulmonary embolism.
- Most infectious causes of chest pain exhibit pleuritic characteristics.
- Diagnostic testing guided by history and physical examination includes the following:
  - Electrocardiogram
  - Computed tomography (CT) of chest
  - Gastrointestinal evaluation
  - Spine, shoulder, or rib radiographs
  - Echocardiogram

EPIDEMIOLOGY
- Chest pain accounts for 5% of emergency department visits.
- Among patients presenting with chest pain, gastroesophageal disease is the most common diagnosis, followed by ischemic heart disease.
- The most common cause of acute mediastinitis is iatrogenic esophageal perforation. The greatest risk for perforation is associated with stricture dilation or sclerotherapy.
- Acute mediastinitis complicates 1.3% of cardiothoracic surgical procedures (from 600–1,200 cases of mediastinitis annually in the US). Reported mortality varies from 20–40%.

- Factors predisposing to development of postsurgical mediastinitis include the following:
  - Duration of the surgical procedure
  - Repeat surgical intervention (within 4 days postoperatively)
  - Previous cardiac surgery
  - Mobilization of one or both internal mammary arteries
  - Diabetes or perioperative hyperglycemia
  - Obesity
  - Vascular disease
  - Tobacco use
  - Prolonged postoperative intensive care
- Acute descending oropharyngeal infections, such as Ludwig's angina give rise to necrotizing mediastinitis, the most aggressive type of acute mediastinitis.
- There are a number of causes of pericarditis, including infection, systemic illness, cardiac disease, trauma, and neoplasm. Iatrogenic causes include surgery, cardiac instrumentation, irradiation, and medications. In a study of 57 patients who underwent surgical treatment because of large pericardial effusions, pericardial fluid and tissue samples were studied cytologically, and cultures for aerobic and anaerobic bacteria, fungi, mycobacteria, mycoplasma, and viruses were done. A diagnosis was made in 53 patients (93%). Malignant disease was the most common finding. 8 patients had an infectious cause, including *Mycoplasma pneumoniae*, cytomegalovirus, herpes simplex virus, *Mycobacterium avium-intracellulare*, and *Mycobacterium chelonae*.

ETIOLOGY
- Infectious causes of chest pain (often with pleuritic characteristics) include viral pleurisy, pleurodynia (Bornholm disease), pneumonia (streptococcal, legionellosis, Chlamydia spp., Mycoplasma spp., *Pneumocystis jirovecii*, tuberculosis, etc.), pulmonary actinomycosis, pneumonic plague, pulmonary histoplasmosis, pulmonary echinococcosis, coccidioidomycosis, infection with the lung fluke Paragonimus, pericarditis, herpes zoster, mediastinitis, biliary disease, and Chagas' disease.
- Noninfectious causes of chest pain include myocardial infarction, angina pectoris, hypertrophic cardiomyopathy, pulmonary embolism, aortic dissection, aortic stenosis, arthritis of the shoulder or spine, cholelithiasis, costochondritis, esophageal reflux, esophageal spasm, malignancy, pancreatitis, peptic ulcer disease, pericarditis, pneumothorax, primary pulmonary hypertension, collagen vascular diseases (including systemic lupus erythematosus, rheumatoid arthritis etc), radiation pneumonitis, familial Mediterranean fever (FMF), and sickle-cell crisis.

- The organisms detected in acute mediastinitis vary with the underlying cause. Mixed infections containing both aerobic and anaerobic organisms are commonly associated with acute mediastinitis resulting from esophageal perforation or spread from oropharyngeal sources. In postoperative mediastinitis the most common microorganisms isolated are *Staphylococcus aureus*, gram-negative bacilli, coagulase-negative Staphylococci, and Streptococci.
- Although most cases of granulomatous or sclerosing mediastinitis have been ascribed to *Histoplasma capsulatum*, other recognized causes include tuberculosis, blastomycosis, actinomycosis, coccidioidomycosis, aspergillosis, and nocardiosis.

DIAGNOSIS
- Patients with aerobic bacterial pneumonia and pleural effusion commonly present with an acute febrile illness consisting of chest pain, sputum production, and leukocytosis. Patients with anaerobic infections usually present with a subacute illness, with weight loss, leukocytosis, mild anemia, and a predisposing history to aspiration.
- Patients with tuberculous pleuritis present with fever, weight loss, dyspnea, and/or pleuritic chest pain. However, pleural pain is absent in about one-fourth of the cases.
- Classically, acute mediastinitis manifests with the sudden onset of fever, chills, and prostration. Patients have severe, usually pleuritic, substernal chest pain, and examination reveals tachycardia, tachypnea, and signs of systemic inflammatory reaction.
- The clinical presentation of pericarditis varies, depending on the cause. Positional pleuritic chest pain radiating to the trapezius muscle and dyspnea are characteristic complaints. Pericardial pain can be aggravated by swallowing, since the esophagus lies just behind the posterior portion of the heart, and is often altered by a change of body position, becoming sharper and more left-sided in the supine position and milder when the patient sits upright, leaning forward.
- Patients with pleurodynia present with an acute onset of fever and muscle spasms of intrapleural or abdominal muscles. Chest pain is more frequent in adults, and abdominal pain is more common in children. Paroxysms of severe, knife-like pain usually last 15–30 min and are associated with diaphoresis and tachypnea. Fever peaks within an hour after the onset of paroxysms and subsides when pain resolves.

- The classic triad of pleuritic chest pain, hemoptysis, and dyspnea occurs in less than 15% of patients with substantiated pulmonary embolism. The most frequent symptoms associated with pulmonary embolism are nonspecific (dyspnea and chest pain); cough, palpitations, syncope, and diaphoresis have also been reported.

DIAGNOSTIC TESTS & INTERPRETATION
Lab
- Electrocardiographic abnormalities, including nonspecific ST-segment and T-wave changes and tachycardia are noted in 70% of patients. Other abnormalities such as right axis deviation, incomplete RBBB, and S1 Q3T3 are infrequent during acute pulmonary embolism.
- Enzyme-linked immunosorbent assay measurement of D-dimers has a reported high sensitivity but is not specific for pulmonary embolism.
- Initial negative troponin test does not exclude acute coronary syndrome.
- BNP level measurement should not be used for the diagnosis of myocardial ischemia.

Imaging
- For the diagnosis of mediastinitis, a Gastrografin swallow study (contrast esophagography) is the modality of choice to reveal the location and extent of extravasation of contrast material when perforation is suspected. A CT scan of the chest may show esophageal wall edema, extraesophageal air, periesophageal fluid with or without gas bubbles, mediastinal widening, and air and fluid in the pleural spaces or in the retroperitoneum.
- The chest radiograph classically demonstrates a widened mediastinum, at times with visible air–fluid levels on the lateral view.
- The chest roentgenographic findings may be normal in 20–30% of patients with pulmonary embolism. Frequently, however, an elevated hemidiaphragm, an infiltrate, or a pleural effusion is detected. Other possible radiologic findings include atelectasis, enlarged pulmonary arteries, or peripheral radiolucency indicative of decreased vascular filling (Westermarck's sign). Hampton's hump is a pyramidal infiltrate peaked toward the hilum, indicating infarction.
- When clinical suspicion exists for pulmonary embolism, helical CT angiography is the test of choice with sensitivity of 90%.

Diagnostic Procedures/Other
- Echocardiography is the most sensitive test for detecting the presence of pericardial effusion.
- Thoracentesis with pleural fluid analysis should be performed in cases of suspected empyema, in conjunction with analysis of pH, protein, lactate dehydrogenase, and glucose, and Gram stain and culture. A bloody effusion would be supportive of the diagnosis of pulmonary embolism.

DIFFERENTIAL DIAGNOSIS
- Fever and pleuritic chest pain after a cardiac operation can be caused by pericardial injury syndrome; the main conditions included under this term are postmyocardial infarction syndrome (Dressler's syndrome), postpericardiotomy syndrome, and traumatic pericarditis
- The radiographic finding of a widened mediastinum in the clinical setting of fever and pleuritic chest pain strongly suggests acute mediastinitis.
- A history of prior upper endoscopy should alert one to the possibility of an esophageal perforation.

 TREATMENT

SURGERY/OTHER PROCEDURES
For patients with acute severe mediastinitis, aggressive open surgical drainage and debridement are necessary to prevent high morbidity and mortality. Percutaneous catheter drainage has been used in less urgent clinical settings, often as a temporizing measure, but open surgical drainage remains the standard of therapy.

ONGOING CARE

FOLLOW-UP RECOMMENDATIONS
- Any form of pericarditis may lead to the development of cardiac tamponade. Malignant effusion is probably the most common single cause.
- Progression of infection during the course of acute mediastinitis can result in mass effect and local tissue injury.
- Initial negative myocardial markers do not exclude acute coronary syndrome. Repeated series of ECG and cardiac markers are necessary to exclude myocardial ischemia.

COMPLICATIONS
- The mortality rate associated with acute mediastinitis from esophageal perforation is 5–30%, even with appropriate treatment.
- Common complications of mediastinitis are a result of the extension of the infectious process into contiguous structures and spaces. Abscess formation and empyema are common complications of acute mediastinitis of any cause. Late complications of acute mediastinitis resulting from esophageal perforation include esophagocutaneous, esophagopleural, and esophagobronchial fistulas.

ADDITIONAL READING
- *Harrison's Principles of internal medicine.* 17th ed. McGraw-Hill.
- Skinner JS, Smeeth L, Kendall JM, et al. NICE guidance. Chest pain of recent onset: Assessment and diagnosis of recent onset chest pain or discomfort of suspected cardiac origin. *Heart* 2010;96:974–978.

CODES

ICD9
- 786.50 Unspecified chest pain
- 786.52 Painful respiration

CLINICAL PEARLS
- While assessing a patient with chest pain, always exclude potentially life-threatening conditions such as acute coronary syndrome, pulmonary embolism, and aortic dissection.
- A patient reporting acute chest pain and fever should be urgently evaluated and if needed transferred to a hospital.

P

POSTOPERATIVE FEVER

Eleni Patrozou

 BASICS

DESCRIPTION

- The term postoperative fever refers to the raised body temperature, usually >38°C (100.4°F), which occurs after an invasive procedure.
- Postoperative fever is categorized based on the timing of the fever as:
  - Immediate:
    - Onset during the operation or within hours afterwards.
  - Acute:
    - Onset within the first week after surgery.
  - Subacute:
    - Onset 1–4 weeks after surgery.
  - Delayed:
    - Onset more than a month after surgery.
- Most cases of postoperative fever are due to the inflammatory stimulus of surgery itself and resolve spontaneously. However, postoperative fevers can also be a manifestation of a serious complication.
- Approach to the patient:
  - The evaluation includes history, physical examination, and appropriate radiologic and laboratory tests, including cultures and Gram stains of body fluids.
  - Fever in the early postoperative period is often noninfectious in origin. However, fever >96 hours postoperative, is likely to represent infection.
  - Keep in mind that the patient might be incubating a community-acquired process prior to the operation.
  - New or persistent fever >4 days after surgery should raise a strong suspicion of persistent pathology or a new complication.
  - It is mandatory to remove the surgical dressing to inspect the wound as well as all previous catheter sites. Also, review other interventions, such as blood transfusions.

EPIDEMIOLOGY

- Drug fever is the most common noninfectious cause of postoperative fever. Antimicrobials and heparin are the drugs most frequently implicated.
- Pneumonia is a common cause of fever after cardiac surgery and may occur in >5% of patients.
- Cardiothoracic surgery with median sternotomy may lead to sternal wound infection in up to 5% of cases. It is detected at a median of 7 postoperative days.
- Aspergillosis after a cardiothoracic procedure shows a mortality of 80%.
- In a study of 284 general surgery patients, fever was used as a predictor of infection and had a sensitivity of 37% and a specificity of 80%.
- Postsurgical mediastinitis has a mortality of up to 47%.
- Bacterial vaginosis might be a risk factor for the development of postoperative infections in obstetrics and gynecology.

GENERAL PREVENTION

Patient should have aggressive pulmonary toilet, including incentive spirometry to reduce the likelihood or extent of atelectasis.

ETIOLOGY

- Urinary or respiratory tract infection is common postoperatively. Other causes include sinusitis, suppurative phlebitis, catheter-related infections, and Clostridium difficile-associated diarrhea. Also, consider noninfectious causes such as deep venous thrombosis, pulmonary embolism, subarachnoid hemorrhage, gout, and fat emboli.
- Surgical site infections are rare in the first 1–3 days after surgery, except for group A streptococcal infections and clostridial infections, which can develop immediately after surgery.
- Postoperative fevers are commonly attributed to atelectasis. Both atelectasis and fever occur frequently after surgery, but their concurrence is probably coincidental rather than causal.

- Other potentially serious causes of postoperative fever include and transplant rejection.
- Among drug categories, fever is most often attributed to antimicrobials (especially beta-lactam drugs) or other drugs such as antiepileptics or heparin.
- Adult respiratory distress syndrome (ARDS) and other inflammatory processes (such as acute myocardial infarction or acute or chronic pancreatitis) could be associated with fever in the absence of infection.
- Endocrine emergencies such as acute adrenal insufficiency and hyperthyroidism can also be associated with fever.

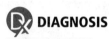 **DIAGNOSIS**

PHYSICAL EXAM

- There is nothing characteristic about the fevers induced by drugs. Fevers do not invariably occur immediately after drug administration and it usually starts days after administration. Eosinophilia and rash are uncommon.
- Malignant hyperthermia is more often identified in the operating room, but onset can be delayed for as long as 24 hours. It can be caused by succinylcholine or halothane and other anesthetics.
- The neuroleptic malignant syndrome is often associated with antipsychotic neuroleptic medications. Haloperidol is the most frequent drug.
- Withdrawal of alcohol, opiates, barbiturates, and benzodiazepines have all been associated with this febrile syndrome. A history of use of these drugs may not be available when the patient is admitted. Withdrawal and related fever may therefore occur several hours or days after admission.

DIAGNOSTIC TESTS & INTERPRETATION
Lab
- Urinalysis and culture should be performed especially among patients with indwelling bladder catheters for >72 hours.
- The role of procalcitonin in defining the bacterial cause of postoperative fever seems to be uncertain.

Imaging
- Clinicians should consider investigating (usually by duplex ultrasonography with color Doppler flow studies) any new swelling of an extremity.
- A chest radiograph is not mandatory during the initial 72 hours postoperatively if fever is the only indication.

Diagnostic Procedures/Other
- Swabbing the wound for culture is rarely helpful unless there is a clear clinical diagnosis of infection.
- Deep abdominal abscesses require surgical exploration if needle aspiration and imaging studies are inconclusive.

TREATMENT
MEDICATION
- Antibiotics are not routinely indicated for most patients with fever in the early postoperative period.
- Patients who require intensive care after a major surgery and patients with hemodynamic instability should be treated with empiric broad-spectrum antibiotics after careful clinical assessment.
- However the empiric antibiotic regimen should be stopped after 48 hours if no source of infection has been identified.
- Treatments for atelectasis include cough and deep breathing, incentive spirometry, percussion and postural drainage, beta-2 agonists, intermittent positive-pressure breathing, and ultrasonic nebulizers.
- Antifungal treatment should not be considered as initial empirical treatment.

ONGOING CARE
FOLLOW-UP RECOMMENDATIONS
- The diagnosis of drug-induced fever is usually established by exclusion and when alternatives are not available.
- Surgical wounds should be examined for infection.

COMPLICATIONS
Infections during the postoperative period can increase morbidity and mortality, lead to sepsis, affect the healing of the surgical wounds, lead to respiratory failure, and so on.

ADDITIONAL READING
- O'Grady NP, Barie PS, Bartlett JG, et al. Guidelines for the evaluation of new fever in critically ill adult patients: 2008 update from the American College of Critical Care Medicine and Infectious Diseases Society of America. *Crit Care Med* 2008;36(4): 1330–1349.
- Lynch BA, Dolan JP, Mann M, et al. Thyrotoxicosis after gastric bypass surgery prompting operative re-exploration. *Obes Surg* 2005;15:883.
- Barone J. Fever: Fact and fiction. *J Trauma* 2009;67: 406–409.

CODES
ICD9
- 780.62 Postprocedural fever
- 998.59 Other postoperative infection

CLINICAL PEARLS
- The presence of fever within 24 hours of patient discharge does not affect the rate of readmission in 30 days.

RASH AND FEVER

Eleni Patrozou

 BASICS

DESCRIPTION
- The term rash describes temporary skin eruptions that accompany localized or generalized infectious diseases.
- Skin manifestations of infectious diseases are discussed throughout this book. In this chapter, the focus is on the differential diagnosis and early recognition of life-threatening, generalized skin eruptions.

Approach to the Patient
- A thorough history should elicit the following information:
  - Immune status
  - Complete medication list
  - Travel history
  - Immunization status
  - Exposure to domestic pets and other animals
  - History of animal or arthropod bites
  - Existence of cardiac abnormalities
  - Presence of prosthetic material
  - Recent exposure to ill individuals
  - Exposure to sexually transmitted diseases
- The thorough history should also include the site of onset of the rash, whether it is pruritic or painful, and its direction and rate of spread.
- A history of associated symptoms (presence of a prodrome, fever, pruritus) should be elicited.
- A careful physical examination determines the type of lesions that make up the eruption (macules, papules, vesicles, plaques, nodules, etc.), including their configuration (i.e., annular or target), the arrangement of their lesions, and their distribution (i.e., central or peripheral).

EPIDEMIOLOGY
- Infectious mononucleosis patients can present with a generalized maculopapular, petechial, or urticarial rash in 10%. The rash most commonly appears after the administration of antibiotics.
- About 20% of erythema infectiosum patients are adults. However, the rash in adults is less characteristic and may be confused with rubella.
- Up to 50% of patients with primary HIV infection will present with a maculopapular rash. The eruption typically occurs 48–72 hours after the onset of fever and can persist for 5–8 days. The upper thorax, collar region, and face are most commonly involved.
- In 2005, CDC declared that rubella has been eliminated from the US.
- Up to 1.5 million cases of cutaneous leishmaniasis occur annually.
- A rash is present in 50% of travelers with dengue fever.
- During the first stage of Lyme disease, a characteristic skin rash, erythema migrans, develops at the site of the tick bite in 80% of the cases.

GENERAL PREVENTION
- Ensure that every woman of reproductive age is immunized against rubella.
- Pregnant women diagnosed with rubella in early pregnancy (before the 16th week of gestation) should be offered termination.

ETIOLOGY
The most common skin eruptions among adults include the following:
- Centrally distributed maculopapular eruptions
  - Adult-onset Still's disease
  - Allergic(drug)-induced eruptions
  - Dengue
  - Ehrlichiosis
  - Endemic (murine) typhus
  - Epidemic typhus
  - Erythema marginatum (rheumatic fever)
  - Infectious mononucleosis
  - Leptospirosis
  - Lyme disease
  - Primary HIV infection
  - Relapsing fever
  - Rubella (German measles)
  - Rubeola (measles)
  - Systemic lupus erythematosus
  - Typhoid fever
- Peripheral eruptions
  - Bacterial endocarditis
  - Chronic meningococcemia
  - Disseminated gonococcal infection
  - Erythema multiforme
  - Rocky Mountain spotted fever (RMSF)
  - Secondary syphilis
- Confluent desquamative erythemas
  - Graft-versus-host disease
  - Kawasaki disease
  - Scarlet fever
  - Staphylococcal and streptococcal toxic shock syndrome
- Vesiculobullous eruptions
  - Disseminated *Vibrio vulnificus* infection
  - Ecthyma gangrenosum
  - Rickettsial pox
- Urticarial vasculitis
- Nodular eruptions
  - Disseminated infections due to fungi and mycobacteria
  - Erythema nodosum
  - Sweet's syndrome
- Purpuric eruptions
  - Acute and chronic meningococcemia
  - Disseminated gonococcal infection
  - Enteroviral petechial rash
  - RMSF
  - Thrombotic thrombocytopenic purpura

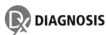 **DIAGNOSIS**

- Rash is the hallmark of RMSF and appears on day 4 (range, 1–15 days) of the illness. Initially, the rash consists of small pink or red macules that blanch with pressure. Over time, the rash evolves into purpura and necrotic areas may develop. Involvement of the scrotum or vulva is a diagnostic clue. Rash may be absent in about 10% of cases and "spotless fever" has a poor prognosis.
- Acute meningococcemia and meningococcal meningitis are caused by Neisseria meningitidis. Classically, the rash appears as a petechial eruption that evolves into the pathognomonic palpable purpura. Urticarial, macular, and papular lesions also may occur. Skin lesions are less common in adults with meningococcal disease.
- Waterhouse-Friderichsen syndrome is fulminant meningococcemia (with disseminated intravascular coagulation).
- Skin lesions are often a clue to the underlying diagnosis of bacterial endocarditis. Peripheral cutaneous or mucocutaneous lesions that can be associated with bacterial endocarditis are divided into vascular phenomena: Petechiae, splinter hemorrhages, Janeway lesions, and immunologic phenomena: Osler's nodes and Roth spots.
- Janeway lesions, Osler's nodes, and Roth spots are more specific for infective endocarditis but less common.
- Lyme disease has been divided into 3 distinct stages: Stage 1, a characteristic macular skin rash, erythema migrans, develops at the site of the tick bite, which resolves spontaneously within 4 weeks; stage 2, neurologic, ocular, or cardiac involvement; and stage 3, arthritis, Lyme encephalopathy, acrodermatitis chronica atrophicans.
- Headache and high fever are prominent in human ehrlichiosis. Rash is not always present and is variable. When it is present, it is usually described as petechial, macular, or erythematous.
- The cutaneous signs of staphylococcal toxic shock syndrome include a sunburn-like diffuse macular erythroderma. The lesions are followed by desquamation, within 5–14 days. Conjunctival injection, mucosal hyperemia, and a strawberry tongue are additional diagnostic signs.

- Streptococcal toxic shock syndrome is discussed on separate chapter, occurs most commonly in the setting of invasive soft-tissue infections, but association with other streptococcal infections (usually of the respiratory track) is less common. Among patients with dengue, rash is usually maculopapular and appears on the second to fifth day of the disease.

DIAGNOSTIC TESTS & INTERPRETATION
Lab
- Gram stain and culture should be performed in infectious material from pustules and bullous lesions.
- Antibodies to *Rickettsia rickettsii* (RMSF) can be detected after the first week of illness.
- Diagnosis of meningococcal disease is made by Gram stain and culture of the blood and cerebrospinal fluid. Microbiologic analysis of biopsied skin lesions may be helpful.
- In contrast to staphylococcal toxic shock syndrome, more than 60% of patients with streptococcal toxic shock syndrome have bacteremia.

Diagnostic Procedures/Other
Skin biopsy from specific lesions and tissue process with culture and histopathologic evaluation may lead to the diagnosis.

DIFFERENTIAL DIAGNOSIS
- Desquamating erythroderma may be present in streptococcal toxic shock syndrome but is less common than in staphylococcal toxic shock syndrome.
- Gonococcemia is frequently associated with a pustular rash, often with a hemorrhagic component. However, other types of lesions such as macules, petechiae, and papules, can also be found.

 TREATMENT

Please see respective chapters for details on the treatment of other causes of skin eruptions caused by infectious causes.

 ONGOING CARE

FOLLOW-UP RECOMMENDATIONS
With the permission of the patient, the physician may follow the progress of the skin eruption with the use of a camera or with ink demarcation.

COMPLICATIONS
The mortality rate of untreated RMSF may be as high as 25–50%.

REFERENCES
1. Levin S, Goodman LJ. An approach to acute fever and rash (AFR) in the adult. *Curr Clin Top Infect Dis* 1995;15:19 [PMID: 7546368].
2. Weber DJ, et al. The acutely ill patient with fever and rash. In: GL Mandell et al, eds. *Principles and practice of infectious diseases,* vol 1, 7th ed, Philadelphia: Elsevier Churchill Livingstone, 2010:791–807.
3. Freedman DO, Weld LH, Kozarsky PE, et al. Spectrum of disease and relation to place of exposure among ill returned travelers. *N Engl J Med* 2006;354:119.
4. Speil C, Mushtaq A, Adamski A, Khardori N. Fever of unknown origin in the returning traveler. *Infect Dis Clin North Am* 2007;21:1091.

ADDITIONAL READING
- Abramson J, Digumarthy S, Ferry JA. A 56-year old woman with fever, rash, and lymphadenopathy. *N Engl J Med* 2009;361:900–911.
- Stevens D, Stevens DL, Bisno AL, Chambers HF. Practice guidelines for the diagnosis and management of skin and soft-tissue infections. *Clin Infect Dis* 2005;41:1373.
- Elaine T. Kaye, Kenneth M. Kaye. Fever and rash. In: *Harrison's principles of internal medicine,* 17th ed, McGraw Hill, 2008.

 CODES

ICD9
- 780.60 Fever, unspecified
- 782.1 Rash and other nonspecific skin eruptions

CLINICAL PEARLS
- Up to 90% of HIV positive patients will develop a dermatologic manifestation in their lifetime.
- Noninfectious processes such as deep venous thrombosis, drug reactions, gouty arthritis, cutaneous lupus erythematosus, graft-versus-host reaction, and generalized pustular psoriasis (von Zumbusch psoriasis) can also cause skin eruptions associated with fevers.

R

RED EYE

Theodoros Filippopoulos

 BASICS

DESCRIPTION

- Serious sight threatening conditions such as uveitis, endophthalmitis, acute angle closure glaucoma, or scleritis can present with redness of the eye (ciliary injection, see: Pathophysiology). In other instances, redness of the eye is secondary to conjunctival hyperemia (see: Pathophysiology) and indicates conjunctivitis, keratitis, dry eye disease, or ocular irritation as the result of a foreign body (including contact lenses), inflammation of the eyelids (blepharitis), or environmental irritants. Finally, ocular trauma can cause localized bleeding under the conjunctiva termed *subconjunctival hemorrhage*. The above entities are not always infectious in nature.
- *Uveitis* refers to inflammation involving the eye; it can be anterior (*iritis* or *iridocyclitis*) or posterior (*posterior uveitis*) or involve both the anterior and posterior segments of the eye (*panuveitis*) (refer to Section II in chapter "Chorioretinitis-Uveitis").
- *Endophthalmitis* is an infectious process involving the ocular (vitreous) cavity (refer to Section II chapter "Endophthalmitis").
- In *acute angle closure glaucoma*, an ophthalmic emergency, the iris assumes a convex configuration and obstructs the ocular outflow pathway (trabecular meshwork), causing an elevation of the intraocular pressure.
- Inflammatory processes of the sclera can be limited to a thin superficial layer of connective tissue between the conjunctiva and sclera (*episcleritis*), or can result in a deeper, more severe inflammatory process (*scleritis*). These may occur alone or in conjunction with keratitis and/or uveitis.
- *Conjunctivitis* is the most common cause of a red eye and is usually accompanied by discharge. *Keratitis* refers to an inflammatory process involving primarily the cornea. Refer to Section II, chapters "Conjunctivitis" and "Keratitis" for details on these conditions.

EPIDEMIOLOGY

Incidence
- The incidence of primary acute angle closure is 9.48 per 100,000 person/years in Asians and 4.14 per 100,000 person/years in Caucasians.
- Please refer to the relevant chapters regarding the incidence of keratitis, conjunctivitis, and uveitis (Section II chapters "Keratitis", "Conjunctivitis", & "Chorioretinitis-Uveitis").

RISK FACTORS

- Risk factors for angle closure include older age, cataract, hyperopia, female gender, a previous episode of acute angle closure glaucoma in the fellow eye, and Asian race. Therefore, fellow eyes of patients with acute angle closure are prophylactically treated with a laser iridotomy to prevent second eye involvement.
- Contact lens use is an established risk factor for the development of bacterial keratitis.
- Subconjunctival hemorrhages occur spontaneously or due to an underlying bleeding disorder, minor blunt trauma, or a sudden increase in intra-abdominal/thoracic pressure (resulting in increased episcleral venous pressure) as in coughing or sneezing.
- Autoimmune connective tissue disorders are associated with ocular inflammation and in some instances uveitis is the first manifestation of such diseases.

GENERAL PREVENTION

- Contact lens use is associated with a wide range of ocular findings ranging from hyperemia, dry eye disease, and allergic reactions to infections such as bacterial keratitis.
- Acute angle-closure glaucoma is preventable with appropriate screening tests (gonioscopy) and preventive measures (laser iridotomy) in individuals at risk.

PATHOPHYSIOLOGY

- Diagnosis in cases of red eyes may be aided by the differentiation between ciliary and conjunctival injection. Ciliary injection involves branches of the anterior ciliary arteries, is located in deeper layers (as in scleritis) and indicates inflammation of the cornea, iris, ciliary body, or sclera. Conjunctival injection is synonymous to hyperemia, is more superficially located, the hyperemic blood vessels are mobile with the conjunctiva, and it improves with topical vasoconstrictors as in episcleritis.
- Pupillary block is the mechanism involved in most cases of acute angle-closure glaucoma. In predisposed eyes the flow of aqueous from the ciliary body through the pupil toward the angle and Schlemm's canal is impeded, which results in a pressure differential between the posterior chamber (posterior to the iris) and the anterior chamber. This pressure differential leads to forward bowing of the iris that in turn obstructs outflow through the trabecular meshwork into Schlemm's canal.

ETIOLOGY

- Please refer to the relevant chapters regarding the etiology of infectious conjunctivitis, keratitis, and chorioretinitis-uveitis.
- Additionally, refer to Section II, chapter "Endophthalmitis", for the etiology of exogenous and endogenous endophthalmitis.
- Acute angle-closure glaucoma and subconjunctival hemorrhage are never infectious in nature.
- Episcleritis is most commonly idiopathic. Rare infectious causes that do not represent pathogen invasion but more of an immunologic reaction include: Herpes simplex virus (HSV) and Varicella zoster virus (Herpes zoster ophthalmicus).
- Scleritis is rarely infectious in nature. If so it can be the result of an immunologic reaction to a systemic infection or represent extension of the infectious process in cases of primarily corneal involvement (keratitis). Infectious causes of scleritis include:
  - *Aspergillus* spp.
  - *Fusarium* spp.
  - Herpes simplex virus (HSV)
  - Leprosy
  - Lyme disease
  - *Nocardia* spp.
  - *Proteus* spp. (associated with retinal detachment surgery [scleral buckle])
  - *Pseudomonas* spp.
  - Syphilis
  - Tuberculosis
  - Varicella Zoster Virus (Herpes Zoster Ophthalmicus)

COMMONLY ASSOCIATED CONDITIONS

- An intraocular surgical procedure is most commonly associated with endophthalmitis.
- Contact lens use should raise a high suspicion for bacterial keratitis.

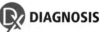 **DIAGNOSIS**

HISTORY

- A subconjunctival hemorrhage is unilateral, asymptomatic, and does not affect the vision.
- In conjunctivitis that can be unilateral but is more commonly bilateral, redness is accompanied by discharge that ranges from watery to mucopurulent and the vision is minimally or not affected at all.
- Keratitis, most commonly unilateral, is associated with conjunctival hyperemia or ciliary injection, foreign body sensation, tearing, and decreased vision due affected corneal clarity.
- In uveitis (unilateral or bilateral), patients may complain about loss of vision, light sensitivity, and periorbital pain.

RED EYE

- Acute angle-closure glaucoma is usually unilateral and presents with pain, decreased vision, and nausea or vomiting.
- In anterior scleritis, patients complain of severe ocular tenderness and pain. With posterior scleritis, the pain and redness may be less pronounced but the vision can be more significantly affected.
- Episcleritis resembles conjunctivitis, is associated with mild pain, and the discharge is absent.
- Endophthalmitis presents with pain and loss of vision.

PHYSICAL EXAM
- Differentiation of the above entities usually requires a slit lamp examination.
- In subconjunctival hemorrhages, a nonmobile fleck of bright red blood can be observed under the conjunctiva.
- In conjunctivitis hyperemia along with discharge, membranes and/or pseudomembranes, a follicular or papillary reaction and preauricular lymphadenopathy can be present.
- In keratitis, disruption of the corneal epithelium along with corneal stromal opacities, discharge and anterior chamber reaction are most commonly encountered.
- The diagnosis of anterior uveitis requires identification of inflammatory cells floating in the aqueous humor or on the corneal endothelium (keratic precipitates). Ciliary injection is usually present.
- A mid-dilated minimally reactive pupil, a cloudy cornea (due to corneal edema), and increased intraocular pressure are characteristic of acute angle closure glaucoma.

DIAGNOSTIC TESTS & INTERPRETATION
Lab
Initial lab tests
- Cultures are not necessary for the diagnosis of conjunctivitis except for the cases of hyperacute conjunctivitis in which Gram stains demonstrate gram-negative diplococci suggestive of *Neisseria gonorrhoeae*.
- Lesions associated with keratitis are routinely sampled and submitted for Gram stains and cultures.

Imaging
Initial approach
- Confocal microscopy is used to confirm the clinical suspicion of *Acanthamoeba keratitis*.
- Neuroimaging modalities are used to diagnose vascular lesions such as carotid-cavernous fistulas or dural-cavernous fistulas (resulting in pulsatile exophthalmos and torturous episcleral and conjunctival blood vessels), arteriovenous malformations, and orbital varices accounting for red eyes.

Diagnostic Procedures/Other
- In cases of keratitis that do not respond to broad spectrum antibiotics, a corneal biopsy can aid in the diagnosis.
- Vitreous samples obtained during pars plana vitrectomy submitted for cytology, cultures, and PCR can aid in the diagnosis of uveitis.

DIFFERENTIAL DIAGNOSIS
Key features for the evaluation of patients with red eye include the following:
- Visual acuity
  - Conjunctivitis: Near normal
  - Subconjunctival hemorrhage: Normal
  - Uveitis: Reduced
  - Keratitis: Reduced
  - Acute angle-closure glaucoma: Reduced
- Discharge
  - Conjunctivitis: Present
  - Subconjunctival hemorrhage: Absent
  - Uveitis: Absent
  - Keratitis: Present
  - Acute angle-closure glaucoma: Absent
- Pain
  - Conjunctivitis: Absent
  - Subconjunctival hemorrhage: Absent
  - Uveitis: Present
  - Keratitis: Present
  - Acute angle-closure glaucoma: Present
- Light sensitivity (photophobia)
  - Conjunctivitis: Absent
  - Subconjunctival hemorrhage: Absent
  - Uveitis: Present
  - Keratitis: Absent/present
  - Acute angle-closure glaucoma: Absent
- Ocular pruritus is suggestive of allergic/atopic/vernal conjunctivitis.

 ## TREATMENT
MEDICATION
First Line
- Viral conjunctivitis requires supportive care with artificial tears and cold compresses and rarely topical steroids (loteprednol 0.5% q.i.d.).
- Mild cases of bacterial conjunctivitis are treated with broad-spectrum topical antibiotics, such as trimethoprim-polymixin B (q.i.d.) or a topical fluoroquinolone (q.i.d.) for 5–7 days (refer to Section II chapter "Conjunctivitis").
- In bacterial keratitis, fortified topical antibiotic eyedrops should be used every 1 hour, such as tobramycin or gentamicin (15 mg/mL) alternating with cefazolin (50 mg/mL) or vancomycin (25 mg/mL) (refer to Section II chapter "Keratitis").
- In acute bacterial endophthalmitis, intravitreal administration of vancomycin (1.0 mg/0.1 mL) for gram-positive coverage and ceftazidime (2.25 mg/0.1 mL) or amikacin (0.4 mg/0.1 mL) in cases of β-lactam hypersensitivity for gram-negative coverage is the recommended treatment (refer to Section II chapter "Endophthalmitis").
- Treatment of anterior uveitis with topical steroids (prednisolone acetate 1%) aims at reducing inflammation. Cycloplegia (cyclopentolate 1% b.i.d.) reduces pain and photophobia and prevents the formation of synechiae. Etiologic treatment is necessary in cases of infectious uveitis (refer to Section II chapter "Chorioretinitis-Uveitis").

- Acute angle-closure glaucoma is treated with acetazolamide (250 mg PO or IV or 500 mg PO, if slow releasing capsules are used) and with mannitol (0.5–2 mg/kg IV administered over 40 min.) to achieve reduction of the intraocular pressure and resolution of the corneal edema. Topical beta blockers (i.e., timolol 0.5%), and weak pilocarpine (1–2%) can be given as well. Eventually, a laser iridotomy is required to relieve the pupillary block.
- Episcleritis is managed with artificial tears, topical steroids such as fluorometholone (0.1% q.i.d.) or loteprednol (0.5% q.i.d.) and oral NSAIDs (i.e., ibuprofen 200–600 mg PO t.i.d.–q.i.d.). Scleritis may require systemic oral prednisone at a dose of 1–1.5 mg/kg per day for 1 week, followed by a slow taper. Immune modulating therapy is also used in cases of scleritis (i.e., methotrexate, cyclophosphamide, cyclosporine, or azathioprine) depending on the systemic association.

ADDITIONAL TREATMENT
SURGERY/OTHER PROCEDURES
- Acute angle-closure requires a laser iridotomy immediately after medical management.
- Infectious scleritis/keratitis can cause melting of the sclera or cornea, requiring a tectonic graft.

 ## ONGOING CARE
PROGNOSIS
- Prognosis depends on etiology and can range from excellent as in subconjunctival hemorrhage to guarded in endophthalmitis.

COMPLICATIONS
- Long standing ocular inflammation leads to cataract formation, to secondary glaucoma, or cystoid macular edema.

ADDITIONAL READING
- Horton JC. Disorders of the eye. In: Fauci A, Braunwald E, Isselbacher K, et al., eds. *Harrison's principles of internal medicine*, 14th ed. New York: McGraw-Hill, 1998:159–172.
- O'Brien TR, Green WR. Conjunctivitis. In: Mandell GL, Bennett JE, Dolin R, eds. *Principles and practice of infectious diseases*, 4th ed. New York: Churchill Livingstone, 1995:1103–1110.
- Cronau H, Kankanala RR, Mauger T. Diagnosis and management of red eye in primary care. *Am Fam Physician*. 2010;81:137–144
- Drancourt M. Management of red eye. In: Cohen J, Powderly WG, Opal SM, eds. *Infectious diseases*, 3rd ed. Philadelphia: Mosby Elsevier, 2010: 204–205.

 ## CODES

ICD9
379.93 Redness or discharge of eye

CLINICAL PEARLS
- Diagnosis of acute angle-closure is frequently delayed as it presents with headache, decreased vision, and nausea and vomiting misleading clinicians toward a neurosurgical emergency.

R

SEPSIS

Luisa M. Stamm

 BASICS

DESCRIPTION

- Bacteremia is the presence of viable bacteria in the blood. Fungemia is the presence of viable fungi in the blood.
- Septicemia is a systemic illness caused by the spread of microbes and their toxins by the bloodstream as a result of bacteremia or fungemia.
- Systemic inflammatory response syndrome (SIRS) is characterized by at least 2 of the following:
  - Oral temperature of >38°C or <35°C.
  - Respiratory rate of >20 breaths/min or $PaCO_2$ of <32 mm Hg.
  - Heart rate of >90 beats/min.
  - Leukocyte count of >12,000/L or <4,000/L or >10% bands.
- Sepsis is SIRS that has a proven or suspected microbial etiology.
- Severe sepsis is sepsis with at least one sign of organ dysfunction, such as metabolic acidosis, alteration in mental status, oliguria, abnormal liver function tests, or adult respiratory distress syndrome.
- Septic shock is severe sepsis with hypotension (i.e., systolic blood pressure <90 mm Hg, or reduction of >40 mm Hg if patient has baseline hypertension) that is unresponsive to fluid resuscitation and requires pressor support.

EPIDEMIOLOGY
Incidence
- Approximately two-thirds of cases occur in patients hospitalized for other illnesses.
- Each year, sepsis develops in more than 650,000 patients in the US, with a mortality rate of 20–50%.

Prevalence
Sepsis presents in 2% of hospitalized patients and up to 75% of ICU patients.

RISK FACTORS
- Factors that predispose to bacteremia, fungemia, and sepsis include very young or advanced age, AIDS, burns, cirrhosis of the liver, hematologic malignancies and neoplasms, high dose glucocorticoids or other immunosuppressive agents, neutropenia, injection drug use, mechanical ventilation,, and presence of indwelling catheters.
- Fungemia occurs most often in immunosuppressed patients with neutropenia.

Genetics
A clear genetic basis for sepsis has not yet been identified. The patients affected are very diverse, but some studies have linked polymorphisms in cytokine genes with hyper- and hypo-inflammatory responses to infection.

GENERAL PREVENTION
- Sepsis can be prevented by earliest removal of indwelling catheters, including central venous lines.
- In pediatrics, sepsis can be prevented by following the recommended vaccination schedule.

PATHOPHYSIOLOGY
- Sepsis is a complicated pathophysiologic entity of inflammation generated by the host in response to bacterial or fungal infection.
- The process is best described for infection with gram-negative bacteria where conserved bacterial components, such as lipopolysaccharide, are sensed by receptors of innate immune, such as toll-like receptor 4, leading to a signaling cascade and eventual release of cytokines.
- Cytokines are host-produced, pleomorphic immunoregulatory peptides. The most widely understood cytokines are tumor necrosis factor-α and interleukin-1β. These pro-inflammatory cytokines cause increased capillary permeability, migration and activation of neutrophils, release of proteases and arachidonate metabolites, and coagulopathy.
- Interleukin-6 and interleukin-10, which are anti-inflammatory cytokines, inhibit the generation of tumor necrosis factor-α, augment the action of acute-phase reactants and immunoglobulins, and inhibit T-lymphocyte and macrophage function.
- In addition, sepsis results in a decrease in anticoagulant factors, such as proteins C and S and anti-thrombin III, leading to disseminated intravascular coagulation.

ETIOLOGY
- In sepsis, the lung is the most common site of infection, followed by the abdomen and the urinary tract.
- Blood cultures yield bacteria or fungi in approximately 20–40% of cases of severe sepsis and in 40–70% of cases of septic shock.

COMMONLY ASSOCIATED CONDITIONS
See Risk Factors

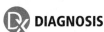 **DIAGNOSIS**

HISTORY
- Patients may report symptoms consistent with antecedent infections such as pneumonia, intra-abdominal infection, or urinary tract infection.
- Patients may develop sepsis post-surgically or following trauma.
- Catheters in place at presentation increase the possibility that they are a source of infection.
- Gastrointestinal manifestations such as nausea, vomiting, and diarrhea can be present.
- Confusion may be an early sign, particularly in the elderly.

PHYSICAL EXAM
- While most septic patients have fever, some have a normal temperature or are hypothermic. Inability to mount a fever has been correlated with a poorer outcome.
- Tachypnea, tachycardia, and altered mental status are common signs.
- The exam may lead to the underlying infection. For example, decreased breath sounds are suggestive of pneumonia, abdominal tenderness of abscess, skin rash of cellulitis or necrotizing fasciitis.

- Skin may appear mottled and digits may have poor capillary refill due to hypoperfusion. Early in sepsis, the skin may be warm but later is most often cool due to vasoconstriction.
- Hypotension and disseminated intravascular coagulopathy predispose to cyanosis and ischemic necrosis of peripheral digits.
- Jaundice may be present as a result of elevated levels of serum bilirubin.

DIAGNOSTIC TESTS & INTERPRETATION
Lab
Initial lab tests
- An initial lab evaluation should include complete blood count with differential cell count. Leukocytosis is most common, but leukopenia is possible. There is often a left shift (with or without toxic granulations) and the percent of band forms is often elevated. Thrombocytopenia may be present.
- A complete chemistry panel, including liver function tests, and a lactate level should be analyzed. Chemistries may indicate renal failure, or shock liver. Patients with sepsis often develop a metabolic acidosis with an anion gap and elevated lactate. An arterial blood gas can help determine the exact cause of metabolic derangement.
- There may be evidence of disseminated intravascular coagulation upon testing of D-dimer, fibrinogen, and prothrombin time.
- At least 2 sets of blood cultures (20–30 mL each) should be obtained as definitive diagnosis requires isolation of a microorganism from the blood. Blood cultures should be drawn through intact, noninfected skin cleaned by 2% chlorhexidine and 1–2% tincture of iodine.
- Urine analysis and urine culture will diagnose urosepsis. Sputum culture, if the patient is able to produce it, and additional cultures from purulent wounds, should also be obtained.

Follow-Up & Special Considerations
Patient thought to have sepsis are critically ill and should be carefully monitored in an ICU setting. Lab tests should be rechecked often to monitor trends and response to therapy.

Imaging
- CT is useful in identifying sources of infection in the chest, abdomen, and sinuses.
- Ultrasound is helpful in evaluating the gallbladder and biliary system for cholecystitis.

Diagnostic Procedures/Other
- Depending on the scenario, many physicians would perform echocardiography to further evaluate for cardiogenic causes of hypotension.
- Urine output should be measured closely to follow renal function.

Pathological Findings
- At death, patients are often found to have necrosis in the liver, brain, and heart.
- Studies at autopsy show global depletion of cells of the adaptive immune system.

DIFFERENTIAL DIAGNOSIS

Noninfectious etiologies of SIRS that need to be considered include adrenal insufficiency, anaphylaxis, burns, bleeding, cardiac tamponade, dissecting or ruptured aortic aneurysm, medication hypersensitivity reaction, drug overdose, myocardial infarction, pancreatitis, pulmonary embolism, and cardiopulmonary bypass syndrome.

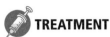 TREATMENT

MEDICATION

Early initiation of intravenous, empiric antibiotics after cultures have been drawn is critical. Selection of antibiotic depends on the patient's history, comorbidities, suspected source of infection, and local resistance patterns. In general, first line therapy is broad-spectrum covering gram-positive and gram-negative organisms.

First Line

- Vancomycin (15 mg/kg q12h) is recommended given the high prevalence and morbidity of methicillin-resistant *Staphylococcus aureus*.
  PLUS
  – Cephalosporin: Ceftriaxone 2 gm IV q24h or cefotaxime 2 gm IV q4h.
  OR
  – Beta lactam-beta lactamase inhibitor: Ticarcillin-clavulanate (3.1 gm q4h) or piperacillin-tazobactam (3.375 gm q4h).
  OR
  – Carbapenem: Meropenem (1 gm q8h) or imipenem (0.5 gm q6h)

Additional Considerations

- In neutropenic patients or in patients suspected to have infection with *Pseudomonas aeruginosa*,
  – substitute an anti-Pseudomonal cephalosporin such as cefepime 2 gm IV q8h or ceftazidime 2 gm IV q8h.
  – consider adding an aminoglycoside such as gentamicin.
- If the patient is allergic to beta-lactam agents
  – fluoroquinolone: Ciprofloxacin 400 mg IV q12h
  – PLUS metronidazole 500 mg IV q8h OR clindamycin (900 mg IV q8h).
- If fungemia is suspected, add amphotericin B.
- Antibiotic regimen should be tailored as microbiological data becomes available.
- Duration is typically 7–10 days and is influenced by factors such as the site of tissue infection, the adequacy of surgical drainage, the patient's underlying disease, and the antimicrobial susceptibility of the pathogen.

ADDITIONAL TREATMENT

General Measures

- The airway should be secured and the patient intubated, if necessary.
- The septic patient should be under continuous monitoring often requiring placement of central venous lines and arterial lines.
- The initial management of hypotension should include the aggressive administration of intravenous fluids (crystalloids or colloids) by early goal-directed therapy. The aim is to maintain a mixed central venous oxyhemoglobin saturation >70 and a mean arterial pressure >65 mm Hg. Other reasonable goals include a central venous pressure of 8–12 mm Hg, urine output >0.5 mL/kg per hour and a hemoglobin of 7–9 g/dL.

- Implement vasopressor treatment if the arterial pressure remains low despite fluid administration.

Issues for Referral

An infectious disease specialist should be consulted if the patient fails to improve on a broad empiric regimen or if they are known to have an infection with a highly resistant organism.

Additional Therapies

- Consider use of recombinant activated protein C in patients with severe sepsis, high risk of death, and no risk of bleeding.
- Hyperglycemia is common. Institute intensive insulin therapy (goal blood glucose 80–110 mg/dL).
- High dose steroids may worsen outcomes by causing further immunosuppression, leading to secondary infections. However, for patients who are not responding to fluids and vasopressors, stress dose hydrocortisone is recommended. It is believed that these patients may have a relative adrenal insufficiency.

SURGERY/OTHER PROCEDURES

- Surgical drainage of focal sources of infection is essential.
- Removal of prior indwelling intravenous catheters is recommended.

IN-PATIENT CONSIDERATIONS

Initial Stabilization

The initial stabilization of the patient and administration of IV fluids as described above is critical.

Admission Criteria

Patient with sepsis should be admitted and monitored in an ICU setting.

Nursing

- The patient's status should be monitored continuously and re-evaluated often to ensure that the patient is responding adequately to therapy.
- Patients should be repositioned often to avoid development of decubitus ulcers.

 ONGOING CARE

FOLLOW-UP RECOMMENDATIONS

- Frequent review of the status of the patient is needed to evaluate for response to therapy.
- To avoid further infectious complications, patients should be extubated and lines should be removed as soon as possible.

Patient Monitoring

As mentioned above, patients with sepsis should be closely monitored in the intensive care setting.

DIET

Enteral feeding, rather than IV nutrition, is preferred in critically ill patients with sepsis.

PATIENT EDUCATION

Patients and their families should be made aware that the patient is critically ill and kept up to date as the patient's condition can change rapidly.

PROGNOSIS

- Prognosis is variable and related to the patient's comorbidities. Mortality rates increase with disease severity.
- Severe sepsis has a fatality rate of 20%. Septic shock has a fatality fate of 50%.
- In general, the more organ systems affected, the higher the likelihood of mortality (basis for scoring systems such as sequential organ failure assessment (SOFA)).

COMPLICATIONS

- Adult respiratory distress syndrome develops in up to half of patients with sepsis.
- Depression of myocardial function develops within 24 hours in most patients with advanced sepsis.
- Renal failure in sepsis occurs due to acute tubular necrosis induced by hypotension or capillary injury, although some patients also have glomerulonephritis, renal cortical necrosis, or interstitial nephritis.
- Thrombocytopenia occurs in up to one-third of patients.
- Prolonged or severe hypotension may induce acute hepatic injury or ischemic bowel necrosis.

ADDITIONAL READING

- Dellinger RP, Levy MM, Carlet JM, et al. Surviving Sepsis Campaign: International guidelines for management of severe sepsis and septic shock: 2008. *Intensive Care Med* 2008;34:17–60.
- Hotchkiss RS, Karl IE. The pathophysiology and treatment of sepsis. *N Engl J Med* 2003;348: 138–150.
- O'Grady NP, Barie PS, Bartlett JG, et al. Guidelines for evaluation of new fever in critically ill adult patient. *Crit Care Med* 2008;36:1330–1349.
- Russell JA. Management of sepsis. *N Engl J Med* 2006;355(16):1699–713.

CODES

ICD9

- 038.9 Unspecified septicemia
- 117.9 Other and unspecified mycoses
- 790.7 Bacteremia

CLINICAL PEARLS

- Patients suspected of having severe sepsis or septic shock should be aggressively resuscitated using early goal-directed therapy.
- Blood cultures should be immediately drawn and empiric broad-spectrum, intravenous antibiotics should be initiated within 1 hour.

SORE THROAT

Eleni Patrozou

 BASICS

DESCRIPTION
- Sore throat is a commonly used term to describe the painful inflammation of the pharynx, especially upon swallowing.
- The most common infectious causes of sore throat are discussed in detail in separate Section II chapters of this book ("Pharyngitis/Tonsillitis," "Laryngitis/Laryngotracheobronchitis (Croup)," and "Infectious Mononucleosis"). In this chapter, the focus is on distinguishing features and other noninfectious causes.

Approach to the Patient
- The first step in evaluating a patient with sore throat is to assess whether the process compromises the airway and to identify whether the symptoms are due to a localized or systemic (usually viral) process.
- The type and duration of symptoms and the presence of hoarseness or fever should be investigated. Based on the clinical situation, history of sick contacts, oral–genital sexual contact, recent weight loss, or other symptoms suggestive of noninfectious causes (neoplasms, etc.) should be elicited.
- Certain clinical findings (e.g., fever, marked tonsillar exudate, enlarged tonsils, tender anterior cervical adenopathy, and myalgias) and epidemiologic findings (e.g., age, season of the year, and prevalence of streptococcal colonization in the community) strongly suggest the diagnosis of streptococcal pharyngitis.
- The presence of conjunctivitis is suggestive of a viral illness.
- When epidemiologic and clinical data suggest the presence of gonococcal pharyngitis or diphtheria, specific microbiologic techniques are indicated and appropriate therapy should be instituted promptly.
- Laryngitis, croup, and other causes of sore throat and hoarseness must be differentiated from epiglottitis.
- In most cases, the pertinent issue is distinguishing group A streptococcal infection from nonstreptococcal causes. The time-honored method of diagnostic confirmation is the throat culture. Commercially produced kits are now available for rapid antigen identification.

EPIDEMIOLOGY
- Most cases of pharyngitis are due to viral agents: Around 90% in adults and 70% in children.
- Group A β-hemolytic Streptococcus pharyngitis is much more common in children (15–30%) than in adults (5–10%).
- 75% of adult patients with pharyngitis are prescribed antibiotics.
- In epidemics with rheumatologic strains of Group A *Streptococcus*, acute rheumatic fever has occurred in up to 1–3% of patients with untreated streptococcal pharyngitis.
- Streptococci of Lancefield groups C and G are now appreciated to produce infections quite similar to Group A *Streptococcus*, although they more commonly cause opportunistic and nosocomial infections
- *Arcanobacterium hemolyticum* has a predilection for adolescents and young adults.
- Parainfluenza virus infection occurs most frequently among children.

GENERAL PREVENTION
- Advise patients with streptococcal pharyngitis to avoid close contact with others.
- Counsel the patient to follow safe sex practices.

ETIOLOGY
- Most cases of acute pharyngitis are viral in etiology (e.g., rhinoviruses, coronaviruses, influenza A and B, and parainfluenza) and can involve the pharynx as well as other parts of the respiratory tract.
- Most cases of acute laryngitis are caused by viruses (e.g., rhinovirus, influenza virus, parainfluenza virus, coxsackievirus, adenovirus, or respiratory syncytial virus).
- Certain viral infections causing sore throat exhibit distinctive clinical manifestations. Examples include enterovirus (herpangina due to coxsackie A), herpes viruses (infectious mononucleosis due to Epstein-Barr virus or Cytomegalovirus and gingivostomatitis due to herpes simplex virus), and adenovirus (pharyngoconjunctival fever, acute respiratory disease of military recruits).
- Primary herpes virus type 1 infection is a cause of acute pharyngitis. Herpes virus type 2 can cause a similar illness as a consequence of oral–genital sexual contact.
- Acute pharyngitis can occur during primary infection with HIV.

- The most important bacterial cause of pharyngitis is group A *Streptococcus*. Other bacterial causes of pharyngitis include the following:
  – Group C and G *Streptococcus*
  – *Arcanobacterium hmolyticum*
  – *Neisseria gonorrhoeae*
  – *Corynebacterium diphtheriae* (diphtheria)
  – *Mycoplasma pneumoniae*
  – *Chlamydophila pneumoniae*
- Sore throat has also been described during the course of acute toxoplasmosis, plague, brucellosis, and leptospirosis. It can accompany infection with *Treponema pallidum* (affecting 15–30% of patients with secondary syphilis), *Yersinia enterocolitica*, *Yersinia pestis*, and *Francisella tularensis*.
- Histoplasma and Blastomyces may cause laryngeal nodules, with or without ulcerations.
- Candida may cause sore throat, along with thrush, in immunosuppressed patients or in patients with mucocutaneous candidiasis.
- West Nile virus, a member of the Japanese encephalitis virus antigenic complex, usually presents as a self-limited febrile illness, commonly associated with malaise, headache, myalgias, rash, and occasionally pharyngitis
- Suppurative thrombophlebitis (Lemierre syndrome) can present with sore throat (see Section II chapter, "Anaerobic Infections").
- Sore throat can be due to abscess formation in the parapharyngeal area:
  – Infection in the lateral pharyngeal space may follow tonsillitis, pharyngitis with adenoid involvement, parotitis, mastoiditis, or periodontal infection.
  – Infection in the retropharyngeal space may result from the spread of lateral pharyngeal space infection or from lymphatic spread of the infection. Retropharyngeal abscess may also follow trauma to the posterior pharynx or may result from anterior extension cervical osteomyelitis.
- Sore throat with foul breath, fever, and chocking sensation can accompany acute necrotizing infections of the pharynx. These infections commonly occur in association with ulcerative gingivitis.

- Submandibular space infection (Ludwig's angina), a periodontal infection usually arising from the tissues surrounding the third molar, produces bilateral submandibular and sublingual rapidly spreading cellulitis without abscess formation or lymphatic involvement that results in marked local swelling of tissues, with pain, trismus, drooling and superior and posterior displacement of the tongue. As the illness progresses, dysphagia and sore throat develop and, if left untreated, airway obstruction.
- Periodic fever with aphthous stomatitis, pharyngitis, and cervical adenitis (PFAPA) syndrome can affect children (2–5 years of age) and is characterized by periodic episodes (usual interval, <4 weeks) of unheralded onset, with a brisk rise to high fever (>39°C) that is sustained over 3–6 days and is unaccompanied by other symptomatology.

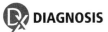 DIAGNOSIS

- With parapharyngeal space infections, most patients appear toxic and have fever, sore throat, dysphagia, and leukocytosis. Rigidity of the neck or torticollis toward the opposite side may develop. Advanced cases present with dyspnea and stridor.
- In acute necrotizing infections of the pharynx, the tonsillar pillars are swollen, red, ulcerated, and covered with a grayish membrane that peels easily. Lymphadenopathy is common.
- In infectious mononucleosis, pharyngitis is most prominent during the first 2 weeks of the illness.
- Herpangina, caused by Coxsackie A virus is characterized by fever, sore throat, myalgias, and a vesicular enanthem on the soft palate between the uvula and the tonsils.
- In tuberculous laryngitis, lesions include mucosal hyperemia and thickening, nodules, and ulcerations.

DIAGNOSTIC TESTS & INTERPRETATION
Lab
- Culture is the presumed "gold standard" but with a delay of 24–72 hours in reporting a diagnosis for *Streptococcus*.
- The current antigen detection tests for *Streptococcus* have a high degree of specificity but variable sensitivity. (See Section II chapter, "Pharyngitis/Tonsillitis").

Imaging
Initial approach
Retropharyngeal space infections may be confirmed by a lateral neck soft-tissue x-ray. However, the source and extent of infection is best evaluated by computed tomography (CT) or magnetic resonance imaging (MRI).

Diagnostic Procedures/Other
In tuberculous laryngitis, biopsy reveals granulomas with acid-fast bacilli. Cultures should be performed to confirm the diagnosis and evaluate the sensitivities of the pathogen.

DIFFERENTIAL DIAGNOSIS
- In most viral cases of pharyngitis, patients have a scratchy or sore throat as well as coryza and cough. The pharynx is inflamed and edematous, but exudate is not usually present. However, exudative pharyngitis may be seen in adenovirus infection and infectious mononucleosis.
- The presence of fever, tender anterior cervical lymphadenopathy, erythematous pharynx with or without tonsillar swelling or exudates, and absence of cough indicate a high probability of streptococcal pharyngitis for both children and adults.
- Most patients with sore throat due to *M. pneumoniae* are young and previously healthy, have mild pharyngitis, and have prominent symptoms of tracheobronchitis.

 TREATMENT

MEDICATION
- A high risk patient with a sore throat (history of rheumatic carditis or valvular disease) should be prescribed immediate antibiotic treatment while awaiting culture results.
- Parapharyngeal space infection treatment includes securing of the airway, surgical drainage in the operating room, and administration of intravenous antibiotics active against streptococci and oral anaerobes (e.g., penicillin 2–4 million units q4–6h IV and metronidazole 500 mg t.i.d IV or cefoxitin 2 g t.i.d. IV or ampicillin-sulbactam 2 gm IV q6h).
- A single intramuscular injection of benzathine penicillin has been shown to be slightly more efficacious than oral penicillin VK for the treatment of streptococcal pharyngitis and ensures compliance.

 ONGOING CARE

FOLLOW-UP RECOMMENDATIONS
- Chronic fatigue syndrome, which may follow a viral infection, can present with debilitating fatigue, fever, sore throat, painful lymphadenopathy, myalgia, arthralgia, sleep disorder, and headache.
- Streptococcal infection from group A streptococci requires appropriate antimicrobial therapy and monitoring to achieve the following:
  - Prevent acute rheumatic fever, glomerulonephritis, and toxic shock, as well as suppurative complications
  - Minimize the possibility of secondary spread
  - Shorten the course of the illness
- Sore throat can be part of the prodrome of nonspecific constitutional symptoms that lead to viral encephalitis.

COMPLICATIONS
- A peritonsillar abscess may complicate untreated streptococcal pharyngitis. Examination reveals pronounced unilateral peritonsillar swelling and erythema, causing deviation of the uvula.
- Potential complications of parapharyngeal pharyngeal space infections include airway obstruction; intraoral rupture of the abscess, causing aspiration pneumonia; jugular vein thrombophlebitis and pulmonary emboli; erosion into the carotid artery; and mediastinitis.

REFERENCES
1. Alcaide ML, Bisno AL. Pharyngitis and epiglottitis. *Infect Dis Clin North Am* 2007;21:449–469.
2. Bisno AL. Acute pharyngitis. *N Engl J Med* 2001;18:205.
3. Linder JA, et al. Evaluation and treatment of pharyngitis in primary care practice. *Arch Intern Med* 2006;166:1374–1379.
4. Wessels MR: Streptococcal pharyngitis. *N Engl J Med* 2011;364:648–655.
5. Gerber MA, Shulman ST. Rapid diagnosis of pharyngitis caused by group A streptococci. *Clin Microbiol Rev* 2004;17:571–580.

ADDITIONAL READING
- Baltimore RS. Re-evaluation of antibiotic treatment of streptococcal pharyngitis. *Curr Opin Pediatr* 2010;22(1):77–82.
- Hayward G, Thompson M, Heneghan C, et al. Corticosteroids for pain relief in sore throat: Systematic review and meta-analysis. *BMJ* 2009;339:b2976.
- Little P. Sore throat in primary care. *BMJ* 2009; 339:b2476.

CODES

ICD9
- 462 Acute pharyngitis
- 464.00 Acute laryngitis without mention of obstruction
- 784.1 Throat pain

CLINICAL PEARLS
- Reduce indiscriminate use of antibiotics to minimize potential adverse effects.
- A symptomatic individual with positive throat culture for *Streptococcus* and a history of recent previous streptococcal pharyngitis should be retreated again with penicillin.

TRAUMA-RELATED INFECTIONS

Rachel P. Simmons

 BASICS

DESCRIPTION

- Trauma-related infections, while not strictly defined, generally refer to infections that directly or indirectly result from wounds or injuries.
- A recently recognized population includes "non-trauma emergency surgery" patients and includes patients presenting with gastrointestinal perforation, obstruction, bleeding, and acute inflammation, which require emergency surgical intervention. This population has been associated with increased mortality due to infections (4).

EPIDEMIOLOGY

Incidence

- In 2005, an estimated 11.8 million wounds were treated in emergency departments in the US.
- More than half a million burns and 7.3 million lacerations are treated annually. In addition, wounds caused by cutting or piercing instruments are responsible for 2 million outpatient visits each year.
- The cumulative incidence of infection of trauma patients ranges from 2% to 37% in different studies.
- Sepsis accounts for 13–50% of all deaths in hospitalized trauma patients (6).

RISK FACTORS

Heavy contamination of wounds, impaired vascular supply as a result of injuries, emergent splenectomy, glucocorticoid administration, delay in treatment, obesity, and severity of injuries are risk factors for trauma-related infections.

GENERAL PREVENTION

- Wounds should be cleaned and irrigated thoroughly with water or normal saline.
- Topical antibiotics and occlusive dressings have been shown to decrease the rates of wound infection for traumatic lacerations (1).
- Tetanus vaccination status should be ascertained. Vaccinate patients who are overdue or cannot recall last tetanus vaccine.
- Highly contaminated wounds may require secondary or delayed primary closure.
- In open fractures of the limbs, prophylactic antibiotics reduce the incidence of early infection.
- Otherwise, the use of antibiotics for severely injured patients with bacterial contamination has not been evaluated in a placebo-controlled, prospective, randomized trial. However, antibiotics are used empirically for victims of penetrating chest or abdominal trauma and severe head wounds.
- Short courses of antibiotics are likely to be equivalent to longer courses in preventing infection in trauma patients.

- Furthermore, a prospective randomized study of patients with penetrating abdominal trauma compared the efficacy of a 24-h regimen to a 5-day regimen and reported no difference in major infection or death rate (5).
- Prophylactic antibiotic levels in trauma patients may be significantly altered by large fluid shifts and hyperdynamic physiologic responses. Data suggest that high doses given for a short duration are more effective than long courses of antibiotics in reducing infections in trauma patients undergoing laparotomy.
- In compound mandibular fractures, a systematic review found decreased rates of infection with short courses of prophylactic antibiotics.
- The risk of early serious infection in adults after splenectomy for trauma is low when isolated splenic injury is present, but this risk is increased by both the degree of injury and the presence of associated injuries. Encapsulated bacteria are frequent pathogens in both early and late infections.
- Following traumatic splenectomy, administer meningococcal and pneumococcal vaccines as soon as the patient is clinically stable.
- Close adherence to accepted infection control practices is recommended to prevent hospital-acquired infections in severely injured patients.

ETIOLOGY

- Trauma patients are at increased risk for infection for a number of reasons:
  - Crush injury and other severe trauma can result in tears of the major vessels and damage to the microcirculation, with resultant ischemia, edema, compartment syndromes, and tissue necrosis.
  - Trauma permits wounds and sterile spaces to be contaminated with bacteria through exposure to soil or water.
  - Post-injury shock leads to impairment in host immunity.
  - Splenectomy sharply reduces IgM response to infection at 7 and 14 days compared with nonsplenectomized infected posttraumatic patients.
  - Corticosteroid administration necessitated by head trauma may further impair immunity.
- Most common types of infection in multiply traumatized patients include the following:
  - Pneumonia and empyema (2)
  - Bacteremia or fungemia (primary or catheter associated)
  - Surgical site infection
  - Intraabdominal infection
  - Meningitis
  - Urinary tract infection
  - Sinus infection
  - Infection at wound site
  - *C. difficile* colitis if previous antibiotics

- *Acinetobacter baumannii* infections have been reported among US military personnel injured in Afghanistan and in the Iraq-Kuwait region with approximately one-third of the isolates being susceptible only to imipenem.

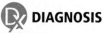 **DIAGNOSIS**

HISTORY

- The diagnosis of infection is difficult in trauma patients because of the following:
  - Fever can be due to noninfectious causes in trauma patients.
  - Patients may be unable to provide a history.
  - The physical examination may be limited.
  - The usual signs and symptoms of infection lose much of their predictive value in the multiply traumatized, critically-ill patient.

PHYSICAL EXAM

- Fever, tachycardia, and hypotension are frequently present after serious injury without infection.
- In the critically ill patient, monitor changes in ventilator settings, sputum production, urine and stool output.
- In the hospitalized trauma patient, a full examination with careful attention to indwelling devices, skin, surgical wounds, abdomen, and the respiratory system is warranted.
- Examine the injured site. Local signs of wound infection include pain, odor, erythema, swelling, purulent drainage, poor healing.

DIAGNOSTIC TESTS & INTERPRETATION

Lab

- Send a complete blood count with differential, serum electrolytes, kidney and liver function tests. Leukocytosis can be present in response to trauma in the absence of infection.
- Obtain culture specimens from sites of presumed infection prior to initiation of antibiotics if possible. Potential specimens include:
  - Blood cultures
  - Sputum cultures
  - Urinalysis and urine cultures
  - CSF cell counts and differential and culture if penetrating head trauma or CNS drain required
  - Wound culture
  - Culture of abscess material
- If watery diarrhea and a history of prior exposure to antibiotics are present, send stool for *C. difficile* testing.

Imaging

- Chest plain film to evaluate for pneumonia especially if the patient is mechanically ventilated.
- Computed tomography (CT) of the chest can demonstrate sites of thoracic infections in septic trauma victims with increased sensitivity compared to chest film. CT has proved helpful in guiding appropriate revisions of malpositioned and occluded thoracostomy tubes.

- The presence of concurrent thoracic pathology (particularly loculated hemothorax or hemopneumothorax and traumatic lung cysts with hemorrhage or surrounding parenchymal consolidation) limits the diagnostic sensitivity and specificity of chest imaging.
- CT of the abdomen can identify sites intraabdominal infection including perforation, colitis, cholecystitis, or intraabdominal abscess.
- In extremity wounds, consider imaging with ultrasound, CT, or MRI of the effected extremity if local infection is suspected to exclude abscess.

Diagnostic Procedures/Other
Image-guided or surgical drainage of abscesses can be both diagnostic and therapeutic. Send abscess fluid for gram stain, bacterial culture, and anaerobic culture. Also send for fungal stain and culture if abdominal or pelvic collection is present. Acid fast bacilli smear and mycobacterial culture may be indicated based on epidemiology.

DIFFERENTIAL DIAGNOSIS
- Among patients with extensive trauma, the differential diagnosis of infection includes the following:
  – Atelectasis
  – Deep vein thrombosis
  – Drug fever
  – Anaphylaxis/allergic reaction
  – Hypovolemia
  – Massive hematoma
  – Noninfectious inflammation
  – Pulmonary contusion
  – Transfusion reactions
  – Central fever in the case of brain injury

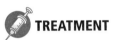 TREATMENT

MEDICATION
- Surgical management of local factors, such as open fractures or perforated abdominal organ, is often more important than antibiotic therapy.
- Among trauma patients, hemodynamic instability in the absence of hypovolemia mandates consideration of empiric antibiotic therapy, even in the absence of other signs of infection.
- The choice of antibiotic regimen should be guided by site or source of presumed infection, local resistance patterns, circumstance of trauma (bite wound, water exposure, soil contamination), duration of hospitalization (pertains to risk of hospital acquired or resistant pathogens), local prevalence of MRSA, and patient allergies.
- If no site is identified, initiate broad-spectrum antibiotics including an antistaphylococcal agent and broad gram-negative and anaerobic coverage.

ADDITIONAL TREATMENT
General Measures
- Monitor response to antibiotic therapy. Tailor regimen to culture results and susceptibilities.
- If diagnostic and interventional workup is negative and the patient is clinically stable, consider discontinuing antibiotics.
- Duration of therapy depends on clinical course and site of infection
- Discontinue central venous catheters and urinary catheters when no longer needed.

Issues for Referral
- Severely injured patients should be emergently evaluated at experienced trauma centers with trauma surgeons, intensivists, and specialty surgeons as needed (3).
- Consider infectious disease consultation to aid in evaluation and treatment of possible infection, especially if the patient is critically ill, giving no response to antibiotics, or the diagnosis of infection remains uncertain.

SURGERY/OTHER PROCEDURES
- Drainage of fluid collections, debridement of necrotic tissues, and repair of open fractures and perforated organs are critical.
- Mobilize respiratory secretions.

IN-PATIENT CONSIDERATIONS
Initial Stabilization
- Assess and stabilize the airway and circulatory system in trauma patients.
- Rapid fluid resuscitation.
- Document location and extent of all injuries.

Admission Criteria
- Patients with penetrating injury, fracture requiring urgent repair, abnormal vital signs, impaired mental status, intractable pain, or severe injuries should be admitted.
- Patients with moderate and major burns (total body surface area ≥10% in adults, ≥5% in elderly, ≥2% for full-thickness burn) require admission to a hospital with expertise in burn care.

Discharge Criteria
Patients may be discharged when fevers have abated for more than 24 h, vital signs have normalized, and follow-up plans for antibiotics and wound care are in place.

 ONGOING CARE

FOLLOW-UP RECOMMENDATIONS
Patient Monitoring
Monitor closely for wound infection and health care-associated infections. Approximately 9% of hospitalized trauma patients develop a hospital-associated infection (7).

DIET
Appropriate nutritional support is essential. Consider evaluation by a nutritionist for severely injured hospitalized patients

PATIENT EDUCATION
- Discuss signs and symptoms of wound infection.
- Provide patient teaching about wound care (packing, frequency of dressing changes, etc.).

PROGNOSIS
Patients with a trauma-related infection have an increased risk of death (HR 1.56) and worse functional status compared to trauma patients without infection in the year following the injury.

COMPLICATIONS
- Septic shock (7)
- Pulmonary insufficiency
- Peritonitis and abdominal abscess
- Osteomyelitis
- Brain abscess
- Acute acalculous cholecystitis

REFERENCES
1. Singer A, Dagum AB. Current management of acute cutaneous wounds. *N Engl J Med* 2008;359: 1037–1046.
2. Evans HL, West MA, Cuschieri J, et al. Inflammation and host response to injury investigators. Inflammation and the host response to injury, a large-scale collaborative project: Patient-oriented research core standard operating procedures for clinical care IX. Definitions for complications of clinical care of critically injured patients. *J Trauma* 2009;67(2):384–388.
3. Velmahos GC, Jurkovich GJ. The concept of acute care surgery: A vision for the not-so-distant future. *Surgery* 2007;141:288–290.
4. Neary WD, Foy C, Heather BP, et al. Identifying high-risk patients undergoing urgent and emergency surgery. *Ann R Coll Surg Engl* 2006;88:151–156.
5. Kirton, et al. Perioperative antibiotic use in high-risk penetrating hollow viscus injury: a prospective randomized, double-blind, placebo-control trial of 24 hours versus 5 days. *J Trauma* 2000;49(5): 822–32.
6. Czaja A, Rivara FP, Wang J, et al. Late outcomes of trauma patients with infections during index hospitalization. *J Trauma* 2009;67:805–814.
7. Lazarus H, Fox J, Lloyd J, et al. Trauma patient hospital-associated infections: Risks and outcomes. *J Trauma* 2005;59:188–194.

 CODES

ICD9
958.3 Posttraumatic wound infection, not elsewhere classified

CLINICAL PEARLS
- The primary goal in the management of wounds is to achieve rapid healing with optimal functional and aesthetic results.
- Antibiotic prophylaxis may be indicated depending on site and extent of injury.
- The diagnosis of infection can be difficult in a trauma patient.
- Thorough physical exam and diagnostic workup is essential to identify a possible source of infection.

URETHRITIS AND URETHRAL DISCHARGE

Eleni Patrozou

 BASICS

DESCRIPTION
- Inflammation of the urethra.
- Urethral discharge is the purulent or mucopurulent excretion from the urethra.
- Urethral syndrome and dysuria with sterile pyuria are used to describe women with dysuria and frequency but few bacteria in the urine.

Approach to the Patient
- Among patients with urethritis or urethral discharge, symptoms can vary from occasional discomfort to continuous.
- Physicians must inquire about the following:
  – The nature, onset, and duration of dysuria
  – Presence of other symptoms
  – Characteristics of urethral discharge
  – Previous sexually transmitted diseases
- Complete physical examination should be performed and the entire genital area must be evaluated.
- The testes and spermatic cord should be palpated for masses, and epididymitis should be excluded.
- Patients should be tested for cystitis, and men should be evaluated for prostatitis.
- Urethral discharge must be "milked" (using the gloved thumb and the forefinger) after the patient has not voided for several hours, preferably overnight (see also section, "Diagnosis").

EPIDEMIOLOGY
- Urethritis is more common in men.
- The most commonly recognized sexually transmitted disease in this population.
- The incidence of nongonococcal urethritis remains high.
- In 2008, 336,742 cases of gonorrhea were reported in the US, a rate of 111.6 cases per 100,000 population, reflecting a small decrease of 5.4% since 2007. Gonorrhea rates have remained relatively stable over the past 12 years.
- In 2008, gonorrhea rates continued to be highest among adolescents and young adults. Among females in 2008, 15- to 19- and 20- to 24-year-old women had the highest rates of gonorrhea.
- More than one-third of the cases of nongonococcal urethritis are caused by *Chlamydia trachomatis*.

- The prevalence of *Neisseria gonorrhoeae* in isolates from men who have sex with men (MSM) slightly decreased from 36.1% in 2007 to 33.6% in 2008. During the same time period, the prevalence of quinolone-resistant *N. gonorrhoeae* in isolates from heterosexuals also decreased from 8.7% in 2007 to 8.2% in 2008.
- Endourethral syphilitic chancre should be considered.

RISK FACTORS
- The risk of acquiring infection depends on the type of contact with an infected person.
- Up to 80% of women in contact with men with urethral gonorrhea develop gonococcal cervicitis, while only one-third of men having sex with infected women develop gonorrhea.
- The highest incidence of gonorrhea is found in young (15–30 years of age) single persons of low socioeconomic and educational status.

GENERAL PREVENTION
- Condoms prevent most sexually transmitted diseases.
- Certain contraceptive foams have anti-gonococcal activity but are of unproved clinical efficacy.
- Sexual partners of patients with gonococcal or nongonococcal urethritis should be evaluated and treated to prevent reinfection and complications to both partners.
- Women with symptoms of urinary tract infection who do not have bacteriuria should have urethral cultures for *N. gonorrhoeae*.
- Patients with urethritis should be screened for other sexually transmitted diseases.

ETIOLOGY
- Infectious urethritis
  – *N. gonorrhoeae*
  – *C. trachomatis*
  – *Ureaplasma urealyticum*
  – *Mycoplasma genitalium*
  – *Trichomonas vaginalis*
  – Herpes simplex virus
  – Adenovirus
- Noninfectious urethritis
  – Stevens–Johnson syndrome
  – Wegener's granulomatosis
  – Urethral irritation (spermicides, chemicals, alcohol, etc.)
  – Reiter's syndrome

 DIAGNOSIS

- 75% of men acquiring urethral gonorrhea develop symptoms within the first 4 days and up to 90% within 2 weeks from exposure.
- The incubation period for nongonococcal urethritis is usually 7–14 days.
- Dysuria is present in 50–75% of patients with nongonococcal urethritis, and in up to 90% of patients with gonorrhea.
- Acute urethral syndrome presents with dysuria, frequency, and urgency.
- The urethral discharge is described as purulent in most cases of gonorrhea urethritis, but in less than one-third of patients with nongonococcal urethritis.

DIAGNOSTIC TESTS & INTERPRETATION
Lab
- Inflammation should be evaluated by examination of a gram-stained smear after passage of a small swab 2–3 cm into the urethra; the presence of 5 or more neutrophils per high-power field in areas containing cells suggests urethritis.
- Gonorrhea is diagnosed by the demonstration of typical gram-negative diplococci within neutrophils.
- A preliminary diagnosis of nongonococcal urethritis is warranted if gram-negative diplococci are not found.
- A gram stain of urethral discharge is 95% sensitive in cases of gonococcal urethritis.
- Alternatively, the centrifuged sediment of the first 20–30 mL of voided urine can be examined for inflammatory cells.
- Culture or genomic detection tests for *N. gonorrhoeae* and culture, antigen, or genomic detection tests for *C. trachomatis*. Genetic amplification is sensitive and highly specific for chlamydial infection and gonorrhea. Diagnostic testing for *C. trachomatis* is recommended, to guide the counseling given to the patient and the management of the patient's sexual partner(s).
- Some investigators consider *Candida* as a possible pathogen among men with urethritis and no other obvious pathogen.

DIFFERENTIAL DIAGNOSIS

- A brief history and examination should exclude systemic complications such as disseminated gonococcal infection and Reiter's syndrome.
- Bacterial prostatitis and cystitis should be excluded.
- Among women with acute dysuria and frequency, costovertebral pain and tenderness or fever suggest acute pyelonephritis.
- A positive urine specimen from a symptomatic woman with pyuria should raise the possibility of bacterial urinary tract infection.
- The evaluation of "sterile pyuria" (in addition to conditions such as tuberculosis, prostatitis, etc.) should include acute urethral syndrome due to *C. trachomatis* or *N. gonorrhoeae*.

 TREATMENT

MEDICATION

- Most patients with gonococcal urethritis should also receive treatment for chlamydial infection.
- Gonococcal urethritis: Ceftriaxone 125 mg intramuscular injection (single dose).
- Nongonococcal urethritis: Doxycycline (100 mg orally twice daily for 7 days) or azithromycin (1 g orally once).

COMPLEMENTARY & ALTERNATIVE THERAPIES

- Gonococcal urethritis: Cefixime (400 mg orally), cefpodoxime (400 mg orally) or spectinomycin (2 g i.v.). Spectinomycin is not currently available in the US.
- Due to rising rates of gonococcal resistance, the CDC no longer recommends the use of fluoroquinolones for the treatment of gonorrhea.
- Nongonococcal urethritis: Erythromycin base (500 mg orally four times daily for 7 days) or ofloxacin (300 mg twice daily orally for 7 days) or levofloxacin (500 mg daily for 7 days).

Treatment Failure

- Patients who present with recurrent urethritis symptoms and have not completed the initial treatment regimen or they have been re-exposed to an untreated sex partner should be retreated with the initially chosen regimen.
- *N. gonorrhoeae* strains resistant to fluoroquinolones have been reported in Asia, the Pacific Islands, and the US. CDC no longer recommends the use of fluoroquinolones for treatment of gonorrhea infections.
- A *T. vaginalis* culture should be collected using either an intraurethral swab or a first-void urine sample.
- Patients with nongonococcal urethritis who do not respond to doxycycline can be infected with doxycycline-resistant *U. urealyticum* or *T. vaginalis*. Empiric treatment with a single 2 g dose of metronidazole, followed by erythromycin 500 mg orally four times daily for 7 days, may be warranted in such cases.
- Patients with recurrent episodes of nongonococcal urethritis occasionally respond to a 3 week course of erythromycin, and require evaluation for prostatic involvement or possible anatomic abnormalities.

 ONGOING CARE

FOLLOW-UP RECOMMENDATIONS

- If patients present with hematuria, especially when it persists after treatment of urethritis, a thorough urologic evaluation is needed.
- Patients who suffer from persistence or recurrence of symptoms after therapy for acute gonococcal urethritis could be experiencing one or more of the following:
  - Coinfection with *Chlamydia* or other bacteria causing nongonococcal urethritis
  - Gonococcal reinfection
  - Treatment failure

COMPLICATIONS

- *C. trachomatis* can lead to acute salpingitis or bartholinitis.
- Babies born to women infected with *C. trachomatis* may develop chlamydial ophthalmia neonatorum or pneumonia.
- Carriage of *U. urealyticum* is associated with infertility.
- *N. gonorrhoeae* and *C. trachomatis* can cause acute epididymitis.

ADDITIONAL READING

- Centers for Disease Control and Prevention. Update to CDC's sexually transmitted diseases treatment guidelines, 2006: Fluoroquinolones no longer recommended for treatment of gonococcal infections. *MMWR* 2007;56(14):332–336.
- Workowski KA, Berman SM. Sexually transmitted diseases treatment guidelines, 2006. *MMWR Recomm Rep* 2006;55(RR11):1–94.

 See Also

- CDC Sexually Transmitted Diseases Surveillance, 2008

 CODES

ICD9

- 099.40 Other nongonococcal urethritis, unspecified
- 597.80 Urethritis, unspecified
- 788.7 Urethral discharge

CLINICAL PEARLS

- If clinic-based diagnostic tools (gram stain microscopy) are not available, patients should be treated for both gonorrhea and chlamydial infections.
- Enteric bacteria have been identified as an uncommon cause of nongonococcal urethritis and might be associated with insertive anal sex.

U

VAGINAL DISCHARGE/VAGINITIS

Eleni Patrozou

 BASICS

DESCRIPTION

- Physiologic or normal vaginal discharge (also referred to as "leukorrhea") that usually consists of cervical mucus and desquamated epithelial cells.
- Usually, the term "vaginal discharge" is used in conjunction with a vaginal infection. Such infections are characterized by the following:
  - Abnormal color of discharge, caused by increased concentration of polymorphonuclear leukocytes
  - Increased volume of discharge
  - Vaginal malodor and/or vulvar pruritus, irritation, burning, or dysuria
  - Dyspareunia
- The most common diseases associated with vaginal discharge are bacterial vaginosis, trichomoniasis, and candidiasis.
- Bacterial vaginosis represents a change of the normal vaginal flora characterized by replacement of hydrogen-peroxide-producing lactobacilli by an overgrowth of anaerobic microorganisms, mycoplasmas, and *Gardnerella vaginalis*.
- Please also see Section I chapter, "Genital Lesions," and Section II chapters, "Cervicitis/Mucopurulent Cervicitis" and "Pelvic Inflammatory Disease."

Approach to the Patient

- Physicians should inquire about the characteristics of the discharge (color, odor, etc.) and the presence of other local or systemic symptoms.
- Previous similar symptoms and a complete sexual history can aid in the diagnosis.
- Examination of the vaginal fluid, using the following tests, can diagnose most cases:
  - Measuring pH, using pH paper that reads from 4.0 to 6.0
  - Detecting an amine ("fishy") odor, which is released upon alkalinizing vaginal fluid by adding one drop of KOH (10%) solution
  - Searching for clue cells (vaginal epithelial cells that are so overladen with adherent bacteria that the cell border is obscured) and for trichomonads and white blood cells in a saline preparation under the microscope
  - Examining a KOH preparation under the microscope for *Candida* filaments

- Investigation of vaginal discharge in sexually active adult women should involve the collection of both endocervical and high vaginal swabs.
- Swabs should be placed in transport medium to prevent drying and to allow the survival of anaerobes.
- Harvesting of endocervical cells from the squamocolumnar junction is required for chlamydial culture, detection of chlamydial antigen, or chlamydial DNA by PCR.
- It is convenient to divide specimens into those requiring a full culture and those requiring a screening culture. A screening culture will include selective plates for *Neisseria gonorrhoeae*, *Candida* spp., and beta-hemolytic streptococci, and microscopy for *Trichomonas vaginalis* and bacterial vaginosis.

EPIDEMIOLOGY

Bacterial vaginosis is the most common cause of vulvovaginal symptoms, followed by vulvovaginal candidiasis. Trichomoniasis is much less common in developed countries.

RISK FACTORS

- The risk of acquiring a vaginal infection depends on the type of contact with an infected person. Up to 80% of women in contact with men with urethral gonorrhea develop gonococcal cervicitis, while only one-third of men having sex with infected women develop gonorrhea.
- Gonorrhea is more common among young (15–30 years of age) single persons of low socioeconomic and educational status.

GENERAL PREVENTION

- Prevention suggestions for vaginal infections:
  - Practice safe sex
  - Limit the number of sex partners
  - Treat infected partners, as indicated
- Weekly oral fluconazole has been found effective in preventing vulvovaginal candidiasis among patients with advanced HIV infection, but this approach is rarely needed and should be based on selective criteria.
- In female patients at high risk of developing yeast infections while on antibiotic therapy, one dose of fluconazole (150 mg orally) at the beginning and at the conclusion of the antibiotic therapy can be used in order to prevent the development of vaginal candidiasis.

ETIOLOGY

- Three etiologies account for over 90% of cases of vaginitis:
  - Bacterial vaginosis (40%)
  - *Trichomonas* (*T. vaginalis*) (25%)
  - *Candida* spp. (25%)
- Bacterial vaginosis is associated with multiple sexual partners and recent intercourse with a new partner.
- Bacterial vaginosis is diagnosed when 3 out of 4 of the following are present:
  - Abnormal, thin, homogeneous vaginal discharge
  - Vaginal pH >4.5
  - Positive amine test
  - Presence of clue cells
- Cervicitis can sometimes cause vaginal discharge.
- Vaginal discharge may be the presenting manifestation of genital herpes and occasionally reflects mucopurulent cervicitis or pelvic inflammatory disease caused by gonorrhea or chlamydial infection.
- Vaginitis may be an early and prominent feature of toxic shock syndrome.

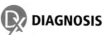 **DIAGNOSIS**

- Although the clinical signs and symptoms are often nonspecific, certain features can suggest the diagnosis of candidal vaginitis:
  - Vulvar pruritus and burning
  - Abnormal vaginal discharge; only 25% have the "typical" thick, curdy discharge
  - Burning on urination at the urethral orifice
  - Vaginal erythema; white or yellow adherent plaques (in 40%)
- Findings and characteristics of the vaginal discharge:
  - Vulvovaginal candidiasis: The vaginal discharge is typically white and scant and sometimes takes the form of white thrush-like plaques adhering loosely to the vaginal mucosa.
  - *T. vaginalis* usually manifests with malodorous vaginal discharge (often yellow), vulvar erythema and itching, dysuria or urinary frequency (in 30–50% of cases), and dyspareunia. These manifestations, however, do not clearly distinguish trichomoniasis from other types of infectious vaginitis.
  - Bacterial vaginosis presents with a thin, homogenous discharge, with a characteristic "fishy" odor, which is usually more noticeable after intercourse.
  - If vulvar inflammation exists in the absence of vaginal pathogens the discharge might be a sign of noninfectious irritation such as chemical or allergic.

DIAGNOSTIC TESTS & INTERPRETATION
Lab
- Detection of motile *Trichomonas* can be done based on microscopy of wet preparations of vaginal secretions. For a wet preparation, vaginal fluid is added to a drop of saline on a slide, and covered with a coverslip. Clue cells are vaginal epithelial cells covered with numerous, short coccobacilli. If clue cells are seen on the wet preparation, a confirmatory Gram stain can be ordered and culture for *T. vaginalis* can yield few additional positives.
- Wet preparations provide an immediate diagnosis. Its sensitivity for the detection of *T. vaginalis* is only about 60% in routine evaluations of vaginal secretions (up to 70–80% among symptomatic patients). Direct immunofluorescent antibody staining is more sensitive (up to 90%) than wet-mount examinations. Culture is the most sensitive means of detection but not generally available.
- The diagnosis of vulvovaginal candidiasis involves the demonstration of fungi by microscopic examination of vaginal fluid in saline or 10% KOH or by Gram stain. Culture does not differentiate between vulvovaginal candidiasis and colonization. The pH of vaginal secretions is usually 4.5, and no amine odor is produced when vaginal secretions are mixed with 10% KOH.
- WBCs in the discharge without evidence of trichomonads or yeast are usually suggestive of cervicitis.
- The absence of trichomonads or pseudohyphae does not rule out these infections that can be demonstrated by culture or PCR.

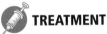

TREATMENT
MEDICATION
- For vaginal trichomoniasis, a single 2 g oral dose of metronidazole is the treatment of choice, and is as effective as more prolonged regimens.
- The standard regimen for the treatment of bacterial vaginosis has been metronidazole (500 mg orally, twice daily for 7 days). Clindamycin (300 mg orally, twice daily for 7 days) is also effective. Intravaginal treatment with 2% clindamycin cream (one applicator each night for 7 nights) or 0.75% metronidazole gel (one applicator twice daily for 5 days) is also effective.
- In most circumstances, therapy for candidal vaginal infection is indicated only if the patient is symptomatic or has signs of vulvovaginitis.

- Intravaginal products, many of which are available over the counter, are the treatments of choice. They should be applied at bedtime.
  - Clotrimazole, 1% vaginal cream, 5 g for 7–14 days; 100 mg vaginal tablet, single tablet for 7 days or two tablets for 3 days; or 500 mg vaginal tablet, single application
  - Miconazole, 2% vaginal cream, 5 g for 7 days; 200 mg vaginal suppository for 3 days; or 100 mg vaginal suppository for 7 days
  - Butoconazole, 2% vaginal cream, 5 g for 3 days
  - Terconazole, 80 mg vaginal suppository for 3 days
  - In pregnancy, intravaginal clotrimazole, miconazole, or terconazole may be used for symptomatic women, but their use should be deferred until the second trimester
  - The newer azoles, fluconazole and itraconazole, can be used as a single oral dose, but they are more expensive
- About 10% of women will have another, or several, attacks of candidal vaginitis after what should be an appropriate treatment course. The definition of "recurrent candidiasis" is 4 or more episodes per year.

 ONGOING CARE

FOLLOW-UP RECOMMENDATIONS
Recurrent or chronic vulvovaginal candidiasis develops with increased frequency among women with systemic illnesses such as diabetes mellitus or HIV infection.

COMPLICATIONS
- Vaginal trichomoniasis and bacterial vaginosis early in pregnancy are independent predictors of premature onset of labor.
- Bacterial vaginosis is a risk factor in the following:
  - Bacterial infection of the upper genital tract
  - Endometritis following caesarean section
  - Neonatal sepsis
  - Preterm labor/late miscarriage
  - Vaginal cuff cellulitis following abdominal hysterectomy
  - HIV acquisition and transmission
  - Acquisition of HSV-2, gonorrhea, and chlamydial infection

ADDITIONAL READING
- Workowski KA, Berman SM. Sexually transmitted diseases treatment guidelines, 2006. *MMWR Recomm Rep* 2006;55:1–94.

 CODES

ICD9
- 616.10 Vaginitis and vulvovaginitis, unspecified
- 623.5 Leukorrhea, not specified as infective

CLINICAL PEARLS
- More than 50% of women with bacterial vaginosis are asymptomatic.
- Pregnant women with BV are at higher risk of preterm delivery. Treatment may reduce the risk for prematurity.

V

ACNE VULGARIS

Michael K. Mansour (E. Mylonakis, Editor)

 BASICS

DESCRIPTION
Acne vulgaris (common acne) is a chronic inflammatory disease of the sebaceous follicles, which are special pilosebaceous units.

EPIDEMIOLOGY
- Acne vulgaris is one of the most common skin diseases, affecting over 85% of persons at some time between the ages of 15 years into the 40s.
- Mean age is 24.
- Accounts for up to 2 million office visits for patients between the ages of 15–19 years old.

RISK FACTORS
- A known risk factor is the hyperresponsiveness of sebaceous cells and keratinocytes to androgenic hormones.
- Androgenic hormones likely play a role in the setting of puberty and women with raised levels of testosterone, dehydroepiandrosterone sulphate, or androstenedione.

GENERAL PREVENTION
- Avoidance of excessive irritants to skin.
- Maintenance of basic hygiene.

PATHOPHYSIOLOGY
Inflammatory changes involving the sebaceous follicles leading to accumulation of lipid-rich sebum and bacterial growth.

ETIOLOGY
- *Propionibacterium acnes* is an anaerobic, Gram-positive bacterium that populates the androgen-stimulated sebaceous follicle and is a normal constituent of the cutaneous flora. Normally in a very low bacterial burden.
- Sebaceous follicles provide sebum, the lipid-rich secretion product of sebaceous glands which is a rich growth medium for *P. acnes*.
- Initial trigger appears to be an overgrowth of *P. acnes* resulting in inflammation, follicular rupture, and extension of the inflammatory process into the surrounding dermis. This results in the formation of papules, pustules, and nodules.

 DIAGNOSIS

HISTORY
- Notable for the presence of closed (whitehead) or open (blackhead) comedones.
- In more advanced cases, comedones undergo inflammatory changes which may lead to painful nodules, pustules, or cellulitis.
- Limited to the area of the body with the most sebaceous glands: Face, neck, chest, upper back, and upper arms.

PHYSICAL EXAM
- An array of characteristics may be present from noninflamed comedones (open or closed) to active nodules and/or pustules.
- Presence of scarring usually indicates a more aggressive acne vulgaris.
- Depending on distribution and severity of inflammation, one can classify acne into mild, moderate, and severe.
  – Mild usually involves noninflammatory comedones.
  – Moderate has an increased number of inflammatory pustules and papules affecting a larger area of skin.
  – Severe acne has large painful nodules and may undergo scar formation.

TREATMENT

- Depends on severity of acne. Mild or moderate acne can respond to topical therapy.
- Mainstay of therapy includes antimicrobial agents, anti-inflammatory drugs, and retinoids for follicular keratinocyte differentiation.

MEDICATION

Retinoids

- Retinoids reduce the size and secretion of sebaceous glands.
- Topical agents are most effective in the prevention of further comedone formation.
- Some topical retinoids, such as tazarotene, will cause severe irritation.
- For more severe acne especially if scarring is suspected, systemic retinoid therapy with oral isotretinoin is indicated.
- Isotretinoin has been shown to also act as an anti-inflammatory agent and inhibits growth of *P. acnes* accounting for its potent activity.
- Common side effects of retinoids, specifically, oral isotretinoin, include birth defects and hypertriglyceridemia. Young women need to be counseled about use of 2 forms of contraception while undergoing oral retinoid therapy.
- Associations between isotretinoin and depression/suicide have been reported.

Antimicrobials

- Indicated if inflammatory component is noted.
- Benzoyl peroxide is a good first-line bactericidal agent with rapid effect.
- Addition of topical antimicrobials is effective when used in conjunction with benzoyl peroxide or retinoids.
- Topical antimicrobials used alone tend to induce high levels of resistance and treatment failure.
- If acne is more severe, oral antimicrobials are indicated.

- Commonly used agents with activity against *P. acnes* include tetracyclines (minocycline, tetracycline, doxycycline), bactrim, erythromycin, and clindamycin.
- Rising resistance has been noted now with more than 50% of *P. acnes* showing full resistance to at least one antimicrobial. Most common resistance is to erythromycin > clindamycin > tetracycline.
- Patient education and drug compliance are critical, and drug resistance should be considered in a failing patient.
- Other cause of clinical failure is overgrowth of Gram-negative bacteria.

Pregnancy Considerations

Oral isotretinoin is highly tretogenic.

ADDITIONAL TREATMENT

Additional Therapies

- In the setting of hyperandrogenism, agents such as spironolactone are useful to prevent overproliferation of androgen-sensitive sebaceous glands.
- Oral contraception has also been shown to reduce rate of acne.
- For severe inflammatory changes, intralesional corticosteroid instillation can be used.

COMPLEMENTARY & ALTERNATIVE THERAPIES

Chemical and physical microabrasion and laser therapy have yet to have defined roles.

ADDITIONAL READING

- James WD. Acne. *N Engl J Med* 2005;352: 1463–1472.
- Leyden JJ. Therapy for acne vulgaris. *N Engl J Med* 1997;336:1156–1162.
- Swerlick RA, Lawley TJ. Eczema, psoriasis, cutaneous infections, acne, and other common skin disorders. In: Fauci AS, Braunwald E, Isselbacher KJ, et al., eds. *Harrison's principles of internal medicine*, 14th ed. New York: McGraw-Hill, 1998:298–303.

 CODES

ICD9
706.1 Other acne

CLINICAL PEARLS

- Acne is an inflammatory state of sebaceous glands due to overproduction of sebum and growth of *P. acnes*.
- Mild forms of acne can be treated with topical agents whereas severe states require oral therapy.
- Combination therapy to include retinoids and anti-inflammatory and antimicrobial agents.
- Other hormonal causes should be investigated as these may be reversible.

ACTINOMYCOSIS

Paschalis Vergidis
Matthew E. Falagas

 BASICS

DESCRIPTION
A chronic, indolent, suppurative, tissue-destructive infection, presenting with lumps and sinus formation, usually involving the head and neck, although it can well affect other parts of the body such as the thorax and abdomen.

EPIDEMIOLOGY
Incidence
- The reported incidence in the general population is about 1:300,000 in the US, and about 1:100,000 in Europe.
- Infection occurs at all ages, with a peak incidence in the middle decades.
- The male-to-female ratio is 3:1.

RISK FACTORS
- Poor oral hygiene, dental procedures, oral surgery, and trauma
- Intrauterine contraceptive devices (all types; increased risk if in place for more than 2 years)
- Abdominal surgery, intraabdominal inflammatory processes (diverticulitis, appendicitis), foreign bodies
- Actinomycosis has been described in the setting of malnutrition and immunodeficiency (HIV infection, chronic granulomatous disease, chronic steroid use).
- Actinomycosis has also been reported in patients with infected osteoradionecrosis and bisphosphonate-associated mandibular osteonecrosis.

GENERAL PREVENTION
- Keep good oral hygiene, including removal of dental plaque.
- Identification of Gupta bodies or ALOs (*Actinomyces*-like organisms) in Papanicolaou cervicovaginal smears may be of help in preventing the development of advanced pelvic disease in women with long-term intrauterine contraceptive devices and symptoms of possible early pelvic actinomycosis such as pain, abnormal bleeding, or abnormal discharge. Removal of the intrauterine device and a 2- to 3-week course of antibiotics are recommended in these cases.
- There is no need for patient isolation.

PATHOPHYSIOLOGY
- Humans are the natural reservoir of actinomycosis pathogens.
- The organisms usually grow as saprophytes in the mouth (mainly in dental plaque and tonsillar crypts).
- Transmission probably occurs from person to person by contact.
- Extraction of teeth or other trauma of the oral mucosa may precipitate actual local infection by *Actinomyces* species.

- The pathogens are probably aspirated and occasionally cause lung actinomycosis.
- Most cases of abdominal actinomycosis originate in the appendix.
- Although the exact incubation period is not known, diagnosis is usually done after long periods of time. Although an acute form has been recognized, chronic disease accounts for the majority of cases.
- Disruption of the mucosal barrier seems to be necessary for the initial establishment of the infection. It subsequently spreads contiguously and/or hematogenously. Aspiration or contiguous spread from the cervical area leads to pulmonary involvement. Foreign bodies and/or bowel perforation secondary to appendicitis or diverticulitis lead to the pathologic process in the abdominal and pelvic disease.
- Depending on the part of the body affected, oral/cervicofacial, thoracic, abdominal, pelvic, central nervous system (CNS), and a disseminated form of the disease are recognized. Muscle and bone involvement is due to direct spread by adjacent tissue infection or (less frequently) follows trauma or dissemination of infection.

ETIOLOGY
- *Actinomyces* are microaerophilic/anaerobic, filamentous, branched, Gram-positive, non-acid-fast rods.
- Among several *Actinomyces* species, *A. israelii* is most commonly found in pus and tissues of patients suffering from actinomycosis (1).
- *A. naeslundii*, *A. meyeri*, *A. odontolyticus*, and *Propionibacterium propionica* (*Arachnia propionica*) have also been reported to cause human actinomycosis.
- *A. viscosus* has been established as a contributing factor to the etiology of periodontal disease.
- *Actinomyces* are oral and female genital tract commensals.
- Nevertheless, in most cases of actinomycosis, careful cultures yield polymicrobial isolates, mostly including anaerobic members of the normal oral flora. These might act as copathogens in the pathologic process.

ⅮⅩ DIAGNOSIS

HISTORY
- Pain, vaginal discharge, and/or bleeding (pelvic disease)
- Headache, focal neurologic symptoms
- Symptoms dependent on the extent of the lesions and the organ/system involved
- Possible pain, low-grade fever, weight loss
- Trismus (oral/cervicofacial disease)
- Chest pain, cough (productive or not), gradually increasing shortness of breath (thoracic disease)
- Abdominal pain, change in bowel habits (abdominal disease)

PHYSICAL EXAM
- Formation of space-occupying lesions of varying sizes, with varying degrees of suppuration and/or fibrosis, is the hallmark of the disease.
  - Spread to the adjacent tissues may occur, as well as drainage to adjacent cavities or to the skin via sinus formation.
  - Sinuses can be self-limited and recurrent.
  - Pus characteristically contains yellowish "sulfur granules," which may be seen macroscopically or microscopically.
- Cervicofacial/oral disease
  - The perimandibular region is most commonly affected, but every part of the head, neck, and oral cavity can be involved, including soft tissues, bones, salivary glands, thyroid, eyes (postoperative canaliculitis and endophthalmitis), and ears (chronic, myringotomy-resistant otitis media).
  - The overlying skin may be purple/red/bluish.
- Thoracic disease
  - Follows aspiration or (more rarely) contiguous spread from the cervical region. Signs are those of a space-occupying lesion or/and pneumonitis, with pleural involvement (thickening, effusion, empyema) in more than 50% of cases.
  - The presence of multiple cavities and the involvement of the chest wall (soft tissues and bones with sinus formation) support the diagnosis.
  - Mediastinal involvement (mainly cardiac structures), as well as spine involvement, may be present.
- Abdominal disease
  - Signs are those of a firm/hard mass lesion, most commonly in the right iliac fossa (following perforated appendicitis).
  - Left iliac fossa disease follows diverticulitis.
  - Perirectal or perianal disease presents as chronic, recurrent abscesses and sinus/fistula formation in the relevant region.
  - Peritonitis is rare.
- Pelvic disease
  - Presents as pelvic masses and abscesses of varying extension, or is diagnosed as frozen pelvis, due to the indolent course of the disease.
- CNS disease
  - Focal neurologic signs and/or signs of chronic meningitis.

DIAGNOSTIC TESTS & INTERPRETATION
Lab
- There is a high degree of suspicion when space-occupying lesions are combined with pus-draining sinus formation and soft-tissue/bone involvement.
- Inspect the bandage covering a draining sinus for sulfur granules.
- Take the specimen before initiating any antimicrobial therapy.

Initial lab tests
- Identification of filamentous, Gram-positive, non-acid-fast organisms in sulfur granules (slide examination) or in material obtained from a normally sterile site (not in sputum, bronchial washings, or vaginal secretions)
- A Gram stain of the specimen is more sensitive than culture.
- Swab cultures are not recommended.
- Anaerobic processing of specimens is necessary.
- Direct immunofluorescence using specific antisera against actinomycosis agents is highly specific and sensitive. It has been mainly used in diagnosis and prevention of intrauterine device-related disease.

Imaging
Initial approach
- CT and MRI are helpful in defining the extent of the disease and the adjacent tissue involvement (2, 3).
- The open bronchus sign – the presence of an aerobronchogram within a mass lesion – is highly suggestive of lung disease.
- A saw-toothed appearance and complete involvement of bones are characteristic of bone disease.
- Single (actinomycetoma) or multiple round or irregular multiloculated brain lesions, surrounded by edema and low-attenuation areas, are the usual mode of CNS disease presentation.

Pathological Findings
Presence of macroscopic or microscopic "sulfur granules" in pus and/or tissue material (other than tonsils), obtained by fine-needle aspiration or biopsy. Tissue Gram and Giemsa stains will reveal the organisms at the periphery of the granule.

DIFFERENTIAL DIAGNOSIS
- Malignant tumors
- Nocardiosis
- Botryomycosis
- Tuberculosis
- Histoplasmosis
- Blastomycosis
- Cryptococcosis

TREATMENT
MEDICATION
First Line
- Penicillin G, 10–24 million units/d i.v. (in divided doses every 4–6 hours) for 2–6 weeks, followed by penicillin V, 2–4 g/d p.o. for 6–12 months, or
- Ampicillin, 50 mg/kg/d i.v. for 2–6 weeks, followed by amoxicillin, 1.5 g/d p.o. for 6–12 months
- Duration of treatment depends on extent of disease and clinical response (4). Mild cases of cervicofacial disease may be treated with oral antibiotics only.

Second Line
- Tetracycline (minocycline)
- Erythromycin (alternative if patient allergic or pregnant)
- Clindamycin

SURGERY/OTHER PROCEDURES
Antibiotic treatment may need to be combined with surgical intervention such as drainage of abscesses, excision of fibrotic tissue, and marsipulation of persisting sinus tracts.

ONGOING CARE
FOLLOW-UP RECOMMENDATIONS
- Emphasize the need for compliance to treatment (long-term drug treatment)
- Observe for drug toxicity

PROGNOSIS
Usually excellent response to antibiotics, no *Actinomyces* resistance (5). In the case of failure, there is a high possibility of an undrained abscess or a resistant bacterial copathogen.

COMPLICATIONS
- Disseminated actinomycosis
- Bowel obstruction due to extensive abdominal/pelvic actinomycosis

REFERENCES
1. Pulverer G, Schutt-Gerowitt H, Schaal KP. Human cervicofacial actinomycoses: Microbiological data for 1997 cases. *Clin Infect Dis* 2003;37(4): 490–497.
2. Lee IJ, Ha HK, Park CM, et al. Abdominopelvic actinomycosis involving the gastrointestinal tract: CT features. *Radiology* 2001;220:76–80.
3. Park JK, Lee HK, Ha HK, et al. Cervicofacial actinomycosis: CT and MR imaging findings in seven patients. *AJNR* 2003;24:331–335.
4. Choi J, Koh WJ, Kim TS, et al. Optimal duration of IV and oral antibiotics in the treatment of thoracic actinomycosis. *Chest* 2005;128:2211–2217.
5. Smith AJ, Hall V, Thakker B, et al. Antimicrobial susceptibility testing of *Actinomyces* species with 12 antimicrobial agents. *J Antimicrob Chemother* 2005;56:407–409.

ADDITIONAL READING
- Acevedo F, Baudrand R, Letelier LM, et al. Actinomycosis: A great pretender. Case reports of unusual presentations and a review of the literature. *Int J Infect Dis* 2008;12(4):358–362.
- Lippes J. Pelvic actinomycosis: A review and preliminary look at prevalence. *Am J Obstet Gynecol* 1999;180:265–269.
- Mabeza GF, Macfarlane J. Pulmonary actinomycosis. *Eur Respir J* 2003;21(3):545–551.
- Smego RA Jr, Foglia G. Actinomycosis. *Clin Infect Dis* 1998;26:1255–1261.

CODES
ICD9
- 039.1 Pulmonary actinomycotic infection
- 039.2 Abdominal actinomycotic infection
- 039.9 Actinomycotic infection of unspecified site

CLINICAL PEARLS
- Actinomycosis is a chronic, indolent, suppurative, tissue-destructive infection, usually involving the head and neck. Pus characteristically contains yellowish "sulfur granules."
- Chronic destructive infection may be mistaken for malignancy.
- Penicillin is the treatment of choice. Surgical intervention may be required.

ADENOVIRUS INFECTIONS

Jatin M. Vyas (E. Mylonakis, Editor)

 BASICS

DESCRIPTION
- Adenovirus infections are caused by double-stranded DNA viruses that measure 70–80 nm in diameter.
- Human adenoviruses belong to the genus *Mastadenovirus*, which includes over 50 serotypes.

EPIDEMIOLOGY
Incidence
- 80% of cases of acute respiratory illnesses are caused by viruses, most commonly rhinovirus, and less often, adenovirus.
- Infections are most common from fall to spring.

RISK FACTORS
- Adenovirus infection can be transmitted by inhalation of aerosolized virus, by inoculation of virus into conjunctival sacs, and, probably, by the fecal–oral route as well.
- Adenoviruses account for up to 5% of acute respiratory infections in children, but for fewer than 2% of respiratory illnesses in adults.

- Certain adenovirus serotypes are associated with outbreaks of acute respiratory disease in military recruits in winter and spring.
- Antibodies develop after infection and are associated with protection against infection with the same serotype.
- Adenoviruses have also been implicated in disseminated disease and pneumonia in immunosuppressed patients, including patients with AIDS and recipients of solid-organ or bone marrow transplants, or children who suffer from congenital immunodeficiency syndromes.

ETIOLOGY
- Adenoviruses have a characteristic morphology consisting of an icosahedral shell composed of 20 equilateral triangular faces and 12 vertices.
- Human adenoviruses have been divided into six subgenera (A through F) on the basis of the homology of DNA genomes and other properties.
- The adenovirus genome is a linear double-stranded DNA that codes for structural and nonstructural polypeptides. The replicative cycle of adenovirus may result either in lytic infection of cells or in the establishment of a latent infection.
- Some adenovirus types can induce oncogenic transformation. Tumor formation has been observed in animals.

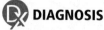 **DIAGNOSIS**

HISTORY
- In children, adenoviruses cause a variety of clinical syndromes. The most common is an acute upper respiratory tract infection with prominent rhinitis.
- On occasion, lower respiratory tract disease, including bronchiolitis and pneumonia, occurs.
- Adenoviruses can cause pharyngoconjunctival fever, a characteristic acute febrile illness of children that occurs in outbreaks, most often in summer camps. Low-grade fever is frequently present for the first 3–5 days, followed by rhinitis, sore throat, and cervical adenopathy. The illness generally lasts for 1–2 weeks and resolves spontaneously.
- Pharyngitis has also been associated with adenovirus infection.
- In adults, the most frequently reported illness has been acute respiratory disease. This illness is marked by a prominent sore throat and the gradual onset of fever, which often reaches 39°C. Cough is almost always present, and coryza and regional lymphadenopathy are frequently seen.

- Adenoviruses can also cause nonrespiratory tract diseases:
  – Acute diarrheal illness in young children
  – Hemorrhagic cystitis
  – Epidemic keratoconjunctivitis
- Immunocompromised patients with adenovirus pneumonia can present with the abrupt onset of fever, rigors, malaise, nonproductive cough, nausea, vomiting, diarrhea, abdominal pain, headache, and arthralgia.

PHYSICAL EXAM
- Physical examination may show pharyngeal edema, injection, and tonsillar enlargement with little or no exudate.
- In immunocompromised patients, localized physical exam findings may not be evident.
  – Patients with ocular disease can show conjunctival irritation with discharge.

DIAGNOSTIC TESTS & INTERPRETATION
Lab
Initial lab tests
- A definitive diagnosis of adenovirus infection is established by culture or detection of the virus from sites such as the conjunctiva and oropharynx or from sputum, urine, or stool.
- Virus may be detected in tissue culture by cytopathic changes, and specifically identified by immunofluorescence or other immunologic techniques.

- Adenovirus types that have been associated with diarrheal disease in children require special tissue-culture cells for isolation or are identified by direct ELISA of stool.
- Serum antibody rises can be demonstrated by complement-fixation or neutralization tests, ELISA, or radioimmunoassay.

Imaging
In adenovirus pneumonia, the chest roentgenogram usually shows bilateral, diffuse, interstitial infiltrates and, occasionally, pleural effusions.

DIFFERENTIAL DIAGNOSIS
In most cases, illnesses caused by adenovirus infection cannot be differentiated from those caused by a number of other viral respiratory agents and *Mycoplasma pneumoniae*.

 TREATMENT

MEDICATION
- Only symptom-based treatment and supportive therapy are available for adenovirus infections.
- Live vaccines have been developed against adenovirus types 4 and 7 (live, unattenuated virus administered in enteric-coated capsules) and are used to control epidemics in military recruits.
- The treatment of adenovirus infections in immunocompromised hosts is usually supportive.
- Severe adenovirus infections in immunocompromised patients can respond to treatment with cidofovir and a single dose of intravenous immunoglobulin.

- Intravenous gamma globulin has been used in the treatment of adenovirus infections in transplant patients and immunocompromised hosts, and type-specific antibody may play a role in the treatment of this infection.
- Ribavirin or ganciclovir has been used successfully for the treatment of adenovirus infections in immunocompromised and immunocompetent hosts, but the evidence of efficacy is limited to case reports.

ONGOING CARE

COMPLICATIONS
In transplant recipients and immunocompromised patients, adenovirus pneumonia is associated with significant morbidity and mortality, which may exceed 60%.

CODES

ICD9
- 008.62 Enteritis due to adenovirus
- 079.0 Adenovirus infection in conditions classified elsewhere and of unspecified site
- 480.0 Pneumonia due to adenovirus

AMEBIASIS

Balaji Veeraraghavan
Paschalis Vergidis
Matthew E. Falagas

 BASICS

DESCRIPTION
- Protozoal infection caused by *Entamoeba histolytica*. Infection with these organisms leads to diarrhea, colitis and, on occasion, extra-intestinal manifestations such as liver abscess.
- Symptomatic disease occurs in <10% of infected individuals. Only a small percentage of those having intestinal infection will develop invasive disease.

EPIDEMIOLOGY
Prevalence
- Ten percent of the global population is estimated to be infected with *E. histolytica*.
- Prevalence ranges from <5% in developed countries to 20–30% in the tropics.
- In the US prevalence is roughly estimated to be <4%.
- Disease is seen at all ages and both sexes are equally affected.

RISK FACTORS
- Risk factors in endemic areas include:
  - Low socioeconomic status
  - Poor sanitation
  - Overcrowding
- In low-prevalence countries:
  - Immigrants or travelers from endemic regions
  - Institutionalized individuals
  - Men who have sex with men
- Risk factors associated with severe disease:
  - Neonates
  - Pregnancy
  - Corticosteroid therapy
  - Malnutrition

GENERAL PREVENTION
- Humans are the only reservoir of the infection.
- Contaminated water or vegetables are often the source for infection in humans.
- Cysts are not eradicated with chlorine; boiling of water is necessary for decontamination.
- Avoid ingestion of contaminated water and food.
- Make sure vegetables are washed well with potable water or be treated with detergent and soaked in acetic acid or vinegar.

PATHOPHYSIOLOGY
- Infection occurs via the fecal–oral route
- The organism exists in two forms:
  - Trophozoite with single nucleus with or without ingested erythrocytes
  - Cyst with four nuclei
- Ingestion of the cyst results in excystation in the small bowel. Trophozoites are formed which infect the colon and result in symptoms.
- During unfavorable conditions, the trophozoite encysts and the cyst form is passed out in feces.
- Cysts remain viable in the moist environment for months.
- Most people infected with the organism have no significant invasion of the colonic mucosa and are asymptomatic (cyst passers).
- Patients with colonic invasion have flask-shaped colonic ulcers.

ETIOLOGY
- *E. histolytica* is one of the several *Entamoeba* species that infect humans.
- Nonpathogenic species include *Entamoeba dispar*, *Entamoeba moshkovskii* (both morphologically identical), *Entamoeba hartmanni* and *Entamoeba coli*.

 DIAGNOSIS

HISTORY
- Patients develop symptoms with invasive disease within 4 weeks of ingestion of the cysts.
- Amebic liver abscess takes about 3 months to develop.
- Some patients carry the organisms for prolonged periods before developing significant clinical manifestations.
- Intestinal disease
  - Asymptomatic infection
  - Symptomatic noninvasive infection
    - Symptoms are mild; diarrhea is the only feature
  - Amebic colitis (or dysentery)
    - Crampy abdominal pain
    - Bloody, mucoid diarrhea
    - Rectal bleeding with diarrhea can occur, especially in children
    - Fevers occur in one-third of patients
    - Weight loss
    - Anorexia

- Extra-intestinal disease
  - Extra-intestinal amebiasis may affect the liver (abscess), spleen, lungs, or brain.
  - Amebic liver abscess presents with fevers and right upper quadrant pain. 50% of the patients with amebic liver abscess have no history of colitis.
  - Rarely, rupture of the abscess may lead to peritonitis.
  - Rupture of the liver abscess into the pleural space leads to empyema. Patients present with fever, shortness of breath, and pleuritic chest pain.
  - Cerebral amebiasis: Nausea, vomiting, headache, mental status changes

PHYSICAL EXAM
- Colitis
  - Diffuse abdominal tenderness
  - Distention, rebound tenderness in fulminant colitis/perforation
- Liver abscess
  - Tenderness to palpation over the liver
  - Hepatomegaly
  - Jaundice is uncommon

DIAGNOSTIC TESTS & INTERPRETATION
Lab
- Stool microscopy, O&P examination
  - Stool leukocytes may be present.
  - Intracytoplasmic red blood cells in trophozoites (seen in *E. histolytica* and *E. dispar*).
  - Wet mount for motile trophozoites and formal-ether concentration followed by iodine stained deposit increase the likelihood of identifying cysts.
  - To improve the yield of microscopic diagnosis multiple samples need to be tested.
- Antigen detection
  - Fecal antigen detected by ELISA. More sensitive than O&P but inferior to PCR. Requires fresh or frozen samples.
  - Can be used in liver abscess fluid.
  - TechLab *E. histolytica* II ELISA allows distinction from nonpathogenic amebae (1).

- Serology
  - Helpful in liver abscess and invasive colonic disease
  - ELISA (most commonly used), indirect immunofluorescent assay, indirect hemagglutination assay
  - Falsely positive early in the course of disease
  - Titers remain high for years
  - In endemic areas, high seropositivity does not allow distinction between active and past infection (2)
- Culture is performed only in research laboratories
- PCR
  - Real-time PCR is technically complex but more sensitive than the stool antigen (3).
  - Can be used in liver abscess fluid.
- Other laboratory tests
  - Leukocytosis without eosinophilia is often seen in patients with invasive amebic disease.
  - Elevated alkaline phosphatase and mildly elevated transaminases in liver abscess.

Imaging
Imaging studies such as ultrasound, CT, MRI scans are helpful in assessing patients with suspected amebic liver abscess. Usually, the amebic abscess is located in the right lobe (right upper, posterior segment of the liver).

Diagnostic Procedures/Other
- Colonoscopy and biopsy for colonic disease
  - Findings may be normal in early disease
  - Friable, ulcerated mucosa with punctate hemorrhages
  - Lateral extension through the submucosal tissues gives rise to the characteristic flask-shaped ulcer of amebic colitis
  - Amebomas present as annular lesions
- Aspiration of liver abscess yields brown, odorless, sterile pus classically described as "anchovy paste" which may show trophozoites. Liver abscess aspiration often fails to recover the organism, since it lives in the walls of the abscess.

Pathological Findings
- Intestinal biopsy specimen taken from the edge of ulcers should be evaluated for motile trophozoites.
- Biopsy shows mucosal thickening, multiple discrete ulcers separated by regions of normal-appearing mucosa.

DIFFERENTIAL DIAGNOSIS
- Ulcerative colitis
- Carcinoma of the colon
- Crohn's disease
- Diverticulitis
- Abdominal abscess
- Irritable bowel syndrome
- Pyogenic abscess
- Hepatoma
- Echinococcal liver cyst

 TREATMENT

MEDICATION
- Asymptomatic disease
  - Intra-luminal carriage should be treated because of the risk of invasive disease
  - Paromomycin 500 mg p.o. t.i.d. for 7 days should be used as first-line agent (4).
  - Diloxanide furoate 500 mg t.i.d. for 10 days
  - Iodoquinol 650 mg p.o. t.i.d. for 20 days
- Colitis
  - Metronidazole 750 mg p.o. t.i.d. for 10 days or tinidazole 1 g b.i.d. for 3 days followed by either of the following:
    ○ Iodoquinol 650 mg p.o. t.i.d. for 20 days
    ○ Paromomycin 500 mg p.o. t.i.d. for 7 days
- Liver abscess
  - Metronidazole 750 mg p.o. or i.v. t.i.d. for 10 days, followed by iodoquinol 650 mg p.o. t.i.d. for 20 days

SURGERY/OTHER PROCEDURES
For a large abscess (>3 cm), aspiration and needle drainage is indicated. Smaller abscesses resolve with medical treatment.

 ONGOING CARE

FOLLOW-UP RECOMMENDATIONS
Patients treated for liver abscess should have follow-up ultrasound to document cyst resolution, which may take several months.

PROGNOSIS
Amebiasis carries substantial morbidity and mortality, especially in developing countries.

COMPLICATIONS
- Fulminant colitis with toxic megacolon, perforation, and peritonitis are rare but well described.
- Amebomas: Mass lesions of the colon, often in the cecum or ascending colon caused by inflammation in the setting of amebic colitis. Amebomas may cause obstruction and can masquerade as colon cancer.
- Ruptured liver abscess with perforation of the diaphragm leading to pleural or pericardial disease.

REFERENCES
1. Haque R, Mollah NU, Ali IK, et al. Diagnosis of amebic liver abscess and intestinal infection with the TechLab *Entamoeba histolytica* II antigen detection and antibody tests. *J Clin Microbiol* 2000;38(9):3235–3239.
2. Stanley SL Jr, Jackson TF, Foster L, et al. Longitudinal study of the antibody response to recombinant *Entamoeba histolytica* antigens in patients with amebic liver abscess. *Am J Trop Med Hyg* 1998;58(4):414–416.
3. Roy S, Kabir M, Mondal D, et al. Real-time-PCR assay for diagnosis of *Entamoeba histolytica* infection. *J Clin Microbiol* 2005;43(5):2168–2172.
4. Blessmann J, Tannich E. Treatment of asymptomatic intestinal *Entamoeba histolytica* infection. *N Engl J Med* 2002;347(17):1384.

ADDITIONAL READING
- Fotedar R, Stark D, Beebe N, et al. Laboratory diagnostic techniques for *Entamoeba* species. *Clin Microbiol Rev* 2007;20(3):511–532.
- Haque R, Huston CD, Hughes M, et al. Amebiasis. *N Engl J Med* 2003;348(16):1565–1573.

 CODES

ICD9
- 006.8 Amebic infection of other sites
- 006.9 Amebiasis, unspecified

CLINICAL PEARLS
- Fecal antigen detection is more sensitive than O&P but less sensitive than PCR in the diagnosis of amebiasis.
- Treat asymptomatic "cyst passers" with luminal agents.
- Amebomas are colonic mass lesions which can be mistaken for colonic carcinoma.

ANAEROBIC INFECTIONS

Bettina Knoll (E. Mylonakis, Editor)

 BASICS

DESCRIPTION
- Anaerobic infections are caused by bacteria that require reduced oxygen for growth.
- Anaerobes associated with human infections are aero-tolerant: They can survive, but not replicate, for up to 72 hours in an oxygenated atmosphere.
- Anaerobic bacteria colonize mucosal membranes and predominate in infections arising from mucosal and adjacent sites.

EPIDEMIOLOGY
Incidence
Anaerobes account for up to 10% of blood culture isolates from patients with clinically significant bacteremia (1). No incidence data is available for anaerobic infections of other sites.

RISK FACTORS
- Mucosal barrier breakdown secondary to neoplasm, chemotherapy, radiation, neutropenia, graft versus host disease, surgery, trauma, inflammatory bowel disease, diverticulitis, appendicitis
- Poor dental hygiene
- Altered mental status, depressed gag reflex, impaired swallowing

GENERAL PREVENTION
- Bowel preparation and perioperative antimicrobial prophylaxis
- Good dental hygiene
- Aspiration precautions

PATHOPHYSIOLOGY
- Translocation of resident flora into sterile sites due to breakdown of mucosal membranes
- Translocation of oral flora into lungs due to aspiration
- Proliferation of obligate anaerobes during polymicrobial infection due to lowered oxidation–reduction potential by aerobic organisms
- Virulence factors enable anaerobic bacteria to induce abscess formation (e.g., *Bacteroides fragilis*: Capsular polysaccharide), to evade host defenses (e.g., *Prevotella*: IgA proteases), to adhere to cell surfaces (e.g., *Porphyromonas gingivalis*: Proteases), and to produce toxins and/or enzymes (e.g., *Fusobacterium necrophorum*: Leukotoxin and endotoxin)

ETIOLOGY
- *B. fragilis* is the most common isolated anaerobic Gram-negative bacillus. Other Gram-negatives are *Fusobacterium*, *Prevotella*, and *Porphyromonas* species.
- *Peptostreptococcus* species are the major Gram-positive cocci, and *Clostridia* is the main Gram-positive rods causing disease.

COMMONLY ASSOCIATED CONDITIONS
- Dental infections
  - Pulpitis
  - Periapical and dental abscess
  - Perimandibular space infection
- Gingivitis
  - Periodontitis
  - Periodontal abscess
- Extension of periodontal infection with maxillary sinus osteomyelitis or submandibular space infection
- Vincent's stomatitis (trench mouth)
- Ludwig's angina: Bilateral infection of the sublingual and submandibular spaces
- Lemierre Syndrome: *F. necrophorum* infection of the posterior compartment of the lateral pharyngeal space complicated by suppurative thrombophlebitis of the jugular vein and secondary metastasis, primarily to the lungs
- Chronic sinusitis and otitis media
- Pleuropulmonary infections
  - Aspiration pneumonia
  - Necrotizing pneumonia
  - Lung abscess
  - Empyema
- Intraabdominal infections
  - Peritonitis
  - Abscesses
  - Neutropenic colitis (Typhlitis)
- Female genital tract infections
  - Pelvic inflammatory disease
  - Pelvic abscess
  - Septic abortion
  - Endometritis
  - Tubo-ovarian abscess
  - Postoperative infection
  - Bacterial vaginosis
  - Pelvic cellulitis
  - Amnionitis
  - Septic thrombosis of pelvic veins

- Central nervous system infections
  - Cerebral abscess
  - Epidural abscess
  - Subdural empyema
  - Anaerobic meningitis: Rare, suggestive of shunt infection or parameningeal collection
- Skin and soft tissue
  - Necrotizing fasciitis
  - Gas gangrene
  - Crepitant cellulitis
  - Bite wounds
  - Surgical wounds
  - Diabetic foot infection
  - Decubitus ulcers
- Bone and joint
  - Osteomyelitis and septic arthritis adjacent to infected soft tissue sites
- Bacteremia
  - Secondary to an intraabdominal/genital tract/respiratory tract/soft tissue infection
  - *B. fragilis* most common isolate

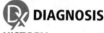 **DIAGNOSIS**

HISTORY
- Sudden onset of tender bleeding gums, halitosis, bad taste, fever, cervical lymphadenopathy
  - Vincent's stomatitis (trench mouth)
- Submandibular and/or sublingual pain, trismus, lateral and posterior tongue displacement causing trouble to swallow and/or airway compromise
  - Ludwig's angina
- Nasopharyngitis or tonsillar abscess followed 1–2 weeks later by high fever, submandibular angel lymphadenopathy, tenderness along the lateral aspect of the sternocleidomastoid muscle, metastasis to the lungs
  - Lemierre's syndrome
- Weight loss, chest wall, or pleuritic pain
  - Empyema
- Chronic malaise, weight loss, fever, chills, foul smelling sputum, and anemia
  - Anaerobic lung abscess
- Poor mental status, difficulty in swallowing, chronic respiratory symptoms, weight loss, fever, and anemia
  - Aspiration pneumonia
- Neutropenia, right lower quadrant abdominal pain, fever, diarrhea
  - Typhlitis
- No improvement of infectious process on antimicrobial regimen without anaerobic activity
  - Suggestive of anaerobes

PHYSICAL EXAM
- Poor dental status
  - Predominance of anaerobic oral flora with risk for translocation
- Gas in tissue, crepitus
  - Infection with gas-forming bacteria
- Foul odor
- Infection adjacent to mucosal surfaces
- Tissue necrosis, abscess formation
  - Indicative of anaerobes

DIAGNOSTIC TESTS & INTERPRETATION
Lab
- Anaerobes are technically difficult to cultivate and identify. In many cases the anaerobic etiology of an infection remains unproven.
- Culture technique
  - Specimens must be collected by avoidance of contamination of indigenous flora of mucosal surfaces.
  - Liquids or tissues are preferable to swab specimens.
  - Air must be expelled from the syringe used to aspirate and needle must be capped.
  - Use of anaerobic transport media.
  - Quick processing of samples.
  - All specimens should be subjected to Gram staining: No growth in culture but Gram-positive and Gram-negative organisms on Gram staining suggest presence of anaerobic organisms.

Imaging
- Radiographs
  - Air–fluid level, cavity formation, gas in tissue
- CT and/or MRI scans
  - Often important to define anatomic location and extent of disease

Diagnostic Procedures/Other
CT- or US-guided aspiration or biopsy

DIFFERENTIAL DIAGNOSIS
Anaerobic lung abscesses have to be differentiated from mycobacterial diseases.

 TREATMENT

- Treatment involves a combination of surgical (resection, debridement, drainage) and antimicrobial therapy.
- Antibiotics used should cover both aerobic and anaerobic flora, given the polymicrobial nature of many of these infections.
- Empiric choice of antibiotic regimen under consideration of type of infection, Gram staining results, compartmental penetration, toxicity. Susceptibility testing difficult due to anaerobic culture techniques, turnaround time, poor quality control.
- Susceptibility testing recommended for patients in need of prolonged antimicrobial therapy: Cerebral abscess, osteomyelitis, prosthetic device associated infection.
- Anaerobic infections arising from below the diaphragm should be treated with specific therapy directed at *B. fragilis*. Organisms belonging to the *B. fragilis* group are resistant to penicillin.
- Antimicrobial agents effective against anaerobes: Carbapenems, β-Lactam/β-lactamase inhibitor combination, metronidazole (metronidazole is inactive against *Actinomyces* spp., *Propionibacterium* spp., peptostreptococci, and microaerophilic streptococci).
- Increasing prevalence of *B. fragilis* antibiotic resistance. Resistance to cephamycins 8–14% (2), clindamycin 26% (2), moxifloxacin 38% (2).

 ONGOING CARE

FOLLOW-UP RECOMMENDATIONS
Patient Monitoring
- Assure adequate drainage of abscesses with follow-up imaging.
- Surgical resection indicated if drainage unsuccessful.
- Repeat sampling if infection unresponsive to antimicrobial therapy to evaluate for drug-resistant organisms.
- Monitoring for antimicrobial drug toxicities.

COMPLICATIONS
Contiguous spread of untreated infections

REFERENCES
1. Lassmann B, Gustafson DR, Wood CM, et al. Reemergence of anaerobic bacteremia. *Clin Infect Dis* 2007;44(7):895–900.
2. Snydman DR, Jacobus NV, McDermott LA, et al. National survey on the susceptibility of *Bacteroides fragilis* group: Report and analysis of trends in the United States from 1997 to 2004. *Antimicrob Agents Chemother* 2007;51(5):1649–1655.

 CODES

ICD9
041.84 Other specified bacterial infections in conditions classified elsewhere and of unspecified site, other anaerobes

ANORECTAL INFECTIONS

Jatin M. Vyas (E. Mylonakis, Editor)

BASICS

DESCRIPTION
- Anorectal infections involve the anus and rectum (the distal part of the large intestine).
- Fournier's gangrene includes any necrotizing infection of the external genitalia and perineum.

EPIDEMIOLOGY
Incidence
Among organ transplant recipients, the prevalence of external anogenital lesions is 1.5–2.3%, and women are more often involved. Most of the lesions are due to anogenital warts, followed by bowenoid papulosis, giant condyloma, and in situ carcinoma.

RISK FACTORS
In Fournier's gangrene, there is often a history of urinary infection and/or urologic instrumentation, or long-standing colorectal disease. Furthermore, most patients are affected by comorbid conditions including diabetes, alcoholism, or intravenous drug abuse, which serve to hinder host defense.

GENERAL PREVENTION
When immunocompromised patients present with abscesses, perianal sepsis must be considered as a possible focus. Perianal fistulas in such patients should be laid open or treated by fistulectomy, and perianal abscesses require adequate drainage, to avoid necrotizing gangrene and metastatic abscesses.

PATHOPHYSIOLOGY
- Among women and men who had sex with men, primary anal or rectal infection develops after receptive anorectal intercourse. In women, rectal infection with lymphogranuloma venereum (or non-LGV) strains of *Chlamydia trachomatis* presumably can also arise by the contiguous spread of infected secretions along the perineum (as in rectal gonococcal infections in women) or perhaps by spread to the rectum via the pelvic lymphatics.

- Both herpes simplex viruses 1 and 2 can cause symptomatic or asymptomatic rectal and perianal infections. Herpes infection proctitis is usually associated with rectal intercourse. However, subclinical perianal shedding of herpes simplex virus (HSV) is detected both in heterosexual men and in women who report no rectal intercourse.
- Perianal warts are common among men who have sex with men, but they develop in heterosexual men as well.
- Perirectal abscesses often represent the tracking down into the anal area of purulent material escaping from the rectosigmoid area. Diverticulitis, Crohn's disease, ulcerative colitis, or previous surgery may be the underlying cause.
- Aerobic bacteria are found in the majority of cases of Fournier's gangrene, but mixed aerobic and anaerobic infections are common.

ETIOLOGY
- Most common anorectal infections include bacterial and parasitic infections (e.g., abscesses or soft-tissue infection) and sexually transmitted diseases. Most of these infections are also discussed in other chapters of the book.
- Among men who had sex with men, most common causes of anorectal infection include the following:
  – Anorectal gonococcal infection
  – HSV
  – Infections with enteric pathogens, usually *Giardia lamblia*, *Entamoeba histolytica*, or *Campylobacter* spp., and *C. trachomatis*
  – Syphilis
  – Rectal lesions are common in HIV-infected patients, particularly the perirectal ulcers and erosions due to the reactivation of HSV infection. Other rectal lesions more commonly seen in HIV-infected patients include condyloma acuminatum, Kaposi's sarcoma, and intraepithelial neoplasia.

COMMONLY ASSOCIATED CONDITIONS
- Diabetes Mellitus Type I
- Diabetes Mellitus Type II

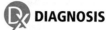

DIAGNOSIS

HISTORY
- Symptoms of herpes simplex proctitis include anorectal pain, anorectal discharge, tenesmus, and constipation.
- Pain out of proportion to skin findings can be seen in Fournier's gangrene.

PHYSICAL EXAM
- The main manifestations of anogenital warts are cauliflower-like condyloma acuminata that usually involve moist surfaces; keratotic and smooth papular warts, usually on dry surfaces; and subclinical "flat" warts, which can be found on any mucosal or cutaneous surface.
- Fournier's gangrene is characterized by localized gangrene and massive swelling of the scrotum and penis, with extension into the perineum or the abdominal wall and legs.
- Blisters
- Bullae
- Erythema

DIAGNOSTIC TESTS & INTERPRETATION
Lab
Initial lab tests
- Anorectal swab samples can help in diagnosing *C. trachomatis* infections with the use of PCR.
- In anorectal infection with HSV, sigmoidoscopy reveals ulcerative lesions of the distal 10 cm of the rectal mucosa. Rectal biopsies show mucosal ulceration, necrosis, polymorphonuclear and lymphocytic infiltration of the lamina propria, and (in occasional cases) multinucleated intranuclear inclusion-bearing cells.
- CBC
- CPK
- ESR
- CRP
- Chem 7
- Glucose
- Arterial blood gas for severely ill patients

Imaging
- CT scan
- MRI

DIFFERENTIAL DIAGNOSIS

- Perianal donovanosis may resemble condylomata lata of secondary syphilis. Other venereal diseases, particularly syphilis, frequently coexist with donovanosis. In countries where donovanosis is endemic, the persistence of suspected condylomata lata after appropriate penicillin therapy for syphilis is highly suggestive of donovanosis.
- The differential diagnosis of anogenital warts includes condylomata lata of secondary syphilis, molluscum contagiosum, hirsutoid papillomatosis (pearly penile papules), fibroepitheliomas, and neoplasms.

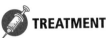 TREATMENT

MEDICATION

- Cryotherapy can be very successful in clearing warts that have failed to respond to podophyllin. Perianal warts, however, do not respond so well. Interferons have been used as adjuvant to other therapy.
- Conservative therapy with local or systemic antibiotics seems appropriate for perianal abscess. For granulomatous lesions, spontaneous resolution is unlikely, and surgery should be the treatment of choice.
- Early and aggressive surgical exploration is essential in patients with Fournier's gangrene and should aim at removing necrotic tissue, reducing compartment pressure, and obtaining material for Gram staining and for aerobic and anaerobic cultures. Empirical antibiotic treatment for mixed aerobic–anaerobic infections could consist of clindamycin (900 mg intravenously t.i.d) ampicillin or ampicillin/sulbactam (2–3 g intravenously q6h), plus gentamicin (1.0–1.5 mg/kg t.i.d). Hyperbaric oxygen treatment may also be useful in gas gangrene due to clostridial species. Duration of therapy varies, but antibiotics should be continued until all signs of systemic toxicity have resolved and all devitalized tissue has been removed.

SURGERY/OTHER PROCEDURES

Early surgery consult is necessary for patients suspected with or have proven Fournier's gangrene.

IN-PATIENT CONSIDERATIONS

Initial Stabilization

Patients with Fournier's gangrene may require admission to the ICU.

 ONGOING CARE

FOLLOW-UP RECOMMENDATIONS

The presence of anal warts and HIV infection are independent risk factors for the development of cytologic abnormalities. Those at highest risk for anal abnormalities include men with anal human papilloma virus infection and a history of intravenous drug use. Some authorities suggest that these groups as well as organ transplant recipients infected with oncogenic human papilloma should be strongly considered as candidates for anal cytology screening to identify and treat potentially precancerous anal disease.

COMPLICATIONS

- Epidermodysplasia verruciformis is a rare autosomal recessive disease characterized by the inability to control human papilloma virus infection. Patients are often infected with unusual human papilloma virus types and frequently develop cutaneous squamous cell malignancies, particularly in sun-exposed areas. The lesions resemble flat warts or macules similar to those of pityriasis versicolor.
- The complications of warts include itching and, occasionally, bleeding. In rare cases, warts become secondarily infected with bacteria or fungi. Large masses of warts may cause mechanical problems, such as obstruction of the birth canal.

- Perianal sepsis must always be kept in mind as a possible focus among HIV-infected patients, especially among those with low CD4 lymphocyte counts.
- Fournier's gangrene can result in septicemia and carries mortality rates as high as 22–66%.

ADDITIONAL READING

- Anaya DA, Dellinger EP. Necrotizing soft-tissue infection: Diagnosis and management. *Clin Infect Dis* 2007;44:705–710.
- Rizzo JA, Naig AL, Johnson EK. Anorectal abscess and fistula-in-ano: Evidence-based management. *Surg Clin North Am*. 2010;90(1):45–68.
- Thwaini A, Khan A, Malik A, et al. Fournier's gangrene and its emergency management. *Postgrad Med J* 2006;82(970):516–519.

 CODES

ICD9

- 078.11 Condyloma acuminatum
- 569.9 Unspecified disorder of intestine
- 608.83 Vascular disorders of male genital organs

ANTHRAX

Irene S. Kourbeti (E. Mylonakis, Editor)

BASICS

DESCRIPTION
- Anthrax is a zoonotic disease of the herbivores and only occasionally infects humans. The term is derived from the Greek word for coal and describes the black eschar of the cutaneous form of the disease.
  – In humans, the disease occurs primarily in three forms: Cutaneous, respiratory, and gastrointestinal.
  – Incubation period:
    ○ Cutaneous disease: 3–10 days
    ○ Pulmonary disease: 3–5 days

EPIDEMIOLOGY
- Anthrax is a rare illness in the US.
- Epidemics have been described in association with importation of wool, hides, and other animal products.
- In developing countries, epidemics occur in humans with their association with disease in animals.
- Foodborne outbreaks have been documented and related to ingestion of tainted meat.
- In 2001, a total of 22 confirmed or suspected anthrax cases (11 cutaneous and 11 inhalational [IA]) related to bioterrorism occurred in the US. 5 of these patients died.
- Since December 2009, a total of 31 cases (including 11 deaths) of a new pattern of the disease, previously described as "injectional," have been reported in Scotland.

ETIOLOGY
Bacillus anthracis is an aerobic gram-positive, spore-forming organism. The endospores are resistant to drying, radiation, and disinfectants, and may remain dormant in soil, at times for years.

RISK FACTORS
- In developing countries, the major risk is with exposure to contaminated soil or sick animals.
- In urban locations, the major risk is through exposure to contaminated hides and animal hairs.

GENERAL PREVENTION
- Vaccination of livestock is indicated in endemic areas.
- Decontamination of imported hides and animal hair would reduce risk.
- Anthrax vaccine is available to individuals with potential exposure to the organism. These include military personnel, veterinarians, and people exposed to imported hides or animal hairs.

PATHOPHYSIOLOGY
The production of two binary toxins (lethal toxin and edema toxin) is essential for the disease process.

DIAGNOSIS

Disease can manifest as cutaneous, respiratory, or gastrointestinal, but cutaneous is the most common form. Meningitis can occur as a complication from bacteremic spread from any of the three primary forms.

PHYSICAL EXAM
- Cutaneous disease: The classic lesion is a circular eschar (1–3 cm) and it can start as an ulcerating papule. Importantly, if left untreated, the infection can progress to bacteremia and sepsis.
- Respiratory disease often presents in two phases. First, a viral-like upper respiratory illness lasts 2–4 days and is followed by a severe fulminant pneumonitis. However, the clinical presentation can be atypical and some patients present without cough, chest pain, or abnormal lung examination.
- Gastrointestinal disease usually presents with abdominal pain, nausea, vomiting, and fever, and can be accompanied with hematemesis and hematochezia.

- Anthrax meningoencephalitis may complicate bacteremia and may have hyperacute onset with rapid progression to coma and death.
- Anthrax disease described in injection drug users is severe and manifests with soft tissue infection with tense edema, intracranial or subarachnoid hemorrhage and gastrointestinal symptoms
- A typical skin lesion should cause suspicion of anthrax. Evaluation of history of exposure to sick or dead animals, hides, or hairs can be helpful.
- The diagnosis of pneumonia or gastroenteritis is difficult to establish because of the nonspecific clinical symptoms.
- A noteworthy finding is that in an advanced pulmonary disease, the mediastinum widens on chest x-ray film. The combination of mediastinal widening, altered mental status, and elevated hematocrit is 100% sensitive in distinguishing IA anthrax from community-acquired pneumonia.
- Hemorrhagic cerebrospinal fluid and gram-positive rods on Gram staining are suggestive of meningeal involvement.

DIAGNOSTIC TESTS & INTERPRETATION
Lab
- Cultures and Gram stains of vesicular lesions should reveal the organism—a large, encapsulated, gram-positive rod in short chains.
- Blood cultures are usually positive in febrile, acutely ill patients with pulmonary or gastrointestinal disease.
- Stool cultures reveal the organism in gastrointestinal disease.

Imaging
Chest x-ray film often reveals diffuse infiltrates and effusions. Widening of the mediastinum is sometimes seen late in the disease.

DIFFERENTIAL DIAGNOSIS

- Cutaneous
  - Tularemia
  - *Staphylococcus aureus*
  - Spider bite
  - Burn lesion
- Pulmonary
  - Wide array of bacterial and viral processes
- Gastrointestinal
  - *Shigella*
  - *Yersinia*
  - *Campylobacter*
- Meningitis
  - Tuberculosis
  - Amebic meningoencephalitis
  - Certain viral infections: Hantavirus, dengue, Ebola

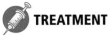 **TREATMENT**

MEDICATION

- Naturally acquired cutaneous anthrax in individuals >2 years:
  - Oral ciprofloxacin (500 mg b.i.d. in adults and 15 mg/kg b.i.d. not exceeding 500 mg in children) for 7–10 days
  - Oral doxycycline (100 mg b.i.d. in adults and 2.2 mg/kg—not exceeding 100 mg—b.i.d. in children) for 7–10 days
  - If susceptibility testing is available, penicillin G 6–8 million units per day IV, penicillin VK 500 mg q.i.d., and 50 mg/kg/d in children <12 years or amoxicillin p.o. 500 mg t.i.d. and 45 mg/kg/d in children may be used to complete the course.
  - Despite the potential of resistance and inducible resistance, probably 7–10 days of penicillin may be sufficient for use in naturally acquired uncomplicated cutaneous anthrax.
- Levofloxacin may be recommended as an additional option.
- For severe forms of naturally occurring cutaneous anthrax:
  - IV ciprofloxacin 400 mg b.i.d. and 10 mg/kg b.i.d. in children
  - IV doxycycline 100 mg b.i.d. in adults and 2.2 mg/kg b.i.d. in children
- Bioterrorism-related cutaneous anthrax: p.o. ciprofloxacin or p.o. doxycycline or p.o. amoxicillin in the above-recommended doses for 60 days to complete a full course of postexposure prophylaxis.

- For IA, gastrointestinal anthrax, and fulminant bacteremia:
  - IV ciprofloxacin is preferred to IV doxycycline.
  - The combination regimens may include IV ciprofloxacin or IV doxycycline plus one or two of the following: Imipenem or meropenem, rifampin, vancomycin, penicillin or ampicillin, chloramphenicol, clindamycin.
- Use at least one agent with good CNS penetration to cover the possibility of subclinical meningitis–Some experts suggest the addition of clindamycin for inhibition of endotoxin production.
- A human IgG1λ monoclonal antibody directed against a component of the anthrax toxin (raxibacumab) improved survival in rabbits and monkeys with symptomatic inhalational anthrax (IA).

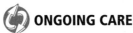 **ONGOING CARE**

FOLLOW-UP RECOMMENDATIONS
Patients should be followed up for evidence of recurrence of disease after therapy.

COMPLICATIONS
- Pulmonary and gastrointestinal diseases are almost always fatal.
- Cutaneous disease often leaves a scar in the area of the eschar.

ADDITIONAL READING

- Arenstein AW. Anthrax: From antiquity to answers. *J Infect Dis* 2007;195:471–473.
- Booth MG, Hood J, Brooks TJ, et al. Anthrax infection in drug users. *Lancet* 2010;17:1345–1346.
- Christie B. Heroin contaminated with anthrax has killed 11 people. *BMJ* 2010;340:c937.
- Holty JEC, Kim RY, Bravata DM. Anthrax: A systematic review of atypical presentations. *Ann Emerg Med* 2006;48:200–211.
- Holty JEC, Bravata D, Hau L, et al. Systematic review: A century of inhalational anthrax cases from 1900 to 2005. *Ann Intern Med* 2006;144:277–280.
- Kyriacou DN, Adamski A, Khardori N. Anthrax: From antiquity and obscurity to a front-runner in bioterrorism. *Infect Dis Clin N Am* 2006;20:227–251.

- Kyriacou DN, Yarnold PR, Stein AC, et al. Discriminating inhalational anthrax from community-acquired pneumonia using chest radiograph findings and a clinical algorithm. *Chest* 2007;131:489–496.
- Migone TS, Subramanian M, Zhong J, et al. Raxibacumab for the treatment of inhalational anthrax. *N Engl J Med* 2009;361:135–144.
- Narayan SK, Sreelakshmi M, Sujatha S, et al. Anthrax meningoencephalitis—declining trends in an uncommon but catastrophic CNS infection in rural Tamil Nadu, south India. *J Neurol Sci* 2009;281:41–46.
- Wu W, Mehta H, Chakrabarty K, et al. Resistance of human alveolar macrophages to *Bacillus anthracis* lethal toxin. *J Immunol* 2009;183:5799–5806.
- Stern EJ, Uhde KB, Shadomy SV, et al. Conference report on public health. *Emerg Infect Dis* 2008;14(4):e1.
- Clinical manifestations and diagnosis of anthrax. www.uptodate.com, Version 18.1.
- Schneemann A, Manchester M. Anti-toxin antibodies in prophylaxis and treatment of inhalation anthrax. *Future Microbiol* 2009;4:35–43.
- Treatment and prevention of anthrax. www.uptodate.com, Version 18.1.
- www.bt.cdc.gov/agent/anthrax/index.asp.

 CODES

ICD9
- 022.0 Cutaneous anthrax
- 022.1 Pulmonary anthrax
- 022.9 Anthrax, unspecified

CLINICAL PEARLS

- The antibiotics cannot prevent the progression of cutaneous anthrax to the eschar phase.
- Because of the potential severity of the disease, several medications that are usually contraindicated in special populations (children, pregnant women, and nursing mothers) may still be used.

ANTIBIOTIC AND *CLOSTRIDIUM DIFFICILE*-RELATED DIARRHEA

Jatin M. Vyas (E. Mylonakis, Editor)

 BASICS

DESCRIPTION
- The term antibiotic-associated diarrhea and colitis is used to describe a variety of clinical syndromes that occur during or within 4–6 weeks after antibiotic therapy that alters the bowel flora. Diagnosis requires that there is no other identifiable cause for diarrhea.
- Based on the degree of colonic involvement, it is divided in 4 categories:
  – Normal colonic mucosa
  – Mild erythema with some edema
  – Granular, friable, or hemorrhagic mucosa
  – Pseudomembrane formation

EPIDEMIOLOGY
- *Clostridium difficile* causes about 3 million cases of diarrhea and colitis in the US every year. Most cases occur in hospitals or long-term care facilities, whereas the incidence of this infection in the outpatient setting is low, but not negligible.
- Transmission of the organism occurs from patient to patient, and the organism can be cultured from many environmental surfaces in rooms of infected patients and from the hands, clothing, and stethoscopes of health care workers.
- Hospital personnel may carry the bacteria from room to room and promote the infection, but fecal carriage by staff is rare.
- Toxigenic *C. difficile* is isolated from stool specimens in approximately 3% of healthy adults, but colonization frequently occurs during hospitalization, and about one-third of patients colonized with *C. difficile* develop clinical symptoms.

RISK FACTORS
- Antibiotics–major risk factor
- Hospitalization
- Advanced age
- Severe illness

GENERAL PREVENTION
- Enteric isolation precautions are recommended for patients with *C. difficile*-associated diarrhea or colitis, and patients should be moved to a private room, if possible.
- Educate personnel to use gloves when in contact with patients with *C. difficile* infection and for the handling of body substances.
- Avoid nonessential antibiotics.

PATHOPHYSIOLOGY
- The first step in development of *C. difficile* colonization is disruption of the normal flora of the colon, usually caused by antibiotics or, in unusual cases, by certain antineoplastic drugs.
- The antibiotics most frequently associated with *C. difficile* infection are clindamycin, ampicillin, amoxicillin, and the cephalosporins. However, all broad-spectrum antibiotics can lead to the infection.
- Some strains of *C. difficile* are non toxigenic, but the majority makes 2 protein exotoxins: Toxin A and toxin B.
- Toxin A is mainly responsible for the disease, but toxin B is a much more potent cytotoxin in tissue culture.

ETIOLOGY
- *C. difficile*, a gram-positive, spore-forming anaerobic bacillus, is the most common identifiable pathogen causing antibiotic-associated diarrhea and colitis.
- Possible pathogens of antibiotic-associated diarrhea in *C. difficile*-negative patients include the following:
  – Salmonella
  – *Clostridium perfringens*
  – *Candida albicans*
  – *Staphylococcus aureus*
  – In most cases of antibiotic-associated diarrhea in which *C. difficile* is not detected, no etiologic agent is identified.

 DIAGNOSIS

HISTORY
- The clinical presentation is variable and includes diarrhea, colitis without pseudomembranes, pseudomembranous colitis, and fulminant colitis.
- Mild to moderate infection is usually accompanied by lower abdominal cramping pain, but no systemic symptoms or physical findings.
- Moderate or severe colitis usually presents with profuse diarrhea, abdominal distention with pain, and, in some cases, occult colonic bleeding. Also, systemic symptoms such as fever, nausea, anorexia, and malaise are usually present.

- A minority of patients have disease primarily in the cecum and right colon, presenting with marked leukocytosis and abdominal pain but little or no diarrhea.

Antibiotic-associated diarrhea not related to *C. Difficile*
- Diarrhea is dose-related, usually mild, and not accompanied by abdominal pain or fever.
- There is often history of diarrhea with the same antibiotic, and symptoms usually resolve quickly after discontinuation of the inciting antibiotic.

PHYSICAL EXAM
- Abdominal tenderness (mild to severe)
- Surgical abdomen
- Patients can appear toxic

DIAGNOSTIC TESTS & INTERPRETATION
Lab
Initial lab tests
- Enzyme immunoassay (EIA) testing for *C. difficile* toxins A and B
- CBC with differential
- Leukocytosis with a left shift and fecal leukocytes in about 50–60% of cases
- The average peripheral count is 12,000–20,000/mm^3, but occasionally the peripheral count is higher and cases of leukemoid reaction have been described.

Follow-Up & Special Considerations
C. difficile can be isolated by anaerobic stool culture, but this test is seldom used because it takes 2–3 days to complete and does not distinguish toxigenic from non-toxigenic strains.

Imaging
- Diffusely thickened or edematous colonic mucosa may sometimes be seen by abdominal CT scan and may be very suggestive of the *C. difficile*-associated diarrhea or colitis.
- Endoscopy for *C. difficile*-associated diarrhea and colitis is reserved for special situations, such as when other diseases need to be ruled out, rapid diagnosis is necessary, or a stool sample cannot be obtained because the patient develops ileus.
- The results of sigmoidoscopy may be normal in patients with mild disease or limited right-sided disease.
- 10% of episodes of colitis involve only the right colon and may be missed by flexible sigmoidoscopy.

Diagnostic Procedures/Other

- Gram stain of fecal specimens is of no value in diagnosing *C. difficile*-associated diarrhea.
- The most sensitive (94–100%) and specific (99%) test for diagnosis of *C. difficile* infection is a tissue culture assay for the cytotoxicity of toxin B. However, the test takes 1–3 days to complete and requires tissue culture facilities.
- Enzyme-linked immunosorbent assays have been developed and have a sensitivity of 71–94% and a specificity of 92–98%. Because of the rapidity of testing and ease of performance, these tests are most frequently used by clinical laboratories for diagnosis of *C. difficile* infection.
- Approximately 20% of patients may require more than one stool assay to detect *C. difficile* toxin. When *C. difficile* infection is suspected, a single stool specimen should be sent. If the results are negative and diarrhea persists, 1 or 2 additional stool samples could be sent.

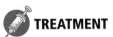 **TREATMENT**

MEDICATION
First Line

- The inciting antibiotic should be discontinued if possible.
- Supportive therapy with fluids and electrolytes should be instituted, as needed.
- Antibiotic-associated diarrhea will resolve without specific antimicrobial therapy in up to one-fourth of patients with infection and in almost all cases of non-*C. difficile*-associated diarrhea due to antibiotics.
- Antiperistaltic and opiate drugs should be avoided in patients with *C. difficile*-associated diarrhea, because they mask symptoms, may worsen the course of the disease, and increase the risk of complications.
- Antibiotic therapy is indicated for patients with moderate or severe infection with *C. difficile*, and antimicrobial therapy can be instituted even before the laboratory results are available.
- Oral metronidazole (500 mg t.i.d) or vancomycin (125 mg q.i.d orally) is the antibiotic most commonly used. The duration of initial therapy is usually 10–14 days (or therapy may be continued until 1 week after completion of the inciting antibiotic, if that therapy cannot be stopped earlier).

- Because of lower cost and avoidance of selective pressure for vancomycin-resistant organisms such as vancomycin-resistant enterococci, initial therapy with metronidazole is currently the preferred initial therapy for *C. difficile* colitis. Vancomycin is the drug of choice for patients with severe disease. Vancomycin is also given to those women who are pregnant or in children <10 years of age, in whom metronidazole should be avoided if possible.

Second Line
- Oral bacitracin (20,000–25,000 U q.i.d)
- For critically ill patients who are unable to take oral antimicrobials, treatment is empirical and includes administration of vancomycin by rectal enema or through long catheters in the small intestine, or, occasionally, surgery (usually subtotal colectomy).
- Mild relapses can be managed without further antibiotic treatment.
- Because the relapses are not related to development of resistance, another 10- to 14-day course of either oral metronidazole or vancomycin can be administered. In cases of recurrent *C. difficile*-associated diarrhea, most clinicians employ tapering oral doses of vancomycin over a 6-week period:
  - Week 1: Vancomycin 125 mg q.i.d
  - Week 2: Vancomycin 125 mg b.i.d
  - Week 3: Vancomycin 125 mg per day
  - Week 4: Vancomycin 125 mg q.i.d
  - Weeks 5 and 6: Vancomycin 125 mg every 3 days

COMPLEMENTARY & ALTERNATIVE THERAPIES
Fecal transplants have been used for severe and recurrent disease.

 ONGOING CARE

FOLLOW-UP RECOMMENDATIONS
- Approximately 2–3% of patients develop fulminant colitis, with ileus, toxic megacolon, perforation, and death.
- The relapse rate among patients with *C. difficile* infection is 10–20%. A smaller number of patients have multiple relapses.

Patient Monitoring
- No diagnostic testing at the end of treatment or during follow-up is needed, unless symptoms recur.
- Clinicians should monitor patients for the development of complications of *C. difficile* infection.
- The development of life-threatening complications (ileus, toxic megacolon, perforation, etc.) might be accompanied by a decrease in diarrhea due to loss of colonic muscular tone and ileus.

COMPLICATIONS
- *C. difficile* diarrhea and colitis can complicate idiopathic inflammatory bowel disease or lead to the following:
  - Hyperpyrexia
  - Fulminant colitis
  - Ileus
  - Perforation
  - Toxic megacolon
  - Reactive arthritis
  - Chronic diarrhea
  - Hypoalbuminemia with anasarca

ADDITIONAL READING

- Cohen SH, Gerding DN, Johnson S, et al. Clinical practice guidelines for Clostridium difficile infection in adults: 2010 update by the society for healthcare epidemiology of America (SHEA) and the infectious diseases society of America (IDSA). *Infect Control Hosp Epidemiol* 2010;31:431.
- Fekety R, McFarland LV, Surawicz CM, et al. Recurrent Clostridium difficile diarrhea: Characteristics of and risk factors for patients enrolled in a prospective, randomized, double-blinded trial. *Clin Infect Dis* 1997;24:324.
- Kelly CP, LaMont JT. Clostridium difficile—more difficult than ever. *N Engl J Med* 2008;359:1932.
- Miller M, Gravel D, Mulvey M, et al. Health care-associated Clostridium difficile infection in Canada: Patient age and infecting strain type are highly predictive of severe outcome and mortality. *Clin Infect Dis* 2010;50:194.
- Zar FA, Bakkanagari SR, Moorthi KM, Davis MB. A comparison of vancomycin and metronidazole for the treatment of Clostridium difficile-associated diarrhea, stratified by disease severity. *Clin Infect Dis* 2007;45:302.

 CODES

ICD9
- 008.45 Intestinal infection due to clostridium difficile
- 787.91 Diarrhea

APPENDICITIS
Luisa M. Stamm (E. Mylonakis, Editor)

 BASICS

DESCRIPTION
- Appendicitis is inflammation of the appendix.
- When the blood supply to the appendix is compromised, then it is called "gangrenous appendicitis."
- When appendicitis is complicated by perforation, it is called "perforating appendicitis."
- When the cause of appendicitis is an obstruction of the lumen, it is called "obstructive appendicitis."

EPIDEMIOLOGY
Incidence
- Appendectomy is the most frequent indication for abdominal surgery.
- Each year in the US there are at least 250,000 cases of appendicitis, requiring >1 million inpatient hospital days.
- The appendix is normal in up to one third of patients who undergo emergency appendectomy.
- Missed appendicitis is among the most frequently successful malpractice claims against emergency department physicians.

RISK FACTORS
- Males have slightly higher rate than females; the male-to-female ratio is 3:2.
- The lifetime risk of appendicitis is 8.5% in men and 6.7% in women.
- Acute appendicitis can occur at any time, but the maximum incidence occurs in the second and third decades.
- Perforation is more common in infants and in the elderly.

PATHOPHYSIOLOGY
- Luminal obstruction is the primary cause of appendicitis.
- Obstruction is most commonly caused by a fecalith but can also be caused by foreign bodies, enlarged lymphoid hyperplasia associated with viral infections (e.g., measles), worms, or tumors (e.g., carcinoid or carcinoma).
- Behind the obstruction, mucus accumulates and luminal bacteria multiply and invade the appendiceal wall resulting in venous engorgement and subsequent arterial compromise and ischemia as a result of the high intraluminal pressures.
- Finally, gangrene and perforation occur.
- Rupture of primary appendiceal abscesses may produce fistulas.
- Occasionally, acute appendicitis may be the first manifestation of Crohn's disease.
- Rarely, recurrent acute appendicitis with complete resolution of inflammation and symptoms between attacks can occur.

ETIOLOGY
- Overgrowth with multiple gastrointestinal bacteria (*E. coli*, *Peptostreptococcus*, *B. fragilis*, Enterobacteriaceae, viridans streptococcus) occurs within the obstructed appendix.
- Chronic infection of the appendix with tuberculosis, amebiasis, and actinomycosis may occur.

DIAGNOSIS

HISTORY
- The onset of pain occurs over several hours. The initial visceral abdominal pain of appendicitis is colicky and usually poorly localized in the periumbilical or epigastric region. As inflammation spreads to the parietal peritoneal surfaces, the pain becomes somatic, steady, and more severe. It is aggravated by movement or cough and localizes in the right lower quadrant (McBurney's point).
- There is often an accompanying urge to defecate or pass flatus, neither of which relieves the distress.
- Anorexia is so frequent that the presence of hunger should arouse suspicion of the diagnosis of acute appendicitis.
- Nausea and vomiting occur in 50–60% of cases, but vomiting is rarely profuse and protracted.
- The development of nausea and vomiting before the onset of pain is extremely rare.
- Urinary frequency and dysuria occur if the appendix lies adjacent to the bladder.

PHYSICAL EXAM
- Physical findings vary with time after onset of the illness and according to the location of the appendix.
- While tenderness is sometimes absent in the early visceral stage of the disease, it ultimately develops and is found in the location corresponding to the position of the appendix. Pregnant women often present with right upper quadrant pain.
- Guarding is due to parietal peritoneal involvement. Tenderness with percussion, rebound tenderness, and referred rebound tenderness are also often present. The rebound tenderness in the right lower quadrant upon palpation of the left lower quadrant is called "Rovsing's sign." Pain elicited on passive flexion of the right hip is called "the psoas sign"; pain elicited on internal rotation of the right hip is called "the obturator sign."
- The temperature is usually normal or slightly elevated, but temperature above 38.3°C (101°F) suggests the presence of perforation.
- A palpable mass in the right lower quadrant suggests an abscess or cecal carcinoma.

DIAGNOSTIC TESTS & INTERPRETATION
Lab
- Leukocytosis of 10,000–18,000 cells per milliliter with a left shift is common, but the absence of leukocytosis does not eliminate the possibility of acute appendicitis.
- A pregnancy test should be performed in all women of childbearing age to rule out uterine or ectopic pregnancy.

Imaging
Initial approach
- Of the noninvasive diagnostic aids, appendiceal CT has proved more precise, with an accuracy of >90%.
- The highest accuracy has been reported with the use of helical CT after the instillation of 3% diatrizoate meglumine (Gastrografin)–saline solution into the colon.
- Appendiceal CT is safe, can be performed in approximately 15 minutes, and requires only one third of the radiation exposure of standard CT of the abdomen and the pelvis.
- Routine appendiceal CT performed in patients who present with suspected appendicitis improves patient care and reduces the use of hospital resources.
- Ultrasound is most useful in women of childbearing age to exclude ovarian cysts, ectopic pregnancy, or tuboovarian abscess. It is also used in pediatrics.
- Normal ultrasonographic findings should not deter the surgeon from performing an appendectomy if the history is indicative of appendicitis and unequivocal tenderness is present in the right lower quadrant.

Follow-Up & Special Considerations
- The management options available to physicians examining patients with suspected appendicitis include observation, diagnostic imaging, laparoscopy, and appendectomy.
- Patients with a history very consistent for appendicitis are often taken to the operating room for laparoscopy regardless of imaging results.
- Patients with a less convincing history are often imaged or observed.

Pathological Findings
Pathology samples from acute appendicitis contain signs of inflammation such as polymorphonuclear cells, edema and vascular congestion within the appendiceal walls.

DIFFERENTIAL DIAGNOSIS
- In the history, the absence of right lower quadrant pain, the absence of the classic migration of pain, and the presence of similar pain previously make appendicitis less likely. In the physical examination, the lack of right lower quadrant pain, rigidity, or guarding makes appendicitis less likely.
- The differential diagnosis of acute appendicitis includes the following:
  - Acute cholecystitis
  - Acute diverticulitis
  - Acute gastroenteritis
  - Acute pancreatitis
  - Acute pelvic inflammatory disease
  - Endometriosis
  - Mesenteric lymphadenitis
  - Perforated ulcer
  - Pyelonephritis
  - Ruptured graafian follicle or corpus luteum cyst
  - Ruptured tubal pregnancy
  - Strangulating intestinal obstruction
  - Twisted ovarian cyst
  - Ureteral calculus
- The differential diagnosis of acute appendicitis is discussed in more detail in the Section I chapter, "Abdominal Pain and Fever."

 TREATMENT

The primary treatment of appendicitis is prompt surgery (see below). Antibiotics are standard preoperative treatment and should be active against gram-negative aerobes and anaerobes.

MEDICATION
- Antibiotic management is the same as in other intra-abdominal infections and is detailed in the Section II chapters, "Peritonitis" and "Intra-abdominal Abscess."
- In brief, options include:
  - Beta-lactam and beta-lactamase inhibitor (ampicillin–sulbactam, piperacillin–tazobactam, ticarcillin–clavulanate)
  - Ceftriaxone and metronidazole
  - Fluoroquinolone and metronidazole
  - Carbapenem (imipenem, meropenem)

ADDITIONAL TREATMENT
Issues for Referral
Surgery should be involved in the care of a patient with suspected appendicitis from the time of initial presentation.

SURGERY/OTHER PROCEDURES
- Prompt surgical evaluation of a patient with a convincing history of appendicitis and/or imaging suggestive of appendicitis is critical.
- Both laparoscopic and open approaches are acceptable. Patients who receive laparoscopic surgery have less wound infections, less pain, and shorter hospital stays than with those who receive an open operation. However, laparoscopic appendectomies are associated with more frequent intra-abdominal abscesses, longer operative times, and higher operative costs.
- If a palpable mass is present 3–5 days after the onset of symptoms, the operation should be delayed, because a phlegmon rather than a definitive abscess will be found. Such patients should be treated with broad-spectrum antibiotics, parenteral fluids, and rest. Appendectomy should be done safely 3 months later. Should the mass enlarge or the patient become more toxic, drainage of the abscess is necessary.

IN-PATIENT CONSIDERATIONS
Initial Stabilization
If unstable, the patient with appendicitis is likely septic or has a perforated appendix and secondary peritonitis. The patient should be resuscitated with IV fluids and pressors should be initiated, if necessary.

Admission Criteria
Any patient with suspected appendicitis should be admitted.

IV Fluids
Preoperatively, patients should be aggressively hydrated and electrolyte abnormalities should be normalized.

Discharge Criteria
Discharge criteria include normalization of white cell count, resolution of fever, and return of bowel function.

 ONGOING CARE

FOLLOW-UP RECOMMENDATIONS
Close follow-up of patients with abdominal pain who do not receive further diagnostic testing is indicated.

DIET
Patients suspected of having appendicitis should not eat.

PROGNOSIS
- The mortality rate has decreased steadily in Europe and the US to <1 per 100,000.
- For a perforated appendicitis, there is an overall mortality rate of 3%, which increases to 15% in the elderly.

COMPLICATIONS
- Delay in the diagnosis of appendicitis increases the risk of appendiceal perforation and perforation is associated with postoperative complications in up to 40% of patients (compared to 5–10% for simple appendicitis).
- Perforation is rare before 24 hours after onset of symptoms, but the rate is as high as 80% after 48 hours.
- The development of intra-abdominal abscesses or phlegmon usually follows perforation with generalized peritonitis and can be avoided by early diagnosis of the disease.
- Wounds should be followed for signs of infection.
- Portal vein thrombophlebitis and pyogenic liver abscess are uncommon.

REFERENCE
1. Sauerland S, Lefering R, Neugebauer EA. Laparoscopic versus open surgery for suspected appendicitis (Cochrane Review). *Cochrane Database Syst Rev* 2002;CD001546.

 CODES

ICD9
- 540.0 Acute appendicitis with generalized peritonitis
- 540.9 Acute appendicitis without mention of peritonitis
- 541 Appendicitis, unqualified

CLINICAL PEARLS
- Acute appendicitis is the most common cause of an acute abdomen.
- The treatment of acute appendicitis is surgery.
- Broad-spectrum antibiotics are an adjunct to proper surgical management.

ASPERGILLOSIS
Jatin M. Vyas (E. Mylonakis, Editor)

 BASICS

DESCRIPTION
- The term "aspergillosis" has been used to describe a wide range of illnesses, from simple colonization or allergic provocation to localized or disseminated invasive disease.
- Although any organ can be involved, the infection usually affects the lungs, and less often the paranasal sinuses and the central nervous system (CNS).

EPIDEMIOLOGY
Incidence
- The number of species of *Aspergillus* causing invasive disease appears to be expanding. While *A. fumigatus* remains the most common species, *A. flavus*, *A. terreus*, *A. niger*, and *A. versicolor* have also been found to cause aspergillosis.
- Invasive aspergillosis is second in frequency to candidiasis among invasive mycoses in most immunosuppressed groups of patients.

RISK FACTORS
- Granulocytopenia (most significant predisposing factor)
- Hematopoietic cell transplant patients
- Solid-organ transplant patients
- Patients with acute leukemia
- Chronic obstructive pulmonary disease (COPD) patients on steroid therapy
- Prolonged corticosteroid or cytotoxic therapy
- Prolonged use of antibiotics
- Liver failure
- Diabetes mellitus
- Chronic granulomatous disease of childhood
- Acquired immunodeficiency syndrome (AIDS) (CD4 count of 50 cells/mm^3 or less)

Genetics
- Polymorphisms in the Toll-like receptor 4 may increase risk of invasive aspergillosis.
- Polymorphisms in the Toll-like receptor 9 may modulate the risk of allergic bronchopulmonary aspergillosis (ABPA).

GENERAL PREVENTION
- Environmental control measures, especially during construction activities, to prevent conidia from reaching patients at risk.
- Air-flow units with high-efficacy particulate air filters.
- Prophylactic use of voriconazole or amphotericin B might be considered in patients with previous invasive disease who could become neutropenic.

PATHOPHYSIOLOGY
- ABPA
  - *Aspergillus* colonization in atopic patients leads to activation of TH2 CD4+ T cells which in turn drive the expression of IgE and promote eosinophilia.
  - This inflammatory environment exacerbates asthma, leading to worsening symptoms.
  - Airway damage and central bronchiectasis can occur.
- Chronic pulmonary aspergillosis including aspergilloma
  - Typically occurs in patients with the following conditions
    - Prior tuberculosis
    - ABPA
    - Lung cancer with resection
    - Bulla formation
- COPD
  - Lesions show chronic inflammatory changes, fibrosis, and necrosis.
  - Invasion is not seen, unless the patient develops an immunocompromised state.
- Invasive aspergillosis
  - Conidia are ubiquitous and are small enough that, when inhaled, they can reach the alveolus.
  - Alveolar macrophages typically phagocytose these pathogens.
  - In the setting of immunocompromised state, macrophages fail to contain the conidia and then they can germinate into hyphae.
  - The presence of hyphal forms triggers influx of macrophages and elicitation of inflammatory cytokines.
  - Vascular invasion and subsequent tissue necrosis can ensue.
  - Dissemination through the bloodstream is possible.

 DIAGNOSIS

HISTORY
- ABPA
  - Occurs in patients with established asthma or cystic fibrosis
  - Bronchial obstruction can be present
  - Malaise
  - Hemoptysis can rarely be seen
- Chronic aspergillosis
  - Weight loss
  - Cough
  - Hemoptysis
  - Shortness of breath
  - Dyspnea on exertion
- Invasive aspergillosis
  - Pleuritic chest pain
  - Cough
  - Hemoptysis
  - Dyspnea

PHYSICAL EXAM
- ABPA
  - Wheezing can be present, but is not required
  - Fever
- Chronic aspergillosis
  - Abnormal pulmonary auscultation
  - Fever
- Invasive aspergillosis
  - Fever
  - Abnormal pulmonary auscultation

DIAGNOSTIC TESTS & INTERPRETATION
Diagnostic Procedures/Other
- ABPA
  - CXR may show parenchymal infiltrates (typically involving the upper lobes)
  - CT scan – bronchial wall thickening, bronchiectasis, ground-glass opacities
  - Peripheral eosinophilia
  - Immediate reaction to skin testing with *Aspergillus*
  - Elevated total serum IgE
  - Serum IgG to *A. fumigatus*
- Chronic aspergillosis
  - CXR and/or Chest CT show one or more cavities
  - Aspergilloma balls can be seen within the cavity, often surrounded by the air-crescent shadow
  - Serum IgG to *A. fumigatus*
  - Elevated CRP or ESR
- Invasive aspergillosis
  - Positive culture from tissue biopsy is gold standard
  - Evidence of fungal invasion in tissue
  - Positive galactomannan level in serum
  - Positive β-glucan level in serum

TREATMENT

MEDICATION

First Line

- ABPA
  - A combination of glucocorticoids and itraconazole is used.
  - Steroids can be tapered over a course of 3–6 months.
  - In some cases, steroids cannot be tapered and maintenance of steroids is required.
- Chronic aspergillosis
  - Aspergilloma typically requires surgical resection in patients who can tolerate the surgery. Some patients benefit from antifungal therapy (most commonly voriconazole).
  - Chronic pulmonary aspergillosis requires long-term antifungal therapy. Embolization is used in patients to reduce risk of hemoptysis.
- Invasive aspergillosis
  - Voriconazole is considered first-line therapy.
  - Surgical debridement is required whenever possible.

Second Line

- For invasive aspergillosis
  - Alternative agents include amphotericin B, itraconazole, and echinocandins.
  - Combination therapy of the above antimicrobials remains unproven.

SURGERY/OTHER PROCEDURES

Aggressive debridement should be considered for patients with chronic disease or invasive disease.

IN-PATIENT CONSIDERATIONS

Initial Stabilization

- Intravenous or oral antifungals should be initiated as soon as possible.
- Hemodynamic parameters should be stabilized.

Admission Criteria

- Hemodynamically unstable patients
- Patients with hemoptysis
- Some patients with fever and immunocompromised state

ONGOING CARE

FOLLOW-UP RECOMMENDATIONS

- Patients with hypersensitivity lung diseases should be monitored for relapses and for the development of pulmonary fibrosis or bronchiectasis.
- Patients with aspergillomas who do not undergo surgery need clinical and radiographic monitoring for extension of the lesion and development of hemoptysis. Patients who undergo surgery for aspergillomas need to be monitored for relapse of the infection, even after initial surgical success.
- Patients with invasive disease need to be monitored for relapses, especially when they become neutropenic.

Patient Monitoring

Drug monitoring for voriconazole levels (trough level) should be done in patients requiring long-term voriconazole treatment.

PROGNOSIS

The overall prognosis in patients with invasive aspergillosis depends on the burden of fungal organisms and degree of immunosuppression.

COMPLICATIONS

- The most feared complication in chronic pulmonary aspergillosis is hemoptysis.
- Dissemination and death are significant complications in patients with invasive aspergillosis.
- Bronchiectasis can complicate ABPA.
- Pulmonary fibrosis can complicate both ABPA and extrinsic allergic alveolitis.
- Hemoptysis (sometimes massive, especially for lesions located close to the hilum) can complicate both invasive and noninvasive pulmonary aspergillosis.
- Pneumothorax might occur in immunocompromised individuals and is usually associated with improvement of the immune system.
- Introduction of Aspergilli to the pleural space (due to pneumothorax or the development of bronchopleural fistula) can lead to empyema.
- In all cases of pulmonary and extrapulmonary invasive aspergillosis, relentless dissemination to other organs and an increase of the lesion can occur, especially among immunocompromised individuals.
- Patients with CNS involvement can have cerebral vessels occluded by *Aspergillus*.

ADDITIONAL READING

- Segal BH. Aspergillosis. *N Engl J Med* 2009;360(18): 1870–1884.
- Walsh TJ, Anaissie EJ, Denning DW, et al. Treatment of aspergillosis: Clinical practice guidelines of the Infectious Diseases Society of America. *Clin Infect Dis* 2008;46:327–360.

CODES

ICD9

- 117.3 Aspergillosis
- 518.6 Allergic bronchopulmonary aspergilliosis

CLINICAL PEARLS

- Invasive aspergillosis is a medical emergency. Prompt treatment is required to optimize outcomes.

ATYPICAL MYCOBACTERIA

Emily P. Hyle (E. Mylonakis, Editor)

 BASICS

DESCRIPTION
Infection by 1 of the species of nontuberculous mycobacteria (NTM).

Pediatric Considerations
- Atypical mycobacteria should be considered in patients with unilateral cervical lymphadenitis (1).
- Most commonly, this infection occurs in children aged 1–5 years.
- Swelling often occurs around the affected nodes, usually in the anterior cervical chain. The adenitis may enlarge rapidly, and fistula formation through the skin is common. Enlarged nodes are often painless.
- Systemic symptoms are rare.
- Most symptoms are caused by MAC; *Mycobacterium scrofulaceum* and *Mycobacterium tuberculosis* are also encountered, but less frequently.

EPIDEMIOLOGY
Incidence
300 cases of MAC lymphadenitis annually in the US.

Prevalence
- 1–7.2 cases/100,000 in the US.
- Highly variable, depending on location.
- ~ 50% of NTM isolates are pathogens.

RISK FACTORS
- Age
- Immunosuppression
- HIV with low CD4 cell counts or other opportunistic infections
- Interferon (IFN)-gamma deficiencies
- Underlying structural pulmonary disease

Genetics
IFNγR1 or IL-12βR1 deficiency

GENERAL PREVENTION
In AIDS patients (CD4 count <100 cells/mm^3), weekly azithromycin 1200 mg is indicated as primary prophylaxis. Other prophylactic regimens include clarithromycin 500 mg t.i.d. or rifabutin 300 mg daily.

PATHOPHYSIOLOGY
- Soil, water, and other environmental exposures; hot tubs and tap water are often implicated.
- Human-to-human transmission has not been documented.
- Primary infection by ingestion or inhalation; no concern for reactivation.
- Granuloma formation results from interplay between macrophages, lymphocytes, and natural-killer cells.
- Disseminated disease originates from localized infection.

ETIOLOGY
- Aerobic, nonspore-forming bacilli with mycolic acid-containing cell walls (2).
- Rapid-growing organisms include the following rapid-growing mycobacteria (RGM) (growth within 7 days):
  - *Mycobacterium fortuitum complex*
  - *Mycobacterium chelonae/abscessus*
  - *Mycobacterium smegmatis*
- Intermediate-growing organisms include the following:
  - *Mycobacterium marinum*
  - *Mycobacterium gordonae*
- Slow-growing organisms (10–21 days) include the following:
  - *Mycobacterium avium* complex (MAC)
  - *Mycobacterium kansasii*
  - *Mycobacterium xenopi*
  - *Mycobacterium scrofulaceum*
  - *Mycobacterium haemophilum*
  - *Mycobacterium ulcerans*

COMMONLY ASSOCIATED CONDITIONS
- Immunosuppression, e.g., AIDS, transplant patients
- TNF-inhibitor use
- Cystic fibrosis
- Pre-existing pulmonary disease: Silicosis, healed tuberculosis, bronchiectasis, or chronic obstructive lung disease

 DIAGNOSIS

CLINICAL SYNDROMES
- Pulmonary
- Lymphadenitis
- Skin and soft tissue
- Osteoarticular
- Catheter-related
- Disseminated

HISTORY
- Pulmonary: Chronic cough usually productive of sputum. More advanced disease is associated with constitutional symptoms (e.g., weight loss, fatigue) and can include dyspnea, hemoptysis, chest pain (2)
- Soft tissue: Often associated with inoculation or recent surgery or instrumentation
- Osteoarticular
- Disseminated: Fevers, fatigue, anorexia.
- Exposures: Water (skin/soft tissue), catheters (bacteremia)
- Immunosuppression

PHYSICAL EXAM
- Pulmonary: Crackles, wheezes, squeaks. Pectus excavatum (27%) and scoliosis (52%) are more common in patients with pulmonary MAC.
- Soft tissue: Small, papular lesions, usually on the extremities; can be ulcerated and spread locally or along lymphatics.
- Lymphadenitis: Painless or mildly painful enlarged but not fluctuant lymph node usually in submandibular or jugular region.

DIAGNOSTIC TESTS & INTERPRETATION
Lab
- Pancytopenia can occur (marrow suppression) in disseminated disease.
- Elevated alkaline phosphatase can be seen in 5% of disseminated MAC (20–40× normal).
- Mycobacterial blood cultures positive in 90% of disseminated cases.

Imaging
Initial approach
Chest x-ray (CXR) or chest CT (pulmonary): Upper lobe cavitary disease, nodular or reticulonodular disease, or adenopathy. Pleural effusions are rare.

Follow-Up & Special Considerations
- Serial imaging to follow for progression (if asymptomatic) or improvement (when on therapy).
- Cavitary disease in 60–90% of MAC pulmonary infections. Cavitations can be 2–4 cm and are typically thin-walled.

Diagnostic Procedures/Other
- Tissue for acid-fast bacillus (AFB) smear, mycobacterial culture, and pathology is essential given that these organisms can be colonizers (2).
- In pulmonary disease, 3 or more sputum samples (or bronchoalveolar lavage) for culture are recommended.
- RNA probes can be used for preliminary identification of *M. tuberculosis*, MAC, and *M. kansasii* from positive cultures.
- Once isolated, mycobacterial cultures should be sent to a specialized center for confirmatory identification and antimicrobial susceptibility testing.

Pathological Findings
- Granuloma with giant cells and acid-fast bacilli evident in localized infection (2).
- In disseminated disease, it is less likely to see well-formed granuloma.

DIFFERENTIAL DIAGNOSIS
- MTb
- Other NTM
- Endemic fungi (histoplasmosis, cryptococcus, blastomycosis, nocardia)
- Underlying structural pulmonary disease

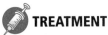

TREATMENT
MEDICATION
First Line
- MAC (pulmonary): Rifampin 600 mg daily, ethambutol 15 or 25 mg/kg daily depending on radiographic pattern, azithromycin or clarithromycin 500 mg with addition of aminoglycoside as needed (2).
- Kansasii (pulmonary): Isoniazid 300 mg daily, rifampin 600 mg daily, ethambutol 15 mg/kg daily.
- RGM (soft tissue): 2 of the following agents for which the isolate is susceptible: Trimethoprim–sulfamethoxazole (TMP-SMX), doxycycline, levofloxacin, clarithromycin.
- *Abscessus* (severe): Amikacin + clarithromycin + cefoxitin or imipenem
- Fortuitum or chelonae (severe): Amikacin or tobramycin + cefoxitin +/– imipenem +/– levofloxacin.
- MAC (disseminated/HIV): Clarithromycin 500 mg p.o. b.i.d. or azithromycin 500–600 mg p.o. b.i.d. and ethambutol 15 mg/kg p.o. daily; consideration of adding rifampin with input of ID.
- *M. marinum* (soft tissue): Clarithromycin 500 mg p.o. b.i.d. and ethambutol 15 mg/kg with the addition of rifampin for osteomyelitis and consideration of surgical debridement. Mild disease could be treated with clarithromycin alone.

Second Line
- Moxifloxacin 400 mg daily
- Amikacin
- *M. abscessus*: Linezolid, doxycycline, TMP–SMX

ADDITIONAL TREATMENT
General Measures
- Susceptibility testing should be obtained for MAC (clarithromycin), *kansasii* (rifampin), and RGM (8 drugs on susceptibility panel) (2).
- Treatment is for long duration; for pulmonary MAC, treat for 12 months after cultures become negative (12–24 months total) and for disseminated MAC, treat for 12 months or 6 months beyond when CD4 is >100 cells/mm^3.
- Skin and soft tissue infections may need 3 months of treatment or more.
- Catheter-based infections requires 6–12 weeks of treatment after catheter removal.

Issues for Referral
Because of the drug resistance of these indolent organisms, specialists with knowledge of these infections are needed for treatment. At times, patients require years of therapy.

SURGERY/OTHER PROCEDURES
- MAC: Lung resection should be considered in those patients with upper lobe disease especially if they cannot tolerate medical therapy or with culture positivity after 6 months of abx.
- MAC lymphadenitis: Resection is associated with 90% cure rate without antimicrobials.
- I&D for soft tissue infections or tenosynovitis, particularly for RGM.

IN-PATIENT CONSIDERATIONS
Admission Criteria
- For diagnostic workup.
- For initiation of parenteral antibiotics.

ONGOING CARE
FOLLOW-UP RECOMMENDATIONS
- Given antimicrobial toxicities, monthly follow-up in initial phases of treatment is often recommended.
- After patients have tolerated medications, can extend intervals of follow-up.

Patient Monitoring
- Safety labs for drug toxicities.
- Screening for drug–drug interactions.
- Therapeutic drug monitoring for antimicrobial peaks and troughs.

PROGNOSIS
Depends on location of disease, identification of NTM, and specific host.

COMPLICATIONS
- Safety labs for drug toxicities.
- Consideration of drug–drug interactions.
- Disseminated MAC: Intussusception, GI bleeding, bowel obstruction can occur but are rare.
- MAC lymphadenitis: Ulceration and fistula formation.

REFERENCES
1. Mandell GL, Bennett JE, Dolin R. *Principles and practice of infectious diseases.* 7th ed. Philadelphia, PA: Churchill Livingstone/Elsevier, 2010.
2. Griffith DE, Aksamit T, Brown-Elliot BA, et al. An official ATS/IDSA Statement: Diagnosis, treatment, and prevention of nontuberculous mycobacterial diseases. *Am J Respir Crit Care Med* 2007;175: 367–416.

ADDITIONAL READING
- Cassidy PM, Hedberg K, Saulson A, McNelly E, Winthrop KL. Nontuberculous mycobacterial disease prevalence and risk factors: A changing epidemiology. *CID* 2009;49:e124–e129.
- Han XY, De I, Jacobson KL. Rapidly growing mycobacteria: Clinical and microbiologic studies of 115 cases. *Am J Clin Pathol* 2007;128:612–621.
- Piersimoni C, Scarparo C. Extrapulmonary infections associated with nontuberculous mycobacteria in immunocompetent persons. *Emerg Infect Dis (CDC website)* http://www.cdc.gov/eid/content/15/9/1351.htm.

 CODES

ICD9
- 031.1 Cutaneous diseases due to other mycobacteria
- 031.8 Other specified mycobacterial diseases
- 031.9 Unspecified diseases due to mycobacteria

CLINICAL PEARLS
- NTM can act as colonizers or pathogens; careful evaluation with cultures and pathology is essential in order to plan appropriate therapy.
- Although severe infection occurs more frequently in the immunocompromised, immunocompetent patients can also have severe disease.
- Antimicrobial therapy is typically for long durations and requires careful monitoring, given toxicities of medications.
- NTM drug-susceptibility testing must be considered carefully because in vitro testing does not have directly applicability to clinical decision making.

BABESIOSIS

Maged Muhammed
Isaac I. Bogoch
Eleftherios Mylonakis

 BASICS

DESCRIPTION
- Babesia is a protozoa with affinity for human red blood cells. It is a common cause of hemolytic disease in endemic areas.
- The main mechanism for transmission of *Babesia microti* is through deer tick bites (Ixodid species). Other less common routes of transmission include blood transfusions and maternally transmitted babesiosis.
- Northeastern and Midwestern US is where most *B. microti* is found. Other Babesia species exist in western US and Europe (1).

EPIDEMIOLOGY
- Babesia is considered an emerging infectious disease as there are an increasing number of reported cases in the last decade (2).
- Increases in deer populations, tick density, and greater human activity in endemic areas are thought to contribute to the rise in Babesia infections.
- Many cases of Babesia are subclinical in younger individuals so the prevalence of this infection is likely underestimated. Data from blood donors demonstrate that 0.5–15% of individuals have been exposed in highly endemic areas.

RISK FACTORS
- Living in/or traveling to endemic regions.
- Asplenic patients.
- Immunosuppression (e.g., HIV, chemotherapy).

GENERAL PREVENTION
- Endemic areas can be avoided in seasons of high transmission (May through October) especially by asplenic and immunocompromised persons who are at risk of severe illness (3).
- Insect repellant is helpful for the prevention of tick bite, specifically products with *N*-diethyl-meta-toluamide (DEET).
- Early removal of ticks is important; the tick must remain attached for at least 24 hours before the transmission occurs. Daily self-examination is recommended for persons who engage in outdoor activities in endemic areas.
- Examining pets for ticks is recommended in endemic areas.
- Clothes can be treated with permethrin to prevent infection.

PATHOPHYSIOLOGY
The life cycle involves transmission of Babesia between vertebrate hosts and Ixodes ticks. Humans are "dead end" and "accidental" hosts as the primary contact points for *B. microti* are between white-footed mice and ticks. Although humans may become ill when infected, humans do not play a role in the transmission of infection. *Ixodes* ticks transmit the sporozoite to host blood. The sporozoites invade the erythrocytes and become trophozoites. The trophozoites replicate asexually by budding, yielding 2–4 merozoites. The merozoites disrupt RBCs and invade other RBCs leading to hemolysis and anemia.

ETIOLOGY
- The most common cause of Babesia in the US is *B. microti* found in New England, coastal New York, and Midwest regions.
- Other common Babesia species that cause disease in humans include *Babesia divergens* in Europe and *Babesia duncani* in Western US.

COMMONLY ASSOCIATED CONDITIONS
- Co-infection with Lyme disease and human granulocytic anaplasmosis is common as both are transmitted by Ixodes ticks in endemic regions (4).
- In the endemic areas, up to 10% of patients with Lyme disease are co-infected with Babesia.

DIAGNOSIS

HISTORY
Patients may be asymptomatic or report the following symptoms:
- Fever
- Chills
- Weakness
- Headache
- Nausea/vomiting
- Abdominal pain
- Diarrhea
- Joint pain
- Shortness of breath/chest pain
- Dark urine
- Also ask about recent Lyme infection, travel/living in endemic areas, outdoor exposures, pets, recent tick bites

PHYSICAL EXAM
- Fever
- Splenomegaly
- Hepatomegaly
- Pallor
- Jaundice
- Absence of lymphadenopathy
- Look for a rash consistent with erythema chronicum migrans in cases of Lyme co-infection

DIAGNOSTIC TESTS & INTERPRETATION
Lab
Initial lab tests
- Thin blood smears to assess for intra-erythrocytic parasites and evidence of hemolysis. Multiple blood smears may be necessary over several days in cases of low parasitemia and in early onset of infection.
- Complete blood count: Anemia and thrombocytopenia.
- Evidence of hemolysis: Elevated reticulocyte count, LDH, and indirect bilirubin. Also low haptoglobin.
- Liver function tests.

Follow-Up & Special Considerations
- If the organism is not detected by blood smear, PCR amplification of 18 srRNA is recommended.
- In patients with a high probability of infection, indirect immunofluorescent antibody testing is recommended when both blood smear and PCR are negative.

Imaging
Usually imaging is not necessary in mild cases. Abdominal ultrasonography will confirm hepatomegaly or splenomegaly.

Pathological Findings
Like malaria, Babesia appears as an intra-erythrocytic parasite. Babesia parasites can be visualized outside of red blood cells in heavy infection – this is not seen in malarial infections. Occasionally, Babesia parasites (in the intracellular merozoite phase) appear in tetrads, known as the "Maltese cross."

DIFFERENTIAL DIAGNOSIS
- Sepsis
- Lyme
- Human granulocytic anaplasmosis
- Hepatitis
- Malaria
- Lymphoma

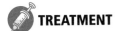

TREATMENT

MEDICATION

First Line
For *B. microti* infection: 7–10 days of oral atovaquone 750 mg 2 times per day plus oral azithromycin 500–1,000 mg/day on day 1, followed by 250 mg/day afterwards.

Second Line
For *B. microti* infection: Oral quinine 650 mg, 3 or 4 times a day plus oral clindamycin 600 mg 3 times a day for 7–10 days. Intravenous formulations can be used. Quinine and clindamycin are used in severe cases.

ADDITIONAL TREATMENT

General Measures
- Asymptomatic individuals who are immunocompetent and have detectable parasites on blood smear for less than 3 months do not require treatment (5).
- Longer treatment courses may be necessary in immunocompromised hosts or in cases of high parasite burden. Treatment should continue for at least 6 weeks, including 2 weeks of therapy after parasites are no longer detectable in blood smears.

Issues for Referral
An infectious disease specialist should be involved if there are signs or symptoms of severe infection or infection in an immunocompromised host.

Additional Therapies
Red blood cell exchange transfusions may be necessary in severe cases where parasitemia is high (>10%) or there are symptoms of shock/ARDS.

ONGOING CARE

FOLLOW-UP RECOMMENDATIONS

Patient Monitoring
Hospitalized patients should have a CBC and blood smear checked daily to monitor hemolysis, anemia, and parasite burden.

PATIENT EDUCATION
Inform patients about risk factors for acquiring Babesia and take precautions to avoid re-infection.

COMPLICATIONS
- DIC
- Anemia
- CHF
- ARDS
- Renal dysfunction
- Hypotension

REFERENCES

1. Vannier E, Gewurz BE, Krause PJ. Human babesiosis. *Infect Dis Clin North Am* 2008;22: 469–488.
2. Krause PJ, McKay K, Gadbaw J, et al. Increasing health burden of human babesiosis in endemic sites. *Am J Trop Med Hyg* 2003;68:431–436.
3. Mylonakis E. When to suspect and how to monitor babesiosis. *Am Fam Physician* 2001;63: 1969–1974.
4. Wormser GP, Dattwyler RJ, Shapiro ED, et al. The clinical assessment, treatment, and prevention of Lyme disease, human granulocytic anaplasmosis, and babesiosis: Clinical practice guidelines by the Infectious Diseases Society of America. *Clin Infect Dis* 2006;43(9):1089–1134.
5. Krause PJ, Gewurz BE, Hill D, et al. Persistent and relapsing babesiosis in immunocompromised patients. *Clin Infect Dis* 2008;46(3):370–376.

CODES

ICD9
088.82 Babesiosis

CLINICAL PEARLS
- Red blood cell exchange transfusion is recommended in case of severe disease with end organ failure.
- Unless the parasitemia has persisted for more than 3 months, there is no need to treat asymptomatic cases of babesiosis in immunocompetent hosts.

BACILLARY ANGIOMATOSIS/PELIOSIS HEPATICA

Paschalis Vergidis
Matthew E. Falagas

 BASICS

DESCRIPTION
- Rare, vascular proliferative infectious disease of the skin and viscera, most commonly seen in the immunosuppressed (T-cell deficiencies), especially HIV-positive individuals.
- The term bacillary angiomatosis (BA) mainly describes the cutaneous/disseminated form, while the term peliosis hepatica (PH) describes the visceral form of this febrile illness related to *Bartonella* species.

EPIDEMIOLOGY
Prevalence
This globally encountered disease is rare; isolated cases have been described from all areas of the world.

RISK FACTORS
- HIV infection (CD4 <100) (1)
- Other forms of immunosuppression
- Poor sanitary conditions, contact with cats

GENERAL PREVENTION
- For HIV-positive or otherwise immunocompromised patients, regarding cats: It is best to obtain a cat over 1 year of age and in good health. The patient should observe careful hand-washing after litter box cleaning. Avoid bites and scratches; hand-wash if they happen. Declawing or testing a cat is not suggested.
- Primary prophylaxis is not recommended. However, prophylaxis using a macrolide is protective against *Bartonella* infection.
- The possible necessity of secondary prophylaxis or life-long continuation of treatment in HIV-positive patients has not been defined.

ETIOLOGY
- *Bartonella henselae* (mainly BA) and *Bartonella quintana* (mainly bacteremia).
- *Bartonella* species are gram-negative organisms of the alpha Proteobacteria family.
- *B. henselae* infection is linked to cat exposure in patients with HIV infection. In contrast, BA caused by *B. quintana* is associated with body louse infestation and homelessness.

 DIAGNOSIS

HISTORY
- The incubation period is of at least 1 week.
- Manifestations range from isolated bacteremia to skin and visceral (PH) disease, as well as multiple organ (skin, bones, central nervous system) involvement.
- If untreated, it can be fatal.
- BA:
  - Constitutional: Fever, malaise, weight loss, anemia
- PH:
  - Constitutional: Persistent fever, malaise, weight loss, abdominal pain
  - Gastrointestinal symptoms: Nausea, vomiting
- Other organ/system symptoms depend on the specific part of the body affected (i.e., bone pain, neurological deficits etc.).

PHYSICAL EXAM
- BA:
  - Cutaneous manifestations (93% of patients):
    ○ Elevated, bright red papules, from one to hundreds in number and from 1 mm to several centimeters in size, in two-thirds of patients.
    ○ Smaller lesions can be covered with an attenuated epidermis, while larger ones tend to erode and bleed easily.
    ○ A surrounding collarette is common.
    ○ Subcutaneous nodular lesions (in one-fourth of patients) are usually large, and there may be no overlying skin change.
    ○ Cellulitic plaque-like lesions (in 5–10% of patients) often overlie deeper osseous lesions.
    ○ Ulcerations and folliculitis lesions are rare.
    ○ Lesions occur in any part of the body; several forms develop concurrently or sequentially.
  - Extracutaneous manifestations: These are mainly bone and visceral (liver, spleen) lesions, but several other organ/system involvements have been reported, with or without vascular proliferation changes, painful or painless lymphadenopathy, and brain abscesses. Bone disease can begin with pain only and can be accompanied, or not, by overlying skin lesions.
- PH:
  - Massive hepatomegaly, developing over weeks or months
  - Splenomegaly
  - Possible skin or other organ involvement

DIAGNOSTIC TESTS & INTERPRETATION
Lab
- Diagnosis is made by demonstration of causative organisms in hematoxylin and eosin-stained tissue sections (granular purple material); it also may be made by the Warthin-Starry or Brown–Hopps tissue stains.
- Organisms appear individually or in clumps and tangles.
- Obtaining culture is difficult and time consuming. The organism can be isolated from the blood in lysis-centrifugation cultures. Incubate for at least 21 days.
- Polymerase chain reaction (PCR) can be used for detection and species identification (2).
- Sensitivity of serologic methods is low in immunocompromised patients.
- Mild elevation of transaminases (average ×2 of normal), moderate-to-severe elevation of alkaline phosphatase (average ×5 of normal), normal or slightly elevated bilirubin.
- Mild-to-moderate pancytopenia may occur in the visceral type of the disease.

Imaging
- Bone disease: Plain bone x-rays show well-circumscribed lytic areas or ill-defined regions of extensive cortical destruction with aggressive periosteal reaction.
- CT scans can show hepatosplenomegaly and intra-abdominal and/or retroperitoneal lymph node enlargement. Visceral parenchyma can appear heterogeneous in consistency.

Pathological Findings
- Skin, liver, and lymph node biopsy or fine-needle aspiration specimens are usually used.
- The pathologic pattern depends on the organ involved.
- Skin: "Epithelioid hemangioma" appearance of lesions, demonstration of organisms.
- PH: In liver biopsy specimens, markedly dilated, blood-filled cystic spaces can be seen within the parenchyma. They are often associated with a myxoid stroma. Foci of necrosis can be seen in advanced cases.

DIFFERENTIAL DIAGNOSIS
- BA:
  - Kaposi's sarcoma
  - Pyogenic granulomas
  - Angiomas
  - Verruga peruana (bartonellosis, endemic in South America)
- PH:
  - Kaposi's sarcoma
- Extracutaneous manifestations:
  - Other space-occurring lesions
  - The possibility of coexistence with Kaposi's sarcoma should always be considered.

 TREATMENT

MEDICATION
First Line
- An initial evaluation is needed to determine the extent of organ involvement.
- Erythromycin 500 mg p.o. q6h or doxycycline 100 mg q12h (AII)
- Duration of treatment: BA 3 months; PH 4 months. Longer treatment for immunocompromised patients.
- Patients may experience a Jarisch–Herxheimer reaction and should be pretreated with antipyretic agents for the first 72 hours of therapy.

Second Line
- For erythromycin/doxycycline intolerance: Azithromycin or clarithromycin have been associated with clinical response (BIII).
- Combination therapy, with the addition of rifampin (300 mg p.o. twice daily) to either erythromycin or doxycycline, is recommended for immunocompromised patients with acute, life-threatening infection or CNS disease.
- TMP-SMX and ciprofloxacin have shown inconsistent clinical response.

IN-PATIENT CONSIDERATIONS
Admission Criteria
Patients can usually be treated on an outpatient basis; inpatient care and intravenous antibiotics are needed for patients with extensive skin disease, lytic bone lesions, and/or visceral lesions or fulminant disease.

 ONGOING CARE

FOLLOW-UP RECOMMENDATIONS
- After initiation of treatment (about 4–7 days of therapy), significant improvement of skin and visceral/other organ lesions is noted frequently.
- There is usually complete resolution by 3–4 weeks.
- Relapses occur in approximately 15% of cases.
- Treatment failure: On relapse, 4 months of continuous suppressive treatment.

Patient Monitoring
- Clinical monitoring is essential.
- Serial biochemical tests (i.e., liver function tests) may help in monitoring response to treatment of visceral disease.
- Use x-rays or bone scans to monitor bone disease.
- The possibility of coexistence with Kaposi's sarcoma should be considered if imaging findings do not reverse after appropriate antibiotic treatment.

COMPLICATIONS
The visceral form of the disease can be complicated by anemia, pancytopenia due to hypersplenism, and splenic rupture with hemoperitoneum.

REFERENCES
1. Koehler JE, Sanchez MA, Tye S, et al. Prevalence of *Bartonella* infection among human immunodeficiency virus-infected patients with fever. *Clin Infect Dis* 2003;37:559–566.
2. Jensen WA, Fall MZ, Rooney J, et al. Rapid identification and differentiation of *Bartonella* species using a single-step PCR assay. *J Clin Microbiol* 2000;38(5):1717–1722.

ADDITIONAL READING
- Kaplan JE, Benson C, Holmes KH, et al. Guidelines for prevention and treatment of opportunistic infections in HIV-infected adults and adolescents: Recommendations from CDC, the National Institutes of Health, and the HIV Medicine Association of the Infectious Diseases Society of America. *MMWR Recomm Rep* 2009;58(RR-4):1–207; quiz CE1–CE4.
- Rolain JM, Brouqui P, Koehler JE, et al. Recommendations for treatment of human infections caused by *Bartonella* species. *Antimicrob Agents Chemother* 2004;48:1921–1933.

 CODES

ICD9
- 088.0 Bartonellosis

CLINICAL PEARLS
- BA mainly describes the cutaneous/disseminated form, while PH describes the visceral form of this febrile illness related to *Bartonella* species.
- Kaposi's sarcoma should be considered in the differential diagnosis.
- Erythromycin or doxycycline for at least 3–4 months is the treatment of choice.

BALANITIS

Irene S. Kourbeti (E. Mylonakis, Editor)

 BASICS

DESCRIPTION
Inflammation and/or infection on the glans penis. Balanoposthitis includes inflammation of the foreskin. In this chapter we will analyze the infectious etiologies.

EPIDEMIOLOGY
Prevalence
- Sexual exposure; increased incidence in men who have women sexual partners with *Candida* vaginitis.
- Balanitis in young boys often occurs in conjunction with diaper dermatitis.

RISK FACTORS
- Uncircumcised men
- Diabetes, especially new-onset diabetes
- For *Candida*, colonization and infection age is an independent risk factor
- Broad-spectrum antibiotics
- Immunodeficiency
- Poor hygiene

GENERAL PREVENTION
- Circumcision
- Good hygiene
- Treatment of sexual partner(s) if they are diagnosed as having *Candida* vaginitis or *Trichomonas*

ETIOLOGY
The pathogens involved in infectious balanitis, include among others:
- *Candida* spp
- *Trichomonas* spp
- Anaerobic bacteria/*Bacteroides* spp/*Gardnerella vaginalis*
- Chlamydia
- *Neisseria gonorrhoeae*
- Human papillomavirus (HPV)
- Herpes simplex virus (HSV)
- *Treponema pallidum*
- Mycoplasma
- Mycobacterium [Bacillus Calmette–Guerin (BCG)]
- Streptococci (group A and B)
- *Staphylococcus aureus*
- *Borrelia burgdorferi* (Lyme disease)
- *Entamoeba histolytica*

 DIAGNOSIS

- Pain, tenderness
- Erosions
- Erythema
- Pruritus
- Pustules
- With anaerobic infections, foul smell of the glans penis
- Edema

DIAGNOSTIC TESTS & INTERPRETATION
Lab
- Fungal preps usually indicate *Candida*.
- Recently, direct impression on CHROMagar Candida medium as a sampling method resulted in highest yield of *Candida* spp compared to the swabs.
- Wet mount may show *Trichomonas*.
- Wet mount slide for *Gardnerella*.
- Test the urethral discharge for sexually transmitted disease.
- Titers or cultures for evidence of HIV, HPV, HSV.
- Glucose testing to rule out diabetes mellitus.

DIFFERENTIAL DIAGNOSIS
- Noninfectious causes of balanitis
  - Irritants, such as soaps
  - Poor hygiene
  - Trauma
  - Contact dermatitis
  - Circinate balanitis
  - Lichen sclerosus
  - Lichen planus
  - Zoon's balanitis
  - Erythroplasia of Queyrat
  - Pemphigus
  - Pemphigoid
  - Bowen's disease
  - Leukoplakia
  - Fixed drug eruption
- Psoriasis, particularly inverse psoriasis
- Paget's disease
- Nummular eczema
- Scabies
- Squamous cell carcinoma

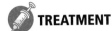 **TREATMENT**

ADDITIONAL TREATMENT

General Measures

- Practice good hygiene, with foreskin retraction and gentle washing of the glans penis.
- For *Candida* balanitis, local treatment includes topical imidazoles. 1% hydrocortisone cream may be used as an adjunct.
- For severe *Candida* balanitis, treat with oral fluconazole.
- *Trichomonas* responds to metronidazole.
- Treat sexual partner(s) simultaneously for *Candida* or *Trichomonas*.
- Treat anaerobic infections with oral metronidazole, oral amoxicillin/clavulanate, or clindamycin topical cream.

 ONGOING CARE

FOLLOW-UP RECOMMENDATIONS

Patients should be followed by a physician for evidence of recurrence or development of diabetes.

COMPLICATIONS

- Phimosis
- Paraphimosis
- Fissure of prepuce
- Scarring

ADDITIONAL READING

- Alsterholm M, Flytstrom I, Leifsdottir R, et al. Frequency of bacteria, Candida and Malassezia species in balanoposthitis. *Acta Derm Venereol* 2008;88:331–336.
- Lisboa C, Santos A, Dias C, et al. Candida balanitis: Risk factors. *J Eur Acad Dermatol Venereol* 2010;24:820–826.
- Lisboa C, Ferreira A, Resende C, Rodrigues AG. Noninfectious balanitis in patients attending a sexually transmitted diseases clinic. *Int J Dermatol* 2009;48:445–446.
- Lisboa C, Santos A, Azevedo F, et al. Direct impression on agar surface as a diagnostic sampling procedure for Candida balanitis. *Sex Transm Infect* 2010;86:32–35.
- Johnson KE, Sherman ME, Scempiija V, et al. Foreskin inflammation is associated with HIV and herpes simplex virus type-2 infections in Rakai, Uganda. *AIDS* 2009;23:1807–1815.

CODES

ICD9

- 112.2 Candidiasis of other urogenital sites
- 607.1 Balanoposthitis

CLINICAL PEARLS

- Be aware of the possibility of sexually transmitted diseases and abuse in children who are diagnosed with balanitis.

BARTONELLOSIS (OROYA FEVER/VERRUGA PERUANA)

Paschalis Vergidis
Matthew E. Falagas

 BASICS

DESCRIPTION
- An infection caused by *Bartonella bacilliformis*, which is transmitted by the sandfly of the genus *Phlebotomus* and presents in endemic areas in two distinct forms:
- Nonimmune persons present with an acute febrile illness associated with profound anemia (Oroya fever).
- After a variable period of time from resolution, a chronic, benign cutaneous form can develop, characterized by angioproliferative skin lesions (verruga peruana). The latter show a striking similarity to bacillary angiomatosis lesions, caused by *Bartonella henselae* and *Bartonella quintana*.

EPIDEMIOLOGY
Prevalence
- The disease is exclusively endemic to the Andes River valleys at altitudes from 600 to 2,500 m (Peru, Ecuador, Colombia).
- Most cases of Oroya fever occur in tourists/visitors who are immunologically naïve. Most cases of verruga peruana occur in the native population.
- Rare cases have been reported in the US.

RISK FACTORS
Life in endemic areas and exposure to the sandfly vector

GENERAL PREVENTION
Prevention requires control of the sandfly vector: The spraying of interiors and exteriors of houses with dichlorodiphenyltrichloroethane (DDT), use of insect repellents, use of bed netting.

PATHOPHYSIOLOGY
- *Bartonella* spp. invade the erythrocytes and endothelial cells.
- They multiply into intracellular vacuoles within the erythrocytes. The latter are subsequently phagocytosed and destroyed by the reticuloendothelial system.

ETIOLOGY
- *B. bacilliformis* is a small, gram-negative bacillus of the class Proteobacteria, closely related to *B. quintana*.
- It is transmitted via an arthropod (sandfly, *Phlebotomus*) vector.

 DIAGNOSIS

HISTORY
- The incubation period of the acute illness (Oroya fever) is about 3 weeks (up to 100 days).
- The onset of symptoms, mainly resulting from high fever and profound anemia, can be either acute or subacute.
- Infectious complications result from transient immunosuppression.
- The acute phase is succeeded by a convalescent phase.
- Verruga skin lesions (nodules) develop in crops over 1–2 months, after a variable time from resolution of Oroya fever.

Acute form (Oroya Fever)
- Subacute onset (low-grade fever, malaise, headache, anorexia).
- Sudden onset (high fever, chills, diaphoresis, headaches, and changes in mental status, followed by sudden development of severe anemia).
- Muscle and joint pains.
- Dyspnea, angina; the patient may have the feeling that the cardiac pulse is transmitted to the head and ears.
- Anasarca is a marker of poor prognosis.
- Insomnia, delirium, decreased level of consciousness, coma.
- During the subsequent convalescent (critical) phase, fever declines and anemia symptoms reverse.

PHYSICAL EXAM
Oroya Fever
- High fever
- Signs of profound anemia
- Generalized, nontender lymphadenopathy
- Splenomegaly not usual; if present, may indicate other concurrent infection
- Thrombocytopenic purpura

Verruga Peruana
- Miliary lesions consist of multiple 1–4 mm papular, erythematous, round lesions, frequently associated with pruritus (1).
- Nodular lesions, usually at the skin and subcutaneous tissues of exposed parts of the body, can also affect mucous membranes and internal organs.

- Mular lesions are typically >5 mm in diameter, erythematous and bleed easily.
- Lesions at varying stages of evolution can be concurrently present.
- There is no local tenderness, unless the patient is secondarily infected.

DIAGNOSTIC TESTS & INTERPRETATION
Lab
- In the acute phase, diagnosis is made by either a positive culture (blood or bone marrow) or demonstration of numerous organisms adhered to red blood cells, in peripheral thin-film blood smears (using Giemsa or Wright stain). The number of bacteria declines abruptly during convalescence.
- Also, in peripheral blood smears, macrocytosis, poikilocytosis, Howell–Jolly bodies, nucleated red blood cells, and immature myeloid cells may be found. The leukocyte differential shifts to the left and the total count may be normal.
- Profound anemia; negative Coombs' test
- In the subacute form, initial peripheral blood smears can be negative; diagnosis can be made by positive blood cultures.
- In the chronic form, diagnosis can be done by the demonstration of the causative agent in cultured material from skin lesions and bone marrow cultures.
- Blood cultures can be positive in apparently healthy individuals.
- Serologic testing (ELISA, indirect fluorescence antibody, western immunoblot) can aid in diagnosis (2,3).

Pathological Findings
- Skin biopsy, bone marrow aspiration, and biopsy specimens from other affected organs are used.
- Increased angiogenesis, Rocha-Lima inclusions in endothelial cells
- Polymerase chain reaction (PCR) to detect *B. bacilliformis* is under development.

DIFFERENTIAL DIAGNOSIS
- The acute phase can be easily differentiated from other endemic febrile illnesses (i.e., malaria, typhoid fever, leptospirosis) by examination of peripheral blood smears and bacterial cultures.
- Verruga peruana lesions resemble those of bacillary angiomatosis and Kaposi's sarcoma, lymphoproliferative diseases, and other neoplasms. The main diagnostic clue is epidemiology.

TREATMENT

MEDICATION

First Line

- Oroya fever:
  - Chloramphenicol (500 mg oral or intravenous every 6 h) plus a second antimicrobial, preferably a beta-lactam (such as penicillin), both for 14 days (AII) (4).
  - Chloramphenicol is active against salmonellosis, the most common secondary infection.
  - The recommendation to add a beta-lactam is based on experience that chloramphenicol alone is not reliable.
- Verruga peruana:
  - Rifampin 10 mg/kg daily, maximum 600 mg daily for 10–14 days (AII) orally (4).

Second Line

- Oroya fever:
  - Doxycycline 100 mg p.o. twice daily for 14 days
  - The organism is commonly resistant to ciprofloxacin; thus, quinolones are not recommended.
- Verruga peruana:
  - Streptomycin 15–20 mg/kg intramuscularly daily for 10 days (AII)

ADDITIONAL TREATMENT

General Measures

Supportive and symptomatic treatment is also necessary in the acute form; use blood transfusion support to reverse anemia.

SURGERY/OTHER PROCEDURES

Large and secondarily infected skin nodules may need surgical excision.

IN-PATIENT CONSIDERATIONS

Admission Criteria

The appropriate health care setting is inpatient in the acute form and outpatient in the chronic form.

 ## ONGOING CARE

FOLLOW-UP RECOMMENDATIONS

- Monitor hydration status and complete blood count during the acute phase.
- Monitor signs of other infections: Splenomegaly, recurrence of fever with leukocytosis in the convalescent phase, diarrheas.
- Monitor verruga lesions for signs of secondary infections.

PROGNOSIS

- Oroya fever, if untreated, can lead to death in 50–88% of cases.
- Fever disappears within 24 hours after appropriate antibiotic treatment, although bacteremia may persist for longer periods of time.

COMPLICATIONS

- Verruga lesions show variable response to antibiotic treatment.
- Bacterial secondary infections, including salmonellosis and other enteric infections, malaria, and tuberculosis are common (45%) during the convalescent phase of Oroya fever.
- Verruga lesions can be secondarily infected and pustulate or ulcerate and bleed.

REFERENCES

1. Maguina C, Garcia PJ, Gotuzzo E, et al. Bartonellosis (Carrion's disease) in the modern era. *Clin Infect Dis* 2001;33:772–779.
2. Chamberlin J, Laughlin L, Gordon S, et al. Serodiagnosis of *Bartonella bacilliformis* infection by indirect fluorescence antibody assay: Test development and application to a population in an area of bartonellosis endemicity. *J Clin Microbiol* 2000;38(11):4269–4271.
3. Mallqui V, Speelmon EC, Verastegui M, et al. Sonicated diagnostic immunoblot for bartonellosis. *Clin Diagn Lab Immunol* 2000;7(1):1–5.
4. Rolain JM, Brouqui P, Koehler JE, et al. Recommendations for treatment of human infections caused by *Bartonella* species. *Antimicrob Agents Chemother* 2004;48:1921–1933.

ADDITIONAL READING

- Maguina C, Gotuzzo E. Bartonellosis. New and old. *Infect Dis Clin North Am* 2000;14(1):1–22, vii.

 ## CODES

ICD9
088.0 Bartonellosis

CLINICAL PEARLS

- Disease endemic to the Andes River valleys of Peru and regions of Ecuador and Colombia.
- The acute phase (Oroya fever) is characterized by fever, profound anemia, and transient immunosuppression. Treatment of choice is chloramphenicol plus a beta-lactam.
- The chronic form is characterized by miliary, nodular, and mular skin lesions (verruga peruana). Treatment of choice is rifampin.

BELL'S PALSY

Irene S. Kourbeti (E. Mylonakis, Editor)

 BASICS

DESCRIPTION
- Bell's palsy is defined as acute, idiopathic, *unilateral* paralysis of the facial nerve.
- About half of the cases of facial nerve palsy qualify as "Bell's palsy".
- Bilateral disease is a rare subcategory (0.3%).

ETIOLOGY
- Herpes simplex
- Herpes zoster, including herpes zoster oticus
- Adverse event following immunization

EPIDEMIOLOGY
Incidence
- Rates average between 13 and 34 cases per 100,000 in the US.
- Incidence is highest in persons aged 20–35 years and over 70 years.
- There is an equal distribution of males and females.
- Bell's palsy is the most common cause of VII nerve palsy in children.

RISK FACTORS
- Pregnancy
- Diabetes mellitus
- Hypertension for ages >40 years

GENERAL PREVENTION
At present, there is no way to prevent Bell's palsy.

DIAGNOSIS
- Acute onset over a day or two, rapid progression of partial or total unilateral paralysis of the facial nerve
- Decreased tear and saliva production on the ipsilateral side
- Hyperacusis
- Dysgeusia
- Retroauricular pain

DIFFERENTIAL DIAGNOSIS
The list of differential diagnoses is long and includes among others:
- Echovirus, enterovirus infection
- Lyme disease
- HIV infection, onset on seroconversion
- Otitis media and mastoiditis
- Mycobacterium tuberculosis
- Syphilis
- Infectious meningitis
- Rubella
- Tetanus
- Mycoplasma
- Cholesteatoma
- Sarcoidosis
- Sjögren's syndrome
- Systemic lupus erythematosus
- Melkersson–Rosenthal syndrome
- Cerebral aneurism
- Tumor of the parotid gland
- Melanoma of head and neck
- Meningioma
- Carcinomatous meningitis
- Granulomatous meningitis of unknown etiology
- Guillain-Barre syndrome
- Pseudobulbar palsy
- Birth trauma
- Petrous bone fractures
- Iatrogenic/ surgery
- Paget's disease
- In bilateral facial nerve paralysis, think of:
  – Lyme disease
  – Sarcoidosis

DIAGNOSTIC TESTS & INTERPRETATION
Lab
- Electrodiagnostic studies:
  - Patients with an incomplete, typical lesion that recovers do not need further study.
  - Electromyograph (EMG)
  - Electroneurography (or evoked electromyography)

Imaging
- Imaging is needed if the clinical picture is atypical, there is slow progression, or there is no improvement at 6 months. A CT or MRI scan may be required to rule out intracerebral pathology or middle ear disease in complicated cases.
- Recently, ultrasound diameter of the distal VII nerve has been shown to be a good predictor of outcome in Bell's palsy at 3 months after disease onset.

 TREATMENT

- Early treatment with prednisolone significantly improves the chances of complete recovery at 3 and 9 months (Recommendation Grade 1A).
- Treatment should begin within 3 days.
- The recommended dose is 60–80 mg/d for 1 week.
- Antivirals are reserved for severe facial palsy (Recommendation Grade 2C).
- Protection of the ipsilateral eye with artificial tears and lubricant ointments at night.
- The issue of surgical decompression is still controversial.

 ONGOING CARE

- Essential for eye care and psychological support.

COMPLICATIONS
- Incomplete recovery in one-third of patients
- Keratitis and corneal abrasions
- Recurrence has been observed in 7–15% of the cases.

REFERENCES

1. Kennedy PGE. Herpes simplex virus type 1 and Bell's palsy – A current assessment of the controversy. *J Neurovirol* 2010;16:1–5.
2. Rath B, Linder T, Cornblath D, et al. All that palsies is not Bell's[1]- The need to define Bell's palsy as an adverse event following immunization. *Vaccine* 2007;26:1–14
3. Wang CH, Chang YC, Shih HM, et al. Facial palsy in children: Emergency department management and outcome. *Pediatr Emerg Care* 2010;26(2): 121–125.
4. Lo YL, Fook-Chong S, Leoh TH, et al. High-resolution ultrasound in the evaluation and prognosis of Bell's palsy. *Eur J Neurol* 2010;17(6):885–889.
5. Sullivan FM, Swan IRC, Donnan PT, et al. Early treatment with prednisolone or acyclovir in Bell's palsy. *N Engl J Med* 2007;357(16):1598–1607.
6. Goudakos JK, Markou KD. Corticosteroids vs corticosteroids plus antiviral agents in the treatment of Bell palsy: A systematic review and meta-analysis. *Arch Otolaryngol Head Neck Surg* 2009;135(6):558–564.

ADDITIONAL READING

- Bell's palsy: Pathogenesis, clinical features, and diagnosis. www.uptodate.com, Version 18.1
- Bell's palsy: Prognosis and treatment. www.uptodate.com, Version 18.1
- Savadi-Oskouei D, Abedi A, Sadeghi-Bazargani H. Independent role of hypertension in Bell's palsy: A case-control study. *Eur Neurol* 2008; 60 (5):253–257.
- Quesnel AM, Lindsay RW, Hadlock TA. When the bell tolls on Bell's palsy: Finding occult malignancy in acute-onset facial paralysis. *Am J Otolaryngol* 2010;31(5):339–342.

 CODES

ICD9
351.0 Bell's palsy

BLASTOMYCOSIS

Emily P. Hyle (E. Mylonakis, Editor)

 BASICS

DESCRIPTION
Acute or chronic infection caused by *Blastomyces dermatitidis*, a dimorphic fungus found in soil.

EPIDEMIOLOGY
Incidence
- Annual incidence 0.3–1.8 cases per 100,000 (1).
- As many as 7.4 hospital admissions per 1 million people in endemic regions (1).

RISK FACTORS
- Location: Endemic in soil near bodies of water in SE US and Mississippi, Ohio, and St. Lawrence River valleys. Also, Mediterranean coast, S. America, Mexico, and Africa.
- Previously considered more prevalent in middle-aged men, but more likely to be caused by environmental exposures.
- Immunocompromised: At risk for more severe disease and worse outcomes.

GENERAL PREVENTION
Prevention of exposure; use of respiratory masks for those at occupational risk (1).

PATHOPHYSIOLOGY
- Inhalation of conidia of *B. dermatitidis* with potential for secondary hematogenous dissemination.
- Immune system is more effective against conidia-form than yeast-form. Blastomyces convert to budding yeast in tissue and then are less susceptible to killing by immune system.
- Reactivation in immunocompromised.

ETIOLOGY
Dimorphic fungi, *B. dermatitidis*

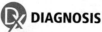 **DIAGNOSIS**

HISTORY
- Acute pneumonia: Sudden onset of symptoms similar to bacterial pneumonia, including (1):
  - Fever, night sweats
  - Productive cough, dyspnea, pleuritic chest pain (60–90%)
  - Rash (60%)
- Chronic pneumonia: Subacute onset of symptoms similar to pulmonary tuberculosis (1)
  - Fever, night sweats, weight loss
  - Mild productive cough, sometimes with chest pain and hemoptysis
- Other (depending on site of infection):
  - Rash
  - Painless soft-tissue swelling
  - Meningitis or focal neurological deficit

PHYSICAL EXAM
- Pulmonary: Crackles and rhonchi.
- Skin lesions: Typically non-tender papules, nodules, or plaques. Can be either verrucous or ulcerated and painful.
- Non-tender soft tissue swelling sometimes with draining tract.

DIAGNOSTIC TESTS & INTERPRETATION
Lab
- No commercially available serologic test bc of cross-reactivity with other endemic mycoses.
- Urine antigen-testing is available but not widely used bc of cross-reactivity (1).

Imaging
Initial approach
Chest x-ray (CXR): Mass, multiple nodules, lobar infiltrate, cavitation. Uncommon to have lymphadenopathy.

Follow-Up & Special Considerations
Other clinical presentations: genitourinary tract, septic arthritis, osteomyelitis, ocular infection, CNS infection (meningitis, intracranial abscess), oropharyngeal abscess (1).

Diagnostic Procedures/Other
- Culture: 86% + sputum; 92% + bronchoalveolar lavage (BAL)
- Wet prep.: 46% sensitivity (multiple specimen using KOH or calcofluor white)
- Characteristics: Large yeast forms (8–15 mm diameter) with single broad-based bud

Pathological Findings
- Pyogranulomas
- Fungal elements seen more easily on methenamine silver stain or Periodic acid-Schiff stain (PAS)

DIFFERENTIAL DIAGNOSIS
- Atypical pneumonia (acute pneumonia)
- Lung cancer or mycobacterial disease (chronic pneumonia)
- Squamous cell cancer (skin lesions)

 TREATMENT

MEDICATION
- Pulmonary or disseminated non-CNS disease (2):
  - Amphotericin B (or lipid/liposomal formulation) × 2 weeks followed by itraconazole 200 mg PO t.i.d. × 3 days, then 200 mg PO b.i.d. × 6–12 months.
  - For mild or moderate disease, itraconazole 200 mg PO t.i.d. × 3 days, then 200 mg PO b.i.d. × 6–12 months.
- CNS disease:
  - Amphotericin B (lipid/liposomal formulation) 3–5 mg/kg IV × 4–6 weeks followed by oral azole therapy × 12 months (minimum).
  - Itraconazole 200 mg PO t.i.d. or b.i.d. OR
  - Fluconazole 800 mg PO daily. OR
  - Voriconazole 200–400 mg PO b.i.d.
- In immunocompromised:
  - Amphotericin B × 2 weeks followed by itraconazole 200 mg PO t.i.d. × 3 days, then 200 mg PO b.i.d. × 12 months.
  - Consider life-long suppression with itraconazole 200 mg PO daily.

Pediatric Considerations
- Rx for milder disease: Itraconazole, 10 mg/kg per day for 6–12 months
- Rx for severe disease: Amphotericin (or liposomal) followed by itraconazole

Pregnancy Considerations
- Rx: Amphotericin B only, given contraindication of azoles in pregnancy

ADDITIONAL TREATMENT
General Measures
Close monitoring for toxicity of anti-fungal agents.

SURGERY/OTHER PROCEDURES
Rare, in cases of CNS mass or abscess.

IN-PATIENT CONSIDERATIONS
Initial Stabilization
- If ARDS develops (1), 50–89% mortality despite appropriate care.
- Close follow-up of neurological exam in CNS disease.

Admission Criteria
- Immunosuppression
- Respiratory distress
- Need for IV therapy

 ## ONGOING CARE

FOLLOW-UP RECOMMENDATIONS
Monitoring of patient post-Rx for ~ 6 months, given risk of relapse.

Patient Monitoring
- Therapeutic drug monitoring is recommended for itraconazole after 2 weeks of therapy: Does not need to be true trough or peak. Goal is >1.0 μg/mL and <10 μg/mL (2).
- Liver function tests (LFTs) while on azoles (every 3 months, minimum)

DIET
Itraconazole should be taken with food.

PATIENT EDUCATION
- Discuss potential for drug–drug interactions with use of itraconazole.
- Concern for relapse despite the existence of appropriate therapy (2).

PROGNOSIS
- Cure without relapse in 90–97% with use of amphotericin in immunocompetent patients.
- 40% mortality in immunocompromised (bone marrow transplant [BMT], AIDS); slightly better outcomes in solid-organ transplant.

Pregnancy Considerations
Outcomes: Can be excellent if diagnosed early; pregnant women at risk for more severe disease given their mild immunosuppression.

REFERENCES

1. McKinnell JA, Pappas PG. Blastomycosis: New insights into diagnosis, prevention, and treatment. *Clin Chest Med* 2009;30:227–239.
2. Chapman SW, Dismukes WE, Proia LA, et al. Clinical practice guidelines for the management of Blastomcyosis: 2008 update by the IDSA. *Clin Infect Dis* 2008;46:1801–1812.

ADDITIONAL READING
- Saccente M, Woods GL. Clinical and laboratory update on blastomycosis. *Clin Microbiol Rev* 2010;23(2):367–381.
- Bariola JR, Perry P, Pappas PG, et al. Blastomycosis of the central nervous system: A multicenter review of diagnosis and treatment in the modern era. *Clin Infect Dis* 2010;50(6):797–804.

 ## CODES

ICD9
- 116.0 Blastomycosis
- 116.1 Paracoccidioidomycosis

CLINICAL PEARLS
- Consider blastomycosis in differential diagnosis of acute or chronic pneumonia or new skin lesions in patients from endemic regions.
- Consider disseminated blastomycosis in any immunosuppressed patient from endemic regions.
- Most diagnoses are made by culture or fungal stain.

BLEPHARITIS AND CHALAZION

Jatin M. Vyas (E. Mylonakis, Editor)

 BASICS

DESCRIPTION

- Blepharitis is an infection of the eyelid and inflammation of lid margins. It includes the following:
  - Anterior – inflammation at the base of the eyelashes
  - Posterior – inner portion of the eyelid
  - Granulomatous
- Chalazion is a painless, granulomatous inflammation of a meibomian gland that produces a nodule within the eyelid.

EPIDEMIOLOGY

Incidence
- Blepharitis is a common condition seen by primary care physicians and ophthalmologists.
- Posterior blepharitis is usually associated with rosacea and seborrheic dermatitis.

RISK FACTORS
More than three-fourths of patients with blepharitis associated with atopic dermatitis have a positive culture for *Staphylococcus aureus*. However, a positive culture does not necessarily mean that there is an ongoing infection, and clinical correlation is important.

PATHOPHYSIOLOGY
- Bacterial organisms may affect meibomian gland secretion.
- There may also be associated changes in the secretions from meibomian glands.

ETIOLOGY
- Almost all infections that affect the skin and colonize the eyelids from nearby areas such as the scalp and nares can cause infectious diseases of the eyelid (1).
- The most common causes are *Staphylococcus* spp, particularly *S. aureus*. Other pathogens include the following:
  - *Bacillus anthracis*
  - *Bacillus cereus*
  - *Blastomyces dermatitidis*
  - *Candida* spp
  - *Clostridium* spp
  - *Cryptococcus neoformans*
  - *Haemophilus ducreyi*
  - Herpes simplex virus
  - Herpes zoster virus
  - *Moraxella* spp
  - Mycobacterium tuberculosis
  - *Mycobacterium leprae*
  - Phthirus pubis
  - *Poxvirus* spp
  - *Proteus mirabilis*
  - *Pseudomonas* spp
  - *Streptococcus* spp
  - Vaccinia virus

COMMONLY ASSOCIATED CONDITIONS
- Rosacea
- Seborrheic dermatitis

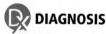 **DIAGNOSIS**

HISTORY
- Usual symptoms include chronic irritation, a burning sensation, mild redness, and occasional pruritus of the eyelids.
- Some patients complain of blurred vision

PHYSICAL EXAM
- In acute blepharitis, there are usually collections of pus and an ulcerative margin.
- In chronic blepharitis, there is usually a loss or misdirection of lashes, telangiectasia, and a swollen lid margin.
- Superficial lid involvement is the most common expression of staphylococcal lid disease and usually presents with hyperemia and telangiectasia of the lid margin.

DIAGNOSTIC TESTS & INTERPRETATION
Imaging
Slit lamp may be done by ophthalmologists.

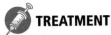

TREATMENT

MEDICATION

- Usually, treatment of blepharitis consists of warm compresses, strict eyelid hygiene, and topical antibiotics (2).
- Firm massage, using a 50:50 mixture of baby shampoo and water and a cotton-tipped applicator, enhances the flow of oily secretions from the meibomian glands.
- Topical ophthalmic preparations for staphylococcal blepharitis include bacitracin or erythromycin (b.i.d. or q.i.d. for 2 weeks), gentamicin, and 1% mercuric oxide.
- In chronic cases of blepharitis, cultures should be obtained when patients have smoldering blepharitis not responding to topical antibiotics. Systemic antibiotics that can be used in such cases are dicloxacillin (500 mg q.i.d.), quinolones, or azithromycin.

- For chalazion, if it persists and is nontender, incision and curettage can be done. Removal of the inflammatory debris can be done by making a vertical or, if necessary, a horizontal conjunctival incision. In the absence of an infection, intralesional injection of corticosteroids may be given.

SURGERY/OTHER PROCEDURES

In the uncommon cases of necrotizing fasciitis that involves the eyelids, prompt surgical debridement is needed.

ONGOING CARE

FOLLOW-UP RECOMMENDATIONS

Basal cell, squamous cell, or meibomian gland carcinoma should be suspected for any nonhealing, ulcerative lesion of the eyelids.

COMPLICATIONS

An external hordeolum (stye) is caused by staphylococcal infection of the superficial accessory glands of Zeis or Moll, located in the eyelid margins. An internal hordeolum occurs after suppurative infection of the oil-secreting meibomian glands within the tarsal plate of the eyelid.

REFERENCES

1. Papier A, Tuttle DJ, Mahar TJ. Differential diagnosis of the swollen red eyelid. *Am Fam Physician* 2007;76(12):1815–1824.
2. Wirbelauer C. Management of the red eye for the primary care physician. *Am J Med* 2006;119(4): 302–306.

CODES

ICD9
- 373.00 Blepharitis, unspecified
- 373.2 Chalazion

BOTULISM

Irene S. Kourbeti (E. Mylonakis, Editor)

BASICS

DESCRIPTION
- Syndrome produced by neurotoxins liberated by Clostridium botulinum. Botulinum neurotoxin (BoNT) is among the most toxic substances known to man.
- There are five epidemiologic forms of botulism:
  - Food borne
  - Infant botulism
  - Wound botulism
  - Intestinal colonization and adult infectious botulism
  - Inhalational botulism
- Incubation: Symptoms develop 12–36 hours after ingestion of the toxin.

EPIDEMIOLOGY
Incidence
- Botulism is a rare but potentially life-threatening syndrome.
- Small outbreaks can be due to either commercially or home-canned foods.
- In the US, most cases occur in infants, approximately one-fourth from foods, and a small number from wounds.

RISK FACTORS
- Homemade fermentation of foods with home canning leads to increased risks.
- The fatality rate is higher among patients >60 years old.
- Ingestion of honey by infants is a risk factor for gastrointestinal colonization and production of toxins.

- Iatrogenic botulism has been reported after injection of unlicensed botulinum toxin A.
- Physicians should be aware of the possibility of wound botulism in intravenous drug users.

GENERAL PREVENTION
- Ensure that care is taken when canning low-acidic foods such as corn, asparagus, beans, and beets.
- If foods have been home canned, boil them for 10 minutes prior to eating.
- Avoid giving honey to infants less than 1 year of age.
- Perform a rapid screening of possible cases in order to stop potential outbreaks.
- Avoid the use of food stored in bulging cans.

ETIOLOGY
- *C. botulinum* is a group of anaerobic gram-positive rods that produce spores and potent neurotoxins.
- The organism is typed A to G by nature of the antibodies to the neurotoxin produced.
- Disease in humans is associated with toxin types A, B, E, and F.
- Type A is often found in the western US and in China.
- Type B is found in the eastern US and in Europe.
- Type F is found in Alaska, is worldwide, and is often associated with fish products.
- Spores are found in soil and in marine sediment.
- Spores are resistant to boiling but can be destroyed by heating to 120°C.
- Due to the high toxicity, BoNT is considered a potential biological warfare agent.

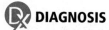

DIAGNOSIS

- Bilateral cranial neuropathies
- Bilateral descending weakness
- Absence of fever
- The patient remains awake and alert as the syndrome progresses
- No sensory abnormalities
- Clinical suspicion remains the cornerstone for the diagnosis

DIAGNOSTIC TESTS & INTERPRETATION
Lab
- Detection of the toxin in serum, stool, or food sample
- The sensitivity of mouse bioassay has been recently determined to be 68% in patients with wound botulism

DIFFERENTIAL DIAGNOSIS
- Myasthenia gravis
- Eaton–Lambert syndrome
- Tick paralysis
- Miller Fisher variant of Guillain–Barré syndrome
- Stroke
- Poliomyelitis
- Heavy metal intoxication

TREATMENT

ADDITIONAL TREATMENT

General Measures
- Supportive care
- Antitoxin available (covers toxin types A, B, and E)
- Antibiotic treatment for wound botulism after antitoxin has been administered
- Intravenous human botulism immunoglobulin (BIG-IV) has been developed and used in infants. It should be used early in the course of illness

 ONGOING CARE

FOLLOW-UP RECOMMENDATIONS
- Patients often need long-term rehabilitation
- Related to controls, the patients who recovered from botulism were more likely to report fatigue, weakness, dizziness, and difficulty breathing.

ADDITIONAL READING

- Barry J, Ward M, Cotter S, et al. Botulism in injecting drug users, Dublin, Ireland, November–December 2008. *Euro Surveill* 2009;14:pii:19082.
- Koepke R, Sobel J, Arnon SS. Global occurrence of infant botulism 1976–2006. *Pediatrics* 2008; 122:e73–e82.
- Wheeler C, Inami G, Mohle-Boetani J, et al. Sensitivity of mouse bioassay in clinical wound botulism. *Clin Infect Dis* 2009;48:1669–1673.
- Sobel J. Diagnosis and treatment of botulism: a century later, clinical suspicion remains the cornerstone. *Clin Infect Dis* 2009;48:1674–1675.
- www.uptodate.com, Version 18.1.
- Torok M. Neurological infections: clinical advances and emerging threats. *Lancet Neurol* 2007;6:16–18.
- Chertow DS, Tan ET, Maslanka SE, et al. Botulism in 4 adults following cosmetic injections with an unlicensed, highly concentrated botulinum preparation. *JAMA* 2006;296:2476–2479.
- Roblot F, Popoff M, Carlier JP, et al. Botulism in patients who inhale cocaine: the first cases in France. *Clin Infect Dis* 2006;43:e51–e52.

 CODES

ICD9
- 005.1 Botulism food poisoning
- 040.41 Infant botulism
- 040.42 Wound botulism

BRAIN ABSCESS

Irene S. Kourbeti (E. Mylonakis, Editor)

 BASICS

DESCRIPTION
Brain abscess is a collection of purulent material within the brain parenchyma caused by an infectious source of bacteria, fungi, or protozoa. The structure can have a defined abscess wall or consist of an inflammatory process (cerebritis).

EPIDEMIOLOGY
Prevalence
- Rare infection, occurring in 0.2–1.3% of large autopsy series, and in 1 of 10,000 hospital admissions
- 25% of brain abscesses develop in children
- Median age of infection: Age 30–45 years

RISK FACTORS
- Sinusitis
- Otitis media
- Poor dental hygiene
- Endocarditis
- Bacteremia from indwelling central lines and intravenous drug use
- Osler–Weber–Rendu disease
- Preexisting brain injury
- Immunodeficiency
- Cyanotic heart disease
- Intrapulmonary shunting in patients with arteriovenous malformations

GENERAL PREVENTION
- Sinusitis and otitis should be treated in all patients.
- Good dental hygiene is needed with treatment of apical abscesses, especially in the upper molars.

PATHOPHYSIOLOGY
- Infection can reach the brain by the following:
  - Direct spread from the sinuses, orbit, tooth, mastoid, middle ear, and meninges
  - Post trauma or neurosurgery
  - Hematogenous spread

ETIOLOGY
- The nature of the organisms found in the infection often relates to the mode of transmission:
- Middle ear, paranasal sinuses, odontogenic infections
  - Mixed infections with anaerobes, microaerophilic streptococci, viridans streptococci, *Streptococcus milleri*, *S. pneumoniae* (rare), *Haemophilus*, *Fusobacterium*, *Prevotella melaninogenica*, *Enterobacteriaceae*, *Pseudomonas*
- Trauma and postoperative:
  - *Staphylococcus aureus*
  - *Pseudomonas*
  - Other gram-negative
  - *Propionibacterium*
- Hematogenous:
  - *S. aureus*
  - *Salmonella*
  - Listeria
  - Streptococci (especially *Streptococcus viridans*)
  - *Klebsiella pneumoniae*
  - *Escherichia coli*, *Proteus* spp.
  - *Pseudomonas*
  - *Bacteroides* spp. (including *Bacteroides fragilis*)
  - Actinomyces
  - Fungi
- Immunocompromised hosts:
  - *Toxoplasma gondii*
  - *Listeria* spp
  - *Rhodococcus equi*
  - *Nocardia asteroides*
  - *Aspergillus* spp., *Cryptococcus neoformans*, *Coccidioides immitis*, *Candida* spp., Zygomycetes, *Cladosporium trichoides*, *Curvularia* spp.
- Immigrants from endemic countries:
  - *Taenia solium*
  - *Entamoeba histolytica*
  - *Schistosoma japonicum*
  - *Paragonimus* spp.

 DIAGNOSIS

The clinical manifestations tend to be subtle and nonspecific:
- Usual symptoms include headache of < 2 weeks' duration (75% of the cases), neck stiffness (25%), mental status changes, nausea, and vomiting
- Low-grade fevers may be present in 45–50%
- Focal neurological deficits in 50%
- Seizures develop in 25% and they may be the initial cause for CT scanning
- Third and sixth cranial nerve deficits and papilledema indicate raised intracranial pressure and cerebral edema
- Diagnosis depends on the location of the abscess, the organism, and the preexisting disease causing it

DIAGNOSTIC TESTS & INTERPRETATION
Lab
- White blood cell count is elevated in 60–70%
- ESR can be increased in 90%
- Lumbar puncture is dangerous, especially in patients with focal signs. If the CSF resembles bacterial meningitis, you may suspect an abscess ruptured into the ventricle
- Microbiological diagnosis
- Positive blood cultures
- Stereotactic abscess aspiration, cultures, and special stains
- 16S ribosomal sequencing of the aspirate
- Serology: Toxoplasmosis, neurocysticercosis

Imaging
- CT and MRI are important diagnostic tools.
- Gadolinium-performed MRI better visualizes the brainstem and diffusion-weighted MRI is used in differentiating brain abscesses from neoplastic lesions
- Serial scans need to be performed, especially when empiric treatment is given.
- Ring lesions can persist for 3–4 months despite adequate therapy.

Diagnostic Procedures/Other
- Stereotactic aspiration: The procedure of choice if the abscess is easily accessible and greater than 2.5 cm in size
- Craniotomy with aspiration in areas where direct visualization of blood vessels is needed and the abscess is greater than 2.5 cm in size

DIFFERENTIAL DIAGNOSIS
- Epidural and subdural empyema
- Septic dural sinus thrombosis
- Mycotic aneurysms
- Septic cerebral emboli with infarcts
- Acute focal necrotizing encephalitis
- Metastatic or primary brain tumors
- Pyogenic meningitis
- Hematoma
- Radiation necrosis

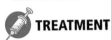

TREATMENT

ADDITIONAL TREATMENT
General Measures
- The antibiotic regimen depends on the likely source of the infection.
- Immediately begin empiric antibiotics after you obtain the appropriate specimens.
- Culture and sensitivity of any isolated organism should help with the choice of antibiotic regimen.
- For empiric treatment for an abscess arising from oral, otogenic, or sinus source: Cefotaxime 2 g i.v. q4h or ceftriaxone 2 g i.v. q12h and metronidazole 7.5 mg/kg i.v. q8h (not to exceed 4 g per day, use 15 mg/kg as a loading dose).
- Alternatively for an oral source, use penicillin G 24 million units per day in divided doses q4h and metronidazole 7.5 mg/kg i.v. q6h.
- For suspected hematogenous spread, use vancomycin (30 mg/kg in 2 divided doses) and metronidazole and cefotaxime or ceftriaxone in the above-mentioned doses.

- Postsurgical infections should be empirically treated with vancomycin 30 mg/kg in 2 divided doses and ceftazidime (2 g i.v. q8h) or cefepime (2 g i.v. q8h). If the cultures reveal Methillicin Sensitive S. aureus (MSSA), replace vancomycin with nafcillin or oxacillin (2 g i.v. q4h) because of better CNS penetration.
- For abscesses following penetrating trauma, treat empirically with vancomycin and ceftriaxone or cefotaxime in the above-mentioned doses. Replace vancomycin with nafcillin or oxacillin if MSSA is confirmed.
- 6–8 or more weeks of intravenous therapy is needed, with follow-up of CT scans.
- Steroids should be used if mass effect is demonstrated and the mental status is depressed.
- Surgical treatment is both diagnostic and therapeutic. Aspiration is a relatively simple procedure performed under local anesthesia and it allows for rapid relief of increased intracranial pressure.
- New techniques in the management of brain abscesses include ioMRI-guided aspiration and ioMRI-guided resection.

COMPLICATIONS
- Cerebral herniation may occur in 15–20% of the patients
- High morbidity is associated with residual neurological deficits in patients with prior brain abscesses. Hemiparesis has been reported in 50%
- Epilepsy occurs in fewer than 50%
- The single most important factor that influences mortality is the neurological status upon presentation

 ONGOING CARE

FOLLOW-UP RECOMMENDATIONS
Patients often require serial CT scans or MRI scans for at least a year following completion of antibiotics.

ADDITIONAL READING

- Wichmann D, Scherpe S, Heese O, et al. If the rumor is tumor, the issue is tissue. *Neurosurgery* 2008; 63:E820.
- Sharma R, Mohandas K, Cooke RPD. Intracranial abscesses: Changes in epidemiology and management over five decades in Merseyside. *Infection* 2009;37:39–43.
- Shachor-Meyouhas Y, Bar-Joseph G, Guilburd JN, et al. Brain abscess in children- epidemiology, predisposing factors and management in the modern medicine era. *Acta Paediatr* 2010; 99:1163–1167.
- Al Masalma M, Armougom F, Scheld WM, et al. The expansion of the microbiological spectrum of brain abscesses with use of multiple 16 S ribosomal DNA sequencing. *Clin Infect Dis* 2009;48:1169–1178.
- Honda H, Warren DK. Central nervous system infections: Meningitis and brain abscess. *Infect Dis Clin North Am* 2009;23:609–623.
- Hall WA, Truwit CL. The surgical management of infections involving the cerebrum. *Neurosurgery* 2008;62:S519–S530.

 CODES

ICD9
324.0 Intracranial abscess

BRONCHIOLITIS

Jatin M. Vyas (E. Mylonakis, Editor)

 BASICS

DESCRIPTION
- Acute bronchiolitis is a disease of the lower respiratory tract and results from inflammatory obstruction of the small bronchioles resulting typically from viral infection though bacterial infections occasionally cause bronchiolitis.
- Bronchiolitis refers to the inflammatory disease primarily involving the terminal and respiratory bronchioles, but in some cases, extending to the adjacent alveolar ducts and alveolar spaces.

EPIDEMIOLOGY
Incidence
- The incidence of bronchiolitis has been shown to be as high as 11 cases per 100 children per year for both the first and second 6 months of life. In the first 6 months of life, 6 children per 1,000 are hospitalized with bronchiolitis per year in the US. The care of hospitalized infants with bronchiolitis is estimated to cost up to $300 million each year.
- In the US, there are at least 675,000 ambulatory and 75,000 hospitalized children (younger than 2 years of age) with bronchiolitis each year.
- In 1995 in New York state, bronchiolitis accounted for 17% of all infant hospitalizations (9 admissions per 1000 child-years).
- Bronchiolitis is the most common cause of hospitalization of infants.
- Bronchiolitis occurs in a seasonal pattern, with peak incidence in the winter to spring months.

RISK FACTORS
- Bronchiolitis usually occurs during the first 2 years of life, with a peak incidence at approximately 6 months of age
- Bronchiolitis is most common among male infants between 3 and 6 months of age who have not been breast fed and who live in crowded conditions
- Infants who are exposed to cigarette smoke are more likely to develop bronchiolitis
- Known causes of bronchiolitis include toxic fume inhalation, tobacco smoke, mineral dust inhalation, penicillamine, collagen vascular diseases, and infections. Bone marrow, heart–lung, and lung transplantation have also been associated with this complication
- Prematurity (gestational age <37 weeks)
- Low birth weight
- Age less than 6–12 weeks
- Chronic pulmonary disease
- Hemodynamically significant congenital heart disease
- Immunodeficiency
- Neurological disease
- Congenital or anatomical defects of the airways
- Passive smoke
- Household crowding
- Child care attendance
- High altitude

PATHOPHYSIOLOGY
Viruses penetrate the bronchiolar epithelial cells, causing direct damage and resulting in inflammation of the small bronchi and bronchioles. Edema, excessive mucus, and sloughed epithelial cells lead to obstruction of small airways and atelectasis.

ETIOLOGY
- Bronchiolitis is most commonly caused by the respiratory syncytial virus (in more than 50% of cases).
- Other viruses, such as parainfluenza, influenza, rhinovirus, rubeola, mumps, parvovirus, enterovirus, coronavirus, coxsackievirus, human metapneumovirus, and varicella zoster, are occasionally isolated.
- In adults, there are occasional reports of viral- or bacterial (*Mycoplasma pneumoniae* and *Legionella pneumophila*)-induced bronchiolitis.
- The histological appearance of bronchiolitis includes inflammatory (cellular) bronchiolitis, constrictive bronchiolitis obliterans, and a proliferative bronchiolitis.

COMMONLY ASSOCIATED CONDITIONS
Otitis media

DIAGNOSIS

HISTORY
- Bronchiolitis is characterized by the following:
  - Air trapping
  - Coryza
  - Cough
  - Expiratory wheezing
  - Fever
  - Grunting
  - Increased respiratory effort
  - Retractions
  - Tachypnea
- Infants with bronchiolitis first have a mild upper respiratory tract infection with serous nasal discharge and sneezing. These symptoms usually last several days and may be accompanied by diminished appetite.
- The fever usually ranges between 38.5°C and 39.0°C.

PHYSICAL EXAM
- Air-flow obstruction is a major clinical finding in patients with constrictive bronchiolitis. Wheezing is expected, but crackles are more common, especially during the first 15% of inspiration.
- An examination may reveal a tachypneic infant often in extreme respiratory distress.

DIAGNOSTIC TESTS & INTERPRETATION
Lab
- The white blood cell and differential cell counts are usually within normal limits.
- For severe cases, viral culture or rapid tests for respiratory viruses is indicated.

Imaging
Chest radiograph usually reveals hyperinflation of the lungs and an increased anteroposterior diameter on lateral view.

DIFFERENTIAL DIAGNOSIS
- The condition most commonly confused with acute bronchiolitis is asthma. Other entities that should be included in the differential include congestive heart failure, foreign body in the trachea, pertussis, organophosphate poisoning, cystic fibrosis, and bronchopneumonias.
- Infants with bronchiolitis are wheezing for the first time, unlike those with asthma, in whom wheezing is recurrent.

TREATMENT

MEDICATION
- The traditional approach to symptomatic management of bronchiolitis has been supportive care with attention to oxygen therapy, hydration, and respiratory support as needed.
- Infants with respiratory distress should be hospitalized. The patients are commonly placed in an atmosphere of cool, humidified oxygen.
- Studies evaluating the effects of bronchodilators on pulmonary mechanics in infants with bronchiolitis have shown mixed results. None of these studies has evaluated the efficacy of patients receiving nebulized albuterol treatments beyond 4 hours or has advocated the use of bronchodilators as a means of reducing hospitalizations or length of stay. The clinical practice guideline of the American Academy of Pediatrics (AAP) recommends that bronchodilators should not be used routinely in the management of bronchiolitis.
- In the outpatient setting, short-term benefit from nebulized beta-adrenergic bronchodilators has been demonstrated through improvements in oxygen saturation or clinical respiratory scores.

COMPLEMENTARY & ALTERNATIVE THERAPIES
Ribavirin has been available for the treatment of respiratory syncytial virus infection since 1985. Its use has been recommended for infants with congestive heart failure and bronchopulmonary dysplasia. However, its use remains controversial.

ONGOING CARE

FOLLOW-UP RECOMMENDATIONS
- Some infants may progress to respiratory failure and require ventilatory support.
- A significant proportion of infants with bronchiolitis have hyperactive airways in late childhood.

COMPLICATIONS
- The case fatality rate is below 1%.
- The mortality rate among infants with high-risk conditions (e.g., congestive heart failure, immune deficiency, cystic fibrosis, etc.) is less than 3.5%.

ADDITIONAL READING
- American Academy of Pediatrics Subcommittee on Diagnosis and Management of Bronchiolitis. Diagnosis and management of bronchiolitis. *Pediatrics* 2006;118:1774.
- Coffin SE. Bronchiolitis: In-patient focus. *Pediatr Clin North Am* 2005;52:1047.

CODES

ICD9
- 466.19 Acute bronciolitis due to other infectious organisms
- 491.8 Other chronic bronchitis

BRONCHITIS

Hanssa Summah
Jieming Qu
Petros I. Rafailidis
Matthew E. Falagas

 BASICS

DESCRIPTION
- Bronchitis is an inflammation of the lining of the tracheobronchial tree. It is usually classified as acute or chronic.
- Acute bronchitis is characterized by cough occasionally associated with sputum production for less than 3 weeks (1).
- Chronic bronchitis is defined clinically as persistent productive cough for at least 3 months during a period of 2 consecutive years.

EPIDEMIOLOGY
Incidence
- Chronic bronchitis affects approximately 9.5 million Americans per year.
- Around 10 million people seek medical care for acute bronchitis each year.

Prevalence
- Acute bronchitis: Found in all age groups. Affects males and females equally.
- Chronic bronchitis: Most prevalent in individuals older than 50. Males more affected than females.

RISK FACTORS
- Acute bronchitis:
  - Smoking
  - Respiratory irritants, for example, exposure to gases, air pollution
  - Upper respiratory tract infections
  - Chronic lung conditions, old age, decreased immunity increase the risk of developing acute bronchitis on exposure to respiratory irritants
- Chronic bronchitis:
  - Smoking
  - Respiratory irritants, for example, exposure to gases, air pollution
  - Frequent upper respiratory tract infections, allergies
  - 50 years old

Genetics
Heritability has a moderate influence on the development of chronic bronchitis.

GENERAL PREVENTION
- Avoid smoking and exposure to second-hand smoke and irritants
- Avoid contact with those who have upper respiratory tract infections
- Annual influenza vaccine
- Pneumococcal vaccine every 5–10 years if aged 65 or older or have chronic disease

PATHOPHYSIOLOGY
- Irritation of bronchial-lining tissue results in mucous membrane becoming hyperemic and edematous
- Excess mucus production
- Bronchial smooth muscle hyperreactivity leading to bronchospasm
- Increased airflow resistance leading to hypoventilation and hence hypercarbia and hypoxemia

ETIOLOGY
- Acute bronchitis:
  - usually caused by viral organisms:
    - Influenza A and B viruses
    - Parainfluenza virus
    - Respiratory syncytial virus
    - Coronavirus
    - Adenovirus
    - Rhinovirus
  - Atypical bacteria are important causes in some cases:
    - *Mycoplasma pneumoniae*
    - *Chlamydia pneumoniae*
    - *Bordetella pertussis*
- Chronic bronchitis:
  - Smoking
  - Environmental pollutants
- Acute exacerbation of chronic bronchitis:
  - Haemophilus influenza
  - *Moraxella catarrhalis*
  - *Pseudomonas aeruginosa* and Enterobacteriaceae more prevalent in patients with severe impairment of lung function
  - *Streptococcus pneumoniae*
  - Viral infections
  - *Chlamydophila pneumoniae*
  - Environmental factors (air pollutants, allergens, temperature changes, irritants like dust and cigarette smoke)

COMMONLY ASSOCIATED CONDITIONS
- Upper respiratory tract infection
- Bronchial asthma
- Bronchitis associated with emphysema in chronic obstructive pulmonary disease

 DIAGNOSIS

HISTORY
- Acute bronchitis:
  - Recent history of a cold or sinus infection
  - Exposure to allergens or irritants
  - Occupational history including exposure to irritants
  - Primary or secondhand smoking
- Chronic bronchitis:
  - As above
  - History of productive cough
- Acute exacerbation of chronic bronchitis:
  - Increased dyspnea
  - Increased sputum production
  - Increased sputum purulence
- Symptoms may include mild *fever*, sore throat, shortness of breath on exertion, wheezing, tightness in the chest, chest pain, fatigue, malaise, and headaches.

PHYSICAL EXAM
- Fever is uncommon
- Tachypnea and tachycardia due to infection
- Signs of upper respiratory tract infection
- Coarse breath sounds/wheezing/prolonged expiration
- Deterioration in respiratory function usually occurs in acute exacerbation of chronic bronchitis

DIAGNOSTIC TESTS & INTERPRETATION
Lab
Initial lab tests
- CBC
- Sputum cultures to rule out the presence of specific causative bacteria
- The use of serum procalcitonin may guide which patients will need antibiotics (2).
- Pulse oximetry and arterial blood gas measurements

Follow-Up & Special Considerations
Spirometry may be performed several weeks after patient recovers to determine lung function and assess airway obstruction

Imaging
Initial approach
Chest x-ray to rule out pneumonia

Follow-Up & Special Considerations
Follow-up chest x-ray usually not required

Diagnostic Procedures/Other
- Pulmonary function tests
- Bronchoscopy

Pathological Findings
- Acute bronchitis:
  - Mucosal/submucosal edema
  - Mucosal and submucosal inflammatory cells
- Chronic bronchitis:
  - Goblet cell hyperplasia
  - Mucosal and submucosal inflammatory cells
  - Mucus plugging
  - Smooth muscle hyperplasia

DIFFERENTIAL DIAGNOSIS
- Asthma
- Bronchiolitis
- Pneumonia
- Pharyngitis
- Bronchiectasis
- Chronic sinusitis
- Pulmonary embolism with infarction
- Congestive heart failure
- Wegener's granulomatosis
- Sarcoid
- Atelectasis
- Chemical pneumonitis
- Gastroesophageal reflux disease

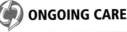

TREATMENT

MEDICATION

First Line
- Acute bronchitis: No treatment unless there is the presence of the following (3–5):
  - Influenza virus:
    - Oseltamivir 75 mg p.o. b.i.d. × 5 days
    - Zanamivir 2 puffs (5 mg/puff) b.i.d. × 5 days
  - B. pertussis:
    - Azithromycin × 5 days at a dose of 500 mg on day 1 and 250 mg on days 2—5
    - Erythromycin 500 mg q.i.d. × 14 days
    - Clarithromycin 500 mg b.i.d. × 7 days
  - M. pneumoniae/C. pneumoniae:
    - No therapy (no compelling data suggestive of improved outcomes as a result of treatment with antibiotic agents)
    - Azithromycin × 5 days at a dose of 500 mg on day 1 and 250 mg on days 2—5
    - Doxycycline 100 mg b.i.d. × 5 days
- Acute exacerbation of chronic bronchitis with acute bacterial infections:
  - Amoxicillin 250–500 mg p.o. q8h;
  - Amoxicillin and clavulanate 500 mg p.o. q8h × 5–10 days;
  - Trimethoprim–sulfamethoxazole 160 mg trimethoprim/800 mg sulfamethoxazole p.o. q12h × 5–10 days
  - Doxycycline100 mg p.o. b.i.d. on day 1, then 100 mg p.o. per day × 5–10 days
  - Short-duration treatment with quinolones or macrolides (for 5 days) is not inferior when compared with longer duration treatment (7–10 days) (6)[A].
  - Levofloxacin 250 mg p.o. b.i.d. or 500 mg p.o. per day × 5 days
  - Ciprofloxacin 250–500 mg p.o. b.i.d. × 5 days
  - Clarithromycin 250–500 mg p.o. b.i.d. × 5 days
  - Azithromycin × 5 days at a dose of 500 mg on day 1 and 250 mg on days 2–5

Second Line
- Acute bronchitis:
  - B. pertussis:
    - Trimethoprim–sulfamethoxazole 1600 mg per day × 14 days or 800 mg b.i.d. × 14 days

ADDITIONAL TREATMENT

General Measures
- Avoidance of environmental irritants
- Bronchodilators for the treatment of dyspnea
- Low-flow oxygen therapy during exacerbation
- Systemic steroids during exacerbation
- Antitussive agents (codeine and dextromethorphan) are effective for short-term symptomatic relief of cough in patients with acute and chronic bronchitis

Issues for Referral
Frequent and severe exacerbations

Additional Therapies
- Pulmonary rehabilitation
- Clinical benefits of postural drainage and chest percussion have not been proven

SURGERY/OTHER PROCEDURES
Lung transplant in those who are severely incapacitated

IN-PATIENT CONSIDERATIONS

Initial Stabilization
- Outpatient treatment of uncomplicated cases
- Low-flow oxygen therapy and bronchodilators in emergency room for acute exacerbations
- Initiation of appropriate antibiotics if required

Admission Criteria
- Presence of high-risk comorbid conditions (pneumonia, cardiac arrhythmia, etc.)
- Inadequate response to outpatient treatment
- Marked increase in dyspnea

IV Fluids
Adequate hydration to help mucus clearance

Nursing
- Monitor intravenous fluids
- Ensure mucus drainage

Discharge Criteria
- Symptoms and oxygenation return to baseline
- Hemodynamic stability
- Ability to ambulate

ONGOING CARE

FOLLOW-UP RECOMMENDATIONS
- Re-evaluation of patient within 4 weeks for assessment of improvement of symptoms and need for oxygenation
- Routine spirometry for patients with chronic bronchitis and inhaled corticosteroid therapy should be offered to stable patients with chronic bronchitis and FEV_1 <50% of predictive value with frequent exacerbations

Patient Monitoring
- Assess patient's ability to cope with environmental needs
- Monitor use of bronchodilators

DIET
No proven specific diet helpful in bronchitis

PATIENT EDUCATION
- Smoking cessation
- Avoidance of exposure to environmental irritants
- Restriction of heavy duties in patients with long-standing chronic bronchitis

PROGNOSIS
- Patients with acute bronchitis generally have a good prognosis
- Smoking cessation has been proven to be associated with slower progression of deterioration in lung function

COMPLICATIONS
- Respiratory failure
- Pulmonary emphysema
- Right heart failure
- Failure to respond to treatment as a result of the following:
  - Disease too far advanced or treatment delayed too long
  - Wrong diagnosis
  - Inadequate dose of antibiotic
  - Compromised or debilitated host
  - Presence of resistant bacteria, for example, Pseudomonas

REFERENCES

1. Wenzel RP, Fowler AA III. Clinical practice. Acute bronchitis. N Engl J Med 2006;355(20): 2125–2130.
2. Schuetz P, Christ-Crain M, Thomann R, et al. Effect of procalcitonin-based guidelines vs standard guidelines on antibiotic use in lower respiratory tract infections: The ProHOSP randomized controlled trial. JAMA 2009;302:1059–1066.
3. Albert RH. Diagnosis and treatment of acute bronchitis. Am Fam Physician 2010;82:1345–1350.
4. Braman SS. Chronic cough due to acute bronchitis: ACCP evidence-based clinical practice guidelines. Chest 2006;129:95S–103S.
5. Blasi F, Ewig S, Torres A, et al. A review of guidelines for antibacterial use in acute exacerbations of chronic bronchitis. Pulm Pharmacol Ther 2006;19:361–369.
6. Falagas ME, Avgeri SG, Matthaiou DK, et al. Short- versus long-duration antimicrobial treatment for exacerbations of chronic bronchitis: A meta-analysis. J Antimicrob Chemother 2008;62: 442–450.

CODES

ICD9
- 466.0 Acute bronchitis
- 490 Bronchitis, not specified as acute or chronic
- 491.9 Unspecified chronic bronchitis

CLINICAL PEARLS
- Antibiotics usually not required in acute bronchitis.
- Patients must be advised that cough may last for 10 to up to 21 days and even longer.

BRUCELLOSIS

Petros I. Rafailidis
Matthew E. Falagas

 BASICS

DESCRIPTION
- Brucellosis is a zoonotic infectious disease of both wild and domestic animals.
- Humans are the accidental host of the pathogen and develop a systemic disease of acute or insidious onset.

EPIDEMIOLOGY
Incidence
Incidence (per million of the general population) varies extensively: Less than 2 new cases in the US and the UK, 2 up to 50 new cases in many countries in the Mediterranean basin, and more than 50 new cases in countries in the Middle East. Approximately 500,000 new cases of brucellosis occur each year (1).

RISK FACTORS
- Brucellosis is an occupational disease. The infection is more common in the following populations:
  – Farm and ranch workers
  – Abattoir workers
  – Veterinarians
  – Meat inspectors
  – Laboratory personnel
- Ingestion of unpasteurized milk or milk products is the most significant risk factor in endemic areas.

GENERAL PREVENTION
- Efforts should be made to eradicate *Brucella* species from cattle, goats, swine, and other animals.
- Vaccination of cattle and identification of sick animals are the mainstay of such an approach.
- Consumption of unpasteurized milk and dairy products should be avoided.
  – If pasteurization of milk is not possible, boiling also is effective.
  – No safe vaccine is available for professions at risk.

PATHOPHYSIOLOGY
A small number of *Brucella* survive in macrophages escaping intracellular destruction. The host–bacterium interaction is characterized by an increase of specific γ/δ lymphocytes and interferon γ and with a decreased body TNF-a response (2).

ETIOLOGY
- Brucellosis is caused by *Brucella* species, which are small, nonmotile, gram-negative coccobacilli.
- Brucella species that infect humans:
  – *Brucella melitensis*
  – *Brucella abortus*
  – *Brucella suis*
  – *Brucella canis*

 DIAGNOSIS

HISTORY
- Brucellosis presents with the following:
  – Fever
  – Chills
  – Rigor
  – Malaise
  – Headache
  – Weight loss
  – Sweating
  – Generalized aches
  – Arthralgias
- Depression is also a common symptom.

PHYSICAL EXAM
- Hepatomegaly, splenomegaly, and lymphadenopathy may be found.
- A significant proportion of patients (20–50%) have osteoarticular involvement. Spondylodiscitis of the spine has to be ruled out.
- Symptoms due to orchitis and/or epididymitis also may be manifestations of brucellosis in a considerable proportion (5–25%) of patients.
- Brucellosis may affect any organ of the body and present occasionally as a localized infection (i.e., pneumonia).

DIAGNOSTIC TESTS & INTERPRETATION
Lab
- Definitive diagnosis of brucellosis is made with the culture of the pathogen from blood, bone marrow, or other tissue specimens.
- The laboratory personnel should be told by the clinician that brucellosis is a diagnostic possibility when cultures are sent. This is because some media that support the growth of *Brucella* species require an environment with 5–10% CO_2 for optimal isolation of the pathogen.
- Cultures should be kept for at least 4 weeks when brucellosis is a possibility.
- Serologic tests (standard tube agglutination test) are also helpful. However, interpretation of the results of these tests should be done carefully.
- False-negative serologic tests for brucellosis may be due to the prozone phenomenon (3).
- False-positive results may be obtained due to cross-reactions with antibodies to other infections, such as *Yersinia enterocolitica*, *Vibrio cholera*, and *Francisella tularensis*. Attention also should be paid to the fact that IgG antibodies against *Brucella* species may be found in all forms of the infection: Acute, recurrent, or chronic brucellosis.
- An ELISA to detect antibodies against *Brucella* is more reliable for the diagnosis.
- A polymerase chain reaction performed on blood or other tissue (bone marrow) may detect *Brucella* spp. DNA. Detection of *Brucella* spp. DNA may last very long even after cure and thus interpretation has to be careful (4)!

Imaging
- An abdominal ultrasound or CT/MRI of the abdomen will detect enlarged lymph nodes and organomegaly.
- An MRI of the afflicted bone area.

Diagnostic Procedures/Other
A liver biopsy may disclose granulomatous hepatitis when performed in a patient with fever of unidentified origin (FUO).

Pathological Findings
Granulomas are the main finding in various tissues. Abscesses may be encountered occasionally.

DIFFERENTIAL DIAGNOSIS

- Brucellosis should come to the mind of a physician when he or she sees a patient from an endemic area with a febrile illness of acute or insidious onset, especially if there are manifestations of osteoarticular involvement.
- Differential diagnosis should be made from several other infectious diseases.
- Brucellosis may present as fever of unknown origin.

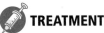

TREATMENT

MEDICATION
First Line

- Streptomycin (1 g/d i.m.) for the first 2–3 weeks of treatment in combination with doxycycline 100 mg p.o. every 12 hours for 6 weeks (5)[A].
- Gentamicin (240 mg/d i.m.) is non-inferior to streptomycin (5)[A].
- Triple regimens (doxycycline plus aminoglycoside plus rifampicin) may be superior.
- Co-trimoxazole and/or rifampicin have been used in pregnant women.

Second Line

- Doxycycline, combined with rifampicin 600–900 mg/d p.o. for 6 weeks, is an alternative option but with less effectiveness for spondylitis, central nervous system involvement, and endocarditis (5)[A].
- Quinolone combinations are suboptimal.

ADDITIONAL TREATMENT
General Measures
Keep strict hygiene measures. *Brucella* is a notorious pathogen (used even as a bioterrorism agent).

Additional Therapies
Prednisone has been used when there is central nervous system involvement.

SURGERY/OTHER PROCEDURES
Valve replacement is usually necessary in cases of *Brucella* endocarditis.

IN-PATIENT CONSIDERATIONS
Admission Criteria
Warranted for endocarditis and meningitis and in the setting of work-up for FUO.

 ONGOING CARE

FOLLOW-UP RECOMMENDATIONS
Careful follow-up is crucial due to the considerable probability of recurrence of symptoms.

Patient Monitoring
Renal and liver function tests have to be monitored during treatment with aminoglycosides and rifampin, respectively.

PATIENT EDUCATION
Urine and body secretions may turn orange when receiving rifampin.

PROGNOSIS
Excellent in general: Endocarditis carries a more severe prognosis. Neurobrucellosis may cause deficits.

COMPLICATIONS

- Recurrence of symptoms is a common problem in brucellosis. It is attributed to the difficulty of eradicating the pathogen due to its sequestration in areas where antibiotics do not accomplish high concentrations and not to the development of resistance of the pathogen to antimicrobial agents.
- Antibiotic regimens of longer duration (several months) must be used in such cases.
- The case-fatality rate for brucellosis is about 2% and is mainly attributable to endocarditis.
- A Jarisch–Herxheimer-like reaction may be seen occasionally, shortly after the initiation of treatment with antibiotics.

REFERENCES

1. Pappas G, Papadimitriou P, Akritidis N, et al. The new global map of human brucellosis. *Lancet Infect Dis* 2006;6:91–99.
2. Pappas G, Akritidis N, Bosilkovski M, et al. Brucellosis. *N Engl J Med* 2005;352:2325–2336.
3. Peiris V, Faser S, Fairhust M, et al. Laboratory diagnosis of *Brucella* infection: some pitfalls. *Lancet* 1992;339:1415–1416.
4. Navarro E, Segura JC, Castaño MJ, et al. Use of real-time quantitative polymerase chain reaction to monitor the evolution of *Brucella melitensis* DNA load during therapy and post-therapy follow-up in patients with brucellosis. *Clin Infect Dis* 2006;42:1266–1273.
5. Skalsky K, Yahav D, Bishara J, et al. Treatment of human brucellosis: Systematic review and meta-analysis of randomised controlled trials. *BMJ* 2008;336:701–704.

 CODES

ICD9
Brucellosis is due to
- 023.0: *Brucella melitensis*
- 023.1: *Brucella abortus*
- 023.9: *Brucellosis, unspecified*

CLINICAL PEARLS

- A bacterium present worldwide.
- Children under 8 years old should be treated with trimethoprim-sulphamethoxazole (± rifampicin).

BURSITIS
Irene S. Kourbeti (E. Mylonakis, Editor)

 BASICS

DESCRIPTION
- Bursitis is inflammation of the bursae and includes pyogenic infections, crystal release secondary to trauma or gout, or arthritis (mainly rheumatoid arthritis). In this chapter, we will discuss septic bursitis
- There are over 150 bursae in the body. They are sac-like structures that protect the soft tissues from the bony prominences
- Septic bursitis mainly involves the superficial bursae
- The most common locations of the disease include the subdeltoid, olecranon, ischial, trochanteric, and prepatellar bursae

RISK FACTORS
- The most important predisposing factor in septic bursitis is trauma (70%)
- Specific associations include ischial bursitis in people with spinal injuries, malleolar bursitis in ice skaters, and subdeltoid bursitis after injections
- Diabetes mellitus, alcohol abuse, and chronic skin conditions may also predispose
- Outbreak of Methicillin-Resistant Stsphylococcus aureus (MRSA) infections has been associated with acupuncture and joint injections
- Intravenous drug use may be associated with septic bursitis

ETIOLOGY
- The most common organism isolated in bursitis is *Staphylococcus aureus*.
- The second most common organism, leading to 5–30% of cases, is *Streptococcus*.
- Disease due to gram-negatives or fungi is rare.
- Recently, *Prototheca wickerhamii*, an algae ubiquitous in nature, has been associated with bursitis in immunocompromised individuals
- In endemic regions, brucellosis should be part of the differential diagnosis
- Tuberculous involvement may occur as part of systemic disease

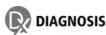 **DIAGNOSIS**

PHYSICAL EXAM
- There may be painful swelling and erythema of the bursae.
- Fevers may be present.
- Evidence of cellulitis may extend from the bursae.
- Systemic signs of infection and bacteremia are more commonly associated with deep bursae infections

DIAGNOSTIC TESTS & INTERPRETATION
Lab
- Aspiration of the infected bursa is the diagnostic procedure of choice
- White blood cell counts, often below 20,000 cells/mm^3, may be consistent with septic bursitis.
- Gram stain positivity ranges from 15% to 100%.
- Aspirate cultures have great sensitivity and specificity. Culture in liquid media may optimize sensitivity
- Crystal analysis should be negative in bacterial bursitis, but both crystal-induced and bacterial bursitis may occur at the same time.

Imaging
- Plain radiograph: Subcutaneous edema and soft tissue swelling
- Ultrasound: Fluid collection
- MRI: Poorly or well-defined fluid collection. After gadolinium administration, a well-defined rim of enhancement of the infected bursa is seen but the surrounding structures are spared

DIFFERENTIAL DIAGNOSIS
- Cellulitis/fasciitis
- Acute monoarthritis
- Gout
- Pseudogout
- Trauma

TREATMENT

MEDICATION

- Aspiration by needle and syringe on a frequent, even daily, basis, until the bursa is no longer fluctuant, may be needed in half of the cases
- Antibiotics:
  - Initial antimicrobial therapy should focus on staphylococci and streptococci.
  - The final choice of antibiotics depends on the culture and sensitivity of the aspirated material. For *S. aureus*, oxacillin or nafcillin (i.v. 2 g q6h). If the organism is methicillin-resistant, vancomycin (i.v. 750–1,000 mg q12h) is indicated.
  - Antibiotics should be given for at least 14 days.
  - Recently, a study suggested that in severe infectious bursitis requiring hospitalization, antibiotic therapy may be limited to 7 days in non-immunosuppressed patients.
  - Use of parenteral versus oral antibiotics depends on the severity of the clinical situation and the amount of systemic toxicity associated with the infection.
  - Immobilization of affected bursae.

- If antibiotics are unable to control the infection, and swelling and pain persist, surgical incision and drainage is indicated. Excision of the bursa is done when the infection is chronic and the fluid has become loculated.

ADDITIONAL TREATMENT

General Measures

Patients require follow-up with rehabilitation services so that limitation of joint movement does not occur.

 ONGOING CARE

ADDITIONAL READING

- Turan H, Serefhanoglu K, Karadeli E, et al. A case of brucellosis with abscess of the iliacus muscle, olecranon bursitis, and sacroiliitis. *Int J Infect Dis* 2009;13:e485–e487.
- Perez C, Huttner A, Assal M, et al. Infectious olecranon and patellar bursitis: Short-course adjuvant antibiotic therapy is not a risk factor for recurrence in adult hospitalized patients. *J Antimicrob Chemother* 2010;65:1008–1014.

- Murray RJ, Pearson JC, Coombs GW, et al. Outbreak of invasive methicillin-resistant *Staphylococcus aureus* infection associated with acupuncture and joint infection. *Infect Control Hosp Epidemiol* 2008;29:859–865.
- Theodorou SJ, Theodorou DJ, Resnick D. Imaging findings of complications affecting the upper extremity in intravenous drug users: Featured cases. *Emerg Radiol* 2008;15:227–239.
- Torralba KD, Quismorio FP Jr. Soft tissue infections. *Rheum Dis Clin North Am* 2009;35:45–62.
- Small LN, Ross JJ. Suppurative tenosynovitis and septic bursitis. *Infect Dis Clin North Am* 2005;19:991–1005.

CODES

ICD9

- 726.19 Other specified disorders of bursae and tendons in shoulder region
- 726.33 Olecranon bursitis
- 727.3 Other bursitis disorders

CAMPYLOBACTER INFECTIONS

Jason B. Harris (E. Mylonakis, Editor)

 BASICS

DESCRIPTION
- *Campylobacter* species are an important food-borne cause of diarrheal illness in both industrialized and developing countries.
- Postinfectious complications of *Campylobacter* infection include Guillain–Barré syndrome and reactive arthritis.

EPIDEMIOLOGY
Incidence
- Campylobacteriosis is a worldwide zoonosis, and *Campylobacter* enteritis is a common form of acute gastroenteritis in North America.
- *C. jejuni* infections occur year-round in the US and other developed countries but with a sharp peak in summer and early fall.
- Up to 90% of broiler chickens are contaminated.
- *Campylobacter* bacteria are easily spread through drinking water and unpasteurized milk. Some cases are associated with the preparation of contaminated food.
- However, the epidemiology of the infection in developing countries is different because *C. jejuni* is often isolated from asymptomatic persons, and is especially common during the first 5 years of life.

RISK FACTORS
- In developed countries, consumption of undercooked poultry is estimated to be responsible for more than half of sporadic *Campylobacter* infection cases.
- HIV-infected patients are at increased risk of infection.

Genetics
A reactive arthritis may occur up to several weeks postinfection in persons with the HLA-B27 histocompatibility antigens.

GENERAL PREVENTION
- *Campylobacter* can be killed by cooking poultry and other meats to an internal temperature of 82°C (180°F). This is the temperature at which the meat is no longer pink and the juice runs clear.
- Poultry and other meats must be prepared separately from other foods, both in restaurants and at home.

- Countertops, utensils, towels, and aprons used in the preparation of poultry and other meats should be washed with hot water and soap before they are used for other foods, particularly foods that will not be cooked.
- Handwashing is also essential.
- Suspected cases, particularly when associated with other cases among family members or acquaintances, should be reported promptly to the local health department.

PATHOPHYSIOLOGY
- The incubation period ranges from 1 to 7 days.
- As few as 500 bacteria may cause disease in some patients.
- The well-established association between *Campylobacter* infection and Guillain–Barré syndrome is thought to be based on the principle of molecular mimicry, as *Campylobacter* and peripheral nerves share structurally similar antigens.

ETIOLOGY
- *C. jejuni* and *C. coli* are the major causes of *Campylobacter* infection in humans.
- *C. fetus* is an important cause of systemic infection and persistent bacteremia in immunocompromised patients, but not a major cause of enteritis in immunocompetent patients.

 DIAGNOSIS

HISTORY
- Acute enteritis is the most common presentation of *C. jejuni* infection.
- Symptoms may last from 1 day to 1 week or longer.
- Often there is a prodrome with fever, headache, myalgia, and malaise.
- The most common symptoms are the following:
  – Abdominal pain (usually cramping)
  – Diarrhea
  – Fever (usually of low grade but can be up to 40°C or more)
  – Malaise

- Diarrhea may vary from loose stools to massive watery stools or grossly bloody stools.
- *C. fetus* infections may cause intermittent diarrhea or nonspecific abdominal pain without localizing signs.
- *C. fetus* may also cause a prolonged relapsing illness characterized by fever, chills, and myalgia, without a source of the infection being demonstrated.

PHYSICAL EXAM
- Physical exam findings in most cases of *Campylobacter* enteritis are nonspecific and include mild abdominal tenderness.
- In some cases, because of severe abdominal pain, the presentation of *Campylobacter* enteritis may mimic appendicitis (pseudoappendicitis); however, classic physical signs of peritonitis, including guarding and rebound tenderness, are rare.

DIAGNOSTIC TESTS & INTERPRETATION
Lab
- In many cases of *Campylobacter* enteritis there is a mild leukocytosis with an increase in neutrophils.
- The diagnosis of *C. jejuni* infection is usually based on a positive stool culture.
- *Campylobacter* species are isolated from fecal specimens, using microaerobic incubation conditions and selective techniques that reduce the growth of competing microorganisms.
- Bacteremia is noted in <1% of patients with *C. jejuni* infection.

DIFFERENTIAL DIAGNOSIS
The diagnosis can be suspected on the basis of symptoms and is easily confirmed by stool culture. See also Section I chapter, "Diarrhea and Fever."

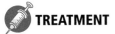
TREATMENT
MEDICATION
First Line
- Because most cases of infection are self-limited, antimicrobial therapy is indicated in patients with severe or persistent symptoms or at risk factors for complications such as pregnancy, immunocompromising conditions, or extremes of age.
- Ciprofloxacin (500 mg p.o. b.i.d. for 5–7 days) is considered a first-line therapy. However, resistance of *Campylobacter* to quinolones is increasing.
- Macrolides, including erythromycin, are another acceptable first-line treatment. The recommended dosage for adults is 250 mg p.o. q.i.d. for 5–7 days; the recommended dosage for children is 30–50 mg/kg/d in divided doses for the same period.
- *Campylobacter* strains acquired in developing countries are more likely to be resistant to erythromycin.
- The necessity for treating septic or bacteremic episodes with agents other than ciprofloxacin has not been established. For those patients who are very toxic-appearing, prolonged treatment with gentamicin or imipenem is indicated.

Second Line
- Most *C. jejuni* and *C. coli* isolates are not susceptible to cephalosporins or penicillin, and these agents should not be used.
- Susceptibility to sulfonamides and metronidazole is variable. Unlike *Salmonella* infections, treatment with antimicrobial agents does not prolong carriage of *C. jejuni*; on the contrary, treatment eliminates carriage within 72 hours in most patients.

ADDITIONAL TREATMENT
General Measures
Assessment of hydration status and appropriate fluid and electrolyte replacement are required.

Additional Therapies
- Use of an antimotility agent can prolong the duration of symptoms, unless it is combined with an antibiotic.
- Antimotility therapies should not be used in children.

IN-PATIENT CONSIDERATIONS
Admission Criteria
- Only a small portion of patients with *Campylobacter* enteritis require hospitalization.
- Potential indications for admission include moderate-to-severe dehydration, severe pain, systemic illness, or complications (discussed below).

IV Fluids
Only isotonic fluids should be used for patients with severe dehydration.

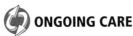
ONGOING CARE
FOLLOW-UP RECOMMENDATIONS
Postinfectious complications of *Campylobacter* enteritis usually occur within 2 months of acute infection.

Patient Monitoring
Patients with frequent diarrhea should be followed with strict recording of intake and output and monitored for signs of dehydration.

DIET
Patients with enteritis can be continued on a regular diet as tolerated.

PROGNOSIS
- The vast majority of patients recover fully after *Campylobacter* enteritis, either spontaneously or after appropriate antimicrobial therapy.
- Although *Campylobacter* infections are the most important recognized antecedent of Guillain–Barré syndrome, it is important to recognize that only 1 of every 1000 patients with *Campylobacter* enteritis subsequently develop GBS so the risk for any single individual is low.
- *C. fetus* infection may be lethal to patients with chronic compensated diseases such as cirrhosis or diabetes mellitus.

COMPLICATIONS
- The major postinfectious complications of *Campylobacter* enteritis in immunocompetent persons are reactive arthritis and Guillain–Barré syndrome as discussed above.
- Among immunocompromised patients, *Campylobacter* infections can be life-threatening.
- *C. jejuni* may cause septic abortion.
- There have been infrequent reports of *C. jejuni* infections manifesting with acute cholecystitis, pancreatitis, and cystitis.

- *C. jejuni* has been associated with an intestinal immunoproliferative syndrome associated with malabsorption and protein-losing enteropathy.
- *C. fetus* infections appear to have a tropism for vascular sites; vascular necrosis occurs in patients with endocarditis and pericarditis.
- CNS infections with *C. fetus* occur in neonates and adults. The prognosis is poor for premature infants, but some full-term neonates have survived infection. Infection is manifested as a meningoencephalitis with a cerebrospinal fluid polymorphonuclear pleocytosis.
- Among immunocompromised patients, especially those with AIDS, bacteremia by the "atypical" *Campylobacter* species appears relatively commonly, and it can continue indefinitely without antibiotic therapy.

ADDITIONAL READING
- Allos BM, Blaser MJ. Campylobacter and related species. In: Mandell GL, Bennett JE, Dolin R, eds. *Principles and practice of infectious diseases*. New York: Churchill Livingstone, 2009:2793–2802.
- Centers for Disease Control and Prevention (CDC). Preliminary FoodNet data on the incidence of infection with pathogens transmitted commonly through food – 10 states, 2009. *MMWR* 2010;59(14):418–422.
- Lecuit M, Abachin E, Martin A, et al. Immunoproliferative small intestinal disease associated with Campylobacter jejuni. *N Engl J Med* 2004;350(3):239–248.
- Nakari UM, Huovinen E, Kuusi M, et al. Population-based surveillance study of Campylobacter infections in Finland. *Epidemiol Infect* 2010;138(12):1712–1718.

CODES
ICD9
008.43 Intestinal infection due to campylobacter

CANDIDIASIS

Maged Muhammed
Isaac I. Bogoch
Eleftherios Mylonakis

 BASICS

DESCRIPTION
- *Candida* is a yeast and is one of the components of normal flora on skin and in the gastrointestinal and genitourinary tracts.
- *Candida* species are an increasing etiology of blood stream infections in immunocompromised patients.
- *Candida* can cause both superficial and systemic infection.

EPIDEMIOLOGY
- Candidal infections can affect patients of all ages, however such infections are more common in the elderly, infants, or pregnant women.
- In a recent study, up to 9% of bloodstream infections in US hospitals were found to be related to candidal infection (1).
  - There are multiple species of *Candida*, and *Candida albicans* is the underlying organism implicated in most infections. Non-albicans *Candida* species are becoming increasingly common. In a recent sample of almost 1400 *Candida* specimens from hospitalized patients, after *C. albicans* the most common species were *C. parapsilosis*, *C. glabrata*, and *C. tropicalis*.

RISK FACTORS
- Immune suppression/neutropenia (2)
- Underlying diseases with immune suppression such as cancer, AIDS, and major burns
- Prolonged use of antibiotics
- Indwelling IV catheter
- Chemotherapy
- Solid organ and bone marrow transplant recipients
- Total parenteral nutrition
- Chronic renal failure and hemodialysis
- Gastrointestinal perforation
- Diabetes mellitus
- Pregnancy
- Glucocorticoid use

GENERAL PREVENTION
- Judicious use of antibiotics.
- Removal of central venous catheters when no longer necessary.

PATHOPHYSIOLOGY
- Candidemia can occur via breaches in mucosal barriers at virtually any point in the gastrointestinal tract.
- Candidemia can also occur through colonization of intravascular catheter devices.

ETIOLOGY
- The genus of *Candida* has more than 150 species; however, the most important clinically related species are: *C. albicans*, *C. glabrata*, *C. parapsilosis*, *C. tropicalis*, *C. krusei*, *C. guilliermondii*, and *C. lusitaniae*.
- *C. albicans* is implicated in more than 50% of candidemia cases.

COMMONLY ASSOCIATED CONDITIONS
Immune suppression with chemotherapy, HIV/AIDS, solid organ or bone marrow transplantation, neutropenia or debilitating underlying diseases, requiring prolonged ICU stays with IV catheters.

 DIAGNOSIS

HISTORY
Clinical presentation and evaluation for risk factors depends on the involved organ (e.g., genitourinary and intestinal tracts, brain, skin) and the extent of disease.
- Vulvovaginal candidiasis: Pruritus, irritation, dysuria, dyspareunia, white "cheesy" discharge.
- Oropharyngeal candidiasis: Occasional pain, loss of taste, sometimes asymptomatic.
- Candida esophagitis: Nausea, vomiting, retrosternal chest pain, odynophagia, dysphagia.
- Invasive candidiasis: History of immunosuppressant medications, HIV/AIDS, concurrent malignancy. May have mental status changes if septic.

PHYSICAL EXAM
- Depends on the involved organ and the extent of disease.
- Vulvovaginal candidiasis: Erythema of the vulva or vagina, white "cheesy" discharge. Sometimes clear discharge.
- Oral candidiasis (thrush) and Candida esophagitis: White plaques covering the tongue, hard and soft palates. Often leaves an erythematous base when scraped off. Patients may have esophageal candidiasis without oral involvement.
- Candidemia: Ranges from fever to signs of severe sepsis such as hypotension, tachycardia, and mental status changes.

DIAGNOSTIC TESTS & INTERPRETATION
Lab
- Vulvovaginal candidiasis: Frequently a clinical diagnosis. The pH of vaginal discharge can range from 4 to 4.5. Yeast will be seen on microscopic exam of KOH preparations or wet mounts (3,4).
- Oral candidiasis (thrush): Also commonly a clinical diagnosis. Can be confirmed by viewing scrapings on KOH preparations under light microscopy.
- Esophageal candidiasis: May require endoscopy and biopsy to make diagnosis.
- Candidemia: Gram stain or growth in blood cultures. *Candida* should never be treated as a contaminant of blood.
- Susceptibility testing to fluconazole should be performed in serious infection or in patients who are not responding to first-line therapies.

Imaging
Initial approach
- Nervous system involvement: CT scan, MRI of the brain.
- Endocarditis: Transesophageal echocardiogram
- Esophagitis: Upper endoscopy with biopsy
- Spleen and liver: MRI is superior to CT
- Pneumonia: CXR, CT
- Peritonitis: CT or ultrasound-guided fluid aspiration

Follow-Up & Special Considerations
- For candidemia: General ICU care for stabilization (mortality can be >30–40%).
- 5–10% of candidemia cases are complicated by endophthalmitis. Ophthalmology should be consulted in all cases of candidemia.

Diagnostic Procedures/Other
Candida esophagitis: Although endoscopy and biopsy are the gold standard for diagnosing Candida esophagitis, many patients are treated empirically if they have compelling symptoms along with risk factors and oral candidiasis. Note that oral candidiasis need not be present for esophageal candidal infections.

Pathological Findings
Yeast with and without pseudohyphae

DIFFERENTIAL DIAGNOSIS
- Oral hairy leukoplakia
- Contact dermatitis
- Atrophic vaginitis
- Bacterial sepsis
- Endocarditis
- Fever of unknown origin
- Cytomegalovirus (CMV) esophagitis

TREATMENT

MEDICATION

First Line

- Vulvovaginal candidiasis: Multiple topical agents available, for example butoconazole cream 5 g/d for 3 days. Oral options are available as well, such as fluconazole 150 mg p.o. × 1 dose. Longer treatment duration is required in severe cases or immunocompromised hosts. 5–7 days of butoconazole cream, or up to 7 days of p.o. fluconazole may be necessary (5–7).
- Oral candidiasis (thrush): Nystatin oral solution (suspension), clotrimazole oral trouche or fluconazole 100–200 mg/day. Duration of therapy is usually 5 days after symptoms resolve.
- Candida esophagitis: Fluconazole 400 mg as a loading dose, then 200–400 mg/day for 7–14 days. This can be given orally, but may be given intravenous in some patients if there is significant dysphagia or odynophagia.
- Candidemia: Choice of empiric therapy depends on the host. *Candida* should be sent for culture and sensitivity testing to triazoles (e.g., fluconazole) (8,9). In stable, non-neutropenic patients without antifungal exposure, fluconazole (800 mg i.v. × 1, then 400 mg i.v. daily) is a reasonable choice. All other patients, including those who are unstable, neutropenic, have previous antifungal exposure, or have recent or prolonged hospitalizations, should be treated empirically with either echinocandin (caspofungin, micafungin, or anidulafungin), or voriconazole, or lipid formulations of amphotericin B. This can be changed to fluconazole if the sample is found to be sensitive.
- *C. krusei* is resistant to fluconazole.
- *C. glabrata* is often resistant to triazoles.
- *C. parapsilosis* isolates have higher minimum inhibitory concentrations (MICs) to echinocandins.
- *C. lusitaniae* is resistant to amphotericin B.
- The recommended duration of antifungal therapy is at least 2 weeks after blood cultures become negative. Ensure there is also appropriate "source control" (e.g., IV lines have been removed and replaced).

Second Line

Candida esophagitis: In fluconazole-resistant cases, other triazoles, such as itraconazole, posaconazole, and voriconazole, are effective. An echinocandin (e.g. caspofungin, micafungin, or anidulafungin) can be used in hospitalized patients, but it is only available in IV form.

ADDITIONAL TREATMENT

Issues for Referral

- Infectious diseases specialists should be consulted for *Candida* infections of the blood stream, and for assistance with the management of neutropenic patients.
- Pharmacists are very helpful as there are many drug interactions with antifungal medications, especially the triazoles. Careful with concomitant use of warfarin, rifampin, anti-seizure medications, and sulfonylureas.

SURGERY/OTHER PROCEDURES

Surgical consultation is warranted to drain fluid pockets infected with *Candida* species, and for the management of candidal endocarditis.

IN-PATIENT CONSIDERATIONS

Admission Criteria

Any patient suspected of candidemia should be admitted to hospital and treated with empiric antifungal therapy.

ONGOING CARE

FOLLOW-UP RECOMMENDATIONS

Patient Monitoring

- QT prolongation should be monitored with ECGs in patients taking triazoles (e.g., fluconazole, voriconazole).
- Pharmacy to assess for drug interactions when using antifungal agents, especially the triazoles.
- Repeat blood cultures daily in patients with candidemia to ensure sterilization.
- Ophthalmology to examine all patients with candidemia for endophthalmitis.

PROGNOSIS

Mortality steadily increases in patients with candidemia who have delayed antifungal therapy. For example those treated at 3 or more days after documented candidemia have mortality rates in excess of 40%.

COMPLICATIONS

- Renal failure
- Esophageal perforation
- Endocarditis
- Endophthalmitis
- Meningitis
- Peritonitis and adhesions
- Pericarditis
- Abscess
- Death

REFERENCES

1. Pfaller MA, Diekema DJ. Epidemiology of invasive mycoses in North America. *Crit Rev Microbiol* 2010;36:1–53.
2. Conica E, Azzini AM, Conti M. Epidemiology, incidence and risk factors for invasive candidiasis in high-risk patients. *Drugs* 2009;69:5–14.
3. Viscoli C. Antifungal prophylaxis and pre-emptive therapy. *Drugs* 2009;69:75–78.
4. Achkar JM, Fries BC. *Candida* infections of the genitourinary tract. *Clin Microbiol Rev* 2010;23:253–273.
5. Pappas PG, Kauffman CA, Andes D, et al. Clinical practice guidelines for treatment of candidiasis: 2009 update by Infectious Diseases Society of America. *Clin Infect Dis* 2009;48:503–535.
6. Aperis G, Myriounis N, Spanakis EK, et al. Developments in the treatment of candidiasis: More choices and new challenges. *Expert Opin Investig Drugs* 2006;15:1319–1339.
7. Spanakis EK, Aperis G, Mylonakis E. New agents for the treatment of fungal infections: Clinical efficacy and gaps in coverage. *Clin Infect Dis* 2006;43:1060–1068.
8. Wisplinghoff H, Bischoff T, Tallent SM. Nosocomial bloodstream infections in US hospitals: Analysis of 24,179 cases from a prospective nationwide surveillance study. *Clin Infect Dis* 2004;39:309–317.
9. Garey KW, Rege M, Pai MP, et al. Time to initiation of fluconazole therapy impacts mortality in patients with candidemia: A multi-institutional study. *Clin Infect Dis* 2006;43:25–31.

CODES

ICD9

- 112.2 Candidiasis of other urogenital sites
- 112.3 Candidiasis of skin and nails
- 112.9 Candidiasis of unspecified site

CLINICAL PEARLS

- In candidemia:
  - Eye assessment by ophthalmology
  - Daily blood culture until sterile
  - Removal of central IV catheters and other foreign materials

CAT-SCRATCH DISEASE (AND *BARTONELLA* INFECTIONS)

Jason B. Harris (E. Mylonakis, Editor)

BASICS

DESCRIPTION
- Cat-scratch disease is typically a self-limited acute illness associated with regional lymphadenopathy with fever and constitutional symptoms caused by *Bartonella henselae*.
- Other presentations of *B. henselae* infection include fever of unknown origin, hepatosplenic granulomatous disease, neuroretinitis, and encephalopathy (1).
- Other medically important *Bartonella* species include:
  - *Bartonella quintana* is the historical cause of trench fever, and is associated with persistent bacteremia, endocarditis, and bacillary angiomatosis.
  - *Bartonella bacilliformis* is the cause of Oroya fever.

EPIDEMIOLOGY
Incidence
- The incidence of cat-scratch disease in the US is approximately 10 cases per 100,000 person years with an estimated 24,000 cases recognized each year.
- Cat-scratch disease occurs worldwide. In temperate climates, it is seasonal, with most cases occurring between August and January.
- Cat-scratch disease occurs in immunocompetent patients of all ages, with 80% being younger than 21 years of age.
- Most cases of cat-scratch disease are self-limited and associated with regional adenopathy.
- *B. quintana* is believed to be globally endemic.
- *B. bacilliformis* infection is transmitted by sand fly bites and occurs only at altitudes of >1 km in areas of the Andes mountains.

RISK FACTORS
- Cats are the natural hosts and reservoir of *B. henselae*.
- Most cases of cat-scratch disease can be directly linked to cat exposure, especially to kittens or cats with fleas:
  - A history of contact with cats is found in 90% of patients.
  - A history of an antecedent cat scratch in 60%.
- Outbreaks of *B. quintana* infection have been reported in homeless and socioeconomically disadvantaged persons. These conditions predispose individuals to *Pediculus humanus* (human body louse), which is a vector for *B. quintana* transmission.
- Patients with advanced HIV infection and other immunocompromised individuals are at high risk of developing chronic infections caused by *B. quintana* and *B. henselae* including bacillary angiomatosis (vascular lesions) and bacillary peliosis (cystic lesions).

GENERAL PREVENTION
- The risk of cat-scratch disease can be reduced by limiting exposures that may lead to a scratch, bite, or lick by cats or kittens.
- The treatment of cat fleas may reduce the risk of transmission, and may be useful in household with immunosuppressed individuals.

PATHOPHYSIOLOGY
- *Bartonella* species are capable of intracellular survival and trigger inflammation in infected tissues.
- The inflammatory response in cat-scratch disease results in local granuloma formation.

ETIOLOGY
- *Bartonella* species are fastidious gram-negative rod-shaped aerobic bacteria.
- The vast majority of cases of cat-scratch disease are caused by *B. henselae*.
- Other medically important *Bartonella* infections include *B. quintana* and *B. bacilliformis*.
- Numerous other *Bartonella* species have been associated with sporadic cases of human infection.

COMMONLY ASSOCIATED CONDITIONS
B. henselae and *B. quintana* cause a distinct spectrum of diseases in HIV infection (see above). Chronic infection may also occur in solid-organ transplant recipients and patients with hematopoietic malignancies.

DIAGNOSIS

HISTORY
- Often, the initial symptom of cat-scratch disease is the formation of a small erythematous papule or pustule at the site of the scratch that persists for several weeks.
- Subsequently, lymph nodes draining the site of inoculation become enlarged and tender.
- Patients with cat-scratch disease do not always have fever. Low-grade fever and malaise are seen in 30% of patients.
- Other manifestations of cat-scratch disease include persistent fever, neuroretinitis (manifested by decreased visual acuity or visual changes), and encephalopathy (manifested by mental status changes).
- *B. henselae* bacteremia in HIV-infected persons is associated with insidious development of fatigue, malaise, body aches, weight loss, recurring fevers of progressively greater duration and elevation, and sometimes headache. Associated hepatomegaly may occur.

- Trench fever is the classic presentation of *B. quintana* infection, and its natural course in normal hosts has been well summarized. Incubation after inoculation may span 3–38 days before the usually sudden onset of chills and fevers. Afebrile infection is the least common form. Associated symptoms and signs (e.g., headache, vertigo, retro-orbital pain, conjunctival infection) are all nonspecific.
- Characteristic of the gross morphology of bacillary angiomatosis, skin lesions are subcutaneous or dermal nodules, and/or single or multiple dome-shaped, skin-colored or red-to-purple papules, any of which may display ulceration, serous or bloody drainage, and crusting. Visceral lesions can be quite dramatic as well, in both their number and heterogeneity of gross appearance.
- Bacillary peliosis involves organs that contain numerous blood-filled cystic structures, the sizes of which can range from microscopic to several millimeters.

PHYSICAL EXAM
- Regional lymphadenopathy is the most common physical finding in cat-scratch disease and occurs in lymph nodes draining the site of inoculation.
- In many cases a small granuloma or lesion can be found at the inoculation site.
- Parinaud's oculoglandular syndrome is reported in approximately 5% of patients with cat-scratch disease; manifestations include conjunctivitis, conjunctival granuloma, and preauricular lymphadenopathy.
- Patients with visceral disease may have hepatosplenomegaly.

DIAGNOSTIC TESTS & INTERPRETATION
Lab
Initial lab tests
- Early in the disease, a total white blood cell count may show mild leukocytosis and an increased number of polymorphonuclear cells, with eosinophilia in 10–20% of patients.
- *B. henselae* and *B. quintana* can be isolated from blood if lysis-centrifugation blood cultures are used, but both species have also been isolated with use of the BACTEC blood culture system.
- Serologic tests for *B. henselae* are becoming standardized. Multiple commercial testing laboratories perform an indirect fluorescence assay. While low positive titers (1:64–1:256) may represent recent or past infection, titers greater than 1:256 ngly suggest active infection (2).

Follow-Up & Special Considerations
In cases where serology is equivocal a repeat serology 2 weeks later may be useful in establishing a diagnosis.

C

Imaging
Sonography of enlarged lymph nodes may be helpful in evaluating other causes of lymphadenopathy, detect early suppuration of the bubo, and to direct needle aspiration, when indicated.

Diagnostic Procedures/Other
In many cases of regional lymphadenopathy excisional biopsy or fine needle aspiration is performed.

Pathological Findings
Pathological findings include nonspecific granuloma formation in affected lymph nodes. A positive Warthin–Starry stain or tissue PCR for *Bartonella* suggest the diagnosis of cat-scratch disease but are not always positive.

DIFFERENTIAL DIAGNOSIS
- The diagnosis of cat-scratch disease in patients with regional lymphadenopathy or a consistent clinical syndrome consistent with cat-scratch disease is suggested by the following:
  - Contact with a cat and the presence of a scratch or primary lesion
  - A positive serologic test for *Bartonella*
  - Characteristic histopathologic findings (the presence of multiple microabscesses or granulomas in a lymph node biopsy specimen)
  - Exclusion of other identifiable causes, especially mycobacteria and suppurative adenitis

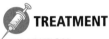 **TREATMENT**

MEDICATION
First Line
- The literature is full of contradictory statements about the role and selection of antibiotics for cat-scratch disease (3).
- Although disease is most often self-limited, antibiotics may hasten resolution and are therefore often used to treat cat-scratch disease.
- Azithromycin (500 mg orally once and 250 mg once daily for the following 4 days) can be used in adults.
- The treatment of cat-scratch neuroretinitis is also controversial but doxycycline plus rifampin has been retrospectively studied and associated with more rapid resolution of symptoms (4).
- For bacillary angiomatosis involving only the skin, 8–12 weeks of oral therapy with erythromycin 500 mg four times daily or doxycycline 100 mg orally twice daily is recommended. Lesions often begin to recede within a week, but usually take considerably longer to involute completely and may leave residual hyperpigmentation. If not resolved by 12 weeks, therapy should be extended.
- For bacteremia, at least 4 weeks of therapy is indicated. Treatment of longer duration (2–3 months) is appropriate in a HIV-infected patient, if fever is persistent or recurrent in the patient, and in the setting of endocarditis.

Second Line
Other oral agents thought to be effective against cat-scratch disease include rifampin, ciprofloxacin, and trimethoprim-sulfamethoxazole.

SURGERY/OTHER PROCEDURES
- If suppuration occurs, aspiration should be considered to relieve the pain and hasten recovery. Needle aspiration is generally preferred to incision and drainage. After washing the skin with an iodophor skin cleanser, aspiration may be accomplished by inserting an 18- or 19-gauge needle tangentially through normal skin at the base of the node. Rarely, reaspiration may be necessary.
- In endocarditis, hemodynamic considerations may require valve replacement (see also chapters in Section II on endocarditis).

 ONGOING CARE

FOLLOW-UP RECOMMENDATIONS
- The lymphadenopathy of cat-scratch disease usually resolves spontaneously within a period of several months.
- One episode of cat-scratch disease appears to confer lifelong immunity. Rarely, a recurrence of sinus tract drainage from the nodes originally involved may occur. If the adenopathy is massive (>5 cm), chronic adenopathy may persist for 1–2 years.
- Remission of fever among patients with bacteremia is usually prompt in non-HIV-infected persons, but may take up to several weeks in HIV-infected patients. Within a week of starting therapy, bacteremia is usually no longer detectable, even if fever persists.

DIET
Normal.

PATIENT EDUCATION
Patients should be educated about the mechanism of transmission and potential risks to immunocompromised members of the household with similar exposure to cats.

PROGNOSIS
Uncomplicated cat-scratch disease has a good prognosis. In immunocompetent individuals lymphadenopathy associated uncomplicated cat-scratch disease resolves illness over a period of weeks to several months. Complications such as retinitis, encephalopathy, or severe systemic disease occur in 5–14% of cases.

COMPLICATIONS
- Encephalopathy usually develops several weeks after the acute illness. Seizures and status epilepticus may herald encephalopathy but are self-limited, with rapid improvement, usually within several days. The cerebrospinal fluid is usually normal, although pleocytosis may occur. The cause of the encephalopathy is uncertain, but direct infection, a toxin, and an autoimmune process have been implicated.
- Inflammatory reactions to *B. henselae* infection in persons with AIDS, without associated angiomatosis or peliosis, have been reported involving liver, spleen, lymph nodes, heart, and bone marrow.

REFERENCES
1. Spach DH, Koehler JE. *Bartonella*-associated infections. *Infect Dis Clin North Am* 1998;12:137.
2. Margileth AM. Recent advances in diagnosis and treatment of cat scratch disease. *Curr Infect Dis Rep* 2000;2(2):141–146.
3. Rolain JM, Brouqui P, Koehler JE, Maguina C, Dolan MJ, Raoult DS. Recommendations for treatment of human infections caused by Bartonella species. *Antimicrob Agents Chemother* 2004;48(6):1921–1933.
4. Reed JB, Scales DK, Wong MT, et al. *Bartonella henselae* neuroretinitis in cat scratch disease: Diagnosis, management, and sequelae. *Ophthalmology* 1998;105:459.

CODE ICD-9-301 CODES

ICD9
- 078.3 Cat-scratch disease
- 088.0 Bartonellosis

CLINICAL PEARLS
- In patients presenting with regional adenopathy, inspect the skin for a primary inoculation lesion and obtain a history of cat exposure.
- Consider cat-scratch disease in the differential diagnosis of patients with fever of unknown origin, neuroretinitis, and encephalopathy.
- The diagnosis of cat-scratch disease is suggested but not made solely on the basis of clinical suspicion. The diagnosis requires positive serologically tested, histologic or microbiologic evidence of *Bartonella* infection.

CERVICITIS

Paschalis Vergidis
Matthew E. Falagas

 BASICS

DESCRIPTION
Sexually transmitted disease manifested as inflammation of the endocervix and/or the ectocervix.

EPIDEMIOLOGY
Prevalence
- Frequent in sexually active adolescent girls under the age of 20 years
- Also found in young adults aged 20–24 years
- In a prospective US cohort study of 14,322 young adults aged 18–26 years (1):
  - Overall prevalence of chlamydial infection was 4.2%. Women (4.7%) were more likely to be infected than men (3.7%). The prevalence was highest among black women.
  - Overall prevalence of gonorrhea was 0.4%.
  - Prevalence of coinfection with both chlamydial and gonococcal infections was 0.03%.

RISK FACTORS
- New sex partner within past 3 months
- More than one sex partner within past 6 months
- Sex partner with multiple other sex partners
- Inconsistent use of barrier contraceptives

GENERAL PREVENTION
- Safe sex practices
- Examination and treatment of sex partners
- When medical evaluation, counseling, and treatment of partners cannot be done, patient-delivered therapy is an option.
- Presumptive treatment if prevalence of *Chlamydia trachomatis* or *Neisseria gonorrhoeae* is high or if compliance with return visits deemed unlikely.
- Annual chlamydial screening is recommended for all sexually active women 25 years of age or younger and also for older women with risk factors (e.g., those who have a new sex partner or multiple sex partners) (2).

ETIOLOGY
- *C. trachomatis*
- *N. gonorrhoeae*
- *Mycoplasma hominis, Ureaplasma urealyticum*
- *Mycoplasma genitalium*
- Herpes simplex virus
- In the majority of cases, no organism is isolated
- Infection of the vagina, due to *Trichomonas vaginalis* or *Candida albicans* can extend to the ectocervix
- Rarely, cytomegalovirus is a cause

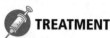 **DIAGNOSIS**

HISTORY
- Frequently asymptomatic
- Abnormal vaginal discharge or vaginal bleeding, particularly after intercourse
- Dysuria or frequency
- Dyspareunia

PHYSICAL EXAM
- Yellow exudate visible in endocervical canal or on an endocervical swab specimen
- Cervical friability

DIAGNOSTIC TESTS & INTERPRETATION
Lab
Initial lab tests
- Culture of cervical discharge, including culture for *N. gonorrhoeae* with a modified Thayer–Martin medium.
- Gram stain
- Cytologic examination of endocervical mucus specimens:
  - Detection of gram-negative, intracellular diplococci in endocervical mucus is highly specific for gonococcal infection.
  - It is only 50% sensitive in mucopurulent cervicitis, in contrast to 95% sensitive in gonococcal urethritis.
- Microscopic examination of ectocervical fluid specimens using normal, wet-mount saline and KOH.
- Leukorrhea (>10 WBC per high power field on microscopic examination of vaginal fluid) has been associated with chlamydial and gonococcal infection of the cervix.
- Nucleic acid amplification testing for *N. gonorrhoeae* and *C. trachomatis*. Can be performed on endocervical sample, vaginal swab specimen, or urine.
- If cervical ulcers or necrotic lesions are present, test for genital herpes (PCR, DFA, viral culture, or type-specific serology).
- Women with cervicitis should be evaluated for bacterial vaginosis, trichomoniasis, and pelvic inflammatory disease.
- Note: Wipe the ectocervix clean with a swab before obtaining the endocervical mucus specimen.

Follow-Up & Special Considerations
- Management of sex partners should be appropriate for the identified or suspected infection.
- To avoid re-infection, patients and their sex partners should abstain from sexual intercourse until therapy is completed (i.e., 7 days after a single-dose regimen or after completion of a 7-day regimen).
- For HIV-infected women, treatment of cervicitis reduces viral shedding and the risk of HIV transmission.

Pediatric Considerations
In pre-adolescent children, sexual abuse must be considered as a cause of chlamydial or gonococcal infection.

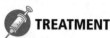 **TREATMENT**

MEDICATION
Presumptive treatment should be undertaken if there is a high prevalence of *C. trachomatis* and *N. gonorrhoeae* in the local population, and there is little likelihood that the patient will comply with return visits. Awaiting test results before treatment is initiated is recommended if prevalence of *C. trachomatis* and *N. gonorrhoeae* is low and compliance with return visits is likely.

First Line
- Chlamydial infection (3):
  - Azithromycin 1 g PO, single dose, or
  - Doxycycline 100 mg PO twice daily for 7 days
- Gonococcal infection: Ceftriaxone 250 mg i.m., single dose
- Specific treatment for other causes of cervicitis is indicated.

Second Line
- Chlamydial infection:
  - Ofloxacin 300 mg PO twice daily for 7 days
  - Levofloxacin 500 mg PO daily for 7 days
  - Erythromycin base 500 mg PO four times daily for 7 days

- Gonococcal infection:
  – Cefixime 400 mg PO, single dose
  – Cefpodoxime 400 mg PO, single dose
  – With oral cephalosporins the bactericidal level is not as high or as sustained as that provided by ceftriaxone.
  – Fluoroquinolones should not be used due to increasing rates of gonococcal resistance.
  – Spectinomycin 2 g i.m., single dose
  – Spectinomycin has poor efficacy in gonococcal pharyngitis.
  – Note: Spectinomycin is currently not manufactured in the US.
  – A single 2 g oral dose of azithromycin is effective against uncomplicated urogenital gonococcal infection. It is not recommended because of gastrointestinal intolerance and cost. Furthermore, sustained low levels of the drug may be favorable for the induction of resistance.

Pregnancy Considerations
First Line
- Chlamydial infection:
  – Azithromycin 1 g PO, single dose (4), or
  – Amoxicillin 500 mg PO three times daily for 7 days
- Theoretically, amoxicillin could induce a persistent chlamydial infection rather than microbiological cure. There are insufficient clinical data to support this concern.
- Gonococcal infection: Ceftriaxone 250 mg i.m., single dose

Second Line
- Chlamydial infection:
  – Erythromycin base 500 mg PO four times daily for 7 days
  – Erythromycin base 250 mg PO four times daily for 14 days
  – Erythromycin ethylsuccinate 800 mg PO four times daily for 7 days
  – Erythromycin ethylsuccinate 400 mg PO four times daily for 14 days:
    ○ Lower dose, if gastrointestinal intolerance
  – Fluoroquinolones and tetracyclines are contraindicated.
  – Erythromycin estolate is contraindicated during pregnancy because of drug-related hepatotoxicity.
- Gonococcal infection: Alternative cephalosporin or spectinomycin

 ONGOING CARE

FOLLOW-UP RECOMMENDATIONS
- Test-of-cure for chlamydial infection is only recommended:
  – If therapeutic compliance is in question
  – If symptoms persist
  – If re-infection is suspected
  – In pregnancy
- Follow-up testing should not be done immediately after clinical resolution. Nonculture tests for *C. trachomatis* performed within 3 weeks of completion of successful treatment may be false-positive as a result of continued excretion of dead organisms.
- Patients with uncomplicated gonorrhea, who received appropriate treatment, do not need a test of cure. Patients with persistent symptoms should be evaluated by culture for *N. gonorrhoeae*, and any gonococci isolated should be tested for antimicrobial susceptibility.
- If persistent cervicitis consider the following:
  – Re-infection (treat partner)
  – Bacterial vaginosis
- Repeat screening should be considered within the first 3–4 months after therapy is completed due to high risk of re-infection, especially in sexually active adolescents.

PATIENT EDUCATION
Advise safe sex practices.

COMPLICATIONS
- Pelvic inflammatory disease
- Ectopic pregnancy
- Infertility
- Chorioamnionitis
- Premature rupture of membranes
- Puerperal infections

REFERENCES

1. Miller WC, Ford CA, Morris M, et al. Prevalence of chlamydial and gonococcal infections among young adults in the United States. *JAMA* 2004;291: 2229–2236.
2. US Preventive Services Task Force. Screening for chlamydial infection: Recommendations and rationale. *Am J Prev Med* 2001;20:90–94.
3. Lau CY, Qureshi AK. Azithromycin versus doxycycline for genital chlamydial infections: A meta-analysis of randomized clinical trials. *Sex Transm Dis* 2002;29:497–502.
4. Adair CD, Gunter M, Stovall TG, et al. Chlamydia in pregnancy: A randomized trial of azithromycin and erythromycin. *Obstet Gynecol* 1998;91:165–168.

ADDITIONAL READING
- Workowski KA, Berman SM. Sexually transmitted diseases treatment guidelines, 2010. *MMWR Recomm Rep* 2010;59(RR-12):1–110.

 CODES

ICD9
- 098.15 Gonococcal cervicitis (acute)
- 099.53 Other venereal diseases due to Chlamydia trachomatis, lower genitourinary sites
- 616.0 Cervicitis and endocervicitis

CLINICAL PEARLS
- The main etiologic agents of cervicitis are *C. trachomatis* and *N. gonorrhoeae*. The disease is frequently asymptomatic.
- Nucleic acid amplification testing is the preferred diagnostic modality.
- Due to increased resistance, fluoroquinolones are no longer recommended for the treatment of gonococcal infection.
- Management of sex partners is key in preventing re-infection.

CHANCROID

Paschalis Vergidis
Matthew E. Falagas

 BASICS

DESCRIPTION
Chancroid is a sexually transmitted disease manifested as tender genital lesions or, later, as genital ulcers. The primary lesion is typically a group of excavated papules or pustules 2–20 mm diameter with undermined, ragged, or irregular edges.

EPIDEMIOLOGY
Incidence
In the US, chancroid usually occurs in outbreaks. 28 cases were reported to the CDC in 2009. The disease may be underdiagnosed.

Prevalence
Prevalent in
- Africa
- Asia
- Latin America
- US, lower socioeconomic groups

RISK FACTORS
- Sex with multiple partners.
- Sex with partner infected with *Haemophilus ducreyi*.
- Sex with persons in countries where chancroid is endemic.
- Transmission of and susceptibility to HIV infection is increased during intercourse in patients with chancroid.

GENERAL PREVENTION
- Avoid sexual contact with a person infected with chancroid or a person who has genital lesions or ulcers.
- Observe safe-sex practices.

ETIOLOGY
H. ducreyi, a small fastidious gram-negative rod

COMMONLY ASSOCIATED CONDITIONS
Approximately 10% of persons who have chancroid that was acquired in the US are coinfected with *Treponema pallidum* or herpes simplex virus (HSV).

DIAGNOSIS

HISTORY
Incubation period: 1–14 days

PHYSICAL EXAM
- Tender papules that become pustular, eroded, and ulcerated within 1–2 days.
- Several lesions can coalesce to form a large ulcer wider than 2 cm.
- Tender inguinal nodes ("buboes") in approximately 40% of patients.
- Inguinal lymph nodes occasionally suppurate and rupture spontaneously.
- Combined painful genital ulcer with suppurative inguinal lymphadenopathy.

DIAGNOSTIC TESTS & INTERPRETATION
Lab
- Initial diagnosis is based on epidemiologic factors and the characteristics of the lesions. History and physical examination alone often lead to misdiagnosis, making laboratory examination of utmost importance.
- Isolation of *H. ducreyi* to provide definitive diagnosis requires special culture media that are not widely commercially available.
- Culture for *H. ducreyi* (80% sensitivity).
- PCR (95% sensitivity) (1). Not FDA approved. Not practical for most clinics.
- No evidence of syphilis by dark-field examination, immunofluorescence test, or a serologic test performed more than 7 days after the onset of ulcers.
- No evidence of genital herpes based on clinical presentation or HSV culture or antigen test.
- Test for HIV at time of diagnosis.

Diagnostic Procedures/Other
- Gently abrade the lesion with sterile gauze pad to provoke oozing, but not gross bleeding.
- Squeeze the lesion between a gloved thumb and forefinger to increase exudate from lesion.
- Apply exudate directly onto a microscope slide if used for dark-field and direct immunofluorescence tests.

Pathological Findings
- Superficial purulent exudate in the epidermis.
- Perivascular and interstitial mononuclear cell infiltrate in the dermis.
- HIV-infected patients tend to have less infiltration with neutrophils.

DIFFERENTIAL DIAGNOSIS
- Infectious diseases
  - Genital herpes
  - Syphilis
  - Acute HIV infection
  - Lymphogranuloma venereum
  - Granuloma inguinale or donovanosis
  - Mycobacteria
  - Fungi
  - Parasites
  - Venereal warts
  - Scabies
  - Molluscum contagiosum
  - Folliculitis
  - Plague
- Noninfectious entities
  - Malignancy
  - Trauma
  - Fixed drug eruption
  - Erythema
  - Dermatitis herpetiformis
  - Behçet's syndrome

TREATMENT

MEDICATION

First Line
- Azithromycin 1 g p.o., single dose (2)
- Ceftriaxone 250 mg i.m., single dose (3)

Second Line
- Ciprofloxacin 500 mg p.o. b.i.d. for 3 days.
- Erythromycin base 500 mg p.o. q.i.d. for 7 days (some experts prefer this regimen for treating HIV-infected patients).
- Worldwide, several isolates with intermediate resistance to either ciprofloxacin or erythromycin have been reported.

Pregnancy Considerations
- Ciprofloxacin is contraindicated for pregnant and lactating women.
- No adverse effects of chancroid on pregnancy outcome have been reported.

ADDITIONAL TREATMENT

General Measures
Evaluate and treat partners who have had sexual intercourse with the patient within 10 days of onset of the patient's symptoms. Use the same drugs and dosages as above.

Additional Therapies
Buboes may require needle aspiration through adjacent intact skin, or incision and drainage. The latter may be preferred because of reduced need for repeat drainage.

 ONGOING CARE

FOLLOW-UP RECOMMENDATIONS
- Reexamine within 3–7 days of initial treatment for signs of improvement of ulcers.
- The time required for complete healing depends on the size of the ulcer; large ulcers might require more than 2 weeks.
- Healing is slower for uncircumcised men who have ulcers under the foreskin.
- Fluctuant lymphadenopathy improves more slowly.
- Failure to improve may suggest:
  - Inaccurate diagnosis
  - Coinfection with another sexually transmitted disease (e.g., syphilis)
  - Reinfection
  - HIV-infected patients are at higher risk of treatment failure
  - Poor patient compliance with treatment
  - Antimicrobial resistance
- Patients should be retested for HIV and syphilis 3 months after the diagnosis of chancroid, if the initial test results were negative.

PATIENT EDUCATION
Educate about safe-sex practices

COMPLICATIONS
- Secondary ulcers or draining fistulas at site of rupture of fluctuant lymphadenopathy.
- Transmission of and susceptibility to HIV infection is increased during intercourse in patients with chancroid.

REFERENCES

1. Morse SA, Trees DL, Htun Y, et al. Comparison of clinical diagnosis and standard laboratory and molecular methods for the diagnosis of genital ulcer disease in Lesotho: Association with human immunodeficiency virus infection. *J Infect Dis* 1997;175(3):583–589.
2. Ballard RC, Ye H, Matta A, et al. Treatment of chancroid with azithromycin. *Int J STD AIDS*. 1996;7(Suppl 1):9.
3. Martin DH, Sargent SJ, Wendel GD Jr, et al. Comparison of azithromycin and ceftriaxone for the treatment of chancroid. *Clin Infect Dis* 1995; 21(2):409.

ADDITIONAL READING
- Workowski KA, Berman SM. Sexually transmitted diseases treatment guidelines, 2010. *MMWR Recomm Rep* 2010;59(RR-12):1–110.
- Lewis DA. Diagnostic tests for chancroid. *Sex Transm Infect* 2000;76(2):137–141.

CODES

ICD9
099.0 Chancroid

CLINICAL PEARLS
- The combination of a painful genital ulcer and tender suppurative inguinal adenopathy suggests the diagnosis of chancroid.
- HIV-infected patients are at higher risk of treatment failure.

C

CHICKENPOX (VARICELLA)

Georgia G. Georgantzi
Petros I. Rafailidis
Matthew E. Falagas

 BASICS

DESCRIPTION
Chickenpox is a febrile, highly contagious illness of the early childhood (usually), due to primary infection by varicella zoster virus (VZV), and characterized by a rash with concurrently present varying stages of evolution (including combinations of macules, papules, vesicles, and pustules).

EPIDEMIOLOGY
Incidence
- It is worldwide in distribution, and occurs in epidemics during late winter and early spring.
- The primary attack rate in susceptible subjects is 90%, and secondary attack rate in the same household is 70–90%.
- Incidence is decreasing due to vaccination program (1).

Prevalence
- In the vaccination era incidence in 2 communities of US where varicella is reported had declined 90% by 2005 in comparison to 1995 (2).
- Also, associated hospitalizations, costs, complications, and deaths have declined (2).
- Predominant sex: Males equal to females.

RISK FACTORS
- Close contact of a nonimmune person with a patient transmitting the virus (exposure to varicella or herpes zoster).
- Predominant age: 90% of cases in children ≤3 years old.
- 90% of subjects aged ≥15 years are immune; 10% remain susceptible.
- In adulthood increasing number of cases.

GENERAL PREVENTION
The patient must be out of school until no longer contagious: A patient is infectious 48 hours prior to the appearance of the rash (at the end of incubation period), until all vesicles are crusted.

Passive Immunization
- Varicella zoster immunoglobulin should be given after exposure to chickenpox or herpes zoster cases to:
  – Susceptible immunocompromised children
  – Susceptible immunocompetent adults and adolescents
  – Susceptible pregnant women
  – Newborn children of mothers who develop chickenpox 5 days before to 2 days after delivery
  – Hospitalized premature infants (≥28 weeks of gestation when mother has no history of chickenpox or <28 weeks of gestation, and/or birth weight of <1000 g, regardless of maternal history)
- It should be administered within 96 hours, preferably within 72 hours, of exposure, intramuscularly. The dose for newborn is 125U and for all the others is 125U/10 kg body weight (maximum of 625U).

Vaccination
- Live attenuated VZV vaccine (Varivax: 0.5 mL s.c.) is licensed in the US since 1995 (1). It is part of the routinely recommended immunization schedule in US for children older than 12 months (2 doses) (3).
- Vaccination with attenuated virus at age 12–15 months and at 4–6 years. The second dose may be administered before age 4 with at least 3 months between doses (3).
- For children aged 12 months to 12 years the minimum interval between doses is 3 months, but the second dose can be considered valid, if the interval is at least 28 days. For children aged ≥13 years the minimum interval between doses is 28 days (3).
- Adults who have not been immunized and have no history of chickenpox should be immunized. Administer 2 doses with at least 28 days between doses, if not previously vaccinated or the second dose, if vaccinated with only 1 dose (3).
- VZV vaccine may also be coadministered as a measles–mumps–rubella–varicella vaccine.

PATHOPHYSIOLOGY
The virus enters the body through the respiratory mucous membranes and replicates in regional lymph nodes. Mononuclear cells of peripheral blood are infected through primary cell associated viremia. A secondary viremia spreads out the virus to cutaneous epithelial cells. It remains latent for life in ganglia (4).

ETIOLOGY
- Varicella zoster virus (HHV-3, DNA virus, family: Herpesviridae, genus: *Varicellovirus*).
- There is no known animal reservoir for VZV. Human is the only reservoir.
- Transmission occurs via person-to-person contact; the virus is spread by the respiratory route and from vesicle fluid and replicates in the nasopharynx or the upper respiratory tract.

DIAGNOSIS

HISTORY
- The incubation period is 10–14 days (range: 10–21 days).
- Systems affected: Skin, disseminated/viremia, CNS, respiratory, other viscera.

Immunocompetent Children
- Prodromal symptoms may occur 1–2 days prior to the rash: Malaise, low-grade fever.
- Constitutional symptoms: Low-grade fever, malaise, pruritus, anorexia, listlessness.
- Rash.

Immunocompromised Patients
- More numerous lesions with hemorrhagic base.
- Healing time 3 times longer.
- At greater risk for visceral complications (30–50% of cases; of those, 15% fatal).

Adults
- More severe illness.
- At greater risk for visceral complications.

Pregnant Women
At greater risk for maternal pneumonia and congenital transmission to the fetus (4).

Perinatal Varicella
- When the mother develops chickenpox 5 days before to 48 hours after delivery, it may result in progressive disease in the newborn, involving viscera, particularly the lung, and death.
- Death rate high (mortality 30%).

Congenital Varicella
Infection of the fetus during the first 2 trimesters of pregnancy may lead to severe malformations (skin scarring, hypoplastic extremities, eye abnormalities, CNS impairment) (teratogenic virus).

PHYSICAL EXAM
- Rash: Begins on the face and trunk and spreads centripetally. It may involve mucous membranes and the vagina. Initially maculopapular; develops into vesicles, full of clear fluid. Fluid turns purulent after a few hours. Lesions are round or oval, with an erythematous base, sized 5–13 mm in diameter. Central umbilication appears as healing progresses. Crust formation follows and coexists with evolution of new lesions. All forms of lesions are concurrently present in varying stages of evolution. The successive crops of lesions generally appear over 2–4 days.
- The crusts fall off within 1–2 weeks of onset and leave a slightly depressed area of skin with no scar unless superinfected.

DIAGNOSTIC TESTS & INTERPRETATION
Lab
- Diagnosis is mainly clinical, but it should be taken into consideration that new physicians have limited experience with chickenpox (1).
- Detection of VZV DNA by PCR from a clinical specimen (1, 5). PCR is the most reliable method.
- VZV isolation from material taken from the bottom of the lesions; needs about 3 days (viral culture).
- Tzanck smear from the bottom of a vesicle shows multinucleated giant cells.
- Detection of VZV in smears by direct immunofluorescence staining (DFA) or other assays.
- Serology: Seroconversion (positive IgM antibody) or fourfold or greater increase in IgG antibody in convalescent serum samples (ELISA test). In vaccinated subjects there might not be a fourfold increase (5).

Imaging
- Abnormalities in chest x-rays appear in 16% of chickenpox patients; only 10% of patients with positive chest x-rays develop clinical symptoms from the respiratory system.
- In pneumonitis, a nodular pattern or increased reticular shadowing can be seen.

DIFFERENTIAL DIAGNOSIS
- Disseminated herpes simplex virus infection in patients with atopic dermatitis.
- Disseminated rashes due to coxsackievirus, echoviruses, scabies, papular urticaria, dermatitis herpetiformis, folliculitis, parapsoriasis, and atypical measles.
- Rickettsialpox ("herald spot" at the site of mite bite, serology).

 TREATMENT

MEDICATION
First Line
- Oral acyclovir is recommended for varicella within 24 hours of onset of the disease.
- Immunocompetent children weighting ≤40 kg (≥2 years old): Orally 80 mg/kg/day divided in 4 doses daily for 5 days; maximum: 3200 mg/day.
- Children weighting >40 kg or adults: Orally 3200 mg divided in 4 doses daily for 5 days.
- Patients need adequate hydration.
- Topical solution in each lesion 6 times daily for 7 days.

Second Line
- Valacyclovir (children 2–18 years: 20 mg/kg; adults: 1 g orally 3 times daily for 7 days) and Famciclovir (adults: 500 mg orally 3 times daily for 7 days; not established for children <18 years old) are active against VZV and have better absorption than acyclovir. Valacyclovir data regarding varicella treatment are sparse.
- Ganciclovir is also active against VZV, but myelosuppression is a major and common adverse effect.

ADDITIONAL TREATMENT
General Measures
- Appropriate health care is usually outpatient, unless complication occurs or the patient is at high risk for complications (i.e., pregnant women, immunocompromised patients).
- General measures are careful bathing, astringent soaks, and closely cropped fingernails to prevent scratching.
- Oral antipruritic drugs.
- Topical administration of antibiotics for bacterial infection.
- Use acetaminophen/paracetamol for fever.
- Do not use aspirin (acetylsalicylic acid) as it predisposes to Reye's syndrome development.

 ONGOING CARE

FOLLOW-UP RECOMMENDATIONS
Patient Monitoring
Monitor respiratory function (% O_2 saturation of hemoglobin) in high-risk groups.

PATIENT EDUCATION
- A vaccinated subject should not be in contact with a pregnant woman for 3 months and should not use aspirin for 6 weeks after the vaccination.
- Vaccination should not be performed during pregnancy.
- Instruct the patient that the disease is highly contagious.

PROGNOSIS
- Most cases are mild.
- The virus remains latent in sensory ganglia, and reactivation (secondary infection) results in herpes zoster.
- Varicella produces almost always lifelong immunity.
- It may be life-threatening for immunocompromised patients, adults, pregnant women and their newborn.

COMPLICATIONS
- The annual average number of deaths in the US during 2003–2005 was 16.
- Secondary bacterial infection mainly due to staphylococci or group A streptococci. This may lead to systemic infection in the neutropenic host.
- Varicella pneumonia especially occurs in adults (1 in 400 cases) and immunocompromised patients. It can be life-threatening in pregnant women during the second or third trimester. It manifests with tachypnea, cough, dyspnea, and fever, usually 3–5 days after the onset of illness. Chest x-ray shows nodular or interstitial pneumonitis. Chest x-ray changes can be apparent in the absence of clinical symptoms.
- Cerebellar ataxia appears in 1 in 4000 cases, usually in patients aged ≤15 years, as late as 21 days after the onset of rash, but usually within 1 week. Symptoms include ataxia, emesis, dysphasia, fever, vertigo, and tremor. Cerebrospinal fluid examination shows lymphocytosis and elevated protein. Usually, it is a benign complication and resolves within 2–4 weeks.
- Encephalitis can be life-threatening in adults and appears in 0.1–0.2% of patients within the first week of illness. It presents with decreased level of consciousness, headache, vomiting, altered thought patterns, fever, and seizures. Mortality ranges from 5 to 20%; neurologic sequelae can be detected in 15% of survivors. The duration is at least 2 weeks.

- Meningitis, transverse myelitis.
- Reye's syndrome appears at the late stages of the illness, and has been epidemiologically associated with the administration of aspirin. It presents with vomiting, restlessness, irritability, progressive decrease in the level of consciousness, progressive cerebral edema, hyperammonemia, bleeding diathesis, hyperglycemia, and elevated transaminases.
- Also, myocarditis, nephritis, bleeding diathesis, hepatitis (rarely).

REFERENCES
1. Leung J, Harpaz R, Baughman AL, et al. Evaluation of laboratory methods for diagnosis of varicella. *Clin Infect Dis* 2010;51:23–32.
2. Marin M, Meissner HC, Seward JF. Varicella prevention in the United States: A review of successes and challenges. *Pediatrics* 2008;122: e744–e751.
3. American Academy of Pediatrics. Immunization schedule USA 2010. www.aap.org/healthtopics/immunizations.cfm Accessed on October 18, 2010.
4. Schimdt-Chanasit J, Sauerbrei A. Evolution and world-wide distribution of varicella–zoster virus clades. *Infect Genet Evol* 2011;11:1-10.
5. Weinmann S, Chun C, Mullooly JP, et al. Laboratory diagnosis and characteristics of breakthrough varicella in children. *J Infect Dis* 2008;197: s132–s138.

 CODES

ICD9
- 052 Chickenpox V01.71, V05.4 Varicella
- 052.1 Varicella (hemorrhagic) pneumonitis
- 052.8 Chickenpox with unspecified complication

CLINICAL PEARLS
- Use acetaminophen, not aspirin.
- It can be life-threatening in pregnant women and immunocompromised patients.
- Don't forget to treat adult immunocompetent patients.
- All forms of lesions are concurrently present in varying stages of evolution.

CHOLECYSTITIS/CHOLANGITIS

Mary L. Pisculli (E. Mylonakis, Editor)

 BASICS

DESCRIPTION
- Cholecystitis is acute or chronic inflammation of the gallbladder.
- Cholangitis is a clinical diagnosis based on symptoms and signs of systemic sepsis originating in the biliary tract.
- Emphysematous (or gaseous) cholecystitis is inflammation of the gallbladder characterized by gas in the gallbladder lumen that can infiltrate the gallbladder wall and/or the surrounding tissues.

EPIDEMIOLOGY
- Acute cholecystitis accounts for 3–10% of all patients with abdominal pain. The frequency increases to 20% among patients over the age of 50.
- Annually, 1–4% of patients with cholelithiasis develop biliary colic. If untreated, 20% of symptomatic patients later develop acute cholecystitis.

RISK FACTORS
- Most cases (90–95%) of acute cholecystitis are due to cholelithiasis.
- Both obesity and extreme dieting increase the risk of cholelithiasis and cholecystitis.
- Hemolytic diseases (sickle cell disease, G6PD deficiency, etc.) increase the risk of pigment stones and subsequent biliary obstruction.
- Certain ethnic groups are at increased risk of stone formation, e.g. Pima Indians.
- Acalculous cholecystitis is a complication associated with other serious medical conditions including diabetes mellitus; ischemia, sepsis, and other low-flow states; motility disorders; serious trauma or burns; direct chemical injury; allergic reactions; prolonged use of total parenteral nutrition; vasculitis; collagen disease; sarcoidosis; infections (including tuberculosis, actinomycosis, ascariasis, and HIV/AIDS); and torsion of the gallbladder.
  - Acalculous cholecystitis in AIDS patients typically occurs at a younger age and is associated with cytomegalovirus (CMV) and cryptosporidium infection.
- Emphysematous cholecystitis is more common in the elderly and patients with diabetes mellitus.
- Infectious complication of endoscopic retrograde cholangiopancreatography (ERCP).

Pregnancy Considerations
Cholelithiasis occurs frequently in pregnancy; however, it is unclear if the incidence of cholecystitis is also increased.

Genetics
- The prevalence of gallstones is more than 2 times higher in women than men, although cholecystitis tends to be more severe in men.
- Acalculous cholecystitis occurs slightly more frequently in men.

GENERAL PREVENTION
A low-fat diet assists in the prevention of gallstone formation. Additionally, the treatment of biliary colic with removal of stones or cholecystectomy has decreased the incidence of acute cholecystitis.

PATHOPHYSIOLOGY
- Acute calculous cholecystitis is caused by gallstone obstruction.
- Acalculous cholecystitis results from gallbladder stasis and stagnant bile.
- Acute cholangitis results from obstruction of the common bile duct with associated increased biliary pressures. Obstruction may lead to translocation of bacteria or endotoxins from the bile ducts into the lymphatic structures and bloodstream, resulting in the signs and symptoms of cholangitis.

ETIOLOGY
- Various medications have been implicated in the development of cholestasis or gallstone formation leading to acute cholecystitis including progesterone, fibrate, estrogen, ceftriaxone, and octreotide. Other medications associated with cholecystitis include narcotics and anticholinergic drugs via altered gallbladder mobility, dapsone via promotion of hemolysis, and erythromycin and ampicillin hypersensitivity.
- Most infections are polymicrobial. The organisms most commonly cultured are *Escherichia coli*, *Klebsiella* spp., *Enterococcus* spp., *Enterobacter* spp., and *Pseudomonas* spp.
  - *Staphylococcus* and *Pseudomonas* may be found after interventional endoscopy or a surgical procedure.
  - Anaerobes are more common in elderly patients and patients with diabetes, and after biliary tract operations.
- Obstructive lesions that predispose to pyogenic bacterial cholangitis include choledocholithiasis, malignant biliary strictures, iatrogenic bile duct injury, stricture of a biliary anastomosis, congenital intrahepatic biliary dilatation (Caroli's disease), primary sclerosing cholangitis, and entry of parasites into the bile duct.
  - Parasites associated with cholangitis include the trematodes (*Clonorchis* and *Opisthorchis*), the nematodes (*Ascaris* and, rarely, *Strongyloides*), and the cestodes (*Echinococcus granulosus* and *Echinococcus multilocularis*).

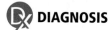 **DIAGNOSIS**

HISTORY
- Biliary tract disease often presents with right upper quadrant abdominal pain which may radiate to the infrascapular area.
- Acute cholecystitis often begins as an attack of biliary colic and fever that progressively worsens.
  - Approximately 60–70% of patients report a history of prior attacks that resolved spontaneously.
  - Unlike biliary colic, the pain of cholecystitis (and cholangitis) is continuous.
- Acalculous cholecystitis may present with unexplained fever or vague abdominal pain. A high index of suspicion is required, especially in unresponsive critically ill patients.
- Acute cholangitis often presents with fever and chills, jaundice, and right upper quadrant pain (Charcot's triad).
  - Only 50–70% of patients present with Charcot's triad.
  - Other additional presenting signs include lethargy or mental confusion and shock (Reynolds' pentad).
  - Other signs of organ failure include renal failure and disseminated intravascular coagulation.

PHYSICAL EXAM
- Right upper quadrant abdominal tenderness is sensitive (98%) for biliary tract disease. Other less sensitive findings include palpation of a right upper quadrant mass. Findings suggestive of biliary tract disease include right upper quadrant abdominal tenderness.
- The presence of a Murphy's sign (pain on palpation of the right subcostal area during inspiration) is sensitive for acute cholecystitis.

DIAGNOSTIC TESTS & INTERPRETATION
Lab
- Patients with acute cholecystitis frequently present with fever and leukocytosis.
  - Temperature >38.5°C or WBC count >12,500 cells/mm³ suggests the presence of infection.
- BUN, Cr, platelet count, and prothrombin time abnormalities indicate disease severity.
- Serum bilirubin is mildly elevated in half of patients, and 25% have modest elevations in serum aminotransferases.
- C-reactive protein is also often elevated.
- Elevated amylase levels suggest concomitant gallstone pancreatitis or gangrenous cholecystitis.
- Biliary cultures are positive in 50% of patients with biliary obstruction and 90% of patients with choledocholithiasis and jaundice. Cultures are positive more often with incomplete versus complete bile duct obstruction. Bile in healthy patients is usually sterile; however, bacterial colonization is usually associated with advanced age (>70 years), previous biliary tract surgery, and common duct stones.

Imaging

- Ultrasonography frequently establishes the diagnosis of cholecystitis.
  - Findings suggestive of acute cholecystitis include gallbladder wall thickening >2 mm; pericholecystic fluid; intramural gas; ductal dilatation or direct tenderness when the probe is placed over the gallbladder (sonographic Murphy's sign).
  - The positive predictive value (PPV) of the presence of stones and a sonographic Murphy's sign is 92%.
  - The PPV of the presence of stones and gallbladder wall thickening is 95%.
  - The negative predictive value of the absence of stones and concomitant normal gallbladder wall or absent Murphy's sign is 95%.

Diagnostic Procedures/Other

- Hepatobiliary scintigraphy tracks the flow of bile using an intravenous injection of technetium-labeled analogues of iminodiacetic acid. The absence of gallbladder filling within 60 minutes after administration indicates obstruction of the cystic duct and is 80–90% sensitive for acute cholecystitis. The false positive rate is 10–20% and is primarily used when ultrasound is not diagnostic.
- CT with intravenous contrast may demonstrate bile duct dilatation and pneumobilia and complement US in the diagnosis of cholangitis.

DIFFERENTIAL DIAGNOSIS

The differential diagnosis of cholangitis and cholecystitis is discussed in the chapters "Abdominal Pain and Fever" and "Jaundice and Fever."

 TREATMENT

MEDICATION

- Antibiotics targeting Enterobacteriaceae should be administered to patients with acute cholecystitis or cholangitis.
- The Infectious Diseases Society of America recommends the use of cefazolin, cefuroxime, or ceftriaxone for mild-to-moderate cases of community-acquired acute cholecystitis.
- Broad-spectrum antibiotic therapy is recommended for acute cholangitis or acute cholecystitis in the setting of advanced age, immune compromise, or severe physiologic disturbance, e.g. imipenem-cilastatin, meropenem, piperacillin-tazobactam, ciprofloxacin, levofloxacin, or cefepime – each in combination with metronidazole.
- The addition of vancomycin is recommended for healthcare-associated biliary infection of any severity.
- Administer antibiotics to patients with diabetes, immunodeficiency, advanced age, or as prophylaxis for cholecystectomy.
- Initiate antibiotics within 1 hour prior to and discontinue antibiotics within 24 hours of cholecystectomy for acute cholecystitis without evidence of infection outside of the gallbladder.

- Anti-enterococcal therapy is not required for community-acquired biliary infection in immunocompetent hosts as the pathogenicity of enterococci in this population has not been demonstrated.
- Intra-operative gallbladder bile cultures may be used to guide antibiotic selection in the event post-operative complications arise.
- The treatment for acute cholangitis is systemic antibiotics and, with more severe disease, biliary drainage.

ADDITIONAL TREATMENT
General Measures

- Eliminate oral intake, initiate nasogastric suction.
- Correct fluid status and electrolyte abnormalities with intravenous fluids.
- Meperidine or pentazocine is usually employed for analgesia.

SURGERY/OTHER PROCEDURES

- Early versus delayed (post-"cooling off") cholecystectomy is preferred due to a lower complication rate, reduced costs, and shortened recovery periods.
- In addition to open or laparoscopic cholecystectomy, biliary decompression may be accomplished via percutaneous transhepatic gallbladder aspiration or endoscopic gallbladder drainage and stenting.
- Urgent cholecystectomy is appropriate when a complication of acute cholecystitis such as emphysematous cholecystitis or gallbladder perforation is suspected or confirmed.
- Biliary drainage in acute cholangitis may be performed via endoscopy (ERCP) or percutaneously. Emergent operative drainage may be required.

 ONGOING CARE

PROGNOSIS

- Of the 75% of patients with acute cholecystitis who undergo remission of symptoms, approximately one-fourth will experience a recurrence of cholecystitis within 1 year, and 60% will have at least one recurrent bout within 6 years.
- Mortality rate of acute cholangitis ranges from 10 to 30%.

COMPLICATIONS

- Repeat occurrences of mild acute cholecystitis or chronic irritation by large gallstones may result in chronic cholecystitis.
- The complication rate for acalculous cholecystitis exceeds that for calculous cholecystitis.
- Empyema of the gallbladder carries a high risk of Gram-negative sepsis and/or perforation.
- Fistulization into an adjacent organ adherent to the gallbladder wall may result from inflammation and adhesion formation.

- The incidence of severe acute cholangitis (with shock or mental confusion) is significantly higher in elderly patients than in younger patients.
- Acute cholangitis can result in hepatic abscess and sepsis.
- An enlarged and tender liver attributable to the abscess may overshadow the underlying cholangitis.

ADDITIONAL READING

- Kimura Y, Takada T, Kawarada Y, et al. Definitions, pathophysiology, and epidemiology of acute cholangitis and cholecystitis: Tokyo guidelines. *J Hepatobiliary Pancreat Surg* 2007;14:15–26.
- Lee SW, Chang CS, Lee TY, et al. The role of the Tokyo guidelines in the diagnosis of acute calculous cholecystitis. *J Hepatobiliary Pancreat Sci* 2010;17:879–884.
- Solomkin JS, Mazuski JE, Bradley JS, et al. Diagnosis and management of complicated intra-abdominal infection in adults and children: Guidelines by the Surgical Infection Society and the Infectious Diseases Society of America. *Clin Infect Dis* 2010;50:133–164.
- Strasberg SM. Acute calculous cholecystitis. *N Engl J Med* 2008;358:2804–2811.

CODES

ICD9

- 575.0 Acute cholecystitis
- 575.10 Cholecystitis, unspecified
- 576.1 Cholangitis

CLINICAL PEARLS

- Ultrasonography frequently establishes the diagnosis of cholecystitis.
- Maintain a high index of suspicion for acalculous cholecystitis in critically ill patients.
- Many patients with acute cholangitis do not present with the complete Charcot's triad.

CHOLERA
Emily P. Hyle (E. Mylonakis, Editor)

 BASICS

DESCRIPTION
Severe watery diarrheal illness caused by *Vibrio cholerae*.

EPIDEMIOLOGY
Incidence
- 3–5 million cases/year (WHO 2010) (2).
- 100,000–120,000 deaths/year.
- Second most common cause of death for children <5 worldwide.

RISK FACTORS
- Immunosuppressed patients have a more severe clinical course.
- Malnutrition.
- Blood group O at risk for severe disease from El Tor subtype.
- Exposure in endemic settings or in epidemics.

Pregnancy Considerations
Increased risk of miscarriage or premature delivery (50% risk in patients who are in third trimester).

GENERAL PREVENTION
- Boiling water or use of filtration, iodine, or chlorine.
- Hand hygiene.
- Vaccination with killed-whole cell vaccine (rBS-WC) is recommended by WHO. Has demonstrated 78% protection in endemic regions but short-lived (~2 years) (2).
- Herd immunity has protective effect in cholera transmission; 50% vaccination in endemic regions may provide 93% reduction in cases (1).

PATHOPHYSIOLOGY
- Fecal–oral contamination; typically contaminated water, food, or undercooked seafood.
- Cholera toxin: 1 A subunit and 5 B subunits; bind to enter enterocytes and increase chloride ion efflux.
- Incubation: 12 hours to 5 days. Can be as quick as hours in high inoculum and high-gastric pH.

ETIOLOGY
- *V. cholerae*, a gram-negative rod.
- 190 serotypes, defined by O-Antigen.
- Only O1 (either El Tor or classical) and O139 produce the epidemic strains; non-O strains produce a mild diarrheal illness.

 DIAGNOSIS

HISTORY
- Watery diarrhea with mucous; described as "rice water stools," often with "fishy" odor (1).
- Diarrhea can be >1 L/hr ("cholera gravis").
- Abdominal cramping but typically without pain.
- No fever.

PHYSICAL EXAM
Dehydration: Poor skin turgor.

DIAGNOSTIC TESTS & INTERPRETATION
Lab
Initial lab tests
- Electrolytes, glucose
- Renal function

Follow-Up & Special Considerations
Close monitoring of acidosis, electrolyte losses, and volume status.

Diagnostic Procedures/Other
- Stool gram stain (motile gram-negative rods).
- Stool culture (on selective media such as Thiosulfate Citrate Bile Sucrose Agar (TCBS) or modified gelatin taurocholate tellurite agar (TTGA)).

DIFFERENTIAL DIAGNOSIS
- Enterotoxigenic *Escherichia Coli*
- Shigellosis, Salmonellosis
- Viral gastroenteritis (e.g., rotavirus)

TREATMENT

MEDICATION
- Adjunctive to rehydration (1).
- Given when PO is tolerated; no benefit to earlier IV therapy.
- Use of antibiotics will reduce stool output (by ~50%) and reduce Vibrio excretion (to 1 day).

First Line
- Tetracycline 500 mg p.o. q.i.d. × 3 days
- Doxycycline 300 mg p.o. × 1 dose

Second Line
- Azithromycin 1 g p.o. × 1 dose
- Ciprofloxacin 250 mg p.o. b.i.d. × 3 days or 1 g p.o. × 1 dose
- Norfloxacin 400 mg p.o. b.i.d. × 3 days

Pediatric Considerations
- Avoid use of quinolones or tetracyclines
- Rx: Erythromycin 12.5 mg/kg p.o. t.i.d. × 3 days or azithromycin 20 mg/kg p.o. × 1 dose

Pregnancy Considerations
Treatment same as in pediatric population.

ADDITIONAL TREATMENT
General Measures
Oral rehydration solutions: Despite cholera toxin, gut will absorb sodium, glucose, and water.

Issues for Referral
If >10% of body weight has been lost from dehydration or patient is unable to take PO (e.g., vomiting or change in mental status).

Additional Therapies
- Zinc supplementation: 30 mg p.o. daily has been shown to decrease stool output and duration of diarrhea (3).
- Concern for increasing resistance (e.g., MARV or multiply antibiotic-resistant *V. cholerae* O1, *gyrA*, *parC*).

IN-PATIENT CONSIDERATIONS
Initial Stabilization
- Rehydration.
- Close monitoring of electrolytes, acidosis, and glucose.
- Initiation of therapy (hydration) should not wait for confirmatory diagnosis.

Admission Criteria
- Hypoglycemia is poor prognostic sign but uncommon.
- Inability to take PO.

IV Fluids
- If PO is not tolerated.
- Should be isotonic with base and potassium (e.g., lactated ringers).

Discharge Criteria
Ability to take adequate POs.

 ONGOING CARE
FOLLOW-UP RECOMMENDATIONS
Antibiotic prophylaxis of household contacts if one member in family of five is affected (WHO) (2).

Patient Monitoring
Diarrhea is usually worst in first 2 days; can last 4–6 days.

DIET
As tolerated; no need to rest gut.

PATIENT EDUCATION
- Many are asymptomatic carriers but not long-term and at low inoculum (as opposed to *Salmonella*).
- Hand hygiene.

PROGNOSIS
- 80% of cases recover with oral hydration alone.
- 50% mortality if untreated.

COMPLICATIONS
- Arrhythmias from electrolyte disturbances.
- Renal failure.

REFERENCES
1. Sack DA, Sack RB, Nair GB, et al. Cholera. *Lancet* 2004;363:223–233.
2. http://www.who.int/mediacentre/factsheets/ fs107/en/index.html. Accessed on July 11, 2010.
3. Nelson EJ, Harris JB, Morris JG, et al. Cholera transmission: The host, pathogen, and bacteriophage dynamic. *Nature Rev Microbiol* 2009;7:693–702.

C

 CODES

ICD9
001.9 Cholera, unspecified

CLINICAL PEARLS
- Rapid onset of watery diarrhea should raise concern for cholera; immediate rehydration should not wait for diagnostics.
- Rehydration and electrolyte management are the mainstay of therapy.
- Antimicrobial therapy reduces time of illness but can occur after volume status is stabilized.
- Must report suspected cases immediately to Infection Control and Department of Public Health.

CHORIORETINITIS (UVEITIS AND RETINITIS)

Theodoros Filippopoulos (E. Mylonakis, Editor)

 BASICS

DESCRIPTION
- Uveitis refers to an inflammation of any part of the uveal tract which includes the choroid, the ciliary body, and the iris, and lies between the outer coat (sclera and cornea) and the inner coat (retina) of the eye.
- Uveitis can be subdivided into:
  - Anterior (confined to iris and anterior chamber termed as iritis or involving the ciliary body as well termed in this case as iridocyclitis)
  - Intermediate (if the inflammatory process arises in the peripheral retina, i.e. pars planitis)
  - Posterior (if the inflammatory process arises in the choroid and vitreous with or without the involvement of retina)
  - Panuveitis (if the inflammation does not respect any anatomic boundaries within the eye)
- Although not a part of the uvea, the retina often becomes primarily (retinitis) or secondarily involved (chorioretinitis) in cases of ocular inflammation. The retina is especially susceptible to neurotropic organisms such as *Toxoplasma gondii* and viruses of the herpes family.
- Uveitis can also be subdivided according to the temporal pattern of ocular involvement into acute, recurrent, and chronic – a distinction that is frequently helpful in making a specific diagnosis.

EPIDEMIOLOGY
Incidence
- The estimated annual incidence of uveitis is estimated between 15 and 50 cases per 100,000 persons.
- In the US, both infectious and noninfectious uveitis accounts for up to 10% of all cases of blindness.
- Anterior uveitis (iritis and iridocyclitis) makes up the majority of uveitis.
- In one-third to one-fifth of cases no etiologic diagnosis can be established (idiopathic uveitis).
- The distribution of uveitis by anatomic location according to population-based studies is as following:
  - Anterior: 73%
  - Posterior: 22%
  - Intermediate: 1%
  - Panuveitis: 5%
- The choroid due to its large blood flow and anatomy often functions as a trap for blood-borne pathogens. Typical choroidal/retinal lesions with concurrent vitreous involvement (endogenous fungal endophthalmitis) occur in about 1–2% of patients with candidemia or invasive *Candida* spp. infections.

Prevalence
The prevalence of both infectious and noninfectious uveitis has been estimated to be about 115 cases per 100,000 persons in the US. Worldwide, prevalence reports range between 75 and 700 cases per 100,000 persons with the higher estimates deriving from developing countries. Prevalence estimates are affected by the duration of the investigation as cases of recurrent uveitis have a higher chance of becoming active the longer a population is studied.

RISK FACTORS
- A decline in the CD4+ T-lymphocyte count below 50 cells/μL is a significant risk factor for CMV retinitis in patients with AIDS or HIV-unrelated immunosuppression.
- AIDS is also a risk factor for a characteristic presentation of a VZV-related necrotizing retinitis termed progressive outer retinal necrosis (PORN).

Genetics
- HLA-typing has been frequently used in diagnosing patients with noninfectious uveitis despite low positive predictive value. HLA-typing should therefore be only applied to confirm a specific clinical suspicion.
- HLA-B27 is associated with anterior uveitis in the context of seronegative spondyloarthropathies.
- Birdshot's chorioretinopathy is a common entity causing posterior uveitis in which 85–95% of patients are HLA-A29 positive.
- HLA-DR2 and HLA-DR15 have been associated with intermediate uveitis, while HLA-B51 is about 9 times more prevalent in patients with Adamantiades–Behçet's disease compared to the general population.

GENERAL PREVENTION
Ocular inflammation is preventable to the degree that the associated condition or infection is preventable. For example, avoidance of consumption of raw or undercooked meat and possibly soil-contaminated fruits and vegetables during pregnancy in women who lack immunity can decrease the rate of vertically transmitted ocular toxoplasmosis.

PATHOPHYSIOLOGY
- In general, uveitis is caused by an immune reaction which may represent a host's response directed against invading organisms or an autoimmune response to a number of uveitogenic ocular antigens (i.e., Retinal S-Antigen).
- Uveitis is frequently diagnosed in association with autoimmune disorders such as seronegative spondyloarthropathies, systemic lupus erythematosus, sarcoidosis, or rheumatoid arthritis. In these cases, uveitis may be due to elements of the immune system that crossreact with loci in the iris epithelium, the retinal pigmented epithelium, the retina, or the ciliary body.

ETIOLOGY
- Infectious etiologies of uveitis include the following:
  - Bacterial
    - Atypical mycobacteria
    - Bejel
    - Brucellosis
    - Cat-scratch disease (*Bartonella henselae*)
    - Leptospirosis
    - Leprosy
    - Lyme disease
    - Nocardiosis
    - Syphilis
    - Tuberculosis
    - Whipple's disease
  - Viral
    - Cytomegalovirus (CMV)
    - Epstein–Barr virus (EBV)
    - Herpes simplex virus (HSV)
    - Varicella zoster virus (VZV)
    - Human immunodeficiency virus (HIV)
    - Human T cell leukemia virus (HTLV)
    - Mumps
    - Rubella
    - Rubeola
    - West Nile virus
  - Fungal
    - Aspergillosis
    - Blastomycosis
    - Candidiasis
    - Coccidiomycosis
    - Cryptococcosis
    - Histoplasmosis (presumed ocular histoplasmosis syndrome [POHS])
    - *Pseudallescheria boydii*
    - Sporotrichosis
  - Parasitic
    - *Acanthamoeba* (causes keratitis and intraocular inflammation)
    - Cysticercosis
    - Onchocerciasis
    - Pneumocystis carinii
    - Toxocariasis
    - Toxoplasmosis (the most common cause of posterior uveitis in western societies)
- CMV retinitis is a common cause of chorioretinitis; it is usually associated with advanced HIV infection and is declining in incidence in the HAART era. Before HAART became available CMV retinitis would develop in up to 30% of patients with AIDS.
- Toxoplasmosis is a surprisingly common cause of uveitis in normal hosts. It is presumed to be a reactivation of a congenitally acquired infection. It is diagnosed on the basis of typical chorioretinal lesions supported by serology. Serologic evidence for previous infection by toxoplasmosis is extremely common in the healthy US population.

- Syphilis accounts for a small fraction of patients with uveitis. It may present in a variety of forms, including posterior uveitis, such as a chorioretinitis or retinal vasculitis. It is critical to recognize syphilis because of its therapeutic implications.
- Tuberculosis is an uncommon cause of uveitis in the western world. It should be considered in the presence of active tuberculosis elsewhere in the body, recent immigration from endemic countries, cachexia, homelessness, a granulomatous appearance of the ocular inflammation, and immunosuppression.
- Cat-scratch disease (*B. henselae*) is increasingly recognized as a cause of uveitis (neuroretinitis).
- HSV and VZV can cause keratouveitis, an inflammation of the cornea along with uveitis that is primarily anterior. Both HSV and VZV can also cause a necrotizing retinitis known as acute retinal necrosis (ARN).
- Histoplasma capsulatum once acquired through inhalation in endemic areas (Ohio–Mississippi river valley) can pass to the choroid through the bloodstream. Exposure has been linked to ophthalmic manifestations such as peripapillary atrophy, small round fundus lesions without significant inflammation, and early in life macular choroidal neovascular membranes that constitute the POHS.
- Geographic considerations are of significance in establishing an etiologic diagnosis. For example in developing countries leptospirosis and tuberculosis are important entities to be considered in cases of uveitis which are otherwise rare in western countries.

COMMONLY ASSOCIATED CONDITIONS
Connective tissue disorders such as seronegative spondyloarthropathies, sarcoidosis, systemic lupus erythematosus, etc., present with or are frequently associated with uveitis.

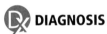 **DIAGNOSIS**

HISTORY
- Anterior uveitis may usually present with dull periorbital pain and light sensitivity (photophobia), with or without decreased vision. Children can suffer from uveitis as in juvenile idiopathic arthritis without significant signs and symptoms but with severe consequences on their vision.
- Posterior uveitis shares similar features along with vitreous opacities (floaters) and usually blurred vision.

PHYSICAL EXAM
- Redness of the eye (conjunctival injection) is usually present in anterior uveitis, and slit-lamp examination reveals inflammatory cells in the anterior chamber.
- The presence of cutaneous vesicles, characteristic corneal changes, decreased corneal sensation, elevated intraocular pressure, and iris atrophy provides clues to the diagnosis of herpetic keratouveitis.
- In posterior and intermediate uveitis there are inflammatory cells or even larger aggregates of cells (snowballs) in the vitreous cavity.
- Immunocompromised individuals often fail to constitute an inflammatory response even in cases of significant ocular involvement.
- Toxoplasma chorioretinitis usually presents as large, smooth, yellow-white retinal lesions with associated vitreous inflammation adjacent to old chorioretinal scars. In immunocompromised patients, lesions can be multiple and bilateral and can be associated with encephalitis.
- CMV retinitis presents as a hemorrhagic necrotizing retinitis without significant inflammation due to the patients' compromised immune status.
- HSV, VZV, and rarely CMV can cause a widespread unilateral or bilateral necrotizing nonhemorrhagic retinitis referred to as acute retinal necrosis in immunocompetent patients. It is often associated with orolabial HSV or trigeminal zoster. Ophthalmologic examination reveals widespread, pale gray peripheral lesions. The lesions spread fast without treatment.
- PORN is a subset of necrotizing rapidly progressing retinitis that occurs mainly among immunocompromised patients. The most commonly isolated viral pathogen is VZV.
- Candida chorioretinitis presents as focal white choroidal lesions that extend into the retina. If the vitreous becomes involved, the term "endogenous fungal endophthalmitis" is more appropriate (see Chapter "Endophthalmitis").
- Initially thought to be idiopathic, *B. henselae* is a cause of neuroretinitis in cat-scratch disease. Neuroretinitis is characterized by swelling of the optic disk, peripapillary and macular hard exudates (macular star), and often vitreous cells.
- In uveitis secondary to tuberculosis, multiple yellow-white choroidal nodules with indistinct borders and sizes up to one-half the disk diameter can be seen. Patients may also have concomitant anterior granulomatous uveitis.
- In Lyme disease a history of a tick bite should be elicited and a variety of ocular manifestations can be expected including intermediate uveitis, conjunctivitis, keratitis, double vision secondary to cranial nerve involvement, or disc edema as a result of optic neuritis.

DIAGNOSTIC TESTS & INTERPRETATION
Lab
Initial lab tests
- The diagnosis of anterior uveitis (iritis and iridocyclitis) requires slit-lamp examination to identify inflammatory cells floating in the aqueous humor and/or deposited on the corneal endothelium (keratic precipitates).
- Posterior involvement (intermediate and posterior uveitis) is best documented with dilated fundus examination.
- Since extensive laboratory workup can be inconclusive in up to one-third of the cases even at tertiary uveitis referral centers, unilateral, nongranulomatous, nonrecurrent cases (first episode) with only anterior involvement should be symptomatically treated with topical steroids and cycloplegics without further workup.
- Patients with posterior uveitis should undergo the following:
  – Complete blood count with differential
  – Serology for syphilis (VDRL and FTA-ABS)
  – Toxoplasma antibodies titer
  – Evaluation for tuberculosis (PPD skin test and chest radiograph)
- Further diagnostic workup should be guided by a comprehensive history and physical examination and according to specific ocular features.
- In tertiary syphilis VDRL can be negative in a significant proportion of patients. False positive nontreponemal screening tests (VDRL& RPR) have also been associated with pregnancy, intravenous drug abuse, tuberculosis, rickettsial infection, nonsyphilis treponemal infection, and endocarditis, among others. Consequently, a reactive nontreponemal test must always be confirmed with a specific treponemal test (FTA-ABS) for proper interpretation.
- IgM-positive and IgG-negative serology are helpful for the diagnosis of primary toxoplasmosis, while, if both IgM and IgG are negative, the diagnosis of toxoplasmosis is unlikely. Toxoplasma IgG titers demonstrate a four-fold increase that peaks 6–8 weeks following infection and declines over the next 2 years, but remains detectable for life which is helpful in diagnosing a reactivation of ocular toxoplasmosis.
- The diagnosis of CMV chorioretinitis is based on clinical grounds in susceptible individuals since serology can be unreliable at times.
- A vitreous biopsy sent for cytology or subjected to PCR for viral pathogens (CMV, HSV, VZV) can be helpful in cases of retinitis but the procedure is not without risk in cases of a necrotizing retinitis which is frequently complicated by spontaneous retinal detachments.

C

- Serum antibody testing can be helpful in a variety of cases (toxocariasis, *B. henselae*, brucellosis, leptospirosis, HSV, CMV, VZV, EBV, HIV, HTLV, Lyme disease, histoplasmosis, etc.).
- Lumbar puncture, neuroimaging, biopsy of skin lesions, ACE levels, chest X-rays, and colonoscopy can assist in the evaluation of certain patients (as in toxoplasmosis, inflammatory bowel disease, neurosyphilis, or sarcoidosis).

Follow-Up & Special Considerations
Frequent follow-up examinations are imperative until a diagnosis is established or a response to treatment is documented.

Imaging
- Chest X-rays or alternatively chest CT scans can provide diagnostic clues for a number of entities (tuberculosis, sarcoidosis, histoplasmosis, tumor, etc.).
- Joint films can be useful among others in rheumatoid arthritis, HLA-B27 associated seronegative spondyloarthropathies, lupus, gonorrhea.
- Gallium scans are employed to confirm suspected sarcoidosis.

Diagnostic Procedures/Other
A vitreous tap can be performed under sterile conditions, and the specimen should be sent for cytology and subject to PCR for specific pathogens (see above).

Pathological Findings
With current diagnostic modalities a diagnostic biopsy is seldom necessary and maybe only limited in cases of necrotizing retinitis (i.e., ARN) which are complicated by retinal detachment, in which case tissue is harvested during surgical repair. In early stages intranuclear inclusions formed by proliferating herpetic viral particles are characteristic.

DIFFERENTIAL DIAGNOSIS
The differential diagnosis of ocular inflammation (uveitis) and chorioretinitis is vast and has been analyzed above under "Etiology."

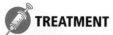

TREATMENT
MEDICATION
First Line
- Treatment of anterior uveitis with judicious use of topical steroids (prednisolone acetate 1%) is aimed at reducing inflammation and scarring. Mydriasis with topical cycloplegic agents (cyclopentolate 1%) reduces pain and photophobia and prevents the formation of synechiae.
- Etiologic treatment is necessary in cases of infectious uveitis. Topical or systemic steroids can be added after antimicrobial treatment has been initiated to limit the inflammatory response.
- In ocular toxoplasmosis no treatment is necessary in immunocompetent patients unless the lesions are present near the macula or the optic nerve threatening the patient's vision. In such cases pyrimethamine (200 mg p.o. loading dose and then 25 mg p.o. per day) with folinic acid (10 mg p.o. twice weekly) along with sulfadiazine (2 g p.o. loading dose and then 1 g p.o. q.i.d.) or clindamycin (150–450 mg p.o. q.i.d.) is recommended. Prednisone may be added (0.5–1 mg/kg p.o. per day) 24 hours after the antibiotic regimen has been initiated.
- Some authors consider any form of ocular inflammation (anterior, intermediate, posterior uveitis, retinitis, or optic neuritis) in syphilis as neurosyphilis and therefore recommend CSF testing and treatment with crystalline penicillin G (2–4 million units i.v. every 4 hours) for 10–14 days followed by benzathine penicillin (2.4 million units i.m. weekly) for 3 weeks. Others believe that only retinal or optic nerve involvement classifies as neurosyphilis. CSF should be obtained and sent for VDRL which can be used to monitor response to treatment. Current CDC recommendation concludes that neurosyphilis is present independent of ocular involvement if CSF VDRL is positive and considers the diagnosis probable if elevated protein or white cell counts are found in the CSF of selected patients. Treatment failures are not uncommon in HIV patients with syphilis, but it has to be noted that HIV patients may demonstrate CSF abnormalities anyway (see relevant chapters).
- In patients with suspected uveitis secondary to tuberculosis a 2 week therapeutic trial of isoniazid (300 mg p.o. per day) may be given along with pyridoxine (10 mg p.o. per day).

- The most important measure in the treatment of CMV retinitis is to initiate HAART to achieve immune recovery which may take a few weeks to achieve. During that period of time CMV-specific treatment is necessary to limit the progression of the necrotizing retinitis and preserve vision.
- Three antiviral agents (ganciclovir, foscarnet, and cidofovir) are effective in treating CMV retinitis. The induction dose for ganciclovir is 5 mg/kg i.v. b.i.d. for 14–21 days; the maintenance dose is 5 mg/kg i.v. per day for 7 days a week or 6 mg/kg i.v. per day for 5 days per week. The induction dose for foscarnet is 90 mg/kg i.v. b.i.d. for 14–21 days; the maintenance dose is 90–120 mg/kg i.v. per day. The induction dose for cidofovir is 5 mg/kg i.v. every week for 2 weeks; the maintenance dose is the same given at 2 week intervals. Recently, an oral prodrug (valganciclovir) became available achieving similar bioavailability as intravenous ganciclovir. Valganciclovir is given at doses of 900 mg p.o. b.i.d. for the first 21 days of induction therapy; after this period, valganciclovir dosing is reduced to 900 mg per day for maintenance therapy. Therapy should be maintained for patients who remain immunosuppressed.
- Anti-CMV treatment can be discontinued once the CD4+ count rises above 100–150 cells/μL for a sustained period of 3–6 months and the CMV retinitis remains quiescent, although continuous monitoring for disease reactivation is recommended.
- Resistant or relapsing CMV retinitis may be treated with intraocular injections (ganciclovir, foscarnet, fomivirsen, cidofovir [used less frequently]) or with the sustained-release ganciclovir implant (Vitrasert®, Bausch and Lomb, San Dimas, CA) which is inserted through the pars plana and releases medication for up to 8 months. The ganciclovir implant is more effective than intravenous ganciclovir in controlling CMV retinitis, making the implant the preferred choice, by most experts, for patients with immediately sight-threatening disease. However, this approach requires intraocular surgery, which may lead to adverse effects. Fomivirsen is a novel anti-sense oligonucleotide that is injected into the eye (0.5 mL) on day 1 and 15 and every month thereafter (330 μg/0.5 mL).
- Local therapy is ineffective in controlling dissemination of the CMV infection to other organs or to the other eye.

- ARN is treated with intravenous acyclovir (1500 mg/m² of body surface area in 3 divided doses) for 10–14 days. Treatment is continued with oral valganciclovir (1 g p.o. t.i.d.) for a total of 6 weeks to prevent second eye involvement. Prophylactic barrier laser photocoagulation should be considered to prevent retinal detachment.
- Cat-scratch disease resolves spontaneously in 6 weeks. Azithromycin (500 mg p.o. q.i.d. followed by 4 doses of 250 mg p.o. per day) can be considered. The long-term prognosis is good but some individuals may suffer from a mild postinfectious optic neuropathy.
- Systemic antifungal medications are not necessary in POHS. Corticosteroids, photocoagulation, and intravitreal anti-VEGF therapy aim at reducing the size and the implications of the macular choroidal neovascularization.

Second Line
- Trimethoprim plus sulfamethoxazole (160/800 mg p.o. b.i.d.) has been shown to be an effective regimen in the treatment of CNS toxoplasmosis in patients with AIDS and can be used in ocular toxoplasmosis for patients unable to tolerate pyrimethamine.
- Aspirin (125–625 mg p.o. per day) can be considered in ARN.
- Fomivirsen is an alternative to the treatment of CMV retinitis in cases of ganciclovir, foscarnet, and cidofovir resistance. It is no longer available in the US.

ADDITIONAL TREATMENT
Issues for Referral
Management decisions are often taken in conjunction with the treating ophthalmologist who can determine the response to therapy.

SURGERY/OTHER PROCEDURES
Surgical interventions are only used for the management of complications such as cataract, retinal detachment, and glaucoma of ocular.

IN-PATIENT CONSIDERATIONS
Initial Stabilization
Most patients with uveitis are managed as outpatients.

Admission Criteria
Only monocular patients with severe ocular involvement, patients out of social considerations, and systemically ill patients are admitted.

 ## ONGOING CARE

FOLLOW-UP RECOMMENDATIONS
Follow-up is individualized.

Patient Monitoring
Patients with recurrent uveitis require lifelong monitoring, while others necessitate chronic immune modulation to keep ocular inflammation under control. Reactivation of ocular inflammation can even occur in cases of infectious uveitis as in toxoplasmosis or herpetic keratouveitis.

DIET
No specific limitations apply that are pertinent to the eye.

PATIENT EDUCATION
Patient education with regard to early recognition of signs and symptoms of ocular inflammation is of great importance especially in cases of recurrent uveitis since prompt treatment is associated with faster recovery and less complications.

PROGNOSIS
Prognosis depends on the specific disease causing uveitis or chorioretinitis. In ocular toxoplasmosis recurrences will develop in 79% of all patients followed for more than 5 years. Legal blindness in one or both eyes has been confirmed for 24% of patients with ocular toxoplasmosis. HAART has increased the CMV retinitis remission duration seven-fold compared to standard anti-CMV therapy alone. The incidence of legal blindness in patients with CMV retinitis has been reduced to about 6–15% per eye-year.

COMPLICATIONS
- Cataract formation and glaucoma are common complications of chronic ocular inflammation in part due to the chronic use of steroids.
- Inflammation can also cause cystoid macular edema that distorts the normal macular architecture and leads to decreased visual acuity.
- Rhegmatogenous retinal detachment can occur in up to one-third of patients with CMV retinitis. The same applies for other forms of necrotizing retinitis such as ARN and PORN.

REFERENCES
1. Zamecki KJ, Jabs DA. HLA typing in uveitis: Use and misuse. *Am J Ophthalmol* 2010;149(2): 189–193.e2.
2. Amaratunge BC, Camuglia JE, Hall AJ. Syphilitic uveitis: A review of clinical manifestations and treatment outcomes of syphilitic uveitis in human immunodeficiency virus-positive and negative patients. *Clin Experiment Ophthalmol* 2010;38: 68–74.
3. Jabs DA, Nussenblatt RB, Rosenbaum JT, et al. Standardization of uveitis nomenclature for reporting clinical data: Results of the first international workshop. *Am J Ophthalmol* 2005;140:509–516.
4. Gritz DC, Wong IG. Incidence and prevalence of uveitis in Northern California: The Northern California Epidemiology of Uveitis Study. *Ophthalmol* 2004;111:491–500.

ADDITIONAL READING
- Nussenblatt RB. Elements of the immune system and concepts of intraocular inflammatory disease pathogenesis. In: Nussenblatt RB, Whitcup SM, eds. *Uveitis fundamentals and clinical practice*, 3rd ed. Philadelphia, PA: Mosby Elsevier, 2004:3–46.

 ## CODES

ICD9
- 360.12 Panuveitis
- 363.20 Chorioretinitis, unspecified
- 364.3 Unspecified iridocyclitis

CLINICAL PEARLS
- A detailed history and physical examination often provides important clues about an etiologic diagnosis of many uveitic entities.
- Uveitis is the most common ocular manifestation of acquired syphilis, and it can take any form of ocular inflammation.
- Do not give pyrimethamine to pregnant or breast-feeding women.
- In patients receiving zidovudine concurrent treatment with ganciclovir can cause severe myelosuppression.
- Probenecid is given before and after treatment with cidofovir to block tubular secretion of the medication.

CHRONIC FATIGUE SYNDROME

Emily P. Hyle (E. Mylonakis, Editor)

 BASICS

DESCRIPTION
- Chronic fatigue syndrome (CFS) is a heterogeneous disorder associated with severe, debilitating fatigue, lasting at least 6 months.

Pediatric Considerations
- Rare in children.
- Absenteeism from school or activities should be monitored as the equivalent of adult disability.

EPIDEMIOLOGY
Prevalence
- 4.0–8.7 per 100,000 people in the US (2).
- 0.6–1% prevalence worldwide.

RISK FACTORS
Gender: 2–3 times more common in women.

Genetics
Ongoing research to determine if specific genes are linked to CFS.

PATHOPHYSIOLOGY
Uncertain.

ETIOLOGY
- Unknown.
- Correlations with EBV, CMV, HHV, HCV, *Borrelia burgdorferi*, and *Brucella* have been postulated but not proven.
- Potential connections with immune disorders or neuroendocrine disorders such as hypothalamic–pituitary–adrenal axis or autonomic nervous system.

COMMONLY ASSOCIATED CONDITIONS
- Depression
- Fibromyalgia

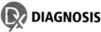 DIAGNOSIS

HISTORY
- Intense fatigue that has not alleviated with rest and has lasted for more than 6 months.
- Four of the following symptoms:
  - Post-exertional malaise
  - Sleep that does not improve fatigue
  - Impaired memory or concentration
  - Pain in muscles
  - Pain in multiple joints without redness or swelling
  - Painful lymph nodes (cervical, axillary)
  - Sore throat
  - Headache

PHYSICAL EXAM
- Tender lymphadenopathy can occur but is not essential for diagnosis.
- Few physical manifestations.

DIAGNOSTIC TESTS & INTERPRETATION
Lab
As needed for consideration of other etiologies for fatigue.

Imaging
None recommended.

Diagnostic Procedures/Other
Diagnosis of exclusion based on clinical history, as guided by 1994 CDC definition (1).

Pathological Findings
None.

DIFFERENTIAL DIAGNOSIS
- Depression
- CMV
- Epstein–Barr virus
- Brucellosis
- Postinfluenza
- Lyme disease
- HIV infection
- Collagen-vascular disorders
- Tumors with paraneoplastic syndrome
- Brain tumor

TREATMENT
Supportive measures as outlined below.

MEDICATION
Antidepressants, in combination with other therapeutic modalities.

ADDITIONAL TREATMENT
General Measures
Emphasis on multiple modalities of treatment with goal of incremental improvement over time.

Additional Therapies
- Cognitive behavioral therapy (CBT) (1,2).
- Graded exercise therapy: A program that carefully increases physical activity for patients with CFS to avoid the "push-crash" cycle common to CFS (i.e., over-exertion followed by post-exertional malaise).
- Activity pacing: Planned shorter episodes of moderate activity throughout the day that reduces risk of "push-crash" cycle. Combines CBT with physical activity.
- Sleep hygiene.
- Sleep studies.

COMPLEMENTARY & ALTERNATIVE THERAPIES
- Massage
- Deep breathing and other relaxation techniques
- Yoga
- Tai Chi
- Healing touch

ONGOING CARE

FOLLOW-UP RECOMMENDATIONS
Frequent follow-up with multi-disciplinary team of providers is recommended.

PROGNOSIS
- Time till diagnosis remains long (average ~ 5 years).
- Improvement in symptoms: 6–63%.
- Resolution of symptoms: 0–37%.

REFERENCES
1. http://www.cdc.gov/cfs/general/case_definition/index.html.
2. Fernandez AA, Martin AP, Martinez MI, et al. Chronic fatigue syndrome: Etiology, diagnosis, and treatment. *BMC Psychiatry* 2009;9(S1):S1.

ADDITIONAL READING
- Peterson DL, Ruscetti SK, Bagni RK, et al. Detection of an infectious retrovirus, XMRV, in blood cells of patients with chronic fatigue syndrome. *Science* 2009;326(5952):585–589.
- Prins JB, Bleijenberg G, Bazelmans E, et al. Cognitive behavior therapy for chronic fatigue syndrome: A multicentre randomized controlled trial. *Lancet* 2001;357(9259):841–847.
- Whiting P, Bagnall AM, Sowden AJ, et al. Interventions for the treatment and management of chronic fatigue syndrome: A systematic review. *JAMA* 2001;286(11):1360–1368.

 ## See Also

- Recommended diagnostic algorithm by CDC: http://www.cdc.gov/cfs/general/diagnosis/diagnosis_process.html

 ## CODES

ICD9
780.71 Chronic fatigue syndrome

CLINICAL PEARLS

- CFS is the diagnosis for a small subset of patients who present for evaluation of fatigue; duration, intensity, and character of fatigue are specific for CFS.
- Further investigation of etiologies and pathogenesis of CFS is needed; infections, immune dysregulation, and hormonal imbalance may be involved.
- A multi-disciplinary approach is necessary to help CFS patients improve their quality of life.

C

COCCIDIOIDOMYCOSIS

Jatin M. Vyas (E. Mylonakis, Editor)

 BASICS

DESCRIPTION
Coccidioidomycosis pulmonary and/or extrapulmonary infection is caused by the dimorphic fungus *Coccidioides immitis*.

EPIDEMIOLOGY
Incidence
- The incidence of coccidioidomycosis in the US is about 91 cases per 100,000.
- *C. immitis* is endemic to the southwestern US (principally, California, Arizona, and Texas) and also to Mexico and Central and South America.
- Increasingly, cases are being recognized outside the endemic areas (travelers or reactivations).
- Periodically, there are sharp increases in the number of cases.

RISK FACTORS
- For patients with immunosuppressive conditions or therapies, such as AIDS, solid-organ transplantation, or lymphoma, it is important to be aware of even distant exposure to endemic regions, because late recrudescence of latent infection is possible in such patients.
- Among patients with AIDS, coccidioidomycosis is particularly likely in patients with CD4 counts under 250 cells/mm^3.
- Patients receiving glucocorticoid and immunosuppressive therapies are at increased risk for coccidioidomycosis though the exact dose of steroids that portends increased risk has not been defined.

PATHOPHYSIOLOGY
- Occasionally, the acute pulmonary infection does not resolve, and a progressive pneumonia or chronic lung infection develops (1).
- Experience with organ transplantation suggests that antifungal therapy should be used in patients with a history of coccidioidomycosis, whether or not they have active infection, at the time of engraftment. Antifungal therapy should also be used in seropositive transplant recipients, even if they are asymptomatic, during episodes of acute rejection.

ETIOLOGY
- The fungus *C. immitis* lives in soil.
- The optimal temperature for the growth of *C. immitis* is 30°C, but the fungus grows well at 37°C.

COMMONLY ASSOCIATED CONDITIONS
- Can occur in immunocompetent patients
- Typically called "Valley fever"
- More invasive disease is seen in immunocompromised patients

 DIAGNOSIS

HISTORY
- Symptoms develop 1–3 weeks after exposure. The typical presentation is a lower respiratory infection accompanied by systemic symptoms, such as the following:
  – Anorexia
  – Arthralgias
  – Chest pain
  – Cough
  – Fever
  – Sputum production
  – Sweating
  – Weakness
  – Erythema nodosum or erythema multiforme may develop.
- About 5% of infected people have asymptomatic residual disease in their lungs, usually nodules or thin-walled cavities.
- Symptomatic extrapulmonary disease develops in about 1 of 200 people infected with *C. immitis*. The common sites are the meninges, bone and joints, skin, and soft tissues.
- Disease outside the lungs usually develops within a year after the initial infection, but may appear much later if immunity is impaired by medication or disease.
- Skin involvement may take a variety of forms, though wart-like nodules are the most common.
- Joint lesions are unilateral in over 90% of patients with joint involvement.

PHYSICAL EXAM
- Special attention should be paid to the skin and nervous system for potential involvement.
- To detect the presence of extrapulmonary infection, a careful review of symptoms and physical examination are usually adequate, because coccidioidal lesions are typically focal and produce localized symptoms, such as discomfort, swelling, or ulceration.

DIAGNOSTIC TESTS & INTERPRETATION
Lab
- In endemic areas, prior *C. immitis* infection is frequently diagnosed when a lung nodule is resected because of suspected carcinoma.
- For patients outside of the endemic regions, prompt diagnosis of coccidioidal infection depends on obtaining an accurate travel history.
- The mainstays of diagnosis are culture, serologic testing, and positive coccidioidal skin test.
- Serologic testing is best performed in experienced laboratories. Serum IgM antibodies can be detected temporarily in 75% of people with primary infections. IgG antibody is present later and usually disappears in several months if the infection resolves. False-positive serologic tests are rare.
- Skin-test reactions to coccidioidal antigens become positive soon after the development of symptoms in virtually all people with primary infections, and cross-reactions with other infections are rare.
- Although cultures are often used to diagnose coccidioidomycosis in patients with disseminated infection, they are often not obtained in patients with primary infections.
- Meningitis usually involves the basilar meninges. Examination of the cerebrospinal fluid shows a mononuclear pleocytosis, with a low glucose level and an elevated protein level.

Imaging
Chest radiographic findings may include infiltrates, a pleural effusion, and hilar adenopathy. Associated conditions that are particularly important risk factors include immunosuppressive diseases or therapies, pregnancy in the late stages, and diabetes.

DIFFERENTIAL DIAGNOSIS
- Lung cancer
- Other disseminated fungal infections

TREATMENT

MEDICATION

First Line

- The role of antifungal therapy in patients with mild or moderate manifestations of early infections is not well established, because randomized comparisons between antifungal and placebo regimens have not been done (2).
- Treatment may hasten symptom resolution. Thus, on a case-by-case basis, physicians should decide whether a patient's circumstances warrant therapy with available oral antifungal agents.
- If treatment is initiated, reasonable dosages are 400 mg/d for fluconazole, and 200 mg twice daily for itraconazole. Courses of typically recommended treatment would range from 3 to 6 months.
- Factors that should be weighed in favor of therapy include the following:
  - A negative skin test
  - Circumstances suggesting a high inoculum of the fungus
  - Concurrent noncoccidioidal disease
  - Elevated antibody titers
  - Inability to work
  - Increased host susceptibility
  - Infiltrates involving more than half of one lung
  - Intense night sweats persisting longer than 3 weeks
  - Loss of body weight greater than 10%
  - Prominent or persistent hilar adenopathy
  - Symptoms that persist for more than 2 months
- In patients with disseminated disease, prolonged chemotherapy is always indicated.
- Pulmonary resection has a role in managing severe hemoptysis or cavities that rupture or enlarge during chemotherapy. Surgery is also indicated to drain empyemas, close persistent bronchopleural fistulas, or expand lungs that are restricted by residual disease.

- Fluconazole and itraconazole are considered the drugs of choice in the treatment of meningeal disease.
- Even if *C. immitis* infection cannot be cured with azole therapy and lifelong suppression is required, the facts that these medications are well tolerated, do not have the toxic effects of amphotericin B, and do not require administration into the cerebrospinal fluid may represent important advantages in patients with an otherwise fatal illness.

Second Line

Once the disease has spread outside the lungs, chemotherapy is almost always indicated. Amphotericin B is used if patients fail therapy with azoles.

ONGOING CARE

FOLLOW-UP RECOMMENDATIONS

- 5–10% of infections result in residual sequelae, many of which have few long-term effects.
- In people with increased susceptibility to *C. immitis* infection, the serologic response to the fungus is usually at least qualitatively intact. A history of travel or residence in endemic areas should alert the physician to the possibility of this diagnosis. Routine serologic testing can prevent a delayed diagnosis.
- Early diagnosis of meningitis is important; without treatment, 90% of patients die within 12 months.
- In some patients, the acute pneumonia does not resolve, but progresses to chronic pulmonary disease. Diabetic patients and patients with compromised immunity are disproportionately overrepresented in this group.

COMPLICATIONS

- The disease is enhanced in immunocompromised patients, particularly if they have extrapulmonary coccidioidal disease. Patients who have received organ transplants are at greatest risk for infection in the first year after the transplantation.
- Meningitis usually occurs within 6 months after the primary infection and may appear acutely almost coincident with it.
- The signs of meningeal irritation common in bacterial meningitis are usually absent. The most common symptom is headache. Fever, weakness, confusion, sluggishness, seizures, abnormal behavior, stiff neck, diplopia, ataxia, vomiting, and focal neurologic defects may occur.

REFERENCES

1. Galgiani JN, Ampel NM, Blair A, et al. Coccidioidomycosis. *Clin Infect Dis* 2005;41:1217.
2. Ampel NM, Giblin A, Mourani JP, et al. Factors and outcomes associated with the decision to treat primary pulmonary coccidioidomycosis. *Clin Infect Dis* 2009;48(2):172–178.

CODES

ICD9

- 114.0 Primary coccidioidomycosis (pulmonary)
- 114.1 Primary extrapulmonary coccidioidomycosis
- 114.9 Coccidioidomycosis, unspecified

COMMON COLD

Hongni Jiang
Jieming Qu
Matthew E. Falagas

 BASICS

DESCRIPTION
Acute upper respiratory tract viral infection

EPIDEMIOLOGY
Incidence
- The average adult reports 2–4 colds per year.
- The average children reports 6–10 colds per year.

Prevalence
An estimated number of about 1 billion colds annually in the US

RISK FACTORS
- Staying in the presence of an infected person in an enclosed area
- Hand contact with an infected person
- Winter season which leads to people clustering indoors
- Children with immature immune system
- Individuals with immunocompromised conditions
- Susceptibility increased by smoking and psychological stress

GENERAL PREVENTION
- Avoid hand-to-eye and hand-to-nose contact
- Wash hands frequently

PATHOPHYSIOLOGY
- A contagious, viral infectious disease of the upper respiratory system
- The virus is transmitted through virus-laden saliva, nasal secretions, or aerosol from infected persons
- Self-limiting

ETIOLOGY
- Rhinovirus (30–50%)
- Coronavirus (10–15%)
- Influenza (5–15%)
- Less common: Parainfluenza, respiratory syncytial virus, adenovirus, enterovirus, and metapneumovirus

COMMONLY ASSOCIATED CONDITIONS
- Rhinitis
- Pharyngitis
- Pharyngolaryngitis
- Acute bronchitis

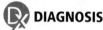 **DIAGNOSIS**

HISTORY
- Rhinorrhea (1–3)
- Sneezing
- Nasal obstruction
- Throat irritation or laryngitis
- Cough
- Chilliness
- Sometimes accompanied by conjunctivitis, muscle aches, fatigue, headaches, shivering, and anorexia

PHYSICAL EXAM
- Fever is characteristically uncommon
- Signs of upper respiratory tract infection

DIAGNOSTIC TESTS & INTERPRETATION
Lab
Initial lab tests
No laboratory tests are required unless differential diagnosis is needed or complications are suspected

Follow-Up & Special Considerations
Usually not required unless differential diagnosis is needed or complications are suspected

Imaging
Initial approach
Not required unless differential diagnosis is needed or complications are suspected

Follow-Up & Special Considerations
Not required unless differential diagnosis is needed or complications are suspected

Diagnostic Procedures/Other
- Usually not required:
  - Virus isolation
  - Direct detection of virus antigen
  - Serology–virus neutralization tests
  - Throat and/or sputum culture
  - Influenza virus testing
  - Culture of nasal discharge

DIFFERENTIAL DIAGNOSIS
- Infectious:
  - Pneumonia
  - Whooping cough
  - Sinusitis
  - Influenza
- Noninfectious:
  - Allergic rhinitis

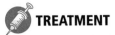 **TREATMENT**

MEDICATION
No antiviral agents with established merits

ADDITIONAL TREATMENT
General Measures
- Aspirin, acetaminophen, and ibuprofen to relieve aches and pains, as well as fever (4)
- Decongestants
  - Nasal: Rebound effect with use greater than 3 days in adults
  - Oral: Benefits questionable
- Ipratropium bromide nasal spray: Recommended for nasal congestion in children and adults
- Dextromethorphan: A treatment option for adults with cough
- Antihistamines: First-generation antihistamines to relieve symptoms in adults

Pediatric Considerations
- Aspirin is not recommended for children or teenagers for the risk of Reye's syndrome
- Codeine, dextromethorphan, and antihistamines: Not recommended for children

Issues for Referral
Severe symptoms

Additional Therapies
Echinacea (5), Vitamin C, and Zinc: Not recommended for active treatment

 ONGOING CARE

FOLLOW-UP RECOMMENDATIONS
A cough persisting longer than 3 weeks could be pneumonia or pertussis

Patient Monitoring
Usually not required

DIET
Plenty of fluids are recommended

PATIENT EDUCATION
- Emphasize that antibiotics are not required for common cold
- Advise against overuse of nasal drops or sprays because they may cause rebound congestion
- Minimize contact with people who have colds
- Wash hands and avoid sharing towels and drink lots of fluids
- Cover nose and mouth with an arm rather than hands when coughing or sneezing to avoid the spread of droplets

PROGNOSIS
The disease is generally mild and self-limiting

COMPLICATIONS
- Pneumonia
- Otitis media
- Sinusitis
- Pharyngitis
- Acute bronchitis
- Exacerbation of chronic bronchitis, asthma, and obstructive sleep apnea

REFERENCES
1. Eccles R. Understanding the symptoms of the common cold and influenza. *Lancet Infect Dis* 2005;5:718–725.
2. Worrall G. Common cold. *Can Fam Physician* 2007;53:1735–1736.
3. Arroll B. Common cold. *Clin Evid (Online)* 2008; pii: 1510.
4. Simasek M, Blandino DA. Treatment of the common cold. *Am Fam Physician* 2007;75:515–520.
5. Barrett B, Brown R, Rakel D, et al. *Echinacea* for treating the common cold: A randomized trial. *Ann Intern Med* 2010;153:769–777.

 CODES

ICD9
460 Acute nasopharyngitis (common cold)

CLINICAL PEARLS
- Common cold is a self-limiting disease without any valid treatment yet.
- Washing hands frequently plays a key role in the prevention of common cold.

CONJUNCTIVITIS
Theodoros Filippopoulos (E. Mylonakis, Editor)

 BASICS

DESCRIPTION
- Conjunctivitis is an inflammatory reaction of the conjunctiva that presents with hyperemia and discharge. Conjunctivitis can be acute or chronic, and can be infectious or non-infectious.
- Trachoma is a chronic conjunctivitis associated with infection by *Chlamydia trachomatis* serotypes A–C.
- Inclusion conjunctivitis is caused by sexually transmitted *C. trachomatis* strains (serotypes D through K) in young adults exposed to infected genital secretions or in their newborn offspring.
- Ophthalmia neonatorum refers to acute mucopurulent conjunctivitis that presents within the 1st month of life.

EPIDEMIOLOGY
Incidence
- The incidence of infectious conjunctivitis presented to general practitioners in the Netherlands has been reported as high as 13.9 cases per 1000 persons-years.
- *Chlamydia* spp. are the most common infectious agents causing ophthalmia neonatorum in the US with a reported incidence of 6.2 per 1000 live births.
- The incidence of gonococcal ophthalmia neonatorum has been reduced dramatically, from 100 per 1000 live births to 3 per 1000 live births.

Prevalence
- Endemic trachoma is still the major cause of preventable blindness in northern Africa, sub-Saharan Africa, Middle East, and parts of Asia.
- In the US, trachoma still occurs in Native American populations and in immigrants from areas where trachoma is endemic.
- In 2003, the WHO estimated that 7.6 million people worldwide were severely visually impaired or blind as a result of trachoma.
- The worldwide incidence and severity of trachoma have decreased in past decades as a result of improving hygienic conditions.

RISK FACTORS
- Trachoma is highly correlated with poverty, limited access to healthcare services, and water.
- Trachoma transmission occurs from eye to eye via hands, flies, towels, etc.

GENERAL PREVENTION
- Promotion of general hygienic measures decreases morbidity associated with trachoma.
- Public health initiatives against trachoma include mass application of tetracycline or erythromycin ointment to eyes of children in endemic areas for 21–60 days, or intermittently, or single-dose oral azithromycin therapy.
- In cases of adult inclusion conjunctivitis, treatment of all sexual partners is mandatory.
- Erythromycin or tetracycline ointment application within 1 hour of delivery markedly decreases the chance of developing chlamydial ophthalmia neonatorum.
- Patients with viral epidemic keratoconjunctivitis (EKC) should be advised to frequently wash their hands, to avoid touching their eyes, sharing towels or pillows with others.

PATHOPHYSIOLOGY
Pathogenesis of bacterial conjunctivitis involves a disruption of the host defense mechanisms such as ocular surface abnormalities, tear film abnormalities, or systemic immunosuppression.

ETIOLOGY
Infectious Causes
- Bacteria (*Bartonella henselae*, *Chlamydia trachomatis*, *Haemophilus* spp., *Neisseria gonorrhoeae*, *Streptococcus* spp., *Staphylococcus* spp., *Treponema pallidum*, etc.)
- Fungi
- Viruses (adenoviruses, Coxsackie virus, echoviruses, enteroviruses, etc.)
- Parasites (*Loa loa worm*, *Onchocerca volvulus*, *Toxocara canis*, *Wuchereria bancrofti*)
- Viral conjunctivitis follows 4 patterns:
  - EKC (caused by adenovirus serotypes 8, 19, and 37)
  - Pharyngoconjunctival fever (caused by adenovirus serotypes 3 and 8) occurring more commonly in children
  - Acute hemorrhagic conjunctivitis (caused by enterovirus type 70 and Coxsackie virus type A24) occurring more commonly in tropical regions
  - In association with systemic viral syndromes such as measles, mumps, influenza
- HSV and VZV ocular involvement can also include a conjunctival reaction (see "Keratitis").
- Cat scratch disease due to *Bartonella henselae* can cause among others conjunctivitis in about 5–10% of patients with the systemic infection. Ocular involvement is termed *Parinaud Oculoglandular Syndrome*.

COMMONLY ASSOCIATED CONDITIONS
- An upper respiratory tract infection or the presence of sick contacts in the household are the most common associated conditions in cases of viral EKC.
- A history of urethritis, vaginitis, or cervicitis may be present with adult inclusion conjunctivitis.

℞ DIAGNOSIS

HISTORY
- Depending on the offending pathogen, patients complain of tearing, mucous or mucopurulent discharge, eyelid edema, conjunctival injection (red eye), and foreign-body sensation. Pain is minimal and visual acuity is only slightly reduced.
- In cases of gonococcal bacterial conjunctivitis, symptoms start both in sexually active young adults and in newborns within a day or two after exposure. Gonococcal ophthalmia neonatorum can have a shorter incubation period in cases of premature rupture of the membranes.
- In cases of viral EKC after an incubation period of up to 1 week, usually one eye becomes affected followed shortly after by second eye. EKC causes watery discharge, mild foreign-body sensation, and light sensitivity (photophobia).

PHYSICAL EXAM
- Clinical findings and course of conjunctivitis are influenced by the offending pathogen.
- Infectious conjunctivitis usually presents with hyperemia, eyelid edema, and discharge. Viral and chlamydial conjunctivitis present with a predominantly follicular conjunctival reaction, whereas bacterial and allergic conjunctivitis usually demonstrate a papillary reaction which represents a lymphoid hyperplasia around a vascular core. The cornea can become secondarily involved, with inflammatory infiltrations and superficial vascularization, especially in viral conjunctivitis.
- Secretions vary from serosanguineous to purulent, depending on the pathogen. Bacterial infections tend to produce more mucopurulent exudates, while *N. gonorrhoeae* produces a profuse, thick, yellow-green purulent discharge.
- Conjunctival membranes and pseudomembranes are among the findings.
- Preauricular lymphadenopathy is commonly encountered in EKC, HSV, gonococcal conjunctivitis, or inclusion conjunctivitis.
- Neonatal chlamydial conjunctivitis has an acute onset (5–14 days postpartum) and often produces a mucopurulent discharge.
- Both trachoma and inclusion conjunctivitis are associated with an early follicular reaction within the conjunctiva. In trachoma after resolution of the follicles, subconjunctival scarring occurs that leads to loss of mucin-producing goblet cells, entropion, trichiasis, and keratitis.
- Inclusion conjunctivitis in adults presents as acute unilateral follicular conjunctivitis with mucopurulent discharge. The conjunctivitis is often chronic lasting for months if untreated.
- Parinaud Oculoglandular Syndrome presents with conjunctival hyperemia, eyelid swelling, fever, granulomatous nodules on the palpebral or bulbar conjunctiva and regional lymphadenopathy. Neuroretinitis can also occur.
- In conjunctivitis due to *F. tularensis*, painful purulent conjunctivitis develops with numerous nodular or ulcerative lesions of the palpebral conjunctiva and regional lymphadenopathy.

DIAGNOSTIC TESTS & INTERPRETATION
Imaging
Initial approach
There are no modalities that are helpful in cases of infectious conjunctivitis.

Follow-Up & Special Considerations
In adult inclusion conjunctivitis, genital examination and tests for genital chlamydial infection are indicated in the affected individuals and their sexual partners.

Diagnostic Procedures/Other
- Microbiologic investigation is only necessary in hyperacute cases suggestive of *N. gonorrhoeae*, in severe, chronic, or unusual cases.
- Gram-stained smears may demonstrate gram-negative intracellular diplococci in gonococcal conjunctivitis or occasional small gram-negative coccobacilli in Haemophilus conjunctivitis, but smears should be accompanied by cultures in blood and chocolate agar.

- Antibodies against *C. trachomatis* can be demonstrated in tear or serum in trachoma. Intracytoplasmic chlamydial inclusions in epithelial cells are found in 10–60% of Giemsa-stained conjunctival smears in such populations, but isolation in cell cultures, ELISA, immunofluorescent monoclonal antibody stains, or chlamydial PCR techniques are more sensitive.
- In adult inclusion conjunctivitis, evidence of chlamydiae by Giemsa- or immunofluorescence-stained smears, by isolation in cell cultures, or by newer non-culture tests are employed.
- Viruses causing viral conjunctivitis can be identified with PCR techniques.

DIFFERENTIAL DIAGNOSIS
- Infectious conjunctivitis must be differentiated from other entities causing red eyes and from cases of non-infectious conjunctivitis. Such entities include dry eye disease, Stevens–Johnson's syndrome, ocular cicatricial pemphigoid (OCP), allergic/atopic/vernal conjunctivitis, exogenous irritation due to pollution and medications (medicamentosa), conjunctival or eyelid tumors and graft-versus-host disease.
- In the newborn, chlamydial conjunctivitis generally has a longer incubation period (5–14 days) than gonococcal conjunctivitis (1–3 days).

TREATMENT
MEDICATION
First Line
- Viral conjunctivitis only requires supportive care with artificial tears and cold compresses. If membranes or pseudomembranes are present, they may be peeled off and a topical steroid (loteprednol 0.5% q.i.d.) may be indicated.
- HSV conjunctivitis is treated with topical antiviral therapy (trifluridine 1% five times a day) to prevent corneal epithelial disease. Topical steroids are contraindicated.
- Mild cases of bacterial conjunctivitis are usually treated empirically with broad-spectrum topical antibiotics, such as trimethoprim-polymyxin B (q.i.d.) or a topical fluoroquinolone (q.i.d.) for 5–7 days. The lowest broad-spectrum antibiotic resistance is observed in the case of fourth-generation fluoroquinolones (gatifloxacin or moxifloxacin).
- *H. influenzae* should be treated with oral amoxicillin/clavulanate (20–40 mg/kg/day in 3 divided doses) because of occasional extraocular involvement (i.e., otitis media, pneumonia, meningitis).
- Gonococcal conjunctivitis with or without keratitis requires systemic treatment with ceftriaxone. If there is no corneal involvement a single dose of ceftriaxone (1 g i.m.) is sufficient; with corneal involvement intravenous ceftriaxone is necessary (1 g i.v. q.d.–b.i.d.) along with a topical fourth-generation fluoroquinolone (gatifloxacin or moxifloxacin every 1 hour around the clock). Duration of treatment depends on clinical response. Treatment for possible chlamydial co-infection with a single dose of oral azithromycin (1 g p.o.) is also recommended.
- Adult inclusion conjunctivitis is treated with a single dose of oral azithromycin (1 g p.o.) along with topical erythromycin or tetracycline ophthalmic ointment b.i.d. or t.i.d. for 2–3 weeks.

- Trachoma is treated with a single dose of azithromycin (20 mg/kg p.o.) and a topical erythromycin, tetracycline or sulfacetamide ointment (b.i.d.–q.i.d.) for 3–4 weeks.
- The course of cat scratch disease is usually self-limited in immune-competent hosts and resolves without therapy. Oral azithromycin (500 mg p.o. q.i.d during the 1st day and subsequently 250 mg p.o. q.d. for 4 days) can be considered. For children the azithromycin dose is adjusted (10 mg/kg p.o. q.i.d. for the 1st day and then 5 mg/kg p.o. q.d. for 4 days). Topical antibiotics such as gentamicin eyedrops (q.i.d.) or bacitracin/polymyxin B ointment (q.i.d.) can be given as well.
- Because concomitant pharyngeal infection is often present, ophthalmia neonatorum should be treated with systemic antimicrobials to prevent systemic involvement:
  – *N. gonorrhoeae*: Systemic ceftriaxone (25–50 mg/kg i.v. or i.m. to a maximum of 125 mg) along with frequent saline irrigations to remove the discharge. A single intramuscular dose of ceftriaxone is sufficient to treat gonococcal ophthalmia neonatorum.
  – *C. trachomatis*: Oral erythromycin (50 mg/kg/day p.o. in 4 divided doses) for 2 weeks plus topical erythromycin ointment (q.i.d.).
  – HSV: In full-term infants intravenous acyclovir (45–60 mg/kg/day i.v. divided in 3 doses) for 2 weeks if the disease is limited to eye, skin, and mouth and for 3 weeks if it involves the central nervous system. Topical treatment with trifluridine eyedrops (1% nine times a day) or vidarabine ointment (3% five times a day) should be also initiated.

Second Line
- Adult inclusion conjunctivitis can also be treated with oral doxycycline (100 mg p.o. b.i.d.) or erythromycin (500 mg p.o. q.i.d.) for 7 days.
- Trachoma can be alternatively treated with doxycycline (100 mg p.o. b.i.d.) or erythromycin (500 mg p.o. q.i.d.) for 2 weeks.
- In penicillin-allergic patients with gonococcal conjunctivitis consider an oral fluoroquinolone (ciprofloxacin 500 mg p.o.) for 5 days. However, emerging resistance is a significant concern.
- Doxycycline (100 mg p.o. b.i.d.) can be given to adults with cat scratch disease.

ADDITIONAL TREATMENT
General Measures
In gonococcal conjunctivitis frequent saline irrigations of the purulent discharge are advisable.

Issues for Referral
In cases of gonococcal or adult inclusion conjunctivitis, an ID consultation should be sought.

SURGERY/OTHER PROCEDURES
On rare occasions a conjunctival biopsy is indicated to diagnose, for example, OCP.

IN-PATIENT CONSIDERATIONS
Admission Criteria
Conjunctivitis is managed on an outpatient basis with the exception of ophthalmia neonatorum and cases requiring intravenous antibiotics.

ONGOING CARE
DIET
No dietary restrictions apply.

PATIENT EDUCATION
Instruct patients on hygienic measures.

PROGNOSIS
With the exception of chlamydial conjunctivitis infectious conjunctivitis rarely lasts >3 weeks.

COMPLICATIONS
- In trachoma, chronic conjunctival inflammation leads to scarring, and distorts the eyelids, causing them to turn inward (trichiasis and entropion). The corneal epithelium may become compromised, with subsequent scarring and opacification.
- In viral EKC subepithelial infiltrates may develop (superficial corneal opacities that are inflammatory in nature) which may require chronic treatment with topical steroids.
- Exposure to pathogens during passage through birth canal puts infants with ophthalmia neonatorum at risk for systemic infections such as rhinitis, stomatitis, arthritis, meningitis, and sepsis (*N. gonorrhoeae*), otitis and pneumonitis (*C. trachomatis*), and encephalitis (HSV).

ADDITIONAL READING
- Adebayo A, Parikh JG, McCormick SA, et al. Shifting trends in *in vitro* antibiotic susceptibilities for common bacterial conjunctivitis isolates in the last decade at the New York Eye and Ear Infirmary. *Graefes Arch Clin Exp Ophthalmol*. 2010;249: 111–119.

CODES
ICD9
- 372.00 Acute conjunctivitis, unspecified
- 372.10 Chronic conjunctivitis, unspecified
- 372.30 Conjunctivitis, unspecified

CLINICAL PEARLS
- The instillation of 1% silver nitrate drops used for prophylaxis against ophthalmia neonatorum can cause a mild chemical conjunctivitis (conjunctival injection and tearing) in newborns lasting for 24–36 hours. Silver nitrate is effective against *N. gonorrhoeae* but ineffective against chlamydial or viral infections.

C

CREUTZFELDT–JAKOB DISEASE

Michael K. Mansour (E. Mylonakis, Editor)

 BASICS

DESCRIPTION
- The transmissible spongiform encephalopathies are chronic, progressive, and always fatal neurodegenerative disorders of animals and humans.
- Animal-transmissible spongiform encephalopathies include the sheep disease (scrapie) and the cow disease (bovine spongiform encephalopathy, BSE).
- Human-transmissible spongiform encephalopathies include Creutzfeldt–Jakob disease (CJD), kuru (first prion disease described from Papua New Guinea), Gerstmann–Straussler–Scheinker syndrome, and fatal familial insomnia.
- CJD, the most common of the prion diseases, is characterized by progressive dementia, muscle atrophy, tremor, and spastic dysarthria.
- CJD can present in different forms such as sporadic, familial, iatrogenic, and variant. Sporadic being the most common.
- Variant CJD (vCJD) was first described in 1996 during the outbreak centered in the United Kingdom and is the only documented animal(BSE)-to-human transmission prion disease.
- To date, three cases of vCJD have been documented in the US.
- In 2008, a new prion disease was described in a series of 11 patients termed "proteinase-sensitive prionopathy" and appears to have a familial distribution.

EPIDEMIOLOGY
Incidence
- Sporadic CJD (sCJD) account for 85% of all spongiform encephalopathies.
- Frequency of sCJD is approximately 1 case per million with mean age ranging from 50 to 60 years.
- Most cases are sporadic, although familial cases with an autosomal dominant pattern of inheritance have been described such as Gerstmann–Straussler–Scheinker syndrome.
- Familial CJD has been reported in higher frequency in North Africa, Middle-East, Italy, and Slovakia.

- Spread of the disease has occurred following transplantation of corneas, dural grafts, or improperly decontaminated neurosurgical instruments and stereotactic intracerebral depth electrodes.
- Approximately 50 cases have been reported in patients with panhypopituitarism who received supplemental cadaveric human growth hormone therapy and in patients who received cadaveric human gonadotropins for treatment of infertility.

RISK FACTORS
A weak correlation exists with prior farm exposure.

Genetics
Certain polymorphism or mutations in the prion gene, PRNP, has been linked to spongiform encephalopathies.

GENERAL PREVENTION
- The consensus is that the current risk of transmission of spongiform encephalopathies in the US is minimal because of the following:
  - Adequate regulations exist to prevent entry of foreign sources of spongiform encephalopathies into the US.
  - Adequate regulations exist to prevent undetected cases of BSE from uncontrolled amplification within the US cattle population.
  - Adequate preventive guidelines exist to prevent high-risk bovine materials from contaminating products intended for human consumption.

PATHOPHYSIOLOGY
Accumulation of abnormal forms of host cell proteins in neuronal tissue related to the prion gene product, PRNP.

ETIOLOGY
- The pathological hallmarks of CJD are spongiform changes (small, round vacuoles) within the neuropil, neuronal loss, hypertrophy, proliferation of glial cells, and absence of significant inflammation or white matter involvement.
- Pathological changes are most severe in the cortex but are often prominent in the basal ganglia, cerebellum, and thalamus as well.
- The finding of prion rods or plaques on electron micrographs of prepared brain material is pathognomonic for prion diseases.

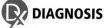 **DIAGNOSIS**

HISTORY
- Kuru, the best known prion disease, has characteristic disease stages including tremors (kuru translates to "shivering" which describes these tremors), ataxia, and finally dementia.
- Incubation time can be as long as 50 years prior to onset of disease.
- Early in the course of the disease, most CJD patients exhibit rapidly progressive dementia, myoclonus, and pyramidal tract dysfunction.
- Mental impairment may be manifested as slowness in thinking, difficulty in concentrating, impaired judgment, and memory loss.
- Mood changes and emotional lability may be combined with visual or other types of hallucinations.
- Almost any combination of cortical, subcortical, cerebellar, and spinal cord findings is possible.
- Myoclonus occurs in more than 90% of patients. Additional motor signs and symptoms can include tremor, clumsiness, and choreoathetosis.
- As the disease progresses, about two-thirds of patients develop a parkinsonian extrapyramidal syndrome with hypokinesia and rigidity. Hyperreflexia, spasticity, and extensor plantar responses occur in about half of patients.
- Autonomic (hyperthermia, hypertension, tachycardia) and endocrine disturbances (hypercortisol, growth hormone) may be seen in prion disease forms such as fatal familial insomnia.
- Cases of a new variant of CJD have recently been identified in certain countries in Europe (mainly the United Kingdom) found to be due to transmission of BSE.
- vCJD patients range in age from 19 to 41 years and develop a progressive illness leading to death within 7–23 months after onset. The clinical features include early and prominent behavioral disturbances and ataxia. Myoclonus and progressive dementia occur in most patients as later features.

PHYSICAL EXAM
- Cognitive decline including dementia, memory loss, behavioral abnormalities, and insomnia are common.
- Myoclonus is present in over 90% of patients.
- Cerebellar signs such as nystagmus and ataxia may be present.
- Spasticity, positive Babinski sign, and hyperreflexia may develop in up to 80% of patients.

DIAGNOSTIC TESTS & INTERPRETATION
Lab
- Definite diagnosis of all forms of CJD is possible only by histological examination of the brain.
- If cerebrospinal fluid (CSF) pleocytosis is unusual this should prompt a thorough search for other processes.
- An abnormal protein, 14-3-3, has been linked to CJD although sensitivity and specificity range from 60 to 90%.
- Other conditions which will also cause 14-3-3 elevations include Alzheimer disease, viral infection (herpes), paraneoplastic syndromes, and vascular dementia.
- Recent molecular genetic studies have established an unequivocal linkage between mutations in the PRNP gene and familial cases of CJD. Several mutations have been described, which may correlate with variations in the clinical phenotype of the disease in individual familial clusters. These include point mutations in codons 178, 200, and 210. Octarepeat inserts in the PRNP gene also occur in several families with CJD.
- Patients with CJD have a median serum concentration of the brain-specific S 100 protein higher than that of controls.
- In vCJD, the typical periodic EEG pattern usually associated with CJD does not occur.
- Prion protein plaques are extensively distributed throughout the cerebrum and cerebellum.
- Laboratory tests are helpful in excluding other causes of rapidly progressing dementia.
- The CSF is typically unremarkable, although the protein level may be mildly elevated.
- Extraneural testing of prion protein is being developed as a rapid diagnostic.

Imaging
- Usually the degree of clinical dementia appears disproportionate to the amount of tissue loss seen on CT and MRI. In some patients, MRI has shown areas of high T2 signal intensity in the striatum.
- Reduced brain cortical perfusion in cases of vCJD disease by single-photon emission computed tomography (SPECT) analysis.

Diagnostic Procedures/Other
- The EEG can be a useful diagnostic in certain forms such as sCJD, where sensitivity has been found to be 64% and specificity 91%.
- A predictive pattern of CJD will show periodic sharp-wave complexes and consists of a generalized slow background interrupted by bilaterally synchronous sharp-wave complexes occurring at intervals of 0.5–2.5 s and lasting for 100–600 ms.
- This classic EEG pattern is found in about 60–95% of cases, although it may not be present very early or in the terminal stages of the disease.
- Kuru, fatal familial insomnia, and variant and familial CJD may not show evidence of sharp-wave complexes.

Pathological Findings
- Multicentric plaques with spicules (cerebellum, mid-brain, cerebrum) that stain for abnormal prion gene protein products, PrPSc, are PAS-positive.
- Small vacuoles form within neuropil producing the characteristic spongiform appearance.

DIFFERENTIAL DIAGNOSIS
The differential diagnosis of dementia is extensive but certain conditions that may also have features of myoclonus and dementia include Alzheimer's disease, frontotemporal dementia, Lewy body dementia, alcoholism, HIV, tubercular meningitis, neurosyphilis, Whipple's disease, progressive multifocal leukoencephalopathy, lymphoma, amyloid angiopathy, metabolic disturbances, and autoimmune disorders.

 TREATMENT

MEDICATION
- CJD is invariably fatal, and no specific therapy is available.
- Amantadine has been reported to slow disease progression in isolated anecdotal case reports; however, the results have not been reproducible.
- Other drugs, such as cytoprotective agents (flupirtine) and inhibitors of PrPSc (chlorpromazine), have been tried with no significant success in survival.
- Immunotherapy and molecular targeting are being investigated.

SURGERY/OTHER PROCEDURES
Consultation with neurosurgical services is required for tissue diagnosis. All services including pathology should be informed of the high suspicion of prion disease.

 ONGOING CARE

FOLLOW-UP RECOMMENDATIONS
In some patients, sequential studies performed at biweekly or monthly intervals may show rapidly progressing loss of brain tissue and ventricular enlargement.

PROGNOSIS
Disease is usually fatal with no available therapies at this time.

ADDITIONAL READING
- Gambetti P, Dong Z, Yuan J, et al. A novel human disease with abnormal prion protein sensitive to protease. *Ann Neurol* 2008;63:697.
- Steinhoff BJ, Zerr I, Glatting M, et al. Diagnostic value of periodic complexes in Creutzfeldt–Jakob disease. *Ann Neurol* 2004;56:702.
- Vanneti S. Prion disease. *Clin Lab Med*. 2010;30(1):293–309.

 CODES

ICD9
- 046.11 Variant Creutzfeldt-Jakob disease
- 046.19 Other and unspecified Creutzfeldt-Jakob disease

CLINICAL PEARLS
- Transmissible spongiform encephalopathy is caused by exposure to prion protein which results in confirmational changes to native prion protein structure resulting in plaque formation and neuronal death.
- Clinically manifests as progressive dementia and spasticity.
- Brain biopsy is the gold standard for diagnosis since laboratory testing (blood and CSF) as well as noninvasive techniques (imaging and EEG) are nonspecific and only suggestive.
- There are no significant treatments for prion diseases and prognosis is poor.

CRYPTOCOCCAL INFECTIONS

Maged Muhammed
Isaac I. Bogoch
Eleftherios Mylonakis

 BASICS

DESCRIPTION
- *Cryptococcus* is a yeast encapsulated by a unique polysaccharide capsule covering the membrane.
- There are over 50 species of *Cryptococcus*; however, the most medically important species are *Cryptococcus neoformans* (primarily infects immunocompromised patients) and *Cryptococcus gattii* (also in immunocompetent hosts).
- Infections with *Cryptococcus* typically involve the lung or CNS in patients with impaired cell-mediated immunity (e.g., AIDS, organ transplantation), but can disseminate to anywhere in the body including bones, skin, prostate, and eyes.
- The primary route of infection is via inhalation. It can then disseminate through the body, and it has a predilection for the CNS.

EPIDEMIOLOGY
- *C. neoformans* is more common in the US and is associated with pigeon feces, although direct transmission from pigeons to humans has not been documented.
- *C. gattii* is primarily found in tropical and subtropical regions, in the vegetation around eucalyptus trees. It has been seen in North America more recently, notably in the Pacific Northwest and British Columbia.
- Respiratory transmission has not been reported between humans, or between other animals to humans. Human-to-human transmission can occur in rare circumstances such as transplantation of an infected organ into a non-infected recipient.
- Among HIV-infected patients, cryptococcal infection has decreased dramatically since the widespread use of antiretroviral therapy.
- For example, a study evaluated the incidence of cryptococcal infection in AIDS patients per 1000 people, and noted a decline from 66 to 7 in Atlanta, and from 24 to 2 in Houston after widespread antiretroviral use (1,2).
- In solid-organ transplant recipients, *Cryptococcus* is the third most common invasive fungal infection, and is responsible for 20–60% of cryptococcal infections in patients without HIV in the US (3).

RISK FACTORS
- AIDS
- Hematologic malignancies
- Solid-organ transplantation
- Immunosuppressive medications: For example, glucocorticoids, cyclosporine, and tacrolimus (4).
- Other: Sarcoidosis, splenectomy, chronic obstructive pulmonary disease, diabetes mellitus, lupus, rheumatoid arthritis

GENERAL PREVENTION
- HIV patients: Reconstitute the immune system with antiretroviral therapy.
- AIDS patients: Reconstitute the immune system with antiretroviral therapy, and in those with CD4 cell count less than 50 cells/μL, fluconazole and itraconazole can help prevent cryptococcal infection; however, due to drug interactions and the lack of survival benefits with this strategy, few HIV providers place patients on primary prophylactic regimens.
- Secondary prophylaxis: Patients with AIDS who have completed treatment for cryptococcal meningitis should stay on fluconazole (200 mg/d PO) lifelong, or until their CD4 count is greater than 200 cells/μL for >6 months.

PATHOPHYSIOLOGY
Yeast spores are inhaled into alveoli. Those with T cell deficiencies are more prone to dissemination of infection. Pneumonia represents primary infection whereas meningitis, skin lesions, or other organ involvement (e.g., bone, prostate, etc.) represents disseminated disease.

ETIOLOGY
Clinically important species include *C. neoformans* and *C. gattii*.

 DIAGNOSIS

HISTORY
- Lung infection: Ranges from asymptomatic to dyspnea, cough, pleuritic chest pain, hemoptysis, fever, and acute respiratory distress syndrome.
- CNS infection: Classically presents with subacute onset of symptoms over 1–3 weeks including headache, fever, irritability and may progress to confusion, nausea, somnolence, and seizures. Only about 25% present with classic symptoms of meningitis such as neck stiffness, fevers, photophonophobia, nausea, and vomiting.

PHYSICAL EXAM
- CNS: Nuchal rigidity is not predominant in most cases. Focal neurologic deficits may be seen in rare cases of cryptococcomas.
- Papilledema is present in almost one third of patients.
- Skin: Painless lesions, papules, or ulcers. Skin findings may have a central umbilication resembling molluscum contagiosum.

DIAGNOSTIC TESTS & INTERPRETATION
Lab
- Blood: Send for cryptococcal antigen. Blood culture may also grow *Cryptococcus*, and the yield of this test is increased if cultures are drawn in fungal isolator tubes.
- Lung infection: Sputum or lung nodule biopsy for culture. Histopathology of lung biopsy may be helpful if there is no growth.
- CNS infection: Culture, India ink staining, and cryptococcal antigen detection in CSF are all important in making a diagnosis.
- CSF opening pressure is typically elevated >200 mm H_2O.
- CSF analysis shows high protein, low glucose, and a lymphocytic pleocytosis.
- Serum for cryptococcal antigen is often helpful in diagnosing meningitis or pneumonia when patients have compatible symptoms.
- Skin biopsy for fungal stains and cultures.

Imaging
- Lung infection: CXR and CT scan is helpful if pulmonary symptoms are present. Interstitial infiltrates are commonly visualized in immunocompromised patients. Solitary or multiple pulmonary nodules can be seen in both immunocompetent and immunocompromised hosts. Rarely there is cavitation. Pleural effusions, hilar or mediastinal lymphadenopathy, and a cryptococcoma may also be visualized (5).
- CNS infection: CT scan or MRI is helpful, especially when focal neurologic deficits are present. Look for nodules, cryptococcomas, or hydrocephalus.

DIFFERENTIAL DIAGNOSIS
- Pneumonia
- *Pneumocystis Carinii* Pneumonia
- TB
- Sarcoidosis
- Histoplasmosis
- Coccidiomycosis
- Meningoencephalitis
- CNS metastases

TREATMENT

MEDICATION

First Line
- Lung infection: Mild-to-moderate infection should be treated with fluconazole 400 mg/d for 6–12 months.
- CNS infection: The initial "induction phase" involves 14 (or more) days of amphotericin B (using a lipid formulation in those at risk of nephrotoxicity) and flucytosine 100 mg/kg/d divided into 4 doses per day. If patients show a clinical response, a "consolidation phase" of fluconazole at 400 mg/d is given for 8 weeks, followed by "maintenance" therapy with fluconazole 200 mg/d.

Second Line
- Alternative active agents for pneumonia include itraconazole, voriconazole, and posaconazole.
- For CNS disease, fluconazole plus flucytosine is an alternative to those who cannot tolerate amphotericin B plus flucytosine during the consolidation phase; however, this is an inferior treatment.

ADDITIONAL TREATMENT

General Measures
Infectious diseases specialists are commonly involved in the care of patients with cryptococcal infections.

SURGERY/OTHER PROCEDURES
Patients may have persistently elevated opening pressures during lumbar puncture. Patients with ongoing neurologic symptoms consistent with raised intracranial pressures (e.g., lower limb clonus, papilledema) should have serial lumbar punctures to relieve increased intracranial pressures. Ventriculoperitoneal shunting should be considered with the input of a neurosurgical service in severe cases that are not responding to serial lumbar punctures.

 ONGOING CARE

FOLLOW-UP RECOMMENDATIONS
- Monitoring BUN and creatinine while on amphotericin and flucytosine.
- Monitoring liver function tests while on fluconazole.

COMPLICATIONS
- Dementia
- Visual impairment
- Hydrocephalus
- Death

ADDITIONAL READING

- Chayakulkeeree M, Perfect JR. Cryptococcosis. *Infect Dis Clin North Am* 2006;20:507–544.
- Mirza SA, Phelan M, Rimland M, et al. The changing epidemiology of cryptococcosis: An update from population-based active surveillance in 2 large metropolitan areas, 1992–2000. *Clin Infect Dis* 2003;36:789–794.
- Pukkila-Worley R, Mylonakis E. Epidemiology and management of cryptococcal meningitis: Developments and challenges. *Expert Opin Pharmacother* 2008;9:1–10.
- Singh N, Dromer F, Perfect JR, et al. Cryptococcosis in solid organ transplant recipients: Current state of the science. *Clin Infect Dis* 2008;47(10): 1321–1327.

- Lindell RM, Hartman TE, Nadrous HF, et al. Pulmonary cryptococcosis: CT findings in immunocompetent patients. *Radiology* 2005;236(1):326–331.

 CODES

ICD9
117.5 Cryptococcosis

CLINICAL PEARLS

- Cryptococcal infections have decreased in patients with HIV due to the greater use of effective antiretroviral therapy. Cryptococcal infections are seen with increasing frequency in the solid-organ transplant population.
- If a serum cryptococcal antigen is positive and there are any neurologic symptoms, a lumbar puncture should be performed with opening pressure measured and CSF sent for culture, India ink staining, and cryptococcal antigen detection.

C

CRYPTOSPORIDIOSIS

Paschalis Vergidis
Matthew E. Falagas

 BASICS

DESCRIPTION
Cryptosporidium, an intracellular protozoan, is responsible for self-limited diarrhea in children and adults and protracted or even fatal diarrhea in patients with HIV infection.

EPIDEMIOLOGY
Incidence
More than 300,000 persons develop the disease in the US each year.

Prevalence
- The organism is ubiquitous and worldwide in distribution.
- Seroprevalence rates are often as high as 25% in industrialized countries and as high as 75% in developing countries.
- In temperate climates, increased transmission is noted during warmer months.
- Large waterborne outbreaks associated with contaminated water supplies have been documented in the US (e.g., Milwaukee, WI).
- Much of the contamination of water supplies has been due to dairy farms or other farms with livestock.

RISK FACTORS
- Chronic diarrhea in patients with AIDS and CD4 count <100 cells/μL
- Other immunosuppression
- Children younger than 5 years in developing countries
- Animal handlers

GENERAL PREVENTION
- For persons with HIV infection, many precautions are recommended, including the following:
  – Avoidance of drinking from rivers, streams, or pools
  – Avoidance of swallowing water while swimming
- Avoidance of contact with human or animal feces. Care must be taken especially when working with farm animals or with soil possibly contaminated with animal feces.
- Pets with diarrhea should have their stools examined for *Cryptosporidium*.
- The organism is resistant to most water purification methods such as chlorination.
- Avoid drinking tap water when visiting developing countries.
- Filtration appears to be the best method of oocyst removal. Drinking water can be filtered to 1 μ or boiled for 1 minute.
- Bottled water may be safer than tap water, but the filtering process may vary with some brands of bottled water, and purity is not guaranteed.
- Carbonated drinks are safe.

PATHOPHYSIOLOGY
- *Cryptosporidium* is an intracellular protozoan, able to infect cells of epithelial origin.
- Cells affected in humans include respiratory and gastrointestinal cells.
- The entire life cycle occurs within one person.
- Infection usually occurs by ingestion of oocysts from fecally contaminated water.
- Oocysts can survive as long as 18 months in the environment.
- Studies have shown that ingestion of less than 1000 oocysts can lead to disease.
- The pathogen is directly transmitted from person to person.
- Other means of infection include transmission via the following:
  – Pets
  – Childcare centers
  – Hospitals
  – Sexual contact
  – Swimming pools

ETIOLOGY
- *C. parvum* (most common)
- *C. hominis*
- *C. meleagridis*

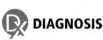 **DIAGNOSIS**

HISTORY
- Incubation is between 7 and 10 days.
- Watery diarrhea in immunocompetent individuals occurs at various degrees of severity from 2 days to 1 month.
- Patients may have crampy abdominal pains.
- Low-grade fever may occur.
- Less likely to cause vomiting than other causes of diarrhea.
- In a minority of patients with immunosuppression, such as HIV infection, voluminous diarrhea with as much as 15 L/d can occur (mainly in those with CD4 count <50 cells/μL).
- Weight loss after protracted diarrhea.
- Disease may recur in up to 40% of patients.
- Respiratory symptoms include dyspnea.

PHYSICAL EXAM
- Nonspecific findings
- Wasting from malabsorption

DIAGNOSTIC TESTS & INTERPRETATION
Lab
- Stool specimens reveal oocysts with Giemsa stains.
- Modified acid-fast stains shows red- or pink-stained round oocysts against a blue-green background.
- Antigen-detection assays are more sensitive: Immunofluorescent antibody stains for stool or tissue specimens have become the gold standard. ELISA or immunochromatographic methods are also available.

- PCR test to detect *C. parvum* DNA.
- Leukocytosis is rare.
- Fecal leukocytes or erythrocytes are not present.
- Fat absorption is impaired.
- D-Xylose tests are abnormal in most patients.
- Liver function tests typically show elevated alkaline phosphatase.
- Vitamin B12 levels may become low.

Imaging
- Radiographs may reveal an ileus pattern along with bowel wall edema. The findings are nonspecific.
- Biliary involvement: Dilated or irregular intrahepatic and extrahepatic bile ducts.
- Respiratory involvement: Bilateral pulmonary infiltrates.

Pathological Findings
Small intestinal biopsy demonstrates an intracellular, extracytoplasmic parasite projecting from the brush border of the mucosal surface.

DIFFERENTIAL DIAGNOSIS
- Enteric bacterial infections such as *Salmonella*, *Shigella*, and *Campylobacter*
- *Clostridium difficile* infection
- Viral gastroenteritis
- Mycobacterial infection
- Enteric protozoal infections such as *Giardia*, *Cyclospora*, *Isospora*, and *Microsporidia*
- Cytomegalovirus colitis

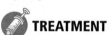 **TREATMENT**

MEDICATION
First Line
- Anti-parasitic drugs have no proven efficacy in the immunocompromised host (1).
- Nitazoxanide is effective in treating diarrhea in non-immunocompromised patients (2). Nitazoxanide is available as 500 mg tablets for use in adults and children >12 years. The dose is 500 mg b.i.d. for 3 days to be taken with food. For children 1–11 years old, nitazoxanide is available as a suspension (powder for reconstitution 100 mg/5 mL). 1–3 years old: 100 mg b.i.d. (5 mL) for 3 days to be taken with food, 4–11 years old: 200 mg b.i.d. (10 mL) for 3 days to be taken with food.
- Nitazoxanide has been used compassionately in AIDS patients (3). In this setting (of compassionate use), treatment is administered for at least 14 days and the doses used for adults ranged from 500 to 1500 mg b.i.d.

- Paromomycin, an oral nonabsorbable aminoglycoside, has been used with variable results (4). For adults 25–35 mg/kg in 2–4 divided doses for 2–4 weeks. Paromomycin has no effect on extraintestinal cryptosporidiosis. Use in combination with antimotility agents (5).
- Macrolides, such as clarithromycin and azithromycin, have some activity against *Cryptosporidium*.

Second Line
- Combination of paromomycin plus azithromycin (5).
- Rifaximin: 600 mg t.i.d. p.o. for 14 days (6).

ADDITIONAL TREATMENT
General Measures
- Patients who are immunocompetent are likely to run a self-limited illness of several days to 6 weeks, for which supportive care is given.
- In HIV-infected individuals, supportive care is critical.

Additional Therapies
- Antimotility agents: Opiates, loperamide, diphenoxylate/atropine.
- Octreotide has been shown to decrease the amount of watery stool produced, without eradication of the organism.
- For patients with AIDS, immune reconstitution with highly active antiretroviral drugs is effective in the treatment of diarrhea. Note: Protease inhibitors have *in vitro* anti-cryptosporidial activity.

SURGERY/OTHER PROCEDURES
Cholecystectomy for acalculous cholecystitis

IN-PATIENT CONSIDERATIONS
Admission Criteria
Hospitalize severely dehydrated patients, especially children.

IV Fluids
Parenteral hydration for severely dehydrated patients. Supplement sodium, potassium, bicarbonate, and glucose.

 # ONGOING CARE

FOLLOW-UP RECOMMENDATIONS
- In patients who are immunocompetent, no special follow-up is required.
- In HIV-infected individuals or other immunocompromised patients, eradication of the organism is less common, and exacerbation and remission is common. Those patients need to be followed closely.

DIET
- Manage malnutrition.
- Avoid lactose-containing foods, as secondary lactose intolerance is common.
- Glutamine supplementation may improve fluid absorption.

PROGNOSIS
Self-limited illness in immunocompetent individuals or patients with AIDS and CD4 count >150 cells/μL.

COMPLICATIONS
- In patients with HIV infection, protracted diarrhea is common and may be life-threatening.
- The organism can involve the bile ducts and the gallbladder, leading to acalculous cholecystitis and sclerosing cholangitis.
- Pancreatitis can occur.
- Tracheitis and bronchitis can occur when the respiratory tract is involved.

REFERENCES
1. Abubakar I, Aliyu SH, Arumugam C, et al. Treatment of cryptosporidiosis in immunocompromised individuals: Systematic review and meta-analysis. *Br J Clin Pharmacol* 2007;63:387–393.
2. Rossignol JF, Kabil SM, el-Gohary Y, et al. Effect of nitazoxanide in diarrhea and enteritis caused by *Cryptosporidium* species. *Clin Gastroenterol Hepatol* 2006;4:320–324.
3. Rossignol JF. Nitazoxanide in the treatment of acquired immune deficiency syndrome-related cryptosporidiosis: Results of the United States compassionate use program in 365 patients. *Aliment Pharmacol Ther* 2006;24:887–894.
4. Hewitt RG, Yiannoutsos CT, Higgs ES, et al. Paromomycin: No more effective than placebo for treatment of cryptosporidiosis in patients with advanced human immunodeficiency virus infection. AIDS Clinical Trial Group. *Clin Infect Dis* 2000; 31:1084–1092.
5. Pantenburg B, Cabada MM, White AC Jr. Treatment of cryptosporidiosis. *Expert Rev Anti Infect Ther* 2009;7:385–391.
6. Amenta M, Dalle Nogare ER, Colomba C, et al. Intestinal protozoa in HIV-infected patients: Effect of rifaximin in *Cryptosporidium parvum* and *Blastocystis hominis* infections. *J Chemother* 1999;11:391–395.

ADDITIONAL READING
- Davies AP, Chalmers RM. Cryptosporidiosis. *BMJ* 2009;339:b4168.
- Pantenburg B, Dann SM, Wang HC, et al. Intestinal immune response to human *Cryptosporidium* sp. infection. *Infect Immun* 2008;76:23–29.

 # CODES

ICD9
007.4 Cryptosporidiosis

CLINICAL PEARLS
- *Cryptosporidium* is associated with waterborne outbreaks of diarrhea in the developed world, and is a common cause of childhood diarrhea in developing countries. The protozoan can cause chronic diarrhea in patients with AIDS or other immunosuppression.
- Antigen-detection assays in stool are more sensitive than detection of oocysts with Giemsa or modified AFB stains.
- Nitazoxanide is effective in the immunocompetent host and can be used in patients with AIDS.

CYSTICERCOSIS

Herman Carneiro (E. Mylonakis, Editor)

🔬 BASICS

DESCRIPTION
- Cysticercosis is a parasitic infection caused by larvae of the pork tapeworm, *Taenia solium* (1–5).
- Clinical syndromes are caused when larvae migrate to subcutaneous tissue, striated muscle, other tissues and vital organs of the body, and form characteristic cysts (cysticerci).
- Organs most often affected include the central nervous system (CNS) (neurocysticercosis), skeletal muscle, heart, eyes, and skin.
- Many infections are asymptomatic.

EPIDEMIOLOGY
Incidence
- *T. solium* is the most common parasite leading to CNS disease (2,4).
- It is the most common cause of seizures in developing countries (2,4).
- In Mexico, up to 10% of all computed tomography (CT) scans in some institutions show evidence of neurocysticercosis (1).

Prevalence
- Worldwide occurrence with over 50 million people infected (2).
- Prevalence highest in Central and South America, sub-Saharan Africa, India, southeast Asia, and eastern Europe.
- In endemic villages 10% or more are seropositive for infection (2).
- Up to 6% of people in endemic villages may harbor adult *T. solium* worms at any time.

RISK FACTORS
- Eating raw or undercooked pork (1–5)
- Living in areas with poor sanitation (1–5)
- Living in areas with pigs, especially where pigs have access to human excrement (1–5)
- Poor hand hygiene leading to fecal–oral infection (1–5)

Genetics
No genetic factors involved

GENERAL PREVENTION
- Health education
  - Prevent fecal contamination of soil, water, human and animal food
  - Cook pork thoroughly
  - Freezing pork below −5°C (23°F) for more than 4 days kills cysticerci
  - Personal hygiene and hygienic food handling
- Screen family members for disease
- Identification of cases and immediate treatment or mass treatment of populations
- Concurrent treatment of pigs
- Immunization of pig populations
- Hand washing
- Improving sanitation
- Strict meat inspection and proper disposal of tainted carcasses

PATHOPHYSIOLOGY
- *T. solium* eggs are ingested and human becomes a host.
- Cysticerci develop within tissue and organs.
- Neurocysticercosis (2)
  - Degenerating cysts cause immune-mediated inflammation, which causes most neurological symptoms.
  - Cysticerci cause mass effect symptoms by taking up space themselves or by blocking the circulation of cerebrospinal fluid.
- Extraneural cysticercosis (2)
  - Ocular cysts usually form in the vitreous humor, but can also be found in the subretinal space. Visual disturbance is related to damage to retinal tissue or the development of chronic uveitis.
  - Cysticerci in the skin present as subcutaneous nodules. Nodules can become tender and inflamed.
  - Skeletal muscle cysts are usually asymptomatic but heavy parasite burden may cause muscular pseudohypertrophy.
  - Cardiac muscle cysts may lead to conduction abnormalities.

ETIOLOGY
- The adult tapeworm is found in the small intestine of humans (definitive host) (3).
- Humans excrete eggs or gravid proglottids in their stool.
  - Proglottids are segments of a tapeworm and contain both male and female reproductive organs. Each segment contains $50–60 \times 10^3$ fertile eggs.
- The pig (intermediate host) ingests the eggs and larvae are formed. The larvae travel via the bloodstream throughout the pig and achieve high concentrations in their muscle.
- Ingestion of undercooked pork (muscle) leads to the evagination of the head, which then attaches to the bowel wall of the new host. This leads to classic intestinal tapeworm infection.
  - Lifespan of the adult *T. solium* is unknown. Estimated from <5 years to 30 years.
- Humans acquire cysticercosis, which is caused by the larval forms, when eggs excreted in the feces are ingested.
- The eggs develop into oncospheres that traverse the small intestine.
- Egg ingestion may occur as autoinfection in a patient with a preexisting tapeworm or from another source.

COMMONLY ASSOCIATED CONDITIONS
- Epilepsy
- Intracranial hypertension
- Hydrocephalus
- Stroke

📋 DIAGNOSIS

HISTORY
- Symptoms of disease include:
  - Insomnia
  - Anorexia and weight loss
  - Abdominal pain
  - Digestive disturbances
  - Chronic headache
  - Nausea and vomiting
  - Seizures
  - Focal neurological complaints
  - Mental status change
  - Visual disturbances or change in vision
  - Skin nodules
- Living in or visiting endemic areas
- Contact with cysticercosis patients
- Consumption of undercooked ham
- Inquire about excreting segments of worm

PHYSICAL EXAM
- Physical findings include the following:
  - Absence of fever
  - Usually nonfocal neurologic signs
  - Papilledema and decreased retinal venous pulsations on ophthalmoscopy
  - Visualization of intraocular larvae on ophthalmoscopy may be diagnostic
  - Meningismus
  - Hyperreflexia
  - Nystagmus or visual deficits
  - Palpable subcutaneous nodules resembling sebaceous cysts
  - Muscular pseudohypertrophy

DIAGNOSTIC TESTS & INTERPRETATION
Lab
- Full blood count; eosinophilia often absent
- Serology (2)
  - Enzyme-linked immunosorbent assay has 74% sensitivity and are highly specific. Sensitivity increases with increasing number of cysts.
  - Enzyme-linked immunoelectrotransfer blot has >95% sensitivity and nearly 100% specificity in patients with multiple cysts. Poor in patients with single cysts.
  - Stool for ova and parasites.

Imaging
- Soft tissue x-ray may show calcified cysts
- Brain CT scan
- MRI of brain as adjunct to CT scan
  - Preferred imaging modality to identify brainstem cysts

Diagnostic Procedures/Other
- Biopsy or fine-needle aspiration of subcutaneous nodules
- Lumbar puncture
  - Neither sensitive nor specific
  - With significant inflammation, cerebrospinal fluid may show lymphocytosis, increased protein, and/or decreased glucose levels

Pathological Findings
Cysts are uniformly round or oval vesicles, from a few millimeters to 1–2 cm in size.

DIFFERENTIAL DIAGNOSIS
- Brain abscess
- Status epilepticus
- Neoplasms, brain
- Encephalitis
- Epidural and subdural infections
- Meningitis
- Tuberculosis
- Stroke, hemorrhagic
- Stroke, ischemic
- Subarachnoid hemorrhage
- Epidural hematoma
- Subdural hematoma
- Endophthalmitis
- Headache, migraine
- Headache, tension
- Coccidioidomycosis
- Toxoplasmosis
- Trichinosis

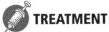

TREATMENT

MEDICATION
First Line
- Anthelmintics (2)
  - Praziquantel 50 mg/kg/d orally in 3 divided doses daily for 2 weeks
- Corticosteroids
  - Prednisone orally or dexamethasone IV
- Anticonvulsants
  - Lorazepam, phenytoin, or phenobarbital

Second Line
Albendazole 15 mg/kg/d orally in 2–3 divided doses daily for 2 weeks (2)

ADDITIONAL TREATMENT
Issues for Referral
- Referral to neurologist
  - Seizures
  - Mental status change
  - Other neurological signs and symptoms
- Referral to ophthalmologist
  - Changes in vision or visual disturbances
- Referral to neurosurgeon
  - For surgical intervention to reduce intracranial pressure

SURGERY/OTHER PROCEDURES
- Burr hole to relieve intracranial pressure
- Interventricular shunt
- Ventriculoperitoneal shunt

IN-PATIENT CONSIDERATIONS
Initial Stabilization
Resuscitation according to Acute Life Support protocol as required

Admission Criteria
- Status epilepticus
- For IV corticosteroid therapy to reduce intracranial pressure
- For surgical interventions to reduce intracranial pressure from obstructive hydrocephalus
- Patients requiring ophthalmic surgery

IV Fluids
Maintenance fluids with Ringers lactate

Nursing
Use appropriate barrier nursing techniques

Discharge Criteria
- Termination of seizures
- Clinically stable

 ONGOING CARE

FOLLOW-UP RECOMMENDATIONS
Long-term anticonvulsant therapy for those with persistent CNS calcifications

Patient Monitoring
Follow-up CT scan or MRI to assess response to treatment

DIET
Pork should be cooked thoroughly prior to consumption

PATIENT EDUCATION
- As above in "General Prevention"
- Patients and their families should be familiar with first-aid management of seizures
- Use of prescribed medications
- Instruction on when to seek medical care, including signs of increasing raised intracranial pressure or focal neurologic complaints
- Patients with recent seizures should not drive, operate heavy machinery, climb ladders, swim, or perform other activities putting them at risk

PROGNOSIS
Prognosis usually excellent with appropriate diagnosis and treatment

COMPLICATIONS
- Intracranial herniation
- Stroke
- Status epilepticus
- Long-term anticonvulsant use
- Intraventricular shunt complications
- Loss of vision

REFERENCES
1. García HH, Gonzalez AE, Evans CA, et al. *Taenia solium* cysticercosis. *Lancet* 2003;362(9383): 547–556.
2. Tenzer R, Blumstein HA. Cysticercosis: eMedicine Emergency Medicine. http://emedicine.medscape.com/article/781845-overview. Accessed on June 4, 2010.
3. Centers for Disease Control and Prevention. DPDx – Cysticercosis. http://www.dpd.cdc.gov/dpdx/html/cysticercosis.htm. Accessed on June 1, 2010.
4. World Health Organization (WHO). Taeniasis/cysticercosis. http://www.who.int/zoonoses/diseases/taeniasis/en/index.html. Accessed on June 1, 2010.
5. The Merck Manuals Online Library. *Taeniasis solium* and cysticercosis: Cestodes (Tapeworms). http://www.merckmanuals.com/professional/sec15/ch195/ch195j.html. Accessed on June 4, 2010.

ADDITIONAL READING
- García HH, Gonzalez AE, Evans CA, et al. *Taenia solium* cysticercosis. *Lancet* 2003;362(9383): 547–556.

 See Also

- Centers for Disease Control and Prevention. DPDx – Cysticercosis. http://www.dpd.cdc.gov/dpdx/html/cysticercosis.htm. Accessed on June 1, 2010.

 CODES

ICD9
123.1 – *Taenia solium* Cysticercosis

CLINICAL PEARLS
- Cysticercosis is the most common cause of seizures in developing countries.

CYSTITIS

Evridiki K. Vouloumanou
Petros I. Rafailidis
Matthew E. Falagas

 BASICS

DESCRIPTION
Cystitis is a lower urinary tract infection (UTI) involving the bladder that occurs in both women and men.

EPIDEMIOLOGY
Incidence
- 7 million cases of UTI annually in the US.
- Approximately one-third of women up to 24 years of age will have at least one episode of UTI requiring antibiotic treatment (1).
- Approximately 50% of the women whose uncomplicated UTIs resolved spontaneously will develop a recurrent UTI within the first year (2).

Prevalence
More prevalent in young women than in young men (20% vs. 0.5%, respectively, ages 16–35 years).

RISK FACTORS
- Premenopausal women: History of UTI, anatomic congenital abnormalities, frequent/recent sexual activity, use of spermicides, diaphragm contraception, increasing parity, diabetes mellitus, pregnancy, obesity, neurologic diseases, medical conditions that require indwelling/repetitive bladder catheterization (3).
- Postmenopausal women: History of UTI, vaginal atrophy, incomplete bladder emptying, rectocele/cystocele/urethrocele/uterovaginal prolapse, diabetes mellitus type 1 (3).
- Men: Prostatic hypertrophy, urethral obstruction, catheterization, surgery, incontinence.

GENERAL PREVENTION
- Maintain good atomic hygiene
- Avoid diaphragm use
- During pregnancy, obtain frequent screenings of urine in third trimester
- In diabetes, avoid glycosuria

ETIOLOGY
- *Escherichia coli* is by far the most common cause (~>80%)
- Other Enterobacteriaceae (*Proteus mirabilis*, *Enterobacter* spp., *Citrobacter* spp., *Serratia* spp., *Klebsiella* spp., *Salmonella* spp., *Morganella morganii*)
- Non-Enterobacteriaceae (*Pseudomonas aeruginosa*)
- The emergence of uropathogens, mainly *E. coli*, which exhibit considerably high resistance due to the production of extended-spectrum β-lactamases (ESBLs), as causes of nosocomial and community-acquired cystitis, is also an issue of major importance (4)
- *Staphylococcus saprophyticus*

 DIAGNOSIS

HISTORY
- Dysuria, urinary frequency, urinary urgency, abrupt onset, turbid urine, sometimes foul-smelling and bloody, suprapubic tenderness or low back pain in 10% of patients
- Children: Nonspecific symptoms (fever, vomiting, diarrhea, etc.)
- Elderly: Paucity of symptoms

PHYSICAL EXAM
Suprapubic tenderness

DIAGNOSTIC TESTS & INTERPRETATION
Lab
- Urinary dipstick testing (identification of nitrites and leukocyte esterase in the urine)
- Urine microscopy
- Urine culture
- Consider whether a pregnancy test is necessary

Imaging
- Ultrasonography in men
- Consider ultrasonography in young women if no response to antibiotic treatment (not explained by in vitro antibiotic susceptibility data) or recurrent episodes not associated with coitus

Diagnostic Procedures/Other
- Urodynamic testing. However, the evidence regarding the usefulness of urodynamic testing in the identification of specific urogynecologic mechanisms that could have potentially contributed to the prevention or improved medical and/or surgical management of recurrent UTI is not supportive (5)
- Urography, cystoscopy, bladder biopsy. However, since anatomical and/or functional abnormalities of the urinary tract are rarely encountered among patients with cystitis, the value of cystoscopy can be considered as rather limited (6)
- Bladder x-rays

DIFFERENTIAL DIAGNOSIS
- Infectious: Pyelonephritis (upper UTI), asymptomatic bacteriuria, urethritis, vaginitis
- Noninfectious: Interstitial cystitis, urolithiasis, bladder tumor, chronic prostatitis/chronic pelvic pain syndrome

 TREATMENT

MEDICATION
Recurrent Cystitis
Continuous prophylaxis with once-daily treatment with norfloxacin, ciprofloxacin, trimethoprim (TMP), trimethoprim–sulfamethoxazole (TMP-SMX), or nitrofurantoin has been suggested to decrease the risk of recurrence by 95% (8). However, in this era of alarmingly high antimicrobial resistance of uropathogens, such an approach has to be individualized.

Acute Uncomplicated Cystitis
- Trimethoprim-sulfamethoxazole (TMP-SMX): TMP: 160 mg-SMX: 800 mg, orally twice daily for 3 days
- TMP: 100 mg orally twice daily for 3 days
- Ciprofloxacin: 250 mg orally twice daily for 3 days
- Levofloxacin: 250 mg orally once daily for 3 days
- Norfloxacin: 400 mg orally twice daily for 3 days
- Fosfomycin tromethamine: 3 g single dose orally (3, 7)
- Nitrofurantoin macrocrystals: 50–100 mg, 4 times daily for 7 days
- Nitrofurantoin monohydrate macrocrystals: 100 mg, twice daily for 7 days (3)

Pregnancy Considerations
- Amoxicillin: 250 mg every 8 hours for 3 days; microcrystalline nitrofurantoin: 100 mg 4 times daily for 3 days; cefpodoxime: 200 mg twice daily for 3 days. Avoid the administration at late pregnancy (38–42 weeks) as well during labor or obstetric delivery due to the potential of inducing hemolysis in the fetus/neonate.
- Fosfomycin may also play a role in the treatment of cystitis during pregnancy, as it seems that adverse events occur significantly less frequently in pregnant patients treated with fosfomycin compared to other antibiotics (7).

COMPLEMENTARY & ALTERNATIVE THERAPIES
- Probiotics: *Lactobacillus rhamnosus* GR-1 and *L. reuteri* RC-14 have been shown to be the most effective among other lactobacilli regarding the prevention of UTIs. *L. casei* shirota and *L. crispatus* CTV-05 have also shown considerable efficacy. On the other hand, *L. rhamnosus* GG has not been shown to be quite as effective as far as the prevention of UTIs is concerned (9).

C

- Cranberry juice: It has been suggested as a potent inhibitor of bacterial adherence that may play a role in the treatment and/or prevention of UTIs (10). Specifically, it has been reported that cranberry juice may potentially result in a reduction of the number of symptomatic UTIs over a period of 12 months, particularly for women with recurrent UTIs (11).
- Methenamine salts (methenamine hippurate): Short-term treatment duration (≤1 week) with methenamine hippurate has been suggested to be associated with a significant reduction in symptomatic UTI in patients without urinary tract abnormalities. However, they do not appear to confer benefit to patients with urinary tract abnormalities or in patients with neuropathic bladder (12).
- Uroanalgesics: The rationale of administration of uroanalgesics such as phenazopyridine to patients with acute cystitis symptoms is the resolution of symptoms associated with acute cystitis. Phenazopyridine has a potential analgesic effect on the mucosa of the urinary bladder. It has also been suggested that when administered in combination with sulfonamides, it enhances its antibacterial activity (13). However, many reports suggested a potential association of phenazopyridine with adverse events including hemolytic anemia (14).
- The evidence regarding the effectiveness of aggressive hydration in the prevention of recurrent cystitis remains insufficient.
- The evidence regarding the effectiveness of oral and vaginal exogenous estrogens in preventing recurrent UTIs in postmenopausal women is also conflicting (15).

SURGERY/OTHER PROCEDURES

Surgical management of anatomical abnormalities of the urinary tract

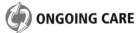 **ONGOING CARE**

PROGNOSIS
- The prognosis for acute uncomplicated cystitis after appropriate antibiotic treatment is excellent for the majority of patients.
- However, recurrent cystitis may occur in patients with risk factors (such as urinary tract abnormalities) or without

COMPLICATIONS
- Urethritis
- Pyelonephritis
- Psychiatric disorders particularly after recurrent cystitis

REFERENCES

1. Foxman B, Barlow R, D'Arcy H, et al. Urinary tract infection: Self-reported incidence and associated costs. *Ann Epidemiol* 2000;10:509–515.
2. Mabeck CE. Treatment of uncomplicated urinary tract infection in non-pregnant women. *Postgrad Med J* 1972;48:69–75.
3. American College of Obstetricians and Gynecologists. ACOG Practice Bulletin No. 91: Treatment of urinary tract infections in nonpregnant women. *Obstet Gynecol* 2008;111:785–794.
4. Zahar JR, Lortholary O, Martin C, et al. Addressing the challenge of extended-spectrum beta-lactamases. *Curr Opin Investig Drugs* 2009;10: 172–180.
5. Athanasiou S, Anstaklis A, Betsi GI, et al. Clinical and urodynamic parameters associated with history of urinary tract infections in women. *Acta Obstet Gynecol Scand* 2007;86:1130–1135.
6. Fowler JE Jr, Pulaski ET. Excretory urography, cystography, and cystoscopy in the evaluation of women with urinary-tract infection: A prospective study. *N Engl J Med* 1981;304:462–465.
7. Falagas ME, Vouloumanou EK, Togias AG, et al. Fosfomycin versus other antibiotics for the treatment of cystitis: A meta-analysis of randomized controlled trials. *J Antimicrob Chemother* 2010;65:1862–1877.
8. Hooton TM. Recurrent urinary tract infection in women. *Int J Antimicrob Agents* 2001;17: 259–268.
9. Falagas ME, Betsi GI, Tokas T, et al. Probiotics for prevention of recurrent urinary tract infections in women: A review of the evidence from microbiological and clinical studies. *Drugs* 2006;66:1253–1261.
10. Sobota AE. Inhibition of bacterial adherence by cranberry juice: Potential use for the treatment of urinary tract infections. *J Urol* 1984;131: 1013–1036.
11. Jepson RG, Craig JC. Cranberries for preventing urinary tract infections. *Cochrane Database Syst Rev* 200823:CD001321.
12. Lee BB, Simpson JM, Craig JC, et al. Methenamine hippurate for preventing urinary tract infections. *Cochrane Database Syst Rev* 2007;17:CD003265.
13. Neter E, Loomis TA. The combined bacteriostatic activity of sulphonamide compound and pyridium upon *E. Coli* in vitro. *Urol Cutaneous Rev* 1941;45:295–297.
14. Jeffery WH, Zelicoff AP, Hardy WR. Acquired methemoglobinemia and hemolytic anemia after usual doses of phenazopyridine. *Drug Intell Clin Pharm* 1982;16:157–159.
15. Brown JS, Vittinghoff E, Kanaya AM, et al. Urinary tract infections in postmenopausal women: Effect of hormone therapy and risk factors. *Obstet Gynecol* 2001;98:1045–1052.

ADDITIONAL READING

- Fihn SD. Clinical practice: Acute uncomplicated urinary tract infection in women. *N Engl J Med* 2003;349:259–266.
- Falagas ME, Kotsantis IK, Vouloumanou EK, et al. Antibiotics versus placebo in the treatment of women with uncomplicated cystitis: A meta-analysis of randomized controlled trials. *J Infect* 2009;58: 91–102.

 CODES

ICD9
- 595.0 Acute cystitis
- 595.1 Chronic interstitial cystitis
- 595.9 Cystitis, unspecified

CLINICAL PEARLS

- Cystitis is a common bacterial infection with a good prognosis after appropriate antibiotic therapy.
- The emergence of nosocomial and community-acquired uropathogens that exhibit considerably high resistance due to the production of ESBLs may have considerable implications in the treatment of cystitis.
- Alternative treatment strategies including probiotics and cranberry juice may also play a role in the prevention and treatment of cystitis.
- Treat asymptomatic bacteriuria in pregnant women.
- In case *Staphylococcus aureus* is cultured from the urine rule out the independent presence of *S. aureus* bacteremia!

CYTOMEGALOVIRUS INFECTION

Paschalis Vergidis
Matthew E. Falagas

 BASICS

DESCRIPTION
A group of infections of different systems and organs caused by cytomegalovirus (CMV)

EPIDEMIOLOGY
Incidence
- In the US, the incidence of infection among individuals aged 10–49 years of age is estimated at 1.6 infections per 100 susceptible persons per year.
- It is estimated that approximately 27,000 new CMV infections occur among seronegative pregnant women each year in the US.

Prevalence
- CMV is a common human pathogen that affects people worldwide.
- Older age and lower socioeconomic status are associated with higher CMV seroprevalence.
- In the US, CMV seroprevalence rate is estimated at 60% among individuals aged older than 6 years (1). The seroprevalence may reach over 90% among those aged older than 80 years.

RISK FACTORS
- Immunosuppression predisposes to severe manifestations of CMV infection.
- The major risk factor for disease in transplantation is having a CMV mismatch status.
  - For solid organ transplant (SOT): When a CMV-seronegative recipient receives an allograft from a CMV-seropositive donor (CMV D+/R–).
  - For allogeneic bone marrow transplant: Higher risk when a CMV-seropositive recipient receives a graft from a CMV-seronegative donor (CMV D–/R+).
- Lung, small intestine, and pancreas transplant recipients are at highest risk for infection. Liver and heart transplant recipients have intermediate risk. Kidney transplant recipients have the lowest risk.
- Use of lymphocyte-depleting agents (such as OKT3, anti-thymocyte globulins, and anti-lymphocyte globulin).
- Acute allograft rejection.
- Graft-versus-host disease.
- HIV infection with CD4 count less than 50/mm^3.

GENERAL PREVENTION
- Antiviral prophylaxis in CMV-seropositive recipients or CMV mismatch. Late-onset CMV disease is an emerging problem among CMV D+/R– patients who received antiviral prophylaxis.
- CMV immunoglobulin is used in some centers for the prevention of disease in high-risk individuals (CMV D+/R– lung and intestinal transplant recipients).
- Blood products from CMV-seronegative donors or leukocyte-depleted blood products should be used in CMV-seronegative allogeneic hematopoietic stem cell transplant recipients (AI).
- Highly active antiretroviral treatment (HAART) has led to a significant reduction of CMV-related diseases in HIV infection.
- There is no available vaccine.

PATHOPHYSIOLOGY
- In SOT recipients, primary CMV infection occurs when a CMV-seronegative recipient receives an allograft from a CMV-seropositive donor (CMV D+/R–).
- Reactivation occurs when the latent virus in a seropositive recipient reactivates during periods of immunosuppression. Disease is less severe due to pre-existing anti-CMV immunity.
- Infection can be classified as asymptomatic (subclinical CMV infection) or symptomatic (CMV disease).
- Disease can be further divided into CMV syndrome (disease without end-organ involvement) or tissue-invasive disease (disease with end-organ involvement).
- The transplanted organ is particularly vulnerable to end-organ disease.

ETIOLOGY
- CMV is a DNA virus that belongs to the herpesvirus group.
- Latent infection after primary infection occurs with CMV, as with other herpes group viruses.

COMMONLY ASSOCIATED CONDITIONS
- Bone marrow transplantation
- Solid organ transplantation
- AIDS
- Patients with severe cancer-related cellular immunity suppression such as lymphoma or leukemia

DIAGNOSIS

HISTORY
- In immunocompetent people, CMV may be asymptomatic or may cause an infectious mononucleosis-like syndrome.
- CMV syndrome is characterized by fever, malaise, myalgias, and arthralgias.
- Colitis is the most common form of end-organ disease and presents with abdominal pain and diarrhea.
- CMV gastritis presents with odynophagia, nausea, and vomiting.
- Pneumonitis presents with fever, cough, and dyspnea.
- Other manifestations include hepatitis and myocarditis.
- Chorioretinitis causes a progressive decrease in visual acuity which may result in blindness. Immune reconstitution syndrome has been reported after initiating HAART.
- Meningoencephalitis presents with severe headache, photophobia, and lethargy.
- Back pain in spinal cord involvement (myelitis, polyradiculitis), which most commonly occurs in HIV-infected patients.

PHYSICAL EXAM
- Pharyngitis
- Lymphadenopathy
- Splenomegaly
- Maculopapular and rubelliform rashes in the setting of CMV mononucleosis.
- Pyramidal tract signs in encephalitis.
- Ascending weakness in the lower extremities with loss of deep tendon reflexes in myeloradiculopathy.
- Funduscopic findings in retinitis: Lesions appear peripherally and progress centrally. Yellow-white areas with perivascular exudates. Hemorrhage may be present.

DIAGNOSTIC TESTS & INTERPRETATION
Lab
Initial lab tests
- Anemia, thrombocytopenia due to myelosuppression or hemolytic anemia.
- Presence of atypical lymphocytes.
- Positive CMV IgG serology suggests antiviral immunity, but is also a marker of latent virus. Helpful in pre-transplant evaluation of transplant candidates and potential donors.
- IgM antibodies against CMV may be found in an acute CMV infection or reactivation.
  - Note: Serology typically not useful in immunosuppressed patients as they cannot mount an immune response.
- Due to rapid turn-around time and high sensitivity, viral nucleic acid detection and antigenemia assays are currently the preferred diagnostic techniques.
- Several real-time PCR platforms are available (2).
- CMV antigenemia assays employ tagged monoclonal antibody that is specific to the CMV pp65 matrix protein in peripheral blood polymorphonuclear leukocytes. Their utility is limited in neutropenic patients due to the absence of leukocytes.
- Viral culture has been used to isolate CMV from blood or other body fluids or tissues. Cytopathic effects are seen after 1–6 weeks.
- A modification of viral culture is the shell vial assay. Results are reported within 24–48 hours.

Follow-Up & Special Considerations
- Consider drug-resistant virus if persistent clinical symptoms and increasing or non-declining viral load after 2 weeks of full-dose treatment.
- Genotypic resistance testing is available:
  - Mutations in UL97 phosphotransferase result in resistance to ganciclovir due to lower levels of active triphosphorylated drug.
  - Mutations in UL54 DNA polymerase are less common and often occur as second-step mutations after exposure to ganciclovir, foscarnet, or cidofovir. Can result in cross-resistance among the three antiviral drugs.

Imaging
- CMV pneumonitis: Interstitial infiltrates on plain radiography
- CMV colitis: Bowel wall thickening on CT imaging
- CMV encephalitis: Periventricular inflammation or meningeal enhancement on brain MRI

Diagnostic Procedures/Other
- Bronchoscopy with bronchoalveolar lavage/biopsy in CMV pneumonitis

- In CMV colitis, colonoscopy shows mucosal erythema, erosions, ulcerations, hemorrhage, nodular or polypoid lesions

Pathological Findings
- CMV viremia does not necessarily correlate with tissue invasion. CMV in tissue can be demonstrated by histopathology, immunohistochemistry, or *in situ* DNA hybridization.
- The typical cytopathic findings are large intranuclear inclusions surrounded by a clear halo. Smaller cytoplasmic inclusions may also be observed.

DIFFERENTIAL DIAGNOSIS
- Infectious mononucleosis
- Toxoplasmosis
- HIV infection (including acute seroconversion)
- Human herpesvirus 6 infection
- Viral hepatitis
- Viral gastroenteritis
- Cryptosporidiosis
- *Clostridium difficile* infection

 ## TREATMENT
- In the immunocompetent host, CMV syndrome is usually self-limited and does not necessitate treatment.
- In immunosuppressed patients, CMV infection should be treated aggressively using antiviral agents.

MEDICATION
First Line
- Ganciclovir is the treatment of choice (AII). Induction dose: 5 mg/kg i.v. twice daily. Dose is adjusted for renal failure.
- Valganciclovir 900 mg p.o. twice daily can be used for induction treatment in mild-to-moderate disease (3).
- Valganciclovir is also used as a step-down oral treatment after an initial induction treatment with intravenous ganciclovir.
- For CMV retinitis, the combination of a systemic agent and a sustained-release intraocular ganciclovir implant is more effective than intravenous treatment alone in patients with AIDS (4).

Second Line
- Foscarnet 60 mg/kg i.v. every 8 hours (or 90 mg/kg i.v. every 12 hours) for ganciclovir-resistant CMV.
- Cidofovir weekly dosing at 5 mg/kg for ganciclovir-resistant CMV. Contraindicated if creatinine clearance <55 mL/min.
- Higher doses of ganciclovir (7.5–10 mg/kg i.v. every 12 hours) have been used in cases of low-level ganciclovir resistance.

ADDITIONAL TREATMENT
General Measures
Reduction in the doses of immunosuppressive regimens

Additional Therapies
CMV immunoglobulin for severe CMV disease, particularly pneumonitis (BIII)

 ## ONGOING CARE

FOLLOW-UP RECOMMENDATIONS
Patient Monitoring
- Weekly monitoring of disease activity by use of molecular assays or antigenemia after initiation of antiviral therapy is helpful.
- It is generally suggested that patients receive treatment for at least 2–4 weeks, and preferably until 2 weeks after clearance of CMV viremia. Lack of clearance is associated with recurrent disease (5).
- The use of maintenance therapy, wherein antiviral drugs are administered at prophylactic doses, has also been recommended in order to complete usually up to 3 months of treatment.

PROGNOSIS
- CMV infection may lead to death, especially in severely immunocompromised persons.
- Pneumonitis is among the most severe forms of CMV infection, especially in bone marrow transplant recipients.
- CMV encephalitis also carries a high mortality.

COMPLICATIONS
- CMV colitis may lead to bowel perforation and peritonitis.
- CMV myocarditis may lead to congestive heart failure.
- HIV-infected patients may develop cauda equina syndrome.
- Indirect CMV effects in transplant recipients:
  – Acute allograft rejection
  – Chronic allograft failure
  – Bronchiolitis obliterans (in lung recipients)
  – Accelerated vasculopathy (in cardiac recipients)
  – Vanishing bile duct syndrome (in liver recipients)
  – Glomerulopathy and tubulo-interstitial fibrosis (in kidney recipients)
- Congenital CMV infection is the most common cause of congenital anomalies in industrialized countries (after the decrease in incidence of rubella due to immunization).
- Congenital CMV infection may cause abortion, fetal jaundice, anemia, and central nervous system damage.

REFERENCES
1. Staras SA, Dollard SC, Radford KW, et al. Seroprevalence of cytomegalovirus infection in the United States, 1988–1994. *Clin Infect Dis* 2006; 43(9):1143–1151.
2. Razonable RR, Brown RA, Espy MJ, et al. Comparative quantitation of cytomegalovirus (CMV) DNA in solid organ transplant recipients with CMV infection by using two high-throughput automated systems. *J Clin Microbiol* 2001;39(12): 4472–4476.
3. Asberg A, Humar A, Rollag H, et al. Oral valganciclovir is noninferior to intravenous ganciclovir for the treatment of cytomegalovirus disease in solid organ transplant recipients. *Am J Transplant* 2007;7(9):2106–2113.
4. Martin DF, Kuppermann BD, Wolitz RA, et al. Oral ganciclovir for patients with cytomegalovirus retinitis treated with a ganciclovir implant. Roche Ganciclovir Study Group. *N Engl J Med* 1999; 340(14):1063–1070.
5. Humar A, Kumar D, Boivin G, et al. Cytomegalovirus (CMV) virus load kinetics to predict recurrent disease in solid-organ transplant patients with CMV disease. *J Infect Dis* 2002;186(6):829–833.

ADDITIONAL READING
- Kotton CN, Kumar D, Caliendo AM, et al. International consensus guidelines on the management of cytomegalovirus in solid organ transplantation. *Transplantation* 2010;89(7): 779–795.
- Humar A, Snydman D. Cytomegalovirus in solid organ transplant recipients. *Am J Transplant* 2009;9(Suppl 4):S78–S86.

 ## CODES

ICD9
- 078.5 Cytomegaloviral disease
- 771.1 Congenital cytomegalovirus infection

CLINICAL PEARLS
- In solid organ transplantation, risk of primary infection is highest when a CMV-seronegative recipient receives an allograft from a CMV-seropositive donor.
- CMV colitis is the most common form of end-organ disease.
- Ganciclovir is the treatment of choice. Foscarnet and cidofovir are alternative options for ganciclovir-resistant virus.

DENGUE
Herman Carneiro (E. Mylonakis, Editor)

 BASICS

DESCRIPTION
Dengue is a mosquito-borne viral illness that causes a severe flu-like illness. At times, the virus causes potentially lethal dengue hemorrhagic fever (DHF) and dengue shock syndrome (DSS), with a patient fatality rate of 1–5%.

EPIDEMIOLOGY
Incidence
- About 2.5 billion people or two-fifths of the world population are at risk of infection (1–4)
- There is increased transmission during the rainy season
- Estimated 50–100 million infections occur annually worldwide, including 500,000 DHF cases and 22,0000 deaths (4)

Prevalence
- The virus is present throughout the tropical and subtropical zones, mostly in urban and suburban areas.
- It is endemic in approximately 100 countries in Asia, the Pacific, the Americas, Africa, and the Caribbean.

RISK FACTORS
Travel to or living in areas where dengue is endemic

Genetics
No genetic factors involved

GENERAL PREVENTION
- Avoid being bitten by mosquitoes
  - Avoid travel to dengue endemic areas
  - Wear mosquito repellent with at least 30% *N,N*-diethyl-3-methylbenzamide (DEET) on exposed skin and clothing
  - Wear long-sleeved clothing, preferably impregnated with permethrin insecticide
  - Aedes are day- biting mosquitoes making the use of bed nets of limited use
- Vector control
  - Use insecticides indoors to eliminate mosquitoes
  - Eliminate mosquito-breeding grounds by clearing pools of stagnant water
  - Use larvicidal agents, e.g. Abate, in stagnant water sources
  - Biological vector control by introducing predatory copepods into stagnant water sources

PATHOPHYSIOLOGY
- Following inoculation, dengue has an incubation periods of 3–14 days, but commonly 4–7 days (1,2,3)
- The virus replicates in dendritic cells
- The virus then infects reticuloendothelial cells including dendritic cells, hepatocytes, and endothelial cells
- Immune mediators released which shape cellular and humoral responses
- Resulting acute febrile illness lasts 5–7 days
- Full recovery in 7–10 days
- Previous infection with another serotype of dengue predisposes to DHF and DSS

- Onset of DHF and DSS is usually around the 3rd to 7th day of illness at the end of febrile period
  - Increased capillary permeability causes plasma leakage resulting in hemoconcentration and possible pleural effusions and ascites
  - Capillary fragility, thrombocytopenia, and disseminated intravascular coagulation (DIC) result in hemorrhages from minor petechiae to life-threatening gastrointestinal (GI) bleeds
  - Liver damage results in deranged liver function tests and coagulopathies
- Dengue hepatitis can be fatal

ETIOLOGY
- Dengue virus is of the family Flaviviridae (ssRNA)
- There are 4 serotypes that are antigenically distinct (types 1–4)
- Human and nonhuman primates are the only reservoirs of infection
- The virus is transmitted by Aedes mosquitoes, most commonly *Aedes aegypti* and *Aedes albopictus*

Pediatric Considerations
Mother-to-child transmission has been documented

COMMONLY ASSOCIATED CONDITIONS
As above in Section Pathophysiology

 DIAGNOSIS

HISTORY
- Symptoms
  - Fever with headache, chills, and myalgias
  - Rash
  - Bone pain after onset of fever
  - Nausea and vomiting
  - Cutaneous hyperesthesia
  - Change in sense of taste
  - Loss of appetite
  - Abdominal pain
  - Hemorrhagic manifestations including bruises, epistaxis, gum bleeding, GI bleeding, menorrhagia
- Travel history

PHYSICAL EXAM
- Fever
- Signs of shock, e.g., tachycardia, hypotension, delayed capillary refill
- Rash
  - Generalized blanching macular rash
  - Second rash is morbilliform maculopapular rash that spares palms and soles
  - Bleeding manifestations such as petechiae, purpura, epistaxis, gum bleeding, GI bleeding
- Conjunctival injection
- Pharyngeal injection—97% of cases
- Bleeding mucosae
- Generalized lymphadenopathy
- Hepatomegaly
- Mental state examination for alternations in mental state due to encephalopathy, which is secondary to cerebral edema and intracranial bleeds

DIAGNOSTIC TESTS & INTERPRETATION
Lab
Initial lab tests
- Serology (ELISA) for IgG and IgM antibodies
- Complete blood count
  - Leucopenia, often with lymphopenia
  - Raised hematocrit
  - Thrombocytopenia
- Liver function tests
  - Raised transaminases
  - Low albumin
- Chemistry panel
  - Hyponatremia
  - Acidosis
  - Elevated blood urea nitrogen (BUN)
- Coagulation screen
  - Raised prothrombin time (PT)
  - Raised activated partial thromboplastin time (APTT)
  - Low fibrinogen and high fibrin degradation products in DIC
- Arterial blood gas in severely ill patients
- Polymerase chain reaction (PCR) methods currently not available in the clinical setting

Follow-Up & Special Considerations
- Blood needs to be cross-matched in case of severe hemorrhage
- Cultures of blood and other bodily fluids should be performed as necessary to exclude other possible causes of illness

Imaging
- Chest radiograph may show pleural effusion
- Ultrasound to evaluate pleural effusions, pericardial effusions, and ascites as required
- Head computed tomography (CT) scan for patients with altered mental state or depressed consciousness

Pathological Findings
As above in Initial Lab Tests

DIFFERENTIAL DIAGNOSIS
- Malaria
- Yellow fever
- Tick-borne Diseases, Rocky Mountain spotted fever
- Hepatitis
- Meningitis
- Leptospirosis
- Rickettsial disease
- Scrub typhus
- Typhoid
- Other viral infections (e.g., influenza, chikungunya, Rift valley fever, and West Nile)
- Bacterial sepsis
- Pre-eclampsia during pregnancy

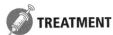

TREATMENT

MEDICATION
There is no specific treatment for dengue fever, DHF, or DSS.

ADDITIONAL TREATMENT
General Measures
- Symptomatic and supportive therapy
- Avoid aspirin, due to the hemorrhagic nature of the illness
- Suggested intake of appropriate analgesia and antipyretics

Issues for Referral
- Infectious disease specialist
- Critical care specialist for patients with DHF or DSS
- Cardiologist for patients with pericardial effusions

IN-PATIENT CONSIDERATIONS
Initial Stabilization
- Resuscitate using advanced life support (ALS) protocol
- Oxygen empirically
- Large-bore intravenous catheter
- Intravenous colloids to maintain systolic blood pressure >90 mm Hg
- Implement therapy for DIC if indicated
- Central venous catheter to measure central venous pressure if indicated
- Arterial line for continuous blood pressure monitoring and serial blood gas measurements if indicated
- Urethral catheter to measure urine output if indicated
- Reverse electrolyte abnormalities and acidosis
- Cross-match blood in the event of major bleed secondary to DHF

Admission Criteria
- Patients with hemodynamic instability
- Patients with DHF or DSS
- Admit to intensive care units (ICUs) if hypotensive or in DIC, otherwise admit to general medicine ward

IV Fluids
- Fluids resuscitation with colloids, e.g., Gelofusine, Dextran, Hetastarch, human albumin solution, etc.
- Maintenance fluids using Ringer's lactate

Nursing
- Maintain strict fluid input–output chart for severely ill patients
- Patients with depressed consciousness may need regular neuro-observations

Discharge Criteria
- Patient is hemodynamically stable
- Preferably full recovery from illness

ONGOING CARE

FOLLOW-UP RECOMMENDATIONS
- No specific follow-up recommendations
- Report cases to department of public health
- Patients should be aware that should they contract dengue of a different serotype they are at higher risk of developing DHF or DSS

DIET
- Encourage oral fluid intake
- No specific diet is necessary

PATIENT EDUCATION
See Section General Prevention

PROGNOSIS
- Prognosis is excellent for dengue fever with most patients making a full recovery
- Patients who survive the critical stages of DHF and DSS usually recover with no lasting sequelae

COMPLICATIONS
- Neurological manifestations
  - Brain damage from prolonged ischemia in shock or intracranial hemorrhage
  - Encephalitis/encephalopathy
  - Seizures
  - Neuropathies
  - Guillain–Barré syndrome
  - Transverse myelitis
- Myocarditis
- Liver failure

REFERENCES

1. Centers for Disease Control and Prevention. CDC—Epidemiology—Dengue. http://www.cdc.gov/dengue/epidemiology/index.html. Accessed on July 2, 2010.
2. Price DD, Wilson SR. Treating the patient with severe dengue infection. http://emedicine.medscape.com/article/781961-overview. Accessed on July 2, 2010.
3. Shepherd SM, Hinfey PB, Shoff WH. Dengue fever: eMedicine infectious diseases. http://emedicine.medscape.com/article/215840-overview. Accessed on July 2, 2010.
4. World Health Organization. WHO. Dengue and dengue haemorrhagic fever. http://www.who.int/mediacentre/factsheets/fs117/en/index.html. Accessed on July 2, 2010.

ADDITIONAL READING
- Kyle JL, Harris E. Global spread and persistence of dengue. *Annu Rev Microbiol* 2008;62:71–92.

 See Also

Price DD, Wilson SR. Treating the patient with severe dengue infection. Available at: http://emedicine.medscape.com/article/781961-media. Accessed on July 2, 2010.

 CODES

ICD9
061 Dengue

CLINICAL PEARLS
Pediatric deaths from dengue most commonly occur in infants younger than 1 year

DIPHTHERIA

Herman Carneiro (E. Mylonakis, Editor)

 BASICS

DESCRIPTION

- Acute upper respiratory tract infection caused by *Corynebacterium diphtheriae* that is characterized by pseudomembrane formation on the tonsils, pharynx, larynx and nasal cavity, or obstructive laryngotracheitis, which can cause difficulty in breathing. Infection may also result in myocarditis, acute tubular necrosis, and peripheral neuropathies.
- *C. diphtheriae* can also cause milder disease restricted to the skin.

EPIDEMIOLOGY

Incidence
- Approximately 0.001 cases per 100,000 population in the US since 1980
- In the pre-vaccination era in the 1920s, there were approximately 100–200 cases per 100,000 population

Prevalence
- Remains endemic in parts of Africa, the Americas, Middle East, Asia, South Pacific, and Europe
- Highest attack rate in preschool-age children
- Recent sporadic outbreaks have mainly affected adults
- In temperate zones, it is more common in colder months
- Seasonal trends less distinct in the tropics

RISK FACTORS
- Low socio-economic status
- Absent or incomplete immunization
- Overcrowded and unsanitary living conditions
- Immunocompromise
- Travel to endemic areas or areas with ongoing epidemics, especially in those without booster of diphtheria toxoid

Genetics
No direct genetic link to disease

GENERAL PREVENTION
- Health education
  - Hazards of diphtheria infection and stressing the importance of immunization
- Immunization with diphtheria toxoid
- Booster of diphtheria toxoid every 10 years
- Government commitment to vaccination and other public health programs
- Strict disease control measures in outbreaks
  - Report cases to Department of Health
  - Isolate and treat cases
  - Disinfect all objects in contact with patient
  - Quarantine patient contacts with jobs in food handling, especially milk, and those in contact with non-immunized children
  - Investigate the source of infection
  - Prophylactic treatment of carriers of infection

PATHOPHYSIOLOGY
- *C. diphtheria* adheres to mucosal epithelial cells and releases exotoxin
- Exotoxin causes local inflammatory reaction followed by tissue destruction and necrosis
- Exotoxin fragment B causes proteolytic cleaving of cell membrane enabling segment A to enter the cell
- Exotoxin fragment A inhibits host cell protein synthesis and leads to cell death
- Lymphatic and hematological exotoxin spread causes systemic disease

ETIOLOGY
- Caused by strains of *C. diphtheriae* infected by a lysogenic bacteriophage virus, which carries a toxin-encoding gene *tox*
- Incubation period 2–5 days (range 1–10 days)
- *C. diphtheriae* are pleomorphic, Gram-positive, aerobic, nonmotile bacilli
- Humans are the main reservoir of infection
- Spread by respiratory droplets, contact with nasopharyngeal secretions and exudates from cutaneous lesions, and fomites
- The organism may colonize the respiratory tract without causing disease

COMMONLY ASSOCIATED CONDITIONS
No commonly associated conditions

DIAGNOSIS

HISTORY
- Symptoms, including:
  - Fevers and chills
  - Malaise and weakness
  - Sore throat, dysphagia, cough, hoarse voice
  - Cervical lymphadenopathy
  - Neck swelling
  - Membrane forming in the nasopharynx
  - Serosanguineous or purulent nasal discharge
  - Headache
  - Dyspnea, wheeze
  - Skin lesions
- Vaccination history, including boosters
- Travel history
- Sick contacts
- Immunocompromising states
- Consumption of unpasteurized milk

PHYSICAL EXAM
- Low-grade fever
- Swollen neck or "bull's neck"
- Tachycardia
- Pseudomembrane (grey and adherent) on tonsils, pharynx or nasal membranes
  - Bleeding in underlying mucosa when pseudomembrane is scraped off
- Halitosis
- Cervical lymphadenopathy
- Features of respiratory distress including stridor, wheeze, cyanosis, and use of accessory muscle
- Signs of heart failure or circulatory collapse
- Dysrhythmias
- Signs of infective endocarditis
- Cranial or peripheral nerve deficits

DIAGNOSTIC TESTS & INTERPRETATION

Lab

Initial lab tests
- Complete blood count (CBC) showing moderate leukocytosis
- Urinalysis showing transient proteinuria
- Serum troponin-I levels
- Definitive diagnosis is based on the isolation of *C. diphtheriae* in culture and identification of the presence of toxin
- Isolation of *C. diphtheriae*
  - Gram stain: Club-shaped, nonencapsulated, nonmotile bacilli in clusters with typical Chinese-character configuration
  - Cultures: Inoculate tellurite or Loeffler media with nasal or throat swabs and identify using colony morphology, microscopic appearance, and fermentation reactions
- Toxin detection
  - Elek test
  - Polymerase chain reaction (PCR) for *tox* gene

Follow-Up & Special Considerations
- Monitor CBC
- 12-lead electrocardiogram

Imaging

Initial approach
- Chest radiograph
- Neck soft tissue radiography, computed topography or ultrasound scan

Follow-Up & Special Considerations
Nil

Diagnostic Procedures/Other
- Patients may require:
  - Endotracheal intubation
- Surgical airway—cricothyroidotomy or tracheostomy
- Laryngoscopy or bronchoscopy
- Electrical pacing for conduction defects

Pathological Findings
- Pseudomembrane on the tonsils, pharynx, larynx and nasal mucosa
- Pseudomembrane may be aspirated into the lungs

DIFFERENTIAL DIAGNOSIS

- Streptococcal pharyngitis
- Infectious mononucleosis
- Viral pharyngitis
- Epiglottitis
- Vincent's angina
- Infective endocarditis
- Herpes simplex virus

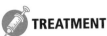# TREATMENT

MEDICATION

First Line

- Diphtheria antitoxin (DAT) should be administered as soon as possible
  - DAT is produced in horses and patients may have a hypersensitivity reaction to horse antiserum. A test dose is required with epinephrine and cardiopulmonary resuscitation facilities close at hand
- Antibiotics
  - Penicillin G
    - 300,000 U/d for patients weighing <10 kg i.m. for 14 days
    - 600,000 U/d for patients weighing >10 kg i.m. for 14 days
  - Erythromycin (for penicillin-allergic patients)
    - Adult: 500 mg p.o./i.v. every 6 h for 14 days
    - Pediatric: 40–50 mg/kg/day p.o./i.v. divided in 6 hourly doses for 14 days
  - Vancomycin
    - Adult: 1 g i.v. infused over 1 h every 12 h
    - Pediatric: 40 mg/kg/d i.v. infused over 1 h divided in 6 hourly doses
- Bronchodilators
- Antipyrexials

Second Line

Pharmacological therapy as above

ADDITIONAL TREATMENT

General Measures

- Isolation of patients promptly
- Early airway management for definitive airway
- Cardiac monitoring
- Insertion of 2 large-bore intravenous cannulae

Issues for Referral

- Anesthetist for airway management
- Surgery for surgical airway
- Cardiology for myocarditis
- Need of renal medicine for acute tubular necrosis
- Neurology for peripheral nerve damage
- Need of respiratory medicine for bronchoscopy for pseudomembrane removal or obstruction

COMPLEMENTARY & ALTERNATIVE THERAPIES

Physiotherapy for neuropathies

SURGERY/OTHER PROCEDURES

May require surgical airway

IN-PATIENT CONSIDERATIONS

Initial Stabilization

Adequately resuscitate patients according to advanced life support (ALS) or pediatric basic life-support protocols

Admission Criteria

Patients with respiratory compromise, septicemia, signs of infective endocarditis, or heart failure

IV Fluids

- Aggressive fluids resuscitation with colloids, e.g., Gelofusin, in patients with septic shock
- Maintenance fluids with Ringer's lactate as required

Nursing

Isolate patients with universal and droplet precautions until 2 nasopharyngeal swab cultures, taken 24 and 48 h after antibiotics are stopped, are negative

Discharge Criteria

- Patients with 2 negative swabs as above
- No signs of respiratory distress
- Hemodynamic stability

ONGOING CARE

FOLLOW-UP RECOMMENDATIONS

- Complete age-appropriate vaccination schedule
- Treat household and close contacts with erythromycin or penicillin for 14 days
- Follow-up nasopharyngeal cultures must be obtained after completing treatment to confirm bacterial eradication

DIET

All dairy products should be pasteurized

PATIENT EDUCATION

- Important of completing age-appropriate immunization schedule
- To seek treatment early with suspected infection

PROGNOSIS

- Cardiac involvement is associated with a very a poor prognosis
- 30–40% mortality with bacteremia
- High mortality rates in patients <5 years and those >40 years of age

COMPLICATIONS

- Respiratory failure
- Myocarditis, cardiac dilatation and failure, mycotic aneurysm, endocarditis
- Cardiac rhythm disturbances
- Secondary bacterial pneumonia
- Cranial nerve dysfunction, peripheral neuropathies, total paralysis
- Optic neuritis
- Acute tubular necrosis
- Septicemia or septic shock
- Septic arthritis, osteomyelitis
- Death occurs in 5–10% of respiratory cases

REFERENCES

1. Guy AM, Silverberg MA. Diphtheria in Emergency Medicine. http://emedicine.medscape.com/article/782051-overview. Accessed June 12, 2010.
2. Centers for Disease Control and Prevention. Disease Listing, diphtheria (Technical Information| CDC Bacterial, Mycotic Diseases). http://www.cdc.gov/ncidod/dbmd/diseaseinfo/diptheria_t.htm. Accessed on June 12, 2010.
3. The Merck Manuals Online Library. Diphtheria: Gram-positive bacilli: Merck Manual Professional. http://www.merck.com/mmpe/sec14/ch172/ch172c.html#sec14-ch172-ch172c-578c. Accessed June 12, 2010.

ADDITIONAL READING

- American Academy of Pediatrics. Diphtheria. In: Pickering LK, Baker CJ, Long SS, McMillan JA, editors. *Red book: 2006 report of the committee on infectious diseases*. 27th ed. Elk Grove Village, IL: American Academy of Pediatrics; 2006:277–281.
- World Health Organization. *WHO vaccine-preventable diseases monitoring system: 2005 global summary*. Geneva, Switzerland: World Health Organization; 2005:333. Report No.: WHO/IVB/2005.
- Galazka A. The changing epidemiology of diphtheria in the vaccine era. *J Infect Dis* 2000;181(Suppl 1): S2–S9.

CODES

ICD9

- 032.1 Nasopharyngeal diphtheria
- 032.3 Laryngeal diphtheria
- 032.9 Diphtheria, unspecified

CLINICAL PEARLS

Major mortality is related to a pseudomembrane on the tonsils, pharynx, larynx and nasal cavity, which causes acute airway obstruction.

DIVERTICULITIS

Michael K. Mansour (E. Mylonakis, Editor)

 BASICS

DESCRIPTION
- A diverticulum is a pouch or sac that results from herniation of the mucous membrane through a defect in the muscular layer of the GI tract.
- Diverticula can occur throughout the GI tract but, most commonly, are encountered in the colon where perforating arteries, the vasa recta, enter.
- The terms diverticulosis and diverticular disease refer simply to the presence of non-inflamed diverticula.
- Diverticulitis is an inflammation of the diverticulum.

EPIDEMIOLOGY
- Prevalence is difficult to accurately measure since only 10–25% of diverticulitis clinically manifests, but it is higher in the Western societies.
- Diverticulitis accounts for over 130,000 admissions annually in the US.
- Male to female ratio is equal.
- Incidence increases with age, with <5% of patients under the age of 40 years and 65–80% over the age of 70 years.
- In the Western world, most diverticulitis occurs in the descending and sigmoid colon, whereas in Asia right-sided diverticulitis is more prevalent.

RISK FACTORS
- Epidemiologic studies have suggested an association with Western diets high in refined carbohydrates and low in dietary fiber.
- Immunocompromised persons such as post-solid organ transplantation have a higher incidence of diverticulitis.
- Obesity and sedentary lifestyles have been associated with increased rates of diverticulitis.

GENERAL PREVENTION
Maintenance of a high-fiber diet has been thought to increase stool bulk and decrease transluminal pressure.

ETIOLOGY
- The etiology of diverticular disease is believed to be increased intraluminal pressure at points of weakness where perforating arteries, the vasa recta, enter the colonic wall.
- This is thought to be secondary to reduced stool bulk due to a decrease in dietary fiber.
- Once diverticula are present, increased intraluminal pressure is thought to cause erosion of the colonic wall resulting in inflammation. In turn, inflammation results in further damage associated with micro- or macroperforations.

- Infection is caused by polymicrobial flora mainly consisting of anaerobes and gram-negative bacilli.
- Complicated diverticulitis involves formation of a fluid collection and can be classified by Hinchey's criteria into 1 of 4 categories:
  - Stage I includes patients with small, confined pericolonic abscesses.
  - Stage II involves larger abscesses.
  - Stage III represents patients with generalized suppurative peritonitis.
  - Stage IV indicates frank fecal peritonitis.

COMMONLY ASSOCIATED CONDITIONS
- Colon cancer
- Inflammatory bowel disease

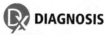 **DIAGNOSIS**

HISTORY
- Acute colonic diverticulitis is a disease of variable severity with the majority of patients being asymptomatic.
- The presentation depends on comorbidities (steroids, chemotherapy, diabetes, etc.) but can be characterized by the following:
  - Low grade fever
  - Abdominal pain (that usually begins in the epigastric region and then localizes to the left lower quadrant)
  - Obstipation
  - Perforation may result in rebound tenderness and guarding
- There may be alterations in bowel habits such as diarrhea.
- If a colovesical fistula is present, pneumaturia, fecaluria, or recurrent urinary tract infections occur.

PHYSICAL EXAM
- Tenderness is usually localized to the left lower quadrant and is often accompanied by peritoneal irritation if perforated (muscle spasm, guarding, and rebound tenderness).
- When generalized peritonitis is present, either rupture of a peridiverticular abscess or free rupture of an uninflamed diverticulum has occurred.
- Rectal examination may reveal a tender mass if the area of inflammation is close to the rectum.
- Rectal bleeding, usually microscopic and may result in trace guaiac positive stool; this is noted in 25% of cases and is rarely massive.

DIAGNOSTIC TESTS & INTERPRETATION
Lab
Polymorphonuclear leukocytosis is common.

Imaging
- Contrast enema can visualize diverticula, but their presence alone does not establish or negate the presence of diverticulitis.
- CT is the safest and most cost-effective diagnostic method, with additional potential for use in the treatment of abscesses. The sensitivity of CT ranges from 93–97% with specificity near 100%.
- Evidence of acute diverticulitis on CT includes the following:
  - Inflammation of the pericolic fat
  - The presence of a single diverticulum or multiple diverticula
  - Thickening of the bowel wall to >4 mm
  - The finding of a peridiverticular abscess
- Several authors advocate the use of ultrasonography in the diagnosis and treatment of acute diverticulitis. However, ultrasonography is more operator-dependent than is CT, abdominal tenderness may preclude the use of the requisite amount of external pressure to visualize the intra-abdominal contents adequately, and the image quality is often poor in obese patients.

Diagnostic Procedures/Other
- Endoscopic evaluation carries a risk of perforation if performed during acute diverticulitis.
- Establishing a possible underlying diagnosis such as carcinoma or inflammatory bowel disease after the acute process has resolved is important.

Pathological Findings
- Lymphoplasmacytic infiltration, crypt abscesses, and ulceration
- Similar in appearance to ulcerative colitis or Crohn's disease

DIFFERENTIAL DIAGNOSIS
- Right-sided diverticulitis is easily confused with appendicitis, because it occurs at a somewhat younger age than left-sided diverticulitis. Sigmoid diverticulitis also may mimic acute appendicitis if a redundant colon is positioned in the suprapubic region or right lower quadrant.
- On barium enema examination or CT study with oral contrast, multiple diverticula along with a segmental sigmoid narrowing or extravasation of contrast material suggest the presence of diverticulitis, although luminal narrowing and extravasation are also consistent with the diagnosis of Crohn's disease.
- See also the Section I chapter, "Abdominal Pain and Fever."

TREATMENT

MEDICATION
- Ciprofloxacin 500 mg PO b.i.d and metronidazole 500 mg PO t.i.d OR
- Trimethoprim-sulfamethoxazole double strength PO b.i.d and metronidazole 500 mg PO t.i.d OR
- Amoxicillin-clavulanate 875 mg PO b.i.d.
- Duration may vary based on clinical response but one should expect to provide about 7–10 days

ADDITIONAL TREATMENT
General Measures
- In patients for whom the diagnosis of diverticulitis can be made with confidence by clinical examination, it is reasonable to begin empirical antibiotic treatment immediately.
- For a patient with a mild first attack, who is able to tolerate oral intake, outpatient treatment may be initiated consisting of broad-spectrum antimicrobial therapy targeting anaerobic and gram-negative microorganisms.

Issues for Referral
If the patient is unable to tolerate oral intake, is not responding to oral antimicrobial therapy, or has high stage diverticulitis, they should be admitted for intravenous antimicrobial treatment. Management of perforated diverticulitis or secondary peritonitis is discussed in the Section II chapter, "Peritonitis."

Additional Therapies
Repeat CT and surgical consultation are advised if the patient is not responding after 2–3 days of therapy.

SURGERY/OTHER PROCEDURES
- For abscesses >4 cm there is lower likelihood of resolution with conservative measures. Often percutaneous drainage can improve chances of resolution without need for emergent surgery.
- After the acute episode resolves, a one-stage resection is recommended to permanently eliminate the chance of recurrence. This should be considered on a case-by-case basis.
- Less than 10% of patients with diverticulitis will require emergent surgical treatment.
- The indications for emergency colonic resection include the following:
  - Peritonitis
  - Perforation with free gas noted on imaging (stage III and IV)
  - Critical illness including Sepsis
- It remains safest to carry out a two-stage procedure in the presence of peritonitis.
- Recent reports advocate the use of radiologically-assisted percutaneous drainage as the initial therapeutic maneuver in patients with peridiverticular abscesses >5 cm in diameter.

- Current trends in the surgical management of diverticular disease include laparoscopic lavage.
- Some authors suggest elective surgery after the first episode of diverticulitis in patients under the age of 40 years since this likely represents a more malignant diverticular process.
- "Immunocompromised patient populations require special attention since clinical presentation may be subtle. Experts recommend considering surgery during the first episode of diverticulitis since progression to sepsis and life-threatening infection can occur quite rapidly."

IN-PATIENT CONSIDERATIONS
Discharge Criteria
- Clinical stability
- Tolerating oral intake

ONGOING CARE

FOLLOW-UP RECOMMENDATIONS
- Once the acute attack has resolved, the patient should be instructed to maintain a diet high in fiber. Previous studies have shown a recurrence rate of at least 50%.
- Colonoscopy is advisable to exclude an underlying colonic cancer.
- About 20–30% of those patients who develop acute diverticulitis will eventually require surgical therapy. However, 70% of elderly patients who have a single uncomplicated episode of diverticulitis will have no further clinical recurrence.

DIET
- Patient should be started on clear diet and transitioned to a low residue diet as tolerated.
- Supplementation of dietary fiber has been shown to increase stool weight, reduce gastrointestinal transit time, and decrease intraluminal pressures, leading to a decrease in the incidence of diverticulosis.

PROGNOSIS
Hinchey's Stage I and II carry an approximate 5% mortality risk, stage III is 13%, and stage IV is 43%.

COMPLICATIONS
- Complications of diverticulitis include free perforation, which results in acute peritonitis, sepsis, and shock, particularly in the elderly.
- The perforation may be walled off by adherent omentum or neighboring structures such as the bladder or small bowel. If nearby organs become involved or if an abscess ruptures into a nearby organ, a fistula may result.
- Colonic obstruction, though relatively uncommon, may develop after repeated episodes of acute diverticulitis. Small-bowel obstruction occurs somewhat more frequently, especially in the presence of a large peridiverticular abscess.

- Severe pericolitis may cause a fibrous stricture around the bowel, which can be associated with colonic obstruction and may mimic a neoplasm.
- Pylephlebitis is a rare but serious complication of diverticular disease and should be suspected in patients with diverticulitis in whom jaundice or hepatic abscesses develop.

ADDITIONAL READING
- Jacobs D. Diverticulitis. *N Engl J Med* 2007;357: 2057–2066.
- Alamili M. Acute complicated diverticulitis managed by laparoscopic lavage. *Dis Colon Rectum*. 2009; 52(7):1345–1349.
- Sarma D. Diagnostic imaging for diverticulitis. *J Clin Gastroenterol*. 2008;42(10):1139–1141 Isselbacher KJ, Epstein A. Diverticular, vascular, and other disorders of the intestine and peritoneum. In: Fauci AS, Braunwald E, Isselbacher KJ, et al., eds. *Harrison's principles of internal medicine*, 14th ed. New York: McGraw-Hill, 1998:1648–1656.
- Margolin D. Timing of elective surgery for diverticular disease. *Clin Colon Rectal Surg*. 2009;22(3): 169–172
- Kotzampassakis N. Presentation and treatment outcome of diverticulitis in younger adults: a different diseases than in older patients? *Dis Colon Rectum*. 2010;53(3):333–338.

CODES

ICD9
- 562.11 Diverticulitis of colon (without mention of hemorrhage)
- 562.13 Diverticulitis of colon with hemorrhage

CLINICAL PEARLS
- Diverticulitis is a polymicrobial infection of gastrointestinal outpouchings or diverticula.
- Multifactorial etiology with some evidence linking decreased stool bulk with increase in diverticular formation.
- CT is the preferred imaging method with high sensitivity and specificity.
- If patient can tolerate PO intake, one can attempt treatment with oral antimicrobials and bowel rest.
- Any complications or lack of response should result in admission and surgical consultation.
- Consider endoscopic evaluation after acute episode resolves to investigate any underlying inflammatory bowel disease or malignancy.

E. COLI INFECTIONS
Michael K. Mansour (E. Mylonakis, Editor)

 BASICS

DESCRIPTION
Escherichia coli are Gram-negative rod-shaped bacteria.

EPIDEMIOLOGY
- *E. coli* is the leading cause of nosocomial bacteremia.
- *E. coli* strains cause >80% of infections in young women with acute uncomplicated cystitis.
- Traveler's diarrhea occurs in individuals from industrialized countries, who visit tropical or subtropical regions.
- Enterotoxigenic *E. coli* is acquired through the fecal–oral route, usually through consumption of unbottled water or uncooked vegetables.
- The typical acute urinary tract infection occurs in a sexually active female following bacterial colonization of the periurethral region and ascension up the urethra.
- The use of diaphragms and spermicides has been associated with recurrence in some patients with urinary tract infection due to *E. coli*.
- Among men, risk factors for urinary tract infections due to *E. coli* include the following:
  - Homosexuality (associated with exposure to *E. coli* through anal intercourse)
  - Sexual intercourse with a partner with vaginal colonization by uropathogens
  - Lack of circumcision (associated with enhanced colonization of the glans and prepuce by *E. coli*)
- Men with HIV infection who have CD4 lymphocyte counts of less than 200 per cubic millimeter may also be at increased risk for urinary infection.

RISK FACTORS
- Defects in anatomy (i.e., stones, incompetent ureteral valves, colitis, colon cancer resulting in translocation).
- Immunocompromised state (steroids, diabetes, HIV, malignancy, advanced cirrhosis).
- *E. coli* is able to bind to uroepithelium from female patients with an inability to secrete blood group antigens.

GENERAL PREVENTION
- Chemoprophylaxis with trimethoprim–sulfamethoxazole (TMP–SMX), or fluoroquinolones, may be reasonable for the prevention of traveler's diarrhea (especially among certain patient populations such as for diabetics, CHF prone to life-threatening fluid shifts, as well as immunocompromised individuals, or persons with underlying inflammatory bowel disease), but because of side effects from the medications and the increasing drug resistance, many authorities do not to recommend chemoprophylaxis for all travelers (see also Section II chapter, "Traveler's Diarrhea").
- Except in selected circumstances (e.g., pregnancy), screening for asymptomatic bacteriuria is unnecessary in adults.

PATHOPHYSIOLOGY
Most *E. coli* strains causing enteric or genitourinary infection have an ability to bind to the surface of host cells and express toxins.

ETIOLOGY
- The most important *E. coli* pathogens are the following:
  - Enterotoxigenic *E. coli*, an important cause of traveler's diarrhea.
  - Enteropathogenic or enteroadherent *E. coli*, an important cause of childhood diarrhea, especially in underdeveloped countries and in nursery outbreaks.
  - Enteroinvasive *E. coli*, which causes a dysentery-like disease and invades the host cell and provokes a significant inflammatory response.
  - Enterohemorrhagic *E. coli* (EHEC), which causes hemorrhagic colitis and has been associated with the hemolytic–uremic syndrome in children (see Section II chapter, "Hemolytic–Uremic Syndrome"). Outbreaks are most often associated with beef contamination since *E. coli* O157 strains colonize the ruminant (predominantly cattle) gastrointestinal tracts (major reservoir). Other outbreaks have involved ingestion of raw dairy products, contaminated foods, petting zoos, and secondary infection via person to person. EHEC may present as severe abdominal pain and lack of fever.
  - Enteroaggregative *E. coli*, the most recent of the diarrheagenic strains appears to affect patients traveling to developing countries. There is also an association with chronic diarrheal state including HIV patients.

- In traveler's diarrhea, the heat-labile toxin of enterotoxigenic *E. coli* leads to elevated cyclic monophosphate levels, stimulates chloride secretion, and inhibits sodium chloride absorption. These effects result in net intestinal secretion.
- Enteropathogenic or enteroadherent *E. coli* strains bind to the membranous cells of Peyer's patches and disrupt the overlying mucus layer of the host cell.
- *E. coli* strains lead to urinary tract infections among women that can range from Gram-negative septicemia to a cystitis-like illness with mild flank pain. Most of the strains are a unique subgroup of *E. coli* (called uropathogenic strains) that possess specific determinants of virulence that enable them to infect the upper urinary tract of normal, healthy persons. These uropathogenic *E. coli* generally have specific adhesins (i.e., pili) that mediate their attachment to uroepithelial cells.
- Uropathogenic strains of *E. coli* can also cause uncomplicated infection (usually cystitis) in young men. These infections often present with symptoms of cystitis, but in some patients they mimic urethritis, causing urethral discharge and urethral leukocytosis.
- *E. coli* can also be associated with intraabdominal abscesses in any location as well as with cholecystitis and ascending cholangitis.
- In industrialized countries, non-O157 Shiga-like toxin-producing *E. coli* strains have been associated with bloody diarrhea and hemolytic–uremic syndrome in up to 30–50% of cases.

COMMONLY ASSOCIATED CONDITIONS
- Infants in their first month of life are predisposed to bacterial meningitis with *E. coli*.
- *E. coli* may also cause the following:
  - Brain abscess
  - Endocarditis
  - Endophthalmitis
  - Osteomyelitis
  - Perinephric abscess
  - Pneumonia
  - Septic arthritis
  - Suppurative thyroiditis

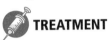

DIAGNOSIS

DIAGNOSTIC TESTS & INTERPRETATION

Lab

- Growth of *E. coli* in a normally sterile location (i.e., bloodstream, cerebrospinal fluid, biliary tract, pleural fluid, etc.) should be assumed to be diagnostic of *E. coli* infection.
- If needed, diagnosis for enteropathogenic *E. coli* can be made with PCR, detection of toxin, or techniques that exploit unique biochemical properties (e.g., sorbitol negativity in EHEC).
- Whether the recovery of *E. coli* from tracheal aspirates in intubated patients indicates colonization or infection must be decided in the context of the patient's clinical state.
- Testing for non-0157 Shiga-like toxin-producing *E. coli* strains should be considered in diarrhea without a recognized cause, particularly if the stool has gross blood.

Imaging

E. coli can commonly result in GI or hepatobiliary infections making right-upper quadrant ultrasound or abdominal CT useful diagnostics to identify collections of infection.

DIFFERENTIAL DIAGNOSIS

- Other bacteria can lead to similar presentations as infection with *E. coli*.
- Bloody diarrhea is more commonly caused by *Campylobacter*, *Salmonella*, or *Shigella*.

TREATMENT

MEDICATION

- The mainstay of treatment for localized *E. coli* infections (e.g., abscess) is twofold: Antimicrobial therapy and elimination of pus, necrotic tissue, and foreign bodies.
- Traveler's diarrhea can be treated with an oral fluoroquinolone (ciprofloxacin 500 mg b.i.d.) or TMP–SMX (1 double-strength tablet b.i.d.) for 3 days. Symptomatic therapy with loperamide can be useful along with the antibiotic.
- Treatment for infection with enteropathogenic or enteroadherent *E. coli* consists of fluid replacement. In severe cases, fluoroquinolones are indicated.
- In the setting of HUS, there is an associated increase in mortality with antimicrobial treatment thought to be related to increased toxin expression.
- Uncomplicated cystitis in a healthy woman is treated for 3 days with oral TMP–SMX (1 double-strength tablet b.i.d.) or a fluoroquinolone (ciprofloxacin 250 mg b.i.d. or ofloxacin 200 mg p.o. b.i.d. or norfloxacillin 400 mg b.i.d. or levofloxacin 250 mg q.d.) for 3 days. Diabetic or pregnant patients require 7 days of treatment.

- For the pregnant patient with urinary tract infection, the choice of oral agents is limited to penicillins, nitrofurantoin, or cephalosporins. If a pregnant patient develops pyelonephritis, admission to the hospital is indicated.
- The patient with mild uncomplicated pyelonephritis can be treated with oral TMP–SMX or a fluoroquinolone for 10–14 days.
- Patients with severe pyelonephritis or other severe infections due to *E. coli* should be given intravenous antibiotics in the hospital. The choices are the following:
  - A fluoroquinolone, such as ciprofloxacin
  - A third-generation cephalosporin, such as ceftriaxone
  - Ampicillin with gentamicin
  - An extended-spectrum penicillin
  - Aztreonam
  - Imipenem/cilastatin
- After acute symptoms resolve, an oral antibiotic should replace the intravenous antibiotic for a total duration of 14–21 days.

SURGERY/OTHER PROCEDURES

- Surgical referral may be required for elimination of foreign body or abscess drainage.
- Development of vaccines to *E. coli* adhesins is being evaluated as a potential therapeutic.

IN-PATIENT CONSIDERATIONS

Admission Criteria

- In the setting of pyelonephritis, patients with inability to maintain sufficient oral hydration or adhere to oral antimicrobial treatment warrant inpatient admission.
- Patients with any concerning signs and symptoms suggesting that a more advanced infection (such as septic physiology) or need for immediate surgical intervention should be admitted to the hospital.

ONGOING CARE

FOLLOW-UP RECOMMENDATIONS

- Patients in whom bacteremia with *E. coli* persists despite adequate therapy often have an undrained abscess, most typically intraabdominal.
- Chronic or relapsing urinary tract infections due to *E. coli* are more common among patients with the following:
  - Anatomic defects involving the urinary tract
  - Foreign bodies of the urinary tract
  - Obstruction of the urinary tract
  - Pregnancy
  - Stones

PROGNOSIS

Hemolytic–uremic syndrome is associated with a 3–5% mortality

COMPLICATIONS

- In diarrhea, dehydration can lead to hypovolemia and shock.
- Patients with ischemia of the bowel or other organs (such as patients with diabetes or atherosclerotic vascular disease) are at high risk of developing acute emphysematous cholecystitis, and *E. coli* is a prominent pathogen in this process.
- Septic shock can complicate *E. coli* infections, especially among patients with poor filtering capacity in the liver (i.e., those with cirrhosis or portosystemic shunts), diminished reticuloendothelial function, or diminished numbers of circulating phagocytic cells.

ADDITIONAL READING

- Dupont HL. Bacterial diarrhea. *NEJM* 2009; 361:1560–1569.

CODES

ICD9

- 008.00 Intestinal infection due to *E. coli*, unspecified
- 009.2 pneumonia due to *Infectious diarrhea*
- 041.4 sepsis due to *Escherichia coli (E. coli) infection in conditions classified elsewhere and of unspecified site*

CLINICAL PEARLS

- *E. coli* infection is a common Gram-negative bacterium which causes a variety of infections.
- Anatomic defects and immunocompromised individuals have the potential to do poorly.
- Goal of treatment is twofold and includes antimicrobial therapy and drainage/removal of foreign bodies or fluid collections (abscess, pus, necrotic tissue).

E

ECHINOCOCCOSIS

Georgios Peppas
Petros I. Rafailidis
Matthew E. Falagas

 BASICS

DESCRIPTION
- Infection caused by *Echinococcus* sp., alternatively called hydatid disease.
  - *Echinococcus granulosus* causes cystic echinococcosis (CE), *Echinococcus multilocularis* alveolar echinococcosis (AE), and *Echinococcus vogeli* causes polycystic echinococcosis

EPIDEMIOLOGY
Incidence
- CE is endemic in Central Asia, South America, North Africa (and probably sub-Saharan Africa); incidence in Southern European countries though is significantly lower in recent years. For 2008, 639 cases of *E. granulosus* were confirmed in the European Union (EU), the majority in Bulgaria, Spain, and Germany. CE is rarely encountered in the US.
- AE is emerging in Central Europe: Fifty cases were confirmed in the EU in 2008, in Germany, Lithuania, France, and Poland. Russian districts and Central Asian countries are also endemic. Rural regions in China remain hyperendemic, with an estimated 16,000 annual cases. Rarely encountered in parts of Alaska and Western Canada.
- Polycystic echinococcosis is rarely encountered in Latin America.

Prevalence
Overall prevalence rates are difficult to evaluate in endemic areas—seroprevalence rates in high-risk populations are not representative

RISK FACTORS
- For CE, direct or indirect contact with infected dogs/dog feces (canines are the definite hosts); recycling of the parasite through sheep and other livestock in endemic areas with inadequate hygienic slaughterhouse practices. Rural populations involved in such practices are at high-risk
- For AE the definite host is foxes and coyote, also domestic cats and dogs are included in this list. Rodents may serve as an intermediate host. Humans in endemic areas who own hunting or free-roaming dogs and farmers are considered at high-risk

Genetics
Ten strains of *E. granulosus* are recognized, with different preferred intermediate hosts and possibly different virulence and drug susceptibility.

GENERAL PREVENTION
- Adequate hygienic practices in slaughterhouses, elimination of stray dogs, and vaccination of preferred intermediate hosts (usually sheep) are the mainstays of preventive campaigns with significant success.
  - In endemic areas, dogs should be kept away from the viscera of slaughtered livestock in order to terminate the parasite lifecycle

PATHOPHYSIOLOGY
- For CE, upon entry through the digestive tract, parasite forms enter circulation and terminate in target organs (liver 65%, lungs 20%, other organs—including kidneys, peritoneum, brain, heart—15%) where they develop a slowly growing multilayered cyst which can evolve to multilocular cysts, development of daughter cysts or calcification and degeneration take place.
  - AE is observed almost exclusively in the liver, is multifocal, destructive to the hepatic parenchyma, mimicking cirrhosis and hepatocellular carcinoma.

ETIOLOGY
E. granulosus causes CE, *E. multilocularis* AE, and *E. vogeli* causes polycystic echinococcosis

 DIAGNOSIS

HISTORY
- Typically CE is an accidental finding. Patients may complain of space-occupying symptoms depending on the organ involved. The patient may present with anaphylactic shock in cases of cyst rupture; rupture to the biliary tract and cholangitis, endobronchial rupture, and rupture of renal cysts in the collecting duct and to the urine are also typical (1).
  - Rural origin of the patient or origin from an endemic country (for immigrants, it may be discovered decades after movement)

PHYSICAL EXAM
Usually insignificant: A mass-like lesion or plain hepatomegaly may be palpable in the right upper abdominal quadrant.

DIAGNOSTIC TESTS & INTERPRETATION
Lab
Initial lab tests
Serology, usually with ELISA, demonstrates antibodies in the majority of cases (but not always). Serology is more reliable in AE. Eosinophilia may be observed in a minority of cases.

Follow-Up & Special Considerations
Follow-up is performed by imaging methods. Serology has not been adequately evaluated as a follow-up tool post treatment

Imaging
Initial approach
- In CE, ultrasonography demonstrates hepatic cystic lesions (or other intraabdominal localizations). Cyst structure is often diagnostic; "pathognomonic" signs include the presence of multilocular cysts, daughter cysts, the "water lily sign" due to internal membrane detachment, and the "snowflake sign." Plain chest X-ray may demonstrate the pneumonic lesions. Computerized tomography and magnetic resonance imaging further assist in fully characterizing the cystic lesions observed.
- In AE, ultrasonography imaging may disorientate towards a diagnosis of cirrhosis or hepatocellular carcinoma.

Follow-Up & Special Considerations
- Ultrasonography may be used to follow-up untreated or conservatively treated lesions, according to a World Health Organization classification system which also evaluates cyst vitality or degeneration.
- Post treatment, ultrasonography in later times may be useful in excluding the presence of secondary or seeded (during surgery) localizations.

Diagnostic Procedures/Other
Cyst puncture is contraindicated due to the significant risk of severe anaphylactic reactions and the smaller risk of parasite seeding (for hepatic cysts, intraperitoneally)

Pathological Findings
In excision specimens, daughter cysts, scolices, and the 3 cyst wall compartments (external-host reactive, internal-parasitic origin, germinal internal layer) may be observed; macroscopically pathognomonic.

DIFFERENTIAL DIAGNOSIS
CE should be differentiated from simple benign cysts, hepatic hemangioma, and malignant cystic lesions. AE should be differentiated from cirrhosis, hepatocellular carcinoma, or metastatic liver involvement.

TREATMENT

MEDICATION
First Line
- Echinococcosis treatment is predominantly surgical.
- Albendazole is the premium pharmaceutical agent used otherwise—typically used in inoperable cases, in polycystic disease, and in multiple-organ involvement (or as adjuvant pre-and post-intervention): Response rates (cyst disappearance, partial size response, cyst degeneration) may reach 60% (2).

Second Line
- Mebendazole is inferior and less convenient.
- Praziquantel may be used as an adjuvant to albendazole, although adequate trial data are missing.

ADDITIONAL TREATMENT
General Measures
Avoidance of any activities predisposing to cyst rupture (through external or intraabdominal pressure exertion)

Issues for Referral
Surgical evaluation is warranted. A cyst may not warrant surgical intervention but only follow-up via ultrasonography.

SURGERY/OTHER PROCEDURES
- Surgery is the mainstay of CE treatment: Interventions may be localized (cystectomy, the most widely used pericystectomy, marsupialization in liver involvement) or more radical (e.g., nephrectomy in renal disease) with usually excellent results. Secondary infections, cyst rupture with anaphylaxis, or parasite seeding are rare complications.
- PAIR (puncture, aspiration, injection, reaspiration) is a novel less invasive approach, with injection referring to scolicidal agents. Encouraging results are seen in selected hepatic cysts. Results are comparable to surgery when combined with albendazole. Its promising role is under further clarification at present. PAIR should not be performed in communicating cysts to avoid sclerosing complications.
- Aggressive surgery with adjuvant pre- and post-operative long-term albendazole is warranted for AE, yet mortality may reach 20%

IN-PATIENT CONSIDERATIONS
Initial Stabilization
Only applicable to cases presenting with cyst rupture-induced anaphylactic shock

Admission Criteria
Only applicable to cases presenting with cyst rupture-induced anaphylactic shock

Discharge Criteria
Post-intervention, according to what is reserved in general for abdominal/thoracic surgery

 # ONGOING CARE

FOLLOW-UP RECOMMENDATIONS
Therapeutic options in pregnancy are limited: Albendazole is contraindicated in pregnancy, as are limited-invasion approaches as PAIR, while planning an adequate invasive procedure may have significant limitations.

Patient Monitoring
As described above

DIET
No dietary modifications needed

PATIENT EDUCATION
Avoidance of exposure, compliance to typical hygienic rules, and compliance to follow-up.

PROGNOSIS
Excellent for CE: In AE survival rates of 80% can be achieved with radical surgery and long-term chemotherapy with albendazole

COMPLICATIONS
- Cyst rupture and anaphylactic shock
- Secondary parasite seeding
- Secondary bacterial infections of cysts
- Metastatic behavior of AE

ADDITIONAL READING
- Falagas ME, Bliziotis IA. Albendazole for the treatment of human echinococcosis: A review of comparative clinical trials. *Am J Med Sci* 2007;334:171–179.
- Moro P, Schantz PM. Echinococcosis: A review. *Int J Infect Dis* 2009;13:125–133.
- Torgerson PR, Keller K, Magnotta M, et al. The global burden of alveolar echinococcosis. *PLoS Negl Trop Dis* 2010;4:e722.

 # CODES

ICD9
- 122.4 Echinococcus granulosus infection, unspecified
- 122.7 Echinococcus multilocularis infection, unspecified
- 122.9 Echinococcosis, other and unspecified

CLINICAL PEARLS
- History dictates the diagnosis: An immigrant from an endemic area may present clinically symptomatic disease decades after immigration
- The "water lily sign", from floating parts of detached membranes, is a commonly observed pathognomonic sign
- A patient who complains for passing grape-like material into his urine may have experienced renal cyst rupture into the collecting duct

EHRLICHIOSIS, ANAPLASMOSIS
Petros M. Karsaliakos (E. Mylonakis, Editor)

 BASICS

DESCRIPTION
The family Anaplasmataceae includes the genera *Ehrlichia, Anaplasma, Neorickettsia*, and *Wolbachia*. They are obligate intracellular pathogens that cause systemic infections to humans and animals.

Approach to the Patient
- Ehrlichiosis and anaplasmosis are transmitted through tick bites especially during summer months when the ticks thrive.
- In immunocompromised patients (AIDS, corticosteroid treatment), it may inflict severe infections with CNS involvement, multiple organ dysfunction syndrome, and death.
- In the immunocompetent patients, they are responsible for mild-to-severe infections with generalized symptoms like fever, malaise, headache, myalgias, nausea, and vomiting.
- These microbes predilect the reticuloendothelial system and, more specifically, monocytes and granulocytes.
- Lymphadenopathy, hepatosplenomegaly, rash are of the commonest signs.
- Leukopenia and thrombocytopenia occur in most cases.
- If left untreated, the infection may progress to a severe disease with multisystemic involvement and high mortality.
- Infections from *Ehrlichia* and *Anaplasma* are frequently underdiagnosed and consequently they require high clinical suspicion.
- The gold standard for the diagnosis is serology with cultivation being less sensitive and PCR demanding a specialized laboratory.
- Tetracyclines are the drugs of choice.

EPIDEMIOLOGY
- Two thirds of affected patients who present with human monocytic ehrlichiosis are male.
- The tick *Amblyomma americanum* is the main vector which is responsible for the transmission of *Ehrlichia chaffeensis* in the Southeastern and the south-central US.
- The tick thrives from May to August especially in rural areas.

- *Ixodes pacificus* and *Dermacentor variabilis* are another tick vectors which transmit ehrlichiosis with cases reported even in Africa, South America, and Eastern Asia.
- Subclinical exposure is common with asymptomatic seroconversion showing that most cases are underdiagnosed.
- About 3500 cases of human monocytic ehrlichiosis have been reported to the centers for disease control and prevention since 1987.
- Human granulocytic anaplasmosis (HGA) due to *Anaplasma phagocytophilum* is commoner during summer months when the tick *Ixodes scapularis* thrives.
- Wisconsin, Minnesota, New England, New Jersey, and New York present with most cases in US. The infection has been also identified in populations of northern Europe as Slovenia, Norway, and Sweden.
- Most cases of HGA which are identified due to seroconversion are subclinical or totally asymptomatic.
- Up to 35% of cases with *A. phagocytophilum* infection are presented with concurrent infection due to *Babesia microti* and *Borrelia burgdorferi*. The common vector *Ixodes* spp. is responsible for the above phenomenon.

GENERAL PREVENTION
- Ehrlichiosis is prevented by avoidance of tick bite and prompt removal of attached ticks.
- It is preferable to wear light-colored clothing to allow early identification of crawling ticks.
- After returning from tick-infested areas, a thorough body search for attached ticks should be performed, with emphasis on areas containing hair.
- If long-sleeved shirts or long pants are not practical, exposed areas of the skin should be covered with insect repellents containing N,N-diethyl-M-toluamide (DEET). This is the most common active agent in insect repellents. Systemic reactions to DEET can occur when concentrations exceeding 35% are used, in patients who repetitively use repellents with lesser concentrations, or in cases of ingestion. Because of these systemic reactions, all DEET-containing compounds should be used with care, and chronic readministration should be avoided.

ETIOLOGY
- The family Anaplasmataceae refers to small, obligatory intracellular Gram-negative bacteria.
- *E. chaffeensis* predilects mostly the macrophages causing the human monocytotropic ehrlichiosis (HME).
- *A. phagocytophilum* inflicts the human granulocytotropic anaplasmosis due to granulocytes entering and infection.
- Both microbes reside in cytoplasmic membrane-lined vacuoles in bone marrow-derived cells and also endothelial cells and are transmitted through tick vectors.
- Neorickettsia is transmitted through raw fish ingestion.
- *Ehrlichia ewingii* affects mainly the immunocompromised, especially the AIDS patients.

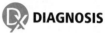 **DIAGNOSIS**

- HME due to *E. chaffeensis* is presented clinically in about a 7 days period after a tick – bite.
- There is a compatible history of outdoor or recreational activities during summer months.
- The infection may cause death to the immunocompromised patient.
- Generalized symptoms with fever, malaise, headache, myalgias, vomiting, weight loss are common.
- Rash may be maculopapular or hemorrhagic.
- Lymphadenopathy implicates 25% of cases.
- Severe untreated infections may drive to multiple organ dysfunction syndrome and ICU admission.
- *E. ewingii* presents with a milder syndrome than HME with less severely complicated cases.
- *Human granulocytotropic anaplasmosis (HGA)* due to *A. phagocytophilum* presents with similar clinical manifestations with HME.
- Rash may be due to concurrent Lyme disease.
- Severe infections may lead to septic shock, acute respiratory distress syndrome (ARDS), and severe CNS involvement.

DIAGNOSTIC TESTS & INTERPRETATION
Lab
- Leukopenia, thrombocytopenia, anemia, elevated aminotransferases, and distorted kidney function may present and are not specific.
- In meningeal and CNS involvement, CSF lymphocytosis may be present.
- Serum samples can be obtained during the acute phase of the illness and during convalescence to test for HGA or *E. chaffeensis*. However, most patients with ehrlichiosis are seronegative for these agents at presentation.
- The CDC case definition for HME requires a clinically compatible history with a minimum antibody titer to *E. chaffeensis* of greater than or equal to 1:64 or a fourfold or greater change in antibody titers from acute and convalescent sera, using indirect fluorescent antibody testing.
- PCR analyses for the organisms associated with HGA and HME show higher sensitivity when the sample contains infected leukocytes.
- Culture of the agents of ehrlichiosis is diagnostic, but the process takes several days and the results are reliable only in a few specialized research laboratories.
- The laboratory diagnosis of HGA is more difficult to establish. Serodiagnosis by indirect immunofluorescence assay, with A. phagocytophilum neutrophils as antigen, is highly sensitive but is useful mainly for retrospective documentation of seroconversion to a titer of 80 or greater during convalescence.
- The sensitivity of the peripheral blood smear as a diagnostic screening tool is low, about 29%

Imaging
Chest X-ray may show infiltrating patches or a radiological appearance compatible with ARDS.

DIFFERENTIAL DIAGNOSIS
- Diseases such as endocarditis, other forms of septicemia, vasculitis, and thrombotic thrombocytopenic purpura must be considered.
- Also, other tick-borne infections such as tularemia, babesiosis, Lyme disease, murine typhus, Rocky Mountain spotted fever, and Colorado tick fever may be considered in the differential diagnosis of patients with ehrlichiosis.

 TREATMENT

MEDICATION
First Line
- Tetracycline drugs such as doxycycline (100 mg b.i.d.) have been shown to shorten the course of HME.
- The issue of the proper medication for HME in children younger than 9 years is not an easy one. Some institutions use doxycycline (4 mg/kg/d b.i.d., with a maximum dose of 100 mg) for the treatment of any patient, regardless of age, with symptomatic HME. If patients are unable to take doxycycline, chloramphenicol (75 mg/kg/d in 4 divided doses) may be used.
- Chloramphenicol appears to shorten the course of illness, some patients do not respond to treatment with this agent, and *E. chaffeensis* is resistant to chloramphenicol in cell culture.
- Doxycycline is also an effective therapeutic drug for HGA. Of 35 HGEA patients treated with doxycycline, 94% are defervesced within 24–48 h. One patient who did not receive doxycycline had the agent of HGA detected by PCR in the blood on day 28 of illness.
- Rifampin has been successfully used in cases of pregnancy and HGA and when an alternative than tetracycline treatment is required.
- The required duration of administration of doxycycline is not known, but most authorities suggest a 7- to 14-day course.

 ONGOING CARE

FOLLOW-UP RECOMMENDATIONS
- Persistent ehrlichial infection has been documented after treatment with tetracycline and chloramphenicol.
- Patients with ehrlichiosis usually have a response to treatment within 24–48 h, and the lack of a response should suggest another diagnosis.
- Expert consultation should be obtained before therapy with a drug other than a tetracycline is considered.

COMPLICATIONS
- Ehrlichial infections can be severe if untreated.
- Over 60% of patients who, at some point, are recognized to have *E. chaffeensis* are hospitalized, 15% of patients have severe infections, and 2–3% of patients die.
- Severe illness due to *E. chaffeensis* may lead to the following:
- Respiratory insufficiency
- Neurological involvement (seizures, coma, etc.)
- Acute renal failure
- Gastrointestinal hemorrhage
- The natural history of untreated HGE in adults is a 3- to 11-week illness with a possibly fatal outcome.
- Among patients with HGA, elderly patients are more likely to have severe disease, but infections also occur in children. The current mortality rate is estimated to be approximately 5%. So far, 51% of patients have been hospitalized, and 7% have been admitted to an intensive care unit.
- Coinfection with *B. burgdorferi* or *B. microti* probably occurs on occasion. It is possible that microbial interactions in this situation lead to more severe disease than infection with a single agent.

ADDITIONAL READING
- Dumler JS, Madigan JE, Pusterla N, et al. Ehrlichioses in humans: Epidemiology, clinical presentation, diagnosis, and treatment. *Clin Infect Dis* 2007;45(Suppl 1):S45–S51.
- Thomas RJ, Dumler JS, Carlyon JA. Current management of human granulocytic anaplasmosis, human monocytic ehrlichiosis and *Ehrlichia ewingii* ehrlichiosis. *Expert Rev Anti Infect Ther* 2009;7(6): 709–722.

CODES

ICD9
- 082.40 Unspecified ehrlichiosis
- 082.41 Ehrlichiosis chafeensis (e chafeensis)
- 082.49 Other ehrlichiosis

CLINICAL PEARLS
- Due to its generalized clinical manifestations with symptoms of low specificity, high suspicion of diagnosis is mandatory.
- Once an ehrlichiosis is suspected on historical and clinical grounds, doxycycline treatment should be initiated concurrently with attempts at etiologic confirmation using laboratory methods such as blood smear examination, polymerase chain reaction, culture, and serologic tests.

E

EMPYEMA

Lili Tao
Jieming Qu
Matthew E. Falagas

 BASICS

DESCRIPTION
- An empyema is defined as the accumulation of purulent fluid in the pleural cavity.
- Empyema is usually a complication of bacterial pneumonia, but may also occur after thoracic surgery, trauma, and many other conditions, such as esophageal perforation, subdiaphragmatic infection.

Pediatric Considerations
- Significant differences exist between empyema in children and in adults in their clinical course and prognosis
- Pediatric empyema has an incidence of 3.3 per 100,000
- Most cases are secondary to underlying bacterial pneumonia
- *Streptococcus pneumoniae* (predominantly serotype 1) accounts for most childhood empyema
- The prognosis in children with empyema is significantly better than in adults although the management does not differ

EPIDEMIOLOGY
Incidence
Pleural effusions occur in up to 57% of patients with pneumonia; approximately 1–2% of simple parapneumonic effusions may evolve into empyema

Prevalence
- Pleural infection affects patients of all ages but is more common in the elderly and in childhood.
- Men are affected twice as often as women.

RISK FACTORS
- Diabetes mellitus
- Alcoholism
- Substance abuse
- Rheumatoid arthritis
- Coincidental chronic lung disease
- Poor dentition
- Risk factors for aspiration are associated with anaerobic infection
- Previous thoracic surgical operation
- Presence of malignancy

Genetics
A variant of the protein tyrosine phosphatase (PTPN22 Trp620) is associated with susceptibility to Gram-positive empyema based on recent genetic studies (1).

GENERAL PREVENTION
- Proper antibiotic treatment of pneumonia
- Adherence to operative regulations
- Use of proper antibiotic surgical prophylaxis
- Pneumococcal vaccine

PATHOPHYSIOLOGY
- The evolution of empyema can be divided into 3 stages
  - Stage 1: Exudative with swelling of the pleural membranes
  - Stage 2: Fibrinopurulent with heavy fibrin deposits
  - Stage 3: Organization with ingrowth of fibroblasts and depositions of collagen

ETIOLOGY
- The bacteriology of community- and hospital-acquired empyema differ substantially, and both differ from pneumonia (2,3)
- Community-acquired empyema:
  - Streptococci (mostly *Streptococcus milleri* group and *S. pneumoniae*) (4)
  - Staphylococci (mostly methicillin-susceptible *Staphylococcus aureus*)
  - Enterobacteriaceae
  - Anaerobes (*Fusobacterium*, *Bacteroides*, *Peptostreptococcus*)
  - Rarely *Mycobacterium tuberculosis* and *Actinomyces* spp.
- Hospital-acquired empyema
  - *S. aureus* (mostly methicillin-resistant)
  - Enterobacteriaceae
  - Enterococci
  - *Pseudomonas aeringosa*
  - *S. milleri* group
  - Anaerobes

COMMONLY ASSOCIATED CONDITIONS
Pneumonia

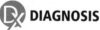 **DIAGNOSIS**

HISTORY
- Preceding pneumonia or thoracic surgery
- Symptoms may include fever, chest pain, dyspnea
- The elderly and immunocompromised: May be asymptomatic or may present with weight loss and anemia

PHYSICAL EXAM
- Stony dull percussion
- Decreased fremitus
- Absent breath sounds over effusion
- Patients with little effusion may not show the signs of effusion

DIAGNOSTIC TESTS & INTERPRETATION
Lab
Initial lab tests
- Complete blood count (CBC), C-reactive protein (CRP)
- Routine chemistry, cytology, and cell count analysis of effusion
- Gram stain and culture of the effusion, blood, and/or sputum
- Pleural fluid pH measured by a blood gas machine: <7.2

Follow-Up & Special Considerations
CRP can be obtained repeatedly to assess the effect of treatments

Imaging
Initial approach
- Chest x-ray (CXR) shows pleural effusion on posteroanterior (PA) or lateral chest radiographs
- Ultrasound (US) enables the exact localization of effusion and guides the insertion of chest tube
- CT with intravenous contrast can differentiate between empyema and lung abscess; empyema is lenticular in shape and the 'split pleura' sign is often noted

Follow-Up & Special Considerations
- Repeated US and CT scan should be taken to evaluate pleural effusion
- Care should be taken to check whether bronchopleural fistula occur or not

Diagnostic Procedures/Other
Thoracentesis: The presence of pus in the pleural cavity confirms the diagnosis

Pathological Findings
Presence of many polymorphonuclear leukocytes, bacteria, and cellular debris in the effusion

DIFFERENTIAL DIAGNOSIS
- Pleural effusion of other causes
- Lung abscess
- Pneumonia

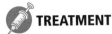

TREATMENT

MEDICATION
- All patients should take antimicrobial therapy when diagnosed.
- Empyema needs prompt drainage usually through chest tube drainage (5). Repeated thoracocentesis procedures have been occasionally used when the fluid has lower viscosity.
- The regimens are different for community and hospital-acquired empyema due to the different etiology.
  - Community-acquired empyema:
    ○ Carbapenems, aminopenicillin + β-lactamase inhibitor
    ○ Second-generation cephalosporin + metronidazole
    ○ Clindamycin monotherapy for patients with a β-lactam allergy
  - Hospital-acquired empyema:
    ○ Carbapenems
    ○ Antipseudomonal penicillin/third- or fourth-generation cephalosporins + metronidazole
    ○ Vancomycin, linezolid, or alternatives should be added for suspected or proven methicillin-resistant *Staphylococcus aureus* (MRSA)

ADDITIONAL TREATMENT
General Measures
- Adequate fluid therapy.
- Nutrition: A key aim of therapy, it should not be overlooked even with adequate antibiotics and drainage.

Issues for Referral
Because empyema has a high mortality and morbidity, referral for complete evacuation of the pleural cavity should be considered immediately upon diagnosis

Additional Therapies
- Intrapleural fibrinolytics
  - Streptokinase 250,000 IU or urokinase 100,000 IU in 30–60 ml sterile saline via chest tube
  - Clamp the tube for 2–4 h before returning to normal drainage
  - Despite the routine use in clinic, the MIST 1 trial (6) failed to substantiate the role of streptokinase in empyema (6). Nevertheless, more data are required to draw final conclusions (7).
- Thoracoscopy, for patients with incompletely drained loculated effusion early in the disease

SURGERY/OTHER PROCEDURES
- Current options of surgery include:
  - Video-assisted thoracoscopic surgery (VATS)
  - Mini-thoracotomy
  - Open thoracotomy with decortications
  - Rib resection with open drainage
  - Open surgical approaches including open window thoracoplasty, open debridement, and thoracomyoplasty are deemed superior to minimally invasive surgery for postsurgical empyema

IN-PATIENT CONSIDERATIONS
Initial Stabilization
- Empirical antibiotic treatment
- Drainage

Admission Criteria
Generally, all patients should be admitted as soon as diagnosed

IV Fluids
- Antibiotics
- Adequate fluid therapy
- Intravenous nutrition in some cases

Nursing
- Monitor intravenous fluids
- Ensure chest tube drainage

Discharge Criteria
- There is no consensus on discharge, the decision is mainly based on personal experiences
- Useful information of clinical improvement may include control of fever, decreased CRP level, and decrease of pleural fluid

ONGOING CARE

FOLLOW-UP RECOMMENDATIONS
- Administer antibiotics intravenously at least for 1 week and then shift to oral formulation
- Patients should receive at least 2–4 weeks of treatment with antibiotics
- The duration of antibiotic treatment depends on the bacteriology, the efficacy of pleural drainage, and the speed of resolution of the patient's symptoms
- The chest tube should be left in place until the volume of the pleural drainage per 24 h is less than 50 ml and until the draining fluid becomes clear yellow

Patient Monitoring
- CBC and CRP to be repeatedly performed during the entire course
- Monitoring the pleural drainage using US or CT
- Assess the ventilation capacity

DIET
High-nutrition diet to be given

PATIENT EDUCATION
- Adherence to the treatment, including medications and drainage
- Lung rehabilitation
- Restriction of workload

PROGNOSIS
- The outcome for empyema varies significantly: Full recovery may require several days of hospitalization and several weeks of at-home recovery
- Mortality rates for empyema vary between 7 and 33% at 1 year but exceed 50% in patients with significant co-morbidity.

COMPLICATIONS
- Pleural thickening
- Pulmonary fibrosis
- Pneumothorax
- Bronchopleural fistula
- Empyema necessitatis
- Respiratory failure
- Septic shock

REFERENCES

ADDITIONAL READING
- British Thoracic Society Standards of Care Committee. BTS guidelines for the management of pleural infection in children. *Thorax* 2005; 60(Suppl 1):i1–i21.
- British Thoracic Society Standards of Care Committee. BTS guidelines for the management of pleural infection. *Thorax* 2003;58(Suppl 2):ii18–ii28.
- Blaschke AJ, Heyrend C, Byington CL, et al. Molecular analysis improves pathogen identification and epidemiologic study of pediatric parapneumonic empyema. *Pediatr Infect Dis J* 2011;30:289–294.
- Cameron R, Davies HR. Intra-pleural fibrinolytic therapy versus conservative management in the treatment of adult parapneumonic effusions and empyema. *Cochrane Database Syst Rev* 2008;(2):CD002312.
- Koegelenberg CF, Diaconi AH, Bolligeri CT. Parapneumonic pleural effusion and empyema. *Respiration* 2008;75:241–250.
- Maskell NA, Batt S, Hedley EL, et al. The bacteriology of pleural infection by genetic and standard methods and its mortality significance. *Am J Respir Crit Care Med* 2006;174:817–823.
- Maskell NA, Davies CW, Nunn AJ, et al. First Multicenter Intrapleural Sepsis Trial (MIST1) Group. U.K. Controlled trial of intrapleural streptokinase for pleural infection. *N Engl J Med* 2005;352:865–874.
- Strachan RE, Cornelius A, Gilbert GL, et al; Australian Research Network in Empyema (ARNiE). A bedside assay to detect *Streptococcus pneumoniae* in children with empyema. *Pediatr Pulmonol* 2011;46:179–183.
- Zahid I, Routledge T, Bille A, et al. What is the best treatment of postpneumonectomy empyema? *Interact Cardiovasc Thorac Surg* 2011;12:260–264.

 # CODES

ICD9
- 510.0 Empyema with fistula
- 510.9 Empyema without mention of fistula

CLINICAL PEARLS
Prompt drainage of the infected pleural space is the most important determinant of outcome and therefore needs to be addressed immediately at the time of diagnosis

ENCEPHALITIS

Erica S. Shenoy (E. Mylonakis, Editor)

 BASICS

DESCRIPTION

Encephalitis is inflammation of the brain parenchyma leading to neurological dysfunction and can be caused by a number of infectious organisms, including viruses, bacteria, fungi, and protozoa. Encephalitis results from infection of the central nervous system with any of these organisms, usually through hematogenous spread. Typical presenting symptoms include fever, confusion, and headache, though seizures can also occur.

EPIDEMIOLOGY
Incidence
- Encephalitis affects the very young and the very old more commonly.
- The most common cause of viral encephalitis in the US is herpes simplex virus (HSV) accounting for 10% of all cases of encephalitis. In neonates, the most common etiology is HSV-2, acquired during delivery.
- The annual incidence of viral encephalitis (the most common etiology) is 3.5–7.4/100,000 person-years with approximately 20,000 new cases per year.

RISK FACTORS
Risk factors include age, season (i.e. arboviruses more common in summer and fall whereas HSV occurs sporadically throughout the year), immune status, as well as possible exposures through travel, activities, and contact with animal and insect.

GENERAL PREVENTION
- Avoidance of tick and mosquito bites may limit transmission.
- Vector control in areas where disease is epidemic should be considered.
- Avoidance of swimming in ponds late in the summer may decrease the risk of enteroviral infections.
- A vaccine is available for Japanese encephalitis and should be given to people who reside in or plan to locate in endemic areas.
- Prevention of mosquito bites is most likely sufficient to prevent disease.
- Vaccination for measles, mumps and rubella, polio, and varicella limits these causes of encephalitis.

PATHOPHYSIOLOGY
The pathophysiology of infection relates in large part to the specific organism. Viremia leads to seeding of the reticuloendothelial system and later distant sites such as the CNS, via hematogenous spread. In the case of rabies encephalitis, infection is caused by retrograde peripheral nerve transmission.

ETIOLOGY
Among infectious etiologies, viral is the most common. In up to 75% of cases, no etiologic agent may be identified.

- Viral
  - Flaviviridae: Japanese encephalitis virus, St. Louis encephalitis, West Nile virus, Central European encephalitis, Russian spring-summer encephalitis, Murray Valley encephalitis, Powassan virus
  - Togaviridae: Eastern equine encephalitis (EEE), Western equine encephalitis, Venezuelan equine encephalitis, Rubella virus
  - Bunyaviridae: California, La Crosse, Rift Valley fever
  - Herpesviridae: HSV, cytomegalovirus (CMV), varicella zoster virus (VZV), HHV6, herpes B virus
  - Paramyxoviridae: Hendra virus, measles virus, mumps virus, Nipah virus
  - Other viruses that are commonly considered: HIV, JC virus, adenovirus, enteroviridae (coxsackievirus, echovirus, poliovirus), influenza, mumps, rabies
- Bacterial: *Listeria monocytogenes, Mycobacterium tuberculosis, Mycoplasma, Tropheryma whippelii* (Whipple's disease), Nocardia, *Bartonella bacilliformis* (Oroya fever), *Bartonella henselae* (cat scratch disease)
- Rickettsiosis and ehrlichiosis: *Anaplasma phagocytophilum* (human granulocytotropic ehrlichiosis), *Coxiella burnetii* (Q fever), *Ehrlichia chaffeensis* (human monocytotropic ehrlichiosis), *Rickettsia rickettsii* (Rocky Mountain spotted fever)
- Spirochetes: *Borrelia burgdorferi* (Lyme Disease), *Treponema pallidum* (syphilis)
- Fungal: *Cryptococcus neoformans,* coccidioidomycosis, Candida, Aspergillus
- Protozoa: *Acanthamoeba, Balamuthia mandrillaris, Toxoplasma gondii, Naegleria fowleri, Plasmodium falciparum* (malaria). *Trypanosoma brucei gambiense* (West African trypanosomiasis), *Trypanosoma brucei rhodesiense* (East African trypanosomiasis)
- Helminths: *Baylisascaris procyonis, Gnathostoma* species, *Taenia solium* (cysticercosis)

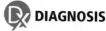 **DIAGNOSIS**

HISTORY
Depending on the organism, the history can be very informative. For example, travel history, and prevalence of particular diseases in the area, recreational activities, insect and animal exposures as well as patient immune status may help narrow the differential.

PHYSICAL EXAM
- Physical exam focuses mostly on the neurological exam, though a careful skin exam should be conducted to look for rashes. Because of meningeal inflammation, signs of meningitis may occur, making it difficult to distinguish between meningitis and encephalitis.
- Focal signs may occur early, and cranial nerve abnormalities may occur with increased intracranial pressure.
- Rashes, when present, are most helpful in diagnosis. Evidence of tick bites or mosquito bites may be lacking.
- Specific etiologies are associated with characteristic physical findings.
  - Japanese encephalitis is associated with a movement disorder similar to Parkinson's disease.
- Lyme disease is associated with cranial nerve abnormalities:
  - HSV tends to localize to the temporal lobes; at times, patients have a prodrome of bizarre behavior.

DIAGNOSTIC TESTS & INTERPRETATION
Lab
Initial lab tests
- Initial laboratory tests, including complete blood count (CBC) with differential, are of limited utility though white blood cell count (WBC) may be low in viral infections and elevated in bacterial infections.
- Once clinical examination or imaging by non-contrast head CT rules out space-occupying lesion, a lumbar puncture should be performed immediately.
- Cerebrospinal fluid (CSF) should be evaluated for: Cell counts, total protein, glucose, viral and bacterial cultures, fungal stain and culture, India ink stain as well as HSV 1 and 2, CMV, and VZV by polymerase chain reaction (PCR).
- In viral encephalitis, the typical CSF profile will demonstrate a lymphocytic pleocytosis, normal glucose, and elevated protein.
- Malaria smears and evaluation of WBCs for morulae in *Ehrlichia* should be considered if there is clinical suspicion that the patient may have malaria or ehrlichiosis.
- Cultures of non-CNS sites (i.e. blood, sputum, nasopharynx, stool) should be performed as indicated and guided by epidemiologic and clinical considerations.

- Often, the diagnosis is based on serology. Both acute and convalescent serologies should be obtained. Serologic tests can also be conducted in the case of West Nile Virus, dengue, Japanese encephalitis.
- A variety of PCR based tests are also available.
- Additional CSF should be held on reserve.

Follow-Up & Special Considerations
Close follow-up with specialists, including those in neurology and infectious diseases, is advised.

Imaging
- Brain imaging should be performed prior to lumbar puncture to rule out impending herniation, hemorrhage, and other complications.
- Brain MRI is the gold standard and should be obtained in all patients. For example, in the case of HSV encephalitis, temporal lobe lesions are a classic finding and can be unilateral or bilateral, and hemorrhagic. MRI in the case of Japanese B encephalitis may reveal gray matter involvement.
- Rhombencephalitis from enterovirus reveals hyperintense lesions in the brainstem.
- Brain CT should be done when MRI is not available. It is a non-specific test and cannot be used to differentiate between etiological agents.

Diagnostic Procedures/Other
- Lumbar puncture as described above.
- EEG can be helpful in some cases. For example, in HSV encephalitis, EEG may reveal focal temporal changes, diffuse slowing, and PLEDS (periodic complexes and periodic lateralizing epileptiform discharges). Japanese B encephalitis is associated with diffuse continuous delta activity, delta activity with spikes, and alpha coma pattern. St. Louis encephalitis is associated with diffuse delta activity.

Pathological Findings
- For viral encephalitis, inflammation of cortical vessels in the gray matter or at the gray–white matter junction is seen. Round cell infiltration, perivascular cuffing, demyelination, and necrosis are common.
- For particular etiologies, there are a variety of specific histopathologic findings, including Cowdry type A inclusion bodies in HSV, Negri bodies in rabies, necrosis in EEE, and Japanese B encephalitis.
- Particular viruses may have specific distribution patterns: While HSV may be classically found in the temporal lobes and pons, there may be widespread lesions. Rabies also has an affinity for the temporal lobes. West Nile virus appears to prefer the brainstem.

DIFFERENTIAL DIAGNOSIS
- Viral meningitis
- Bacterial meningitis
- Brain abscess
- Acute disseminated encephalomyelitis (ADEM)
- Encephalopathy
- Reye's Syndrome
- Toxic metabolic abnormalities
- Aseptic meningitis caused by medications such as trimethoprim–sulfamethoxazole, ibuprofen, metronidazole
- Vasculitis
- Collagen vascular diseases
- Paraneoplastic syndromes

 TREATMENT

Until bacterial meningitis is ruled out, empiric therapy should include treatment for bacterial meningitis as well as HSV. If rickettsial or *Ehrlichia* infection is considered, doxycycline should be added to the empiric regimen.

MEDICATION
- Acyclovir 10 mg/kg intravenously every 8 h for 14–21 days is used for treatment of HSV encephalitis. Higher doses, at 20 mg/kg intravenously every 8 h is recommended in neonates.
- Ganciclovir alone or in combination foscarnet is used to treat CMV encephalitis.
- Ganciclovir or foscarnet is used to treat HHV6 in immunocompromised hosts.
- Highly active antiviral therapy (HAART) is indicated as adjunctive therapy in the setting of HIV.
- Other specific therapies depend on the etiologic agent.

IN-PATIENT CONSIDERATIONS
Admission Criteria
Patients with encephalitis require admission to the hospital and specialized care, which may include ICU-level care.

IV Fluids
Patients should be well-hydrated, especially while undergoing treatment with acyclovir, which is associated with renal toxicity.

 ONGOING CARE

FOLLOW-UP RECOMMENDATIONS
Patients should be monitored closely for response to therapy. Of note, as in the case with HSV encephalitis, recovery may be slow or may not occur.

Patient Monitoring
The nature and extent of patient monitoring depends on clinical circumstances. Neuropsychological testing may reveal long-term sequelae of the initial infection.

PROGNOSIS
- Varies based on the etiological agent. For example, in the case of HSV encephalitis, prompt diagnosis and initiation of therapy can greatly improve prognosis. Delays in appropriate therapy are associated with poorer outcomes.
- The mortality rate of untreated HSV encephalitis is 70%; with treatment, 6–19% with about half of survivors suffering from moderate or severe neurological impairment. Younger age (less than 30 years) is associated with better outcomes.

COMPLICATIONS
Include seizures, permanent neurological deficits, and death. In the case of HSV encephalitis, relapse has been shown to occur in 5–26% of patients, some of which may be due to inadequate treatment, though there is some debate as to whether or not relapse represents recurrent viral infection or the host immune response to infection.

REFERENCES
1. Beckham JD, Tyler KL. Encephalitis. In: Mandell, Douglas, Bennett, eds. *Principles and practice of infectious diseases*, 7th ed. Philadelphia, PA: Elsevier Churchill Livingstone, 2009.
2. Gondim FAA, Olivera G, Thomas FP. Viral encephalitis. *EMedicine neurology*, 2008. http://emedicine.medscape.com/article/1166498-overview. Accessed August 2, 2011.
3. Tunkel AR. Approach to the patient with central nervous system infection. In: Mandell, Douglas, Bennett, eds. *Principles and practice of infectious diseases*, 7th ed. Philadelphia, PA: Elsevier Churchill Livingstone, 2009.
4. Tunkel AR, Glaser CA, Bloch KC, et al. The management of encephalitis: Clinical practice guidelines by the Infectious Diseases Society of America. *Clin Infect Dis* 2008;47:303–327.
5. Carson PJ, Konewko P, Wold KS, et al. Long-term clinical and neuropsychological outcomes of West Nile virus infection. *Clin Infect Dis* 2006;43:723–730.
6. Pritz T. Herpes simplex encephalitis. *EMedicine neurology*, 2010. http://emedicine.medscape.com/article/791896-overview. Accessed August 2, 2011.

E

 CODES

ICD9
- 049.9 Unspecified non-arthropod-borne viral diseases of central nervous system
- 058.20 and 058.29 Other human herpesvirus encephalitis
- 323.9 Unspecified cause of encephalitis, myelitis, and encephalomyelitis

CLINICAL PEARLS
- HSV is the most common cause of viral encephalitis in the US.
- Epidemiologic history is important in providing clues to the diagnosis.
- Empiric treatment should include acyclovir, with the addition of doxycycline if there is concern for rickettsial or *Ehrlichia* disease.
- The cause of encephalitis may remain unknown in up to 75% of patients.

ENDOCARDITIS (NATIVE VALVES)

Rachel P. Simmons (E. Mylonakis, Editor)

 BASICS

DESCRIPTION
- Endocarditis is an infection of the heart valves or endocardium with bacteria or fungi, or rarely chlamydiae, or rickettsiae
- The mitral valve (41%) or aortic valve (38%) is involved most commonly in native valve infective endocarditis (NVIE). Tricuspid valve endocarditis occurs with greater frequency in intravenous drug users. Pulmonic valve endocarditis is very rare. Multiple valves may be infected.

EPIDEMIOLOGY
Incidence
The incidence of NVIE is approximately 1.7–6.2 cases per 100,000 patient years. In intravenous drug users, the incidence is estimated at 1500–3300 cases per 100,000 patient years.

RISK FACTORS
Predisposing conditions include current intravenous drug use, previous endocarditis, chronic intravascular access, implantable cardiac device, congenital heart disease, bicuspid aortic valve, rheumatic heart disease, and degenerative valve disease (1).

GENERAL PREVENTION
- Prevention of endocarditis with antibiotics is recommended for patients with the following:
  - Prosthetic cardiac valve or valve repair prosthetic material
  - Previous endocarditis
  - Congenital heart disease (unrepaired cyanotic CHD, repaired CHD with persistent defect)
  - Cardiac transplant recipients with cardiac valvulopathy (2)
- Prophylaxis is recommended for dental procedures that include disruption of the oral mucosa and manipulation of the gingiva.
- Prophylaxis is also reasonable for patients with high risk conditions listed above who undergo procedures of the respiratory tract, skin soft tissue, or muscle. Antibiotics for prevention of IE are not recommended for GI or GU procedures.
- Antibiotic regimens include amoxicillin 2 g or clindamycin 600 mg given for a single dose 30–60 minutes prior to the procedure.

ETIOLOGY
- The most common causative pathogens are gram-positive bacteria. *Staphylococcus aureus* has recently become the most common cause of NVIE (3).
- The common microbiologic etiologies for NVIE are listed below:
  - *S. aureus* (25–35%)
  - Coagulase negative staphylococcus (3–11%)
  - Viridans group streptococci (17–40%)
  - *Streptococcus bovis* (6%)
  - Other streptococcus (6–19%)
  - *Enterococcus* spp. (10–18%)
  - HACEK (2–5%) - Haemophilus species, *Aggregatibacter actinomycetemcomitans*, *Cardiobacterium hominis*, *Eikenella corrodens*, and *Kingella* spp.
  - Fungi/yeast (2–4%)

- Culture negative endocarditis (10%)
  - The most common cause is antibiotics within the last 7 days.
  - Other possible causes include slow growing fastidious anaerobes, fungi (non-*Candida* species), *Bartonella* spp., *Coxiella burnetii* (Q fever), *Legionella* spp., *Tropheryma whippelii*, *Chlamydia* spp., and *Brucella* spp.
- In intravenous drug users, polymicrobial NVIE is more common.

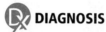 **DIAGNOSIS**

HISTORY
- The clinical features of NVIE are highly variable and are comprised of symptoms and signs due to the infected valve itself, to embolic phenomena, to metastatic sites of infection, and due to circulating immune complexes.
- Fever is present in over 90% of patients with NVIE. Nonspecific symptoms such as weakness, chills, sweats, anorexia, weight loss, nausea, and malaise may be present (3).
- The modified Duke criteria are widely used diagnostic criteria for NVIE.
- Major criteria:
  - Microbiologic (1) 2 sets of blood cultures positive for typical microorganisms including *Viridans streptococci*, *S. bovis*, HACEK group, *S. aureus*; or community-acquired enterococci without a primary focus; or (2) microorganism consistent with IE from persistently positive blood cultures; or (3) single positive blood culture for *Coxiella burnetii* or anti–phase 1 IgG antibody titer >1:800
  - Evidence of endocardial involvement (1) Positive echocardiogram (oscillating intracardiac mass on valve, abscess, or new partial dehiscence of prosthetic valve) (2) new valvular regurgitation (worsening or changing or preexisting murmur not sufficient)
- Minor criteria
  - Predisposition, predisposing heart condition, or IDU
  - Fever
  - Vascular phenomena: Major arterial emboli, septic pulmonary infarcts, mycotic aneurysm, intracranial hemorrhage, conjunctival hemorrhages, and Janeway's lesions
  - Immunologic phenomena: Glomerulonephritis, Osler's nodes, Roth's spots, and rheumatoid factor
  - Microbiological evidence: Positive blood culture but does not meet a major criterion as noted above or serological evidence of active infection with organism consistent with IE
- Definitive endocarditis (clinical criteria): 2 major criteria; or 1 major criterion plus 3 minor criteria; or 5 minor criteria
- Definitive endocarditis (pathologic criteria): Microorganisms identified by culture or pathologic examination of vegetation, embolized vegetation, or intracardiac abscess; or vegetation or intracardiac abscess demonstrating active endocarditis by histological examination.

- Possible endocarditis: 1 major criteria plus 1 minor criteria; or 3 minor criteria
- Rejected: Firm alternative diagnosis; resolution of symptoms in less than 4 days with antibiotics; no pathologic evidence of IE at surgery with less than 4 days of antibiotics; does not meet clinical criteria for possible IE.

PHYSICAL EXAM
- Clinical signs of IE include a new or changing murmur in up to 85%.
- Petechiae are found in 20–40% of patients. Other cutaneous findings (Osler nodes, Janeway lesions, splinter hemorrhages) or Roth spots are present in a minority of patients.
- To identify other sites of infection (epidural abscess, psoas abscess, septic arthritis) or to identify embolic events (stroke), a thorough examination should be performed.

DIAGNOSTIC TESTS & INTERPRETATION
Lab
Initial lab tests
- In suspected NVIE, initial laboratory evaluation includes complete blood count with differential, electrolytes, blood urea nitrogen, creatinine, liver function tests, multiple sets of blood cultures, urinalysis, and ESR.
- In the first 24 hours, obtain at least 3 sets of blood cultures. Draw several sets of blood cultures before administering antibiotics to maximize the possibility of identifying the causative organism. The first 2 sets are positive in up to 90% of patients.
- Leukocytosis is common. More than half of patients have elevated serum markers of inflammation (ESR, C-reactive protein).
- The urinalysis is frequently positive for proteinuria or microscopic hematuria.

Follow-Up & Special Considerations
- In cases of culture negative endocarditis, serologic evaluation for rare organisms such as Q fever and Bartonella spp. may be indicated.
- Obtain 2 sets of blood cultures every 24–48 hours until endovascular infection has cleared.

Imaging
Initial approach
- Echocardiography is the imaging test of choice and should be performed as soon as possible in all cases of suspected NVIE.
- The sensitivity of transthoracic echocardiography (TTE) for detecting left-sided vegetations ranges from 40–63% (specificity 91–98%). The sensitivity for right-sided lesions is higher as the tricuspid and pulmonic valves sit closer to the chest wall. TTE may be limited due to obesity, chronic lung disease, or chest wall deformity.
- Transesophageal echocardiography (TEE) has a sensitivity of 90–100% and specificity of 91–98% for detecting vegetations. TEE is also more sensitive than TTE in identifying valvular perforation, pacemaker associated IE, and myocardial abscess.
- TEE as the initial test is recommended if the TTE is likely to be of poor quality, clinical suspicion of IE is high, or perivalvular extension is suspected. If initial TTE is negative and clinical concern for IE remains moderate to high, obtain a TEE.

Follow-Up & Special Considerations
Additional imaging of chest, abdomen, spine, or brain is warranted if emboli, abscesses, or mycotic aneurysm are suspected.

Diagnostic Procedures/Other
Obtain an EKG to establish a baseline cardiac rhythm and identify any conduction disease. Repeat EKG is warranted for change in clinical status, bradycardia, syncope, or presyncope.

Pathological Findings
- On histopathologic examination, vegetations consist of fibrin, platelet aggregates, and bacterial or fungal masses.
- PCR-based tests on blood or vavlular tissue for organisms such as *Bartonella* spp. and *T. whippleii* are available at some laboratories.

DIFFERENTIAL DIAGNOSIS
Noninfective endocarditis, other systemic infection, bacteriemia, or fungemia without IE.

 ## TREATMENT

MEDICATION
- Prolonged bactericidal therapy is required to penetrate the vegetation and prevent relapse. Identification of the causative organism and drug susceptibilities are paramount.
- Empiric therapy is based on patient risk factors for various pathogens, severity of illness, and local resistance patterns.
- Recommended treatment regimens for select pathogens are listed below (1).
- Penicillin susceptible *Viridans streptococci*, *S. bovis*, or other streptococci (minimum inhibitory concentration ≤0.12 µg/mL)
  – Penicillin G 12–18 million U/24 h (dosed continuously or in 4–6 doses) or ceftriaxone 2g IV daily for 4 weeks
  – Penicillin G 12–18 million U/24 h (dosed continuously or in 4–6 doses) or ceftriaxone 2 g IV daily plus gentamicin 3 mg/kg/d in 1 dose for 2 weeks
  – Vancomycin 30 mg/kg/d in 2 divided doses for 4 weeks if PCN & ceftriaxone intolerant or allergic
- Streptococci relatively resistant to penicillin (MIC >0.12 µg/mL or ≤0.5 µg/mL)
  – Penicillin G 24 million U/24 h (dosed continuously or in 4–6 doses) or ceftriaxone 2 g IV daily for 4 weeks plus gentamicin 3 mg/kg/d in 1 dose for 2 weeks
  – Vancomycin 30 mg/kg/d in 2 divided doses for 4 weeks if PCN & ceftriaxone intolerant or allergic
- Streptococci resistant to penicillin (MIC >0. 5 µg/mL) and enterococci
  – Ampicillin 12 g/d in 6 divided doses plus gentamicin 3 mg/kg/d in 3 divided doses for 4–6 weeks
  – Vancomycin 30 mg/kg/d in 2 divided doses plus gentamicin 3 mg/kg/d in 3 divided doses for 6 weeks if ampicillin allergic
- Methicillin susceptible *S. aureus*
  – Nafcillin 12 g/d IV in 4–6 divided doses for 6 weeks ± gentamicin 3 mg/kg/d in 2 or 3 divided doses for 3–5 days
  – If penicillin allergic (no anaphylactoid) but tolerant of cephalosporins, cefazolin 6 g/d in 3 divided doses for 6 weeks

- Methicillin resistant *S. aureus*
  – Vancomycin 30 mg/kg/d in 2 divided doses for 6 weeks
- Goal vancomycin trough is 15–20 µg/mL.
- Doses above are based on normal renal function.

ADDITIONAL TREATMENT
Issues for Referral
Native valve infective endocarditis and its sequelae can be life-threatening, and complex management issues are common. A multidisciplinary approach with cardiology, cardiovascular surgery, and infectious diseases input is recommended.

SURGERY/OTHER PROCEDURES
- Approximately 30–50% of patients with NVIE undergo combined antimicrobial and surgical treatment for IE.
- Patients with decompensated heart failure should be evaluated quickly for potential early surgery.
- The timing and necessity of valve replacement is individualized to each patient with NVIE.
- Other potential indications for valve replacement include significant valvular dysfunction, uncontrolled infection, multiple serious systemic emoboli, inadequate antimicrobial therapy (highly resistant pathogens), cardiac complications such as perivalvular or myocardial abscesses.

IN-PATIENT CONSIDERATIONS
Initial Stabilization
Assess and stabilize respiratory and cardiac systems in suspected acute endocarditis. Prompt evaluation of volume status and cardiac rhythm is warranted.

Admission Criteria
Patients with endocarditis should be admitted to the hospital for monitoring, initiation of intravenous antibiotics, and expedited workup.

Discharge Criteria
Patients may be discharged when fevers have abated for more than 24 hours, vital signs are normal, and antibiotic and follow-up plans are in place.

 ## ONGOING CARE

FOLLOW-UP RECOMMENDATIONS
- In the short term, follow patients closely for complications or relapse of endocarditis and adverse events related to antimicrobial therapy.
- At completion of therapy for IE, a TTE is recommended to document new baseline valve and cardiac function.

Patient Monitoring
For patients receiving intravenous antibiotics, send weekly monitoring labs per guidelines (http://www.idsociety.org/content.aspx?id=4428#opat) or package insert.

PATIENT EDUCATION
Patients with IE require information about the importance of good oral hygiene, how to prevent IE associated with dental procedures, and symptoms and signs of valvular dysfunction,

PROGNOSIS
- Congestive heart failure, extension of the infection beyond the valve annulus, presence of comorbid conditions, increasing age, immunosuppression, and *S. aureus* infection have been associated with higher mortality rate. Infection with Viridians group streptococci has been associated with lower mortality.
- In-hospital mortality associated with IE is lower in patients who are drug abusers (10% vs. 17% in a recent study). Mortality approaches 40% at 1 year for all comers with IE.

COMPLICATIONS
Congestive heart failure, cerebral emboli, stroke, kidney infarctions, immune complex glomerulonephritis, mycotic aneurysm, meningitis, cerebritis, splenic infarctions, splenic abscess, and pulmonary embolism with or without infarction in right-sided endocarditis.

REFERENCES

1. Baddour LM, Wilsom WR, Bayer AS, et al. Infective endocarditis: Diagnosis, antimicrobial therapy, and management of complications: A statement for healthcare professionals from the Committee on Rheumatic Fever, Endocarditis, and Kawasaki Disease, Council on Cardiovascular Disease in the Young, and the Councils on Clinical Cardiology, Stroke, and Cardiovascular Surgery and Anesthesia, American Heart Association: Endorsed by the Infectious Diseases Society of America. *Circulation* 2005;111(23):e394–e434.
2. Wilson W, Taubert KA, Gewitz M, et al. Prevention of infective endocarditis: Guidelines from the American Heart Association: A guideline from the American Heart Association Rheumatic Fever, Endocarditis, and Kawasaki Disease Committee, Council on Cardiovascular Disease in the Young, and the Council on Clinical Cardiology, Council on Cardiovascular Surgery and Anesthesia, and the Quality of Care and Outcomes Research Interdisciplinary Working Group. *Circulation* 2007;116(15):1736–1754.
3. Murdoch, et al. Clinical presentation, etiology, and outcome of infective endocarditis in the 21st century: the International Collaboration on Endocarditis-Prospective Cohort Study. *Arch Intern Med* 2009;169(5):463–473.

 ## See Also

- Prosthetic valve endocarditis

CODES

ICD9
- 394.9 Other and unspecified mitral valve diseases
- 421.0 Acute and subacute bacterial endocarditis
- 424.90 Endocarditis, valve unspecified, unspecified cause

CLINICAL PEARLS

- *S. aureus* is the most common cause of native valve IE.
- Obtain multiple sets of blood cultures prior to the administration of antibiotics.

E

ENDOCARDITIS (PROSTHETIC VALVE)

Rachel P. Simmons (E. Mylonakis, Editor)

 BASICS

DESCRIPTION
Prosthetic valve endocarditis is an infection of prosthetic heart valves or prosthetic material with bacteria, fungi, or rarely chlamydiae, or rickettsiae.

EPIDEMIOLOGY
Incidence
The incidence of prosthetic valve infective endocarditis (PVIE) is approximately 0.3–1% per patient-year.

RISK FACTORS
- The most important predisposing conditions for the development of prosthetic valve IE are health-care associated infections.
- Predisposing conditions also include chronic intravascular access and hemodialysis.

GENERAL PREVENTION
- Prevention of endocarditis with antibiotics is recommended for patients with the following (2):
  – Prosthetic cardiac valve or valve repair prosthetic material
  – Previous endocarditis
  – Congenital heart disease (unrepaired cyanotic CHD, repaired CHD with persistent defect)
  – Cardiac transplant recipients with cardiac valvulopathy
- Prophylaxis is recommended for dental procedures that include disruption of the oral mucosa and manipulation of the gingiva.
- Prophylaxis is also reasonable for patients with high risk conditions listed above, who undergo procedures of the respiratory tract, skin soft tissue, or muscle. Antibiotics for prevention of IE are not recommended for GI or GU procedures.
- Antibiotic regimens include amoxicillin 2 g or clindamycin 600 mg given for a single dose 30–60 minutes prior to the procedure.

PATHOPHYSIOLOGY
The development of prosthetic valve endocarditis can develop from contamination of the device during implantation, from secondary infection by hematogenous spread, or due to contiguous spread of infection.

ETIOLOGY
- Staphylococci are the most common causes of prosthetic valve IE.
- Prosthetic valve IE is characterized as early-onset (within 60 days of surgery) or late-onset (occurring thereafter).
- Early-onset PVIE is commonly due to hospital-acquired pathogens, whereas late-onset PVIE is caused by similar pathogens to native valve IE.
- The common microbiologic etiologies for early onset IE are *Staphylococcus aureus* (20–35%) including MRSA, coagulase negative staphylococcus (17–30%), *Streptococcus* spp. (1–4%), *Enterococcus* spp. (5–10%), fungal (5–10%), gram-negative bacilli (6–15%), or culture-negative IE (3–17%).

- The common microbiologic etiologies for late onset IE are *S. aureus* (15–20%), coagulase negative staphylococcus (10–20%), *Streptococcus* spp. (20–30%), *Enterococcus* spp. (8–13%), fungal (1–3%), gram-negative bacilli (4–7%), or culture-negative (3–12%) IE.
- Possible causes of culture negative endocarditis include antibiotics within the last 7 days, slow growing fastidious anaerobes, fungi (non-Candida species), *Bartonella* spp., *Coxiella burnetii* (Q fever), *Legionella* spp., *Tropheryma whippelii*, *Chlamydia* spp., or *Brucella* spp.

 DIAGNOSIS

HISTORY
- The clinical features of PVIE are highly variable. It may present as a subacute indolent illness or as an acute, toxic illness with high fevers.
- In patients with prosthetic valves and unexplained fever, a thorough workup for endocarditis is warranted.
- Fever is present in over 70% of patients with PVIE. Nonspecific symptoms such as weakness, chills, sweats, anorexia, weight loss, nausea, and malaise may be present.
- Collect a detailed history including recent travel, animal exposures, and dietary habits such as consuming unpasteurized dairy products.
- The modified Duke criteria are widely used diagnostic criteria for IE. They combine clinical features, microbiologic data, echocardiography, and pathologic data to classify endocarditis as definite or possible or to reject the diagnosis altogether. (Adapted from Li et al).
- Major criteria:
  – Microbiologic (1) 2 sets of blood cultures positive for typical microorganisms including *Viridans streptococci*, *Streptococcus bovis*, HACEK group, *S. aureus*; or community-acquired enterococci without a primary focus; or (2) Microorganism consistent with IE from persistently positive blood cultures; or (3) Single positive blood culture for *Coxiella burnetii* or anti–phase 1 IgG antibody titer >1:800
  – Evidence of endocardial involvement (1) Positive echocardiogram (oscillating intracardiac mass on valve, abscess, or new partial dehiscence of prosthetic valve) (2) New valvular regurgitation (worsening or changing or preexisting murmur not sufficient)
- Minor criteria
  – Predisposition, predisposing heart condition, or IDU
  – Fever
  – Vascular phenomena: Major arterial emboli, septic pulmonary infarcts, mycotic aneurysm, intracranial hemorrhage, conjunctival hemorrhages, and Janeway's lesions
  – Immunologic phenomena: Glomerulonephritis, Osler's nodes, Roth's spots, and rheumatoid factor
  – Microbiological evidence: Positive blood culture but does not meet a major criterion as noted above or serological evidence of active infection with organism consistent with IE

- Definitive endocarditis (clinical criteria): 2 major criteria; or 1 major criterion plus 3 minor criteria; or 5 minor criteria
- Definitive endocarditis (pathologic criteria): Microorganisms identified by culture or pathologic examination of vegetation, embolized vegetation, or intracardiac abscess; or vegetation or intracardiac abscess demonstrating active endocarditis by histological examination.
- Possible endocarditis: 1 major criteria plus 1 minor criteria; or 3 minor criteria
- Rejected: Firm alternative diagnosis; resolution of symptoms in less than 4 days with antibiotics; no pathologic evidence of IE at surgery with less than 4 days of antibiotics; does not meet clinical criteria for possible IE.

PHYSICAL EXAM
- The cardiac examination may include a changed or new murmur or an evidence of congestive heart failure.
- To identify other sites of infection (epidural abscess, psoas abscess, septic arthritis) or to identify embolic events (stroke), a thorough examination should be undertaken.

DIAGNOSTIC TESTS & INTERPRETATION
Lab
Initial lab tests
- In suspected IE, initial laboratory evaluation includes complete blood count with differential, electrolytes, blood urea nitrogen, creatinine, liver function tests, multiple sets of blood cultures, urinalysis, and ESR.
- In the first 24 hours, obtain at least 3 sets of blood cultures. Draw several sets of blood cultures before administering antibiotics to maximize the possibility of identifying the causative organism. The first 2 sets are positive in up to 90% of patients.
- Leukocytosis and elevation of serum markers of inflammation (ESR, CRP) are common.

Follow-Up & Special Considerations
- In cases of culture-negative endocarditis, serologic evaluation for rare organisms such as Q fever and *Bartonella* spp. may be indicated.
- Obtain 2 sets of blood cultures every 24–48 hours until endovascular infection has cleared.

Imaging
Initial approach
- Transesophageal echocardiography (TEE) is the imaging test of choice. TEE is preferred over transthoracic echocardiography due to artifact from mechanical prostheses, high rates of paravalvular complications, and small vegetation size. TEE has a sensitivity of 86–94% and specificity of 91–100% for detecting vegetations
- A TEE should be performed as soon as possible in cases of suspected prosthetic valve IE.

Follow-Up & Special Considerations
Additional imaging of lungs, abdomen, spine, or brain is warranted if emboli or abscesses or mycotic aneurysm are suspected.

Diagnostic Procedures/Other
Obtain an EKG to establish a baseline cardiac rhythm and identify any conduction disease. Repeat EKG is warranted for change in clinical status, bradycardia, syncope, or presyncope.

Pathological Findings
- On histopathologic examination, vegetations consist of fibrin, platelet aggregates, and bacterial or fungal masses.
- PCR-based tests on blood or valvular tissue for difficult to culture organisms such as *Bartonella* spp. and *T. whippleii* are available at some laboratories and may be indicated in select cases of culture negative endocarditis.

DIFFERENTIAL DIAGNOSIS
Noninfective endocarditis, other systemic infections such as malaria, bacteriemia, or fungemia without IE.

TREATMENT
MEDICATION
- Prolonged bactericidal therapy is required to penetrate the vegetation and prevent relapse. Identification of the causative organism and drug susceptibilities are paramount.
- Empiric therapy is based on patient risk factors for various pathogens, severity of illness, and local resistance patterns.
- Recommended treatment regimens for select pathogens are listed below (1).
- Penicillin susceptible *Viridans streptococci, S. bovis,* or other streptococci (minimum inhibitory concentration ≤0.12 μg/mL)
  – Penicillin G 24 million U/24 h (dosed continuously or in 4–6 doses) or ceftriaxone 2g IV daily for 6 weeks plus gentamicin 3 mg/kg/d in 1 dose for 2 weeks
  – Vancomycin 30 mg/kg/d in 2 divided doses for 6 weeks if PCN & ceftriaxone intolerant or allergic
- Streptococci relatively resistant to penicillin (MIC >0.12 μg/mL or ≤0.5 μg/mL)
  – Penicillin G 24 million U/24 h (dosed continuously or in 4–6 doses) or ceftriaxone 2g IV daily plus gentamicin 3 mg/kg/d in 1 dose for 6 weeks
- Streptococci resistant to penicillin (MIC >0.5 μg/mL) and enterococci
  – Ampicillin 12 g/d in 6 divided doses plus gentamicin 3 mg/kg/d in 3 divided doses for 6 weeks
  – Vancomycin 30 mg/kg/d in 2 divided doses plus gentamicin 3 mg/kg/d in 3 divided doses for 6 weeks if ampicillin allergic
- Methicillin susceptible staphylococci
  – Nafcillin 12 g/d IV in 6 divided doses plus rifampin 900 mg/d in 3 divided doses for ≥6 weeks plus gentamicin 3 mg/kg/d in 2 or 3 divided doses for 2 weeks
- Methicillin resistant staphylococci
  – Vancomycin 30 mg/kg/d in 2 divided doses plus rifampin 900 mg/d in 3 divided doses for ≥6 weeks plus gentamicin 3 mg/kg/d in 2 or 3 divided doses for 2 weeks
- Goal vancomycin trough is 15–20 μg/mL
- It may be prudent to delay the start of rifampin by a few days given its low barrier to resistance.
- Doses above are based on normal renal function.

ADDITIONAL TREATMENT
General Measures
For IDU patients, refer to drug treatment programs when clinically stable.

Issues for Referral
Prosthetic valve infective endocarditis and its sequelae can be life-threatening, and complex management issues are common. A multidisciplinary approach with cardiology, cardiovascular surgery, and infectious diseases input is paramount.

SURGERY/OTHER PROCEDURES
- Patients with prosthetic valve endocarditis should be evaluated quickly for potential surgery. The timing and necessity of valve replacement is individualized to each patient.
- Indications for consideration of valve replacement include valve dehiscence, perforation, fistula, rupture, large abscess, or inadequate antimicrobial therapy (highly resistant pathogens).

IN-PATIENT CONSIDERATIONS
Initial Stabilization
Assess and stabilize respiratory and cardiac systems in suspected acute endocarditis. Prompt evaluation of volume status and cardiac conduction is warranted.

Admission Criteria
Patients with endocarditis should be admitted to the hospital for monitoring, initiation of intravenous antibiotics, and expedited workup.

Discharge Criteria
Patients may be discharged when fevers have abated for more than 24 hours, vital signs are normal, and an antibiotic and follow-up plans are in place.

ONGOING CARE
FOLLOW-UP RECOMMENDATIONS
- In the short term, follow patients closely for complications or relapse of endocarditis and adverse events related to antimicrobial therapy.
- At completion of therapy for IE, a TTE is recommended to document new baseline valve and cardiac function.

Patient Monitoring
For patients receiving intravenous antibiotics, send weekly monitoring labs per guidelines (http://www.idsociety.org/content.aspx?id=4428#opat) or package insert.

PATIENT EDUCATION
Patients with IE require information about the importance of good oral hygiene, how to prevent IE associated with dental procedures, and symptoms and signs of valvular dysfunction.

PROGNOSIS
- Health care-associated infection, congestive heart failure, increasing age, *S. aureus* infection, persistent bacteremia, stroke, and intracardiac abscess have been associated with higher mortality rate.
- In-hospital mortality associated with PVIE was 22.8% in a recent study.

COMPLICATIONS
Periprosthetic leak, ring abscess, congestive heart failure, cerebral emboli, stroke, kidney infarctions, immune complex glomerulonephritis, mycotic aneurysm, meningitis, cerebritis, splenic infarctions, splenic abscess, heart block, and pulmonary embolism with or without infarction in right sided endocarditis.

REFERENCES
1. Baddour LM, Wilsom WR, Bayer AS, et al. Infective endocarditis: Diagnosis, antimicrobial therapy, and management of complications: A statement for healthcare professionals from the Committee on Rheumatic Fever, Endocarditis, and Kawasaki Disease, Council on Cardiovascular Disease in the Young, and the Councils on Clinical Cardiology, Stroke, and Cardiovascular Surgery and Anesthesia, American Heart Association: Endorsed by the Infectious Diseases Society of America. *Circulation* 2005;111(23):e394–e434.
2. Wilson W, Taubert KA, Gewitz M, et al. Prevention of infective endocarditis: Guidelines from the American Heart Association: A guideline from the American Heart Association Rheumatic Fever, Endocarditis, and Kawasaki Disease Committee, Council on Cardiovascular Disease in the Young, and the Council on Clinical Cardiology, Council on Cardiovascular Surgery and Anesthesia, and the Quality of Care and Outcomes Research Interdisciplinary Working Group. *Circulation* 2007;116(15):1736–1754.

ADDITIONAL READING
- Li JS, Sexton DJ, Mick N, et al. Proposed modifications to the Duke criteria for the diagnosis of infective endocarditis. *Clin Infect Dis* 2000;30(4):633–638.

 See Also

- Endocarditis (Native Valves)

 CODES

ICD9
- 424.90 Endocarditis, valve unspecified, unspecified cause
- 996.61 Infection and inflammatory reaction due to cardiac device, implant, and graft

CLINICAL PEARLS
- In patients with prosthetic valves and unexplained fever, investigate for endocarditis.
- Health care-associated infection is an important risk factor for prosthetic valve endocarditis.
- TEE is the imaging test of choice.
- Prolonged antibiotic therapy and prompt surgical evaluation are indicated.

ENDOPHTHALMITIS

Theodoros Filippopoulos (E. Mylonakis, Editor)

 BASICS

DESCRIPTION
- Endophthalmitis is an infectious process involving the ocular (vitreous) cavity.
- Panophthalmitis is inflammation involving all structures of the eye.

EPIDEMIOLOGY
Incidence
The incidence of endophthalmitis after cataract surgery varies between 0.1 and 0.3%, while the incidence after penetrating ocular trauma is estimated between 3 and 30% and tends to be higher in cases of retained intraocular foreign bodies.

RISK FACTORS
- The presence of untreated eyelid disease (blepharitis), inadequate surgical technique and intraoperative complications/increased operative time are the most important risk factors for acute post-operative endophthalmitis.
- Chronically ill, diabetic, or immunocompromised patients, especially those with indwelling intravenous catheters and/or positive blood cultures, are at greatest risk for endogenous endophthalmitis with a reported incidence of 1 in 5.000 to 10.000 hospitalizations.

GENERAL PREVENTION
- Routine post-operative use of topical fluoroquinolones is considered the standard of care after cataract surgery despite the lack of evidence demonstrating a reduction in the incidence of post-operative endophthalmitis.
- The intracameral use of cefuroxime has been recently shown to decrease the incidence of post-operative endophthalmitis after cataract surgery (1).
- Many authorities recommend systemic intravenous prophylaxis with vancomycin (1 g i.v. b.i.d.) or moxifloxacin (400 mg p.o. per day) for cases of penetrating ocular injuries with high risk for infection, as in cases of intraocular foreign bodies.
- For trauma limited to the anterior segment, i.e. corneal laceration, frequent fortified (vancomycin 25–50 mg/mL or cefazolin 50 mg/mL and/or tobramycin 15 mg/mL) topical antibiotics or a topical fluoroquinolone and/or subconjunctival injections at the end of the surgical procedure can produce therapeutic levels of antimicrobials in the anterior chamber.
- Patients with infectious foci and especially those with fungemia due to *Candida* spp. should be monitored for the development of endogenous endophthalmitis.

PATHOPHYSIOLOGY
- Inadequate wound construction during cataract surgery may allow eyelid and conjunctival flora to gain access to the anterior chamber and cause post-operative endophthalmitis.
- Dissemination of pathogens via the bloodstream in patients with infectious processes elsewhere can initially affect the choroid and cause endogenous endophthalmitis.

ETIOLOGY
- Infectious endophthalmitis can be bacterial, fungal, or parasitic in origin. The most common causes in alphabetical order include the following:
  – Bacteria (*Acinetobacter* spp., *Actinomyces israelii*, *Bacillus* spp., *Clostridium* spp., *Corynebacterium* spp., *Enterobacter* spp., *Enterococcus* spp., *Escherichia coli*, *Haemophilus influenzae*, *Klebsiella* spp., *Listeria monocytogenes*, *Neisseria meningitides*, *Proteus* spp., *Propionibacterium acnes*, *Pseudomonas aeruginosa*, *Salmonella typhimurium*, *Serratia marcescens*, *Streptococcus* spp., *Staphylococcus* spp.)
  – Fungi (*Aspergillus* spp., *Blastomyces dermatitidis*, *Candida* spp., *Coccidioides immitis*, *Fusarium* spp., *Penicillium* spp., *Rhizopus* spp., *Sporothrix schenckii*)
  – Parasites (*Taenia solium*, *Toxocara canis*, *Toxoplasma gondii*)
- Endophthalmitis occurs:
  – After ocular surgery or an intravitreal injection within 6 weeks after the intervention termed acute post-operative endophthalmitis or up to months or even years after the intervention due to less virulent organisms (i.e. *Propionibacterium acnes*) termed in this case chronic endophthalmitis
  – After penetrating ocular trauma to the globe
  – Late after a glaucoma filtering procedure due to the inability of the thinned and stretched conjunctiva to function as a barrier to bacterial invasion
  – In rare cases due to hematogenous seeding from a remote site, including septic emboli from a diseased heart valve that lodge into the choroidal circulation termed endogenous endophthalmitis
- Gram-positive organisms constitute the majority of identified isolates in cases of acute post-operative endophthalmitis after cataract surgery.
- Bacteria such as streptococcal and Gram-negative organisms cause infections with worse prognosis.
- Mixed flora infections occur more frequently after trauma, with an incidence as high as 42% in open globe injuries from rural areas where organic matter is inflicting the injury to the globe.
- Parasites commonly cause chorioretinal lesions and a more indolent inflammatory response that can be more destructive than the actual pathogen itself (see Uveitis-Chorioretinitis).

COMMONLY ASSOCIATED CONDITIONS
A history of recent ocular surgery or penetrating trauma is the most common associated condition.

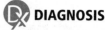 **DIAGNOSIS**

HISTORY
- Most patients with endophthalmitis present with ocular pain and conjunctival injection (redness). Photophobia (light sensitivity) is an associated symptom. Conjunctival chemosis and eyelid edema may also be present. However, visual loss is sometimes the only symptom.
- In some instances, a seemingly mild injury may not lead the patient to seek care until the signs and symptoms of an infection have developed days or weeks later, revealing an occult penetrating injury, particularly when the infecting organism is a fungus.
- In other cases, notably with *Bacillus cereus* infections, the onset of pain and profound visual loss are signs of an aggressive course.
- Pain with movement of the eye is a feature of panophthalmitis.

PHYSICAL EXAM
- Vitreous opacities are essential in establishing the diagnosis.
- Hypopyon, the layering of white blood cells (WBCs) in the anterior chamber, is a common feature.
- Chorioretinal infiltrates with secondary vitreous involvement are typical of hematogenous spread of pathogens.

DIAGNOSTIC TESTS & INTERPRETATION
Lab
Initial lab tests
- In cases of suspected endophthalmitis, aqueous and vitreous aspiration for microbial cultures and smear should be performed but can be inconclusive at times (cultures are positive in about 70% of suspected cases of post-operative infectious endophthalmitis).
- Smears should be stained with Gram, Giemsa, and methenamine-silver and cultured for aerobic and anaerobic bacteria, mycobacteria, and fungi (blood, chocolate, thioglycolate, Sabouraud, etc.).

Follow-Up & Special Considerations
- Cultures results are typically positive within 48 h but should not delay treatment.
- Negative results may be due to inadequate sampling, fastidious organisms or because of sterile post-operative inflammation.
- Vitreous aspiration material during vitrectomy, which is performed for diagnostic or therapeutic reasons, is routinely collected and can be centrifuged and smeared or passed through a filter that can be stained and cultured.

Imaging
Imaging with ultrasonography or computer tomography can be useful in cases of suspected retained intraocular foreign bodies especially when visualization is suboptimal due to hazy media.

Diagnostic Procedures/Other
Aqueous humor should be obtained with a 25–30 G needle and sent for culture in an office procedure under local anesthesia. Vitreous samples can be obtained with a 23 G needle through pars plana.

Pathological Findings
Acute endophthalmitis is characterized by the presence of neutrophils.

DIFFERENTIAL DIAGNOSIS
- Other intraocular inflammatory syndromes that can mimic infectious endophthalmitis include:
  - Idiopathic or non-idiopathic uveitis
  - Postoperative sterile inflammation due to intraocular use of pharmacologic agents (i.e. toxic anterior segment syndrome TASS)
  - Postoperative sterile inflammation due to retained lens fragments in cases of complicated cataract surgery

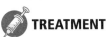 TREATMENT

MEDICATION
First Line
- Acute post-operative bacterial endophthalmitis represents a true ophthalmologic emergency, and therapy should be initiated promptly.
- Intravitreal administration (0.1 mL of each respectively) of vancomycin (1.0 mg/0.1 mL) for Gram-positive coverage and ceftazidime (2.25 mg/0.1 mL) or amikacin (0.4 mg/0.1 mL) in cases of β-lactam hypersensitivity for Gram-negative coverage is the currently recommended treatment strategy. Antibiotic selection is limited by the potential toxic effect on the retina of certain agents.
- Hourly administration of fortified topical antibiotic preparations (cefazolin 50 mg/mL or vancomycin 25–50 mg/mL and/or tobramycin 15 mg/mL) or a topical fluoroquinolone may achieve sufficient concentrations in the anterior chamber and should be considered in cases of exposed sutures or wound leaks.
- Systemic administration of antibiotics after cataract surgery-related infections is not supported by the endophthalmitis vitrectomy study. This conclusion is methodologically limited by the selection of aminoglycosides in this specific study for the management of an infection caused predominantly by Gram-positive isolates.
- Systemic 4th-generation fluoroquinolones (i.e. moxifloxacin 400 mg p.o. per day) should be considered due to the high intraocular concentration that these antibiotics achieve, despite the lack of prospective evidence.
- In cases of bacterial endogenous endophthalmitis, empiric systemic treatment of the suspected source in addition to intravitreal vancomycin and ceftazidime as above is recommended. The antibiotic regimen should be tailored based on culture results.
- For post-operative or traumatic fungal endophthalmitis, most treatment protocols recommend intravitreal administration of 0.1 mL of amphotericin B (5–10 μg/0.1 mL). The potential of retinal toxicity, however, should be kept in mind. Systemic administration of amphotericin B does not appear to achieve sufficient intraocular concentrations. Nevertheless, systemic treatment is necessary for endogenous cases.

- In cases of traumatic endophthalmitis or endogenous endophthalmitis in intravenous drug abusers, systemic administration of clindamycin (150–300 mg i.v. t.i.d.) or intravitreal clindamycin (0.1 mL of a 1 mg/0.1 mL preparation) instead of vancomycin is recommended by some authorities to offer coverage against *B. cereus* which is associated with a very aggressive course.

Second Line
Systemic fluconazole (400–600 mg i.v. or p.o. loading dose per day followed by 200–400 mg p.o. or i.v. per day) for endogenous endophthalmitis due to *C. albicans* may be less toxic than systemic amphotericin B, but no comparative data are available. Voriconazole and caspofungin are additional options.

ADDITIONAL TREATMENT
General Measures
Management of the associated pain with adequate oral medications and topical cycloplegic eye drops (atropine 1% per day or b.i.d.) is necessary.

Issues for Referral
Once the diagnosis is suspected or made, the patient should be referred to ophthalmology.

COMPLEMENTARY & ALTERNATIVE THERAPIES
Topical (prednisolone acetate 1% eye drops) or periocular corticosteroids are widely accepted to modulate the host immune response. The systemic or intravitreal use of steroids (prednisone 60 mg p.o. or triamcinolone acetate 4 mg/0.1 mL [1 mL]) is controversial.

SURGERY/OTHER PROCEDURES
Pars Plana vitrectomy is beneficial if visual acuity at presentation is light perception or worse according to the endophthalmitis vitrectomy study in cataract surgery-associated cases. Early vitrectomy can decrease the bacterial burden and remove toxins and necrotic tissue from the eye.

IN-PATIENT CONSIDERATIONS
Initial Stabilization
Post-operative endophthalmitis can be treated on an outpatient basis.

Admission Criteria
Hospital admission may become necessary out of social considerations or in monocular patients.

 ONGOING CARE

FOLLOW-UP RECOMMENDATIONS
Re-administration of the intravitreal antibiotics with or without vitrectomy should be considered if the condition of the patient is worsening 48 h after initiation.

Patient Monitoring
The patient should be followed on a daily basis by the treating ophthalmologist.

PROGNOSIS
- Visual prognosis of traumatic endophthalmitis is worse than postoperative endophthalmitis, in part, because the spectrum of involved microorganisms and the associated direct tissue damage.
- After elective cataract surgery, culture-proven infected eyes achieved visual acuity of 20/40 or better 50% of the time and 20/400 or better 85% of the time, while in a recent combined series of post-traumatic endophthalmitis, only 30% of eyes were 20/400 or better. In the endophthalmitis vitrectomy study, 74% of patients had visual recovery of 20/100 or better.
- The outcome of *B. cereus* endophthalmitis is almost uniformly poor.

COMPLICATIONS
Loss of vision due to a direct effect of the inflammatory response to the retina and tissue necrosis is the most common. Retinal detachment, secondary glaucoma, and phthisis can follow.

REFERENCE
1. Endophthalmitis Study Group, European Society of Cataract & Refractive Surgeons. Prophylaxis of postoperative endophthalmitis following cataract surgery: Results of the ESCRS multicenter study and identification of risk factors. *J Cataract Refract Surg* 2007;33:978–988.

ADDITIONAL READING
- Endophthalmitis Vitrectomy Study Group. Results of the Endophthalmitis Vitrectomy Study. A randomized trial of immediate vitrectomy and of intravenous antibiotics for the treatment of postoperative bacterial endophthalmitis. *Arch Ophthalmol*. 1995;113:1479–1496.
- Read RW. Endophthalmitis. In: Yanoff M, Duker JS, eds. *Ophthalmology*, 3rd ed. York: Mosby Elsevier, 2009:815–819.
- Sternberg P, Martin DF. Management of endophthalmitis in the post-endophthalmitis vitrectomy study era. *Arch Ophthalmol* 2001;119: 754–755.

CODES

ICD9
- 360.00 Purulent endophthalmitis, unspecified
- 360.01 Acute endophthalmitis
- 360.19 Other endophthalmitis

CLINICAL PEARLS
- Early recognition is crucial for visual recovery.
- Intravitreal aminoglycosides have been associated with macular infarction.
- PCR of vitreous samples can be helpful especially in cases of culture negative endophthalmitis.
- Penetrating ocular injuries require tetanus prophylaxis if immunization is not up to date.
- Judicious use of steroids is recommended whenever a fungus is suspected.

E

EPIDEMIC PLEURODYNIA (BORNHOLM DISEASE)

Alejandro Restrepo
Eleftherios Mylonakis

 BASICS

DESCRIPTION
Epidemic pleurodynia is an acute, febrile infection that is characterized by the abrupt onset of chest or abdominal pain and spasms. It is also known as epidemic myalgia and/or Bornholm disease (named after the Danish island Bornholm) or devil's grip.

EPIDEMIOLOGY (3)
Incidence
- Usually occurs in small or large epidemics, and multiple family members develop symptoms.
- Symptoms of the other family members can start at the same time or in succession, separated by several days.
- Enteroviral infections (coxsackievirus groups A and B, echoviruses, and the newer numbered enteroviruses) are common causes, especially in late summer and early fall.
- Because the peak incidence of enteroviral illness coincides with the football and soccer seasons, it has been postulated that close contact either on the playing field or in the locker room facilitates person-to-person transmission. Another explanation is that water and common containers become contaminated through direct oral contact by infected individuals and serve as a source of virus.
- Intense physical exertion during the incubation period may result in more severe symptomatic infection, making illness among athletes more readily identifiable.
- Children have milder disease than adults.
- Infections can occur in neonates (1)

GENERAL PREVENTION
- Specific control measures recommended to avoid outbreaks include the following:
  – Avoid oral contact
  – Use of disposable cups or individual drinking containers
  – Use of ice packs rather than ice cubes from a team ice chest for injuries
  – Provision of education and information for students, school nurses, and coaching staff

PATHOPHYSIOLOGY
Probably results from direct viral invasion of thoracic and abdominal muscles

ETIOLOGY
- As its name suggests, the disease often occurs in localized epidemics; it is generally caused by coxsackievirus B.
- Other viruses, such as echoviruses 1, 6, 9, 16, and 19, and group A coxsackieviruses 4, 6, 9, and 10 have been associated (2).

 DIAGNOSIS

HISTORY
- Usually has no prodrome and begins with the abrupt onset of fever and spasms of pleuritic chest or upper abdominal pain.
- Fever is usually up to 38.0–39.5°C, peaks within an hour after the onset of paroxysms, and subsides when pain resolves and is associated with headaches.
- Chest pain is more frequent in adults, and abdominal pain is more common in children. Paroxysms of severe, sharp, knifelike and rib pain usually last 15–30 minutes and are associated with diaphoresis and tachypnea. The involved muscles are tender to palpation, and a pleural rub may be detected.
- Periumbilical pain and pain in the lower abdominal quadrants can occur, especially among children.
- Cases of pain limited to the neck and limbs have been reported.
- Illness lasts 4–6 days in most of the cases (2).

PHYSICAL EXAM
- Pain can be elicited by pressure on the involved muscles in most cases.
- Swelling of the muscles is seen or felt in some cases.

DIAGNOSTIC TESTS & INTERPRETATION
Lab
- The white blood cell count is usually normal (1).
- Virologic diagnosis can be achieved by isolating group B coxsackievirus from throat washings or feces, or by demonstrating an increase in antibody titers.

Imaging
Chest radiographs are normal, although, rarely, small pleural effusions can occur.

DIFFERENTIAL DIAGNOSIS
The differential diagnosis includes pneumonia, pulmonary infarct, myocardial ischemia, pulmonary embolism, herpes zoster, or any cause of acute abdominal pain, particularly acute appendicitis or renal colic (see Section chapters I, "Pleuritic and Chest Pain and Fever" and "Abdominal Pain and Fever").

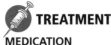 **TREATMENT**

MEDICATION
First Line
- Administration of nonsteroidal anti-inflammatory agents, and application of heat to the affected muscles has been seen beneficial.
- Opiate analgesics are indicated in severe cases.

ADDITIONAL TREATMENT
General Measures
Application of heat to the affected muscles (2).

 ONGOING CARE

FOLLOW-UP RECOMMENDATIONS
Based on clinical and recurrence of the symptoms

PROGNOSIS
- Illness usually lasts for 4–7 days and is rarely fatal.
- Relapses can occur.

COMPLICATIONS
- Symptoms resolve in a few days (usually 4–6 days; range, 12 hours to 3 weeks), and recurrences are rare.
- Aseptic meningitis and orchitis can occur (each in fewer than 10% of cases), while pericarditis and pneumonia are even less common.

REFERENCES
1. Tang JW, Bendig JW, Ossuetta I. Vertical transmission of human echovirus 11 at the time of Bornholm disease in late pregnancy. *Pediatr Infect Dis J* 2005;24(1):88–89.
2. Modlin JF. Coxsackieviruses, echoviruses, newer enteroviruses, and parechoviruses. In: Mandell GL, Bennett JE, Dolin R, eds. *Principles and practice of infectious diseases*, 7th ed. New York: Churchill Livingstone, 2009:2356–2357.
3. Ikeda RM, Kondracki SF, Drabkin PD, et al. Pleurodynia among football players at a high school. An outbreak associated with coxsackievirus B1. *JAMA* 1993;270:2205–2006.

 CODES

ICD9
074.1 Epidemic pleurodynia

E

EPIDIDYMITIS

Renato Finkelstein
Matthew E. Falagas

 BASICS

DESCRIPTION
- An inflammatory reaction of the epididymis due to various infectious agents, but also due to uncommon noninfectious diseases or local trauma.
- Epididymitis may be classified as acute and chronic, the latter characterized by a 3-month or longer history of symptoms.

EPIDEMIOLOGY
Incidence
- Epididymitis is the fifth most common urologic diagnosis in men aged 18–50 years (1). The majority of patients are 20–39 years old (43%), followed by those 40–59 years old (29%) (2).
- Epididymitis accounts for more loss of man-hours in the US military than any other urologic diagnosis (3).
- In a review of 121 patients with epididymitis in an ambulatory setting, a bimodal distribution was noted with the peak incidence occurring in men 16–30 years of age and 51–70 years of age (4).
- Increased frequency in homosexual men who engage in unprotected anal intercourse.

RISK FACTORS
- Bacteriuria
- Sexual activity
- Strenuous physical activity
- Bicycle or motorcycle riding
- Prolonged periods of sitting (e.g., during travel, sedentary job)
- Patients >35 years and prepuberty
- Recent urinary tract surgery or instrumentation
- Prostatic obstruction (elderly) and posterior urethral valves or meatal stenosis (prepuberty)

GENERAL PREVENTION
Prevention of sexually transmitted diseases (STDs) by abstaining from sexual intercourse, or being in a long-term mutually monogamous relationship with a partner who has been tested and is known to be uninfected. Latex condoms, when used consistently and correctly, can reduce the risk of transmission of STDs.

PATHOPHYSIOLOGY
- Retrograde ascent of pathogens.
- High voiding pressures might predispose to epididymitis by promoting urethrovasal reflux. In about half of the patients voiding dysfunction is caused by proximal urethral strictures, bladder neck abnormalities, and detrusor external sphincter dyssynergia (5).

ETIOLOGY
- Infective
  – Common specific clinical conditions
    ○ STDs: The most common cause among young men. Common: *Neisseria gonorrhoeae* or *Chlamydia trachomatis* (peak incidence between ages 14–35) (6). Less common: *Ureaplasma urealyticum*
    ○ Associated with urinary tract infection – Common: *Escherichia coli*, *Klebsiella pneumoniae*, *Proteus* spp., *Pseudomonas aeruginosa*. Uncommon: *Salmonella* spp., Staphylococci, Streptococci
  – Nonspecific and uncommon clinical conditions
    ○ Bacterial: *Mycobacterium tuberculosis*, *Brucella* spp., *Nocardia* spp. Several iatrogenic cases of epididymitis after Calmette-Guérin bacillus therapy for transitional cell carcinoma of the bladder have been reported
    ○ Fungal: *Blastomyces dermatitidis*, *Histoplasma capsulatum*, *Candida* spp.
    ○ Parasitic: *Schistosoma haematobium*, *Wuchereria bancrofti*
- Noninfective
  – Vasculitides: Behçet's disease, Polyarteritis nodosa, Henoch-Schönlein purpura
  – Drugs: Amiodarone
  – Trauma
- Idiopathic

COMMONLY ASSOCIATED CONDITIONS
Orchitis

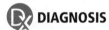 **DIAGNOSIS**

HISTORY
- Gradual onset of scrotal pain and swelling, often developing over several days (as opposed to hours such as in testicular torsion).
- Usually unilateral.
- Pain is localized posterior to the testis and occasionally radiates to the lower abdomen.
- Pain is often unilateral but it can spread to the adjacent testis.
- Symptoms of lower urinary tract infection, such as fever, frequency, urgency, hematuria, and dysuria, may be present.
- Fever and chills (25% of adult patients but in up to 71% of children).
- Preceding urethral discharge is an important diagnostic clue that epididymitis is caused by STDs.
- In chronic epididymitis the patient has a long-standing history of constant or intermittent pain (>6 weeks).

PHYSICAL EXAM
- Urethral discharge may be apparent on inspection or stripping of the urethra.
- Localized epididymal tenderness progressing to testicular swelling and tenderness.
- Normal cremasteric reflex (i.e., ipsilateral cremasteric muscle contraction producing unilateral testis elevation).
- Pain relief with testicular elevation (Prehn's sign).
- The scrotum is not usually swollen.
- May progress to reactive hydrocele and scrotal wall erythema.

DIAGNOSTIC TESTS & INTERPRETATION
Lab
Initial lab tests
- Gram stain and culture of swabbed urethral discharge may detect urethritis. Avoid bladder emptying <2 h of taking urethral tests.
- If urethritis is diagnosed the patients should be also evaluated for other STDs.
- Urinalysis and urine culture, preferably on first-void urine samples.
- C-reactive protein levels and erythrocyte sedimentation rate are useful in differentiating from testicular torsion.
- The presence of leukocyte esterase and white blood cells is suggestive of urethritis.
- Polymerase chain reaction (PCR) assays for *C. trachomatis* and *N. gonorrhoeae* should be performed on urethral swab or urine specimens.
- Blood culture may be diagnostic when epididymitis is associated with urosepsis.

Follow-Up & Special Considerations
- Cultures, histopathologic examination, and PCR assays (if available) should be performed in all surgically removed tissue specimens.
- Brucellar epididymitis is diagnosed by blood cultures and serologic tests.

Imaging
Initial approach
Color Doppler ultrasonography particularly to rule out testicular torsion. An increased Doppler wave pulsation (increased blood flow) suggests epididymitis.

Follow-Up & Special Considerations
If tuberculosis is considered, chest X-rays and appropriate urine cultures should be performed. Scrotal draining sinuses, if present, should also be cultured.

DIFFERENTIAL DIAGNOSIS
- Testicular torsion
- Neoplasms (rarely)

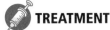 # TREATMENT

MEDICATION

First Line

- Medical management is appropriate for most patients with bacterial epididymitis.
- Empiric treatment of epididymitis should be initiated based on likely pathogens, before laboratory testing is complete.
- Bed rest, scrotal elevation and support, and analgesics are recommended, and nonsteroidal anti-inflammatory drugs (NSAIDs) may be helpful (7).
- Empiric antibiotic selection should be based on age, sexual history, recent instrumentation or catheterization, and local knowledge of antibiotic sensitivities of the major sexual and urinary pathogens.
- Empiric therapy for sexually transmitted epididymitis consists of treatment for *N. gonorrhoeae* and *C. trachomatis* infections with a one-time dose of ceftriaxone, 250 mg i.m., followed by oral doxycycline, 100 mg twice a day for 10 days. A single 1 g dose of azithromycin is an alternative to doxycycline, which may improve compliance. For acute epididymitis most likely caused by enteric organisms or for patients allergic to cephalosporins and/or tetracyclines, ofloxacin 300 mg orally twice a day for 10 days or levofloxacin 500 mg orally once daily for 10 days may also be given (6).
- For acute epididymitis most likely caused by urinary pathogens the use of fluoroquinolones (ofloxacin 300 mg orally twice a day for 10 days, or levofloxacin 500 mg orally once daily for 10 days or ciprofloxacin 500 mg twice daily for 10 days) was shown to be effective (6).

ALERT

HIV Infection: Same regimens as those who are HIV-negative. Fungi and mycobacteria, however, are more likely to occur in these patients.

SURGERY/OTHER PROCEDURES

Surgery may be necessary for the management of complications of acute epididymal infections such as testicular infarction, abscess, or pyocele of the scrotum.

IN-PATIENT CONSIDERATIONS

Admission Criteria

In severe infections with systemic disturbance or features suggesting bacteremia, initial intravenous therapy is indicated.

 # ONGOING CARE

PATIENT EDUCATION

- Patients who have acute epididymitis caused by *N. gonorrhoeae* or *C. trachomatis* should be instructed to refer sex partners for evaluation and treatment if their contact with the index patient was within the 60 days preceding onset of the patient's symptoms.
- Patients should be instructed to avoid sexual intercourse until they and their sex partners are cured (i.e., therapy is completed and patient and partners are without symptoms).

COMPLICATIONS

- Bacteremia
- Testicular infarction
- Scrotal abscess
- Pyocele
- Chronic draining scrotal sinus
- Chronic epididymitis
- Infertility

Pediatric Considerations

- Differential diagnosis with testicular torsion is particularly important.
- Epididymitis diagnosed in only 15% of 113 consecutive cases of painful scrotum at a children's hospital in Canada (8).
- In most cases a specific etiology is not found.

REFERENCES

1. Collins MM, Stafford RS, O'Leary MP, et al. How common is prostatitis? A national survey of physician visits. *J Urol* 1998;159:1224–1228.
2. Tracy CR, Costabile RA. The changing face of epididymitis from 1965 to 2005. Abstract presentation, 53rd James C. Kimbrough Urological Seminar, Savannah, GA, 2006.
3. Moore CA, Lockett BL, Lennox KW, et al. Prednisone in the treatment of acute epididymitis: A cooperative study. *J Urol* 1971;106:578.
4. Kaver I, Matzkin H, Braf ZF. Epididymo-orchitis: A retrospective study of 121 patients. *J Fam Pract* 1990;30(5):548–552.
5. Thind P, Brandt B, Kristensen JK. Assessment of voiding dysfunction in men with acute epididymitis. *Urol Int* 1992;48:320–322.
6. Workowski KA, Berman S. Centers for Disease Control and Prevention (CDC). Sexually transmitted diseases treatment guidelines, 2010. *MMWR Recomm Rep* 2010;59(RR-12):1–110.
7. Luzzi GA, O'Brien TS. Acute epididymitis. *BJU Int* 2001;87:747–755.
8. Anderson PAM, Giacomantonio JM. The acutely painful scrotum in children: Review of 113 consecutive cases. *Can Med Assoc J* 1985;132:1153–1155.

ADDITIONAL READING

- Trojian TH, Lishnak TS, Heiman D. Epididymitis and orchitis: An overview. *Am Fam Physician* 2009;79:583–587.
- Tracy CR, Steers WD, Costabile R. Diagnosis and management of epididymitis. *Urol Clin North Am* 2008;35:101–108.

 # CODES

ICD9

- 604.90 Orchitis and epididymitis, unspecified
- 604.99 Other orchitis, epididymitis, and epididymo-orchitis, without mention of abscess

CLINICAL PEARLS

- Among sexually active men aged <35 years, acute epididymitis is most frequently caused by *C. trachomatis* or *N. gonorrhoeae*.
- When not related to STDs, epididymitis is generally a complication of urinary tract infection (UTI) and is caused by the Enterobacteriaceae flora (e.g., *E. coli*).
- Testicular torsion is the most important differential diagnosis. If the diagnosis remains unclear and testicular torsion is suspected, surgical exploration of the scrotum is warranted.

E

EPIGLOTTITIS

Petros I. Rafailidis
Matthew E. Falagas

 BASICS

DESCRIPTION
Rapidly progressive infection of the epiglottis and adjacent supraglottic structures.

EPIDEMIOLOGY
Incidence
- The incidence has decreased dramatically in countries with widespread use of vaccination against Haemophilus influenzae type b (1)[A].
- 0.9–3.1 per 100,000 adults general population.
- The mean age of a patient with epiglottitis is 44.9 years (2).

RISK FACTORS
- Age under 4 years old
- In the vaccination era mean age of pediatric patients has doubled approximately to 11.6 years
- Unvaccinated children
- Immunodeficiency
- Post-splenectomy
- Nonimmune adults!

GENERAL PREVENTION
- Immunization against *H. influenzae* type b (1)[A].
- If the patient with *H. influenzae* epiglottitis has household contacts that include an unvaccinated child under age 4, rifampin prophylaxis given once daily for 4 days in a dose of 20 mg/kg/d (maximum of 600 mg/d) by mouth is recommended for all members of the household and the patient to eradicate the carriage of *H. influenzae*.

ETIOLOGY
- *H. influenzae* type b is still responsible for the majority of pediatric cases (more than 90%) and is frequently isolated from the blood. In adult patients, blood cultures are positive in about 25% of cases.
- Other pathogens isolated from the pharynx of adults with epiglottitis include the following:
  – *Haemophilus parainfluenzae*
  – *Streptococcus pneumoniae*
  – Group A *Streptococcus*
  – *Staphylococcus aureus*
- In immunosuppressed patients other pathogens such as *Candida* spp. and even *Aspergillus* spp. may be culprits.
- Viral infections such as varicella zoster, infectious mononucleosis, HIV and herpes simplex infections can be complicated by epiglottitis.

 DIAGNOSIS

HISTORY
- Symptom onset is usually acute.
- Young children usually present within 24 hours of the onset of symptoms with fever, dysphonia, dysphagia, and irritability.
- Fever may not be present in adults.

PHYSICAL EXAM
- Respiratory distress, inspiratory stridor, and a muffled (like having hot food in the mouth) voice may occur.
- Up to one-third of pediatric patients are in shock, with cyanosis and loss of consciousness on admission.
- The patient prefers to sit leaning forward with accompanying extension of the upper limbs.
- There is frequently drooling of oral secretions.
- The direct examination of the pharynx in a child, using a tongue blade, should not be attempted because of the possibility of laryngospasm and complete airway obstruction.
- Adolescents and adults may have a less fulminant presentation; sore throat is the most prominent symptom without signs of pharyngitis.
- In the adult patient neck tenderness and tenderness over the hyoid bone (3) may also point to the diagnosis.

DIAGNOSTIC TESTS & INTERPRETATION
Lab
- It cannot be emphasized enough that once there is a possibility that a pediatric patient has epiglottitis, diagnostic testing should be performed after securing the airway.
- Moderate leukocytosis with a left shift.
- Positive cultures of blood and epiglottis.

Imaging
- A lateral neck film may show an enlarged epiglottis (the thumb sign), ballooning of the hypopharynx, and normal subglottis structures.
- Radiography should not be performed unless physicians who are able to manage acute airway obstruction are present.
- In the adult patient the use of ultrasound to depict the swollen epiglottis has been used occasionally in emergency departments in adult patients (4).
- A chest X-ray film may show pneumonia or atelectasis in up to 50% of cases.

Diagnostic Procedures/Other
- The patient should be transferred to an operating room for visualization of the epiglottis with a fiberoptic laryngoscope after all preparations for immediate airway control.
- The diagnosis is established by visualizing an edematous "cherry-red" epiglottis.

Pathological Findings
Edema of the epiglottis and infiltration with leucocytes. Abscess may be present.

DIFFERENTIAL DIAGNOSIS
- Croup syndrome
  – Usually has a more gradual onset.
  – Is more frequently preceded by an upper respiratory tract infection.
  – Involves younger children (ages 3 months to 3 years).
  – Has a viral etiology.
  – Children with croup do not have prominent drooling or dysphagia and are more likely to lie supine.
- Diphtheria
  – A pseudomembrane is visible in the pharynx.
  – Smear and culture of the membrane demonstrate typical gram-positive rods.
- Allergic laryngeal edema
  – Patients usually appear less toxic and have no fever.
- Foreign-body aspiration
- Lingual tonsillitis
- Peritonsillar abscess, retropharyngeal abscess

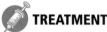 **TREATMENT**

MEDICATION
First Line
- Acute epiglottitis constitutes a medical emergency, as airway obstruction may occur suddenly.
- Observation without intubation of children with epiglottitis is not recommended because mortality may exceed 25% with a watchful waiting approach.
- An uncuffed endotracheal or nasotracheal tube should be inserted, and the child must be monitored in an intensive care unit (5).
- Tracheostomy (or needle cricothyrotomy as an interim measure) should be performed if an intact airway cannot be maintained otherwise. In the adult patient a less aggressive treatment approach is elected at times (intubation in some patients only) (6,7). If such an approach is followed, one must remember that the presence of respiratory distress, stridor, muffled voice, or laryngoscopic evidence of less than 50% visualization of the vocal cords are factors that have been associated with the need of securing the airway (8).

- Intravenous antibiotic therapy directed at *H. influenzae* should be given.
  - Cefotaxime 100–200 mg/kg/d in 4 divided doses (maximum adult daily dose: 12 g)
  - Ceftriaxone 50–100 mg/kg/d in 1 or 2 divided doses (maximum adult daily dose: 2 g)
  - Ampicillin/sulbactam 200–300 mg/kg/d (of ampicillin) in 4 divided doses (maximum adult daily dose: 12 g)
- Duration of therapy is 10 days.

Second Line
Due to the potential for toxicity the use of chloramphenicol (50–100 mg/kg/d in 4 divided doses), in addition to ampicillin, has become much less frequent.

ADDITIONAL TREATMENT
Additional Therapies
There are no controlled data to support the use of corticosteroids or epinephrine for the treatment of acute epiglottitis.

SURGERY/OTHER PROCEDURES
Tracheostomy, if intubation is not possible.

IN-PATIENT CONSIDERATIONS
Initial Stabilization
Airway patency maintenance is the top priority.

Admission Criteria
All patients with the diagnosis of epiglottitis should be admitted.

IV Fluids
Frequently needed. Don't try to establish intravenous access in a child before the airway is secured.

Nursing
Do not cause anxiety to the child.

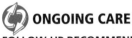 ONGOING CARE

FOLLOW-UP RECOMMENDATIONS
- Patients with epiglottitis usually improve rapidly, that is, within 12–48 hours after starting appropriate antimicrobial therapy.
- Patients can be extubated once they are afebrile, alert, clinically improved, and have laryngoscopic evidence of resolution of edema.

Patient Monitoring
In the adult patient, who is elected not to proceed to intubation, monitoring in the ICU is mandatory.

PROGNOSIS
- Depends on whether the airway is secured at an early stage. Hypoxia resulting from airway obstruction is the key determinant of prognosis.
- A mortality rate of 0.89% has been reported in the US.
- Extremely rare, a recurrence may occur.

COMPLICATIONS
- Complete airway obstruction with resulting hypoxia/anoxia of many organs (anoxemic encephalopathy is the most severe complication).
- Rarely, *H. influenzae* bacteremia has been associated with metastatic infections such as meningitis and arthritis.
- Iatrogenic complications (mostly associated with intubation)
  - Aspiration
  - Endotracheal tube dislodgment
  - Tracheal erosion
  - Pneumomediastinum
  - Pneumothorax
  - Pulmonary edema

REFERENCES

1. Adams WG, Deaver KA, Cochi SL, et al. Decline of childhood *Haemophilus influenzae* type b (Hib) disease in the Hib vaccine era. *JAMA* 1993;269:221–226.
2. Shah RK, Stocks C. Epiglottitis in the United States: National trends, variances, prognosis, and management. *Laryngoscope* 2010;120:1256–1262.
3. Ehara H. Tenderness over the hyoid bone can indicate epiglottitis in adults. *J Am Board Fam Med* 2006;19:517–520.
4. Bektas F, Soyuncu S, Yigit O, et al. Sonographic diagnosis of epiglottal enlargement. *Emerg Med J* 2010;27:224–225.
5. Acevedo JL, Lander L, Choi S, et al. Airway management in pediatric epiglottitis: A national perspective. *Otolaryngol Head Neck Surg* 2009;140:548–551.
6. Mayo-Smith MF, Spinale JW, Donskey CJ, et al. Acute epiglottitis. An 18-year experience in Rhode Island. *Chest* 1995;108:1640–1647.
7. Park KW, Darvish A, Lowenstein E. Airway management for adult patients with acute epiglottitis: A 12-year experience at an academic medical center (1984–1995). *Anesthesiology* 1998;88:254–261.
8. Katori H, Tsukuda M. Acute epiglottitis: Analysis of factors associated with airway intervention. *J Laryngol Otol* 2005;119:967–972.

ADDITIONAL READING

- Friedman M, Toriumi DM, Grybauskas V, et al. A plea for uniformity in the staging and management of adult epiglottitis. *Ear Nose Throat J* 1988;67:873–874, 876–877, 880.
- Ng HL, Sin LM, Li MF, et al. Acute epiglottitis in adults: A retrospective review of 106 patients in Hong Kong. *Emerg Med J* 2008;25:253–255.

 CODES

ICD9
- 041.5 Hemophilus influenzae (H. influenzae) infection in conditions classified elsewhere and of unspecified site
- 464.30 Acute epiglottitis without mention of obstruction

CLINICAL PEARLS
- While this was mainly a childhood disease, adults are the main victims in the post-vaccine era!
- A small percentage of vaccinated children may still be afflicted by the disease.
- Physicians capable of maintaining the airway should be summoned without hesitation!
- Don't make the child cry!
- In splenectomized patients keep their vaccination status against *H. influenzae* up to date!

ERYTHEMA NODOSUM

Anastasios M. Kapaskelis
Petros I. Rafailidis
Matthew E. Falagas

 BASICS

DESCRIPTION
Erythema nodosum is the commonest type of panniculitis. Its clinical manifestation consists of inflammatory, tender, nodular lesions. The lesions are mainly located on the lower extremities.

EPIDEMIOLOGY
Incidence
- Peak incidence occurs between the ages of 18 and 34 years (1).
- Annual incidence rate of biopsy-proven erythema nodosum in hospitalized patients aged 14 years and older was estimated as 52 cases per million of persons (2).
- Most common in females.

Prevalence
- 2.4 per 1000 population per year.
- Seasonal clustering of sarcoidosis that presents with erythema nodosum has been reported, as well. Peak clustering was observed in August, September, and October (3).

RISK FACTORS
Genetics
Specific types of human leukocyte antigens, HLA-B8 and HLA-DR3, were found to be associated with the presence of erythema nodosum in sarcoidosis (4).

PATHOPHYSIOLOGY
Erythema nodosum may be regarded as a type IV delayed hypersensitivity response to various antigens (5).

ETIOLOGY
Various etiologic factors have been associated with erythema nodosum:

- Bacterial infections: Streptococcal infections (Group A beta-hemolytic *Streptococcus*) are the commonest infectious causes of erythema nodosum, mycobacterial infections (Hansen's bacillus, tuberculosis), brucellosis, cat-scratch disease, *Yersinia enterocolitica*. Syphilis, as well as infections due to *Salmonella* spp. (*S. enteritidis* and *S. typhi*), *Mycoplasma* spp., *Chlamydia* spp. (including *C. psittaci*, *C. pneumoniae*, and *C. trachomatis*), *Neisseria meningitidis*, *N. gonorrhoeae*, *Francisella tularensis*, and *Rickettsiae* spp. may also cause erythema nodosum (6)

- Viral infections: CMV, EBV, HIV, HBV, HSV
- Fungal infections: Coccidioidomycosis, aspergillosis, histoplasmosis
- Protozoal infections: Amebiasis, toxoplasmosis, giardiasis
- Drugs: Sulphonamides, sulfones, bromides, oral contraceptives
- Malignancies: Hodgkin's disease, non-Hodgkin's lymphoma, leukemia, pancreatic carcinoma, colon adenocarcinoma
- Other pathological conditions: Sarcoidosis, Adamantiades–Behçet's disease, Crohn's disease, ulcerative colitis, Sweet's syndrome, lupus erythematosus, Sjögren's syndrome
- Pregnancy
- Idiopathic (probably the most common cause)

DIAGNOSIS

HISTORY
- Careful medical history-taking is of major importance
- Sudden onset of tender, erythematous nodules and raised plaques commonly located on shins, ankles, and knees
- Erythema nodosum is often accompanied by fever of ~3–39°C, fatigue, and arthralgias
- Self-limiting within a few weeks

PHYSICAL EXAM
- Erythematous, tender red nodules and raised plaques located on the shins, ankles, knees, and rarely on the extensor aspects of the arms, neck, or face.
- At first, the nodules have a bright red color and are raised, but in a few days, they become flat and have a livid red or purplish color. Finally, they become yellow or greenish and often have an appearance like a deep bruise ("erythema contusiformis"). The nodules heal without atrophy or scarring. Ulceration is never observed.

DIAGNOSTIC TESTS & INTERPRETATION
Lab
- Complete blood count
- Erythrocyte sedimentation rate
- Antistreptolysin O titer
- Streptococcal rapid antigen test

- Polymerase chain reaction to detect streptococcal DNA
- Throat culture
- Urinalysis
- Intradermal tuberculin test

Imaging
Chest roentgenogram (tuberculosis, bilateral hilar lymphadenopathy [Lofgren's syndrome])

Diagnostic Procedures/Other
- Consider stool culture and examination for parasites or their ova if abdominal pain, bloating, or diarrhea
- Punch biopsy of the skin
- Transbronchial lung biopsy for histologic confirmation of sarcoidosis
- Biopsy of the gastrocnemius muscle (because myopathy is commonly encountered in Lofgren's syndrome)
- Interferon-γ release assay
- Colonoscopy may be performed to rule out inflammatory bowel disease

Pathological Findings
- Histopathologic hallmark is the presence of "Miescher's radial granulomas." It consists of small, well-defined nodular aggregations of small histiocytes around a central cleft (7).
- Infiltration of polymorphonuclear leukocytes is also another histopathologic finding.

DIFFERENTIAL DIAGNOSIS
- Erythema induratum of Bazin:
  - Histopathologic differences: The erythema induratum of Bazin is mainly lobular panniculitis, whereas erythema nodosum is mainly septal panniculitis.
  - Clinical differences: The nodules of erythema induratum of Bazin are mainly located on the posterior surface of the legs, they are more persistent and ulceration may also be observed.
- Cutaneous lesions of superficial thrombophlebitis:
  - The lesions are mainly located on the sides of the legs and are hard, irregular, and fibrotic cords or plaques.
  - The biopsy reveals little or no evidence of inflammatory infiltrate and a more vasculitic rather than panniculitic process.
- Lyme disease
- Causes of panniculitis (i.e. systemic lupus erythematosus [SLE], acute pancreatitis)

TREATMENT

MEDICATION

First Line
- Erythema nodosum is self-limiting for the majority of patients over the duration of a few weeks.
- Treatment should be specified according to the underlying disease.
- Symptomatic treatment may include nonsteroidal anti-inflammatory drugs (NSAIDs): Indomethacin 100–150 mg daily, naproxen 500 mg daily (8). Don't use NSAIDs if inflammatory bowel disease is the cause.
- Steroids can be used in severe cases if infectious causes or cancer have been ruled out.
- Prednisone at a dose of 1 mg/kg tapered over several days.
- Potassium iodide: The maximum dose for adults is 300 mg three times daily. However, severe secondary hyperthyroidism may occur.
- Hydroxychloroquine (particularly for chronic erythema nodosum; 200 mg twice a day) (9).
- Colchicine (useful in erythema nodosum associated with Adamantiades–Behçet's disease; 1–2 mg daily, divided in 2 doses).
- Erythema nodosum leprosum: There is some evidence regarding the benefit of thalidomide and clofazimine. Moreover, significantly fewer minor adverse events were found to be associated with a low-dose thalidomide regimen compared to a high-dose thalidomide regimen (10).

Second Line
Infliximab: In erythema nodosum associated with inflammatory bowel disease.

ADDITIONAL TREATMENT

General Measures
- Bed rest
- Regular elevation
- Compression (11)

 ONGOING CARE

PROGNOSIS
- The majority of the cases resolve within 3–4 weeks.
- Relapse is rare, however more common in idiopathic cases of erythema nodosum as well as in erythema nodosum associated with upper respiratory tract infections (either streptococcal or non-streptococcal) (2).

COMPLICATIONS
- Optic nerve neuritis has bee reported in a patient during an acute episode of erythema nodosum (12).

REFERENCES

1. Bohn S, Büchner S, Itin P. Erythema nodosum: 112 cases. Epidemiology, clinical aspects and histopathology. *Schweiz Med Wochenschr* 1997;127:1168–1176.
2. García-Porra C, González-Gay MA, Vázquez-Caruncho M, et al. Erythema nodosum: Etiologic and predictive factors in a defined population. *Arthritis Rheum* 2000;43:584–592.
3. Wilsher ML. Seasonal clustering of sarcoidosis presenting with erythema nodosum. *Eur Respir J* 1998;12:1197–1199.
4. Smith MJ, Turton CW, Mitchell DN, et al. Association of HLA B8 with spontaneous resolution in sarcoidosis. *Thorax* 1981;36: 296–298.
5. Requena L, Yus ES. Panniculitis. Part I. Mostly septal panniculitis. *J Am Acad Dermatol* 2001;45:163–183; quiz 184–186.
6. Schwartz RA, Nervi SJ. Erythema nodosum: A sign of systemic disease. *Am Fam Physician* 2007;75: 695–700.
7. Sánchez Yus E, Sanz Vico MD, de Diego V. Miescher's radial granuloma. A characteristic marker of erythema nodosum. *Am J Dermatopathol* 1989;11:434–442.
8. Ubogy Z, Persellin RH. Suppression of erythema nodosum by indomethacin. *Acta Derm Venereol* 1982;62:265–266.
9. Jarrett P, Goodfield MJ. Hydroxychloroquine and chronic erythema nodosum. *Br J Dermatol* 1996; 134:373.
10. Van Veen NH, Lockwood DN, Van Brakel WH, et al. Interventions for erythema nodosum leprosum. A Cochrane review. *Lepr Rev* 2009;80:355–372.
11. Gilchrist H, Patterson JW. Erythema nodosum and erythema induratum (nodular vasculitis): Diagnosis and management. *Dermatol Ther* 2010;23:320–327.
12. Tanaka M, Inoue K, Yamasaki Y, Hatano H. Erythema nodosum complicated by retrobulbar optic nerve neuritis. *Clin Exp Dermatol* 2001;26:306–307.

ADDITIONAL READING

- Gheith O, Al-Otaibi T, Tawab KA, et al. Erythema nodosum in renal transplant recipients: Multiple cases and review of literature. *Transpl Infect Dis* 2010;12:164–168.

 CODES

ICD9
- 695.2 Erythema nodosum
- 729.30 Panniculitis, unspecified site

CLINICAL PEARLS
- A meticulous medical history-taking is of major importance in the management of erythema nodosum.
- Many of the etiologic factors are infections.
- Treatment of erythema nodosum should be directed according to the underlying disease (when known).
- The majority of the erythema nodosum cases resolve within 3–4 weeks without relapse or persistence.

E

ESOPHAGITIS, INFECTIVE

Paschalis Vergidis
Matthew E. Falagas

 BASICS

DESCRIPTION
Infection of the esophagus by a variety of fungi, viruses, and bacteria

EPIDEMIOLOGY
Incidence
- Infectious esophagitis is rare in individuals whose immune system is normal but is frequent in immunocompromised patients, in individuals who receive medications that affect the normal esophageal microflora or the immune status, and in the presence of abnormalities that delay the clearance of the esophageal lumen.
- Primary cytomegalovirus (CMV) infections are common in preschool children and young adults. However, they cause esophagitis very rarely in immunocompetent persons.

RISK FACTORS
- Immune defects
- Medications that may alter immune status or esophageal microflora
- Esophageal anatomic abnormalities or motility disorders

GENERAL PREVENTION
- Avoidance of risk factors, if possible
- Appropriate antiretroviral treatment to decrease the level of immunosuppression in HIV-infected patients

ETIOLOGY
- The most common causes of infectious esophagitis in immunocompromised and immunocompetent individuals are one or a combination of the following three organisms: *Candida* spp., herpes simplex virus (HSV), and CMV.
- Most cases of *Candida* esophagitis are caused by *C. albicans*. Symptomatic diseases due to *C. glabrata* and *C. krusei* have also been described.
- Other pathogens that may rarely cause infectious esophagitis are the following:
  – *Aspergillus* species
  – *Histoplasma* species
  – *Blastomyces dermatitidis*
  – Varicella zoster virus
  – Epstein–Barr virus
  – Human papillomavirus
  – *Mycobacterium tuberculosis* and *Mycobacterium avium*
  – Normal oropharyngeal flora (very rarely) such as *Staphylococcus aureus*, *Staphylococcus epidermidis*, *Streptococcus viridans*, and *Bacillus* species
  – Acute HIV infection

DIAGNOSIS

HISTORY
- Dysphagia, odynophagia, or both are the most frequent complaints.
- Persistent chest pain is also common.
- Other nonspecific clinical manifestations (e.g., weight loss) may occur as a result of these symptoms or as a manifestation of an underlying illness that is responsible for the esophagitis.
- Local complications (e.g., hemorrhage, perforation of the esophagus, or the formation of fistulas) may occur if deep esophageal ulcerations due to infectious esophagitis are present.
- Infectious esophagitis may be asymptomatic. The frequency of asymptomatic esophageal infections is unknown.

PHYSICAL EXAM
CMV esophagitis may present with systemic symptoms (e.g., fever, nausea, vomiting, or abdominal pain), whereas *Candida* and HSV esophagitis tend to develop oral lesions. However, these occasional differences are not distinctive. The absence of thrush does not rule out *Candida* esophagitis.

DIAGNOSTIC TESTS & INTERPRETATION
Lab
- Hematologic profile
- Serologic tests for HSV, CMV, and HIV
- CMV antigenemia assays or CMV molecular amplification techniques
- Brush cytology specimens obtained by endoscopy for the diagnosis of *Candida* and HSV esophagitis
- Tissue culture for the diagnosis of HSV and CMV esophagitis. Culture is not routinely recommended for the diagnosis of *Candida* esophagitis. It is reserved for cases with clinical features suggesting the presence of a pathogen resistant to standard antifungal therapy

Imaging
Radiographic examination after a barium swallow shows an irregular, shaggy appearance of the esophageal mucosa in cases of *Candida* esophagitis. Sometimes, the picture is indistinguishable from that seen in cases of HSV and CMV esophagitis.

Diagnostic Procedures/Other
- Endoscopy and tissue sampling for histologic examination or brush cytology.
- The typical endoscopic appearance of *Candida* esophagitis includes white plaques on the mucosa, which often bleed when removed by the endoscope.
- Endoscopy in HSV esophagitis reveals small, demarcated ulcers with a yellowish base. The esophageal mucosa between them may often be normal appearing.
- Shallow, elongated ulcerations, surrounded by mucosa that appears to be normal, may be the endoscopic appearance of CMV esophagitis.
- However, the endoscopic features of *Candida*, HSV, or CMV esophagitis may be indistinguishable.

Pathological Findings
- Tissue specimens obtained by endoscopy may demonstrate:
  – Budding yeast cells, hyphae, or pseudohyphae in *Candida* esophagitis
  – Multinucleated giant cells and intranuclear inclusion bodies in HSV esophagitis
  – Cytomegaly of fibroblasts and endothelial cells with intranuclear and cytoplasmic inclusion bodies in CMV esophagitis

DIFFERENTIAL DIAGNOSIS
- Esophageal cancer (primary or metastatic).
- Systemic illnesses such as:
  – Crohn's disease
  – Sarcoidosis
  – Collagen vascular diseases
- Pill esophagitis, after use of certain antibiotics (e.g., tetracycline, doxycycline, clindamycin, ciprofloxacin, and others), potassium chloride, nonsteroidal anti-inflammatory drugs, and quinidine.
- Chemotherapy-induced esophagitis (dactinomycin, bleomycin, cytarabine, methotrexate, and other medications).
- Esophagitis due to radiation or concomitant use of radiation and chemotherapy.
- Inflammation due to sclerotherapy of esophageal varices.
- Idiopathic (aphthous) esophageal ulcers in HIV infection.
- Oral lesions are commonly encountered in patients with *Candida* and HSV esophagitis, whereas CMV esophagitis is rarely associated with stomatitis.

TREATMENT

MEDICATION
First Line
- For *Candida* esophagitis, systemic antifungal treatment is always required (A-II).
- A diagnostic trial of antifungal therapy is appropriate before performing an endoscopic examination (B-II).
- Oral fluconazole 200–400 mg (3–6 mg/kg) daily for 14–21 days is recommended (A-I). For patients who cannot tolerate oral therapy: Intravenous fluconazole 400 mg (6 mg/kg) daily, deoxycholate amphotericin B 0.3–0.7 mg/kg daily, or an echinocandin (B-II).
- For fluconazole-refractory disease: Itraconazole solution 200 mg daily (1), posaconazole suspension 400 mg twice daily (2), or voriconazole 200 mg twice daily administered intravenously or orally for 14–21 days (A-III).
- For recurrent infections: Suppressive therapy with fluconazole 100–200 mg 3 times weekly (3) (A-I).
- In patients with AIDS, treatment with HAART is recommended to reduce recurrent infections (A-I).
- HSV esophagitis usually resolves spontaneously in the immunocompetent host (4).
- Immunocompromised individuals should be treated with antiviral agents for 14–21 days. Acyclovir 400 mg p.o. 5 times daily, valacyclovir 1 g p.o. 3 times daily, famciclovir 500 mg p.o. 3 times daily. For patients who cannot tolerate oral therapy: Acyclovir 5 mg/kg i.v. every 8 hours for 7–14 days, followed by an orally administered antiviral for at least 1 more week.
- Prophylactic therapy (acyclovir 200–400 mg/d orally or 5 mg/kg b.i.d. i.v.) may be indicated if there is high risk for HSV reactivation.
- CMV esophagitis is treated with ganciclovir 5 mg/kg i.v. twice daily for at least 2 weeks (5).
- Maintenance therapy (valganciclovir 900 mg p.o. daily) may be necessary to avoid recurrence of CMV esophagitis in severely immunocompromised persons.
- In order to prevent CMV infection, CMV seronegative hosts receiving transplants from seropositive donors should receive antiviral prophylaxis.
- Idiopathic (aphthous) esophageal ulcers in HIV infection are treated with prednisone or thalidomide.

Second Line
- For fluconazole-refractory *Candida* esophagitis: Micafungin 150 mg daily, caspofungin 50 mg daily, anidulafungin 200 mg daily, or deoxycholate amphotericin B 0.3–0.7 mg/kg daily (B-II).
- The echinocandins are associated with higher relapse rates compared to fluconazole.
- For HSV or CMV esophagitis resistant to ganciclovir: Foscarnet.

IN-PATIENT CONSIDERATIONS
Admission Criteria
Outpatient care is appropriate, unless the patient's immune status is severely compromised or the infection is very severe. In those cases, hospitalization may be necessary.

IV Fluids
If the patient experiences severe odynophagia or the esophagitis is accompanied by oral lesions that make chewing or swallowing impossible, the administration of intravenous fluids may be necessary.

 ONGOING CARE

FOLLOW-UP RECOMMENDATIONS
- The expected course and prognosis depend on the underlying disease and pathogen; if the patient is severely immunosuppressed, prolonged treatment with effective medications is necessary.
- Patients with infectious esophagitis should have a follow-up appointment 2 weeks after resolution of symptoms.
- Most patients with *Candida* esophagitis will have resolution of their symptoms within 7 days of treatment.
- Myelosuppression is the main side effect of ganciclovir treatment. Concurrent administration of zidovudine may worsen myelosuppression.

COMPLICATIONS
- Complications are uncommon. If deep esophageal ulcers occur, serious local complications may develop, such as:
  – Massive hemorrhage
  – Perforation of the esophagus
  – Esophagobronchial or esophagomediastinal fistulas

REFERENCES
1. Phillips P, De Beule K, Frechette G, et al. A double-blind comparison of itraconazole oral solution and fluconazole capsules for the treatment of oropharyngeal candidiasis in patients with AIDS. *Clin Infect Dis* 1998;26:1368–1373.
2. Vazquez JA, Skiest DJ, Tissot-Dupont H, et al. Safety and efficacy of posaconazole in the long-term treatment of azole-refractory oropharyngeal and esophageal candidiasis in patients with HIV infection. *HIV Clin Trials* 2007;8:86–97.
3. Goldman M, Cloud GA, Wade KD, et al. A randomized study of the use of fluconazole in continuous versus episodic therapy in patients with advanced HIV infection and a history of oropharyngeal candidiasis: AIDS Clinical Trials Group Study 323/Mycoses Study Group Study 40. *Clin Infect Dis* 2005;41:1473–1480.
4. Ramanathan J, Rammouni M, Baran J Jr, et al. Herpes simplex virus esophagitis in the immunocompetent host: An overview. *Am J Gastroenterol* 2000;95:2171–2176.
5. Wilcox CM, Straub RF, Schwartz DA. Cytomegalovirus esophagitis in AIDS: A prospective evaluation of clinical response to ganciclovir therapy, relapse rate, and long-term outcome. *Am J Med* 1995;98:169–176.

ADDITIONAL READING
- Pappas PG, Kauffman CA, Andes D, et al. Clinical practice guidelines for the management of candidiasis: 2009 update by the Infectious Diseases Society of America. *Clin Infect Dis* 2009;48:503–535.

 CODES

ICD9
- 112.84 Candidal esophagitis
- 530.10 Esophagitis, unspecified

CLINICAL PEARLS
- The most common causes of infectious esophagitis are: *Candida* spp., HSV, and CMV.
- For *Candida* esophagitis fluconazole is the preferred agent.
- For fluconazole-refractory disease, itraconazole, voriconazole, or posaconazole are recommended.
- For patients who cannot tolerate oral therapy due to dysphagia or odynophagia, intravenous treatment is indicated.

E

EXANTHEM SUBITUM (ROSEOLA INFANTUM)

Georgia G. Georgantzi
Petros I. Rafailidis
Matthew E. Falagas

 BASICS

DESCRIPTION
- Exanthema subitum is a benign, self-limiting childhood viral illness caused by human herpesvirus 6B (HHV-6B) in most cases or by human herpesvirus 7 (HHV-7).
- It is also known as roseola infantum or sixth disease.

EPIDEMIOLOGY
Incidence
- It is worldwide.
- Infections occur from 6 months to 3 years, mostly (90%) before the age of 2 years.
- Human herpesvirus 7 causes illness in older children and may be associated with higher incidence of febrile seizures.
- Antibody prevalence is as high as 100% in the US population that is older than 3 years.
- Antibody titers are high in the newborn (maternal antibodies), fall until the age of 6 months, and then rise again.
- Antibody levels may be detectable at high levels until the age of 60 years.

Prevalence
Human herpesvirus 6B causes approximately 10–45% of all febrile illnesses in young children.

RISK FACTORS
Genetics
In the US, 1% of subjects are born with inherited chromosomally integrated HHV-6 infection, which was first described in 1993 and has unknown clinical implications until now (1).

GENERAL PREVENTION
- Currently, there is no way to prevent initial infection or reactivation with human herpesvirus 6.
- Prophylaxis may be necessary for patients undergoing bone marrow transplantation.

PATHOPHYSIOLOGY
- The virus persists in a latent state in secondary lymphoid organs (2), in saliva, and in the CNS (3) following primary infection by a different mechanism in comparison with other human herpesviruses (1).
- It may be found in activated CD4+ T-lymphocytes, monocytes, macrophages, endothelial cells, epithelial cells, astrocytes, and B cells, as well as in tissues throughout the body (1).
- Reactivation of the infection occurs mostly in immunocompromised patients (1).

ETIOLOGY
- Human herpesvirus 6 is closely related to cytomegalovirus (CMV) (50% homology, in the same group: Beta 2 herpesvirus).
- Human herpesvirus 6A and 6B should be considered as different viruses, because they are sufficiently different (1).
- The presence of human herpesvirus 7.

COMMONLY ASSOCIATED CONDITIONS
- This virus may be associated with transplantation.
- The implication of this virus in many diseases, such as AIDS, lymphoma, leukemia, chronic fatigue syndrome, drug-induced hypersensitivity syndrome, and multiple sclerosis in adults, is under discussion.

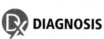 **DIAGNOSIS**

HISTORY
Incubation period is 10–14 days.
Pediatric Patients
- It is a benign illness in children with upper respiratory symptoms, fever, and rash.
- Fevers reaching 41°C have been associated with this illness.
- The child is otherwise mildly ill except for the high fever.

- A maculopapular rash typically (10%) occurs following the febrile period, though disease without a rash occurs more often. Rash without fever may also occur.
- Upper respiratory symptoms (involvement of pharynx, tonsils, and ears) without conjunctivitis and pharyngeal exudates.
- Cervical lymphadenopathy is often present.
- Illness lasts 3–5 days.
- Gastrointestinal symptoms (diarrhea, vomiting) may occur.
- Febrile seizures in 10%.
- It is a rare cause of encephalitis in nontransplant patients (4).
Adults
- Mononucleosis-like illness.
- This may cause upper respiratory illness or pneumonia with hepatitis.
Transplant Patients
- Exanthem subitum must be considered as a possible diagnosis in organ transplant patients.
- Human herpesvirus 6 is an important cause of bone marrow suppression and interstitial pneumonitis after bone marrow transplant.

PHYSICAL EXAM
- Fever: Up to 41°C with abrupt onset and abrupt resolution.
- Rash: Macular or maculopapular, pink, transient, nonpruritic, without pigmentation and desquamation, appears when the fever subsides, begins on the trunk, then spreads to the face, neck, limbs, and disappears in 1–2 days.
- Lymphadenopathy: Cervical.
- General good condition of the patient.
- Anterior fontanelle in infants may be bulging.

DIAGNOSTIC TESTS & INTERPRETATION
Lab
- Leukopenia
- Mononucleosis
- Lymphocytopenia
- Atypical lymphocytes
- Hepatitis, especially in adults
- Erythrocyte sedimentation rate is normal
- Cerebrospinal fluid is normal
- Diagnosis is via viral isolation, PCR, and serology.
- Viral isolation by rapid antigen detection from a specimen or tissue culture.
- Serology: IgG and IgM antibodies, antibody avidity, ELISA test
- The current serological assays cannot distinguish between HHV-6A and 6B (1).
- Detection via PCR or real-time PCR on cells or plasma
- Rapid shell vial assay is used for transplant patients.

Imaging
Magnetic resonance imaging in suspicion of CNS involvement (5).

DIFFERENTIAL DIAGNOSIS
- CMV
- Viral upper respiratory infection
- Adenovirus
- Hepatitis A, B, and C
- Measles, rubella
- Serious bacterial infections: The well-being of the child despite the fever, the rash after the febrile episode, normal erythrocyte sedimentation rate, and normal cerebrospinal fluid are in favor of the diagnosis of exanthema subitum.
- In cases of antibiotics use, the rash may be considered as drug allergy.

 TREATMENT

MEDICATION
- There is no specific treatment, and in most cases the treatment is supportive.
- The disease responds to ganciclovir or foscarnet, but treatment is usually limited to patients who are ill following bone marrow transplantation or in severe cases (4).

ADDITIONAL TREATMENT
General Measures
- Medical care is usually outpatient. Cases of febrile seizures or CNS involvement require hospitalization.
- Use acetaminophen/paracetamol and baths for fever.
- Ensure adequate hydration.

 ONGOING CARE

PROGNOSIS
It is benign and self-limited with good prognosis in general.

COMPLICATIONS
- Occur mainly in immunocompromised patients:
- Pneumonia
- Hepatitis
- Bone marrow suppression
- Encephalitis, meningoencephalitis, aseptic meningitis

REFERENCES

1. Flamand L, Komaroff A, Arbuckle J, et al. Review, part 1: Human herpesvirus-6 – Basic biology, diagnostic testing, and antiviral efficacy. *J Med Virol* 2010;82:1560–1568.
2. Comar M, Grasso D, dal Molin G, et al. HHV-6 infection of tonsils and adenoids in children with hypertrophy and upper airway recurrent infections. *Int J Pediatr Otorhinolaryngol* 2010;74:47–49.
3. Laina I, Syriopoulou V, Daikos G, et al. Febrile seizures and primary human herpesvirus 6 infection. *Pediatr Neurol* 2010;42:28–31.
4. Olli-Lähdesmäki T, Haataja L, Parkkola R, et al. High-dose ganciclovir in HHV-6 encephalitis of an immunocompetent child. *Pediatr Neurol* 2010;43:53–56.
5. Sauter A, Ernemann U, Beck R. Spectrum of imaging findings in immunocompromised patients with HHV-6 infection. *AJR Am J Roentgenol* 2009;193:W373–W380.

ADDITIONAL READING
- Cameron B, Flamand L, Juwana H, et al. Serological and virological investigation of the role of the herpesviruses EBV, CMV and HHV-6 in post-infective fatigue syndrome. *J Med Virol* 2010;82:1684–1688.
- Jaskula E, Dlubek D, Sedzimirska M, et al. Reactivations of cytomegalovirus, human herpes virus 6, and Epstein–Barr virus differ with respect to risk factors and clinical outcome after hematopoietic stem cell transplantation. *Transplant Proc* 2010;42:3273–3276.
- Singh N, Carrigan DR. Human herpesvirus-6 in transplantation: An emerging pathogen. *Ann Intern Med* 1996;124:1065–1071.

 CODES

ICD9
- 058.1 Roseola infantum
- 058.10 Roseola infantum, unspecified
- 058.11 Roseola infantum due to human herpesvirus 6

CLINICAL PEARLS
- Consider HHV-6 in a first febrile episode in a young child.
- The rash occurs after the fever subsides abruptly.
- Use acetaminophen, not aspirin.
- Consider HHV-6 in a child with first episode of febrile seizures (3).
- Consider HHV-6 in transplant patients who are ill.

E

FILARIASIS
Herman Carneiro (E. Mylonakis, Editor)

 BASICS

DESCRIPTION
- Filariasis is a parasitic tropical disease caused by thread-like nematode worms in the superfamily Filarioidea, which are transmitted by vectors.
- 9 filarial worms are known to use humans as a definitive host and live within lymphatics, skin and connective tissue, serous cavities, and blood vessels.
- Adult worms may live in the host for over 20 years.

EPIDEMIOLOGY
- Bancroftian and Malayan filariasis
  - Endemic in 83 countries in tropical and sub-tropical regions of Asia, Africa, Central and South America, and Pacific Island nations.
  - Estimated 1.3 billion people worldwide at risk of infection (1).
  - 120 million people already infected (1).
  - 40 million people have disabling or disfiguring disease (1).
- Loiasis
  - Confined to the rain forest belt of western and central Africa.
  - Humans are the only known reservoir.
- Onchocerciasis ("river blindness")
  - About 18 million people are infected (1).
  - About 270,000 are blind and an additional 500,000 are visually impaired. Second leading cause of blindness worldwide after trachoma (1).
  - Disease seen in South America and Africa.
- Dracunculiasis (Guinea worm)
  - Infection occurs mainly within a narrow belt of African countries and Yemen (1).
- Dirofilariasis (Dog heartworm)
  - Symptomatic infection rare (1)
  - Worldwide distribution
- Mansonelliasis
  - Disease found in Africa, Central and South America, and the Caribbean (1).

RISK FACTORS
- Living in or traveling to endemic areas
- Low socio-economic status

Genetics
No genetic factors involved

GENERAL PREVENTION
- Health education
- Vector control methods
- Sleep under a mosquito net
- Use insect repellent with at least 30% DEET (N,N-Diethyl-meta-toluamide) on exposed skin and on clothing
- Long-sleeved clothing to prevent insect bites
- Prophylaxis with diethylcarbamazine 300 mg/wk orally to prevent Loiasis

- Dracunculiasis
  - Drink clean boiled water
  - Filter copepods from drinking water
  - Prevent people with Guinea worm ulcers from entering drinking water sources
  - Treat contaminated water sources with chemicals, e.g. Abate, to kill copepods
  - Introduce copepod-eating fish into contaminated water sources

PATHOPHYSIOLOGY
- Bancroftian and Malayan Filariasis
  - Adult worms cause hypertrophy and dilatation of lymphatic vessels causing loss of valvular function, which leads to massive irreversible lymphoedema ("elephantiasis").
- Loiasis
  - Larvae enter with the bite of a red fly, which molt and move under the skin causing transient migratory angioedema ("Calabar" swellings), pain, pruritus, and urticaria, which are local hypersensitivity responses.
- Onchocerciasis
  - Larvae enter with the bite of a blackfly, mature, and mate producing microfilariae about a year after being bitten. Adult worms live in nodules in the dermis and deep fascia. Microfilariae migrate through the skin and can enter the eye causing inflammation that can cause blindness ("river blindness"), skin nodules, and onchodermatitis.
- Dracunculiasis
  - Larvae are ingested in drinking water via infected copepods. Larvae are released. They penetrate the bowel, mature the abdominal cavity, and mate. Males die and gravid females migrate to the lower extremities, where they produce a papule which eventually ulcerates. The worm emerges to release larvae on contact with water. Worms that do no reach the skin die and become calcified.
- Dirofilariasis
  - Worms produce a subtle granulomatous reaction in subcutaneous tissue or wedge in a pulmonary artery and cause a single, small, pulmonary infarct.
- Mansonelliasis
  - Dying worms release antigenic material causing an inflammatory response resulting in focal abscesses and granulomas.

ETIOLOGY
- Lymphatic filariasis
  - Infection with *Wuchereria bancrofti*, *Brugia malayi*, and *Brugia timori*
  - Transmitted by mosquitoes (*Anopheles*, *Aedes*, *Culex*, and *Mansonia* species)
- *Loa loa* transmitted by red tabanid flies (*Chrysops* species)
- *Onchocerca volvulus* transmitted by blackflies (*Simulium* species)

- *Dracunculus medinensis* is ingested in drinking water with infected microcrustaceans (copepods)
- *Dirofilaria* species transmitted by mosquitoes (*Culex* species)
- *Mansonella streptocerca* transmitted by midges (*Culicoides* species)
- *Mansonella perstans* and *Mansonella ozzardi* cause serous cavity filariasis

COMMONLY ASSOCIATED CONDITIONS
No commonly associated conditions

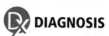 **DIAGNOSIS**

HISTORY
- Bancroftian and Malayan filariasis
  - Acute symptoms including fever, lymphadenitis, lymphangitis, funiculitis, and epididymitis
  - Chronic symptoms including abscesses, hyperkeratosis, polyarthritis, hydroceles, lymphoedema, and elephantiasis
  - Bronchospasm
- Loiasis
  - Transient swellings, usually of wrists and ankles, pruritus, paraesthesias, and hives
  - Worm migration across the eye
- Onchocerciasis
  - Subcutaneous nodules, pruritus, rashes, lymphadenopathy, lymphatic obstruction, chronic skin disease, eye lesions
- Dracunculiasis
  - Painful, inflamed skin lesion containing a worm and arthritis
- Dirofilariasis
  - Chest pain, cough, and hemoptysis
- Mansonelliasis
  - Localized swellings, pruritus, fever, headaches, arthralgias, neurologic manifestations, and hydroceles
- Ask about travel to endemic areas

PHYSICAL EXAM
- Bancroftian and Malayan filariasis
  - Lymphangitis and lymphadenitis
  - Femoral/inguinal lymphadenopathy
  - Enlarged epididymis and spermatic cord
  - Hydrocele, lower extremity lymphoedema
  - May cause monoarticular arthritis
- Loiasis
  - Adult worms may pass under the conjunctiva or through the skin.
  - Calabar swelling is often seen in the wrists and ankles; swelling may last only hours but can be recurrent for years.

- Onchocerciasis
  - Skin changes vary from papular rashes to areas of hyper- or hypopigmentation.
  - Patients may have eczematoid dermatitis and thickening of the skin.
  - Nontender subcutaneous nodules.
  - May have decreased visual acuity.
- Dracunculiasis
  - White, filamentous adult worm appears at cutaneous ulcer in distal extremities.
- Dirofilariasis
  - Usually no signs of infection
- Mansonelliasis
  - Angioedema, pruritus, popular rash, skin pigment change, fever, headaches, arthralgias, lymphadenopathy, hepatomegaly, and neurologic manifestations

DIAGNOSTIC TESTS & INTERPRETATION
Lab
- Bancroftian and Malayan filariasis
  - Blood smears show filarial worms.
  - Serological tests are nonspecific in filariasis.
  - Eosinophilia is often absent.
  - PCR-based assays for DNA of *W. bancrofti* and *B. malayi* are available in research settings.
- Loiasis
  - Blood smears, skin snips, or skin biopsy
- Onchocerciasis
  - Microscopy of skin biopsy shows worms
  - Dracunculiasis
  - Diagnosis is clinical
- Dirofilariasis
  - Histologic examination
- Mansonelliasis
  - Blood smears show filarial worms.
  - Microscopy of skin biopsy shows worms.
  - Eosinophilia is prominent.

Imaging
- Bancroftian and Malayan filariasis
  - Adult worms can be visualized in dilated lymphatics using ultrasound.
- Onchocerciasis
  - Skin and deep nodules detected using ultrasound and magnetic resonance imaging.
- Dracunculiasis
  - Plain radiographs show calcified worms.
- Dirofilariasis
  - Larvae may become encapsulated in infarcted lung tissue and produce well-defined pulmonary nodules, which may be visible on computed tomography scans.

DIFFERENTIAL DIAGNOSIS
- Bancroftian and Malayan filariasis
  - Bacterial lymphangitis, thrombophlebitis, idiopathic hydrocele, congestive heart failure, cirrhosis, nephrotic syndrome
- Loiasis
  - Cutaneous larva migrans, dracunculiasis, gnathostomiasis, myiasis, onchocerciasis
- Onchocerciasis
  - *M. streptocerca*, scabies, leprosy, eczema, glaucoma, loiasis

- Dracunculiasis
  - Cutaneous larva migrans, loiasis, rat bite infection, gnathostomiasis, myiasis
- Dirofilariasis
  - Asthma, allergies, lung cancer
- Mansonelliasis
  - Loiasis, onchocerciasis

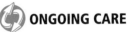 TREATMENT
MEDICATION
First Line
- Bancroftian and Malayan filariasis
  - *Wolbachia* spp., a type of *Rickettsia*, are required for filarial development. Treat *Wolbachia* with Doxycycline 100 mg orally twice daily for 4–6 weeks. 4 months after starting treatment one dose each of albendazole 400 mg orally and ivermectin 150 mg/kg orally.
- Loiasis
  - 1 dose diethylcarbamazine citrate (DEC) 6 mg/kg orally
- Onchocerciasis
  - 1 dose ivermectin 150 mcg/kg orally (does not kill adult worms). Repeat at 6 months.
  - If eyes involved, start prednisone 1 mg/kg/d orally 1 week before ivermectin.
- Dracunculiasis
  - Slow and careful extraction of emerging worm. Metronidazole 250 mg orally 3 times a day may reduce inflammatory response, facilitating worm removal. Mebendazole 400–800 mg/d for 6 days may kill worm.
- *M. perstans*
  - Albendazole 400 mg orally twice daily for 10 days
- *M. streptocerca* and *M. ozzardi*
  - 1 dose ivermectin 200 mcg/kg
- Dirofilariasis
  - No effective pharmacological therapy

Second Line
- Bancroftian and Malayan filariasis
  - DEC, as above for *M. streptocerca*. DEC should not be used in area with endemic lymphatic filariasis and loiasis/onchocerciasis.

ADDITIONAL TREATMENT
General Measures
Treatment is mainly for the microfilarial stage of infection. Adult worms are rarely affected by one dose of medication. Repeat therapy is often needed for cure.
Issues for Referral
- Infectious disease specialists
- Ophthalmologist for eye examination in onchocerciasis

SURGERY/OTHER PROCEDURES
- Nodulectomy of palpable nodules in onchocerciasis
- Surgical removal of dirofilariasis from lung

IN-PATIENT CONSIDERATIONS
Initial Stabilization
Resuscitation according to advanced life support protocol as required

Admission Criteria
- Patients with septicemia from open wounds
- Admission overnight to obtain blood samples at night for diagnostic tests
IV Fluids
- Fluid resuscitation with colloids, e.g. Gelofusine, if septicemic
- Maintenance fluids with Ringers lactate
Nursing
Patients with elephantiasis may need intensive nursing of affected body part.
Discharge Criteria
Resolution of septicemia

 ONGOING CARE
FOLLOW-UP RECOMMENDATIONS
Every 4–6 weeks to monitor treatment and for symptomatic control
Patient Monitoring
Regular eye examinations
PROGNOSIS
Disability and disfigurement is limited with appropriate diagnosis and treatment
COMPLICATIONS
- Bancroftian filariasis
  - Elephantiasis
  - Septicemia secondary to bacterial infection of open wounds
- Onchocerciasis
  - Blindness

REFERENCE
1. World Health Organization (WHO). Filariasis. http://www.who.int/topics/filariasis/en/. Accessed on May 24, 2010.

ADDITIONAL READING
- Centers for Disease Control and Prevention. Filariasis. http://www.dpd.cdc.gov/dpdx/HTML/Filariasis.htm. Accessed on May 24, 2010.

CODES
ICD9
- 125.0 Bancroftian filariasis
- 125.1 Malayan filariasis
- 125.9 Unspecified filariasis

CLINICAL PEARLS
Adult worms are rarely affected by one dose of medication. Repeat therapy is often needed for cure.

FOOD-BORNE DISEASES

Paschalis Vergidis
Matthew E. Falagas

 BASICS

DESCRIPTION
Infection arising from consumption of food contaminated with a pathogenic organism, microbial toxin, or chemical

EPIDEMIOLOGY
Incidence
- It is estimated that more than 75 million episodes of food-borne illnesses occur yearly in the US (1).
- Food-borne outbreaks are most commonly caused by noroviruses, followed by *Salmonella* (2).

RISK FACTORS
- Infants, elderly, and immunocompromised patients are at higher risk.
- *Vibrio vulnificus*: More common in patients with chronic liver disease or other immunosuppression.

GENERAL PREVENTION
- Avoid certain foods:
  - Food containing raw or undercooked eggs
  - Unpasteurized dairy products
  - Raw or undercooked meat, poultry, and seafood
  - Soft cheeses
- Avoid cross-contamination in food preparation
- Hand washing before handling food
- Immunization for hepatitis A
- Infant immunization for rotavirus

ETIOLOGY
Bacterial
- *Salmonella*: Contaminated eggs, poultry, cheese, raw fruits and vegetables (alfalfa sprouts, melon). *S. typhi* outbreaks related to contaminated water supplies
- *Shigella*: Food or water contaminated with human feces. Usually person-to-person spread
- Enterohemorrhagic *Escherichia coli* including *E. coli* O157:H7 and other Shiga toxin-producing *E. coli*: Undercooked beef, especially hamburger, unpasteurized milk and juice, raw fruits and vegetables, contaminated water
- Enterotoxigenic *E. coli*: Water or food contaminated with human feces
- *Campylobacter jejuni*: Raw and undercooked poultry, unpasteurized milk, contaminated water
- *Vibrio cholerae*: Contaminated water, fish, shellfish
- *Vibrio parahaemolyticus*: Undercooked or raw seafood
- *Vibrio vulnificus*: Undercooked or raw seafood (especially oysters)
- *Yersinia enterocolitica, Yersinia pseudotuberculosis*: Undercooked pork, unpasteurized milk, tofu, contaminated water
- *Clostridium perfringens*: Beef, turkey, chicken precooked, then reheated before serving
- *Staphylococcus aureus* (preformed enterotoxin): Food with high salt content (ham, canned meat) or high sugar content (cream, custard), potato and egg salads

- *Bacillus cereus*: Meats, vegetables, and sauces. Fried rice is implicated in almost all cases of an emetic form of bacterial infection
- *Clostridium botulinum*: Fish products and home-canned food, honey in infant botulism
- *Listeria monocytogenes*: Raw and unpasteurized milk, soft cheeses, coleslaw, raw vegetables

Viral
- Norovirus (formerly Norwalk virus): Shellfish, fecally contaminated food, ready-to-eat food touched by infected persons
- Rotavirus: Fecally contaminated food, ready-to-eat food touched by infected persons
- Hepatitis A: Contaminated seafood (especially shellfish), contaminated drinking water, food not reheated after contact with infected food handler

Parasitic
- *Giardia lamblia*: Fresh water, uncooked food, or food contaminated by an infected handler
- *Entamoeba histolytica*: Water, uncooked food, or food contaminated by an infected handler
- *Cryptosporidium*: Water, uncooked food, or food contaminated by an infected handler
- *Cyclospora cayetanensis*: Imported berries, lettuce, other fresh products

Noninfectious
- Ciguatera toxin produced by large reef fish: Barracuda, red snapper, amberjack, grouper, found in tropical and subtropical regions
- Scombroid toxin (histamine) produced by fish: Bluefin, tuna, skipjack, mackerel, marlin, escolar, mahi mahi
- Tetrodotoxin produced by puffer fish
- Shellfish toxins
  - Diarrheic, neurotoxic, amnesic: Variety of shellfish, primarily mussels, oysters, scallops, and shellfish from the Florida coast and the Gulf of Mexico
  - Paralytic: Scallops, mussels, clams, cockles
- Heavy metals (cadmium, arsenic, zinc, copper, mercury, antimony)
- Mushroom toxins (especially *Amanita* species)
- Pesticides
- Monosodium L-glutamate: Additive in Chinese cooking; soups contain greatest quantity

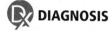 **DIAGNOSIS**

HISTORY
Bacterial
- *Salmonella* (incubation 1–3 days): Diarrhea, fever, cramps, vomiting. Lasts 4–7 days
- *S. typhi* and *S. paratyphi* produce typhoid (fever, chills, headache, constipation, myalgias; diarrhea is uncommon)
- *Shigella* (24–48 hours): Abdominal cramps, fever, diarrhea (blood, mucous in stool). Lasts 4–7 days
- Enterohemorrhagic *E. coli* (1–8 days): Severe diarrhea (often bloody), abdominal pain, vomiting. Low-grade or no fever. Lasts 5–10 days
- Enterotoxigenic *E. coli* (1–3 days): Watery diarrhea, cramps, some vomiting. Lasts 3 to more than 7 days
- *C. jejuni* (2–5 days): Diarrhea (may be bloody), cramps, fever, vomiting. Lasts 2–10 days
- *V. cholerae* (24–72 hours): Profuse watery diarrhea and vomiting which can lead to dehydration and death. Lasts 3–7 days
- *V. parahaemolyticus* (2–48 hours): Watery diarrhea, cramps, nausea, vomiting. Lasts 2–5 days
- *V. vulnificus* (1–7 days): Vomiting, diarrhea, abdominal pain. Lasts 2–8 days
- *Y. enterocolitica, Y. pseudotuberculosis* (24–48 hours): Appendicitis-like symptoms (diarrhea, vomiting, fever, abdominal pain), scarlatiniform rash with *Y. pseudotuberculosis*. Lasts 1–3 weeks
- *C. perfringens* (8–16 hours): Watery diarrhea, nausea, cramps. Rarely fever. Lasts 24–48 hours
- *S. aureus* (1–6 hours): Sudden onset of severe nausea and vomiting, cramps, diarrhea and fever may be present. Lasts 24–48 hours
- *B. cereus*:
  - Preformed enterotoxin (1–6 hours): Sudden onset of severe nausea and vomiting. Diarrhea may be present. Lasts 24 hours
  - Diarrheal toxin (10–16 hours): Abdominal cramps, watery diarrhea, nausea. Lasts 24–48 hours
- *C. botulinum* (12–72 hours, preformed toxin): Vomiting, diarrhea, blurred vision, diplopia, dysphagia, descending muscle weakness. Lasts from days to months
- *L. monocytogenes* (9–48 hours for gastrointestinal symptoms): Fever, myalgias, nausea, or diarrhea. Flu-like illness in pregnant women

Viral
- Norovirus (incubation 12–48 hours): Nausea, vomiting, cramping, diarrhea, fever, myalgias, some headache. Diarrhea more prevalent in adults, vomiting more prevalent in children. Lasts 12–60 hours
- Rotavirus (1–3 days): Vomiting, watery diarrhea, low-grade fever. Lasts 4–8 days
- Hepatitis A (15–50 days): Diarrhea, dark urine, jaundice, flu-like symptoms. Lasts 2 weeks to 3 months.

Parasitic
- *G. lamblia* (incubation 2 days to 4 weeks): Diarrhea, cramps, gas. May last weeks to months
- *E. histolytica*: Diarrhea (often bloody), lower abdominal pain
- *Cryptosporidium*: Diarrhea (usually watery), stomach cramps, mild fever
- *C. cayetanensis*: Diarrhea (usually watery), loss of appetite, loss of weight, nausea, vomiting

Noninfectious
- Ciguatera toxin:
  - Gastrointestinal (2–6 hours): Abdominal pain, nausea, vomiting, diarrhea
  - Neurologic (3 hours): Paresthesias, reversal of hot or cold sensations, pain, weakness
  - Cardiovascular (2–5 days): Bradycardia, hypotension, T-wave abnormalities
    ○ Symptoms last for days to weeks to months
- Scombroid toxin (1 minute to 3 hours): Flushing, rash, paresthesias, dizziness, urticaria. Symptoms last for 3–6 hours
- Tetrodotoxin (less than 30 minutes): Paresthesias, vomiting, diarrhea, abdominal pain, ascending paralysis, respiratory failure. Death usually in 4–6 hours
- Shellfish toxins:
  - Diarrheic (30 minutes to 2 hours): Nausea, vomiting, diarrhea, abdominal pain accompanied by chills, headache, fever
  - Neurotoxic (few minutes to hours): Tingling and numbness of lips, tongue, throat, muscular aches, dizziness, diarrhea, vomiting
  - Amnesic (24–48 hours): Vomiting, diarrhea, abdominal pain, memory loss, disorientation, confusion, seizure, coma
    ○ Symptoms last for hours to 2–3 days
- Paralytic shellfish toxins (30 minutes to 3 hours): Diarrhea, nausea, vomiting, paresthesias, weakness, dysphonia, dysphasia, respiratory paralysis
  - Symptoms last for days

PHYSICAL EXAM
- Signs of volume depletion: Dry mucosae, decreased urine output, hypotension, tachycardia
- Abdominal tenderness
- Bullous skin lesions in *V. vulnificus* infection

DIAGNOSTIC TESTS & INTERPRETATION
Lab
Bacterial
- *Salmonella*, *Shigella*, *E. coli*: Stool culture
  - *E. coli* O157:H7 requires special media.
  - Enterotoxigenic *E. coli* requires special techniques for identification.
- *C. jejuni*: Stool culture (*Campylobacter* requires special media and incubation at 42°C).
- *Vibrio* spp.: Stool culture with special media.
- *Yersinia* spp.: Stool, vomitus, blood culture. Special media required. Serology available in reference laboratories.
- *S. aureus*: Clinical diagnosis. Stool, vomitus, food can be tested for toxin and cultured.
- *B. cereus*: Clinical diagnosis. Test food and stool for toxin in outbreaks.
- *C. perfringens*: Stool for enterotoxin and culture. Organism normally found in stool; thus quantitative cultures must be done.

- *C. botulinum*: Stool, serum, food for toxin. Stool and food can be cultured. Send specimens to state health laboratory.
- *L. monocytogenes*: Blood or cerebrospinal fluid culture. Asymptomatic fecal carriage occurs; stool culture not helpful.

Viral
- Norovirus: Clinical diagnosis, negative bacterial cultures, no fecal leukocytes
- Rotavirus: Identification in stool via immunoassay
- Hepatitis A: Positive IgM antibody

Parasitic
- *G. lamblia*: Stool for oocysts. Enzyme immunoassay (EIA) in stool
- *E. histolytica*: Stool for cysts and parasites
- *Cryptosporidium*: Stool for ova and parasites. EIA in stool
- *C. cayetanensis*: Stool for oocysts

Noninfectious
- Ciguatera toxin: Radioassay for toxin in fish
- Scombroid toxin: Detection of histamine in food
- Tetrodotoxin: Detection in fish
- Shellfish toxins: High-pressure liquid chromatography

TREATMENT
Most forms of food-borne diseases are treated supportively. For specific treatment, see below.

MEDICATION
Bacterial
- *S. typhi* and *S. paratyphi*: Cefixime, ceftriaxone, quinolones. Note: Resistance to quinolones in Southeast Asia.
- *E. coli* O157:H7: Supportive care. Antibiotics may promote the development of hemolytic-uremic syndrome.
- Enterotoxigenic *E. coli*: Supportive care. Trimethoprim-sulfamethoxazole (TMP-SMX), quinolones in severe cases.
- *C. jejuni*: Erythromycin, quinolones in severe cases.
- Cholera: Tetracycline or doxycycline for adults. TMP-SMX for children <8 years.
- *C. botulinum*: Trivalent equine antitoxin to prevent further paralysis. Botulism immune globulin for infants (antitoxin not recommended for infants).
- *L. monocytogenes*: Ampicillin alone or with gentamicin for serious infections.

Parasitic
- *G. lamblia*: Metronidazole
- *E. histolytica*: Metronidazole
- *Cryptosporidium*: Nitazoxanide
- *C. cayetanensis*: TMP-SMX

Noninfectious
- Ciguatera toxin: Intravenous mannitol. Amitriptyline and fluoxetine may alleviate chronic fatigue, depression.
- Scombroid toxin: Anti-histamines.

ADDITIONAL TREATMENT
General Measures
- Cholera: Aggressive oral or intravenous rehydration.
- Tetrodotoxin and paralytic shellfish toxin poisoning may need respiratory support.

ONGOING CARE
PROGNOSIS
- In general, protracted course of illness and prolonged viral shedding in immunocompromised patients.
- Cholera causes life-threatening dehydration.
- Diarrheic, neurotoxic, amnesic shellfish toxins generally cause self-limiting disease.
- Paralytic shellfish toxin and tetrodotoxin are life-threatening.

COMPLICATIONS
- Temporary lactose intolerance, especially after rotavirus infection.
- *C. jejuni* associated with reactive arthritis, Guillain–Barré syndrome.

REFERENCES
1. Mead PS, Slutsker L, Dietz V, et al. Food-related illness and death in the United States. *Emerg Infect Dis* 1999;5:607–625.
2. Surveillance for foodborne disease outbreaks – United States, 2007. *MMWR* 2010;59:973–979.

ADDITIONAL READING
- Foodborne Illness Primer Work Group. Foodborne illness primer for physicians and other health care professionals. *Nutr Clin Care* 2004;7:134–140.

CODES
ICD9
- 003.9 Salmonella infection, unspecified
- 005.9 Food poisoning, unspecified
- 008.63 Enteritis due to Norwalk virus

CLINICAL PEARLS
- Norovirus and *Salmonella* are the most common causes of food-borne outbreaks in the US.
- Infants, elderly, and the immunocompromised patients are at higher risk of disease.
- Food-borne illnesses due to noninfectious causes include fish or shellfish toxin, mushroom toxin, and heavy metal poisoning.

F

FUNGAL INFECTIONS OF THE HAIR, NAILS, AND SKIN
Herman Carneiro (E. Mylonakis, Editor)

 BASICS

DESCRIPTION
- These infections are collectively referred to as "dermatophytosis" or "tinea," which is a fungal infection of keratinized areas of the body (hair, skin, and nails) (1–5).
- Dermatophytosis is very common and categorized according to the site of infection.

EPIDEMIOLOGY
Incidence
- Highest incidence of Tinea capitis in children (5)
- Young adult males commonly have Tinea pedis (1)
- Patients with immunodeficiency often have extensive disease, especially Tinea pedis
- Incidence of onychomycosis estimated between 2–13% in North America (2)

Prevalence
- 70% of the population will be infected with Tinea pedis at some point in their lives (1).
- Tinea corporis common in hot, humid climates (2,3).
- Tinea cruris is also common in hot, humid climates – 3 times more common in men than women (3)
- Tinea capitis is widespread in some urban areas in the US particularly in Afro-Caribbean children. It is also common in parts of Africa and India (5).
- Onychomycosis is the most common nail disease in adults.
- Species such as *Trichophyton verrucosum* (cattle) and *Microsporum canis* (cats and dogs) can cause disease in people.

RISK FACTORS
- Obesity – Tinea cruris
- Diabetes mellitus – Tinea cruris
- Tight-fitting clothing – Tinea cruris
- Wet clothing or undergarments – Tinea cruris
- Immunodeficiency – Tinea pedis

Genetics
No genetic factors involved

GENERAL PREVENTION
- Tinea pedis, onychomycosis
  - Wear sandals in communal showers
  - Avoid communal showers if susceptible or being treated for a fungal infection
  - Treat the inside of shoes with antifungal powder to prevent reinfection
- Tinea corporis
  - Avoid close contact between patients and those not infected
  - Avoid sharing fomites, e.g. towels, hats

- Tinea cruris
  - Keep groin area dry
  - Avoid tight-fitting clothing
  - Put on socks before undergarments to prevent fungal transfer from feet to groin
  - Use antifungal powders in groin
  - Laundry of cloths frequently

PATHOPHYSIOLOGY
- Tinea pedis
  - Dermatophyte fungi use keratinase enzymes to invade superficial layer of skin. Cell wall mannans inhibit host immune response.
- Tinea corporis/Tinea cruris
  - Inhabits cornified layers of the skin, hair, and nails. Uses keratinases and other enzymes to invade deeper into the stratum corneum.
  - Incubation period is 1–3 weeks, following which the fungus invades laterally. The advancing border of infection has increased epidermal proliferation and scaling used as a defense mechanism to shed infected skin.
  - Cell-mediated immunity clears infection.
- Tinea capitis
  - Infection and invasion as above but growth continues into hair. Infection visible on the surface around day 12. Infected hair is brittle and breaks.
- Onychomycosis
  - Fungus extends from plantar skin to invade nail bed causing inflammation and nail signs in distal lateral subungual onychomycosis.
  - In white superficial onychomycosis there is direct invasion from the surface to the nail bed.
  - Invasion is via the nail fold in proximal subungual onychomycosis.

ETIOLOGY
- Infections of the hair are termed Tinea capitis (scalp) or Tinea barbae (beard). Infections of the skin are termed Tinea corporis. The infections are frequently due to *Trichophyton* and *Microsporum* species.
  - Tinea corporis is spread through contact with desquamated skin.
- Tinea manuum occurs on the hand.
- Tinea pedis, commonly referred to as Athlete's Foot, occurs between the toes and on the soles of the feet.
  - The most common cause worldwide is *T. rubrum*. *T. mentagrophytes* and *Epidermophyton floccosum* also cause infection.
  - Tinea pedis is spread through contact within showers or bathroom facilities.
- Infection of the nails is referred to as onychomycosis. *Trichophyton* and *Candida* species are often responsible.

COMMONLY ASSOCIATED CONDITIONS
No commonly associated conditions.

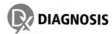 **DIAGNOSIS**

HISTORY
- Tinea pedis
  - Blisters or fissuring in the interdigital spaces or under the toes. Spread of infection to the sole of the foot is common.
  - The lesions are pruritic, and maceration may occur as a result of scratching.
  - Secondary infection with bacteria may lead to cellulitis.
- Tinea corporis
  - Multiple or single round lesions with prominent edges and marked scaling.
  - Some lesions may contain pustules.
  - Some of the lesions may appear nodular, especially on the legs.
- Tinea cruris
  - Rash that may contain pustules in the groin. At times, the infection causes itching or burning.
- Tinea capitis
  - Infection invades the hair shafts, leading to circular patches of erythema, scaling, and alopecia. The lesions are pruritic.
- Onychomycosis
  - The nail becomes discolored, and thickening may occur.
  - Infection often creeps across the nail from the distal and lateral margins.
- Contacts with dermatophyte infections
- Travel to or living in hot, humid climates

PHYSICAL EXAM
- Tinea pedis
  - Interdigital erythema, maceration, fissuring, and scaling, often with pruritus.
  - Plantar erythema, scaling due to hyperkeratosis, pruritus vesicles or bullae, pustular lesions, and ulceration.
  - Patients often develop cellulitis, lymphangitis, adenopathy, and pyrexia.
- Tinea corporis/tinea cruris
  - Annular lesions with erythema and scaly plaques that may rapidly enlarge.
  - Papules, vesicles, and bullae can develop.
  - Tinea cruris occurs in the groin and perianal area.
- Tinea capitis
  - Red papules turning into ring-shaped lesions.
  - Pustules containing matted infected hairs and other debris may form.
  - Progresses to patchy hair loss with scarring alopecia.
- Onychomycosis
  - Nails may show subungual hyperkeratosis, onycholysis, change in color including yellow, brown, and white, brittle nails, roughened nail surfaces, and thickened nails.

DIAGNOSTIC TESTS & INTERPRETATION

Lab

Initial lab tests
- Diagnosis can be made by microscopic evaluation of skin scrapings, skin biopsy, hair pluckings, nail fragments and nail bed samples obtained by curettage.
- Scrapings and other samples can also be cultured on Sabouraud agar.
- A Woods light can pick up infections with Microsporidia, which fluoresces green.
- Polymerase chain reaction for fungal DNA identification.

Follow-Up & Special Considerations
- Tinea corporis/tinea cruris
  - If initial treatment is unsuccessful repeat samples and cultures may be indicated.
- Tinea capitis
  - Household contacts, children's playmates and classmates should be screened for clinically silent infection on scalp and treated.
- Onychomycosis
  - Upon completion of antifungal therapy disease-free nail growth should be measured regularly.

Pathological Findings
- Histological examination of samples may show fungal elements and inflammatory cells.
- Hyperkeratosis and nail changes may be seen.

DIFFERENTIAL DIAGNOSIS
- Cutaneous candidal infections can mimic dermatophyte infections.
- Psoriasis
- Contact dermatitis
- Superficial bacterial infections
- Acanthosis nigricans
- Granuloma annulare
- Alopecia areata
- Lichen planus

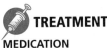 **TREATMENT**

MEDICATION

First Line
- Tinea corporis, Tinea cruris, and Tinea pedis
  - Topical tolnaftate, undecylenic acid, or terbinafine cream for 2–4 weeks alone or in combination with oral antifungals (1–4)
  - Terbinafine 250 mg orally daily for 14 days has had excellent results
  - Ketoconazole 200 mg orally daily for 4 weeks
- Tinea capitis
  - Antifungal shampoo such as selenium sulfate for 2 weeks, with griseofulvin 500 mg to 1 g orally daily (5)
- Onychomycosis
  - Terbinafine 250 mg daily for 6 weeks, or itraconazole 200 mg daily for 3 months (2)
  - Fingernail infection is treated for 2 months
  - Toenail infection is treated for 3–4 months

Second Line
- Tinea corporis, Tinea cruris, and Tinea pedis
  - Fluconazole 150 mg orally once a week for 1–4 weeks should be considered for refractory cases (3)
- Tinea capitis
  - Fluconazole or terbinafine orally (5)

ADDITIONAL TREATMENT

General Measures
As above in "General Prevention"

Issues for Referral
- Dermatologist to treat infection
- Infectious disease specialist if patients develop cellulites and/or sepsis

Additional Therapies
- Tinea pedis
  - Soak feet in aluminum acetate solution
  - Apply ammonium lactate lotion to affected areas

SURGERY/OTHER PROCEDURES
- Onychomycosis
  - Consider surgical removal of nail plate as an adjunct in patients taking oral therapy

IN-PATIENT CONSIDERATIONS

Initial Stabilization
Resuscitate according to advanced life support protocol as required

Admission Criteria
Sepsis secondary bacterial infection of open wound sites for intravenous antibiotic treatment

IV Fluids
- Fluid resuscitation with colloids, e.g. Gelofusine
- Maintenance fluids with Ringers lactate

Nursing
Keep open wound sites clean and dress daily if necessary

Discharge Criteria
Sepsis fully resolved and patient hemodynamically stable

 ONGOING CARE

FOLLOW-UP RECOMMENDATIONS
Recurrent disease is common; close follow-up after therapy is needed.

Patient Monitoring
Monitor response to treatment as required

DIET
No specific diet necessary

PATIENT EDUCATION
As above in "General Prevention"

PROGNOSIS
- Prognosis is usually excellent with appropriate diagnosis and treatment.
- Tinea capitis has resulted in severe hair loss and scarring alopecia.

COMPLICATIONS
Secondary bacterial cellulitis, lymphangitis, and even osteomyelitis can complicate dermatophyte infection, especially on the foot. This is a constant concern in patients with diabetes or peripheral vascular disease.

REFERENCES
1. Robbins CM, Elewski BE. Tinea pedis: eMedicine dermatology. http://emedicine.medscape.com/article/1091684-overview. Accessed on July 4, 2010.
2. Ameen M. Epidemiology of superficial fungal infections. *Clin Dermatol* 2010;28(2):197–201.
3. Lesher JL. Tinea corporis: eMedicine dermatology. http://emedicine.medscape.com/article/1091473-overview. Accessed on July 4, 2010.
4. Wiederkehr M, Schwartz RA. Tinea cruris: eMedicine dermatology. http://emedicine.medscape.com/article/1091806-overview. Accessed on July 4, 2010.
5. Kao GF. Tinea capitis: eMedicine dermatology. http://emedicine.medscape.com/article/1091351-overview. Accessed on July 4, 2010.

 CODES

ICD9
- 110.0 Dermatophytosis of scalp and beard
- 110.1 Dermatophytosis of nail
- 110.8 Dermatophytosis of other specified sites

CLINICAL PEARLS
- Cutaneous fungal infection of the stratum corneum or the nails is very common and is present worldwide. These infections are commonly encountered in clinical practice.

F

GAS GANGRENE

Herman Carneiro (E. Mylonakis, Editor)

 BASICS

DESCRIPTION
Gas gangrene is a life-threatening infection of muscle and soft tissue caused by toxin- and gas-producing *Clostridium* species, causing rapid onset of muscle necrosis with muscle swelling, severe pain, gas production, and sepsis.

EPIDEMIOLOGY
Incidence
- Trauma accounts for half of all cases. Historically, this disease is seen most commonly with wartime injuries (1–3).
- In wounds, as many as 40% may be contaminated with potential pathogens, but a fraction of a percentage will become infected (1,2).
- The annual number of cases in the US is 1,000–3,000 (1,2).
- Illness typically occurs 1–4 days following trauma. At times, incubation may be much longer.

Prevalence
- Patients with gas gangrene have an average age of 35–40 years.
- Gas gangrene is 2–3 times more common in men.

RISK FACTORS
- Atherosclerosis
- Burns
- Chronic alcoholism
- Corticosteroid use
- Diabetes mellitus
- Gastrointestinal malignancy
- HIV/AIDS
- Hypoalbuminemia
- Intravenous drug use
- Malnutrition
- Obesity
- Open fractures
- Peripheral vascular disease
- Surgery
- Trauma – major or minor (insect bites, injection sites)

Genetics
No genetic factors involved.

GENERAL PREVENTION
Irrigation and debridement of wounds and leaving them open when possible reduces the incidence of gas gangrene.

PATHOPHYSIOLOGY
- Wounds with compromised blood supplies create an anaerobic environment ideal for *Clostridium* to proliferate.
- *C. perfringens* produces at least 20 toxins, the most important of which is alpha-toxin (3).
- Alpha-toxin has phospholipase-C activity, which causes cell destruction by hydrolysis of key components of the cell membrane (3).
- It is responsible for lysis of erythrocytes, leukocytes, platelets, fibroblasts, and muscle cells leading to necrosis of muscle and surrounding tissue, hemolysis, and shock (3).
- Kappa-toxin, a collagenase, causes destruction of blood vessels (3).

ETIOLOGY
- Infection with *Clostridium* species, which are gram-positive, spore-forming, anaerobic rods.
- They are normally found in soil and the gastrointestinal tract of humans and animals.
- Infection usually occurs from direct inoculation of surgical and traumatic wounds, but can also occur spontaneously with hematological spread.
- 80% of cases are caused by *Clostridium perfringens* (1,3).
- The other 20% of cases may be caused by *Clostridium septicum* and *Clostridium novyi* amongst other clostridia (1–3).
- Some infections may be due to mixed aerobic and anaerobic organisms.

COMMONLY ASSOCIATED CONDITIONS
No commonly associated conditions.

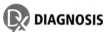 **DIAGNOSIS**

HISTORY
- Pain is usually the first symptom:
  - Increasing pain after surgery or trauma (including minor trauma)
  - Sudden onset
  - May be severe
- Skin changes
- Risk factors including:
  - Prior surgery or trauma
  - Diabetes mellitus
  - Chronic alcohol excess
  - Peripheral vascular disease
  - Intravenous drug use
  - Corticosteroid use
  - Immunocompromised states including steroid use, malnutrition, malignancy, and HIV/AIDS.

PHYSICAL EXAM
- Vital signs: May indicate degree of systemic involvement and include no fever or low-grade fever, and a spectrum from tachycardia to outright septic shock.
- Examination of involved body part:
  - Severe tenderness
  - Violaceous skin changes progress to weeping bullae within hours.
  - A brownish, foul-smelling discharge runs from the bullae.
  - Crepitans may be palpated over the affected area and in areas remote from the origin.
  - Patients usually remain conscious despite hypotension.
  - Massive hemolysis may lead to profound jaundice and black urine.
  - Mental state depressed in early disease.

DIAGNOSTIC TESTS & INTERPRETATION
Lab
- Complete blood count: Anemia.
- Blood film: Signs of intravascular hemolysis.
- Clotting: Deranged clotting and thrombocytopenia.
- Electrolytes: Hyperkalemia from cell breakdown and hypocalcemia secondary to fat necrosis.
- Renal: Hemoglobinuria, myoglobinuria, and signs of renal failure.
- Liver function tests: Hyperbilirubinemia and deranged liver function secondary to toxins.
- Arterial blood gas: Metabolic acidosis secondary to lactic acidosis.
- A Gram stain of discharge from the bullae will show the gram-positive rods (boxcars).
- Blood cultures: Less than 1% yield *Clostridium* species.
- ELISA for rapid detection of alpha-toxin using wound exudate, tissue samples, or serum.
- PCR detection of *Clostridium* species, although not widely available in clinical practice.

Imaging
- X-rays of the affected area will show gas within the striated muscle.
- Ultrasound can also be used to demonstrate gas in tissues.
- A computed tomography (CT) scan or magnetic resonance imaging (MRI) may be needed when gas is deep in the pelvic walls or uterus.

Diagnostic Procedures/Other
- Tissue biopsy with Gram stain and culture.
- Surgical exploration reveals pale, necrotic muscle that does not contract with stimulation.

Pathological Findings
Histopathologic analysis reveals widespread necrotic muscle, destruction of connective tissue, clostridia, and a minimal inflammatory infiltrate.

DIFFERENTIAL DIAGNOSIS
- Cutaneous anthrax
- Pyomyositis (muscle abscess)
- Cellulitis
- Rhabdomyolysis
- Deep venous thrombosis and thrombophlebitis
- Streptococcal (pyogenes) myositis
- Necrotizing fasciitis
- Vibrio vulnificus infection

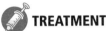 TREATMENT

MEDICATION
First Line
- Clindamycin 600–1200 mg IV/IM every 6–8 hours, depending on severity of infection; use in combination with Penicillin G 10 million units every 6 hours (1–3)

Second Line
- Ceftriaxone 2 g IV every 12 hours
- Metronidazole 7.5 mg/kg IV every 6 hours
- Tetracycline 1 g IV every 12 hours
- Linezolid 400–600 mg PO/IV every 12 hours for 10–28 days
- Gentamicin 3–5 mg/kg/day IV/IM every 8 hours depending on severity of infection (NB: based on normal renal function)
- Vancomycin 500 mg IV every 6 hours for 7–10 days
- Erythromycin 1 g IV every 6 hours
- Chloramphenicol 500–1000 mg IV every 6 hours

ADDITIONAL TREATMENT
General Measures
- Hyperbaric oxygen is effective in reducing the toxin production of the organism, but its clinical utility has not been proved.
  - Note: Arranging a chamber should not delay surgical debridement or antibiotics.
- Toxoids to induce active immunity
  - Tetanus toxoid
- Immunoglobulins for passive immunity
- Appropriate analgesia

Issues for Referral
- General surgeon – surgical debridement
- Orthopedic surgeon – amputations
- Infectious disease specialist – antibiotic recommendations and other issues
- Hematologist – hemolytic anemia
- Oncologist – spontaneous gas gangrene secondary to malignancy
- Gastroenterologist – colonic polyps, diverticuli, or malignancy leading to hematological spread.

SURGERY/OTHER PROCEDURES
Surgical debridement is the most important life-saving procedure. Rapid surgical debridement may avert the need for radical amputations.

IN-PATIENT CONSIDERATIONS
Initial Stabilization
- Resuscitate according to Advanced Life Support (ALS) as required.
- Frequent assessment of circulatory status.
- Good intravenous access.

Admission Criteria
- Pain out of proportion to overlying skin changes.
- Any patient with suspected gas gangrene.

IV Fluids
Aggressive fluid resuscitation with Ringers lactate

Nursing
- Nurse patient in isolation
- Use appropriate barrier nursing techniques

Discharge Criteria
Patient stable following surgical debridement, treatment of infection with antibiotics, and other necessary procedures

 ONGOING CARE

FOLLOW-UP RECOMMENDATIONS
- Patients with spontaneous infection, especially with *C. septicum*, should, at some point, be evaluated for colonic polyps, diverticulitis, or malignancy (1).
- Reconstructive surgery
- Physical rehabilitation

DIET
Avoid foods with high potassium content if patient has hyperkalemia

PATIENT EDUCATION
- Alert patients with spontaneous gas gangrene to the possibility of occult malignancy
- Educate intravenous drug users of the risk of gas gangrene and its complications

PROGNOSIS
- Early diagnosis and aggressive treatment decreases mortality
- Better prognosis if incubation period <30 hours
- Better prognosis in patients without comorbidities or complications of infection
- Worse with spontaneous gas gangrene

COMPLICATIONS
- Hemolysis requiring blood transfusions
- Disseminated intravascular coagulation
- Acute renal failure
- Acute respiratory distress syndrome
- Shock
- Death
- Amputation
- Permanent deformity or disability

REFERENCES
1. Shukla A, Rosen CL, Wong JK. Gas Gangrene: eMedicine Emergency Medicine. http://emedicine.medscape.com/article/782709-overview. Accessed June 28, 2010.
2. Revis DR Jr. Clostridial Gas Gangrene: eMedicine Infectious Diseases. http://emedicine.medscape.com/article/214992-overview. Accessed June 28, 2010.
3. Ho H, Aragon LB, Tcheng JW, et al. Gas Gangrene: eMedicine Infectious Diseases. http://emedicine.medscape.com/article/217943-overview. Accessed June 28, 2010.

ADDITIONAL READING
- Headley AJ. Necrotizing soft tissue infections: A primary care review. *Am Fam Physician* 2003;68(2): 323–328.
- Kaide CG, Khandelwal S. Hyperbaric oxygen: Applications in infectious disease. *Emerg Med Clin North Am* 2008;26(2):571–595, xi.

 See Also
- Shukla A, Rosen CL, Wong JK. Gas Gangrene: Multimedia – eMedicine Emergency Medicine. Available at: http://emedicine.medscape.com/article/782709-media. Accessed 28 June 2010.

 CODES

ICD9
040.0 Gas gangrene

CLINICAL PEARLS
- Suspect gas gangrene in cases where pain is out of proportion to the overlying skin changes.

G

GENITAL HERPES

Paschalis Vergidis
Matthew E. Falagas

 BASICS

DESCRIPTION
Sexually transmitted disease manifested with vesicles and caused by herpes simplex virus (HSV).

EPIDEMIOLOGY
Prevalence
- At least 50 million persons in the US have genital HSV infection. Overall age-adjusted HSV-2 seroprevalence decreased from 21% in 1988–1994 to 17% in 1999–2004 (1).
- Seroprevalence of HSV-1 has decreased but the incidence of genital herpes caused by HSV-1 may be increasing.
- Higher rates of HSV-2 among African Americans may reflect patterns of sexual networking rather than high-risk sexual behavior.
- Higher seroprevalence in adults of lower socioeconomic status.

RISK FACTORS
- Sexual intercourse with partner infected with HSV.
- Women are at higher risk of HSV-2 acquisition than men.

GENERAL PREVENTION
- If >6 recurrences occur in a 12-month period, suppressive therapy is recommended.
- Sexual transmission can occur during asymptomatic periods. Asymptomatic viral shedding is more frequent in HSV-2 than HSV-1 infection and is most frequent during the first 12 months after acquiring HSV-2.
- All persons with genital herpes should remain abstinent from sexual activity with uninfected partners when lesions or prodromal symptoms are present.
- Consistent condom use has been associated with 50% reduction in HSV-2 transmission.
- Circumcision, which decreases HIV acquisition, may have less effect on risk of HSV-2 acquisition.
- Suppressive therapy with valacyclovir reduces the risk of transmission among heterosexual, HSV-2-discordant couples (2).

ETIOLOGY
- Caused by HSV-2 in 70% of cases.
- Recurrences and subclinical shedding are much more frequent for genital HSV-2 than for genital HSV-1.
- Acquisition of genital HSV-1 appears to be increasing.
- Persons with HSV-1 infection, regardless of the site of infection, remain at risk for HSV-2 acquisition.

DIAGNOSIS

HISTORY
- Incubation period: 2–7 days (range, 1 day to 3 weeks)
- Signs and symptoms during primary infection are more prominent and last longer (up to 3 weeks) than during recurrent episodes of genital herpes.
- Local symptoms: Itching, pain, dysuria, and vaginal or urethral discharge.
- Constitutional symptoms: Fever, headache, malaise, and myalgias in approximately 40% of men and 70% of women who seek medical advice.
- Recurrent genital herpes is preceded by tenderness, pain, and burning at the site of eruption lasting from 2 hours to 2 days.
- The frequency and severity of recurrences decrease with time.

PHYSICAL EXAM
- Multiple superficial vesicles, 1–2 mm in diameter, with a serous, erythematous base
- In women:
  - Lesions on the external genitalia, labia majora, labia minora, vaginal vestibule, and introitus. Vesicles leave exquisitely tender ulcers after rupture. The vaginal mucosa is inflamed and edematous.
  - The cervix is involved in 70–90% of cases and is characterized by ulcerative or necrotic cervical mucosa. Cervicitis may be the only manifestation in some patients.
- In men:
  - Lesions in the glans penis, the prepuce, the shaft of the penis, and sometimes on the scrotum, thighs, and buttocks. In dry areas, the lesions progress to pustules and then encrust.
  - Herpetic urethritis occurs in 30–40% of affected men.
  - Proctitis may occur in men who engage in receptive anal intercourse.
- Tender regional lymphadenopathy is common.
- History and physical examination alone often lead to an inaccurate diagnosis. Typical lesions are frequently absent.

DIAGNOSTIC TESTS & INTERPRETATION
Lab
Initial lab tests
- Viral culture has low sensitivity, especially for recurrent lesions.
- Multinucleated giant cells are seen in Tzanck smears. Has low sensitivity and specificity.
- Direct fluorescent antibody: Used in specimens obtained from ulcer bases or in tissue culture cells.

- PCR assays for HSV DNA are more sensitive (Not FDA cleared for testing genital specimens). Can distinguish between HSV-1 and HSV-2.
- HSV antibodies develop during the first several weeks after infection and persist indefinitely. Type-specific HSV serologic assays are based on the HSV-specific glycoprotein G2 for HSV-2, and glycoprotein G1 for HSV-1. Sensitivity varies from 80–98%.

Follow-Up & Special Considerations
- Consider HSV type-specific serologies in HIV-positive persons during their initial evaluation.
- For infants exposed to HSV during birth, as documented by maternal virologic testing or presumed by observation of maternal lesions, consider surveillance cultures of mucosal surfaces to detect HSV infection before development of clinical signs.

Diagnostic Procedures/Other
- Gently abrade the lesion with a sterile gauze pad to provoke oozing but not gross bleeding.
- Squeeze the lesion between a gloved thumb and forefinger to increase exudate from the lesion.
- Apply the exudate directly onto the microscope slide, if used for dark-field and direct immunofluorescence tests.

DIFFERENTIAL DIAGNOSIS
Infectious
- Syphilis
- Chancroid
- Acute HIV infection
- Mycobacteria (rare)
- Fungi (rare)
- Parasites (rare)
- Lymphogranuloma venereum (rare)
- Granuloma inguinale (rare)
- Donovanosis (rare)

Noninfectious
- Malignancy
- Trauma
- Fixed drug eruption
- Erythema multiforme
- Dermatitis herpetiformis
- Behçet's syndrome

TREATMENT

MEDICATION

Systemic Antivirals
- Valacyclovir is the valine ester of acyclovir and has enhanced absorption after oral administration.
- Famciclovir also has high oral bioavailability.
- Antivirals have no effect on risk, frequency, or severity of recurrences.
- Topical therapy with antivirals is not recommended.

PRIMARY INFECTION
- Treatment reduces severity and shortens the course of disease if administered within 72 hours of onset of lesion. Therapy should be offered even after 72 hours if ongoing symptoms persist.
- Acyclovir 400 mg orally 3 times a day for 7–10 days.
- Acyclovir 200 mg orally 5 times a day for 7–10 days.
- Famciclovir 250 mg orally 3 times a day for 7–10 days.
- Valacyclovir 1 g orally twice a day for 7–10 days.
  - Treatment may be extended if healing is incomplete after 10 days of therapy.
  - Immunocompromised patients may require longer treatment.
  - Parenteral therapy indicated if central nervous system (CNS) disease, pneumonitis, hepatitis, or disseminated disease. Administer acyclovir 5–10 mg/kg IV every 8 hours for 2–7 days or until clinical improvement, followed by oral antiviral therapy to complete at least 10 days of total therapy.

RECURRENT GENITAL HERPES

Episodic Treatment
Effective if administered within 1 day of lesion onset or during the prodrome.
- Acyclovir 400 mg orally 3 times a day for 5 days.
- Acyclovir 800 mg orally twice a day for 5 days.
- Acyclovir 800 mg orally 3 times a day for 2 days.
- Famciclovir 125 mg orally twice daily for 5 days.
- Famciclovir 1000 mg orally twice daily for 1 day.
- Valacyclovir 500 mg orally twice a day for 3 days (3).
- Valacyclovir 1 g orally once a day for 5 days.

Suppressive Treatment
If >6 recurrences per year.
- Acyclovir 400 mg orally twice a day.
- Famciclovir 250 mg orally twice a day.
- Valacyclovir 500 mg orally once a day. May be less effective than other valacyclovir or acyclovir dosing regimens if >10 episodes per year.
- Valacyclovir 1 g orally once a day
  - Safety and efficacy have been documented among patients receiving daily therapy with acyclovir for as long as 6 years and with valacyclovir or famciclovir for 1 year.
  - Frequency of recurrent genital herpes outbreaks diminishes over time. Consider discontinuation of suppressive treatment.

HIV INFECTION
Immunocompromised patients may have prolonged or severe episodes with increased viral shedding.

Episodic Treatment
- Acyclovir 400 mg orally 3 times a day for 5–10 days.
- Famciclovir 500 mg orally twice a day for 5–10 days.
- Valacyclovir 1 gram orally twice a day for 5–10 days.
- Intravenous acyclovir for severe genital herpes.
- If no improvement, consider resistance to acyclovir and treat with foscarnet 40 mg/kg IV every 8 hours until clinical resolution.

Suppressive Treatment
- Acyclovir 400–800 mg orally 2–3 times a day.
- Famciclovir 500 mg orally twice a day.
- Valacyclovir 500 mg orally twice a day.

Pregnancy Considerations
- The safety of acyclovir, valacyclovir, and famciclovir therapy has not been definitively established in pregnancy. Available data do not indicate an increased risk for major birth defects during the first trimester (4). Data for the use of valacyclovir or famciclovir are limited.
- Acyclovir treatment late in pregnancy reduces the frequency of cesarean section among women who have recurrent genital herpes.
- Antiviral therapy among HSV seropositive women without a history of genital herpes is not recommended.

Pediatric Considerations
- Known or suspected neonatal herpes: Treat with acyclovir 20 mg/kg body weight IV every 8 hours for 21 days for disseminated and CNS disease, or for 14 days for disease limited to the skin and mucous membranes.
- Consider empiric use of acyclovir for infants born to women who acquired HSV near term because of the high risk of neonatal herpes.

ALERT
Thrombotic thrombocytopenic purpura/hemolytic uremic syndrome occurs in patients with advanced HIV disease and other immunosuppressing conditions receiving high doses of valacyclovir.

ADDITIONAL TREATMENT

General Measures
- Evaluation and counseling of sex partners, even if asymptomatic. Type-specific serologic testing of asymptomatic partners is recommended to determine risk for HSV acquisition.
- Analgesics for patients with primary HSV infection and several painful lesions.
- Sitz baths for women with multiple ulcerations.

ONGOING CARE

PATIENT EDUCATION
- Patients with genital herpes should be educated concerning the natural history of the disease, with emphasis on the potential for recurrent episodes, asymptomatic viral shedding, and risk of sexual transmission.
- Asymptomatic persons diagnosed with HSV-2 infection by type-specific serologic testing should receive the same counseling messages as for persons with symptomatic infection.

PROGNOSIS
Neonatal herpes is associated with a 70% mortality rate if untreated.

COMPLICATIONS
- Complications during primary genital herpetic infection: Secondary yeast infections, aseptic meningitis, extragenital herpetic lesions, and sacral autonomic neuropathy.
- Genital ulcers associated with increased susceptibility and transmission of HIV infection during intercourse.
- Neonatal HSV infection is usually the result of intrapartum HSV transmission.
- There is an increased risk of spontaneous abortion and prematurity in cases of primary HSV infection during pregnancy.

REFERENCES
1. Xu F, Sternberg MR, Kottiri BJ, et al. Trends in herpes simplex virus type 1 and type 2 seroprevalence in the United States. *JAMA* 2006;296(8):964–973.
2. Corey L, Wald A, Patel R, et al. Once-daily valacyclovir to reduce the risk of transmission of genital herpes. *N Engl J Med* 2004;350(1):11–20.
3. Leone PA, Trottier S, Miller JM. Valacyclovir for episodic treatment of genital herpes: A shorter 3-day treatment course compared with 5-day treatment. *Clin Infect Dis* 2002;34(7):958–962.
4. Pasternak B, Hviid A. Use of acyclovir, valacyclovir, and famciclovir in the first trimester of pregnancy and the risk of birth defects. *JAMA* 2010;304(8):859–866.

ADDITIONAL READING
- Workowski KA, Berman SM. Sexually transmitted diseases treatment guidelines, 2010. *MMWR Recomm Rep* 2010;59(RR-12):1–110

 CODES

ICD9
- 054.10 Genital herpes, unspecified
- 054.11 Herpetic vulvovaginitis
- 054.13 Herpetic infection of penis

CLINICAL PEARLS
- Signs and symptoms during primary infection are more prominent and last longer than during recurrent episodes.
- Antiviral treatment reduces the severity and shortens the disease course but has no effect on risk, frequency, or severity of recurrences.
- Suppressive therapy is recommended if >6 recurrences occur in a 12-month period.

G

GIARDIASIS

Paschalis Vergidis
Matthew E. Falagas

 BASICS

DESCRIPTION
An infection of the upper small bowel with *Giardia lamblia*, which may cause diarrhea. Mode of transmission include from person to person, water-borne, and less commonly food-borne.

EPIDEMIOLOGY
Incidence
- Globally distributed parasitosis.
- Commonest where standards of sanitation are low.
- In a survey from 2003 to 2006 it was estimated that 20,000 cases occur in the US annually.
- Infection is usually sporadic and spreads from person to person directly by the fecal–oral route or indirectly by ingestion of fecally contaminated water or food.
- Epidemics mainly occur where gross *Giardia* cyst contamination of water supplies occurs.
- Humans are the principal reservoir of infection, but wild beavers and other animals have also been found to be infected in North America.

RISK FACTORS
- Epidemics resulting from person-to-person transmission sometimes occur in childcare centers, in institutionalized individuals, and among men who have sex with men.
- Overland travelers to the Far East are at high risk for infection.

GENERAL PREVENTION
- Implementation of high standards of environmental sanitation and personal hygiene.
- Avoidance of consumption of raw vegetables and tap water in endemic areas.
- Boiling destroys cysts rapidly, and appropriate filtering removes them effectively.
- Institution of prevention measures in day care centers, residential communities of children and the mentally handicapped, and among men who have sex with men.

PATHOPHYSIOLOGY
Infection occurs after ingestion of cysts. After excystation, trophozoites colonize the upper small bowel. Diarrhea results mainly from disruption of the brush border.

ETIOLOGY
- A flagellate protozoon, *G. lamblia* (*Giardia intestinalis*), that exists in trophozoite and cyst forms. The infective form is the cyst of the parasite.
- Cysts are infective as soon as passed and remain infective in water for a few months.
- When ingested by a new host, they excyst in the upper gastrointestinal tract and liberate trophozoites, which attach with their suckers to the surface of the duodenal or jejunal mucosa and multiply by binary fission.
- When trophozoites drop off the duodenal and jejunal mucosa, they are carried on with the contents in the gut and encyst.

COMMONLY ASSOCIATED CONDITIONS
- Hypochlorhydria (e.g., prior gastric surgery)
- IgA deficiency
- Cystic fibrosis

 DIAGNOSIS

HISTORY
- Infection may be asymptomatic.
- The ratio of asymptomatic to symptomatic cases is high.
- Children usually acquire the infection but exhibit a high degree of tolerance.
- Symptoms develop a few days to several weeks (average, 9 days) after ingestion of cysts.
- Severe infection may develop in immunodeficient hosts.
- Infection may become chronic.
- The main symptom is diarrhea, usually of subacute onset, although sometimes of acute onset; diarrhea may continue for weeks or months if untreated.

- Stool frequency: Usually 3–8 bowel motions daily.
- Stool: Pale, offensive, bulky, with much flatus but no blood or mucus.
- Crampy abdominal pain, urgent call to stool; no tenesmus, but perianal soreness may develop.
- Bloating, borborygmi, steatorrhea.
- Anorexia and possibly vomiting in each stage of symptomatic infection; loss of weight.
- Unusual features: Urticaria, arthritis, biliary tract disease, gastric infection.
- Abdominal distention (typical), flatulence.
- Development of anemia is uncommon.

DIAGNOSTIC TESTS & INTERPRETATION
Lab
- Search in a direct saline smear of stool for characteristic cysts.
- Repeat 3 times for up to 90% success of identifying the cysts, versus 50–70% on single stool specimen examination.
- Cyst: Oval, 8 to 14 μm long, 5 to 10 μm wide; contains 4 small nuclei and a central retractile axostyle.
- The number of cysts found bears no relationship to severity of symptoms.
- Occasionally, trophozoites are found in fresh diarrheal stools. Sometimes, in patients with intense symptoms, no cysts are detected in stool, probably because of high concentrations of trophozoites adhering to mucosa.
- Trophozoite: Pear-shaped, 15 μm long, 9 μm wide, 3 μm thick; possesses 4 pairs of flagella.
- *Giardia* antigen detection by immunofluorescence or ELISA (sensitivity 90–100%, specificity 95–100%) are commonly employed.
- Serologic methods are mainly used in epidemiologic studies.

Diagnostic Procedures/Other
In difficult cases with a high suspicion index for diagnosis, employ the "hairy string test" (Entero-Test), which may recover trophozoites by duodenal aspiration. This is now rarely used.

Pathological Findings
Intestinal biopsy reveals partial villous atrophy with mild lymphocytic infiltration of the duodenum or jejunum. Trophozoites may be seen on the surface of the bowel.

DIFFERENTIAL DIAGNOSIS
- Secondary disaccharidase deficiency.
- Tropical sprue
- Enteropathogenic *E. coli* infection.
- Cryptosporidiosis, isosporiasis.
- Crohn's ileitis

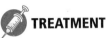 TREATMENT

MEDICATION

First Line
- Symptomatic patients should be treated. Treatment of asymptomatic children prevents the spread of infection.
- Metronidazole (with efficacy up to 80–95%):
  – In adults (50 kg body weight and above): Either 250–500 mg (400 mg in the United Kingdom) t.i.d by mouth for 5 days, or 2.0–2.5 g by mouth once daily for 3 days.
  – Avoid alcohol intake, as it may produce side effects such as headache and flushing.
  – In children, dosage modified: 5 mg/kg t.i.d for 7 days.
- Tinidazole (with efficacy up to 90%): In adults a single dose of 2 g is usually effective (1).
- Nitazoxanide at 500 mg twice daily for 5 days, has equal or superior efficacy to metronidazole (2).

Second Line
- Albendazole 400 mg by mouth daily for 5 days (3,4).
- Quinacrine (mepacrine):
  – In adults (with efficacy up to 90%): 100 mg 3 times daily by mouth for 5–7 days
  – In children: 2 mg/kg bid for 5–7 days.
  – Not available in the US.

- Furazolidone (with efficacy up to 80%):
  – Caution: Hemolysis in patients with G-6PD deficiency.
  – In adults: 100 mg 4 times daily by mouth for 7–10 days.
  – In children: 2 mg/kg daily 4 times daily for 7–10 days.
- A failure rate of about 10–20% is expected.
- Repeating treatment for a longer course or changing to another appropriate drug usually eradicates infection. A combination of 2 drugs (i.e., metronidazole plus mepacrine) may be helpful when failure to a classical one drug regimen fails.
- Repeated relapses may be due to infection from another family member or close contact with a person with an asymptomatic infection.
- Treat all suspected cases simultaneously.
- Diarrhea may persist after treatment and may be attributed to secondary lactose intolerance or concomitant tropical sprue.

Pregnancy Considerations
- Metronidazole is avoided due to possible teratogenic effect.
- For mild disease avoid treatment until after delivery.
- If necessary, use paromomycin 25–35 mg/kg PO daily in 3 divided doses for 7 days.

 ONGOING CARE

PROGNOSIS
- Monitor symptoms, body weight, and stool examinations.
- Patients with a high degree of tolerance have asymptomatic infection.
- If symptomatic, diarrhea may last for weeks or months and can be self-limiting.
- Patients may have concomitant bacterial infection of the small bowel.

COMPLICATIONS
- Steatorrhea
- Malabsorption
- Weight loss
- Hypogammaglobulinemia

REFERENCES
1. Speelman P. Single-dose tinidazole for the treatment of giardiasis. *Antimicrob Agents Chemother* 1985;27:227–229.
2. Ortiz JJ, Ayoub A, Gargala G, et al. Randomized clinical study of nitazoxanide compared to metronidazole in the treatment of symptomatic giardiasis in children from Northern Peru. *Aliment Pharmacol Ther* 2001;15:1409–1415.
3. Misra PK, Kumar A, Agarwal V, et al. A comparative clinical trial of albendazole versus metronidazole in children with giardiasis. *Indian Pediatr* 1995;32:779–782.
4. Solaymani-Mohammadi S, Genkinger JM, Loffredo CA, et al. A meta-analysis of the effectiveness of albendazole compared with metronidazole as treatments for infections with *Giardia duodenalis*. *PLoS Negl Trop Dis* 2010;4:e682.

ADDITIONAL READING
- Rossignol JF. *Cryptosporidium* and *Giardia*: Treatment options and prospects for new drugs. *Exp Parasitol* 2010;124:45–53.
- Gardner TB, Hill DR. Treatment of giardiasis. *Clin Microbiol Rev* 2001;14:114–128.

 CODES

ICD9
007.1 Giardiasis

CLINICAL PEARLS
- Giardiasis is a parasitosis of the upper small bowel that can cause diarrhea. There is a high rate of asymptomatic infection.
- Treatment options: Metronidazole, tinidazole, or nitazoxanide. Paromomycin for pregnant women.
- Relapse may be due to infection from a close contact with asymptomatic infection.

G

GINGIVITIS

Alejandro Restrepo
Eleftherios Mylonakis

 BASICS

DESCRIPTION
- Inflammation of the gingiva, which may lead to localized bleeding, systemic fevers, or tooth loss secondary to periodontitis.
- Classification:
  – Dental plaque induced
  – Non-dental plaque induced

EPIDEMIOLOGY
Incidence
- There is an increased incidence of disease in immunodeficient states and pregnancy.
- Most common in adults more than 35 years old (1).

RISK FACTORS
- Poor dental hygiene
- Diabetes mellitus
- Coronary artery disease
- Mal occlusion
- Pregnancy
- Medications: Like OCPs, Dilantin
- Leukemia
- HIV
- Malnutrition

GENERAL PREVENTION
- Oral hygiene
- Stannous fluoride
- Regular visits with a dental care provider.

PATHOPHYSIOLOGY
Acute and chronic inflammation of gingiva with hyperemia, neutrophils infiltration, and accumulation of bacteria with accumulation of the plaque in the gingival margin (1).

ETIOLOGY
A number of organisms are responsible for gingivitis. Especially: *Streptococcus* spp., actinomycetes, spirochetes, and anaerobes (2).

 DIAGNOSIS

HISTORY
- Bleeding of gums with brushing is the first manifestation.
- Halitosis may occur.

PHYSICAL EXAM
- Erythema, edema, plaque, and calculus with bleeding in the gingival area.
- Then can become necrotic.
- With more severe disease, termed Vincent's angina, pain, edema, fever, and adenopathy may develop.

DIAGNOSTIC TESTS & INTERPRETATION
Lab
Initial lab tests
Gingivitis is a clinical diagnosis.

Follow-Up & Special Considerations
Needs close follow up with dental provider.

DIFFERENTIAL DIAGNOSIS
- Periodontitis
- Glossitis
- Pericoronitis

 TREATMENT

MEDICATION
First Line
- Debridement of plaque
- Chlorhexidine rinses
- Antibiotic use in severe cases. Use antibiotics against mouth flora. These include the following: Metronidazole, penicillins, and clindamycin.

Second Line
Other antibiotics based on the culture results (2).

ADDITIONAL TREATMENT
The antibiotic regimen can be changed based on cultures results and sensitivities in cases that do not respond to therapy

General Measures
- Remove irritating factors
- Good oral hygiene
- Regular dental checkups
- No smoking

SURGERY/OTHER PROCEDURES
Debridement of the teeth and gingival area by a professional is needed (3).

ONGOING CARE

FOLLOW-UP RECOMMENDATIONS
Follow up with a dental provider is mandatory.

Patient Monitoring
Until symptoms resolve

DIET
Appropriate diet is important.

PATIENT EDUCATION
- Good dental hygiene is needed to prevent disease.
- Regular teeth brushing and flossing.

PROGNOSIS
Good prognosis responds well to appropriate treatment (4).

COMPLICATIONS
- Tooth loss
- Severe periodontal disease
- Recurrence of gingivitis
- Abscess of the gingiva or bone area
- Some studies indicate that gingivitis might be associated with coronary artery disease.

ADDITIONAL READING

- Chow AW, Roser SM, Brady FA. Orofacial odontogenic infections. *Ann Intern Med* 1978;88:392.
- Coventry J, Griffiths G, Scully C, et al. ABC of oral health: periodontal disease. *Br Med J.* 2000;321: 36–39.

- Loesche W. Dental caries and periodontitis: Contrasting two infections that have medical implications. *Infect Dis Clin N Am* 2007;21: 471–502.
- Tanner A, Stillman N. Oral and dental infections with anaerobic bacteria: Clinical features, predominant pathogens and treatment. *Clin Infect Dis* 1993;16(Suppl 4):S304.

 CODES

ICD9
- 523.00 Acute gingivitis, plaque induced
- 523.01 Acute gingivitis, non-plaque induced
- 523.10 Chronic gingivitis, plaque induced

G

GRANULOMA INGUINALE (DONOVANOSIS)

Paschalis Vergidis
Matthew E. Falagas

 BASICS

DESCRIPTION
Sexually transmitted disease manifested as a single lesion or multiple nodules; also known as donovanosis.

EPIDEMIOLOGY
Prevalence
- Endemic in tropical and developing countries (India, Papua New Guinea, central Australia, and southern Africa)
- Rare in developed countries. In the US, fewer than 100 cases are reported annually.

RISK FACTORS
Geographic location (endemic in tropics), residence, work, and travel

GENERAL PREVENTION
Use of barrier contraceptives

ETIOLOGY
Klebsiella granulomatis (formerly known as *Calymmatobacterium granulomatis*)

 DIAGNOSIS

HISTORY
Incubation period: 2–3 weeks.

PHYSICAL EXAM
- Nodules on the genitals that slowly enlarge and ulcerate.
- The ulcerative lesions are painless without regional lymphadenopathy. Subcutaneous spread of the lesions can cause pseudobuboes.
- Verrucous form likely to occur in the perianal area.
- Elongated ulcer with elevated papillary edges.
- Ulcer edge is white, on a beefy-red, hypertrophic base. Bleeds easily on contact
- Rectal lesions associated with receptive anal intercourse.
- Scar formation and deformities in late stages.

DIAGNOSTIC TESTS & INTERPRETATION
Lab
Initial lab tests
- Usually based on clinical appearance.
- Can identify intracellular "Donovan bodies" (rod-shaped oval organisms) from lesion scrapings (1).
- The organism is very difficult to culture.
- No FDA-cleared PCR tests for the detection of *K. granulomatis* DNA exist.

Follow-Up & Special Considerations
- The disease may coexist with other sexually transmitted infections.
- The lesions can develop secondary bacterial infection.

Diagnostic Procedures/Other
- Gently abrade the lesion with a sterile gauze pad to provoke oozing but not gross bleeding.
- Squeeze the lesion between a gloved thumb and forefinger to increase exudate from the lesion.
- Apply the exudate directly onto a microscope slide if used for dark-field and direct immunofluorescence tests.

Pathological Findings
Histologic examination of crush or biopsy preparations of the lesion that show typical intracytoplasmic organisms (Donovan bodies)

DIFFERENTIAL DIAGNOSIS
Infectious
- Genital herpes
- Syphilis
- Chancroid
- Acute HIV infection
- Lymphogranuloma venereum (rare)
- Mycobacteria (rare)
- Fungi (rare)
- Parasites (rare)

Noninfectious
- Malignancy
- Trauma
- Fixed drug eruption
- Erythema multiforme
- Dermatitis herpetiformis
- Behçet's syndrome

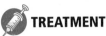 TREATMENT

MEDICATION
First Line
Doxycycline 100 mg orally twice a day for at least 3 weeks and until all lesions have completely healed.

Second Line
- Azithromycin 1 g orally once per week (2,3).
- Ciprofloxacin 750 mg orally twice a day.
- Erythromycin base 500 mg orally 4 times a day.
- Trimethoprim–sulfamethoxazole: One double-strength tablet twice daily.
- Treatment is given for at least 3 weeks and until all lesions have completely healed.
- Some specialists recommend the addition of an aminoglycoside (e.g., gentamicin 1 mg/kg IV every 8 hours) if improvement is not evident within the first few days of therapy. Addition of an aminoglycoside should also be considered in patients with HIV infection.

Pregnancy Considerations
- Doxycycline and ciprofloxacin are contraindicated.
- Pregnancy is a relative contraindication to the use of sulfonamides.
- Pregnant and lactating women should be treated with erythromycin.
- Addition of an aminoglycoside can be considered.
- Azithromycin might be useful, but data are lacking.

 ONGOING CARE

FOLLOW-UP RECOMMENDATIONS
- Follow-up clinically until signs and symptoms have resolved.
- Healing typically proceeds inward from the ulcer margins. Relapse can occur 6–18 months after apparently effective therapy.
- Persons who have had sexual contact with a patient who has granuloma *inguinale* within the 60 days before onset of the patient's symptoms should be examined and offered therapy. The value of empiric therapy in the absence of clinical signs and symptoms has not been established.

PROGNOSIS
Failures of treatment and relapses have been reported even with first-line medications.

COMPLICATIONS
- Genital pseudoelephantiasis
- Extremely rare: Psoas abscess

REFERENCES
1. Richens J. Donovanosis (granuloma inguinale). *Sex Transm Infect* 2006;82(Suppl 4):iv21–iv22.
2. Bowden FJ, Mein J, Plunkett C, et al. Pilot study of azithromycin in the treatment of genital donovanosis. *Genitourin Med* 1996;72(1):17–19.
3. Workowski KA, Berman SM. Sexually transmitted diseases treatment guidelines, 2010. *MMWR Recomm Rep* 2010;59(RR-12):1–110.

ADDITIONAL READING
- O'Farrell N. Donovanosis. *Sex Trans Infect* 2002;78(6):452–457.

 CODES

ICD9
099.2 Granuloma inguinale

CLINICAL PEARLS
- Donovanosis is characterized by chronic, progressive, painless ulcers of the genital region.
- Diagnosis is based on epidemiologic history and clinical appearance of the lesions.
- Treatment is necessary until all lesions have completely healed.

G

HANTAVIRUS PULMONARY SYNDROME

Alejandro Restrepo
Eleftherios Mylonakis

 BASICS

DESCRIPTION
Hantavirus pulmonary syndrome (HPS) is a cardiopulmonary illness with high mortality.

EPIDEMIOLOGY
Prevalence
- First described in a cluster of patients in 1993 in the southwestern US
- There are a total of 541 cases reported in humans in 31 states from 1993 until February 2010
- The incidence of disease seems to correlate to changes in the deer mouse populations
- In 1993, at the time the disease was first discovered, the mouse population in the southwestern US had dramatically increased, and indoor invasion of homes by field mice has been implicated for some illness.
- There also confirmed cases in Central and South America

RISK FACTORS (1)
- Exposure to deer mice, cotton rat, rice rat, and white-footed mouse. Contact with infected rodents, mainly urine and droppings
- Exterminators, farm laborers, sleeping on ground, people who work in construction, and pest control workers are at risk
- Field mice infestation at home, also campers and hikers
- People opening and cleaning previously unused cabins or buildings

GENERAL PREVENTION
- At the present time, no vaccine is available
- Rodent control in and around home is important
- Avoidance of areas inhabited by large numbers of mice
- Protecting houses from the habitation of field mice may be effective.
- Exterminators and others who deal with large numbers of dead mice should use respirators.
- Air-borne and universal isolation is needed for patients with HPS in the hospital

PATHOPHYSIOLOGY
Hantaviral antigens are detected in pulmonary microvasculature and dendritic cells. The hantavirus mainly causes functional impairment of vascular endothelium and permeability associated with pneumonitis and shock.

ETIOLOGY
Sin Nombre virus is an RNA virus of the genus Hantavirus of the family Bunyaviridae
- Sin Nombre hantavirus was found to be the etiology of HPS; however, many classes have been identified, causing similar symptoms in North and South America
- The reservoir of this zoonotic infection is the rodents. The hosts are deer mice (*Peromyscus maniculatus*), white-footed mice (*Peromyscus leucopus*), rice rat (*Oryzomys palustris*), and cotton rats (*Sigmodon hispidus*)
- Infection is by inhalation of virus-containing aerosols of rodent feces, urine, or saliva
- Rare person-to-person spread has been reported but is rare and usually associated with exposure to infected body fluids
- The Andes virus was reported in South America and there have been outbreaks in Argentina and Chile. Also have had cases of human–human transmission (2)

[Rx] DIAGNOSIS

HISTORY
- Incubation: Between 8 and 28 days
- Prodrome: 4–10 days
- Following the prodrome, patients abruptly develop cough and shortness of breath. This progresses to respiratory failure within hours
- Often patients present with fever, myalgia, fatigue, headache, and other nonspecific flu-like symptoms and gastrointestinal symptoms
- Tachypnea is the most common finding on hospital admission.

PHYSICAL EXAM
- Dyspnea and respiratory distress
- Cyanosis, pulmonary rales, and rhonchi
- Patients develop pulmonary edema, pneumonitis, and shock during the acute phase of the illness.
- Death is usually due to shock and ventricular arrhythmia

DIAGNOSTIC TESTS & INTERPRETATION
Lab
Initial lab tests
- Leukocytosis (with left shift) along with thrombocytopenia and atypical lymphocytes
- Hemoconcentration is common
- Elevated creatine phosphokinase (CPK) consistent with myositis, elevated liver functions tests, LDH, and amylase are seen. Acute hypoalbuminemia is common
- Very mild azotemia with proteinuria occurs early in the course of the disease; however, renal failure is an uncommon complication.
- Hypoxemia
- Can cause disseminated intravascular coagulation (DIC)

Follow-Up & Special Considerations
Needs close follow-up in the hospital

Imaging
Initial approach
- Chest x-rays reveal interstitial or alveolar infiltrates, pulmonary edema, and pleural effusion.
- Chest tomography shows interstitial infiltrates with pleural effusions

Follow-Up & Special Considerations
The state health department should be contacted (1)

Diagnostic Procedures/Other
- Serologic testing for hantavirus, mainly detection of IgM, and/or rising titers of IgG
- Detection of Hantavirus PCR in blood or tissue
- Detection of hantavirus antigen by immunohistochemistry in tissue (2)

Pathological Findings
Hantaviral viremia produces capillary leak syndrome with pneumonitis, shock, and respiratory failure

DIFFERENTIAL DIAGNOSIS
- Other viral pneumonia
- Bacterial and fungal pneumonia including: Chlamydia, Mycoplasma, Legionnaire's disease, anthrax, tularemia, pneumonic plague, leptospirosis, group A streptococcus, coccidioidomycosis, and histoplasmosis
- Pulmonary edema
- Pneumocystis jiroveci pneumonia
- Hypersensitivity pneumonitis

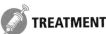 TREATMENT

MEDICATION
First Line
- Supportive care is crucial
- May need mechanical ventilation and oxygenation in severe cases
- Start broad spectrum antibiotics while awaiting the confirmation of Hantavirus infection (1)

Second Line
- Ribavirin has not been shown to be effective for treatment of HPS
- Extracorporeal membrane oxygenation (ECMO) has been used in the past

IN-PATIENT CONSIDERATIONS
Initial Stabilization
Needs admission to the hospital and may need transfer to ICU if severe hypoxemia

Admission Criteria
Dyspnea and respiratory distress with history of exposure to rodents

Discharge Criteria
Until infection is cleared and patient hemodynamically stable

 ONGOING CARE

PROGNOSIS
- Prognosis is poor in patients with fulminant illness due to HPS
- Earlier management in intensive care may improve survival
- Mortality rate is around 35–40%

COMPLICATIONS
- Respiratory failure requiring mechanical ventilation
- Adult respiratory distress syndrome
- Myocardial depression
- Shock and death

REFERENCES
1. Jonsson CB, Figueiredo LT, Vapalahti O. A global perspective on Hantavirus ecology, epidemiology, and disease. *Clin Microbiol Rev.* 2010;23(2):412–441.
2. Simpson SQ, Spikes L, Patel S, et al. Hantavirus pulmonary syndrome. *Infect Dis Clin North Am* 2010;24:159–173.

ADDITIONAL READING
- http://www.cdc.gov/ncidod/diseases/hanta/hps/index.htm. Accessed June 8, 2010.

 CODES

ICD9
079.81 Hantavirus infection

H

HELICOBACTER PYLORI INFECTION

Mary L. Pisculli (E. Mylonakis, Editor)

 BASICS

DESCRIPTION

Helicobacter pylori, a gram-negative, spiral microaerophilic bacterium, is the most common cause of gastritis and of its associated disease, gastric cancer and gastric mucosa complications – gastric and duodenal ulcer-associated lymphoid-tissue (MALT) lymphoma.

EPIDEMIOLOGY

Incidence
- 0.5% in industrialized countries
- 4–15% in developing countries

Prevalence
- *H. pylori* colonizes more than half of the world's population with an increased prevalence among poorer countries and communities.
- The prevalence of *H. pylori* infection is about 30% in the US and other developed countries. Rate of infection is 50% among those over 60 years of age and 25% among those 30–59 years old. Infection rate in children is 5%.
- In most developing countries, the prevalence of *H. pylori* is 80%, with high rates among children and adolescents.

RISK FACTORS

Most infections are acquired in early childhood. Risk factors include low socioeconomic status, household crowding during childhood, and no fixed hot water supply. In adults, the risk increases with the number of children living in the home.

Genetics
- In the US, the prevalence of infection is significantly higher in African-Americans and Hispanics compared to whites and may reflect socioeconomic factors rather than genetic predisposition.
- Polymorphisms in the human *IL-1B* gene increase the risk for atrophic gastritis and gastric adenocarcinoma.

GENERAL PREVENTION
- Improved standards of living including sanitation and overall hygiene have been shown to reduce *H. pylori* transmission.
- Testing and treating first degree relatives of patients with gastric cancer may reduce their risk of gastric cancer.

PATHOPHYSIOLOGY
- *H. pylori* has an efficient urease that protects it against acid by catalyzing urea to produce ammonia.
- Colonization of the stomach leads to chronic active gastritis which may damage the gastric and duodenal mucosa causing ulceration and intestinal metaplasia.
  - Neoplasia occurs in only a small proportion of colonized hosts and may be dependent on strain-specific bacterial factors [e.g., cytotoxin-associated gene A (cagA+)] and host traits.

ETIOLOGY
- *H. pylori* is a gram-negative, spiral, flagellated microaerophilic bacterium.
- The primary mode of infection is unknown although person-to-person transmission seems most likely, possibly via an oral–oral, oral–gastro or oral–fecal route.

COMMONLY ASSOCIATED CONDITIONS
- Duodenal or gastric ulcers develop in 1–10% of infected patients.
- Gastric cancer develops in 1–3%. *H. pylori* is the strongest known risk factor for gastric adenocarcinoma and is considered a group 1 carcinogen by the World Health Organization (WHO).
- Gastric mucosa-associated lymphoid-tissue (MALT) lymphoma (<0.01%).
- *H. pylori* infection is associated with iron deficiency anemia and idiopathic thrombocytopenic purpura (ITP).

 DIAGNOSIS

HISTORY
- The majority of patients with *H. pylori* infection are asymptomatic and do not develop complications.
- Dyspepsia symptoms may include pain centered in the upper abdomen, early satiety, bloating, or nausea.
  - Features concerning for malignancy or ulcer disease (red flag) include unexplained weight loss, early satiety, GI bleeding, anemia, progressive dysphagia, odynophagia, persistent vomiting, anorexia, as well as previous esophagogastric malignancy or a family history of gastric cancer.

PHYSICAL EXAM
Assess for rectal bleeding, jaundice, or an abdominal mass possibly indicative of peptic ulcer disease (PUD) or gastrointestinal malignancy.

DIAGNOSTIC TESTS & INTERPRETATION
Lab
Initial lab tests
- Diagnosis can be made either with esophagogastroduodenoscopy (EGD) with biopsy for urease testing, histology, and culture; via non-invasive tests (urea breath test [UBT], fecal antigen test [FAT]); or through serum antibody detection.
- A "test and treat" strategy utilizing non-endoscopic testing for *H. pylori* is appropriate for adult patients presenting with dyspepsia under the age of 45–55 and without "red flag" features.
- Other indications for "test and treat" include: Confirmed gastric or duodenal ulcers and gastric MALT disease; after resection of early gastric cancers; and in persons with a history of PUD not previously treated for *H. pylori* infection.

- The American College of Gastroenterology recommends the UBT or the FAT for the initial diagnosis of active *H. pylori* infection and as a test of cure.
  - UBT: The patient ingests a small amount of isotope-labeled (13C or 14C) urea and the urease of *H. pylori* rapidly converts the urea to bicarbonate which is expired as labeled CO_2. UBT are >95% sensitive and specific for diagnosis and eradication.
  - FAT: Detects *H. pylori* antigen in the stool using an enzyme immunoassay with either a mono- or polyclonal antibody. Sensitivity and specificity of the monoclonal antibody assay for diagnosis and post-treatment are excellent (95–97%) and is a reasonable alternative to UBT for test of eradication and superior to the polyclonal assay due to the latter's lower sensitivity (86%) and specificity (92%) post-treatment.
  - Serum antibody: Widely available and inexpensive but has a low diagnostic accuracy (sensitivity 85%, specificity 79%). Lacks specificity as patients colonized with *H. pylori* (in particular older persons) may have positive results. Antibody testing can also remain positive 4–6 months post-successful treatment and are then only helpful if negative.

Follow-Up & Special Considerations
- The sensitivity of the UBT and FAT may be reduced by concomitant medication use that may suppress infection or in the setting of acute upper gastrointestinal bleeding.
  - To avoid false-negative results, proton-pump inhibitors (PPIs) should be discontinued 2 weeks prior to testing, H2 receptor antagonists 24 hours, and bismuth and antimicrobial agents 4 weeks before diagnostic testing or test of cure.
  - Serology may be helpful in the setting of low bacterial density (gastric atrophy or MALT lymphoma), an actively bleeding ulcer or when the UBT or FAT may be falsely negative.
- NSAIDs independently increase the risk of PUD. The risk increases significantly in the presence of *H. pylori* infection. Patients on long-term aspirin therapy with ulcer disease and/or bleeding should be tested and treated if positive.

Imaging
Imaging procedures are rarely necessary.

Diagnostic Procedures/Other
- EGD with biopsy for urease testing and histology should be performed in adults older than age 45–55 (depending on local rate of gastric cancer) with new-onset dyspepsia and in patients with persistent and severe upper abdominal pain.
  - Urease testing: Sensitivity, 93–97%, specificity >95%; as with UBT, sensitivity reduced by medications suppressing *H. pylori* activity.
  - Histology: >95% sensitive, 100% specific.
  - Microbiologic culture (sensitivity 70–80%, specificity 100%) is expensive but may be useful to guide antibiotic selection, particularly after treatment failure.
  - Endoscopic evaluation should also be performed in persons recently treated with a PPI, antibiotics, or bismuth.
- Infection with *H. pylori* can be patchy, and several gastric mucosal biopsy specimens may be necessary for diagnosis.

Pediatric Considerations
- Children with recurrent upper abdominal pain or iron deficiency anemia refractory to replacement should undergo endoscopy with biopsy for diagnosis.
- Avoid treatment with tetracycline in children below 8 years of age (risk of tooth discoloration).

Pathological Findings
- Acute *H. pylori* infection is characterized by neutrophil infiltration in the surface epithelium. Progression to chronic active gastritis consists of surface epithelial degeneration, persistent neutrophil infiltration of the epithelium and lamina propria, and mononuclear infiltration (lymphocytes and plasma cells) of the lamina propria.
- Atrophic gastritis may result from longstanding infection and is characterized by glandular atrophy, intestinal metaplasia, and sparse inflammatory cells.

DIFFERENTIAL DIAGNOSIS
- PUD
- Non-ulcer dyspepsia
- Gastroesophageal reflux disease (GERD)
- Gastric malignancy
- Pancreatitis
- Biliary tract disease
- In the absence of NSAID use or acid hypersecretory states such as Zollinger–Ellison syndrome, as many as 90% of patients with duodenal ulcer and 80% of patients with gastric ulcer are infected by *H. pylori*

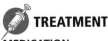 **TREATMENT**

MEDICATION
First Line
- The American College of Gastroenterology recommends clarithromycin plus amoxicillin or metronidazole and a PPI for 14 days (clarithromycin-based triple therapy), or bismuth, metronidazole, tetracycline, and a PPI or H2 receptor antagonist for 10–14 days (bismuth quadruple therapy).
  – Bismuth quadruple therapy is preferred in patients with a penicillin allergy or prior macrolide exposure.
  – These regimens have yielded eradication rates of 70–80% in the US. Treatment failures are largely due to rising antibiotic resistance.
- Sequential therapy (5 days of a PPI and amoxicillin followed by 5 days of a PPI, clarithromycin, and a nitroimidazole) has resulted in high eradication rates internationally, although data are lacking in the US.

Second Line
- Bismuth quadruple therapy as salvage therapy is associated with eradication rates <80%.
- Levofloxacin-based regimens (with a PPI and amoxicillin) may prove effective in the US, depending on underlying resistance.
- Treatment history is useful to avoid potential antimicrobial resistance from a previously used agent. When available, culture and sensitivity data may help guide treatment selection.

 ONGOING CARE

FOLLOW-UP RECOMMENDATIONS
- Confirmation of eradication should be performed in patients with the following: Those with persistent dyspeptic symptoms after treatment, an *H. pylori*-associated ulcer, *H. pylori*-associated MALT lymphoma, a history of resection of early gastric cancer, or an *H. pylori*-associated ulcer.
  – UBT and FAT s may be used to confirm eradication post-treatment, whereas serology tests may remain positive for months following eradication.

PATIENT EDUCATION
Encourage compliance with treatment regimens as shorter courses have yielded higher rates of failure.

PROGNOSIS
- PUD: *H. pylori* eradication significantly reduces the risk of ulcer recurrence and rebleeding.
- Non-ulcer dyspepsia: *H. pylori* eradication may provide a small and highly variable symptomatic benefit.
- Gastric cancer: Several studies suggest that eradication therapy in patients with documented gastric ulcer may decrease the likelihood of developing gastric adenocarcinoma, although this remains controversial.
- Gastric MALT lymphoma: Eradication of *H. pylori* infection causes regression of most localized gastric MALT lymphomas.

COMPLICATIONS
- Recurrence is defined as a positive UBT result after 6 or more months of documented successful eradication therapy. Recurrence is rare in developed settings and primarily due to recurrence within the first year (annual recurrence rate, 1.45%); recurrence in developing areas is more common (annual recurrence rate, 12%) and likely represents reinfection.
- The most commonly reported adverse effects associated with *H. pylori* therapy are nausea, vomiting, and diarrhea. Regimens including clarithromycin or metronidazole may cause a bitter or metallic taste in the mouth. Tetracycline is also associated with photosensitivity and bismuth compounds with darkening of the tongue and stool.

ADDITIONAL READING
- Ables AZ, Simon I, Melton ER. Update on *Helicobacter pylori* treatment. *Am Fam Physician* 2007;75(3):351–358.
- Chey WD, Wong BCY; Practice Parameters Committee of the American College of Gastroenterology. American College of Gastroenterology guideline on the management of *Helicobacter pylori* infection. *Am J Gastroenterol* 2007;102:1808–1825.

- Duck WM, Sobel J, Pruckler JM, et al. Antimicrobial resistance incidence and risk factors among *Helicobacter pylori*-infected persons, United States. *Emerg Infect Dis* [serial on the Internet]. 2004 Jun [August 30, 2010]. http://www.cdc.gov/ncidod/EID/vol10no6/03–0744.htm.
- Everhart JE, Kruszon-Moran D, Perez-Perez GI, et al. Seroprevalence and ethnic differences in *Helicobacter pylori* infection among adults in the United States. *J Infect Dis*. 2000;181:1359–1363.
- Graham DY, Fischbach L. *Helicobacter pylori* treatment in the era of antibiotic resistance. *Gut* 2010;59:1143–1153.
- Malfertheiner P, Megraud F, O'Marain C, et al. Current concepts in the management of *Helicobacter pylori* infection: The Maastricht III Consensus Report. *Gut* 2007;56:772–781.
- Malfertheiner P, Selgrad M. *Helicobacter pylori* infection and current clinical areas of contention. *Curr Opin Gastroenterol* 2010;26:618–623.
- Mccoll K. Clinical practice: *Helicobacter pylori*. *N Engl J Med* 2010;362:1597–1604.
- Niv Y. H pylori after successful eradication. *World J Gastroenterol* 2008;14(10):1477–1478.
- Polk DB, Peek PM. *Helicobacter pylori*: Gastric cancer and beyond. *Nat Rev Cancer* 2010;10(6):403–414.
- Versalovic J. *Helicobacter pylori*: Pathology and diagnostic strategies. *Am J Clin Pathol* 2003;119(3):403–412.

 CODES

ICD9
041.86 Helicobacter pylori [H. pylori]

CLINICAL PEARLS
- UBT is non-invasive and highly accurate, although false-negative results may be obtained in patients taking PPIs or antibiotics.
- Resistance to antibiotic treatment regimens is increasing and confirmation of eradication should be performed.
- *H. pylori* eradication in PUD reduces the risk of ulcer recurrence and rebleeding.

H

HEMOLYTIC–UREMIC SYNDROME

Jatin M. Vyas (E. Mylonakis, Editor)

 BASICS

DESCRIPTION
- The hemolytic–uremic syndrome (HUS) is defined by the following:
  - Acute renal insufficiency
  - Microangiopathic hemolytic anemia
  - Thrombocytopenia

EPIDEMIOLOGY
Incidence
- In industrialized countries, the annual incidence of infection with enterohemorrhagic *Escherichia coli* 0157.H7 (EHEC) ranges from 1 to 5 cases per 100,000 people and is highest in young children under 5 years (1). This frequency is likely an underestimate as it is not reportable in all states.
- In the US, EHEC is estimated to cause more than 70,000 infections.
- The rate of EHEC infection follows a seasonal pattern, with a peak incidence from June through September.
- It is estimated that 0.6–2.4% of all cases of diarrhea and 15–36% of cases of bloody diarrhea or hemorrhagic colitis are associated with EHEC.
- During outbreaks of EHEC infection, about 8% of patients develop HUS.

RISK FACTORS
- Transmission of the infection is primarily linked to undercooked ground beef, the drinking of contaminated water or unpasteurized milk, and working with cattle.
- Hamburger is a major vehicle, associated with food-borne outbreaks of EHEC infection. Other vehicles include apples, cider, cantaloupe, and contaminated drinking water.
- EHEC can be recovered from the intestines in about 1% of healthy cattle. Cattle may harbor the organisms asymptomatically in the intestinal tract and are an important reservoir for the pathogen.
- Beef can also be contaminated during slaughter, and the process of grinding beef may transfer pathogens from the surface of the meat to the interior of it.
- Water-borne transmission and secondary person-to-person contact can be additional important ways of spread in institutional settings, especially in daycare centers and nursing homes.
- Increased susceptibility to this infection has been described after gastrectomy.

GENERAL PREVENTION
- The Food and Drug Administration has recommended a minimum internal temperature of 155°F (86.1°C) for cooked hamburgers. Also, patients should be instructed to do the following:
  - Cook ground beef thoroughly, until its interior is no longer pink and the juices run gray.
  - Always use pasteurized milk.
  - Keep food refrigerated or frozen.
  - Thaw frozen food in a refrigerator or microwave.
  - Keep raw meat and poultry separate from other foods.
  - Wash hands carefully with soap before cooking is begun.
  - Wash the working surfaces (including cutting boards), utensils, and hands after touching raw meat or poultry.
  - Keep hot foods hot.
  - Refrigerate leftovers immediately or discard them.
  - Never taste small bits of raw ground beef during meal preparation.
  - Never place cooked hamburgers back on the unwashed plate that had previously held the raw ground beef.

PATHOPHYSIOLOGY
The pathophysiology is incompletely understood. Bacterially derived toxin acts directly on endothelial cells, which causes inflammation and presumably creates a procoagulant effect, resulting in microvascular thrombosis.

ETIOLOGY
HUS can be due to the following:
- Infectious causes
- Enterohemorrhagic *Escherichia coli* 0157.H7 (EHEC)
- *Aeromonas enterocolitis*
- *Campylobacter* spp.
- HIV infection
- Rotavirus
- *Shigella* spp.
- *Streptococcus pneumoniae*
- *Yersinia* spp.
- Sporadic, noninfectious causes
- Autoimmune diseases (systemic lupus erythematosus, scleroderma, etc.)

- Autologous stem-cell transplantation
- Familial
- Idiopathic
- Malignancy
- Medications (mitomycin, cyclosporin, high doses of valacyclovir, etc.)
- Pregnancy
- Radiation
- EHEC, most commonly serotype 0157:H7 in the US, is the most common cause of HUS. EHEC produces a Shiga-like (vero) cytotoxin. The toxin blocks protein synthesis, leading to cell death (2). Colonic vascular damage by Shiga-like toxin may allow lipopolysaccharides and other inflammatory mediators to gain access to the circulation, thus initiating the HUS.
- Non-0157 *E. coli* organisms that produce Shiga toxin are more difficult to detect than *E. coli* 0157 and can cause uncomplicated diarrhea, hemorrhagic colitis, and HUS.
- An association of younger age with HUS might be explained on the basis of increased toxin available per body weight.

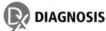 **DIAGNOSIS**

HISTORY
- Infection with EHEC presents with a wide spectrum of clinical manifestation, including asymptomatic carriage and non-bloody diarrhea. However, bloody diarrhea is the most common symptom and is present in 60–90% of cases.
- The infection usually begins with sudden onset of severe abdominal cramps, which are followed within hours by watery diarrhea. Usually within 24 hours after the onset of symptoms, watery diarrhea progresses to grossly bloody stools.
- On presentation, nausea and vomiting may be prominent.
- Bloody diarrhea usually lasts 2–4 days and lasts longer among children.

PHYSICAL EXAM
- The incidence of fever ranges from none to 32%.
- Abdominal cramps and diffuse tenderness sometimes accompany infection with EHEC and may lead to misdiagnosis and even result in unnecessary surgical procedures.
- Oliguria and a marked drop in hematocrit are the first signs of HUS.

DIAGNOSTIC TESTS & INTERPRETATION
Lab
- Routine stool cultures do not identify EHEC, and the presence of fecal leukocytes should not dissuade the clinician from considering the diagnosis of EHEC.
- Because the rate of recovery of *E. coli* 0157:H7 may decline rapidly after the first 4–6 days of illness, special stool cultures should be obtained as early in the course of the illness as possible.
- Unlike other *E. coli* serotypes, *E. coli* 0157:H7 does not rapidly ferment D-sorbitol. When plated on MacConkey and sorbitol agar, *E. coli* 0157:H7 appears sorbitol-negative at 24 hours. These colorless, sorbitol-negative colonies can then be screened for agglutination in 0157:H7.
- In HUS, laboratory findings can reveal the following:
  – Severe-to-moderate anemia associated with red-cell fragmentation and numerous schistocytes on peripheral smear
  – Decreased plasma haptoglobin and an elevated LDH level
  – Negative Coombs' test
  – Thrombocytopenia
  – Elevated creatinine level
  – Hematuria, proteinuria, and granular or hyaline casts

Imaging
- In patients with EHEC, barium enema studies can show marked thickening of the mucosa and, in some cases, thumbprinting of the colon.
- At endoscopy, the colonic mucosa appears edematous and hyperemic, sometimes with superficial ulcerations.

Diagnostic Procedures/Other
Renal biopsy is reserved for patients with atypical presentation of HUS.

DIFFERENTIAL DIAGNOSIS
Other causes of bloody diarrhea include the following:
- Shigellosis
- Amebiasis
- Campylobacteriosis
- Enteroinvasive *E. coli* infection
- Patients with EHEC infection are usually afebrile, and, when fever is present, it is usually mild, unlike that seen with other causes of bloody diarrhea (see also the Section I chapter, "Diarrhea and Fever").

- Other causes are hematochezia hemorrhoids, inflammatory bowel disease, diverticulosis, angiodysplasia, neoplasm, intestinal ischemia
- The differential diagnosis of HUS includes the following:
  – Sepsis with or without disseminated intravascular coagulation (usually due to gram-negative pathogens)
  – Thrombotic thrombocytopenic purpura
  – Dengue
  – Malaria
  – Hantavirus infection
- Although skin petechiae and purpura occur frequently with thrombotic thrombocytopenic purpura, they are uncommon with HUS unless there is profound thrombocytopenia.

 TREATMENT

MEDICATION
- Management is supportive, and no specific treatment for EHEC currently exists.
- Antimicrobial agents have not been shown to modify the course of the illness, and it has been postulated that antibiotics can worsen the clinical course of EHEC infection. Especially, the use of trimethoprim–sulfamethoxazole in EHEC infection has also been questioned, because subinhibitory concentrations of that agent increase the production of Shiga-like toxin in vitro.
- The antimotility agents are contraindicated because they can lead to bowel stasis and increased toxin absorption.
- Patients with HUS are treated with plasmapheresis, dialysis, and transfusions.
- The efficacy of glucocorticoids and heparin in HUS is uncertain.

 ONGOING CARE

FOLLOW-UP RECOMMENDATIONS
- Even with advanced therapy, 5–20% of patients with HUS die of the acute illness, and the mortality rate is even higher among elderly patients.
- Renal damage progresses slowly over several decades in survivors, an estimated 50% of whom develop significant renal failure and most of whom require long-term dialysis or renal transplantation.

COMPLICATIONS
- Infection with EHEC, besides HUS, can lead to hemorrhagic colitis or thrombotic thrombocytopenic purpura.
- HUS can lead to the following:
  – Hypoglycemia
  – Hyponatremia
  – Leukemoid reactions
  – Renal failure (that may require hemodialysis)
  – Rhabdomyolysis
  – Severe anemia (that may require transfusions)
  – Thrombocytopenia

ADDITIONAL READING
- Johannes L, Römer W. *Nat Rev Microbiol* 2010; 8(2):105–116.
- Pennington H. *Escherichia coli* O157. *Lancet* 2010;376(9750):1428–1435.

 CODES

ICD9
- 008.00 Intestinal infection due to e. coli, unspecified
- 283.11 Hemolytic-uremic syndrome

CLINICAL PEARLS
- Antibiotics should not be given to patients with *E. coli* O157 infection
- Supportive care including renal replacement therapy, when indicated, is the mainstay of therapy for HUS

H

HERPES SIMPLEX VIRUS INFECTIONS

Paschalis Vergidis
Matthew E. Falagas

 BASICS

DESCRIPTION
Herpes simplex virus (HSV) can cause a group of infections of various organs. Disease may be severe, especially in the immunocompromised host.

EPIDEMIOLOGY
Prevalence
- HSV has a worldwide distribution.
- In the US, the overall age-adjusted HSV-2 seroprevalence was 17% and HSV-1 seroprevalence was 58% in 1999–2004 (1).
- Prevalence is inversely correlated with socioeconomic status.
- There is higher prevalence of HSV-2 in women than in men.
- HSV encephalitis has a bimodal distribution by age, with the first peak occurring in those younger than 20 years and a second peak in those older than 50 years.

RISK FACTORS
- Neonates and immunosuppressed individuals are predisposed to severe, systemic herpes simplex infections.
- Vaginal delivery in a woman with active genital herpes places the newborn at risk for severe HSV infection.
- Reactivation of HSV may be precipitated by several forms of physical or psychological stress, including fever, trauma, sunlight, menstruation, stress-provoking situations.

GENERAL PREVENTION
- Sexual transmission can occur during asymptomatic periods.
- All persons with genital herpes should remain abstinent from sexual activity with uninfected partners when lesions or prodromal symptoms are present.
- Cesarean section in pregnant women with active genital tract herpetic infection decreases the probability of HSV infection in the newborn.

PATHOPHYSIOLOGY
- At primary infection, HSV initially replicates in cells of the dermis and the epidermis.
- Oral infection most commonly spreads to the trigeminal ganglion. Genital infection spreads to the sacral ganglia.
- Reactivation and replication of latent HSV can be induced by various stimuli. This occurs in the area supplied by the ganglia in which latency was established.

ETIOLOGY
HSV is a double-stranded DNA virus. There are 2 types: HSV type 1 and HSV type 2.

DIAGNOSIS

HISTORY
- Acute herpetic gingivostomatitis
  - Usually results from primary infection and occurs in children
  - Incubation period: 3–6 days. Lasts 5–7 days
  - Abrupt onset with fever
- Acute herpetic pharyngotonsillitis
  - Usually results from primary infection and occurs in young adults
  - Fever, malaise
  - Sore throat
  - Headache
  - Severe infection with extension into deeper layers, bleeding and necrosis may be seen in immunosuppressed individuals.
- Herpes labialis
  - Most common manifestation of recurrent infection
  - Herpetic lesions are preceded by pain, tingling, burning at the site
- Genital herpes
  - Incubation period: 2–7 days
  - Symptoms are more prominent during primary infection that during reactivation
  - Fever, malaise, headache in primary infection
  - Pain, burning at site in recurrence
- Herpetic whitlow (HSV infection of the finger)
  - May be a complication of oral or genital infection with inoculation of the virus to the finger
  - May be the result of occupational exposure (e.g. dentists, anesthesiologists, and other healthcare workers exposed to infected secretions)
- Herpes gladiatorum (herpetic skin infection in wrestlers)
- Herpetic keratoconjunctivitis
- Acute retinal necrosis (potentially sight-threatening)
- Herpetic meningoencephalitis
  - Overt meningitis, most commonly with HSV-2
  - Fever, headache
  - Photophobia
  - Nausea, vomiting
  - Meningismus
- Transverse myelitis/sacral radiculopathy
- Herpetic esophagitis
  - Odynophagia, dysphagia, retrosternal pain
- Hepatitis
  - Fever, anorexia, nausea/vomiting, abdominal pain
- Pneumonitis

PHYSICAL EXAM
- Acute herpetic gingivostomatitis
  - Erythematous, swollen, painful gums
  - Vesicular lesions on the oral mucosa and lips. These may rupture and form ulcers
  - Tender cervical lymphadenopathy
- Acute herpetic pharyngotonsillitis
  - Painful vesicular lesions can form ulcers with grayish exudates.
- Herpes labialis
  - Vesicles on an erythematous base, usually on the lips or elsewhere on the face. Lesions may rupture and ulcerate.
- Genital herpes
  - Multiple superficial vesicles, 1–2 mm in diameter, with a serous, erythematous base
  - Tender inguinal lymphadenopathy
- Herpetic whitlow
  - Single or multiple vesicular lesions on the distal parts of fingers
- Herpes gladiatorum
  - Lesions usually occur on face, neck, and arms
- Herpetic keratoconjunctivitis
  - Chemosis, decreased corneal sensation, and characteristic dendritic lesions of the cornea
- Acute retinal necrosis
  - Retinitis and peripheral areas of necrosis with discrete borders
- Herpetic meningoencephalitis
  - Confusion, lethargy, stupor, coma
  - Nuchal rigidity
- Transverse myelitis/sacral radiculopathy
  - Decreased muscle strength and decreased deep tendon reflexes in the lower extremities.
- Herpetic esophagitis
  - Coalescing lesions that form ulcers with volcano-like appearance
  - Ulcers are usually less than 2 cm in depth
- Hepatitis and pneumonitis may be accompanied by mucocutaneous lesions

DIAGNOSTIC TESTS & INTERPRETATION
Lab
- Isolation of HSV in tissue culture. Sensitivity is higher in vesicular compared to ulcerative lesions. Specimens should be placed in viral culture media and the cytopathic effect is demonstrated in 48–96 h.
- HSV DNA detection by polymerase chain reaction (PCR) is more sensitive than tissue culture and is the preferred diagnostic method for specimens from mucocutaneous lesions, genital ulcers, and cerebrospinal fluid (CSF) (2).
  - Note: HSV recovery from respiratory tract secretions may be due to viral contamination of the lower tract after instrumentation, local viral reactivation without parenchymal involvement, or true pneumonitis.

- The Tzanck smear exhibits characteristic cytopathic effects (multinucleated giant cells or intranuclear inclusions). This technique has low sensitivity and does not differentiate between HSV and varicella-zoster virus.
- Immunofluorescence staining: Detection of HSV antigens in specimens prepared from scrapings.
- Type-specific serologic assays are available. The Western Blot assay is the most accurate. Acute and convalescent-phase serum can be used to demonstrate seroconversion.
- Herpetic encephalitis: CSF-elevated opening pressure. CSF analysis: 100–1,000 cells/μL with lymphocytic predominance. Mildly elevated protein. Glucose more than 50% of blood glucose.

Imaging
MRI is more sensitive and specific than CT scan to detect herpetic encephalitis. Lesions are typically unilateral and involve the temporal lobe. There may be associated mass effect.

Diagnostic Procedures/Other
- Gently unroof the alcohol-wiped vesicle with a sterile needle and collect specimen.
- Upper endoscopy for herpetic esophagitis.
- Electroencephalogram in herpetic encephalitis: Prominent intermittent high-amplitude slow waves (delta and theta slowing), and, occasionally, continuous periodic lateralized epileptiform discharges in the affected region.
- Brain biopsy for diagnosis of herpetic encephalitis if diagnosis in doubt or failure of antiviral treatment.

Pathological Findings
A Tzanck preparation of scrapings from the base of HSV lesions commonly demonstrates multinucleated giant cells.

DIFFERENTIAL DIAGNOSIS
- Oropharyngeal lesions: Bacterial pharyngitis, candidiasis, mucositis due to chemotherapy, Stevens–Johnson syndrome
- Genital lesions: Syphilis, genital warts, chancroid, granuloma inguinale, lymphogranuloma venereum, and neoplasms
- Esophagitis: Cytomegalovirus (CMV), candida, idiopathic aphthous ulcers in HIV-infected patients
- Encephalitis: Other viral causes (such as VZV, CMV, enterovirus), brain abscess, subdural empyema, acute demyelinating encephalomyelitis

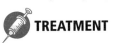 TREATMENT

MEDICATION
First Line
- Orolabial infections
  - First episode: Acyclovir 15 mg/kg p.o. (up to 200 mg) 5 times daily or 400 mg p.o. t.i.d. Famciclovir 500 mg p.o. b.i.d. Valacyclovir 1000 mg p.o. b.i.d. All for 7 days.
  - Recurrent episodes: Acyclovir 400 mg p.o. 5 times daily for 5 days. Valacyclovir 2000 mg p.o. b.i.d. for 1 day (3). Famciclovir 1500 mg p.o. once. Self-initiated therapy with topical 1% penciclovir cream every 2 h during waking hours. Topical acyclovir cream 5%, 5 times daily for 4 days.

- Chronic suppression: Consider for patients with more than 6 episodes per year or in immunocompromised patients. Acyclovir 400 mg p.o. b.i.d. or valacyclovir 500 mg daily or 1000 mg p.o. daily. Famciclovir 500 mg p.o. b.i.d.
- Genital infections
  - First episode: Acyclovir 200 mg p.o. 5 times daily or 400 mg p.o. t.i.d. for 7–10 days. Valacyclovir 1000 mg p.o. b.i.d. for 7–10 days. Famciclovir 250 mg p.o. t.i.d. for 7–10 days. All given for 7–10 days.
  - Recurrent episodes: Acyclovir 200 mg p.o. 5 times daily for 5 days, 400 mg p.o. t.i.d. for 5 days, 800 mg p.o. t.i.d. for 2 days (4) or b.i.d. for 5 days. Valacyclovir 500 mg p.o. b.i.d. for 3–5 days or 1 g p.o. daily for 5 days or 1 g p.o. b.i.d. for 1 day. Famciclovir 125 mg p.o. b.i.d. for 5 days, 500 mg p.o. b.i.d. for 5 days, 1 g p.o. b.i.d. for 1 day (5), or 500 mg once and then 250 mg p.o. b.i.d. for 3 doses.
  - Suppression: Consider for patients with more than 6 episodes per year or immunosuppressed patients. Acyclovir 400 mg p.o. b.i.d. Famciclovir 250 mg p.o. b.i.d. Valacyclovir 500 mg p.o. daily. For persons with >10 episodes per year, valacyclovir 1000 mg p.o. daily.
- Herpetic keratitis
  - Topical trifluorothymidine, vidarabine, idoxuridine, acyclovir, penciclovir, interferon
  - Herpetic encephalitis
  - Acyclovir 10 mg/kg i.v. every 8 h for 14–21 days. Shorter courses have been associated with relapse
- Visceral infections (pneumonitis, hepatitis)
  - Acyclovir 10 mg/kg i.v. every 8 h

Second Line
- Acyclovir-resistant HSV may cause infection, especially in immunosuppressed patients.
  - Foscarnet 40 mg/kg i.v. every 8 h until lesions heal.
  - For mucocutaneous lesions: Application of trifluorothymidine or 5% cidofovir gel.

ADDITIONAL TREATMENT
Additional Therapies
Corticosteroids have been used to reduce cerebral edema in herpetic encephalitis. Their role is uncertain.

 ONGOING CARE

FOLLOW-UP RECOMMENDATIONS
Careful follow-up is necessary after a serious HSV infection due to the risk of recurrence and the high probability of residual abnormalities.

PROGNOSIS
The mortality of untreated herpetic encephalitis can approach 70%. Even with treatment, mortality may be as high as 30%

COMPLICATIONS
- Herpetic keratitis may lead to corneal destruction.
- Serious neurologic abnormalities may be the result of the infection in survivors of herpetic encephalitis.

REFERENCES
1. Xu F, Sternberg MR, Kottiri BJ, et al. Trends in herpes simplex virus type 1 and type 2 seroprevalence in the United States. JAMA 2006;296:964–973.
2. Whiley DM, Mackay IM, Syrmis MW, et al. Detection and differentiation of herpes simplex virus types 1 and 2 by a duplex LightCycler PCR that incorporates an internal control PCR reaction. J Clin Virol 2004;30:32–38.
3. Spruance SL, Jones TM, Blatter MM, et al. High-dose, short-duration, early valacyclovir therapy for episodic treatment of cold sores: Results of two randomized, placebo-controlled, multicenter studies. Antimicrob Agents Chemother 2003;47:1072–10780.
4. Wald A, Carrell D, Remington M, et al. Two-day regimen of acyclovir for treatment of recurrent genital herpes simplex virus type 2 infection. Clin Infect Dis 2002;34:944–948.
5. Abudalu M, Tyring S, Koltun W, et al. Single-day, patient-initiated famciclovir therapy versus 3-day valacyclovir regimen for recurrent genital herpes: A randomized, double-blind, comparative trial. Clin Infect Dis 2008;47:651–658.

ADDITIONAL READING
- Cernik C, Gallina K, Brodell RT. The treatment of herpes simplex infections: An evidence-based review. Arch Intern Med 2008;168:1137–1144.
- Spruance S, Aoki FY, Tyring S, et al. Short-course therapy for recurrent genital herpes and herpes labialis. J Fam Pract 2007;56:30–36.

CODES

ICD9
- 054.3 Herpetic meningoencephalitis
- 054.9 Herpes simplex without mention of complication
- 054.10 Genital herpes, unspecified

CLINICAL PEARLS
- HSV can cause a group of infections of various organs. Disease may be severe, especially in the immunocompromised host.
- HSV DNA detection by PCR is more sensitive than tissue culture and is the preferred diagnostic method.

H

HERPES ZOSTER

Constantinos Sgouros
Petros I. Rafailidis
Matthew E. Falagas

BASICS

DESCRIPTION
Herpes zoster (shingles) is a local manifestation on the skin of reactivation of the varicella zoster virus (VZV)

EPIDEMIOLOGY
Incidence
- VZV affects people worldwide
- The incidence of herpes zoster was 6.3 per 1000 persons. About 63.7% of persons who developed herpes zoster were older than 50 years in this study (1)

Prevalence
- About 90% of people have serologic evidence of past infection by young adulthood.
- Herpes zoster afflicts about 20% of the population overall at some time during their lifetime.

RISK FACTORS
- The elderly are more likely than younger people to develop herpes zoster.
- Immunosuppressed patients, due to medications (2), neoplasms (especially lymphoproliferative disorders), or infections (e.g., HIV), are predisposed to develop herpes zoster.

Genetics
VZV is a DNA virus that belongs to the herpes viruse group

GENERAL PREVENTION
- Use of varicella zoster immunoglobulin (VZIG) is recommended for immunocompromised patients who have no history of chickenpox or herpes zoster and who were substantially exposed to a patient with varicella or herpes zoster. As far as quantification of exposure to a patient with herpes zoster is concerned, intimate contact (e.g., touching or hugging) with a person deemed contagious with herpes zoster is necessary to warrant VZIG administration.
- The lack of this specific immunoglobulin in many centers has forced physicians to resort to acyclovir or valganciclovir after exposure as a preventive measure. There is no consensus regarding optimal timing of administration after exposure: 7–10 days after exposure for a duration of 7 days or alternatively from day 3 up to day 28 after exposure (3).
- Antiviral medications such as acyclovir or valganciclovir are used as primary prevention in the early post-transplant period. Currently suggested regimens suggested as prophylaxis against CMV or HSV will likely prevent herpes zoster virus infection in the posttransplant period (3).

- Acyclovir, ganciclovir, and famciclovir have been also used successfully to prevent herpes zoster infections in patients receiving bortezomib therapy for multiple myeloma (4).
- VZV vaccine in persons with no previous VZV infection prevents chickenpox and herpes zoster (5 [A]). Furthermore, data also suggest that postherpetic neuralgia incidence is decreased as well (6).
- VZV vaccine may be used also in the pretransplant period if there are no contraindications (3).
- Vaccination although generally is avoided if history of immunosuppression has been present in patients with leukemia while in remission and in HIV-infected patients.

ETIOLOGY
- Primary infection with VZV leads to a subclinical condition or clinically apparent varicella (chickenpox).
- The virus remains latent for years after primary infection.
- After a variable period of time (usually many years), basically undetermined factors permit reactivation of VZV, which is manifested by herpes zoster.

COMMONLY ASSOCIATED CONDITIONS
Rule out the presence of immunosuppression in cases of multiple dermatomal involvement

DIAGNOSIS

HISTORY
Pain in any body area either isolated or in addition to skin lesions usually in a half-belt distribution.

PHYSICAL EXAM
- Herpes zoster is manifested with vesicles on an erythematous base, with a characteristic distribution of a dermatome (usually unilaterally).
- Severe pain and paresthesia at the area of lesions are common symptoms.
- Thoracic and lumbar dermatomes are most commonly affected.
- However, herpes zoster may affect any dermatome of the body.
- When the 1st or 2nd branch of the 5th cranial nerve (trigeminal) is affected, herpes zoster may involve the eyelids.

- Herpes zoster ophthalmicus is manifested by keratitis, which may be followed by iridocyclitis and secondary glaucoma.
- The involvement of the maxillary or mandibular branch of the 5th cranial nerve may result in herpes zoster lesions in the mouth.
- Involvement of the geniculate ganglion may lead to Ramsay Hunt syndrome, with pain and vesicular lesions on the external auditory meatus, loss of taste in the anterior two-thirds of the tongue, and ipsilateral facial palsy.
- In case of central nervous system affliction, the rash may be absent (6)!

DIAGNOSTIC TESTS & INTERPRETATION
Lab
Serologic and molecular biology (PCR) tests are available to help establish diagnosis of herpes zoster, but it is emphasized that these tests are not necessary to be performed in clinical practice (because clinical diagnosis usually suffices).

Imaging
CT or MRI of the brain if involvement is deemed possible.

Diagnostic Procedures/Other
Lumbar puncture if central nervous system disease suspected.

Pathological Findings
A Tzanck smear of skin lesions (performed by scraping the base of the lesion) may demonstrate multinucleated giant cells, which are more common in herpes simplex virus infection

DIFFERENTIAL DIAGNOSIS
- The appearance of characteristic herpes zoster skin lesions with a typical dermatomal distribution should suffice for a clinical diagnosis.
- Other viral infections, including herpes simplex virus or coxsackievirus, may very rarely present with lesions with a dermatoma-like distribution.

TREATMENT

MEDICATION
First Line
- Acyclovir 800 mg p.o. 5 times a day (q4h, except a dose that is missed during night sleep) for 7 days is the recommended treatment.
- Acyclovir intravenously (10 mg/kg q8h) is recommended in immunosuppressed patients with severe herpes zoster on multiple dermatomes.

Second Line
- Valacyclovir 1000 mg p.o. q8h or famciclovir 500 mg p.o. q8h for 7 days may be used to treat patients with herpes zoster.
- Steroids in combination to antiviral medications may lead to somewhat accelerated healing and decrease of acute pain.

ADDITIONAL TREATMENT
General Measures
Steroid treatment does not decrease the probability of subsequent postherpetic neuralgia according to a recent meta-analysis (7).

Issues for Referral
Ophthalmic involvement mandates referral to an ophthalmologist. Even the sole presence of eye pain must alert the physician to ask for ophthalmological consultation (8).

Additional Therapies
- Capsaicin 0.025–0.075% ointments applied to healed intact skin may help patients with postherpetic neuralgia
- Gabapentin 300 mg p.o. o.d. (9)
- Lidocaine 5% patch applied to healed intact skin
- Sympathetic block or spinal cord stimulation has been used when medical treatment fails

IN-PATIENT CONSIDERATIONS
Initial Stabilization
Required in cases of CNS or other severe organ involvement (i.e., pneumonitis)

Admission Criteria
In cases where parenteral treatment is deemed necessary, i.e., central nervous system affliction (6) or immunocompromised host.

 ONGOING CARE

FOLLOW-UP RECOMMENDATIONS
Not required usually. If postherpetic neuralgia develops ask patient to arrange follow-up.

PROGNOSIS
- A significant proportion of patients develop postherpetic neuralgia, especially the elderly (up to 30%). The management of these patients should start with simple analgesics, such as paracetamol, and proceed to small doses of opiates and/or amitriptyline, if necessary.
- The impact of postherpetic neuralgia on the quality of life of patients cannot be emphasized enough. Some of these patients may go on to develop frank depression.
- Recurrent attacks of herpes zoster may occur.

COMPLICATIONS
- An immunocompromised host may be manifested by a generalized infection with rash distributed very extensively on the skin. In addition, systemic manifestations may appear with pneumonitis, hepatitis, and central nervous system abnormalities.
- Central nervous system involvement, manifested by granulomatous cerebral angiitis, may follow herpes zoster ophthalmicus.
- Secondary bacterial infection may develop on skin lesions due to herpes zoster.
- Postherpetic neuralgia and its impact on the quality of life (i.e. depression). Pain intensity at presentation, age, smoking, and missed antiviral prescription are all associated with postherpetic neuralgia).
- Blindness.

REFERENCES

1. Gialloreti LE, Merito M, Pezzotti P, et al. Epidemiology and economic burden of herpes zoster and post-herpetic neuralgia in Italy: A retrospective, population-based study. *BMC Infect Dis* 2010;10:230.
2. Salmon-Ceron D, Tubach F, Lortholary O, et al; for the RATIO group. Drug-specific risk of non-tuberculosis opportunistic infections in patients receiving anti-TNF therapy reported to the 3-year prospective French RATIO registry. *Ann Rheum Dis* 2011;70(4):616–623.
3. Pergam SA, Limaye AP; AST Infectious Diseases Community of Practice. Varicella zoster virus (VZV) in solid organ transplant recipients. *Am J Transplant* 2009;9(Suppl 4):S108–S115.
4. Vickrey E, Allen S, Mehta J, et al. Acyclovir to prevent reactivation of varicella zoster virus (herpes zoster) in multiple myeloma patients receiving bortezomib therapy. *Cancer* 2009;115: 229–232.
5. Oxman MN, Levin MJ; Shingles Prevention Study Group. Vaccination against herpes zoster and postherpetic neuralgia. *J Infect Dis* 2008; 197(Suppl 2):S228–S236.
6. Pahud BA, Glaser CA, Dekker CL, et al. Varicella zoster disease of the central nervous system: Epidemiological, clinical, and laboratory features 10 years after the introduction of the varicella vaccine. *J Infect Dis* 2011;203(3):316–323
7. Chen N, Yang M, He L, et al. Corticosteroids for preventing postherpetic neuralgia. *Cochrane Database Syst Rev* 2010;12:CD005582.
8. Adam RS, Vale N, Bona MD, et al. Triaging herpes zoster ophthalmicus patients in the emergency department: Do all patients require referral? *Acad Emerg Med* 2010;17:1183–1188.
9. Van Wijck AJ, Wallace M, Mekhail N, et al. Herpes zoster and post-herpetic neuralgia. *Pain Pract* 2011;11:88–97
10. Parruti G, Tontodonati M, Rebuzzi C, et al. Predictors of pain intensity and persistence in a prospective Italian cohort of patients with herpes zoster: Relevance of smoking, trauma and antiviral therapy. *BMC Med* 2010;8:58.

ADDITIONAL READING

- Harpaz R, Ortega-Sanchez IR, Seward JF; Advisory Committee on Immunization Practices (ACIP) Centers for Disease Control and Prevention (CDC). Prevention of herpes zoster: Recommendations of the Advisory Committee on Immunization Practices (ACIP). *MMWR Recomm Rep* 2008;57(RR-5):1–30.
- Taweesith W, Puthanakit T, Kowitdamrong E, et al. The immunogenicity and safety of live attenuated varicella-zoster virus vaccine in human immunodeficiency virus-infected children. *Pediatr Infect Dis J* 2010;30(4):320–324.
- Lawrence R, Gershon AA, Holzman R, et al. The risk of zoster after vaccination in children with leukemia. *N Engl J Med* 1988;318:543–548.

 CODES

ICD9
- 053.9 Herpes zoster without mention of complication
- 053.29 Herpes zoster with other ophthalmic complications

CLINICAL PEARLS
- Beware of making a diagnosis of new onset "migraine" in an elderly person without looking for skin lesions in his face
- Multiple dermatomes may be afflicted in the immunocompromised host, and internal organs may be affected concurrently.
- In your first encounter with a patient over 60 years of age, suggest vaccination against varicella zoster virus in the absence of contraindications.

H

HISTOPLASMOSIS

Paschalis Vergidis
Matthew E. Falagas

BASICS

DESCRIPTION
An inhalation-acquired endemic mycosis mainly affecting the lungs.

EPIDEMIOLOGY
Incidence
- Five hundred thousand individuals become infected annually in the US, especially within the Ohio and Mississippi River valleys.
- Children under age 1 year and men over age 50 years are more susceptible.
- Even though the skin test with antigens of *Histoplasma capsulatum* has the same rate of positivity in males and females (suggesting same rate of asymptomatic acute infection in both sexes), disseminated histoplasmosis is about 5 times more common in males than in females.

RISK FACTORS
- Living in an endemic region: North and Latin America for *H. capsulatum* and Central Africa for African histoplasmosis
- Impaired immunologic status

GENERAL PREVENTION
- An individual is more likely to be exposed to *H. capsulatum* inside caves (soil contaminated from bat droppings), from chicken coops, in bamboo canebrakes, and from decayed wood piles. Avoidance of activity in these areas is advisable for immunosuppressed persons.
- Prophylaxis with itraconazole (200 mg daily) is recommended in patients with HIV infection with CD4 cell counts <150 cells/mm^3 in specific areas of endemicity (A-I).

PATHOPHYSIOLOGY
- Disruption of the soil by excavation or construction releases infectious elements that can be inhaled.
- Pulmonary histoplasmosis is almost never transmitted from person to person.
- In nature the mold bears microconidia (2–5 μm), which is the infectious form of the organism. When inhaled, it is multiplied intracellularly and transforms to the yeast form.

ETIOLOGY
- The etiologic agent is *H. capsulatum*, a dimorphic fungus, with 2 varieties: Var. *capsulatum* and var. *duboisii*.

COMMONLY ASSOCIATED CONDITIONS
- HIV infection, AIDS
- Hematological malingnancies
- Organ transplantation
- Tumor necrosis factor-alpha blockers
- Other immunosuppression

DIAGNOSIS

HISTORY
The lungs are the mainly involved tissue. There are the following clinical forms:
- Acute primary pulmonary histoplasmosis
  - 90% of cases are asymptomatic. After heavy exposure, patients are likely to develop symptomatic infection. Most symptomatic patients (incubation period, 3–21 days) develop a flu-like syndrome that resolves without treatment.
  - Fever, chills, headache, anorexia, nonproductive cough, and retrosternal or pleuritic pain may develop. Symptoms last for 2 weeks, then resolve. Fatigability and malaise may persist for months.
- Chronic pulmonary histoplasmosis
  - Occurs usually in men more than 50 years old with chronic obstructive pulmonary disease.
  - Cough, pleuritic pain, night sweats, erythema nodosum or multiforme, sputum production, weight loss, and intermittent hemoptysis.
  - Untreated cases may resolve spontaneously, but they usually progress.
- Mediastinal granuloma and fibrosis
  - Extension of infection to paratracheal, hilar, and subcarinal lymph nodes causes nodal enlargement, caseating necrosis, and perilymphadenitis.
  - Resolution of lymphadenitis progresses to extensive fibroplastic proliferation that surrounds caseated nodes.
  - Rarely, progressive fibrosis that invades the mediastinal structures occurs.
  - Large cystic lesions to the mediastinum can cause cough, postobstructive pneumonia, bronchiectasis, and atelectasis. Heavier forms of mediastinal infection may lead to cor pulmonale, respiratory failure, vena cava syndrome, stenosis of esophagus, and/or fistula formation between the esophagus and the respiratory tract.
  - Broncholithiasis is an unusual condition that results from injury to the bronchial tree by the compressive or erosive effects of calcified mediastinal lymph nodes.
- Progressive disseminated disease
  - Acute progressive disseminated histoplasmosis: Fever, weight loss, malaise, cough, dyspnea, hepatosplenomegaly, and cutaneous lesions (erythematous, maculopapular eruptions on the face, trunk, and extremities). HIV patients may present with an acute syndrome, such as septic shock or meningitis.
  - Subacute progressive disseminated histoplasmosis: Focal lesions in gastrointestinal tract, endovascular structures, central nervous system (CNS), adrenal glands.
    - Heart valves can be infected (large vegetations in mitral or aortic valves).
    - Patients with CNS infection may have symptoms of chronic meningitis or a cerebral mass lesion.
    - Adrenal insufficiency occurs in 10% of cases.
  - Chronic progressive disseminated histoplasmosis: Diarrhea, weight loss, abdominal pain, carpal tunnel syndrome, headache, confusion.

PHYSICAL EXAM
- Acute primary pulmonary histoplasmosis
  - Hepatosplenomegaly, erythema nodosum, or erythema multiforme may occur.
  - Acute pericarditis, frequently with concurrent pleural effusions.
  - Arthritis.
- Progressive disseminated disease
  - Hepatosplenomegaly and cutaneous lesions (erythematous, maculopapular eruptions on the face, trunk, and extremities) are seen in acute disease. The most common physical finding in the chronic form is an oropharyngeal ulcer that is typically well-circumscribed, indurated, deep, and painless.
- Ocular histoplasmosis syndrome: Chorioiditis.

DIAGNOSTIC TESTS & INTERPRETATION
Lab
Initial lab tests
- Cultures need 4–6 weeks to grow at 30°C.
- For blood cultures, lysis centrifugation is indicated.
- *Histoplasma* polysaccharide antigen can be detected in the urine in >90% of patients and in the serum in 80% of patients who have disseminated histoplasmosis.
- Serology: Complement fixation (CF), Immunodiffusion (ID) (M band for early or chronic infection, H band for active infection).
  - Antibodies develop within 4–6 weeks after exposure. CF is most sensitive, and the result becomes positive earlier than with the ID test. ID is more specific.
- Cerebrospinal fluid (CSF): Cells, 10–500/mm^3 (mostly neutrophils); protein, greater than 45 mg/dL; glucose, less than 40 mg/dL
- Specific DNA probes are available.

Imaging
- Acute primary pulmonary histoplasmosis: Patchy pulmonary infiltrates. In cases of heavy exposure, soft, nodular infiltrates with irregular outlines, enlarged hilar, or mediastinal lymph nodes, and, rarely, pleural effusions may be seen.
- Small calcifications of uniform size are sometimes seen in cases of healed histoplasmosis.
- Mediastinal granuloma and fibrosis: Mild subcarinal or superior mediastinal widening; calcified debris into bronchi.

- Histoplasmoma: Coin lesion. Large pulmonary lesion that heals to become a residual nodule (1–4 cm), usually in the subpleural regions.
- Chronic pulmonary histoplasmosis: Nodules (initial phase), infarct-like necrosis (median phase), linear scar formation (final phase); interstitial infiltrates of upper lobes, mediastinal or pulmonary calcifications; if cavities: Pleural thickening, hilar retraction, air-fluid levels.
- Subacute progressive disseminated histoplasmosis: Diffuse interstitial infiltrates (70%), mediastinal lymphadenopathy (20%); CT scan or Computed Tomography scan: Bilateral enlargement of adrenals, with a low attenuation center.

Pathological Findings
Well-organized granulomas that contain lymphocytes, epithelioid cells, giant cells, and variable amounts of caseating necrosis. Yeast forms may be sparse.

DIFFERENTIAL DIAGNOSIS
- Tuberculosis
- Blastomycosis
- Coccidioidomycosis
- Paracoccidioidomycosis
- Sarcoidosis

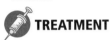

TREATMENT

MEDICATION
First Line
- First line: Lipid formulations of amphotericin B (1) and itraconazole (2).
- Mild-to-moderate acute pulmonary histoplasmosis: Treatment is usually unnecessary (A-III). For patients who have symptoms for more than 1 month: Itraconazole 200 mg 3 times daily for 3 days and then 200 mg twice daily for 6–12 weeks (B-III).
- Moderately-severe to severe pulmonary histoplasmosis: Lipid formulation of amphotericin B (i.v. 3.0–5.0 mg/kg daily for 1–2 weeks) followed by itraconazole 200 mg 3 times daily for 3 days and then 200 mg once or twice daily, for a total of 12 weeks (A-III).
- Chronic cavitary pulmonary histoplasmosis: Itraconazole 200 mg 3 times daily for 3 days and then 200 mg once or twice daily for at least 1 year (A-II).
- Mediastinal lymphadenitis, mediastinal granuloma: Antifungal treatment is usually unnecessary (A-III).
- Mediastinal fibrosis, broncholithiasis, and histoplasmomas: Antifungal treatment not recommended (A-III).
- Mild-to-moderate progressive disseminated histoplasmosis: Itraconazole (200 mg 3 times daily for 3 days and then twice daily) for at least 12 months (A-II).
- Moderately-severe to severe progressive disseminated histoplasmosis: Lipid formulation of amphotericin B (3.0 mg/kg daily) for 1–2 weeks, followed by oral itraconazole (200 mg 3 times daily for 3 days and then 200 mg twice daily) for a total of at least 12 months (A-I).

- CNS histoplasmosis: Liposomal amphotericin B (5.0 mg/kg daily for a total of 175 mg/kg given over 4–6 weeks) followed by itraconazole (200 mg 2 or 3 times daily) for at least 1 year and until resolution of CSF abnormalities, including *Histoplasma* antigen levels (B-III).
- Lifelong suppressive therapy with itraconazole (200 mg daily) may be required in immunosuppressed patients.
- Discontinuation of treatment in HIV patients may be considered if the following are fulfilled: At least 1 year of therapy, negative blood cultures, *Histoplasma* serum, and urine antigen level <2 ng/mL, receiving highly active antiretroviral therapy, CD4 cell count >150 cells/mm³ (3).
- Itraconazole concentrations are higher with use of the solution given on an empty stomach than with capsules. Hence, the solution should be used whenever possible.
- Antacids, H_2 blockers, and proton pump inhibitors decrease the absorption of itraconazole capsules.

Second Line
- Deoxycholate amphotericin B (0.7–1.0 mg/kg daily intravenously) is an alternative for patients at low risk for nephrotoxicity.
- Fluconazole is less effective than itraconazole. Other triazoles (i.e., voriconazole, posaconazole) are also second-line agents.
- Echinocandins should not be used.

ADDITIONAL TREATMENT
Additional Therapies
- For severe respiratory complications, methylprednisone is recommended during the first 1–2 weeks of treatment (B-III).
- Inflammatory complications (pericarditis, arthritis or arthralgia with erythema nodosum): Nonsteroidal anti-inflammatory therapy is recommended in mild cases (B-III). Prednisone in tapering doses over 1–2 weeks is recommended for patients with hemodynamic compromise or unremitting symptoms (B-III).

SURGERY/OTHER PROCEDURES
- Take surgical measures if vena cava syndrome or other obstructive complications occur.
- Pericardial fluid drainage is indicated for patients with pericarditis and hemodynamic compromise (A-III).

ONGOING CARE

FOLLOW-UP RECOMMENDATIONS
The status of the infection should be evaluated every 2–3 weeks in patients with chronic disease.

Patient Monitoring
- Blood levels of itraconazole should be obtained after steady state (approximately 2 weeks). Random concentrations of at least 1.0 μg/mL are recommended. When measured by high-pressure liquid chromatography, both itraconazole and its bioactive hydroxyl-itraconazole metabolite are reported.
- Antigen levels should be measured before treatment is initiated, at 2 weeks, at 1 month, then approximately every 3 months during therapy, and for at least 6 months after treatment is stopped.

PROGNOSIS
- The disseminated form of the disease can be lethal, not only in immunosuppressed but also in healthy individuals.
- In chronic disease, death may be the result of cor pulmonale, bacterial pneumonia, or respiratory failure.

REFERENCES
1. Johnson PC, Wheat LJ, Cloud GA, et al. Safety and efficacy of liposomal amphotericin B compared with conventional amphotericin B for induction therapy of histoplasmosis in patients with AIDS. *Ann Intern Med* 2002;137(2):105–109.
2. Dismukes WE, Bradsher RW Jr, Cloud GC, et al. Itraconazole therapy for blastomycosis and histoplasmosis. NIAID Mycoses Study Group. *Am J Med* 1992;93(5):489–497.
3. Goldman M, Zackin R, Fichtenbaum CJ, et al. Safety of discontinuation of maintenance therapy for disseminated histoplasmosis after immunologic response to antiretroviral therapy. *Clin Infect Dis* 2004;38(10):1485–1489.

ADDITIONAL READING
Wheat LJ, Freifeld AG, Kleiman MB, et al. Clinical practice guidelines for the management of patients with histoplasmosis: 2007 update by the Infectious Diseases Society of America. *Clin Infect Dis* 2007; 45(7):807–825.

CODES

ICD9
115.90 Histoplasmosis, unspecified without mention of manifestation

CLINICAL PEARLS
- In the US, histoplasmosis is endemic within the Ohio and Mississippi River valleys.
- HIV infection, organ transplantation, use of TNF-alpha blockers or other immunosuppressants are predisposing factors. Disease can occur in otherwise healthy individuals.
- Severe infection is treated with lipid formulations of amphotericin B, followed by step-down therapy with itraconazole.

H

HIV INFECTION

Jennifer A. Johnson (E. Mylonakis, Editor)

BASICS

DESCRIPTION
- Infection with human immunodeficiency virus (HIV) is a chronic infection resulting in immunodeficiency with numerous infectious and some non-infectious complications, usually fatal without treatment.
- HIV-1 is the predominant cause of HIV infection worldwide. HIV-2 is endemic in West Africa, with limited impact outside this region at present. HIV-2 infection has a lower associated mortality and lower risk of severe immunodeficiency than HIV-1 infection, and there are fewer clinical data regarding optimal diagnostics and treatment of HIV-2 infection. This chapter deals primarily with information relative to HIV-1 infection; the terms HIV and HIV-1 will be used interchangeably.
- Acquired immunodeficiency syndrome (AIDS) is the spectrum of disorders resulting from advanced HIV infection.

EPIDEMIOLOGY
- At present, more than 1 million individuals in the US, and more than 30 million individuals worldwide, are infected with HIV. The incidence of HIV infection in the US is now estimated at 50,000 cases per year, with mortality declining in recent years due to advances in antiretroviral therapy (ART).
- In 2007, the largest proportion of new HIV infections in the US was among men who have sex with men (MSM), followed by individuals with heterosexual exposure, and less frequently by those with injection drug use. Over half the new HIV diagnoses in 2007 were in black/African-American individuals, followed by whites and then Hispanics/Latinos.

RISK FACTORS
- HIV is transmitted by sexual intercourse (anal, vaginal, or rarely oral), blood exposure (needle-sharing during injection drug use, or rarely by occupational exposure or transfusion of blood products), or maternal–fetal transmission. The risk of transmission of HIV via all of these routes depends on multiple factors, including the circulating HIV viral load of the source patient, the use of ART, and the exact mechanism of exposure.
- In general, the highest risk of transmission from an HIV-infected source is with blood-borne exposure, estimated at 1 in 150 for needle-sharing, and 1 in 300 for occupational percutaneous blood exposure. Receptive anal intercourse has the highest risk of HIV transmission via sexual exposure, estimated at 1 in 200–1000, with lower rates of transmission for receptive vaginal intercourse (1 in 500–1250), insertive vaginal intercourse (1 in 1000–3000), insertive anal intercourse (1 in 3000), and oral intercourse (1 in 10,000–20,000).
- Maternal–fetal transmission of HIV, previously estimated at 25–30% without ART, has been greatly reduced (now around 1–2% in optimal conditions) by advances in ART and perinatal care.

Pregnancy Considerations
- HIV screening should be performed for all pregnant women as a part of routine prenatal testing and repeated in the third trimester for high-risk patients.

- Combination ART with a fully active regimen is initiated in the antepartum period, often after nausea decreases around 10–12 weeks of gestation. Commonly used regimens are combivir (co-formulated zidovudine and lamivudine) with ritonavir-boosted atazanavir or ritonavir-boosted lopinavir. Efavirenz should not be used due to risk of teratogenicity. Other antiretroviral agents have limited safety data during pregnancy, but case reports of safe and effective treatment with other regimens are increasing. The goal of antepartum ART is to fully suppress the plasma HIV RNA prior to delivery.
- Based on early studies, intravenous zidovudine is administered by continuous infection through delivery, in addition to continuation of other components of the antepartum ART regimen. Additional agents, such as single-dose nevirapine, may be given for HIV-infected women who present in active labor with virologic failure or without having received antepartum ART.
- Scheduled cesarean section is recommended for women who have not achieved virologic suppression prior to delivery (especially if HIV RNA is >1000 copies/mL) to decrease the risk of transmission.
- In the postpartum period, women continue combination ART if indicated based on maternal clinical status. Infants are treated with oral zidovudine, or other agents in the case of maternal infection with drug-resistant HIV, for the first 6 weeks of life. If clean water and formula are available, breastfeeding is not recommended as HIV may be transmitted via breast milk.

GENERAL PREVENTION
- Blood-borne transmission of HIV may be prevented by careful screening of blood products for transfusion (transmission by blood transfusion is extremely rare in the US), using safety devices in healthcare settings, and providing injection drug users with access to clean needles and injection paraphernalia.
- Sexual transmission may be prevented by use of condoms.
- Circumcised males have a decreased risk of acquisition of HIV infection via heterosexual intercourse as compared to uncircumcised males.
- Recent studies indicate that novel therapies such as vaginal microbicides and pre-exposure prophylaxis (PrEP) with antiretrovirals may also be safe and effective at reducing transmission of HIV in high-risk populations. Vaccines to prevent HIV have been, and continue to be, studied in laboratory and clinical trials, but none are currently approved for clinical use.
- Maternal–fetal transmission of HIV, previously estimated at 25–30% without ART, has been greatly reduced (around 1–2% in optimal conditions) by advances in ART and perinatal care.

Post-Exposure Prophylaxis
- Although rates of transmission after occupational exposure to HIV-infected blood are low (approximately 0.3% for percutaneous exposure and 0.09% for mucosal exposure), transmission can be further reduced with the use of antiretroviral PEP.

- HIV testing of the source patient should be performed whenever possible. Antiretroviral PEP is generally not indicated for exposures to source patients with unknown HIV status unless the source patient has known HIV risk factors.
- Antiretroviral PEP may also be effective at reducing the risk of HIV transmission after nonoccupational exposures such as needle-sharing and sexual exposures (both consensual and nonconsensual).
- Individuals initiating PEP should undergo evaluation including baseline HIV testing and pregnancy testing for women. In cases of sexual exposure, patients should have screening and prophylaxis for hepatitis B, gonorrhea, chlamydia, and screening for syphilis and hepatitis C.
- Antiretroviral PEP should be initiated as soon as possible after an exposure (ideally within hours) since efficacy decreases over time and is likely minimal at more than 72 h after an exposure. PEP should be continued for 4 weeks.
- Choice of ART regimen for PEP is based on patient-related factors and the type of exposure. Two-drug regimens (e.g. co-formulated tenofovir + emtricitabine or Truvada) are recommended for lower-risk exposures, and 3 drug regimens (e.g. Truvada with ritonavir-boosted lopinavir, ritonavir-boosted atazanavir or raltegravir) are recommended for higher-risk exposures.
- For exposures to source patients with known HIV infection, the HIV treatment and resistance history of the source patient should be considered when selecting a PEP regimen.

ETIOLOGY
- HIV belongs to the family of human retroviruses and the subfamily of lentiviruses.
- The HIV envelope glycoproteins bind to the CD4+ T-lymphocyte via the CD4 receptor and 1 of 2 co-receptors, CCR5 or CXCR4, and the HIV nucleoprotein complex enters the cytoplasm. The RNA viral genome undergoes transcription by the virally encoded reverse transcriptase. The double-stranded viral DNA enters into the nucleus, where integration of the DNA provirus into the host chromosome is catalyzed by integrase (another retroviral enzyme).
- When a CD4 cell with integrated provirus is activated, viral genes are transcribed and viral proteins are cleaved by the viral protease enzyme. Viral particles are assembled and virions are released from the cell by budding. Productive viral replication is lytic to infected T cells. A decrease in function as well as number of CD4 cells is central to the immune dysfunction.
- Rapid production and turnover of CD4 cells occur throughout the course of HIV infection. Although a highly dynamic, complex equilibrium between HIV and CD4 cells may be maintained for several years, eventually a decline in circulating CD4 cells occurs in almost all HIV-infected individuals.

COMMONLY ASSOCIATED CONDITIONS
Common Opportunistic Infections
- HIV-infected individuals are at risk for different opportunistic infections depending on the current CD4 cell count (thresholds are only approximated):
  - CD4 cell count >500 cells/mm^3: Some increased risk of bacterial pneumonia and sinusitis, herpes zoster and tuberculosis, but generally infections are similar to those in HIV-negative individuals.

- CD4 cell count 200–500 cells/mm^3: Recurrent vaginal candidiasis, increased risk of bacterial infections (especially pneumococcal pneumonia), and cutaneous Kaposi's sarcoma.
- CD4 cell count 50–200 cells/mm^3: Thrush (oral candidiasis) *Pneumocystis jiroveci* pneumonia (PJP), cryptococcal meningitis, and central nervous system (CNS) toxoplasmosis.
- CD4 cell count <50 cells/mm^3: Disseminated *Mycobacterium avium* complex (MAC), cytomegalovirus (CMV) colitis, CMV retinitis, Progressive multifocal leukoencephalopathy (PML) and neurological complications of HIV (encephalopathy, neuropathy)

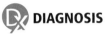 **DIAGNOSIS**

- Acute HIV
  - Approximately 1–6 weeks after viral transmission, many patients will experience symptoms of acute HIV, associated with the rapid viral replication and decrease in CD4 cell count that occurs early in the course of infection. As many as 50–90% of HIV-infected individuals experience symptoms of acute HIV, but these symptoms are nonspecific and are often mistaken for other viral syndromes such as flu or other respiratory viral illnesses or mononucleosis.
  - Signs and symptoms of acute HIV usually last between 3 days and 3 weeks and include: fever, pharyngitis, maculopapular rash, arthralgias, myalgias, lymphadenopathy, diarrhea, weight loss, nausea, vomiting, and headache. Meningoencephalitis and other neurological complications are less common, but may be present in acute HIV infection.
  - Laboratory findings of acute HIV may include lymphopenia or lymphocytosis, thrombocytopenia, and elevated transaminases.
  - Testing for HIV antibody is usually negative in acute HIV infection; seroconversion to a positive HIV antibody test usually occurs within 4–12 weeks of acute infection. Clinicians considering a diagnosis of acute HIV should always send HIV RNA PCR (viral load) testing. The HIV RNA is usually high (>100,000 copies/mL) in acute HIV.
- Asymptomatic infection
  - After acute infection, an asymptomatic phase follows, often lasting around 8–10 years.
  - During asymptomatic infection, the CD4 cell count slowly declines while the viral load often remains stable.
  - A small percentage of patients do not develop symptoms of HIV infection or significant HIV viremia even after prolonged HIV infection. Depending on the duration of infection with minimal HIV viremia, the nadir CD4 cell count and the plasma HIV RNA level (viral load), these patients may be categorized as long-term nonprogressors, elite controllers, or immune controllers.
- Symptomatic infection
  - Early symptomatic HIV infection is often characterized by mucocutaneous infections such as recurrent thrush or vaginal candidiasis, recurrent genital herpes simplex virus (HSV) infections, varicella zoster virus (VZV) infection, and oral hairy leukoplakia. Systemic symptoms such as fevers and weight loss may also be present.

- Individuals with advanced HIV infection or AIDS (CD4 cell count <200 cells/mm^3) may develop fever, cough, diarrhea, headache, or other signs or symptoms of AIDS-related opportunistic infections (as described above in the definition of AIDS).
- Independent of any opportunistic infections, HIV infection may cause hematologic abnormalities (e.g., anemia or idiopathic thrombocytopenic purpura), pulmonary and vascular complications (e.g., pulmonary hypertension or pulmonary embolism), endocrine abnormalities (e.g., adrenal insufficiency or hypogonadism), renal disease (e.g., HIV-associated nephropathy), dermatologic complications (e.g., seborrheic dermatitis or eosinophilic foliculitis), and neurologic disease (e.g., peripheral neuropathy or cognitive disorders).
- Malignancies such as Kaposi's sarcoma, non-Hodgkin's lymphoma, primary CNS lymphoma, anal cancer, and cervical cancer may develop as HIV infection progresses.
- Approximately 10–15% of individuals with advanced HIV infection may develop HIV-associated neuro-cognitive disorder (HAND), characterized by memory loss, confusion, depression/apathy, gait disorders, urinary incontinence, and other neurologic deficits.
- HIV-2 infection usually yields a much longer asymptomatic incubation period than HIV-1 infection, and progression to AIDS is less common with HIV-2.

DIAGNOSTIC TESTS & INTERPRETATION

- Routine HIV screening is critically important to diagnose infection prior to the development of advanced immunosuppression, thereby improving prognosis.
- The Centers for Disease Control (CDC) currently recommends HIV screening for patients in all healthcare settings, and annual screening is recommended for high-risk patients. HIV screening is recommended as a part of routine prenatal testing, and re-screening in the third trimester is recommended in settings with a high burden of HIV infection among pregnant women.
- Although the CDC recommends HIV screening after the patient is notified that the test will be performed unless the patient declines (opt-out screening), some states still require separate written informed consent for HIV testing. Clinicians should check the local requirements prior to testing, but written consent and pre-test counseling should not be considered an impediment to routine HIV testing.

Lab
Initial lab tests
- Screening and initial diagnostic testing are performed via enzyme-linked immunosorbent assay (ELISA) for HIV antibody. The ELISA is >99% sensitive and >98% specific for HIV infection.
- If the ELISA is negative, then no further HIV testing is warranted unless acute HIV infection is suspected, in which case testing for HIV RNA PCR (viral load) should be performed.
- If the ELISA is reactive, then the test is repeated in duplicate. If either or both repeat tests are reactive, then the sample is considered positive and a Western blot (WB) is performed.
- The WB is read as positive if at least 2 of the following bands are present: p24, gp41, and gp160/120. If the WB is positive then the diagnosis of HIV infection is confirmed.

- The WB is read as negative if no bands are positive, in which case the HIV test is considered negative. Further testing after a negative WB should be performed if considering acute HIV (check HIV RNA PCR), or HIV-2 infection (check HIV-2 specific Western Blot).
- The WB is read as indeterminate if any bands are present but they do not meet criteria for positivity. This occurs with between 4 and 20% of reactive ELISAs, often due to a single p24 band. Indeterminate WB may be due to early seroconversion, advanced immunosuppression with loss of antibody, HIV-2 infection (requires specific confirmatory testing), or non-infectious causes (autoantibodies from autoimmune diseases, organ transplantation, pregnancy, and receipt of HIV vaccination). Repeat antibody testing (ELISA and WB) and HIV RNA testing is recommended for patients with indeterminate WB.
- Plasma HIV RNA (viral load) testing should be performed for individuals with positive antibody testing (by both ELISA and WB), indeterminate WB, or suspected acute HIV infection.
- Positive testing for plasma HIV RNA usually confirms the diagnosis of HIV infection in these settings, but false-positive test results for HIV RNA (usually with low positive results, e.g., <1000 copies/mL) may occur.
- Negative testing for plasma HIV RNA in patients with indeterminate WB usually indicates that HIV infection is not present. Antibody testing and HIV RNA testing should be repeated for these patients after approximately 3 months to ensure that seroconversion is not in progress.
- In rare cases, a negative test for plasma HIV RNA in combination with positive HIV antibody testing may indicate an HIV long-term nonprogressor or controller.
- Rapid tests are available that can be performed in 30 min or less from blood or oral mucosal swabs, used primarily in urgent or inconvenient settings (e.g. pregnant women in labor without prior HIV testing or source testing for occupational exposures). However, high rates of false positive results have been reported with some tests using oral samples, so confirmatory testing is important.

Follow-Up & Special Considerations
- Clinicians should perform a panel of baseline laboratory tests for all patients with confirmed HIV infection to determine the extent of immunosuppression, pace of HIV infection, indications for ART, complications of HIV infection and active or latent co-infections. Initial tests should include: CD4 cell count and HIV RNA (viral load), HIV resistance genotype (this is needed to determine appropriate therapy), complete blood count (CBC) with differential, chemistry panel, including renal function tests and liver function tests, hepatitis A serology (HAV Ab), hepatitis B serologies (HBsAb, HBcAb, HBsAg), hepatitis C serology (HCV Ab), syphilis serology (rapid plasma reagin [RPR], Venereal Disease Research Laboratory [VDRL] or treponemal tests such as the TP-PA), tuberculin skin test (Purified Protein Derivative, or PPD), toxoplasma serology (IgG), CMV serology (IgG), VZV serology (IgG). If dapsone or primaquine therapy is used, then G6PD testing should be performed. If abacavir therapy is used, then HLA-B*5701 testing should be performed to identify patients at risk for abacavir hypersensitivity reaction.

H

- Further testing should be guided by any findings on careful history and physical exam that may indicate opportunistic infections or other complications of HIV infection.

 TREATMENT

MEDICATION

Timing of Initiation of ART

- Advances in antiretroviral medications have decreased the drug-related toxicities associated with ART and improved the prognosis of HIV infection, such that with early initiation and maintenance of effective ART, the mortality among HIV-infected individuals may approach mortality in the general population.
- In addition to decreasing mortality and complications due to HIV infection, ART reduces the risk of transmission of HIV.
- The goals of ART are suppression of plasma HIV RNA to an undetectable level (<20–75 copies/mL, depending on the RNA assay) and reconstitution or preservation of immune function.
- The current guidelines from the US Department of Health and Human Services (DHHS) recommend:
  - ART should be initiated for all patients with a CD4 cell count <350 cells/mm^3 or a history of any AIDS-defining illness.
  - ART is also recommended (with controversial strength of recommendation) for all patients with a CD4 cell count between 350 and 500 cells/mm^3.
  - The DHHS panel split over recommendations for patients with CD4 cell count >500 cells/mm^3, with half recommending initiation of ART at this stage and half recommending that ART should be optional at this stage.
  - ART should be initiated regardless of CD4 cell count for all pregnant women for prevention of mother-to-child transmission (PMTCT), patients with HIV-associated nephropathy (HIVAN), and patients with hepatitis B co-infection for whom treatment of hepatitis B has been indicated.
- Interruptions in ART have been associated with increased mortality and complications of HIV infection, and lapses in adherence promote the development of drug-resistance. So, patients should be prepared to continue ART for a lifelong course, and initiation of ART may be postponed on a case-by-case basis for management of clinical or psychosocial factors that are obstacles to ART adherence.

Initial ART Regimens for ART-Naïve Patients

- The following 3 types of regimens are recommended as initial ART for treatment-naïve patients, and the DHHS-preferred antiretroviral agents for each regimen structure are included:
  - Non-nucleoside reverse transcriptase inhibitor (NNRTI) + 2 nucleos(t)ide reverse transcriptase inhibitors (NRTIs) (preferred regimen: Efavirenz + tenofovir + emtricitabine)
  - Protease inhibitor (PI, preferably with ritonavir-boosting) + 2 NRTIs
    ○ Preferred regimen: Ritonavir-boosted atazanavir + tenofovir + emtricitabine
    ○ Preferred regimen: Ritonavir-boosted darunavir + tenofovir + emtricitabine
  - Integrase strand transfer inhibitor (INSTI) + 2 NRTIs (preferred regimen: Raltegravir + tenofovir + emtricitabine)

- Selection of the optimal ART regimen for each individual patient depends on results of resistance testing, dosing schedule, pill burden, toxicity profile, drug–drug interactions and co-morbidities.

Antiretroviral Agents

- These antiretroviral drugs are currently used in the US, listed with the abbreviated and names and some selected important considerations:
- NRTIs:
  - Tenofovir (TDF, Viread) and emtricitabine (FTC, Emtriva) are available as separate pills or co-formulated in the once-daily combination pill Truvada (the preferred NRTI combination for initial therapy per DHHS guidelines). Both medications are generally well-tolerated, but tenofovir may cause nephrotoxicity and should be dose-reduced or avoided in patients with baseline renal insufficiency.
  - Abacavir (ABC, Ziagen) and lamivudine (3TC, Epivir) are available as separate pills or co-formulated in the once-daily combination pill Epzicom. HLA-B*5701 screening virtually eliminates the risk of abacavir hypersensitivity reaction, which can be fatal. Abacavir may be associated with increased risk of cardiovascular disease, but the data are unclear. Lamivudine is generally well-tolerated.
  - Zidovudine (AZT or ZDV, Retrovir) and lamivudine (3TC, Epivir) are available as separate pills or co-formulated in the twice-daily combination pill Combivir. Zidovudine can cause bone marrow suppression, gastrointestinal toxicity, and lipoatrophy.
  - Didanosine (ddI, Videx) and stavudine (d4T, Zerit) are both infrequently used in the US due to multiple toxicities including gastrointestinal intolerance, peripheral neuropathy, lipoatrophy, and mitochondrial toxicities including pancreatitis, hepatitis, and lactic acidosis.
- NNRTIs:
  - Efavirenz (EFV, Sustiva) is available as a single-drug formulation or co-formulated with tenofovir and emtricitabine in the once-daily pill Atripla (the preferred NNRTI-based initial regimen per DHHS guidelines). Atripla was the only available one pill once-daily 3-drug ART regimen until the recent approval of Complera (tenofovir, emtricitabine, and rilpivirine). Efavirenz causes central nervous system toxicity with sleep and mood disturbances that usually improve or resolve after several weeks on therapy, and may also cause rash. Efavirenz is potentially teratogenic in the first trimester of pregnancy, so should not be used during pregnancy or for women of childbearing potential without concurrent effective contraception.
  - Nevirapine (NVP, Viramune) is commonly used worldwide, but less frequently used in the US due to the risk of serious hepatic toxicity which may be fatal, particularly in women with higher CD4 cell counts.
  - Etravirine (ETR, Intelence) is used as a second-line NNRTI for patients with drug resistance, including some resistance to other NNRTIs. Etravirine has a high pill burden with 4 pills total per day, causes drug–drug interactions (particularly with some PIs), can cause rash and hepatic dysfunction, and rarely causes a serious hypersensitivity reaction.

  - Rilpivirine (RPV, Edurant) is the newest NNRTI. Rilpivirine has fewer toxicities than Efavirenz and no known teratogenicity, but also has an increased rate of virologic failure for patients with high baseline viral load, and high rates of resistance at time of virologic failure. It is also now available co-formulated with tenofovir and emtricitabine in the newest one pill once-daily ART regimen – Complera.
  - Delavirdine (DLV, Rescriptor) is infrequently used due to high pill burden (6 pills per day), drug–drug interactions, and associated rash, headaches, and hepatic toxicity.
- PIs:
  - Ritonavir (RTV, Norvir) is now primarily used at a low dose (100 mg in the capsule or in heat-stable tablet) as a pharmacokinetic booster for other PIs. Even at the lower dose, ritonavir causes drug–drug interactions (also seen with other PIs, though to a lesser extent) with many other medications due to its effects on the cytochrome P450 family. Drugs that interact with ritonavir (and other PIs) include: Lipid-lowering agents – "statins", rifamycins, oral contraceptives, inhaled fluticasone, benzodiazepines, antidepressants, anticonvulsants, methadone, immunosuppressants, and azole antifungals. Ritonavir also causes gastrointestinal adverse effects and hyperlipidemia.
  - Atazanavir (ATV, Reyataz) may be dosed once-daily and is one of the DHHS-preferred components for initial ART when used with ritonavir-boosting. Atazanavir may cause asymptomatic indirect hyperbilirubinemia, PR interval prolongation, and has been associated with nephrolithiasis. Acid-reducing medications (H2 blockers and proton pump inhibitors) decrease effective atazanavir concentrations and should be used with careful consideration of the atazanavir product insert instructions if used in combination. Atazanavir may also be used without ritonavir-boosting in certain situations.
  - Darunavir (DRV, Prezista) may be dosed once-daily and is one of the DHHS-preferred components for initial ART when used with ritonavir-boosting. Darunavir is generally well-tolerated and may cause rash.
  - Lopinavir (LPV) is the only PI that is available co-formulated with the ritonavir booster, as the heat-stable tablet Kaletra. Kaletra has a higher pill burden (4 pills per day), increased gastrointestinal adverse effects, and increased hyperlipidemia as compared with ritonavir-boosted atazanavir or darunavir.
  - Fosamprenavir (FPV, Lexiva) is given in a variety of doses both with and without ritonavir, with similar efficacy and adverse effect profile to ritonavir-boosted lopinavir.
  - Saquinavir (SQV, Invirase) is used less frequently due to twice-daily dosing and high pill burden (4 pills per day).
  - Nelfinavir (NFV, Viracept) is infrequently used in the US due to inferior efficacy and side effects including hyperlipidemia, hyperglycemia, diarrhea, and fat maldistribution.
  - Indinavir (IDV, Crixivan) is rarely used in the US due to difficult dosing schedule and significant toxicities, including gastrointestinal adverse effects, nephrolithiasis, hyperlipidemia, headache, rash, metallic taste, dizziness, and others.

- Tipranavir (TPV, Aptivus) is primarily used as a component of therapy for treatment-experienced patients with significant drug-resistance. Tipranavir is not used as a component of initial ART due to inferior efficacy for initial ART, multiple drug–drug interactions, and multiple side effects including hepatotoxicity, hyperlipidemia, hyperglycemia, and possibly intracranial hemorrhage.
- Integrase inhibitor or INSTI:
  - Raltegravir (RAL, Isentress) is currently dosed as one pill twice daily and is one of the DHHS-preferred regimens for initial ART. Raltegravir is generally well-tolerated, but may cause headache, nausea, diarrhea, or CPK elevation.
- CCR5 antagonist:
  - Maraviroc (MVC, Selzentry) is dosed twice-daily with variable dosing depending on interactions with the other antiretroviral agents in the regimen. An HIV tropism assay should be performed prior to initiation of maraviroc and maraviroc should only be used for patients with CCR5-tropic virus. At present, maraviroc is primarily used as a component of therapy for treatment-experienced patients. Maraviroc can cause dizziness, abdominal pain, cough, and rash.
- Fusion inhibitor:
  - Enfuvirtide (T-20, Fuzeon) is not used in initial ART regimens because it requires twice-daily subcutaneous administration and causes injection site reactions. Enfuvirtide is now almost exclusively used as a component of therapy for treatment-experienced patients with extensive drug-resistance.
- Therapeutic studies of patients infected with HIV-2 are limited. HIV-2 is intrinsically resistant to NNRTIs, so these agents should not be used in ART patients with HIV-2 infection.

COMPLEMENTARY & ALTERNATIVE THERAPIES
Prophylaxis of Opportunistic Infections
- Prophylaxis of opportunistic infections with antimicrobial agents is recommended with the following guidelines:
  - For patients with CD4 cell count <200 cells/mm^3: Trimethoprim–sulfamethoxazole for prophylaxis for pneumocystis.
  - For patients with CD4 cell count <100 cells/mm^3 with toxoplasma IgG positivity: Trimethoprim–sulfamethoxazole (or alternative) for prophylaxis for toxoplasmosis.
  - For patients with CD4 cell count <50 cells/mm^3: Azithromycin for prophylaxis for MAC.
  - For patients with PPD >5 mm (current or past) or exposure to active tuberculosis infection: Isoniazid.

ONGOING CARE

FOLLOW-UP RECOMMENDATIONS
- Plasma HIV RNA testing is usually repeated approximately 2–4 weeks after the initiation of ART to confirm appropriate virologic response. Once stable on effective ART, plasma HIV RNA and CD4 cell count should be monitored at 3–6 month intervals. "Safety labs" including CBC with differential and chemistry panel (with renal and liver function tests) are often repeated at the same interval to monitor for new complications of HIV infection or of ART. Monitoring of fasting lipid panel, and other cardiovascular risk factors, is important.

- Patients with advanced HIV infection may experience signs and symptoms of immune reconstitution inflammatory syndrome (IRIS) after initiation of ART, often due to underlying opportunistic infections such as M. avium complex and CNS toxoplasmosis.
- Depending on risk factors, patients should intermittently (e.g. annually) undergo repeat screening for additional infections such as hepatitis C and syphilis.
- Vaccinations are important to prevent additional infections among HIV-infected individuals. All HIV-infected patients should be vaccinated for hepatitis A, hepatitis B (if non-infected and non-immune), tetanus (with diphtheria booster on one occasion) and Streptococcus pneumoniae (ideally when CD4 cell count is >200 cells/mm^3), have annual influenza vaccination, and may have vaccination for VZV (if VZV IgG is negative and CD4 cell count is >200–350 cells/mm^3).
- Age-appropriate cancer screening is of particular importance for HIV-infected patients because of increased risks of many malignancies during HIV infection. Cervical Pap smears should be performed regularly (ideally annually after 2 normal Pap smears at 6-month intervals) due to a high prevalence of cervical dysplasia among HIV-infected women. Although anal dysplasia and malignancies are also more prevalent among HIV-infected patients, data and recommendations regarding the optimal use of anal Pap smears for screening are controversial at present.

COMPLICATIONS
Treatment Failure
- In instances of treatment failure, virologic failure (inability to achieve or maintain suppression of plasma HIV RNA) usually occurs first, followed by immunologic failure (inability to increase CD4 cell count from low baseline or decrease in CD4 cell count during therapy), and then clinical failure with the development of HIV-related complications while on ART.
- Poor medication adherence is the most common cause of virologic failure. Adherence should always be assessed and discussed in detail at the time of virologic failure.
- Virologic failure may also be associated with the development antiretroviral drug-resistance, so HIV drug-resistance testing with a genotypic assay should be performed for all patients at the time of virologic failure. Phenotypic drug-resistance testing is used primarily with extensive PI-resistance. Tropism assays are used for patients who may initiate therapy with a CCR5 antagonist.
- Interpretation of HIV resistance testing is beyond the scope of this chapter and can be complex. HIV specialists should be consulted for questions of interpretation of HIV resistance testing results and selection of ART regimen for highly treatment-experienced patients.

ADDITIONAL READING
- HIV/AIDS in the United States, and other factsheets: Factsheets | CDC HIV/AIDS. Available at: http://www.cdc.gov/hiv/resources/factsheets/.
- Gray RH, Wawer MJ, Brookmeyer R, et al. Rakai Project Team. Probability of HIV-1 transmission per coital act in monogamous, heterosexual, HIV-1-discordant couples in Rakai, Uganda. Lancet 2001;357(9263):1149–1153.

- Centers for Disease Control and Prevention. Revised recommendations for HIV testing of adults, adolescents, and pregnant women in health-care settings. MMWR Recommendations and Reports 2006;55(No. RR-55):11–17.
- Panel on antiretroviral guidelines for adults and adolescents. Guidelines for the use of antiretroviral agents in HIV-1-infected adults and adolescents. Department of Health and Human Services. January 10,2011;1–166. Available at http://www.aidsinfo.nih.gov/ContentFiles/AdultandAdolescentGL.pdf.
- Centers for Disease Control and Prevention. Guidelines for prevention and treatment of opportunistic infections in HIV-infected adults and adolescents. MMWR.Morbidity and mortality weekly report. 2009 April 10;58(No. RR–4).
- Panel on treatment of HIV-infected pregnant women and prevention of perinatal transmission. Recommendations for use of antiretroviral drugs in pregnant HIV-1-infected women for maternal health and interventions to reduce perinatal HIV transmission in the United States. May 24, 2010; pp1-117. Available at http://aidsinfo.nih.gov/ContentFiles/Perinatal GL.pdf.
- Centers for Disease Control and Prevention. Updated U.S. Public Health Service guidelines for the management of occupational exposures to HIV and recommendations for Postexposure Prophylaxis. MMWR 2005;54(No. RR-9).
- Centers for Disease Control and Prevention. Antiretroviral postexposure prophylaxis after sexual, injection-drug use, or other nonoccupational exposure to HIV in the United States: recommendations from the U.S. Department of Health and Human Services. MMWR 2005;54(No. RR-2).
- Molina JM, Cahn P, Grinsztejn B, et al. ECHO study group. Rilpivirine versus efavirenz with tenofovir and emtiricitabine in treatment-naïve adults infected with HIV-1 (ECHO): a phase 3 randomised double-blind active-controlled trial. Lancet 2011;378(9787):238–246.
- Cohen CJ, Andrade-Villanueva J, Clotet B, et al. THRIVE study group. Rilpivirine versus efavirenz with two background nucleoside or nucleotide reverse transcriptase inhibitors in treatment-naïve adults infected with HIV-1 (THRIVE): a phase 3 randomised, non-inferiority trial. Lancet 2011; 378(9787):229–237.

 See Also

DHHS guidelines: http://www.aidsinfo.nih.gov/Guidelines/Default.aspx

 CODES

ICD9
042 Human immunodeficiency virus (HIV) disease

INFECTIOUS MONONUCLEOSIS

Ioanna M. Zarkada
Petros I. Farafilidis
Matthew E. Falagas

 BASICS

DESCRIPTION
Infectious mononucleosis (IM, also called "glandular fever") is a common self-limiting clinical syndrome, characterized by acute onset of fever, sore throat, lymphadenopathy, and atypical lymphocytosis, following infection by the Epstein–Barr virus (EBV).

EPIDEMIOLOGY
Incidence
- IM is a common cause of pharyngitis, with a current incidence of 5 cases per 1000 persons-years (in the US) (1). In industrialized countries, half the cases of primary EBV infection happen during early childhood (usually running a subclinical course), with a second peak during late adolescence.
  - Primary EBV infection is rare during the first year of life due to the passively transferred maternal antibodies (1).
  - In developing countries, most EBV infections happen in children at an early age and symptomatic IM is less common (2).

Prevalence
By adulthood, 90–95% of people worldwide are expected to infected with EBV and have antibodies to the virus (2).

RISK FACTORS
- Close contact with a person with EBV infection.
- Immunosuppressed patients such as transplant recipients are highly susceptible to EBV infection.

Genetics
In males with selective immunodeficiency to EBV (a recessive genetic defect), EBV infection may run a life-threatening course (X-linked lymphoproliferative disease or Duncan's syndrome) (1).

GENERAL PREVENTION
- Avoid drinking beverages from a common container, to decrease contact with saliva of an affected person.
- Avoid intimate contact with EBV shedders.
- Patients with a recent history of IM should not donate blood products.
- Efforts are made to develop an EBV vaccine, but none is clinically available yet.

PATHOPHYSIOLOGY
- The virus is transmitted through salivary secretions. The incubation period is about 4–6 weeks. It is estimated that the median duration of shedding the virus is 32 weeks after onset of the illness (3), (4).
- EBV infects the epithelium of the oropharynx and then the B-lymphocytes.

- The virus spreads through the bloodstream; meanwhile, the shedding of EBV from the oropharynx is very high.
- Activated B-lymphocytes produce antibodies against viral antigens.
- The infection of B-cells causes a proliferation of T-lymphocytes, which are cytotoxic to EBV-infected cells, leading to the control of primary EBV infection and also the onset of the clinical syndrome of IM.
- CD8+ T lymphocytes are increased and enlarged and predominate among the atypical mononuclear lymphocytes that characterize IM.
- Despite the immune response and the control of the primary infection, EBV results in a lifelong infection (2).

ETIOLOGY
- The cause of IM is the EBV, which belongs to the family of Herpesviridae.
- EBV is primarily transmitted through oral secretions (also called "the kissing disease"). Rarely, it may be transmitted by blood transfusion.
- Clinical syndromes similar to that of IM are also caused by CMV, Human herpesvirus type 6 (HHV-6), HIV, *Toxoplasma gondii*, *Toxoplasma pallidum*, hepatitis B virus (HBV), and drugs (phenytoin).
- Humans are the only reservoir of EBV.

It is of importance that EBV has been associated with Burkitt's lymphoma (90% of cases in Africa are associated with EBV) and nasopharyngeal carcinoma. EBV DNA has been also detected in Hodgkin's disease (in 50% of cases, EBV DNA is detected in Reed–Sternberg cells) and non-Hodgkin lymphoma (in about 50% of cases in HIV patients, EBV DNA is also found) as well as in HIV patients with oral hairy leucoplakia (2).

DIAGNOSIS

HISTORY
- Young children are usually asymptomatic. Mild pharyngitis or tonsillitis is less common.
- Young adults usually complain of fatigue, malaise, and myalgia during the first week, accompanied by fever and sore throat the following weeks.
- Based on observations from large series of patients with infectious mononucleosis, the following symptoms may be manifested (with indicative proportion of patients who had the various symptoms):
  - Fever (>90%)
  - Sore throat (82%)
  - Malaise (57%)
  - Headache (51%)
  - Abdominal pain, nausea, or vomiting (5%)
  - Anorexia (21%), myalgias (20%), chills (16%), cough (5%), arthralgias (2%) (2)

PHYSICAL EXAM
- The physical examination may reveal the following signs (percentages are indicative):
  - Lymphadenopathy (94%), usually cervical but may also be generalized.
  - Pharyngitis or tonsillitis (84%), sometimes with white or grey exudate.
  - Splenomegaly (52%), hepatomegaly (12%)
  - Periorbital edema (13%), rash (10%), palatal petechiae (7%), jaundice (9%).
- Maculopapular, urticarial, or petechial rash usually presents after the administration of beta-lactams (more often ampicillin or amoxicillin)

DIAGNOSTIC TESTS & INTERPRETATION
Lab
- Absolute or relative lymphocytosis (>50% of total leukocyte number) is a common laboratory finding.
- Atypical lymphocytosis (>10%)
  - Atypical lymphocytes are large lymphocytes with abundant cytoplasm, vacuoles, irregular nuclei, which tend to be indented by surrounding RBCs (red blood cells).
  - In a symptomatic patient, lymphocytosis and >10% atypical lymphocytes has 75% sensitivity and 92% specificity for IM (1).
- Mild thrombocytopenia.
- Elevated transaminases, alkaline phosphatase, and bilirubin may be found (2).

Imaging
Initial approach
Ultrasonography can be used to confirm splenomegaly (1).

Follow-Up & Special Considerations
- Patients with abnormal tests should be monitored on a weekly basis until laboratory values return to normal.
- Splenic enlargement usually subsides within 3 weeks (for athletic patients, ultrasonography should be performed before returning to sports).

Diagnostic Procedures/Other
- Heterophile antibodies (HA) tests are used to detect HAs induced by EBV infection that cross-react with antigens of sheep (Paul Bunnell test) and horse RBCs (monospot test). The HA test in symptomatic patients has 85% sensitivity and 94% specificity but may be negative early in the course of IM and in children <5 years old. (1),(2)
- EBV-specific antibodies can also be detected. These are IgM and IgG antibodies against viral capsid antigen (VCA, elevated in >90% of patients), anti-D and anti-R against early antigen and anti-Epstein–Barr nuclear antigen (EBNA) (becomes detectable 3–6 weeks after the onset of symptoms) (2).
- EBV DNA can be detected in the serum with PCR (2).

DIFFERENTIAL DIAGNOSIS
- Other causes of an infectious mononucleosis-like syndrome include the following:
  - CMV
  - *T. gondii*
  - HHV-6
  - Viral hepatitis (HBV)
  - Human immunodeficiency virus (HIV)
  - Especially in the acute infection phase
  - Rubella
  - Measles
  - Mumps
  - Adenoviral infections
  - Syphilis
  - Coxsackievirus
  - Drug hypersensitivity reactions

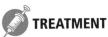

TREATMENT
MEDICATION
First Line
- The majority of cases of IM require only supportive treatment based on:
  - Acetaminophen and nonsteroid antiinflammatory agents to resolve headache, fever, and malaise (1).

Second Line
- Corticosteroids may be used for severe complications such as impeding or established upper airway obstruction, myocarditis, pericarditis, massive splenomegaly, autoimmune hemolytic anemia, severe thrombocytopenia, and nervous system abnormalities.
  - Rarely, they may also be used in neurological abnormalities, pericarditis, myocarditis, and severe malaise.
  - The preferred regimen is prednisone 40–60 mg/d for 2–3 days, quickly tapering over 1–2 weeks (2).
- Antivirals, in conjunction with corticosteroids, may be considered for use in severe forms of the disease; however, final conclusions regarding their role cannot be drawn (5).

ADDITIONAL TREATMENT
General Measures
- Adequate fluid intake and nutrition
- Avoid intense physical exercise (especially contact sports) at least during the first 3 weeks of the disease (and longer if splenomegaly persists), mainly due the risk for splenic rupture. Splenomegaly may persist for several weeks at times (1).
- Avoid beta-lactams (especially amoxicillin or ampicillin) as they are inappropriate to treat a viral disease and may cause a severe rash.

Issues for Referral
- In CNS complications such as meningitis or cranial nerve palsy, consider consulting a neurologist.
- If myocarditis or pericarditis is suspected, consulting a cardiologist might be necessary.

SURGERY/OTHER PROCEDURES
In the rare case of splenic rupture, splenectomy may be indicated for hemodynamically unstable patients.

IN-PATIENT CONSIDERATIONS
Initial Stabilization
Patients with excessive tonsillar enlargement are at high risk of upper airway obstruction, and steroids may be needed to be administered to them.

Admission Criteria
- Dehydration (severe pharyngitis leading to poor oral intake of fluids).
- CNS complications, pericarditis, myocarditis, hemolytic anemia, thrombocytopenia, or splenic rupture.

 ONGOING CARE

FOLLOW-UP RECOMMENDATIONS
- Follow-up is not necessary for patients with mild infectious mononucleosis who had a full recovery.
- Careful follow-up is needed for those with moderate or severe infectious mononucleosis to promptly detect and appropriately manage potential complication

PATIENT EDUCATION
Refrain from active physical exercise for 3–4 weeks.

PROGNOSIS
- IM usually runs a self-limited course, resolving in 1–2 weeks.
  - Sometimes, fatigue and malaise may persist for more than 6 months in patients with chronic fatigue syndrome (2).
  - Rarely, complications may occur.

COMPLICATIONS
- Autoimmune hemolytic anemia (occurs in about 2% of patients)
- Severe thrombocytopenia
- Airway obstruction due to severe tonsillar enlargement
- Neurological complications (encephalitis, Guillain–Barré syndrome, myelitis, and others.)
- Splenic rupture (caution in palpation of spleen during examination and avoidance of contact sports are recommended)
- Severe hepatitis
- Myocarditis or pericarditis
- Pneumonia
- Lymphoproliferative disorders in susceptible patients (patients who receive immunosuppressive agents, severe immunodeficiency due to HIV, or genetic predisposition, such as individuals with Duncan's syndrome).

REFERENCES
1. Luzuriaga K, Sullivan JL. Infectious mononucleosis. *N Engl J Med* 2010;362:1993–2000.
2. Cohen JI. Epstein–Barr virus infection. *N Engl J Med* 2000;343:481.
3. Balfour HH Jr, Holman CJ, Hokanson KM, et al. A prospective clinical study of Epstein–Barr virus and host interactions during acute infectious mononucleosis. *J Infect Dis* 2005;192:1503.
4. Fali-Kremer S, Morand P, Brion JP, et al. Long-term shedding of infectious Epstein–Barr virus after infectious mononucleosis. *J Infect Dis* 2005; 191:985.
5. Rafailidis PI, Mavros MN, Kapaskelis A, et al. Antiviral treatment for severe EBV infection in apparently immunocompetent patients. *J Clin Virol* 2010;49:151–157.

ADDITIONAL READING
- Auwaerter PG. Infectious mononucleosis in middle age. *JAMA* 1999;281:454–459.
- Alpert G, Fleisher GR. Complications of infection with Epstein–Barr virus during childhood: A study of children admitted to the hospital. *Pediatr Infect Dis* 1984;3:304–307.

CODES
ICD9
075 Infectious mononucleosis

CLINICAL PEARLS
- Complications may sometimes arise, including airway obstruction, splenic rupture, and CNS complications.
- Treatment is usually supportive, except for the more severe cases, where corticosteroids may be of benefit.

INFLUENZA

Mary L. Pisculli (E. Mylonakis, Editor)

 BASICS

DESCRIPTION
Influenza virus typically causes a mild, self-limited respiratory infection; however, certain groups including the elderly, the very young, and those with associated medical comorbidities may experience severe or life-threatening disease.

EPIDEMIOLOGY
- 5–20% of the population is typically infected by influenza each year, and an estimated 36,000 deaths occur in the US as a result of influenza-related complications.
- Seasonal variation occurs, with most infections occurring during the winter months. "Flu season" in the US usually lasts from November to March.
- Pandemics occur when new subtypes of influenza A virus are introduced into the population which are capable of causing serious illness in humans and spreading easily from person to person in a sustained manner.

RISK FACTORS
- Elderly persons, very young persons, and persons with underlying medical conditions, such as cardiopulmonary diseases, immune compromise, and diabetes, are at increased risk for severe disease or death secondary to influenza infection.
- Pregnant women are also at higher risk for severe complications of infection or death.

GENERAL PREVENTION
- Viral transmission occurs by direct contact with infected persons, contact with contaminated surfaces, or inhalation of virus-containing respiratory droplets. Viral shedding may occur within the first day of infection and typically continues for 5–10 days. Young children may shed virus for longer periods of time.
- Detergents are effective at inactivating influenza viral particles and hand-washing can decrease rates of transmission.
- Vaccination is the best method for preventing influenza infection. All persons older than 6 months should be vaccinated annually. Two formulations are available: A trivalent inactivated virus (TIV) administered intramuscular and a live attenuated influenza vaccine (LAIV) administered via an intranasal spray.

- TIV is indicated for all persons 6 months of age or older, and in particular for the following groups at high risk of influenza-related complications:
  - Pregnant women
  - Patients with an immunodeficiency or chronic medical condition such as diabetes, or cardiac, pulmonary, renal, or hematologic disease
  - Persons aged 50 years and older
  - Health care workers
  - Household contacts of children younger than 5 years (and especially if younger than 6 months), or of other persons of high risk
- LAIV may be administered to healthy immunocompetent persons aged 2–49 who are not pregnant.
- Vaccination is contraindicated in patients with a severe allergy to chicken eggs or a prior severe reaction to an influenza vaccine, or during a moderate-to-severe illness with associated fever.

PATHOPHYSIOLOGY
- The influenza virion consists of a lipid envelope containing multiple glycoproteins, including hemagglutinin (HA) and neuraminidase (NA) surrounding a central core.
  - HA facilitates binding of viral particles to sialic-acid-containing receptors on the surface of respiratory epithelial cells while NA enables the release of viral progeny from infected cells.
  - Symptoms are believed to result from the release of proinflammatory cytokines from infected cells. Cytokine storm may occur and cause direct cellular injury with possible neural injury, disseminated intravascular coagulation, and multiple organ failure.

ETIOLOGY
- Influenza viruses are RNA viruses belonging to the family Orthomyxoviridae. Human infection may be caused by influenza A, B, or C virus. Type C virus is associated with mild infection while influenza virus types A and B occur in seasonal outbreaks and may cause more severe disease.
  - Influenza A viruses may be classified into subtypes (e.g., H1N1) based on antibody responses against the HA and NA glycoproteins.
  - Novel viruses may evolve as the result of genetic mutations or reassortments. Antigenic drift refers to small mutations in the genes for HA or NA, resulting in new strains that may not be recognized by antibodies to previously circulating strains. Antigenic shift is due to reassortment and results in major genetic changes rendering the virus nonsusceptible to previous immunity-enabling pandemic outbreaks.
  - The 2009 H1N1 pandemic resulted from an influenza strain that combined human, avian, and swine genetic elements.

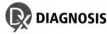 **DIAGNOSIS**

HISTORY
- Influenza infection is associated with a variety of symptoms that may vary by age and underlying medical conditions, but the illness is most commonly characterized by acute onset of fever, cough, nasal congestion, myalgias, and headaches.
  - During periods of influenza activity, abrupt onset of fever with cough carries a >70% sensitivity for influenza infection.
  - Bacterial superinfection leading to pneumonia often occurs 5–7 days after onset of viral symptoms. This is associated with re-emergence of fevers and worsening of cough.

PHYSICAL EXAM
- Exacerbation of chronic diseases such as asthma, chronic obstructive pulmonary disease, and congestive heart failure is common.
- Severe nonpulmonary manifestations include encephalitis, myocarditis, rhabdomyolysis, and hypovolemic shock.
- Severe infections may be associated with fever or hypothermia.

DIAGNOSTIC TESTS & INTERPRETATION
Lab
Initial lab tests
- Respiratory tract specimens (nasopharyngeal aspirates and swabs) should be obtained as close to illness onset as possible while viral shedding is still occurring. The following influenza tests are recommended by the Centers for Disease Control and Prevention:
  - RT-PCR: Most sensitive and specific assay for influenza with results usually available within 4–6 hours.
  - Immunofluorescence: Carries a slightly lower sensitivity and specificity than viral culture but provides results in a more timely fashion; assay depends heavily on the quality of specimen collected.
  - Rapid influenza diagnostic tests: Provides results within 30 minutes of specimen collection but exhibits decreased sensitivity (70–90% in children, <40–60% in adults); confirmatory testing is recommended.
  - Viral culture: Not useful as a screening test but may be useful as a confirmatory test, especially in settings when the prevalence of influenza is low.

Follow-Up & Special Considerations
Screening tests are more likely to be accurate during periods of peak influenza activity.

Imaging
In severe infections, chest x-ray may reveal evidence of bacterial superinfection or pneumonia, or diffuse air-space disease.

Pathological Findings
Autopsy results demonstrate necrosis and desquamation of infected mucosal epithelium and diffuse alveolar damage within the lung parenchyma consisting of edema and thrombosis.

DIFFERENTIAL DIAGNOSIS
- Viral upper respiratory illness
- Respiratory syncytial virus
- Adenovirus
- Pneumococcal pneumonia
- Atypical pneumonias such as *Legionella* and *Mycoplasma*

 ## TREATMENT

MEDICATION
- Two classes of antiviral therapies are commonly used to treat influenza; however, viral susceptibility patterns may change rapidly.
- NA inhibitors include oseltamivir and zanamivir and are generally effective against both influenza A and B. Oseltamivir is administered as a 75 mg dose orally twice a day for 5 days. Zanamivir is administered as 2 inhalations twice a day for 5 days.
- Adamantines (amantadine and rimantadine) block the M2 viral ion channel and prevent viral entry into epithelial cells. Influenza B viruses do not possess M2 channels. Amantadine is given orally at a dose of 75 mg twice a day, rimantadine at a dosage of 100 mg orally twice a day and discontinued 24–48 hours after symptoms abate.

Pregnancy Considerations
Although oseltamivir and zanamivir have not specifically been studied in pregnancy, their use is recommended in any trimester for suspected or confirmed influenza infection given the associated increased risk of severe complications during pregnancy.

ADDITIONAL TREATMENT
General Measures
- The Infectious Diseases Society of America guidelines recommend antiviral treatment for adults and children at high risk of developing complications with laboratory-confirmed or highly suspected infection within 48 hours after symptom onset. Persons requiring hospitalization should be treated regardless of timing of symptom onset.
- Treatment should not be delayed for laboratory confirmation of infection.
  - Consider treatment for persons not at increased risk of complications if they present within 48 hours of symptom onset and wish to shorten their duration of illness or if they are in close contact with persons at high risk for complications.

Additional Therapies
- Antiviral chemoprophylaxis should be considered in adults and children who are exposed to influenza and are at high risk for developing complications and have not received vaccination, or for whom influenza vaccination is contraindicated or expected to have low effectiveness (due to either very recent vaccine administration or underlying immunodeficiency).
  - The infectious period is from 24 hours prior to fever onset to 24 hours after fever resolves.
- Pre- and post-exposure chemoprophylaxis should also be considered for health care providers and public health workers.
- Chemoprophylaxis regimen selection is based on the circulating influenza strain.

IN-PATIENT CONSIDERATIONS
Initial Stabilization
Hypoxia is the most common reason for admission to an ICU, and acute respiratory distress syndrome (ARDS) may rapidly ensue and require mechanical ventilation or extracorporeal membrane oxygenation.

Admission Criteria
Approximately 10% of patients infected with pandemic 2009 influenza A (H1N1) required hospitalization, most of whom possessed an underlying condition such as asthma, diabetes, or cardiopulmonary diseases.

 ## ONGOING CARE

PROGNOSIS
- Most people with influenza illness will recover without complications with only supportive care; however, an estimated average of 36,000 deaths and >200,000 hospitalizations occur each year in the US as the result of influenza infection.
- Children under the age of 2 and persons younger than 19 who are receiving long-term aspirin therapy are at increased risk for complications.

COMPLICATIONS
- Complications include bacterial pneumonia, myocarditis, and ARDS. A variety of neurologic complications may occur including encephalopathy, seizures, and Guillain–Barré syndrome.
  - 29% of patients who died during the 2009 H1N1 pandemic exhibited bacterial pneumonia superinfection, with *Streptococcus pneumoniae* as the most common pathogen.

ADDITIONAL READING
- Baker WH, Mullooly JP. Pneumonia and influenza deaths during epidemics: Implications for prevention. *JAMA* 1982;142:84–89.
- Del Rio C, Guarner J. The 2009 influenza A (H1N1) pandemic: What we have learned in the past 6 months. *Trans Am Clin Climatol Assoc* 2010; 121:128–137.
- Douglas RG. Prophylaxis and treatment of influenza. *N Engl J Med* 1990;322:443–450.
- Glezen WP, Payne AA, Snyder DN, et al. Mortality and influenza. *J Infect Dis* 1982;146:313–321.
- Harber SA, Bradley JS, Englund JA, et al. Seasonal influenza in adults and children-diagnosis, treatment, chemoprophylaxis, and institutional management: Clinical practice guidelines of the Infectious Diseases Society of America. *Clin Infec Dis* 2009;48:1003–1032.
- Sullivan SJ, Jacobsen RM, Dowdle WR, et al. 2008 H1N1 influenza. *Mayo Clin Proc* 2010;85(1): 64–76.

 ## CODES

ICD9
- 487.0 Influenza with pneumonia
- 487.1 Influenza with other respiratory manifestations
- 488.02 Influenza due to identified avian influenza virus with other respiratory manifestations

CLINICAL PEARLS
- All persons older than 6 months should receive the influenza vaccine.
- Bacterial pneumonia may complicate influenza infection and present with re-emergence of fever 5–7 days after onset of viral symptoms.

INTRAABDOMINAL ABSCESS

Alejandro Restrepo
Eleftherios Mylonakis

 BASICS

DESCRIPTION
- An intraabdominal abscess is a localized collection of microorganisms and neutrophils in a fibrous capsule associated with tissues, organs, or confined spaces of the abdomen.
- Abscesses may invade the peritoneal cavity, and localize in the omentum or mesentery. They can develop in any abdominal organ, such as liver, spleen, or kidney, and can extend to the pelvic area and psoas.
- Based on their location, the abscesses are divided into the following:
  - Intraperitoneal (subphrenic, subhepatic, paracolic, lesser sac, interloop, etc.)
  - Visceral
  - Retroperitoneal

EPIDEMIOLOGY
- Men are more common than women to develop intraabdominal abscesses.
- Highest incidence is in the third to fifth decade.
- Of all intraabdominal abscesses, 74% are retro- or intraperitoneal and are not visceral, and only 26% are located in an organ.
- Appendicitis is the cause of 50% of subphrenic abscesses in children. In adults perihepatic abscesses are usually associated with surgical complications.
- *Candida* infections can produce abscesses and lesions in the liver and/or spleen and are more commonly seen in immunocompromised hosts. Lesions are multilocular in >90% of cases.
- Bacterial splenic abscesses are usually solitary collections in 70% of the cases.
- *Salmonella* spp can cause abscesses in the spleen, which are more commonly seen in patients who have sickle cell disease.
- Diabetes mellitus patients are more at risk to develop splenic and perinephric abscesses.
- Up to 9% of patients who develop acute pancreatitis can have pancreatic abscesses as a complication.

RISK FACTORS
Factors associated with failure to control intraabdominal infection: High APACHE score, hypoalbuminemia, malnutrition, degree of peritoneal involvement or peritonitis, inadequate debridement or control of drainage, presence of malignancy.

GENERAL PREVENTION
- Early diagnosis and management of the peritonitis
- Appropriate medical and surgical management of the predisposed conditions to intraabdominal abscesses

PATHOPHYSIOLOGY
- Generally the infection is due to enteric microorganisms entering the peritoneal cavity through a defect in the wall of the intestine or any other viscera as a result of direct trauma, obstruction, or infarction. It can also be produced through introduction of chemically irritating materials such as gastric acid or bile.
- A synergistic relationship between aerobic and anaerobic bacteria occurs.
- There is an inflammation of the serosal membrane of the abdominal cavity and organs.

ETIOLOGY
- Intraperitoneal abscesses may result from:
  - Primary or spontaneous infection
  - Secondary peritonitis related to pathologic process in a visceral organ (appendicitis, diverticulitis, necrotizing enterocolitis, pelvic inflammatory disease, and tubo-ovarian infection, surgery, or trauma)
  - Tertiary peritonitis due to recurrent or persistent infection after adequate initial treatment. It is frequent in immunocompromised patients
  - Spread of infection from an adjacent organ
  - In neonatal period there can be a complication of necrotizing enterocolitis, and also meconium ileus or spontaneous rupture of the stomach or intestine
- Liver abscesses usually develop from:
  - Adjacent foci of infection (such as biliary tract disease and/or other organs)
  - Hematogenous spread
  - Bile obstruction due to stone disease, malignancy, stricture, and congenital diseases
- Splenic abscesses are associated with:
  - Endovascular infections such as bacterial endocarditis
  - Contiguous spread from gastric or colonic perforation, pancreatic pseudocysts, and subphrenic abscesses
  - Patients with hemoglobinopathies
  - Immunocompromised hosts
  - Intravenous drug abuse
  - Patients with malignancies (common: Myeloproliferative diseases)
  - Primary spleen disease
  - Septicemia
  - Trauma in the spleen
- Perinephric and renal abscesses result from:
  - Kidney and ureteral stones
  - Patients with history of urologic procedures
  - Patients with previous structural abnormalities of the urinary tract (e.g., reflux)
  - Trauma in the urinary tract
  - H/o urinary tract infections
  - Patients with hematogenous spread (common: *Staphylococcus*)
- Some reviews on intraabdominal abscesses also include discussion on pelvic and psoas abscesses, pelvic inflammatory disease, and myositis.

Most Common Pathogens
- Intraperitoneal abscesses
  - *Bacteroides fragilis* (found in 65% of overall intraabdominal infections)
  - Enterobacteriaceae (usually *Escherichia coli*, *Proteus* spp, and *Klebsiella* spp)
  - Anaerobic cocci
  - Enterococci
  - *Staphylococcus aureus*
  - Fungal and mycobacterial infections
- Hepatic abscesses: Enterobacteriaceae, *B. fragilis*, anaerobic and microaerophilic Streptococci, *Actinomyces* spp, *S. aureus* (from hematogenous spread), Enterococci, *Entamoeba histolytica*, *Candida* spp, *Aspergillus* spp

- Splenic abscesses from endocarditis or hematogenous spread: Staphylococci (usually *S. aureus*), Streptococci, Enterococci, *Candida* spp, *Fusobacterium* spp
- Splenic abscesses from intraabdominal site, pancreatic abscesses, and perinephric abscesses: Enterobacteriaceae, *Proteus mirabilis*, *B. fragilis*, Enterococci, Streptococci, Staphylococci, Anaerobes, *Salmonella* spp, *Candida* spp
- There is an increased bacterial resistance; it could be hospital acquired, but there is also an increased resistance in the community (1)

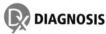 **DIAGNOSIS**

HISTORY
- Intraabdominal abscesses frequently manifest with fever, diffuse abdominal pain, nausea, and vomiting, followed by signs of peritoneal inflammation, and shock and toxemia later. However, since the presentation is often nonspecific, clinical suspicion must be high.
- Patients with liver abscesses associated with active biliary tract disease may show symptoms and signs localized to the right upper quadrant, including pain, guarding, and tenderness. Nonspecific symptoms, such as chills, anorexia, malaise, sweats, weight loss, nausea, and vomiting, may develop.
- Fever of unknown origin may be the only presenting manifestation of liver abscess and abdominal infections, especially in the elderly.
- 50% of the splenic abscesses present with abdominal pain, and can be localized to the left upper quadrant.
- Flank pain is common in perinephric and renal abscesses. Pain can be referred to the inguinal area or leg. At least 50% of patients are febrile.
- Clinical findings do not distinguish pancreatitis itself from complications such as pancreatic pseudocysts, pancreatic abscesses, or intraabdominal collections of pus.

PHYSICAL EXAM
- Only half of patients with liver abscesses have localized signs (epigastric or right upper quadrant tenderness, hepatomegaly, or jaundice).
- Half of patients with splenic infections have splenomegaly.
- *Candida* spp may spread to the kidney via the hematogenous route or by ascension from the bladder. The hallmark of the latter route is ureteral obstruction with large fungal balls.

DIAGNOSTIC TESTS & INTERPRETATION
Lab
- If suggestive of amebic abscess, the amebic serologic testing gives positive results in >95% of cases; thus, a negative result helps to exclude this diagnosis.

- Laboratory findings associated with liver abscesses/infections include the following:
  - Elevated alkaline phosphatase
  - Leukocytosis
  - Elevated bilirubin, mainly direct bilirubin
  - Anemia
  - Elevated aminotransferases (AST and ALT)
  - Hypoalbuminemia
  - Bacteremia
- Patients with splenic abscesses usually have leukocytosis, and about half of them have positive blood cultures.

Imaging
- Liver abscess is sometimes suggested by chest x-ray, and especially shows an elevation of the right hemidiaphragm.
- An air-fluid level outside the intestinal lumen, localized ileus, and right quadrant mass suggest an appendiceal abscess.
- Abdominal and pelvic computerized tomography (CT) has the highest yield in the diagnosis of intraabdominal abscesses.
- Ultrasonography is especially useful for the liver, biliary tract, and kidneys.
- Gallium- and indium-labeled white blood cell scans may be useful in finding an abscess.
- In splenic abscesses, chest x-ray demonstrates elevation of the left hemidiaphragm and a left pleural effusion.

Diagnostic Procedures/Other
- A diagnostic aspirate of abscess contents should be ideally obtained before the initiation of empiric therapy.
- Some authors have advocated early fine needle aspiration of pancreatic collections under CT guidance or endoscopic ultrasound as a means of distinguishing pancreatic pseudocysts from abscesses.
- Exploratory laparotomy is sometimes needed, although this procedure has been less commonly used since the use of percutaneous drainage.

DIFFERENTIAL DIAGNOSIS
See section "Abdominal Pain and Fever."

TREATMENT
MEDICATION
First Line
- The treatment involves:
  - Establishment of the initial focus of infection
  - Administration of broad-spectrum antibiotics targeted at organisms involved in the associated infection
  - Performance of a drainage procedure
- Agents for initial empiric treatment of intraabdominal infections are: Cefoxitin, carbapenems (ertapenem, meropenem, imipenem), ticarcillin-clavulanate, piperacillin-tazobactam, third- or fourth-generation cephalosporins (cefepime, ceftriaxone, cefotaxime, ceftazidime) in combination with metronidazole, also aminoglycosides in combination with metronidazole or clindamycin. Other combination is fluoroquinolone (moxifloxacin (alone), or levofloxacin, ciprofloxacin) in combination with metronidazole (1).

- Antifungal therapy is recommended if *Candida* spp is growing from cultures. Fluconazole and echinocandins are appropriate choices for the treatment of *Candida* infections.
- Antimicrobial therapy should be individualized, based on culture and sensitivity results.
- Empiric antibiotic management of intraperitoneal or liver abscesses should be directed against Enterobacteriaceae and *B. fragilis*. Aminoglycosides, carbapenems, piperacillin-tazobactam, and third- or fourth-generation cephalosporins are effective against Enterobacteriaceae, while metronidazole is the most widely used agent against *B. fragilis*.
- The duration of therapy should be individualized based on location, successful drainage, clinical course, and follow-up imaging studies.
- The complete therapy could be given orally if patient tolerates oral antibiotics and if bacterial susceptibility studies do not demonstrate resistance.
- Antibiotics should be adjusted when resistant Enterobacteriaceae are the possible culprits, and carbapenems would be the first line therapy.
- If ameba serology is positive, monotherapy with metronidazole may suffice (see chapter "Amebiasis").
- Liver abscesses due to *Candida* spp usually require lengthy administration of amphotericin B or fluconazole or echinocandins. Patient can receive fluconazole whose infected isolate is susceptible to this drug.
- When splenic or perinephric abscess is due to endocarditis or bacteremia, gram-positive coverage should be used.
- Sometimes you need splenectomy for the treatment of splenic abscesses.
- Pancreatic abscess requires early surgical treatment or CT-guided drainage. Carbapenems, ticarcillin-clavulanic acid, piperacillin-tazobactam are the most often used antibiotics.
- Antibiotics for the management of perinephric abscesses associated with urinary tract infection should be directed against Enterobacteriaceae (see chapter "Urethritis and Urethral Discharge").

Second Line
- Selected cases, such as those with amebic liver abscess or intraabdominal abscess associated with diverticulitis, can be managed medically but under close combined medical and surgical monitoring.
- Percutaneous drainage with antibiotic administration has been successful in selected cases of splenic, hepatic, renal, and pancreatic abscesses.
- Imipenem and piperacillin-tazobactam are active against *B. fragilis*.

SURGERY/OTHER PROCEDURES
- The following factors favor primary surgical intervention against percutaneous drainage:
  - An abscess that is inaccessible via the percutaneous route
  - Associated disease that requires surgery
  - Lack of a clinical response to percutaneous drainage in 4–7 days
  - Lack of an experienced radiologist or adequate surgical backup
  - Multilocular or vascular abscess
  - Large or multiple abscesses
  - Viscous abscess contents that tend to plug the catheter

IN-PATIENT CONSIDERATIONS
Initial Stabilization
- Patients should undergo rapid stabilization if shock is suspected, and intravenous fluid should be started if there is evidence of volume depletion.
- Antibiotics should be started rapidly in patients with septic shock and/or diagnosis of intraabdominal infection.
- Surgical consultation is necessary (1).

ONGOING CARE
FOLLOW-UP RECOMMENDATIONS
- Always give vaccination to patients who undergo splenectomy. Splenectomized patients should receive pneumococcal, Haemophilus influenza, and meningococcal vaccines (encapsulated organisms).
- If a renal abscess or perinephric abscess is diagnosed, nephrolithiasis should be excluded. Kidney stones are associated with a high pH in the urine and suggest the presence of a urea-splitting organism. Urology should be consulted.
- The patient would need a close medical and surgical monitoring. Imaging such as ultrasound or tomography follow-up is sometimes necessary in cases of intraabdominal abscesses.
- In case of suspected treatment failure, appropriate investigation is needed, including imaging and adequate empiric antibiotic therapy.

PROGNOSIS
- Mortality due to liver abscesses averages 15% despite treatment.
- Mortality due to splenic abscesses is high, in around 37% of the cases. You need to have a good clinical suspicion due to high mortality if not treated.

ADDITIONAL READING
- Brook I. Microbiology and management of abdominal infections. *Dig Dis Sci* 2008;53: 2585–2591.
- Solomkin JS, Mazuski, JE, Bradley JS, et al. Diagnosis and management of complicated intra-abdominal infection in adults and children. *Clin Infec Dis* 2010;50:133–164.

CODES
ICD9
567.22 Peritoneal abscess

KAPOSI SARCOMA

Paschalis Vergidis
Matthew E. Falagas

 BASICS

DESCRIPTION
Kaposi sarcoma (KS) is a multifocal systemic tumor of endothelial origin associated with human herpesvirus-8 (HHV-8) infection.

EPIDEMIOLOGY
Incidence
• Approximately 2,500 cases of KS occur yearly in the US.
• Incidence has decreased after introduction of highly active antiretroviral therapy (HAART).

Prevalence
• There are 4 clinical variants:
  – Classic (sporadic) KS:
    ○ Affects elderly males of Eastern European background (Mediterranean and Ashkenazi Jewish). Peak incidence after sixth decade. More common in males than females. Disease is slowly progressive and often indolent.
  – Endemic African KS:
    ○ Affects young adults, mean age 35 years; and children, mean age 3 years. Equal frequency between males and females.
  – Immunosuppressive-therapy related KS:
    ○ Occurs in solid-organ transplant recipients and other patients on immunosuppressive drugs. Occurs in an average 16.5 months after transplantation. Resolves after cessation of immunosuppression.
  – AIDS-related KS:
    ○ Between 1981 and 1983, KS was the AIDS-defining illness in 50% of homosexual men in some locales. Incidence fell sharply after the introduction of HAART (1). Rapidly progressive with systemic involvement.

RISK FACTORS
• Men who have sex with men and their female partners.
• HIV/AIDS. Risk higher in men who have sex with men than other HIV-infected patients.
• Solid organ transplantation.
• Other immunosuppressive therapy.

GENERAL PREVENTION
• It is likely that HHV-8 is transmitted sexually; therefore, patients should continue to use a barrier method with any sexual activity.
• At present, screening for HHV-8 is not available.

PATHOPHYSIOLOGY
• KS is caused by a neoplastic proliferation of spindle cells and other vascular structures.
• Infection with HHV-8, in association with profound defects in cell-mediated immunity, leads to a complex mechanism that results in malignant transformation of spindle cells and the development of KS.

ETIOLOGY
• HHV-8 has been isolated from KS lesions, as well as peripheral blood mononuclear cells of affected patients.
• HHV-8 is sexually transmitted, with viral detection noted in the semen.

 DIAGNOSIS

HISTORY
Clinical course ranges from minimal cutaneous disease to widespread organ involvement.

PHYSICAL EXAM
• KS lesions begin as ecchymotic-like macules that evolve into patches, papules, plaques, nodules, and tumors, which are violaceous, red, pink, or tan and become purple–brownish as they age. Lesions are palpable and painless unless they ulcerate or bleed.
• Classic KS lesions in elderly men are noted mainly on the lower legs or hands, but also in lymph nodes.
• Patients with AIDS often present with multiple, painless, firm, purple skin nodules. In dark-skinned patients, the nodules appear brown or black.
• Often, the lesions are <2 cm, but may increase in size and coalesce with neighboring lesions.
• Lesions can appear anywhere over the entire body, in the conjunctivae, and in the oral cavity. Lesions can be found on the hard palate or gingiva.
• Facial edema or edema of the extremities suggests lymph node involvement. Lymphedema may be massive and lead to recurrent infections and marked morbidity.

• In HIV-infected people, the course of KS is quite variable. It appears to be most aggressive with lower CD4 counts. At times, spontaneous remission or regression is noted. This is much more likely after initiation of highly active antiretroviral therapy.
• Involvement of the gastrointestinal tract or the lung and airways is common in AIDS.
• On rare occasions, perforation, bleeding, or obstruction of the gastrointestinal tract may occur; however, these side effects are rare.
• Pulmonary involvement leads to bronchospasm, cough, and dyspnea. Respiratory failure can occur rapidly in some cases.

DIAGNOSTIC TESTS & INTERPRETATION
Lab
• Diagnosis is confirmed with biopsy.
• Check CD4 count and HIV viral load in AIDS-related KS.
• Isolation of HHV-8 in bronchoalveolar lavage fluid is specific for pulmonary KS.

Imaging
• Chest x-ray shows a variable pattern in patients with pulmonary involvement. Pleural effusions and hilar adenopathy are frequently seen. Nodular infiltrates are often present; however, a diffuse interstitial infiltrate can be seen in one-third of cases.
• Thallium and gallium scans can be useful in determining the nature of the pulmonary involvement. Infections are thallium negative but gallium avid. KS lesions demonstrate intense thallium uptake but produce a negative gallium scan.

Diagnostic Procedures/Other
• Diagnosis is made with histologic examination of biopsy material.
• In the gastrointestinal tract, lesions may be submucosal and less apparent.
• In the respiratory tract, lesions are often endobronchial and appear violaceous. Biopsy of the lesions may lead to bleeding, and the procedure is risky.

Pathological Findings

Proliferation of spindle cells, prominent vascular spaces, and extravasated erythrocytes with hemosiderin deposition.

DIFFERENTIAL DIAGNOSIS

- Dermatofibroma
- Pyogenic granuloma
- Ecchymosis/Hematoma
- Hemangioma
- Bacillary angiomatosis

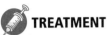 TREATMENT

MEDICATION

First Line

- **Local treatment:**
  - Local treatment of lesions is used for cosmesis or for the management of bulky lesions or lymphedema.
  - Injection of small lesions with vinblastine has had good results.
- **Chemotherapy:**
  - Systemic therapy is used for advanced disease (extensive cutaneous disease, symptomatic visceral involvement), rapid disease progression, or unresponsive cutaneous disease.
  - Pegylated liposomal doxorubicin and daunorubicin are recommended as first line treatment (2).

ALERT

Steroids increase immunosuppression and may enhance proliferation of the tumor.

Second Line

- **Local treatment:**
  - Vincristine and vinblastine have been used for intralesional chemotherapy
  - Alitretinoin gel for limited cutaneous disease.
- **Chemotherapy:**
  - Paclitaxel is more toxic than the liposomal anthracyclines but has had good results (3).
  - Other agents that may be effective are vinorelbine, oral etoposide, and interferon-alfa.

ADDITIONAL TREATMENT

Additional Therapies

- Initiation of HAART often leads to remission of disease and accompanying regression of lesions. Antiretrovirals may have antiangiogenic properties.
- Immune reconstitution inflammatory syndrome after initiation of HAART has been associated with progression of KS.
- Decrease immunosuppression in immunosuppressive-therapy related KS.

SURGERY/OTHER PROCEDURES

- Radiation treatment for large lesions.
- Cryosurgery for deeply pigmented, protruding lesions.
- Laser surgery for small superficial lesions.
- Photodynamic therapy.
- Electrosurgery for ulcerated, bleeding nodular lesions.
- Excisional surgery for small lesions.

 ONGOING CARE

FOLLOW-UP RECOMMENDATIONS

- Patients should follow up with both infectious disease specialists and oncologists.
- Every effort should be made to continue HAART in patients in remission.

PROGNOSIS

Treatment of KS with pegylated liposomal doxorubicin in HIV-infected patients is followed by a low relapse rate (4).

COMPLICATIONS

- Painful and bulky lesions can occur throughout the body.
- Lymph node involvement can lead to marked lymphedema beyond the affected areas.
- Gastrointestinal complications include hemorrhage, obstruction, and protein-losing enteropathy.
- Pulmonary involvement can lead to rapid respiratory failure if not treated promptly.

REFERENCES

1. Franceschi S, Maso LD, Rickenbach M, et al. Kaposi sarcoma incidence in the Swiss HIV Cohort Study before and after highly active antiretroviral therapy. *Br J Cancer* 2008;99:800–804.
2. Cooley T, Henry D, Tonda M, et al. A randomized, double-blind study of pegylated liposomal doxorubicin for the treatment of AIDS-related Kaposi's sarcoma. *Oncologist* 2007;12:114–123.
3. Tulpule A, Groopman J, Saville MW, et al. Multicenter trial of low-dose paclitaxel in patients with advanced AIDS-related Kaposi sarcoma. *Cancer* 2002;95:147–154.
4. Martin-Carbonero L, Palacios R, et al. Long-term prognosis of HIV-infected patients with Kaposi sarcoma treated with pegylated liposomal doxorubicin. *Clin Infect Dis* 2008;47:410–417.

ADDITIONAL READING

- Dezube BJ, Pantanowitz L, Aboulafia DM. Management of AIDS-related Kaposi sarcoma: Advances in target discovery and treatment. *AIDS Read*. 2004;14:236–238, 243–244, 251–253.

 CODES

ICD9

- 176.0 Kaposi's sarcoma, skin
- 176.1 Kaposi's sarcoma, soft tissue
- 176.9 Kaposi's sarcoma, unspecified site

CLINICAL PEARLS

- KS is associated with HHV-8 infection.
- Intralesional chemotherapy can be used locally. For advanced disease, systemic therapy with pegylated liposomal doxorubicin and daunorubicin is recommended.
- For AIDS-related KS, initiation of HAART is recommended.

K

KAWASAKI SYNDROME

Ata Nevzat Yalçin
Petros I. Rafailidis
Matthew E. Falagas

BASICS

DESCRIPTION
An acute, rare, self-limited systemic vasculitis of childhood. Synonyms for Kawasaki syndrome include Kawasaki disease (KD) and mucocutaneous lymph node syndrome (MCLS, MLNS, or MCLNS).

EPIDEMIOLOGY
Incidence
- Large nationwide epidemics occurred in 1979, 1982, and 1985–1986 in Japan.
- Approximately 85% of children with Kawasaki disease are <5 years old.
- The incidence of Kawasaki syndrome varies throughout the world and reflects primarily the racial composition of various countries.
- Reported incidence rates vary from 3 per 100,000 in South America to 134 per 100,000 in Japan.

Prevalence
The syndrome occurs year round but is most prevalent in winter and spring with peaks usually occurring in December or January.

RISK FACTORS
- Higher rate of antecedent respiratory tract illness,
- Exposure to recent carpet cleaning, shampooing, house dust, mites (chiefly *Dermatophagoides farnae*, *D. pteronyssinus*),
- Residence near bodies of water.

Genetics
- Alteration of the caspase –3 gene leads to susceptibility to KD (1).
- Alterations in the TGF-beta pathway also lead to susceptibility to the disease (2).

PATHOPHYSIOLOGY
- Small arterioles, larger arteries, capillaries, and veins are affected.
- In the early stages of the vasculitis of Kawasaki disease, edema of endothelial cells with nuclear degeneration and mild adventitial inflammation are seen.
- In the acute stage of the disease, systemic inflammatory changes are evident in many organs, including myocardium, pericardium, cardiac valves, cerebrospinal fluid, lung, lymph nodes, pancreas, spleen, joints, and liver.
- Cardiac death generally occurs in the subacute or convalescent stages of illness.

ETIOLOGY
- The origin of the syndrome remains unknown.
- Clinical and epidemiologic features strongly suggest that the disease has an infectious cause.
- Two major theories to explain the etiology; respiratory pathogen theory and the superantigen theory.

DIAGNOSIS

HISTORY
A history of fever along with an exanthem should be sought.

PHYSICAL EXAM
- Fever for at least 5 days duration.
- In addition to fever, presence of 4 of the following clinical criteria:
  - Polymorphous exanthem
  - Bilateral conjunctival injection
  - Oropharyngeal erythema, lips cracking, strawberry tongue
  - Extremity changes as erythema, edema, and induration of hands and feet, and periungual desquamation
  - Cervical lymphadenopathy
- Beware of incomplete criteria satisfaction as "incomplete manifestations" of the syndrome are not infrequent and may lead to inappropriate delay in treatment (3).
- Other associated clinical findings: Arthritis, arthralgia, coronary artery ectasia or aneurysms, pericarditis, myocarditis, aseptic meningitis, facial nerve palsy, marked irritability, sensorineural hearing loss, pulmonary infiltrates, nodules, preceding respiratory illness, hepatitis, pancreatitis, diarrhea, urethritis, meatitis, peripheral gangrene, desquamating groin rash, erythema, and anterior uveitis (3).

DIAGNOSTIC TESTS & INTERPRETATION
Lab
- Anemia (normocytic, normochromic) (3)
- Leukocytosis with neutrophilia and band forms
- Thrombocytosis
- Elevated erythrocyte sedimentation rate, C-reactive protein and procalcitonin levels
- Hypoalbuminemia
- Hyponatremia
- Elevated serum transaminases, gamma-glutamyltransferase
- Plasma lipid abnormalities
- Cerebrospinal fluid pleocytosis
- Synovial fluid pleocytosis

Imaging
Initial approach
- Electrocardiographies show tachycardia, along with ST, T, and QT changes.
- Three-dimensional echocardiography reveals aneurysms in the coronary arteries in 25% of children who are untreated (4).

Follow-Up & Special Considerations
Magnetic resonance imaging, and ultrafast computed tomography scans are also helpful in the diagnosis of coronary aneurysms, occlusions, and stenosis.

Diagnostic Procedures/Other
- Stress test with evaluation of myocardial perfusion
- Coronary angiography

DIFFERENTIAL DIAGNOSIS
- Viruses: Measles, Echovirus, Adenovirus, and Epstein-Barr virus
- Bacteria: *Staphylococcus aureus*, *Streptococcus pyogenes*, *Rickettsia rickettsii*, *Leptospira interrogans*
- Drug reactions: Serum sickness, Stevens-Johnson syndrome
- Rheumatologic disease: Systemic-onset juvenile idiopathic arthritis

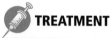

TREATMENT

MEDICATION
First Line

- Intravenous immunoglobulin (IVIG) is the mainstay of therapy, and is given as a single infusion of 2 g/kg over 10–12 hours (3)[A]. Most experts recommend a second dose of IVIG for patients who remain febrile 36–48 hours after their first infusion. Side effects of IVIG depend on the infused product and range from fever, chills, and hypotension to increased blood viscosity and therefore, risk of thromboembolism.

- A second dose of IVIG of 2 g/kg can be used if fever persists or recurs for over 36 hours after the initial IVIG administration (3)[C].

- In addition to IVIG, acetylsalicylic acid 80–100 mg/kg/day in 4 divided doses until at least 72 hours afebrile, then 3–5 mg/kg/day for 6–8 weeks (3).

- Continue acetylsalicylic acid long-term (minimum duration is up to regression of the aneurysm) if evidence of coronary aneurysm (>3 mm) (3)[B].

- If there is a giant coronary aneurysm (>6 mm), add warfarin to acetylsalicylic acid and maintain an INR of 2–2,5. Substitute low molecular weight heparin for warfarin if blood monitoring of prothrombin time is difficult.

Second Line
- Intravenous pulse methylprednisolone 30 mg/kg administered over 3 hours, daily for 1–3 days.
- Infliximab has been used successfully in cases refractory to IVIG (5,6).

ADDITIONAL TREATMENT

Issues for Referral

- Referral to a cardiologist for coronary angiography if coronary artery thrombosis is present.
- Referral to a cardiothoracic surgeon may be necessary.

Additional Therapies

Various agents such as pentoxifylline, cyclophosphamide, ulinastatin, and plasmapheresis have been used, but their potential benefit has to be verified from more data. Beta-blockers are used if coronary artery obstruction is present.

SURGERY/OTHER PROCEDURES

Coronary artery bypass surgery is the recommended surgical therapy upon evidence of reversible ischemia (3,7). Catheter intervention is also indicated in this situation.

IN-PATIENT CONSIDERATIONS

IV Fluids

Careful to avoid overload

Discharge Criteria

- Lack of fever and lack of signs of congestive heart failure.
- Lack of coronary ischemia signs (chest pain, angina equivalent).
- Normalization of inflammatory markers.

 ONGOING CARE

FOLLOW-UP RECOMMENDATIONS

Patient Monitoring

- Children with a coronary aneurysm need to have an ECG and an echocardiogram every 6–12 months along with a cardiology consult.
- Annual stress test with evaluation of the myocardial perfusion may also be necessary every 1–2 years. This will help guide the decision whether to participate in noncontact sports by ruling out exercise-induced myocardial ischemia.
- Children without coronary aneurysm need follow-up every 3–5 years.
- Coronary angiography for children with giant coronary aneurysm is indicated at 6–12 months or sooner if evidence of myocardial ischemia. For children with smaller coronary aneurysm, perform coronary angiography if noninvasive tests point to myocardial ischemia.

PATIENT EDUCATION

Education regarding physical activities is of paramount importance (to avoid bleeding) in patients receiving antiplatelet drugs and/or anticoagulants. Suggest avoidance of contact sports in these patients.

PROGNOSIS

- Coronary aneurysms occur in 20–25% of those untreated or in those treated late in the disease (after 10 days).
- Early treatment with IVIG reduces the incidence of coronary aneurysms.
- About half of all children with documented aneurysms and appropriate treatment have regression of the aneurysms over time.

COMPLICATIONS

- Cardiovascular complications
- Coronary artery stenosis
- Myocardial infarction is the most common cause of death in Kawasaki disease.
- Myocarditis (8)
- Pericarditis
- Mitral valvulitis
- Non-cardiovascular complications
- Pneumonitis
- Transient unilateral facial nerve palsy
- Sensorineural hearing loss
- Hemophagocytic syndrome
- Macrophage activation
- Painful arthritis, arthralgia

REFERENCES

1. Onouchi Y, Ozaki K, Buns JC, et al. Common variants in CASP3 confer susceptibility to Kawasaki disease. *Hum Mol Genet* 2010;19:2898–2906.
2. Shimizu C, Jain S, Davila S, et al. Transforming growth Factor-{beta} signaling pathway in patients with kawasaki disease. *Circ Cardiovasc Genet* 2011;4:16–25.
3. Newburger JW, Takahashi M, Gerber MA, et al. Diagnosis, treatment, and long-term management of Kawasaki disease: A statement for health professionals from the Committee on Rheumatic Fever, Endocarditis and Kawasaki Disease, Council on Cardiovascular Disease in the Young, American Heart Association. *Circulation* 2004;110:2747–2771.
4. Miyashita M, Karasawa K, Taniguchi K, et al. Usefulness of real-time 3-dimensional echocardiography for the evaluation of coronary artery morphology in patients with Kawasaki disease. *J Am Soc Echocardiogr* 2007;20:930–933.
5. Son MB, Gauvreau K, Burns JC, et al. Infliximab for intravenous immunoglobulin resistance in Kawasaki Disease: A retrospective study. *J Pediatr* 2011;158:644–649.
6. Yellen ES, Gauvreau K, Takahashi M, et al. Performance of 2004 American Heart Association recommendations for treatment of Kawasaki disease. *Pediatrics* 2010;125:e234–e241.
7. Tsuda E, Kitamura S, Kimura K, et al. Long-term patency of internal thoracic artery grafts for coronary artery stenosis due to Kawasaki disease: Comparison of early with recent results in small children. *Am Heart J* 2007;153:995–1000.
8. Printz BF, Sleeper LA, Newburger JW, et al. Noncoronary cardiac abnormalities are associated with coronary artery dilation and with laboratory inflammatory markers in acute Kawasaki disease. *J Am Coll Cardiol* 2010;57:86–92.

ADDITIONAL READING

- Rowley AH, Baker SC, Orenstein JM, et al. Searching for the cause of Kawasaki disease–cytoplasmic inclusion bodies provide new insight. *Nat Rev Microbiol* 2008;6:394–401.

 CODES

ICD9

446.1 Acute febrile mucocutaneous lymph node syndrome (mcls)

CLINICAL PEARLS

- If you have administered IVIG, postpone immunization against varicella and measles for 11 months; if risk of exposure is very high, immunize at the earliest time but repeat immunization after 11 months.
- Reye syndrome may manifest after high dose aspirin treatment.
- Keep these eponymous diseases always in mind. This is not a medical rarity and treatment may be life-saving.
- Keep always a high index of suspicion for the disease when it manifests itself with fewer criterions to fulfill a formal diagnosis (atypical Kawasaki).
- Avoid the concurrent use of ibuprofen and aspirin as the former antagonizes the latter regarding platelet inhibition!

K

KERATITIS

Theodoros Filippopoulos (E. Mylonakis, Editor)

 BASICS

DESCRIPTION
- The term keratitis is used in cases of corneal inflammation due to infectious or noninfectious etiologies. Infectious keratitis can be caused by bacteria, viruses, fungi, or parasites. Keratitis secondary to a bacterial infection is termed corneal ulcer.
- Chlamydia trachomatis (serotypes A-C) causes a chronic follicular conjunctivitis that leads to in-turning of the eyelashes (trichiasis) and corneal scarring. Trachoma is currently the leading cause of infectious blindness worldwide.

EPIDEMIOLOGY
Incidence
Annual incidence estimates of bacterial keratitis vary among studies. A fair estimate is an annual incidence of 0.63 cases per 10,000 population, which escalates to 3.4 cases per 10,000 population in contact lens wearers.

Prevalence
In 2003, the WHO estimated that 7.6 million people worldwide were severely visually impaired or blind as a result of trachoma.

RISK FACTORS
- A breach in the integrity of the epithelial surface as in ocular surface disease is an important risk factor for the development of bacterial keratitis.
- In the US, contact lenses play a major role in development of bacterial keratitis. Important risk factors include the following:
  – Poor contact lens hygiene
  – Overnight continuous contact lens wear
  – Use of homemade saline (risk factor for *Acanthamoeba* keratitis)
- For critically ill patients, risk factors may be different and include the inability to shut the eyes (lagophthalmos), inadequate blinking, underlying dry eye disease (keratoconjunctivitis sicca), and intermittent positive-pressure ventilation.
- Fungal infections are more common in warm, humid climates, especially after corneal trauma by vegetable matter.
- Trachoma is highly correlated with poverty and limited access to healthcare services and water.

GENERAL PREVENTION
- Contact lenses should not be worn by anyone with an active eye infection. Instructions provided by the manufacturer regarding the time intervals for replacement and overnight wear should be strictly followed.
- Among critically ill patients, frequent eye examinations, instillation of artificial tears and/or lubricating ointments, and prevention of exposure by maintaining proper eyelid closure at all times are important preventive measures.

- Hospital personnel that care for critically ill patients should avoid the following:
  – Touching the ocular surface or eyelashes with the tip of ointment tubes or drop applicators
  – Using the same ointment tube or drop applicator across patients
  – Applying patches on eyes with discharge
  – Suctioning respiratory tract secretions across the head of patients without covering patient's eyes
  – Leaving contact lenses in situ
- A vaccine has been approved by the FDA for people >60 years to decrease the incidence and the severity of herpes zoster ophthalmicus (HZO).

PATHOPHYSIOLOGY
- Interruption of corneal epithelium integrity permits entrance of microorganisms into the corneal stroma, where they proliferate. Several bacteria display adhesins, molecules that allow adherence to host corneal cells.
- Primary Herpes simplex virus (HSV-1) infection usually occurs in the mucocutaneous distribution of the trigeminal nerve. After primary infection, the virus spreads from the infected epithelial cells to nearby sensory nerve endings and is transported along nerve axons to cell bodies located in the trigeminal ganglion. There, the virus genome is incorporated into the human genome, where it persists indefinitely in a latent state. Reactivation and interneuronal spread of HSV-1 can lead to recurrent ocular disease.
- Following primary Varicella zoster virus (VZV) infection, virus particles remain in the dorsal roots or sensory ganglia where they may lay dormant for years. As a result of aging, immunosuppression, or medical treatment (steroids), cell-mediated immune responses decline which allows reactivation of VZV and results in a localized cutaneous rash erupting in a single dermatome. Involvement of the first division of the trigeminal nerve results in a disease process termed herpes zoster ophthalmicus (HZO).

ETIOLOGY
- Worldwide, the two leading causes of blindness from keratitis are trachoma due to *Chlamydia* spp. and vitamin A deficiency related to malnutrition. The infectious causes of keratitis include the following:
  – Bacteria:
    ○ *Acinetobacter calcoaceticus*
    ○ *Aeromonas hydrophila*
    ○ *Bacillus* spp.
    ○ *Bartonella henselae*
    ○ *Borrelia burgdorferi*
    ○ *Brucella* spp.
    ○ *Chlamydia trachomatis*
    ○ *Clostridium* (*C. perfringens* and *C. tetani*)
    ○ *Corynebacterium diphtheriae*
    ○ *Enterococcus* spp.
    ○ *Escherichia coli*

    ○ *Klebsiella pneumoniae*
    ○ *Moraxella* spp.
    ○ *Morganella morganii*
    ○ *Mycobacterium tuberculosis* and atypical Mycobacteria
    ○ *Neisseria gonorrhoeae*
    ○ *Nocardia* spp.
    ○ *Pasteurella multocida*
    ○ *Proteus mirabilis*
    ○ *Pseudomonas* spp.
    ○ *Serratia marcescens*
    ○ *Staphylococcus aureus*
    ○ *Staphylococcus epidermidis*
    ○ *Streptococcus* spp. (particularly *S. pneumoniae*)
    ○ *Treponema pallidum*
  – Viruses:
    ○ Adenovirus
    ○ Cytomegalovirus (CMV)
    ○ Epstein-Barr virus (EBV)
    ○ Herpes simplex virus (HSV type 1 rather than type 2)
    ○ Molluscum contagiosum
    ○ Rubeola
    ○ Varicella zoster virus (VZV)
  – Fungi:
    ○ *Aspergillus* spp.
    ○ *Candida* spp.
    ○ *Fusarium* spp.
    ○ *Penicillium* spp.
  – Parasites:
    ○ *Acanthamoeba* spp.
    ○ *Leishmania* spp.
    ○ *Microsporidia* spp.
    ○ *Trypanosoma* spp.
- Corneal ulcers due to *P. aeruginosa* may advance rapidly to involve the entire cornea in a few days.
- Many entities start with primarily conjunctival involvement with secondary infectious or inflammatory corneal sequelae as in adenoviral epidemic keratoconjunctivitis.
- *Neisseria gonorrhoeae* causes a hyper purulent conjunctivitis and keratitis. The associated inflammation can lead to corneal perforation.
- Fungal keratitis tends to be insidious and slowly progressive.
- The most common primary HSV ocular manifestation is a follicular blepharoconjunctivitis. HSV corneal involvement can range from isolated epithelial disease to stromal involvement (immune stromal and interstitial keratitis) and uveitis. The classic herpetic corneal lesion consists of a linear branching epithelial lesion with terminal bulbs (dendrite). Recurrent episodes of HSV keratitis with stromal involvement can lead to extensive corneal scarring requiring corneal transplantation.

- HZO sequelae include the following:
  - Conjunctivitis
  - Anterior uveitis (iridocyclitis)
  - Keratitis ranging from epithelial disease to stromal or neurotrophic keratitis
  - Ophthalmoplegia
  - Postherpetic scarring and neuralgia
  - Increased intraocular pressure

COMMONLY ASSOCIATED CONDITIONS
Contact lens wear and/or a history of ocular trauma are the most frequently associated conditions in cases of bacterial keratitis.

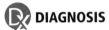 DIAGNOSIS

HISTORY
- The most common symptoms are eye pain, conjunctival injection (redness), and foreign body sensation. Other symptoms include:
  - Blepharospasm
  - Mucopurulent discharge
  - Photophobia (light sensitivity)
  - Tearing
  - Visual loss
- Severe pain, often out of proportion to the clinical picture, is a feature of *Acanthamoeba* keratitis.
- HSV (and VZV) can result in corneal hypoesthesia as a result of which subsequent episodes may lack pain or foreign body sensation.
- HZO usually begins with an influenza-like prodrome. Ocular symptoms due to VZV can occur after vesicle eruption in dermatomes associated with any branch of the trigeminal nerve, but are particularly common when vesicles form on the tip of the nose, reflecting nasociliary nerve (CN V1) involvement (Hutchinson's sign). Cutaneous lesions typically respect the vertical midline.

PHYSICAL EXAM
- Slit-lamp examination shows disruption of the corneal epithelium, a cloudy infiltrate or abscess in the stroma, and an inflammatory cellular reaction in the anterior chamber in cases of bacterial keratitis. The breakdown in corneal epithelium is best seen with cobalt blue light after installation of fluorescein.
- In severe cases of keratitis, inflammatory cells may settle at the bottom of the anterior chamber, giving rise to a hypopyon.

- *P. aeruginosa* keratitis usually starts as a small ulcer that spreads concentrically to involve a large portion of the cornea, sclera, and underlying stroma. A history of contact lens use is highly indicative of *P. aeruginosa* keratitis. Clinical manifestations of *P. aeruginosa* keratitis include the following:
  - A rapidly expanding infiltrate at the bed of an epithelial breakdown
  - Surrounding corneal edema
  - An anterior chamber reaction
  - Mucopurulent discharge adherent to the ulcer's surface
- Clinical characteristics of bacterial corneal ulcers are not specific enough to diagnose one pathogen over the other.
- Feathery indistinct borders of a corneal infiltrate and/or satellite lesions suggest fungal keratitis.
- In late stages of *Acanthamoeba* keratitis, the infiltrate may become ring shaped.
- A branching dendritic pattern of corneal epithelial breakdown (revealed by fluorescein staining) is characteristic for herpetic infections (HSV & VZV). With Zoster (VZV), pseudodendrites (which are usually raised mucous plaques that do not stain well with fluorescein) without terminal bulbs may initially form and can coalesce at later stages.

DIAGNOSTIC TESTS & INTERPRETATION
Lab
Serologic testing is rarely employed in the diagnosis of infectious keratitis. A rare example is VDRL/FTA-ABS in cases of interstitial keratitis (corneal stromal inflammation with vascularization).

Imaging
In vivo confocal microscopy can be helpful in diagnosing *Acanthamoeba* keratitis allowing the visualization of pear-shaped cysts and trophozoites.

Diagnostic Procedures/Other
- Corneal scrapings are obtained for Gram stain, Giemsa stain, Calcofluor white stain (if *Acanthamoeba* is suspected) and cultures. Routine culture media include blood agar, Sabouraud, thioglycolate, and chocolate agar. Lowenstein-Jensen medium (mycobacteria, *Nocardia* spp.) is employed if there is a history of corneal refractive surgery or an atypical ulcer appearance.
- A corneal biopsy can also be obtained if initial smears and cultures are inconclusive with a disposable skin punch or a small corneal trephine. The material is plated directly onto culture media and a portion is sent for histopathology.

- The irregular polygonal cysts of Acanthamoeba may be identified in corneal scrapings or biopsy material, and trophozoites can be grown on special media (non-nutrient agar with *E. coli* overlay).
- Corneal or cutaneous vesicular swabs and scrapings can be used for the diagnosis of herpetic disease (HSV or VZV). Culture, DNA testing (real-time PCR), and Fluorescent Antibody testing are used for that purpose. Giemsa stains (Tzanck preparation) demonstrate multinucleated giant cells.

Pathological Findings
In cases of bacterial keratitis, inflammatory cells (mainly neutrophils) surround the ulcer causing necrosis of the stromal lamellae. A deep stromal abscess may coalesce, resulting in thinning of the cornea.

DIFFERENTIAL DIAGNOSIS
- For a differential diagnosis of entities associated with a red eye (keratitis, conjunctivitis, uveitis, endophthalmitis etc.), please refer to the Section I of chapter, "Red Eye," and the Section II of chapter, "Endophthalmitis" and "Chorioretinitis-Uveitis."
- Sterile corneal thinning can occur in association with systemic autoimmune disorders as in peripheral ulcerative keratitis.
- It is very important in cases of HSV keratitis to differentiate between only epithelial involvement which is associated with actively replicating viral particles on the corneal surface and deeper stromal/endothelial involvement as management decisions may differ.
- Keratoconjunctivitis due to a HSV can be easily confused with adenoviral epidemic keratoconjunctivitis, unless vesicles appear on the periocular skin.
- Peripheral corneal infiltrates often with overlying epithelial defect with a clear zone between the limbus and the infiltrate can represent a hypersensitivity reaction to staphylococcal antigens in patients with coexisting blepharitis.

K

TREATMENT

MEDICATION
First Line

- If there is clinical suspicion of bacterial keratitis, empiric, topical broad antibiotic coverage should be initiated promptly. Ulcers and infiltrates should be treated as bacterial unless a very high index of suspicion for other pathogens exists until Gram stains are back.
- Fortified topical antibiotic eyedrops should be used every 1 hour round the clock such as tobramycin or gentamicin (15 mg/mL) for gram-negative coverage alternating with cefazolin (50 mg/mL) or vancomycin (25 mg/mL) for gram-positive coverage.
- All patients with vision-threatening ulcers should be treated with loading doses with 1 antibiotic drop every 5 minutes for the first 1/2 hour.
- Alternatively, for smaller, peripheral and vision non-threatening ulcers, a commercially available fourth generation fluoroquinolone such as gatifloxacin or moxifloxacin can be used starting at a frequency every 1 hour round the clock.
- Duration and frequency of treatment are tailored based on clinical response.
- Cycloplegic eyedrops (i.e., cyclopentolate 1% b.i.d. or atropine 1% b.i.d.) can be used for pain management and prevention of synechiae whenever there is significant anterior chamber reaction.
- Systemic antibiotic therapy is mainly indicated in cases of severe suppurative keratitis (i.e., due to *Neisseria gonorrhoeae*) or for infections that involve the sclera. Consider also oral clarithromycin (500 mg PO b.i.d.) in cases of atypical mycobacteria.
- Fungal keratitis is treated with topical natamycin 5% eyedrops in cases of filamentous fungi (i.e., Fusarium spp. or Aspergillus spp.) and with amphotericin B 0.15% in cases of non-filamentous organisms (i.e., Candida spp.). Eyedrops should be used hourly initially and treatment is usually extended to 4–6 weeks. Oral antifungal agents such as voriconazole (200 mg PO b.i.d) or fluconazole (200–400 mg PO loading dose and then 100–200 mg PO per day) should be considered in cases of deep corneal ulcers or suspected secondary fungal endophthalmitis.

- *Acanthamoeba* keratitis is often misdiagnosed. Cysts of *Acanthamoeba* can be difficult to eradicate with available drugs.
- Polyhexamethyl biguanidine 0.02% (PHMB) eyedrops used hourly is the first line of treatment.
- Topical chlorhexidine 0.02% can be used as well.
- Dibromopropamidine isethionate ointment 0.1% (Brolene) is also available for *Acanthamoeba* keratitis.
- Treatment is usually continued for 3 months after resolution of inflammation. Corneal transplantation should be delayed for at least 6–12 months.
- HSV keratitis is treated according to the type of corneal involvement. Eyelid cutaneous involvement extending to the lid margin is treated with acyclovir ointment 5 times a day to the skin and trifluridine 1% eyedrops 5 times a day to prevent corneal epithelial disease. Vidarabine 3% ointment is an alternative that can be used in children if eyedrop installation is difficult. Therapy is continued for 7–14 days until resolution of cutaneous vesicles.
- Herpetic keratitis with only corneal epithelial involvement is treated with topical antiviral agents (trifluridine 1% 1 drop 9 times daily or vidarabine 3% ointment 5 times daily for 1–2 weeks) and cycloplegics. Gentle epithelial debridement of corneal dendrites decreases the viral load. All topical steroids should be discontinued. Oral acyclovir (400 mg PO 5 times a day) does not prevent development of stromal disease and should be reserved for cases where drops cannot be given due to corneal toxicity.
- HSV stromal disease requires topical cycloplegics (i.e., cyclopentolate 1% b.i.d.) and topical steroids (prednisolone acetate 1% q.i.d.). Antiviral prophylaxis with topical trifluridine 1% q.i.d. or oral acyclovir 400 mg PO b.i.d. is also recommended.
- In cases where recurrent episodes of stromal disease result in scarring and visual disability, long term suppression with oral acyclovir (400 mg PO b.i.d.) for up to 1 year should be considered.

- HZO is treated with oral antiviral agents (acyclovir 800 mg PO 5 times per day or famciclovir 500 mg PO t.i.d. or valacyclovir 1 g PO t.i.d.) for 10 days. Antiviral therapy is not of significant benefit in cases that present late (more than 1 week after vesicle eruption). Systemically ill patients may require hospitalization and intravenous acyclovir (5–10 mg/kg IV t.i.d.). Bacitracin or erythromycin ointment may prevent secondary superinfection of cutaneous lesions. Corneal epithelial involvement only requires supportive measures with artificial tears or lubricating ointments. Immune stromal keratitis and/or uveitis are treated with topical steroids (prednisolone acetate 1% q.i.d.) and topical cycloplegics. Retinitis, optic neuritis, or ophthalmoplegia require intravenous acyclovir (5–10 mg/kg IV t.i.d.) and oral prednisone (refer to acute retinal necrosis [ARN] Section II chapter "Chorioretinitis-Uveitis").
- Amitriptyline (25 mg PO t.i.d.) may be helpful in the treatment of postherpetic neuralgia and depression that can follow HZO.
- Epidemic keratoconjunctivitis due to adenovirus and ocular involvement in infectious mononucleosis usually requires only symptomatic care.
- Trachoma is treated with a single dose of azithromycin (20 mg/kg PO) and topical erythromycin or sulfacetamide ointment (b.i.d.–q.i.d.) for 3–4 weeks.
- Gonococcal conjunctivitis with or without keratitis requires systemic treatment with ceftriaxone. If there is no corneal involvement, a single dose of ceftriaxone (1 g i.m.) is sufficient; with corneal involvement, intravenous ceftriaxone is necessary (1 g IV per day– b.i.d.) along with a topical fourth generation fluoroquinolone (gatifloxacin or moxifloxacin every 1 hour round the clock). Treatment for possible chlamydial (serotypes D-K) co-infection with a single dose of oral azithromycin (1 g PO) is also recommended.

Second Line
- Alternatively, fungal keratitis can be treated with topical fortified voriconazole (0.5 mg/mL) every 1 hour round the clock.
- Trachoma can be alternatively treated with doxycycline (100 mg PO b.i.d.) or erythromycin 500 mg PO q.i.d.) for 2 weeks.

ADDITIONAL TREATMENT
Additional Therapies
In cases of bacterial keratitis, topical corticosteroids (prednisolone acetate 1% q.i.d.) can be added to control the inflammatory response once the infection is under control.

SURGERY/OTHER PROCEDURES
- Bacterial keratitis complicated by corneal perforation may require a corneal tectonic graft to maintain ocular integrity.
- Treatment failure is not uncommon in cases of *Acanthamoeba* keratitis requiring penetrating keratoplasty. Re-occurrence in the corneal graft is a possibility since *Acanthamoeba* cysts are difficult to eradicate.

IN-PATIENT CONSIDERATIONS
Admission Criteria
Bacterial and viral keratitis is managed on an outpatient basis unless social or other limitations interfere with adherence to the strict treatment protocol.

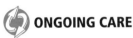 ONGOING CARE

FOLLOW-UP RECOMMENDATIONS
Frequent slit-lamp examinations are mandatory until signs of improvement are obvious.

DIET
No dietary restrictions apply.

PATIENT EDUCATION
Patients should be instructed on proper contact lens use.

PROGNOSIS
- Prognosis in cases of bacterial keratitis depends on location, size of the initial infiltrate, and delay in initiation of proper antibiotic coverage.
- PKP results for HSV keratitis are uniformly poor with a high rate of graft rejection and HSV reactivation respectively.

COMPLICATIONS
- Infiltration of the corneal stroma by neutrophils in bacterial keratitis can lead to keratolysis with the development of corneal thinning and therefore irregular astigmatism, and in extreme cases, can even lead to corneal perforation when treatment is inadequate or delayed. Corneal perforation may result in secondary endophthalmitis and possible loss of the eye.
- Scar formation (corneal leukoma) with the presence of corneal vascularization may be the end result of a bacterial keratitis or recurrent episodes of HSV stromal keratitis. Depending on the location and depth of stromal involvement, the resulting corneal leukoma may be visually significant and necessitate corneal surgery for visual rehabilitation (including phototherapeutic keratectomy [PTK] or penetrating keratoplasty [PKP]).
- As a late sequelae of severe keratitis, inflammation can lead to invasion of the corneal stroma by blood vessels (neovascularization).

ADDITIONAL READING
- Holz HA, Espandar L, Moshirfar M. Herpes zoster ophthalmicus. In: Yanoff M, Duker JS, eds. *Ophthalmology*, 3rd ed. Philadelphia, Mosby Elsevier, 2009:222–225.
- Lam DSC, Houang E, Fan DSP, et al. Incidence and risk factors for microbial keratitis in Hong Kong: Comparison with Europe and North America. *Eye* 2002;16:608–618.
- Mariotti SP, Pascolini D, Rose-Nussbaumer J. Trachoma: Global magnitude of a preventable cause of blindness. *Br J Ophthalmol* 2009;93:563–568.
- Tuli SS. Herpes simplex keratitis. In: Yanoff M, Duker JS, eds. *Ophthalmology*, 3rd ed. Philadelphia, Mosby Elsevier, 2009:279–284.

 CODES

ICD9
- 370.00 Corneal ulcer, unspecified
- 370.8 Other forms of keratitis
- 370.9 Unspecified keratitis

CLINICAL PEARLS
- If *P. aeruginosa* is suspected based on history (contact lens use), clinical picture or Gram stain double antibiotic coverage is recommended. Fortified topical tobramycin or gentamicin (15 mg/mL) along with a commercially available fourth generation fluoroquinolone is a reasonable option.
- Corticosteroids can worsen keratitis caused by fungi or atypical mycobacteria.
- *Neisseria gonorrhoeae* organisms can penetrate intact epithelium. In addition to antibiotic treatment, frequent irrigation of the ocular surface is required to remove inflammatory cells and mediators.
- In patients with gonococcal conjunctivitis with or without concurrent keratitis, screening and/or treatment for other sexually transmitted diseases (Chlamydia, HIV, syphilis) is highly advisable. An infectious diseases consultation should be obtained.
- Tetracyclines are contraindicated in children younger than 8 years, pregnant, or nursing women.
- Topical antivirals can cause a toxic or allergic reaction (conjunctivitis) upon which oral medications should be employed.
- HZO can be the initial manifestation of HIV in patients younger than 40 years without any other immune-compromising pathology.

K

LARVA MIGRANS SYNDROMES

Padma Srikanth
Paschalis Vergidis
Matthew E. Falagas

 BASICS

DESCRIPTION
Wide spectrum of syndromes caused by larvae of helminthes migrating through the skin, soft tissues, or visceral organs

EPIDEMIOLOGY
Incidence
- In the US, about 10,000 cases of *Toxocara* infection are reported in humans each year.
- Most commonly occurs in children <6 years

Prevalence
- Cutaneous larva migrans
  - Cutaneous larva migrans is mainly found in tropical and subtropical geographic areas and the southern US.
  - It is the most common tropical acquired dermatosis.
  - More frequently seen in children.
- Visceral, ocular larva migrans
  - Almost 14% of the US population has been infected with *Toxocara* (1).
  - Toxocariasis is found in many countries. Seroprevalence rates can be 40% or higher.

RISK FACTORS
- Contact with soil contaminated with dog feces
- Contact with dogs and cats
- Lack of hand hygiene prior to eating food.
- Geophagia

GENERAL PREVENTION
- Avoidance of direct skin contact with fecally contaminated soil (wearing shoes, protective clothing)
- Regular anthelmintic care in dogs and cats.

PATHOPHYSIOLOGY
- Visceral, ocular larva migrans
  - The roundworm eggs are deposited in dog feces, become infectious after 3–4 weeks, and can infect humans.
  - The eggs hatch in the human stomach and the larvae migrate through mesenteric vessels to the liver.
  - The larvae then enter the circulation and disseminate throughout the body.
  - Larvae may persist for years in the human host.

ETIOLOGY
- Cutaneous larva migrans
  - *Ancylostoma braziliense*, a dog and cat hookworm, can cause cutaneous larva migrans (creeping eruption) in humans.
  - Other helminths that can cause a larva migrans syndrome include:
    - *Ancylostoma caninum* (Australia)
    - *Uncinaria stenocephala* (Europe)
    - *Bunostomum phlebotomum*
    - *Gnathostoma spinigerum*
    - *Strongyloides stercoralis* (Larva currens caused by rapid migration)
    - *Fasciola gigantica* (Vietnam)
    - *Spirulina* spp. (Japan)
- Visceral, ocular larva migrans
  - *Toxocara canis*, a dog roundworm, and less commonly *Toxocara cati*, a feline roundworm, can cause visceral or ocular larva migrans (toxocariasis) in humans by ingestion.
  - Another form of visceral larva migrans is caused by *Ascaris suum*.

COMMONLY ASSOCIATED CONDITIONS
With toxocariasis: Lead poisoning among those with pica and where soil is contaminated with lead paint.

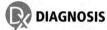 **DIAGNOSIS**

HISTORY
- Cutaneous larva migrans
  - History of sunbathing, walking barefoot on the beach, or similar activity in a tropical location
  - Intense pruritus. Begins shortly after the larvae start penetrating.
  - Symptoms last for few weeks, but may recur.
- Visceral larva migrans
  - Mild infection may be asymptomatic
  - Fever
  - Malaise, fatigue
  - Anorexia, weight loss
  - Abdominal pain
  - Cough, dyspnea
  - Abdominal pain
  - History of convulsions
- Ocular larva migrans
  - May present without visceral involvement
  - Seeing floaters or bubble-like images
  - Decreased visual acuity
  - Blindness

PHYSICAL EXAM
- Cutaneous larva migrans
  - Erythematous, serpiginous, slightly elevated, pruritic, cutaneous eruption.
  - Eruption moves forward in an irregular pattern.
  - Most patients have a single larval track
  - The larvae causing the tracks can migrate a few millimeters to several centimeters per day depending on parasite species.
  - Vesicles with serous fluid may be seen along the track
  - Folliculitis is an uncommon manifestation
  - Primarily the distal lower extremities are affected. Other sites: Buttocks, anogenital area, abdomen, and hands
- Visceral larva migrans
  - Hepatomegaly, right upper quadrant tenderness
  - Splenomegaly (less common)
  - Lymphadenitis
  - Rales, Wheezing
  - Skin nodules, Chronic urticaria
- Ocular larva migrans
  - Inflammation is typically unilateral (2).
  - Decreased visual acuity
  - Leukocoria
  - Whitish elevated granuloma in the posterior pole of the retina
  - Peripheral retinal exudates
  - Chorioretinitis
  - Uveitis
  - Secondary retinal detachment
  - Optic neuritis

DIAGNOSTIC TESTS & INTERPRETATION
Lab
- Cutaneous larva migrans
  - A minority of patients with cutaneous larva migrans demonstrate peripheral eosinophilia.
- Visceral, ocular larva migrans
  - Leukocytosis with marked eosinophilia
  - Increased total IgE
  - Serology may be positive (ELISA, immunoblot)
  - Smaller worm burden in ocular disease: Eosinophilia may be absent, antibody titers are lower.
  - In pulmonary involvement: Eosinophilia in bronchoalveolar lavage fluid

Imaging
- Visceral larva migrans
  - Hepatic involvement: Liver ultrasound may show hypoechoic areas. CT scan may show single or multiple ill-defined, oval or elongated, small, low-attenuating lesions (3).
  - Pulmonary involvement: CXR may show pulmonary nodules, infiltrates, or pleural effusion. Chest CT scan shows nodules with surrounding ground-glass opacities
  - Meningeal/cerebral involvement: CT/MRI of brain may show presence of granulomas (hyperintense lesions on T2-weighted images)

Diagnostic Procedures/Other
- Skin biopsy is not useful in the diagnosis of cutaneous larva migrans. The helminth is rarely identified by biopsy.
- Similarly, larvae are usually not found in visceral larva migrans.
- Funduscopic exam in ocular larva migrans

Pathological Findings
- In the skin: The larva is unable to penetrate beneath the epidermis, therefore the larva migrates forming a tunnel with accompanying local eosinophilic infiltration
- In the liver and other organs: Granulomatous reaction, producing nodular lesions
- In the eye: Subretinal masses

DIFFERENTIAL DIAGNOSIS
- Cutaneous larva migrans
  - Tinea pedis
  - Contact dermatitis
  - Impetigo
  - Migratory myiasis
- Visceral larva migrans
  - Strongyloidiasis
  - Schistosomiasis
  - Ascariasis
  - Echinococcosis
  - Acute hepatitis
  - Pulmonary eosinophilia
  - Allergic bronchopulmonary aspergillosis
- Ocular larva migrans
  - Retinoblastoma
  - Retinal tuberculosis
  - Toxoplasmosis

 TREATMENT

MEDICATION
- Cutaneous larva migrans
  - Albendazole 200 mg orally twice daily for 3 days
  - Ivermectin 150 μg/kg orally (single dose) (4)
  - For localized lesions, topical 15% thiabendazole cream applied 2–3 times a day for 5 days
- Visceral larva migrans
  - Most patients recover without specific treatment. Consider anthelmintic treatment for severe disease.
  - Albendazole 400 mg orally twice daily for 5 days
  - Mebendazole 200 mg orally twice daily for 5 days
- Ocular larva migrans
  - Anthelmintic treatment with albendazole or mebendazole at the same doses as for visceral disease may be beneficial for active disease.

ADDITIONAL TREATMENT
Additional Therapies
- Antihistamines to relieve pruritus in cutaneous larva migrans
- Corticosteroids for neurologic or cardiac disease in visceral larva migrans.
- Local and systemic steroids for ocular larva migrans. Note that anthelmintic therapy alone may exacerbate ocular inflammation.

SURGERY/OTHER PROCEDURES
- Ocular larva migrans
  - Surgical intervention to prevent further damage due to chronic inflammation in quiescent disease.
  - Laser treatment for retinal detachment.

 ONGOING CARE

FOLLOW-UP RECOMMENDATIONS
Patient Monitoring
- Symptoms persist for 8 weeks, or sometimes even 1 year in untreated patients
- Those on therapy should be monitored for improvement of symptoms

PATIENT EDUCATION
- Avoid walking barefoot on beaches
- Use gloves while gardening
- Treatment of puppies and dogs with anthelmintics

PROGNOSIS
- Cutaneous: Benign, self-limited disease. Most patients recover when the larva dies.
- Visceral: Usually good prognosis. Marked organ damage or rarely death may occur.
- Ocular: Variable, loss in vision of affected eye may occur.

COMPLICATIONS
- Cutaneous larva migrans
  - Secondary bacterial infections (*Staphylococcus aureus*, Streptococci)
  - Löffler syndrome (pulmonary involvement)
  - Eosinophilic enteritis (*Ancylostoma caninum*)
- Visceral larva migrans
  - Meningitis, encephalitis
  - Myocarditis
  - Respiratory distress
- Ocular larva migrans
  - Unilateral blindness

REFERENCES

1. Won KY, Kruszon-Moran D, Schantz PM, et al. National seroprevalence and risk factors for zoonotic *Toxocara* spp. infection. *Am J Trop Med Hyg* 2008;79(4):552–557.
2. Stewart JM, Cubillan LD, Cunningham ET Jr. Prevalence, clinical features, and causes of vision loss among patients with ocular toxocariasis. *Retina* 2005;25(8):1005–1013.
3. Chang S, Lim JH, Choi D, et al. Hepatic visceral larva migrans of *Toxocara canis*: CT and sonographic findings. *AJR Am J Roentgenol* 2006;187(6):W622–W629.
4. Caumes E, Carriere J, Datry A, et al. A randomized trial of ivermectin versus albendazole for the treatment of cutaneous larva migrans. *Am J Trop Med Hyg* 1993;49(5):641–644.

ADDITIONAL READING

- Caumes E. Treatment of cutaneous larva migrans. *Clin Infect Dis* 2000;30(5):811–814.
- Heukelbach J, Feldmeier H. Epidemiological and clinical characteristics of hookworm-related cutaneous larva migrans. *Lancet Infect Dis* 2008;8(5):302–309.

CODES

ICD9
- 126.9 Ancylostomiasis and necatoriasis, unspecified
- 128.0 Toxocariasis

CLINICAL PEARLS
- The diagnosis of cutaneous larva migrans is made on clinical grounds and is supported by a relevant exposure history.
- Cutaneous larva migrans is characterized by an erythematous, serpiginous, intensely pruritic eruption.
- Young children in contact with puppy/dog litters are at highest risk for toxocariasis.
- A whitish elevated granuloma in the posterior pole of the retina is the typical finding in ocular toxocariasis. This might be confused with retinoblastoma.

LARYNGITIS/LARYNGOTRACHEOBRONCHITIS (CROUP)

Petros I. Rafailidis
Matthew E. Falagas

 BASICS

DESCRIPTION
Laryngitis
Inflammation of the mucosa of larynx.

Laryngotracheobronchitis
Inflammation of the mucosa of the subglottic area of the respiratory tract.

EPIDEMIOLOGY
Incidence
Laryngitis
- Usually occurs in association with episodes of respiratory tract infections in midwinter.

Laryngotracheobronchitis
- Parainfluenza type 1 virus causes outbreaks of infection in the fall, influenza virus types A and B and respiratory syncytial virus in the winter to early spring, and enterovirus in the summer to early fall.
- Sporadic cases are commonly associated with parainfluenza type 3 virus and less frequently with adenoviruses, rhinoviruses, and *Mycoplasma pneumoniae*.
- Croup is a relatively common infection in young children under 6 years of age.
- Most cases occur between 3 months and 3 years of age.
- In several series of cases of croup, boys predominated.

RISK FACTORS
Laryngitis
- Close quarters
- Occurs in all age groups; more frequent in children
- Smoking
- Excess alcohol consumption
- Immunosuppression
- Equal occurrence in males and females

Laryngotracheobronchitis
- Age (particularly the second year of life)
- Probably a defect in the regulation of the immune response

GENERAL PREVENTION
- Avoid contact with infected people.
- Wash your hands after contact.

PATHOPHYSIOLOGY
Parainfluenza virus infected patients have higher concentrations of interleukin-6, CX-chemokine ligands 8 and 9, as well as chemokine (C-C motif) receptors 3, 4, and 5 in nasal wash, in comparison with control patients without parainfluenza virus infection (1).

ETIOLOGY
Laryngitis
- Viral
  - Influenza virus
  - Rhinovirus
  - Adenovirus
  - Parainfluenza virus
  - Respiratory syncytial virus
  - Coxsackievirus
  - Coronavirus
- Bacterial
  - *Streptococcus pyogenes*
  - *Moraxella catarrhalis*
- Unusual causes
  - Tuberculosis
  - Syphilis
  - Diphtheria
  - Candidiasis
  - Histoplasmosis
  - Blastomycosis

Laryngotracheobronchitis
- Several viruses may cause croup.
- Parainfluenza viruses are the major causative agents for all ages (most common, type 1; second most common, type 3; and least common, type 2)
- Influenza viruses are important causes in children >5 years of age.
- Respiratory syncytial virus is a frequent cause in the first few months of life.
- Adenoviruses, rhinoviruses, and enterovirus are less frequent causes.
- *M. pneumoniae* may cause croup, mainly in older ages.

 DIAGNOSIS

HISTORY
Acute upper respiratory tract infection.

PHYSICAL EXAM
Laryngitis
- Hoarseness
- Lowering of the normal pitch of voice; occasionally aphonia
- Stridor if airway obstruction occurs
- Examination of the larynx reveals hyperemia, edema, and vascular injection of the vocal cords, and there may be mucosal ulcerations.

Laryngotracheobronchitis
- Fever (range, 38°C–40°C) precedes usually the other symptoms and signs and abates as they become established
- Hoarseness
- A "sears bark" cough (deepening, not productive, with a striking brassy tone)

- Inspiratory stridor
- Tachypnea
- Often, retractions of the chest wall, usually in the supraclavicular and suprasternal areas and tracheal tug.
- In more severe cases, there is stridor on expiration and marked tachypnea and, in auscultation, rales, rhonchi, wheezing, or diminished breath sounds. Pulsus paradoxus and marked tachycardia may be present (2).

DIAGNOSTIC TESTS & INTERPRETATION
Lab
Initial lab tests
- Diagnosis is clinical.
- WBC and differential counts are normal.
- In severe cases, hypoxemia is usually present without or with hypercapnia.

Follow-Up & Special Considerations
For etiologic diagnosis, special serologic or other tests may be used, although they do not have any practical value.

Imaging
Helpful is the anterior–posterior neck x-ray, which shows the characteristic subglottic swelling, the "hourglass" or "steeple" sign.

DIFFERENTIAL DIAGNOSIS
The syndrome of acute viral laryngitis should be distinguished from the following:
- Bacterial laryngitis
- A rare cause of laryngitis, such as tuberculosis, syphilis, diphtheria, or fungal infections
- Acute epiglottitis
- Acute laryngotracheobronchitis
- Traumatic aphonia
- Tumors and other noninfectious chronic diseases of the larynx (laryngoscopic examination should be done if hoarseness persists longer than 10–14 days)
- Acute epiglottitis: The course is much more rapidly progressive, the patient appears to be more toxic, and there is no history of previous upper respiratory illness. The characteristic cough of croup is absent, and the patient has dysphonia and dysphagia. In croup, the anterior–posterior neck x-ray shows the characteristic subglottic swelling, and, in epiglottitis, the lateral neck x-ray shows an enlarged epiglottis (the thumb sign) and normal subglottic structures.
- Foreign-body aspiration: History is helpful.
- Allergic reaction: History, other signs of allergy, and no symptoms of infection are helpful.
- Anatomic airway obstruction: Children with a long-standing history of stridor or those (under 3 months of age) with "croup" should be carefully evaluated for anatomic airway obstruction.
- Bacterial tracheitis: Dramatic clinical picture with high fever, toxic appearance, stridor, dyspnea, and cough with purulent sputum. It is caused by *S. aureus*, group A β-hemolytic streptococci, and *H. influenzae* type B. The lateral soft-tissue x-ray reveals a normal epiglottis with subglottic narrowing.

TREATMENT

MEDICATION

First Line

Laryngitis
- The outpatient health care setting is appropriate.
- Hospitalization is necessary when airway obstruction occurs.
- General measures
  – Inhalation of moistened air
  – Medications are not indicated unless bacterial laryngitis is established.

Laryngotracheobronchitis
- In mild to moderate cases, nebulized budesonide (where available) or dexamethasone (oral or intramuscular) in a dose of 0.15–0.6 mg/kg results in acute clinical improvement in outpatients, reducing the need for hospitalization (3,4[A]). Nebulized racemic epinephrine 2.25% (0.5 mL in 2.5 mL of normal saline) or nebulized L-epinephrine (4–5 mL of an undiluted 1:1000 solution) provides temporary clinical improvement to many children with marked stridor, but such patients should be observed for at least 4 hours because of the possibility of rebound edema and dyspnea (5[A]). Children requiring two epinephrine treatments should be hospitalized.
- In moderately severe or severe croup, corticosteroid therapy (0.3–0.6 mg/kg dexamethasone or its equivalent every 6 hours for 2–4 doses) may result in significant clinical improvement and decrease the need for intubation.
- Children with hypoxemia (without hypercapnia) respond to low concentrations of supplemental oxygen. If hypercapnia occurs, mechanical ventilation should be considered. Nasotracheal intubation is the preferred method.

Second Line
- Antihistamines, decongestants, and antibiotics have no proven efficacy in uncomplicated viral croup.
- Despite the extensive use of humidified air and mist, these do not seem to be effective (6[A]).

ADDITIONAL TREATMENT

General Measures

Allow the child to resume the posture that provides comfort for respiration.

Additional Therapies

Heliox treatment is of potential benefit to patients with severe croup (7[A]).

IN-PATIENT CONSIDERATIONS

Admission Criteria
- Nonresponse to a corticosteroid dose and 2 doses of epinephrine
- Hypercapnia or hypoxemia
- Agitation, confusion, or lethargy
- Marked signs of cardiorespiratory exhaustion

 ONGOING CARE

FOLLOW-UP RECOMMENDATIONS
- High fever, significant shortness of breath, and a large amount of respiratory tract secretions may suggest bacterial tracheitis. In this case, antibiotics are needed.
- The diseases are usually self-limited, with a fluctuating course.
- They last about 3–4 days, although cough may persist for a longer period.
- Some children have repeated episodes of croup; allergic diathesis or hyperreactivity of the airway may contribute.

PATIENT MONITORING

Oxygen saturation is mandatory in moderate to severe cases.

PATIENT EDUCATION

Educate the parents when to return to hospital in case of recurrence, that is, stridor, changes in mental state, difficulty in breathing or talking or eating, and cyanosis.

PROGNOSIS

Generally very good. However, some children will necessitate mechanical ventilation. Mortality is extremely rare.

COMPLICATIONS

Laryngitis
- Airway obstruction

Laryngotracheobronchitis
- Acute complications
  – Airway obstruction leading to acute respiratory failure, often necessitating mechanical ventilation
  – Pneumothorax
  – Noncardiac pulmonary edema
  – Aspiration pneumonia
  – Spontaneous pneumomediastinum
  – Long-term complications (usually after severe croup early in life)
  – Increased frequency of hyperreactivity of the airway
  – Probable altered pulmonary function
  – Occasional occurrence of subglottic stenosis after intubation

REFERENCES

1. El Feghaly RE, McGann L, Bonville CA, et al. Local production of inflammatory mediators during childhood parainfluenza virus infection. *Pediatr Infect Dis J* 2010;29:e26–e31.
2. Steele DW, Santucci KA, Wright RO, et al. Pulsus paradoxus: An objective measure of severity in croup. *Am J Respir Crit Care Med* 1998;157: 331–334.
3. Dobrovoljac M, Geelhoed GC. 27 years of croup: An update highlighting the effectiveness of 0.15 mg/kg of dexamethasone. *Emerg Med Australas* 2009;21:309–314.
4. Klassen TP, Craig WR, Moher D, et al. Nebulized budesonide and oral dexamethasone for treatment of croup: A randomized controlled trial. *JAMA* 1998;279:1629–1632.
5. Kristjanson S, Berg-Kelly K, Winso E. Inhalation of racemic adrenaline in the treatment of mild and moderately severe croup. Clinical symptom score and oxygen saturation measurements for evaluation of treatment effects. *Acta Paediatr* 1994;83:1156–1160.
6. Scolnik D, Coates AL, Stephens D, et al. Controlled delivery of high vs low humidity vs mist therapy for croup in emergency departments: A randomized controlled trial. *JAMA* 2006;295:1274–1280.
7. Weber JE, Chudnofsky CR, Younger JG, et al. A randomized comparison of helium-oxygen mixture (Heliox) and racemic epinephrine for the treatment of moderate to severe croup. *Pediatrics* 2001; 107:E96.

ADDITIONAL READING

- Bjornson CL, Johnson DW. Croup. *Lancet* 2008;371: 329–339.

 CODES

ICD9
- 464.00 Acute laryngitis without mention of obstruction
- 490 Bronchitis, not specified as acute or chronic

CLINICAL PEARLS
- Don't underestimate mild cases. Steroids are of value even in these cases.
- If there is stridor or chest wall retractions at presentation, don't discharge the patient until 4 hours have elapsed.
- When the child is exhausted there may be no stridor and the heart rate may start falling.

L

LEGIONNAIRES DISEASE
Erica S. Shenoy (E. Mylonakis, Editor)

 BASICS

DESCRIPTION
- Legionnaires' disease (LD) refers to pneumonia caused by gram-negative bacteria of the *Legionellaceae* family.
- LD was discovered in 1976 in Philadelphia when 182 members of the American Legion, attending an annual convention developed pneumonia thought to be spread by the hotel's contaminated air conditioning system. The bacteria isolated from lung tissue samples were named *L. pneumophila*.
- Pontiac fever is an acute, febrile, self-limited illness that has been serologically linked to the *Legionella* species.
- Together, LD and Pontiac fever are considered to be Legionellosis.

EPIDEMIOLOGY
- The annual incidence of Legionnaire's diseases is estimated to be 8,000–18,000 cases per year, though only 5–10% of cases are reported.
- Legionella pneumonia accounts for between 1–9% of patients hospitalized for community acquired pneumonia (CAP).
- Since 2003, an increase in the number of cases reported, especially along the East Coast of the US. It is not clear if this reflects an actual increase in the number of cases or changes in detection or reporting methods. In addition to an absolute increase in the number of cases reported, there was shift to a younger population with more reported cases in individuals aged 45–64 years than those over 65 years of age.
- Outbreaks of Legionnaires disease in hotels, cruise ships, spas, hospitals, nursing homes, decorative fountains, office buildings, and sporadic clusters of nosocomial cases have been reported.

RISK FACTORS
Older age, cigarette smoking, chronic lung disease, immunosuppression (i.e., malignancy, HIV, immunosuppressive medications), surgery (i.e., transplant), renal or hepatic disease, diabetes are risk factors. Additionally, recent travel,exposure to whirlpool spas, and recent water or soil exposure are all risk factors.

GENERAL PREVENTION
The Centers for Disease Control and Prevention (CDC) have published guidelines on the prevention of transmission through careful planning of water supplies, maintenance of these supplies, and appropriate investigations in the case of Legionella transmission.

PATHOPHYSIOLOGY
- Legionella is an aerobic, gram-negative organism that requires buffered charcoal yeast extract (BCYE) agar for isolation. It is an obligate or facultative intracellular parasite that is able to infect and replicate within protozoa. It is found in aquatic bodies in nature in small amounts but once it contaminates aquatic reservoirs such as water distribution systems, cooling towers, whirlpools, and air conditioning systems, it can proliferate.
- Transmission occurs by inhalation of contaminated water for the most part in the summer months when air-conditioning systems are used frequently.
- Once inhaled, the bacteria infect and replicate within alveolar macrophages and monocytes. The host response is mediated by activated T cells that stimulate the activity of macrophages.

ETIOLOGY
- Although 42 different Legionella species and 64 serogroups have been identified, less than half of these species have been linked to disease in humans. *Legionella pneumophila* is the most pathogenic, accounting for 90% of the cases of legionellosis, followed by *Legionella micdadei*.
- Serogroup 1 accounts for 80% of the reported cases of legionellosis caused by *L. pneumophila*.

DIAGNOSIS

HISTORY
- Patients with LD may present with fever (>40 C/100.4F), malaise, myalgias, anorexia, and headache. Initially, they may have a dry cough which subsequently may become more productive. Pleuritic or non-pleuritic chest pain may be present. Gastrointestinal symptoms, including nausea, vomiting, abdominal pain, and watery, non-bloody diarrhea are common. Symptoms may progress to mental status changes, encephalopathy, stupor, respiratory failure, and multiorgan system failure.
- The incubation period is 2–10 days. If a patient has been hospitalized for 10 days or more and develops LD, this is considered definite nosocomial LD. LD that develops 2–9 days after admission should be considered a possible case of nosocomial disease.
- A diagnostic algorithm based on clinical features and laboratory tests has been developed which allows for designation of likelihood of LD as very likely, likely, or unlikely.

- Extrapulmonary legionellosis is rare, but the clinical manifestations are often dramatic. The most common site is the heart, with numerous reports of myocarditis, pericarditis, postcardiotomy syndrome, and prosthetic valve endocarditis. Legionella spp. have been implicated in cases of sinusitis, cellulitis, pancreatitis, peritonitis, hip-wound infection, and pyelonephritis.
- Pontiac fever is a self-limiting, illness with a 24- to 48-hour incubation period. Malaise, fatigue, and myalgias are the most frequent symptoms. Fever develops in 80–90% of cases, and headache in 80%. Other symptoms include arthralgias, nausea, cough, abdominal pain, and diarrhea.

PHYSICAL EXAM
May reveal fever, hypotension, relative bradycardia, tachypnea, changes in mental status, rales or evidence of consolidation on pulmonary exam, pancreatitis, peritonitis, and acute renal failure.

DIAGNOSTIC TESTS & INTERPRETATION
Lab
- May reveal hyponatremia (secondary to SIADH), hypophosphatemia, elevated liver enzymes, increased CPK, increased CRP, microscopic hematuria, and proteinuria.
- Gram stain and culture of respiratory secretions, including sputum, lung fluid or pleural fluid, should be obtained. This should be plated on BCYE agar at 35–37°C. Cultures may take 5 days to produce colonies. Sputum cultures have a sensitivity of 80% and specificity of 100%. Direct fluorescent antibody (DFA) of sputum has decreased sensitivity and becomes negative within 4 days of the onset of illness.
- Blood cultures should be obtained prior to initiation of antibiotics.
- Serological tests are most commonly used. Because they take several weeks to demonstrate a change in titer, they are not useful clinically. Of note, 1–16% of healthy adults may have a positive titre.
- In Pontiac fever, modest leukocytosis with a neutrophilic predominance is sometimes detected. The diagnosis is established by antibody seroconversion.
- The urinary antigen test is positive in 80% of patients on days 1–3 of illness, though it can remain positive for months after acute illness. It detects only the serogroup 1 of *L. pneumophila*. Patients requiring admission to an ICU, patients who have experienced failure of antimicrobial therapy, and those with history of recent travel, active alcohol abuse, and pleural effusion should be tested with the urinary antigen assay.
- Polymerase chain reaction (PCR) of urine, serum, and bronchial alveolar lavage (BAL) fluid is specific but not sensitive.

Imaging
Initial approach
Chest x-ray almost always demonstrates abnormalities, including patchy infiltrates or consolidations. Findings are usually unilateral and found in the lower lobes. Up to one-third of patients may have pleural effusions.

Follow-Up & Special Considerations
Resolution of chest x-ray abnormalities may take months.

Diagnostic Procedures/Other
Diagnostic/therapeutic thoracentesis may be indicated in patients with pleural effusions.

DIFFERENTIAL DIAGNOSIS
- Atypical pneumonia including those caused by:
  - *Chlamydia pneumonia*
  - *Chlamydia psittaci*
  - *Mycoplasma pneumonia*
  - *Coxiella burnetii*
  - Tularemia
  - Viruses

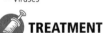 TREATMENT

MEDICATION
- Current recommendations for first line antimicrobial therapy include quinolones and azithromycin. doxycycline and other macrolides. Erythromycin had been the drug of choice in the past, but this is no longer the case.
- Fluoroquinolones are recommended in severe disease.
- Parenteral therapy should be instituted until there is an objective clinical response; most patients become afebrile within 3 days; then, oral therapy can be substituted. The total duration of therapy is 10–14 days, but a 21-day course has been recommended for immunosuppressed patients or for those with extensive evidence of disease on chest radiographs.

ADDITIONAL TREATMENT
General Measures
Detailed history should be obtained to determine whether or not the index case is part of an outbreak.

Issues for Referral
Infectious disease consultation is recommended.

IN-PATIENT CONSIDERATIONS
Admission Criteria
Most patients require admission for parenteral antibiotic therapy.

 ONGOING CARE

FOLLOW-UP RECOMMENDATIONS
- Patients should complete the entire course of antibiotics and should be monitored closely for evidence of recovery.
- Cases of LD should be reported to the state health department and the CDC.

Patient Monitoring
Patients should be monitored in the hospital during the transition from parenteral to oral therapy to ensure continued improvement, and then post-hospitalization to document complete recovery.

PROGNOSIS
The mortality rate for LD ranges from 5–30% and depends in large part on patient comorbidities.

COMPLICATIONS
- Respiratory failure.
- Multiorgan system failure.
- Extrapulmonary manifestations—almost always in immunocompromised patients and include myocarditis, pericarditis, prosthetic valve endocarditis, pancreatitis, peritonitis, acute renal failure.
- Death.

ADDITIONAL READING
- Edelstein PH, Cianciotto NP. "Legionella". In: Mandell GL, Douglas RG, and Bennett JE eds. *Principles and Practice of Infectious Diseases*, 7th Edition. Philadelphia: Churchill Livingstone, 2009;2969–2984.
- Smeeks FC. Legionnaires Disease in Emergency Medicine. *eMedicine*. http://emedicine.medscape.com/article/783656-overview. Accessed March 31, 2011.
- Cunha BA, Sullivan LE. Legionnaires Disease. *eMedicine*. http://emedicine.medscape.com/article/220163-overview. Accessed February 5, 2008.
- BA Cunha. Severe Legionella pneumonia: Rapid diagnosis with Winthrop-University Hospital's weighted point-score system (modified). *Heart Lung* 2008;37:312–321.
- Neil K, Berkelman R. Increasing incidence of legionellosis in the United States, 1990–2005: changing epidemiologic trends. *Clin Inf Dis* 2008;47:591–599.
- Sehulster L, Chinn RYW. Guidelines for environmental infection control in health-care facilities. *MMWR Recomm Rep* 2003;52:1–42.

- Edelstein PH. Antimicrobial chemotherapy for legionnaires' disease: Time for a change. *Ann Intern Med* 1998;129:328–330.
- Lieberman D, Porath A, Schlaeffer F, et al. Legionella species community-acquired pneumonia. A review of 56 hospitalized adult patients. *Chest* 1996;109:1243–1249.
- Mulazimoglu L, Yu VL. Legionella infection. In: Fauci AS, Braunwald E, Isselbacher KJ, et al., eds. *Harrison's principles of internal medicine*, 14th ed. New York: McGraw-Hill, 1998:928–933.
- Sopena N, Sabria-Leal M, Pedro-Botet ML, et al. Comparative study of the clinical presentation of Legionella pneumonia and other community-acquired pneumonias. *Chest* 1998;113:1195–1200.
- Stout JE, Yu VL. Legionellosis. *N Engl J Med* 1997;337:682–687.
- Sehulster L, Chinn RYW. Guidelines for Environmental Infection Control in Health-Care Facilities: Recommendations of the CDC and Healthcare Infection Control Practices Advisory Committee (HICPAC). *MMWR* 2003;52:1–42.
- Mandell LA, et al. Infectious Diseases Society of America/Thoracic Society consensus guidelines on the management of community-acquired pneumonia in adults. *Clin Inf Diseases* 2007;44:S27–S72.

 See Also

- CDC Legionellosis Case Report Form: http://www.cdc.gov/legionella/files/legionella_case_report.pdf

CODES

ICD9
482.84 Legionnaires' disease

CLINICAL PEARLS

- LD disease should be considered in patients with both CAP and hospital-acquired pneumonia occurring after 10 days of admission and in those with epidemiologic and clinical risk factors.
- Most patients with LD will require admission.
- LD is a reportable disease.

L

LEISHMANIASIS

Michael K. Mansour (E. Mylonakis, Editor)

 BASICS

DESCRIPTION

- Leishmaniasis is a disease caused by the protozoa *Leishmania* and transmitted by the sandfly vector.
- Clinically, leishmaniasis is divided into cutaneous, mucosal, and visceral syndromes.
- There is a controversy considering the taxonomy of *Leishmania*. Taxonomy is being continuously updated.
- There are over 20 species of Leishmanial species, which are divided into 2 groups, New (South America) and Old world (Africa, Middle East).
- Clinical presentations can be varied depending on each individual's immune response.

EPIDEMIOLOGY

- *Leishmania* infections are among the most common parasitic diseases, with about 12 million infected persons and 2 million new infections every year.
- Approximately over 350 million people worldwide are at risk of being infected by *Leishmania* spp.
- Visceral leishmaniasis involves the species *L. infantum* and *L. donovani* in South America as well as near the Ganges river in the eastern India, southern Nepal, Bangladesh, and the Sudan.
- Visceral leishmaniasis predilects immunocompromised people, especially AIDS patients as an opportunistic infection.
- The majority of cutaneous leishmaniasis exist in the Middle East (Iran, Saudi Arabia, and Syria), in Central Asia (mainly in Afghanistan), and in Brazil and Peru from Latin America.
- Most mucosal leishmaniasis cases are found in Latin America, specifically Bolivia, Brazil, and Peru.
- There is high prevalence of cutaneous leishmaniasis among American soldiers serving in Iraq or Afghanistan.
- In Europe, infections with *L. major* or *L. tropica* are increasingly encountered due to travel and immigration.
- Besides sand flies, rarer routes of transmission are blood transfusions, sexual intercourse, organ transplantation, IVDU, and congenital routes.

GENERAL PREVENTION

Insect repellents and bed nets may provide protection to sand flies.

ETIOLOGY

- *Leishmania* spp. have a dimorphic life cycle. In most areas, the *Leishmania* spp. are inoculated when the sandfly vector attempts to feed.
- Promastigotes, which exist within the female sandfly's digestive tract, are injected into the skin where they are phagocytosed by macrophages and transformed to amastigotes.
- The parasite is not sexually reproduced.
- *Leishmania* spp. predilects the cells of reticuloendothelial system.
- Endogenous parasite factors (invasiveness, tropism, and pathogenicity) and the patient's cell-mediated immune status determine the manifestations of the disease.
- An oligoparasitic infection with intact immunity may present as a mild mucosal leishmaniasis. A high parasite-burden infection with distorted immunity may lead to diffuse cutaneous leishmaniasis. The main agents of New-world cutaneous leishmaniasis include *L. braziliensis* and *L. Mexicana*. Old world agents include *L. tropica*, *L. infantum*, and *L. major*.
- The incubation period of visceral leishmaniasis varies and depends on the type of the infection, but it can be up to 8 months to years. The incubation period of cutaneous leishmaniasis varies from a few weeks to several months or, in some cases, up to years.
- Visceral leishmaniasis is usually caused by *L. donovani* (New World) and *L. infantum* (Old World, common in the Mediterranean), and are clinically indistinguishable (unlike cutaneous Leishmaniasis).
- Malnutrition, genetic background, and cachexia are well-established risk factors for visceral leishmaniasis.
- Kala-azar is a most concerning form of visceral leishmaniasis with marked hepatosplenomegaly as high numbers of parasitic organisms replicate in the reticuloendothelial system.

 DIAGNOSIS

- Old World cutaneous leishmaniasis is a local lesion that starts as a papule at the site where promastigotes are inoculated. The papule gradually increases in size, becomes crusted, and finally ulcerates. The ulcer is usually shallow and circular with well-defined, raised, erythematous borders and a bed of granulation tissue. It gradually increases in size and may reach a diameter of 2 cm or more.
- A wide variety of skin manifestations, ranging from small, dry, crusted lesions to large, deep, mutilating ulcers, are seen in American cutaneous leishmaniasis. In localized cutaneous disease, the initial lesion usually appears 1–8 weeks after the sandfly bite. The ulcer may persist for months to years.
- Mucosal leishmaniasis commonly due to *L. braziliensis* may affect the nose, the oral cavity, the pharynx, and the larynx.
- Nasal septum and soft palate perforation are common clinical findings.
- Voice change should lead to a thorough larynx examination.
- Fever, weight loss, weakness, splenomegaly, hepatomegaly, cytopenia, and hypergammaglobulinemia are findings that altogether raise the sensitivity for diagnosing visceral leishmaniasis in an endemic area.
- Clinical features of Kala-azar include fever, weight loss, wasting, edema, hypoalbuminemia, and anemia as the marrow is progressively infiltrated.
- "Acute kala-azar" is characterized by the abrupt onset of fever and rigors as early as 2 weeks after infection.
- Kala-azar has been noted to cause spontaneous abortions when occurring in pregnancy.
- Kala-azar carries a high fatality rate without treatment.

DIAGNOSTIC TESTS & INTERPRETATION
Lab
- Anemia, leukopenia, eosinopenia, and hypergammaglobulinemia are present in persons with visceral leishmaniasis.
- A definitive diagnosis depends on the demonstration of amastigotes in tissue or isolation of the organism in culture.
- Cultures of bone marrow, liver, spleen, lymph node, and, in some cases, blood may reveal the parasite in the promastigotic stage. Specimens can be inoculated into Novy- McNeal-Nicolle (NNN) medium.
- Splenic and hepatic aspiration has some of the highest sensitivity for detecting the protozoa but carries a high risk of internal hemorrhage.
- Bone marrow aspiration (Wright- and Giemsa-stained smears) is the most common diagnostic procedure for the diagnosis of visceral leishmaniasis.
- PCR of aspirated material or blood may define also the *Leishmania* spp.
- Smears, scrapings, aspirates, or punch biopsies from a cutaneous lesion may be sent for culture or PCR.
- Enzyme-linked immunosorbent assay (ELISA) and the indirect immunofluorescent antibody assay are positive in a patient with visceral leishmaniasis and intact immunity.
- Serology in cutaneous or mucosal involvement is typically negative.
- The leishmanin skin test (Montenegro) is useful only in epidemiologic studies in case of visceral leishmaniasis but is a high yield test for cutaneous and mucosal leishmaniasis.
- A urinary leishmanial antigen test is available but has a poor sensitivity of <70%.

DIFFERENTIAL DIAGNOSIS
- The differential diagnosis of cutaneous leishmaniasis includes the following:
  - Fungal infections
  - Lupus vulgaris (skin tuberculosis)
  - Mycobacterial infections of the skin (due to atypical mycobacteria, tuberculosis, or leprosy)
  - Neoplasms
  - Syphilis
  - Sporothrix
- Visceral leishmaniasis can present as organomegaly, fever of unclear etiology, or unexplained chronic anemia, or can mimic other infectious diseases (malaria, typhoid fever, brucellosis, histoplasmosis), or lymphoma.

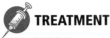

TREATMENT
MEDICATION
- Mainstay of therapy has been amphotericin, pentamidine, and pentavalent antimonial compounds, although resistance has been noted.
- Depending on the clinical scenario and region of the world, different regimens are used.
- Liposomal amphotericin B is the first choice treatment for visceral leishmaniasis.
- Pentavalent antimony has an unclear mechanism of action. It is available in 2 forms, sodium antimonylgluconate, and N-methylglucamine antimonate.
- Addition of pentoxifylline to antimony agents has been shown to increase cure rates of cutaneous leishmaniasis.
- Liposomal AmBisome is considered safe in case of pregnancy. Antimony compounds are contraindicated due to spontaneous abortion.
- Miltefosine is a new oral drug originally marked as a cancer therapeutic now showing good results for the treatment of visceral and cutaneous leishmaniasis.
- Most cutaneous lesions heal spontaneously.
- Intralesional treatment has been tested in some cases with positive response.
- Alternative treatments for cutaneous leishmaniasis include cryotherapy, thermotherapy, paromomycin, imiquimod, and oral azoles.
- Antimony is the treatment of choice for mucosal leishmaniasis, but new data is building in support for oral miltefosine.

ADDITIONAL TREATMENT
General Measures
Treatment Failure
- Diffuse cutaneous leishmaniasis is a difficult medical disorder in which treatment failure is common.
- The immunocompromised and especially the AIDS patients present frequently with relapses.

ONGOING CARE
FOLLOW-UP RECOMMENDATIONS
- The response to treatment is rapid.
- The spleen may return to its normal size in a few weeks.
- Post-kala-azar dermal leishmaniasis is a macular rash that may resemble leprosy following leishmanial treatment but has no sensorineural manifestations.

COMPLICATIONS
- Mucosal leishmaniasis due to *L. braziliensis* is the only form of American cutaneous leishmaniasis that carries a significant mortality.
- Side effects of pentavalent antimonials include:
  - Arthralgias
  - Gastrointestinal symptoms
  - Electrocardiographic changes
  - Headache
  - Pancreatitis

ADDITIONAL READING
- Banuls AL, Hide M, Prugnolle F. Leishmania and the leishmaniases: A parasite genetic update and advances in taxonomy, epidemiology and pathogenicity in humans. *Adv Parasitol* 2007;64: 1–109.

CODES

ICD9
- 085.0 Leishmaniasis visceral (kala-azar)
- 085.5 Mucocutaneous leishmaniasis, (american)
- 085.9 Leishmaniasis, unspecified

CLINICAL PEARLS
- Leishmaniasis is a common protozoal infection worldwide with a varied clinical presentation depending on the individual's immune response.
- Each clinical manifestation carries a specific morbidity and mortality, with visceral patient's leishmaniasis being the most severe.
- There are mainly treatment options that need to be tailored to the patient and the epidemiology of that region of the world.

L

LEPROSY

Emily P. Hyle (E. Mylonakis, Editor)

 BASICS

DESCRIPTION
Infection caused by *Mycobacterium leprae*.

EPIDEMIOLOGY (1)

Incidence
- 249,000 new cases reported in 2008.
- Incidence was reduced by 4% when compared to 2007.

Prevalence
- 213, 036 active cases as reported from 121 countries.
- A marked decrease in cases from 5.2 million cases in 1985.
- 14 million cases cured in the past 20 years.

RISK FACTORS
- Close contacts
- Age: 5–15 years and >30 years.
- Immunocompromise: Especially with impaired cell-mediated immunity.
- Regions of endemicity (83% of cases): Brazil, India, Myanmar, Nepal, Indonesia, Madagascar. Also endemic in central Africa (1).

Genetics (2)
- Tuberculoid leprosy has been linked to HLA-DR3; lepromatous leprosy to HLA-DQ1.
- Susceptibility appears to be linked to non-MHC-linked loci, including NOD2-mediated regulation of innate immunity.

GENERAL PREVENTION
Efforts at global eradication are ongoing.

PATHOPHYSIOLOGY
- Average incubation time is 5–7 years.
- Likely respiratory transmission by close contact with untreated patients; also by direct contact with skin lesions (2).
- Tropism for Schwann cell of peripheral nerves, and infection triggers cellular immune response, which determines disease progression and classification.

ETIOLOGY
- *Mycobacterium leprae*, an acid-fast obligate intracellular organism that grows very slowly and at cooler temperatures (27–33°C).
- Cannot be cultured on media; animal model is the armadillo.

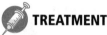 **DIAGNOSIS**

HISTORY
- Sensory loss in the setting of skin lesions.
- Less common subtype of purely neural disease without skin lesions (5–10%, especially Nepal and Indian).
- WHO Classification into paucibacillary (PB) with ≤5 smear-negative lesions versus multibacillary (MB) with >5 lesions that can be smear-positive.
- Ridley-Jopling classification system: Range from Tuberculoid (less smear-positive disease) to lepromatous (high smear-positive disease).
- Vision, respiratory tract, and testes can be affected in severe disease.

PHYSICAL EXAM
- Skin lesions: Range from small hypopigmented or erythematous lesions (tuberculoid) to mixed erythematous or scaly macules, papules, or nodules (lepromatous).
- Enlarged, thickened peripheral nerves, especially in tuberculoid disease.
- Peripheral nerve loss can be motor or sensory or both.
- In localized disease (tuberculoid), nerve changes occur in distribution of skin lesions, whereas lepromatous disease can be more diffuse.
- Can result in anesthetic skin patches.
- Advanced lepromatous disease can result in saddle nose deformity (collapse of cartilage), loss of hair (on skin, eyebrows), and hoarseness (laryngeal nerve).

DIAGNOSTIC TESTS & INTERPRETATION

Lab

Initial lab tests
As baseline for antimicrobial use.

Follow-Up & Special Considerations
LFTs and CBC as indicated for use of rifampin.

Diagnostic Procedures/Other
- Remains a clinical diagnosis.
- Skin smear: If obtained, take entire sample from within the lesion.

Pathological Findings
- Tuberculoid: Granuloma with rare bacilli.
- Lepromatous: Foamy histiocytes with abundant bacilli.

DIFFERENTIAL DIAGNOSIS
- Syphilis
- Cutaneous T-cell lymphoma
- Sarcoidosis
- Dermal lupus

TREATMENT

MEDICATION (3)

First Line
- Multidrug therapy for multibacillary disease: Dapsone 100 mg PO daily
  - Rifampin 600 mg PO daily (US) or monthly (WHO)
  - Clofazimine 50 mg PO daily
- In US, MDT is for 2 years, whereas WHO recommends 1 year.
- Two-drug therapy for paucibacillary disease: Rifampin 600 mg PO monthly
  - Dapsone 100 mg PO daily
  - × 6 months
- Some choose to continue daily dapsone after completion of treatment to prevent relapse.

Second Line
- Quinolones (Levofloxacin, Moxifloxacin, Ofloxacin)
- Macrolides: Only Clarithromycin
- Tetracyclines: Only Minocycline

Pregnancy Considerations
- Concern for type I and II reactions with clinical worsening.
- Avoid Class C, D, or X antibiotics in treatment regimens.

ADDITIONAL TREATMENT
General Measures
Issues for Referral
In the US, for initiation of therapy and access to clofazimine.

Additional Therapies
- Consideration of IFN-G therapy: Intent to trigger change to TH1 response that would prompt tuberculoid form; still experimental at this time.
- Bacillus Calmette-Guerin (BCG) revaccination has shown ~50% protection with higher rates.

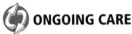 ONGOING CARE

FOLLOW-UP RECOMMENDATIONS
- Pregnant women are most at risk for both Type I and II complications and should be monitored carefully.
- If concern for drug-resistance, mouse foot-pad model can be used to assess for *rpoB* (rifampin resistance) or *folP1* (dapsone resistance).

PATIENT MONITORING
- Antibiotic regimens include supervised therapy.
- Skin and foot care, especially for anesthetic areas.
- Close clinical follow-up, especially for those with baseline neural dysfunction and during early therapy given the potential for immune-mediated reactions and paradoxical worsening with antimicrobial therapy.

PATIENT EDUCATION
- Infants can be infected, especially by mothers in lepromatous or borderline stage.
- Studies of prophylaxis of close-contacts are ongoing; single-dose rifampin has been shown to reduce new infection for at least 2 years.
- Rifampin will have multiple drug–drug interactions.
- Clofazimine will result in bluish-tint to skin but will improve after medication is discontinued.

PROGNOSIS
- Excellent with treatment.
- Concern that misclassification will lead to undertreatment, given the limited correlation between WHO and Ridley-Jopling classification.
- Relapse is associated with high bacillary burden initially and can occur 5–10 years after treatment.

COMPLICATIONS (2) and (4)
- Type I reaction: Also known as "reversal." When treatment prompts lepromatous disease to revert to tuberculoid, it can provoke a delayed hypersensitivity reaction associated with worsened peripheral nerve loss and exacerbation of skin lesions. Especially common among patients with borderline disease.
- Severe Type I reactions should be treated with prednisolone × 3–6 months to reduce long-standing nerve damage (TRIPOD trial). Cyclosporine is a second-line agent.
- Type II reaction (erythema nodosum leprosum): Occurs more often in lepromar borderline lepromatous disease and is likely due to immune complex deposition. Clinically, presents with evidence of inflammation (e.g., fevers and erythematous, tender nodular lesions, neuritis, iritis).
- Severe Type II reactions can be treated with prednisone, clofazimine, or thalidomide.

REFERENCES
1. http://www.who.int/mediacentre/factsheets/fs101/en/.
2. Walsh DS, Protaels F, Meyers WM. Recent advances in leprosy and Buruli ulcer (*Mycobacterium ulcerans* infection). *Curr Opin Infect Dis* 2010;23(5):445–55.
3. World Health Organization (WHO). WHO Expert Committee on Leprosy: 7th report. WHO Technical Report Series, no. 874. Geneva: World Health Organization, 1998.
4. Ustianowski AP, Lockwood DNJ. Leprosy: Current. diagnostic and treatment approaches. *Curr Opin Infect Dis* 2003;16:421–427.

ADDITIONAL READING
- Moet FJ, Pahan D, Oskam L, et al. Effectiveness of single dose rifampicin in preventing leprosy in close contacts of patients with newly diagnosed leprosy: Cluster randomized controlled trial. *Br Med J* 2008; 336:761–764.
- National Hansen's Disease Programs Center (Baton Rouge, LA). 800/642–2477.
- Pardillo FEF, Fajardo TT, Abalos RM, et al. Methods for the classification of leprosy for treatment purposes. *CID* 2007;44:1096–1099.
- Moet FJ, Pahan D, Schuring RP, et al. Physical distance, genetic relationship, age, and leprosy classification are independent risk factors for leprosy in contacts of patients with leprosy. *J Infect Dis* 2006;193(3):346–353.

 CODES

ICD10
- 030.0

ICD9
- 030.0 Lepromatous leprosy (type l)
- 030.1 Tuberculoid leprosy (type t)
- 030.9 Leprosy, unspecified

CLINICAL PEARLS
- Common nerve findings include claw hand (median nerve), foot drop (common peroneal nerve) and claw toes (posterior tibial nerve), as well as facial nerve.
- Classification is essential to determine treatment regimen and duration.

L

LEPTOSPIROSIS

Constantinos Sgouros
Petros I. Rafailidis
Matthew E. Falagas

 BASICS

DESCRIPTION
An infectious zoonotic disease caused by pathogenic leptospire

EPIDEMIOLOGY
Incidence
- Leptospirosis is a worldwide infection and the incidence is higher than usually suspected (1).
- Most infections are asymptomatic.
- Leptospirosis is an underdiagnosed cause of encephalitis and aseptic meningitis worldwide.
- Serologic evidence for leptospirosis is found in about 10% of cases of meningitis and encephalitis with unclear etiology.
- Leptospirosis is more common in males than females due to epidemiologic reasons related to occupation and preference of recreational activities.

Prevalence
- In the United Kingdom and Oceania, *L. interrogans* serovar hardjo seems to be the most common cause of leptospirosis among individuals in close contact with infected livestock.
- In the US, *L. interrogans* serovars icterohaemorrhagiae (rats), canicola (dogs), autumnalis, australis, bratislava, Pomona (cattle and swine), and hebdomidis are the most common causes of leptospirosis.

RISK FACTORS
- The main mode of transmission of leptospirosis is through contact of the abraded skin or of mucous membranes with water, vegetation, or soil contaminated with urine of infected animals, but, also food and drink consumption.
- Farmers
- Abattoir workers
- Miners
- Sewer workers
- Veterinarians
- Military troops
- Bathers
- Campers
- Strawberry harvesters
- Triathlon participants
- Flooding
- Urban slum area

GENERAL PREVENTION
- Control of the rodent population decreases the incidence of human leptospirosis.
- Exposure to *Leptospira* related to occupation or recreational activities is decreased by wearing protective boots, gloves, and clothing.
- A doxycycline dose of 200 mg per week may be useful in travelers and military personnel likely to be exposed to *Leptospira*, as a preventive measure. However, data are scarce to employ this as a widespread strategy (2).

PATHOPHYSIOLOGY
- *Leptospira* bind to the skin through elastin with their transmembrane protein OmpL37 (3). Pathogenic leptospira may disrupt the endothelial barrier after adhering to it and thus permit the dissemination of leptospira in the various organs of the patient (4). The direct endothelium affliction may lead to hemorrhage.
- Of note, hemorrhage in leptospirosis is due to this direct effect, in contrast to other infections where the disseminated intravascular coagulation is the mechanism of bleeding.

ETIOLOGY
- Leptospirosis is caused by one pathogenic leptospire species (*Leptospira interrogans*), which is subdivided into more than 200 serovars.
- There are 24 serogroups of *L. interrogans* that have been found to cause leptospirosis.
- Wild and domestic animals are the reservoir for leptospirosis.
- Rats are the main reservoir for *L. interrogans* serovar icterohaemorrhagiae.
- The incubation period between infection and development of symptoms is usually 1–2 weeks (range, 2–25 days)

DIAGNOSIS

HISTORY
- Elicit history of exposure to Leptospira either through work or through leisure. Keep a high index of suspicion.
- The protean manifestations of the disease may mimic a variety of viral diseases!

PHYSICAL EXAM
Anicteric leptospirosis
- Fever and chills (fever may be biphasic)
- Headache
- Severe myalgia, especially the calf muscles
- Conjunctival suffusion
- Neck stiffness
- Rash (with palatal enanthem), sometimes hemorrhagic
- Symptoms from CNS disease, including depression, changes in behavior, and confusion
- Symptoms from the respiratory tract, including shortness of breath, cough, and hemoptysis
- Gastrointestinal tract symptoms

Icteric leptospirosis (Weil's syndrome)
- In addition to the above mentioned symptoms, icteric leptospirosis is characterized by jaundice and renal failure and is the most severe form of the disease.

DIAGNOSTIC TESTS & INTERPRETATION
Lab
Initial lab tests
- Leptospira organisms may be seen in the urine, CSF, and blood of infected patients using a dark-field microscope
- After 2–3 days of patient improvement, Leptospira may be absent from blood or CSF but, they are still present in kidney.
- Renal function tests may be abnormal
- Thrombocytopenia may be present
- Abnormal liver function tests are common, whereas increased bilirubin levels signify the severity of the disease
- Increased cretinophosphokinase levels
- Leptospira can be isolated from blood, CSF, and tissues.
- Cultures from the urine are more likely to be positive when obtained during the first week while those from blood and CSF after the first week up to the fourth week of the disease.
- Culture of *Leptospira* needs special media and requires prolonged incubation (rarely up to 4 months!)
- Cultures may be positive if obtained during the first week regarding

Follow-Up & Special Considerations
- Serologic tests are helpful in the diagnosis of leptospirosis.
- The microscopic agglutination test is the reference serological method for diagnosis: Either a fourfold increase or a transition from seronegative to 1:100 have been regarded as useful criteria.
- IgM antibodies against *Leptospira* are a valuable tool for diagnosis. A problem related to these tests is the fact that may be present for a long time (several months to 1 or 2 years) after an acute leptospirosis infection. Thus, caution is needed in the interpretation of serologic tests.
- Polymerase chain reaction for the detection of *Leptospira* spp. DNA is a useful laboratory method (5).
- Pulsed field gel electrophoresis helps to detect the various Leptospira serovars (6)

Imaging
Initial approach
Only if respiratory symptoms are present
Follow-Up & Special Considerations
A chest x-ray or a CT of the chest may be necessary if pulmonary symptoms are present.

Diagnostic Procedures/Other
Lumbar puncture

Pathological Findings
Leptospira organisms may be seen in tissue biopsy specimens.

DIFFERENTIAL DIAGNOSIS
- Leptospirosis is an underdiagnosed disease.
- Leptospirosis should come to the mind of the physician as a diagnostic possibility in every febrile patient at risk for the infection due to occupation or recreational activities.
- Cases of leptospirosis are frequently misdiagnosed as a viral infection, including influenza.
- Hemolytic uremic syndrome
- Rickettsioses
- Hantavirus fever
- Viral hemorrhagic fevers (including Crimean–Congo) (7)
- Acute meningitis
- Consider leptospirosis when encountering fever in the returning traveler

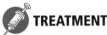 TREATMENT

MEDICATION
First Line
- Penicillin is the drug of choice. The dose may be smaller compared with the dose needed to treat other serious infections. 4–10 million units of intravenous penicillin G (divided in 4–6 doses) is sufficient.
- Ceftriaxone 1g intravenously daily is not inferior to penicillin G for severe leptospirosis (8)
- Duration of treatment is 7 days.

Second Line
- Several other antimicrobial agents also are efficient against leptospirosis.
- Doxycycline 100 mg PO every 12 hours for 7 days may be given in mild cases of leptospirosis.
- Azithromycin is effective for mild disease.

ADDITIONAL TREATMENT
Issues for Referral
A nephrologist's opinion should be sought in case of acute renal failure.

Additional Therapies
Steroids have been used in severe case of leptospirosis especially when the respiratory or the renal system has been afflicted but there is no consensus on this use.

IN-PATIENT CONSIDERATIONS
Admission Criteria
Presence of jaundice or renal failure or thrombocytopenia

Discharge Criteria
Clinical and laboratory improvement

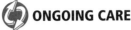 ONGOING CARE

FOLLOW-UP RECOMMENDATIONS
- Patients with mild leptospirosis syndrome who were treated appropriately and had full recovery need no follow-up.
- Patients with severe leptospirosis should have a follow-up visit about a week after the discontinuation of treatment.

PATIENT EDUCATION
In patients who due to profession have a high probability of exposure discuss about the symptoms of the disease and the significance of wearing protective clothing.

PROGNOSIS
- The case fatality rate is 20% for severe leptospirosis with liver and kidney dysfunction treated with appropriate antibiotics.
- Mortality for untreated sever disease may reach ~50%

COMPLICATIONS
- Patients may rarely develop a Jarisch–Herxheimer reaction during treatment
- Main causes of death include the following:
  – Hepatorenal syndrome
  – Adult respiratory distress syndrome
  – Arrhythmias due to myocarditis
  – Vascular dysfunction with severe bleeding
- Recovery of untreated cases may take several months.
- Severe leptospirosis with jaundice is known as Weil's syndrome.
- A leptospirosis syndrome presenting with fever and pretibial rash is known as Fort Bragg fever.
- Keep a high index of suspicion in pregnant women: If leptospirosis occurs in the first months of pregnancy, abortion may ensue. However, congenital infection is rare and thus should not necessarily lead to pregnancy termination (9).

REFERENCES
1. Bharti AR, Nally JE, Ricaldi JN, et al. Leptospirosis: A zoonotic disease of global importance. *Lancet Infect Dis* 2003;3:757–771.
2. Brett-Major DM, Lipnick RJ. Antibiotic prophylaxis for leptospirosis. *Cochrane Database Syst Rev* 2009;(3):CD007342.
3. Martinez-Lopez DG, Fahey M, Coburn J. Responses of human endothelial cells to pathogenic and non-pathogenic Leptospira species. *PLoS Negl Trop Dis* 2010;4:e918.
4. Pinne M, Choy HA, Haake DA. The OmpL37 surface-exposed protein is expressed by pathogenic Leptospira during infection and binds skin and vascular elastin. *PLoS Negl Trop Dis* 2010;4:e815.
5. Ahmed A, Engelberts MF, Boer KR, et al. Development and validation of a real-time PCR for detection of pathogenic Leptospira species in clinical materials. *PLoS One* 2009;4:e7093.
6. Turk N, Milas Z, Mojcec V, et al. Molecular analysis of Leptospira spp. isolated from humans by restriction fragment length polymorphism, real-time PCR and pulsed-field gel electrophoresis. *FEMS Microbiol Lett* 2009;300:174–179.
7. Papa A, Bino S, Papadimitriou E, et al. Suspected Crimean Congo haemorrhagic fever cases in Albania. *Scand J Infect Dis* 2008;40:978–980.
8. Panaphut T, Domrongkitchaiporn S, Vibhagool A, et al. Ceftriaxone compared with sodium penicillin g for treatment of severe leptospirosis. *Clin Infect Dis* 2003;36:1507–1513.
9. Shaked Y, Shpilberg O, Samra D, Samra Y. Leptospirosis in pregnancy and its effect on the fetus: Case report and review. *Clin Infect Dis* 1993;17:241–243.

ADDITIONAL READING
- Gochenour WS Jr, Smadel JE, Jackson EB, et al. Leptospiral etiology of Fort Bragg fever. *Public Health Rep* 1952;67:811.
- Lau CL, Smythe LD, Craig SB, et al. Climate change, flooding, urbanization and leptospirosis: Fuelling the fire? *Trans R Soc Trop Med Hyg* 2010;104:631–638.
- Pappas MG, Ballou WR, Gray MR, et al. Rapid serodiagnosis of leptospirosis using the IgM-specific dot-ELISA: Comparison with the microscopic agglutination test. *Am J Trop Med Hyg* 1985;34:346–354.

 CODES

ICD9
- 100.0 Leptospirosis icterohemorrhagica
- 100.89 Other specified leptospiral infections
- 100.9 Leptospirosis, unspecified

CLINICAL PEARLS
- Asymptomatic disease is very frequent!
- Consider the diagnosis in the differential of a viral disease and in the returning traveler.
- Fever is not necessarily a sign of deterioration but may be part of the Jarisch–Herxheimer reaction.

L

LICE

Georgios Pappas
Petros I. Rafailidis
Matthew E. Falagas

 BASICS

DESCRIPTION
Human infestation by ectoparasitic insects of the order Phthiraptera. Classified as head lice (pediculosis capitis), body lice (pediculosis corporis), and pubic lice (pediculosis pubis), depending on the body site of infestation.

EPIDEMIOLOGY
Incidence
- For head lice, intra-country variations according to the populations studied and detection methods used preclude any generalized incidence rate–related conclusions. It is estimated that up to 6 million children are annually infested in the US, with lower incidence observed in African Americans, possibly due to hair characteristics.
- Body lice and pubic lice incidence unknown–limited reports of incidence in localized settings exist.

Prevalence
- For head lice, prevalence varies from <1% to >50%, according to different studies (1). Not related to socioeconomic status, but related to household population and crowding. Point prevalence may be a more accurate determinant of the extent of infestation burden.
- Prevalence is undetermined for body lice and pubic lice. Prevalence has been studied in localized settings (homeless or patients with sexually transmitted diseases, STD, respectively) or in rare outbreaks in enclosed settings (i.e., refugee camps and prisons). Pubic lice incidence may reach 3.5% in STD clinics; prevalence of both body and pubic lice may exceed 5% in related reports of certain developing countries.

RISK FACTORS
- For head lice, overcrowding is a risk factor, but not the socioeconomic status. Controlled studies have demonstrated that only household size was associated with increased prevalence. Typically observed in schoolchildren, predominance in girls has not been systematically reproduced.
- Body lice have been traditionally associated with low hygiene situations, particularly with homeless individuals and refugees.
- Pubic lice are essentially an STD.

GENERAL PREVENTION
Personal hygiene for body lice; typical STD precautions are not applicable to pubic lice; a "no-nit" policy for readmission of schoolchildren with head lice has been advocated by certain schools to inhibit further infestations: Not unanimously accepted as effective though.

PATHOPHYSIOLOGY
An initial egg harboring an embryo releases a nymph in 7–10 days, which matures sexually in 10 days and lays up to 10 eggs daily (with a life expectancy of 15–20 days).

ETIOLOGY
Head lice (pediculosis capitis): Pediculus humanus capitis, body lice (pediculosis corporis): Pediculus humanus humanus, and pubic lice (pediculosis pubis): Phthirus pubis. Lice is an infestation and NOT an infection.

COMMONLY ASSOCIATED CONDITIONS
- Pediculus humanus serves as a vector for *Bartonella quintana* (and less often Rickettsia prowazekii).
- Pubic lice may be associated with other STDs in up to 30% of cases.

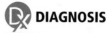 **DIAGNOSIS**

HISTORY
- Pruritus is the predominant symptom, localized according to the syndrome present.
- Secondary bacterial infections may develop.

PHYSICAL EXAM
- Inspection is diagnostic, by observation of lice or their viable eggs (nits). Inspection may require a magnifying lens for visualization. For head lice, combing of wet hair with special brushes allows for more sensitive recognition of lice on the comb teeth. Pubic lice may involve the eyelids.
- Self-induced excoriations and hypersensitivity rash (pediculid) may be observed; rarely regional lymphadenopathy also. Chronic body lice infestation may lead to skin thickening and hyperpigmentation areas. Maculae cerulae are reactive eruptions to pubic lice bites with characteristic gray–blue color, also observed in the lower abdomen.

DIAGNOSTIC TESTS & INTERPRETATION
Lab
Initial lab tests
Not warranted–Diagnosis is by inspection.

Follow-Up & Special Considerations
Patients with pubic lice should be evaluated for STDs. Patients with body lice, according to other symptoms present, may be candidates for *Bartonella quintana* infection.

Imaging
Not warranted.

DIFFERENTIAL DIAGNOSIS
- Head lice: Black and white piedra, hair casts, debris of hair spray or seborrheic dermatitis, and trichodystrophies.
- Body lice: Numerous forms of dermatitis, scabies (scabies often coexists with body lice).
- Pubic lice: Trichomycosis, white piedra, scabies, and allergic dermatitis.

TREATMENT

MEDICATION

First Line

- Therapeutic applications are similar for all types of lice infestation.
- Pyrethroid agents, topically applied, sold over the counter. Permethrin 1% is considered first-line treatment: Application to dry hair, potential reapplication in 7–10 days (2,3). Permethrin 5% is more active in pubic lice. Pyrethrin and piperonyl butoxide are also used. Evolving resistance to pyrethroids has been observed.

Second Line

- Malathion lotion is equally effective but potentially inconvenient in its use.
- Lindane shampoos are slower-acting and public caution exists regarding their potential neurotoxicity.
- Oral ivermectin, administered once and re-administered in 7–10 days is effective, but not FDA-labeled, neither endorsed by the expert community.

ADDITIONAL TREATMENT

General Measures

- Adherence to application guidelines is essential for treatment success.
- Any clothing (including bed sheets) or comb that has come in contact with an infested person should be put in hot water (60°C) for decontamination; essential, particularly for body lice treatment.
- Application of insecticides to clothing is warranted in body lice.
- Decontamination of inanimate objects that may carry head lice is not warranted.
- Pubic lice involving eyelids should be treated with topical application of Vaseline petroleum jelly.

Additional Therapies

- Head shaving is partly effective.
- Manual removal of lice and nits alone is associated with lower success rates.
- Wet combing by specialized personnel and equipment, repeated every 3–4 days, for a period of 2 weeks, has been partly effective.

COMPLEMENTARY & ALTERNATIVE THERAPIES

- Numerous available herbal preparations, not adequately tested.
- Vinegar application has been popular in rural areas in the past.

ONGOING CARE

FOLLOW-UP RECOMMENDATIONS

Inspection for therapeutic success should be performed after 24 hours; presence of viable lice equals treatment failure, due to resistance or improper agent application.

Patient Monitoring

The presence of nits only post-treatment is not a marker of treatment failure: If viable embryos are visualized inside them, reapplication in 7–10 days is warranted.

PROGNOSIS

Excellent in adherence to treatment guidelines.

COMPLICATIONS

- Secondary bacterial infections in the sites of infestation.
- Transmission of *Bartonella quintana* (and less often *Rickettsia prowazekii*) through *Pediculus humanus*.
- Psychological stress in parents and schoolchildren in the case of head lice.

ADDITIONAL READING

- Anderson AL, Chaney E. Pubic lice (Pthirus pubis): History, biology and treatment vs. knowledge and beliefs of US college students. *Int J Environ Res Public Health* 2009;6:592–600.
- Falagas ME, Matthaiou DK, Rafailidis PI, et al. Worldwide prevalence of head lice. *Emerg Infect Dis* 2008;14:1493–1494.
- Flinders DC, De Schweinitz P. Pediculosis and scabies. *Am Fam Physician* 2004;69:341–348.
- Ko CJ, Elston DM. Pediculosis. *J Am Acad Dermatol* 2004;50:1–12.

CODES

ICD9

- 132.0 Pediculus capitis (head louse)
- 132.1 Pediculus corporis (body louse)
- 132.9 Pediculosis, unspecified

CLINICAL PEARLS

- Differential diagnosis of body lice includes scabies, but due to the common epidemiologic background of both, scabies and body lice may coexist in a significant percentage of patients.
- Pubic lice has been utilized in forensic medicine/law, for human DNA extraction.

L

LISTERIOSIS

Jatin M. Vyas (E. Mylonakis, Editor)

 BASICS

DESCRIPTION
- Listeriosis is an infection caused by the gram-positive rod *Listeria monocytogenes*.
- 7 common clinical syndromes have been described:
  - Febrile gastroenteritis
  - CNS infection
  - Infection during pregnancy
  - Focal infections
  - Infection in immunocompromised patients
  - Bacteremia, endocarditis
  - Infection in neonates

EPIDEMIOLOGY
- Listeriosis can present as sporadic or as outbreaks. The incidence of laboratory-confirmed cases of listeriosis in 2009 was 0.34 per 100,000 persons. It is usually attributed to food-borne transmission of *L. monocytogenes* and is associated with a variety of foods such as milk, cheese, meat products, and raw vegetables. 1–5% of humans are asymptomatic intestinal carriers, providing a reservoir for the pathogen.
- Listeriosis can occur throughout life, even among individuals without predisposing factors. The lack of predisposing factors does not rule out listeriosis.

RISK FACTORS
The following populations are at higher risk for listeriosis:
- Neonates: *L. monocytogenes* is the third most common cause of neonatal sepsis and meningitis after *Escherichia coli* and group *B. streptococci*.
- Individuals above 50 years
- Pregnant women: One-third of all listeriosis cases are related to pregnancy. In this population, listeriosis mainly predisposes to non-CNS listeriosis, and it can occur at any time during pregnancy, but more often during the third trimester.
- Glucocorticoid therapy
- Hematologic or solid-organ malignancy
- Chemotherapy
- Solid-organ or bone marrow transplantation
- Liver disease including alcoholism
- HIV/AIDS: There is a more than 100-fold increase in incidence among patients with AIDS, but incidence can be reduced by the use of prophylactic trimethoprim-sulfamethoxazole.
- Diabetes mellitus
- Splenectomy
- Autoimmune disorders
- Hemochromatosis
- Treatment with immunomodulatory agents including TNF-antagonists.
- End-stage renal disease (including patients requiring dialysis).

GENERAL PREVENTION
- The following recommendations are based on guidelines published by the CDC:
  - Do not drink raw (unpasteurized) milk or foods that contain unpasteurized milk.
  - Wash raw vegetables thoroughly before eating.
  - Keep the refrigerator temperature at 40°F (4.4°C) or lower; the freezer at 0°F (−17.8°C) or lower.
  - Eat precooked, perishable, or ready-to-eat foods as soon as possible.
  - Keep raw meat, fish, and poultry separate from cooked foods, ready-to-eat foods, and also from other foods that will not be cooked.
  - Wash hands, knives, and cutting boards after handling uncooked food.
  - Thoroughly cook raw food from animal sources to a safe internal temperature: Ground beef 160°F (71°C); chicken 170°F (77°C); turkey 180°F (82°C); and pork 160°F (71°C).
- For patients at higher risk, the following recommendations should also be followed:
  - Avoid delicatessen meats unless they are reheated.
  - Avoid soft cheeses unless they are clearly made from pasteurized milk.

PATHOPHYSIOLOGY
- Febrile gastroenteritis
  - Typically self-limited febrile non-bloody gastroenteritis in normal hosts.
  - Mean incubation period is 24 hours.
  - Typical duration of symptoms is ≤2 days.
- CNS Infection:
  - Typically, *Listeria* causes meningoencephalitis. Cerebritis, focal brain abscess, and rhombencephalitis are less common.
  - Meningoencephalitis occurs most commonly in neonates, immunocompromised patients, and elderly adults.
  - Presents with mild fever and mental status changes rarely present fulminantly with coma.
  - Up to 15% of patients have symptoms for 5 days or more before hospitalization, and 42% lack meningeal signs on admission.
  - Symptoms of cerebritis can resemble CVA, stroke.
  - Rhombencephalitis may follow a biphasic course with headache and fever and then develop into with cranial nerve palsies, cerebellar signs, and seizures.
- Infection in pregnancy:
  - Occurs most commonly during the third trimester.
  - Non-specific flu like syndrome, including fever and chills are common symptoms.
  - Infection in pregnant women can lead to fetal death, premature birth, or infected newborns.
  - If bacteremia is present, it rarely leads to CNS infection.
- Focal Infections:
  - Skin and eye infections in persons working with animals or lab workers.
  - Other sites include lymph nodes, lungs, pleural space, heart, joints, bone, soft tissues, and prosthetic grafts.

- Infection in immunocompromised patients:
  - Most common cause of bacterial meningitis in this patient population.
  - Bacteremia in this group of patients has an increased risk of CNS infection.
- Bacteremia, endocarditis:
  - Fever and chills are common presenting symptoms.
  - Up to one-fourth of the patients have gastrointestinal symptoms (nausea, vomiting, diarrhea, or abdominal pain).
  - *Listeria* is an infrequent cause of (usually subacute) endocarditis, usually involving the left side of the heart. It is more common among patients with preexisting valve lesions.
- Infection in neonates (0–28 days of life):
  - Neonates in the first 7 days of life usually present with signs of sepsis or pneumonia. Sepsis, CNS infection, and focal infections are the most common syndromes after the first 7 days of life.
  - In utero-infected neonates can develop granulomatosis infantiseptica. These infants might appear very sick, develop cardiopulmonary collapse, or just appear weak.

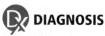 **DIAGNOSIS**

HISTORY
- For patients with increased risk for *Listeria* infections, a detailed history of any neurologic symptoms is required.
- There is no specific history that will establish the diagnosis of listeriosis.

PHYSICAL EXAM
- No specific physical exam findings establish the diagnosis of listeriosis.
- In patients with suspected focal infection, careful examination of affected area is indicated.

DIAGNOSTIC TESTS & INTERPRETATION
Lab
- In immunocompetent patients with non-bloody diarrhea caused by *Listeria*, no tests are required.
- In patients with suspected invasive disease or patients with increased risk for listeriosis, the following tests should be considered:
  - CBC with differential:
    - Despite its name, *Listeria* does not cause monocytosis.
  - Stool culture is not typically helpful.
  - Blood cultures
  - LP with measurements of opening pressure, CSF glucose, CSF protein, CSF cell counts, CSF gram stain, and CSF bacterial culture:
    - Despite its name, monocytes do not predominate in the CSF of patients with CNS infection.

Imaging
Brain MRI should be performed in patients with listerial meningitis, patients with *Listeria bacteremia* and CNS symptoms.

DIFFERENTIAL DIAGNOSIS
- Febrile gastroenteritis (Salmonella, Campylobacter, Shigella, *Escherichia coli* O157:H7, *Clostridium difficile*, Rotavirus, Cryptosporidium, Giardia, Cyclospora, *Entamoeba histolytica*).
- CNS infection:
  - Infection due to *Streptococcus pneumoniae*, *Haemophilus influenzae*, and *Neisseria meningitidis* in adults. *Cryptococcus neoformans* should also be considered in immunocompromised individuals.
  - Metabolic encephalopathy
  - Psychiatric illnesses
  - Brain abscess
  - CNS tumor
  - CVA, stroke
- Infection in pregnancy:
  - Influenza, congenital syphilis or toxoplasmosis, pyelonephritis, and septic abortion
- Focal infections:
  - Other bacteria causing infection in affected anatomic area
- Infection in immunocompromised patients:
  - Other bacteria causing bacteremia
  - See CNS DDx for other causes of CNS infection
- Bacteremia, endocarditis:
  - Other causes of bacteria causing bacteremia
  - See endocarditis for review of agents causing endocarditis
- Infection in neonates:
  - Meningitis due to *E. coli* or group B *Streptococci*
  - Bacteremia and sepsis
  - *Granulomatosis infantiseptica*
  - Pneumonia

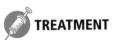
TREATMENT
MEDICATION
First Line
Treatment depends on the clinical syndrome.
- Febrile gastroenteritis:
  - Generally immunocompetent patients do not require antibiotic therapy.
  - Immunocompromised patients can be treated with oral amoxicillin or trimethoprim-sulfamethoxazole for several days.
- CNS Infection:
  - In adults, Ampicillin or Penicillin G IV are the antibiotics of choice, though no controlled trials have been published.
  - Duration of therapy is 2–4 weeks in immunocompetent patients and 4–8 weeks in immunocompromised patients.
  - When given, gentamicin should be given until patient improves (typically 7–14 days) or does not respond up to 3 weeks and if patient tolerates the therapy.
  - Trimethoprim-sulfamethoxazole can be used as an alternative. The dose is 10–20 mg/kg (based on the trimethoprim component) divided every 6 hours. The higher dose should be used for ill patients or patients with CNS infection.

- Infection in pregnancy: Amoxicillin or trimethoprim-sulfamethoxazole for several days.
- Focal infections:
  - Should be individualized based on location of infection and immune status of patient.
- Infection in immunocompromised patients:
  - Immunocompromised patients with febrile gastroenteritis should be given oral amoxicillin or trimethoprim-sulfamethoxazole for several days.
  - Immunocompromised patients with bacteremia should be treated with IV ampicillin or trimethoprim-sulfamethoxazole for 3–6 weeks.
  - Immunocompromised patients with CNS infections should be treated with IV ampicillin or trimethoprim-sulfamethoxazole for 4–8 weeks.
- Bacteremia, endocarditis:
  - Immunocompetent patients with bacteremia should be treated with IV ampicillin or trimethoprim-sulfamethoxazole for 2 weeks.
  - Immunocompromised patients with bacteremia should be treated with IV ampicillin or trimethoprim-sulfamethoxazole for 3–6 weeks.
  - Endocarditis should be treated for a minimum of 6 weeks of IV antibiotics.
- Infection in neonates:
  - Should be individualized based on location of infection and immune status of patient.

ADDITIONAL TREATMENT
Issues for Referral
- ID consultation should be considered for patients with invasive infection.
- Consultation with an appropriate specialist should be considered for patients with focal infection.
- Collaboration with high-risk obstetrician should be considered for pregnant patients.
- Collaboration with neonatologist should be considered for infected neonates.

SURGERY/OTHER PROCEDURES
If abscess is present, consideration of draining should be considered.

IN-PATIENT CONSIDERATIONS
Initial Stabilization
- Antibiotics for patients suspected with bacterial meningitis should be given within 60 minutes of arrival to the ER.

Admission Criteria
Patients suspected of having invasive listeriosis should be admitted to the hospital.

ONGOING CARE
FOLLOW-UP RECOMMENDATIONS
- Patients with positive blood cultures should have follow-up blood cultures to document sterility.
- Immunocompromised patients should be closely followed after cessation of antibiotics therapy to assess for relapse of infection.

Patient Monitoring
Immunocompromised patients should be closely followed for signs of infection.

DIET
Patients with listeriosis should be given recommendations to prevent bacterial infection.

PATIENT EDUCATION
Patients with listeriosis should be given recommendations to prevent bacterial infection.

PROGNOSIS
The prognosis of listeriosis depends on the clinical syndrome.
- Febrile gastroenteritis:
  - Excellent prognosis in immunocompetent patients.
- CNS Infection:
  - The mortality rate of meningitis/meningoencephalitis is the highest among all causes of bacterial meningitis (>27%). Mortality is higher among immunocompromised patients and those who develop seizures.
  - The mortality rate of cerebritis and CNS abscess secondary to Listeria is even higher (~50%).
- Infection in pregnancy:
  - The exact morbidity and mortality of the pregnancy-associated listeriosis is unclear, but treatment of maternal bacteremia and antibiotic therapy of the newborn can improve outcome.
- Focal infections:
  - The mortality rate of cerebritis and CNS abscess due to Listeria is even higher (~50%).
- Infection in immunocompromised patients:
  - Increased risk of relapse of infection.
- Bacteremia, endocarditis:
  - The mortality rate of endocarditis due to Listeria is even higher (~50%).
- Infection in neonates:
  - *Granulomatosis infantiseptica* carries the worst prognosis.

COMPLICATIONS
- CNS infection can lead to seizures or severe neurologic compromise (ataxia, personality changes, coma, etc.).
- Bacteremia might lead to CNS infection.
- Listeriosis during pregnancy can lead to amnionitis, premature labor, recurrent abortion, premature rupture of membranes, and stillbirth.

ADDITIONAL READING
- Mylonakis E, Hohmann EL, Calderwood SB. Central nervous system infection with Listeria monocytogenes: 33 years' experience at a general hospital and review of 776 episodes from the literature. *Medicine (Baltimore)* 1998;77:313–336.

CODES
ICD9
- 027.0 Listeriosis
- 771.2 Other congenital infections specific to the perinatal period

LUNG ABSCESS

Jing Zhang
Jieming Qu
Matthew E. Falagas

 BASICS

DESCRIPTION
- A cavity containing necrotic lung tissue and pus resulting from microbial infection. Secondary lung abscesses can occur due to bacteremia (right-sided bacterial endocarditis or jugular vein thrombophlebitis [Lemierre's syndrome]).
- There may be a single abscess, generally >2 cm in diameter, or multiple small abscesses; the latter condition is known as necrotizing pneumonia.
- Presentation may be acute or chronic (symptoms for > 4–6 weeks).
- Lung abscess can be classified as primary, occurring in a previously healthy person, or secondary, related to an underlying condition such as pulmonary neoplasm, bronchiectasis, prior surgery in the lung, or an immunocompromising illness (1).

EPIDEMIOLOGY
Incidence
- Predominant age: Mainly 4th-6th decades.
- Predominant gender: Male > Female (4:1).

Prevalence
Lung abscess was common in the pre-antibiotic era but is currently rare.

RISK FACTORS
- Present in 80–90% of primary lung abscess cases.
- Periodontal infection with pyorrhea or gingivitis; dental abscess, dental surgery.
- Conditions that predispose to aspiration, for example, altered state of consciousness, dysphagia, general anesthesia with surgery, tracheal/nasogastric tube, epilepsy, and severe gastroesophageal reflux disease.
- Airway obstruction, for example, foreign body and enlarged lymph node.
- Immunocompromised status, for example, HIV, chronic corticosteroid use, and diabetes mellitus.

Genetics
No known genetic pattern.

GENERAL PREVENTION
- Treatment of predisposing diseases
- Prevention of aspiration
- Treatment of periodontal diseases

PATHOPHYSIOLOGY
- Most frequently, microorganisms may reach the lung through aspiration of oropharyngeal contents and mouth anaerobes. The patients who develop lung abscess are predisposed to aspiration and commonly have periodontal disease.
- Other mechanisms for lung abscess formation include hematogenous seeding from an extrapulmonary focus, such as bacteremia or tricuspid valve endocarditis causing septic emboli (usually multiple) to the lung.

ETIOLOGY
- Lung abscess are usually caused by pure anaerobic bacteria (40–50%) or a mixture of aerobes and anaerobes (40–50%). Aerobic or facultative bacteria alone account for 10–20% of cases. The major anaerobic isolates are:
  - Peptostreptococcus
  - Fusobacterium
  - Prevotella
  - Bacteroides spp.
- The major aerobic/facultative bacteria are:
  - Staphylococcus aureus, including methicillin-resistant Staphylococcus aureus (MRSA) (rare, but serious and becoming more common). Suspect with recent or concurrent influenza illness or evidence of necrotizing pneumonia and shock in young adults or adolescents.
  - Streptococcus pyogenes
  - Streptococcus milleri
  - Gram-negative bacteria, especially Klebsiella sp.
  - Pseudomonas aeruginosa
- Rare causes include Legionella, Nocardia, Actinomyces, and fungi.
- In patients with HIV, Rhodococcus, Salmonella, Pneumocystis jiroveci, Cryptococcus, and Aspergillus may also cause lung abscess.

Pediatric Considerations
Occurs in children; Staphylococcus is the most common organism.

COMMONLY ASSOCIATED CONDITIONS
- Periodontal diseases
- Pneumonia
- Alcoholism
- Empyema
- Tuberculosis
- Immunosuppression

 DIAGNOSIS

HISTORY
- Cough with purulent, foul-smelling, putrid, sour-tasting sputum
- Fever
- In the more common chronic form, symptoms of fatigue, malaise, night sweat, productive cough, weight loss, and pleuritic pain lasting for weeks or months.

PHYSICAL EXAM
- Tachypnea and tachycardia
- May include crackles, wheezing, dullness to percussion, consolidation by auscultation, cavernous breath sounds, and decreased breath sounds.
- Clubbing of digits can be seen in chronic lung abscess (2).

DIAGNOSTIC TESTS & INTERPRETATION
Lab
Initial lab tests
- A complete white blood cell count with differential may reveal leukocytosis and a left shift. Leukopenia is common with MRSA.
- Sputum smear and Gram stain: Neutrophils, mixed bacteria.
- Sputum culture and sensitivity test: Often negative.
- Blood culture: Often negative in anaerobic abscess. Pay details to transferring the sample to the microbiology laboratory.

Follow-Up & Special Considerations
- Anemia and hypoalbuminemia can be seen in chronic lung abscess.
- Prior antibiotics may alter culture results.
- If tuberculosis is suspected, request acid-fast bacilli stain and polymerase chain reaction (PCR) for the detection of mycobacterial DNA and culture.
- Anti-neutrophil cytoplasmic autoantibodies (c-ANCA).

Imaging
Initial approach
- Chest radiograph shows a pulmonary infiltrate along with a cavity that may have an air–fluid level, usually confined to a single segment or lobe. One-third of patients have coexistent empyema.
- CT scan provides best anatomical definition. The most common sites are those liable to aspiration, for example, the superior segments of the lower lobes and the posterior segments of the upper lobes.

Follow-Up & Special Considerations
- CT scan can help to find out obstructing lesion in suspected patients.
- CT scan is recommended for cases of uncertain cause and for cases that do not respond to antibiotic therapy.
- A transesophageal ultrasound may be needed to rule out right-sided endocarditis in case of multiple abscesses (3).

Diagnostic Procedures/Other
- Bronchoscopy, if atypical presentation or failure to respond:
  - To check for obstruction.
  - Brushing and bronchoalveolar lavage for microbiological test.
- Transthoracic needle aspiration for microbiological test.

Pathological Findings
- Solitary or multiple abscesses.
- Cavitation with necrosis.
- Effusion/Empyema

DIFFERENTIAL DIAGNOSIS

- Infectious: Pneumonia, bronchitis, infected pulmonary bulla, and parasitic lung infections.
- Bronchiectasis
- Lung cancer
- Aspirated foreign body
- Wegener's granulomatosis (Note any presence of nasal bleeding or nasal ulcer or pyoderma gangrenosum or hematuria that may indicate Wegener's granulomatosis).
- Pulmonary embolism leading to pulmonary infarct.
- Endocarditis with associated septi emboli (Listen specifically for the presence of a cardiac murmur that may indicate right-sided endocarditis).

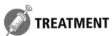 **TREATMENT**

MEDICATION

Antibiotic treatment should be started intravenously, but can be switched to the oral route after the fever and toxicity have abated. Duration is usually 3 weeks to several months, based on cavity closure and reduction of the pulmonary infiltrate. Antibiotics should be used according to culture and drug sensitivity results.

First Line

- Clindamycin 600 mg IV q8h, followed by 300 mg q6h PO.
- Ampicillin/sulbactam 1.5–3g q6h (4,5), followed by amoxicillin-clavulanate 875 mg PO BID or clindamycin 300 mg PO q6h.
- Moxifloxacin 400 mg IV OD (6).
- Carbapenems: Meropenem 1g IV q8h or imipenem/cilastatin 500 mg IV q6–8h

Second Line

- Piperacillin-tazobactam 3.375 g IV q6h
- Ticarcillin-clavulanate 3.0 g IV q6h
- Metronidazole is often recommended as an adjunctive therapy (500 mg IV q6h).
- MRSA: Linezolid 600mg IV q12h or vancomycin 15mg/kg IV q12h

ADDITIONAL TREATMENT

General Measures

- Postural drainage and pulmonary physiotherapy.
- Prolonged course of antibiotics.
- Nasotracheal suctioning or bronchoscopy with selective therapeutic lavage if needed (7).

SURGERY/OTHER PROCEDURES

- Surgical drainage is needed in about 10% of cases that are refractory to antibiotics alone.
- Drainage can be accomplished by a percutaneous needle-guided approach.
- Resectional surgery is only considered if prolonged antibiotic therapy fails or neoplasm or congenital lung malformation is suspected.

IN-PATIENT CONSIDERATIONS

Initial Stabilization

- Evaluation and management of patient's respiratory status. .
- Oxygen supplementation should be given to patients who have concomitant hypoxia.
- Analgesia

Admission Criteria

- Admit all patients with lung abscess for administration of intravenous antibiotics.
- Drainage of the abscess or empyema.

Nursing

- Pain assessment
- Sputum drainage

 ONGOING CARE

FOLLOW-UP RECOMMENDATIONS

- Clinical improvement with decrease in fever expected 3–4 days after starting antibiotics.
- Defervescence expected in 7–10 days.
- For patients with poor response to antibiotic therapy, bronchial obstruction with a foreign body or neoplasm, or infection with resistant bacteria, mycobacteria, or fungi should be considered.

Patient Monitoring

Serial radiographs or CT scan until resolution of cavity and resolution of the infiltrate to a stable scar.

DIET

High energy and high nutrition.

PATIENT EDUCATION

Pulmonary physiotherapy techniques.

PROGNOSIS

- Overall mortality is 5–15%.
- Risk factors for a poor prognosis include cavity size >6 cm, persistence of symptoms >8 weeks before diagnosis, anatomic obstruction, elderly and/or debilitated patient, underlying diseases or immunosuppression, certain bacteriological etiology (S. aureus, Klebsiella, Pseudomonas), and nosocomial acquisition.

COMPLICATIONS

- Obstructed bronchus and/or large abscess can produce failures of medical management, with contiguous involvement of other segments of lung.
- Empyema
- Massive hemoptysis
- Pneumothorax
- Brain abscess

REFERENCES

1. Gadkowski LB, Stout JE. Cavitary pulmonary disease. Clin Microbiol Rev 2008;21:305–333.
2. Schiza S, Siafakas NM. Clinical presentation and management of empyema, lung abscess and pleural effusion. Curr Opin Pulm Med 2006;12(3): 205–211.
3. Que YA, Muller O, Liaudet L. Images in cardiovascular medicine. Rapid resolution of massive lung abscesses complicating tricuspid-valve endocarditis. Circulation 2006;114(14): e523–e524.
4. Allewelt M, Schüler P, Bölcskei PL. Ampicillin + sulbactam vs clindamycin +/− cephalosporin for the treatment of aspiration pneumonia and primary lung abscess. Clin Microbiol Infect 2004;10: 163–170.
5. Mandell LA, Wunderink RG, Anzueto A, et al. Infectious Diseases Society of America/American Thoracic Society consensus guidelines on the management of community-acquired pneumonia in adults. Clin Infect Dis 2007;44(Suppl 2):S27–S72.
6. Ott SR, Allewelt M, Lorenz J, et al. Moxifloxacin vs ampicillin/sulbactam in aspiration pneumonia and primary lung abscess. Infection 2008;36:23–30.
7. Herth F, Ernst A, Becker HD. Endoscopic drainage of lung abscesses: Technique and outcome. Chest 2005;127:1378–1381.

 CODES

ICD9

513.0 Abscess of lung

CLINICAL PEARLS

- The posterior segment of the right upper lobe is the most common location for abscess.
- Prolonged antibiotic treatment is needed.
- For those failing medical therapy, percutaneous drainage, surgical resection, or bronchoscopic drainage must be considered.
- Rule out Wegener's granulomatosis before proceeding to surgery.

LYME DISEASE

Paschalis Vergidis
Matthew E. Falagas

BASICS

DESCRIPTION
- Lyme disease is a multisystemic, tick-borne disease. The infection begins at the site of a hard-bodied tick bite, followed by local dissemination of the organism in the skin and subsequent spread by blood or lymph to other skin sites, joints, cerebrospinal fluid, heart, muscle, bone, retina, spleen, liver, and brain. Stages of the disease are classified as early localized, early disseminated, and late.
- First described in 1977 following the investigation of a cluster of arthritis cases among children living near Lyme, Connecticut.

EPIDEMIOLOGY
Incidence
- The most common tick-borne infection in North America and Europe.
- The number of reported cases in the US increased from 9,908 in 1992 to 19,931 in 2006 (1).
- The 10 reference states with the highest incidence (92.6% of overall cases) are Maryland, Delaware, Pennsylvania, New Jersey, New York, Connecticut, Rhode Island, and Massachusetts along the Atlantic seaboard, as well as Minnesota and Wisconsin in the upper Midwest.

RISK FACTORS
Outdoor work or activities in endemic areas.

GENERAL PREVENTION
- Protective clothing, long sleeves and long pants, in endemic areas; light-colored clothing makes dark ticks easier to see.
- Application of tick repellants containing N,N-Diethyl-meta-toluamide (DEET) to clothing and exposed skin. Application of acaricides to clothing; not for use on skin.
- A Lyme disease vaccine, approved in 1998, had poor acceptance and is not marketed anymore.
- Single dose of doxycycline should be considered for prophylaxis in persons aged >8 years who have been bitten by *Ixodes scapularis* or *I. pacificus* tick in an area in which at least 20% of ticks are thought to be infected with *Borellia burgdorferi*. The tick must have been attached for ≥36 hours and prophylactic antibiotic administered within 72 hours of tick removal.

ETIOLOGY
- Spirochete, *B. burgdorferi* in the US.
- Primarily *B. afzelii* and *B. garinii* in Europe and Asia.
- Restricted to certain members of the Ixodes species complex.

DIAGNOSIS

HISTORY
Ticks transmit disease to humans only if they are attached for more than 36 hours. Most patients do not recall a tick bite.

PHYSICAL EXAM
Early Localized
- Expanding rash, erythema migrans (EM), at site of tick bite 3 days to 1 month later (70%).
- A red macule or papule expands to a larger round or oval patch or erythema, 3–68 cm.
- Frequently, the ring has central clearing with a flat, occasionally raised, intensely erythematous outer border; lesion fades within 1 month.
- Rash can be anywhere on the body, most commonly the groin, thigh, axilla, and popliteal fossa.

Early Disseminated
- Dermatologic:
  - There are secondary annular skin lesions in up to 5% of untreated patients with EM within several days to a few weeks after onset of primary EM.
  - Lesions are smaller than in primary EM, may coalesce, and do not have an indurated center.
- Intermittent symptoms of fever, headache, fatigue, malaise, generalized achiness, migratory musculoskeletal pain, regional or generalized lymphadenopathy, or splenomegaly.
- Musculoskeletal:
  - Symptoms develop in 60% of patients with untreated EM.
  - After intermittent episodes of arthralgia or migratory musculoskeletal pain, arthritis develops approximately 6 months after the onset of infection.
  - Most patients experience swelling and pain in 1 or 2 large joints, especially the knee, lasting several days to a few weeks.
  - Some patients experience pain in the temporomandibular joints, the small joints of the hands and feet, and the periarticular structures, including tendons, bursae, and muscle.
- Neurologic:
  - Symptoms are common; approximately 15% of patients with untreated EM develop frank neurologic abnormalities weeks to months after the onset of infection.
  - In the US, it is manifested most commonly as subacute, basilar, lymphocytic meningitis with or without unilateral or bilateral facial palsy or peripheral neuritis.
  - In Europe, it is most commonly manifested as Bannwarth's syndrome, which consists of radiculitis, lymphocytic pleocytosis in cerebrospinal fluid, and sometimes cranial neuritis.

- Cardiac:
  - Symptoms develop in 5% of patients with untreated EM, 1 week to 7 months after the onset of infection.
  - The most common cardiac manifestations are atrioventricular conduction defects: First-degree, second-degree, Wenckebach, and complete block.
  - Duration is usually brief—a few days to 6 weeks.
- Ocular:
  - Follicular conjunctivitis in 10% of patients.
- Mild hepatitis occurs in 20% of patients.

Late
- Musculoskeletal:
  - Arthritis becomes more persistent, lasting months.
  - Arthritis becomes chronic—at least 1 year of continuing joint inflammation—in 10% of untreated patients.
- Neurologic:
  - Subacute encephalopathy, characterized by cognitive defects and disturbances in sleep or mood, occurs months to years after onset of infection in a small percentage of patients.
  - Chronic polyneuropathy (rare)
  - Encephalomyelitis, characterized by cognitive defects, ataxia, spastic paraparesis, and bladder dysfunction (more common in Europe, rare in US) can occur.
- Dermatologic:
  - Acrodermatitis chronica atrophicans: Appears on extremities as a doughy, violaceous skin infiltration that gradually becomes indurated, thickened, and hyperpigmented
  - Borrelial lymphocytoma: Appears in the dermis, subcutis, or both, as a bluish-red, tumor-like skin infiltration (common in Europe, rare in the US)
- Cardiac:
  - Chronic cardiomyopathy is possible, but evidence suggests that it is rare.

Post-Lyme Disease syndrome
- Pain, neurocognitive, or fatigue symptoms after appropriate antibiotic treatment without any residual or new objective findings.

DIAGNOSTIC TESTS & INTERPRETATION
Lab
Initial lab tests
- Diagnosis is based on characteristic clinical symptoms, history of exposure in an endemic area, and laboratory tests. Note the limitations of laboratory testing.
- Misdiagnosis occurs as a result of misinterpretation, overuse, and suboptimal performance and standardization of laboratory tests for the disease.
- A two-test approach is recommended: Sensitive enzyme immunoassay or immunofluorescent assay, followed by a Western immunoblot. Specimens that are negative by enzyme immunoassay or immunofluorescent assay do not need to be confirmed by Western immunoblot, only those that are positive or equivocal.

- PCR has been used to isolate *B. burgdorferi* from cerebrospinal or synovial fluid. The test should be performed in a reliable laboratory.
- Culture is not available in most clinical laboratories.
- Cautions:
  - Serology tests may have negative results in patients with early Lyme disease; most patients seroconvert within the first 4 weeks after onset of infection.
  - A positive IgM test result late after the onset of Lyme disease does not, by itself, mean that the disease is active.
  - False-positive results for Lyme disease can occur in patients with syphilis, oral infection with other spirochete species, or seronegative spondyloarthropathy due to the low sensitivity and specificity of some tests for Lyme disease.
  - Antibiotics administered early in the disease course may prevent seroconversion.

DIFFERENTIAL DIAGNOSIS
Infectious
- Fungal skin infections
- Cellulitis
- Erythema annulare centrifugum
- Guillain-Barré syndrome and sarcoidosis (bilateral facial palsy)
- Insect or spider bites
- Plant dermatitis
- Erysipelas
- Granuloma annulare
- Fibromyalgia (neurologic symptoms)
- Chronic fatigue (neurologic symptoms)
- Coinfection with *Babesia microti* or *Anaplasma phagocytophilum* or both may occur in patients with early Lyme (usually patients with EM) in endemic areas.
- Consider coinfection in patients who present with severe initial symptoms, especially high fever for >48 hours, despite receiving appropriate antibiotic therapy, or those who have unexplained leukopenia, thrombocytopenia, anemia, or elevated transaminases.

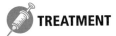 TREATMENT
MEDICATION
First Line
- Oral regimens:
  - Amoxicillin 500 mg PO 3 times per day
  - Doxycycline 100 mg PO twice per day
  - Cefuroxime axetil 500 mg PO twice per day.
    - Note: Doxycycline treats coinfection with anaplasmosis.
- Parenteral regimen:
  - Ceftriaxone 2 g IV single dose daily.

Second Line
- Oral regimens
  - Azithromycin 500 mg PO per day for 7–10 days.
  - Clarithromycin 500 mg PO twice per day for 14–21 days, if the patient is not pregnant.
  - Erythromycin 500 mg PO 4 times per day for 14–21 days.

- Parenteral regimens
  - Cefotaxime 2 g IV every 8 hours.
  - Penicillin G 18–24 million units per day IV divided every 4 hours.

Recommended Therapy
- Erythema migrans. Oral regimen for 14 days (14–21 days) (A-I) (2)
- Early neurologic disease (3)
  - Meningitis or radiculopathy. Parenteral regimen for 14 days (10–28 days) (B-I)
  - Cranial nerve palsy. Oral regimen for 14 days (14–21 days) (B-III)
- Cardiac disease. A parenteral regimen is recommended at the start of therapy for hospitalized patients; an oral regimen may be substituted to complete a course of therapy or to treat ambulatory patients. Duration 14 days (14–21 days) (B-III).
- Borrelial lymphocytoma. Oral regimen for 14 days (14–21 days) (B-II).
- Late disease (4).
  - Arthritis without neurologic disease. Oral regimen for 28 days (B-I).
  - Recurrent arthritis after oral regimen. Oral regimen for 28 days or parenteral regimen for 14 days (14–28 days) (B-III).
  - Antibiotic-refractory arthritis. Symptomatic therapy (B-III).
  - Central or peripheral nervous system disease. Parenteral regimen for 14 days (14–28 days) (B-II).
  - Acrodermatitis chronica atrophicans. Oral regimen for 21 days (14–28 days) (B-II).
- Post–Lyme disease syndrome. Consider and evaluate other potential causes of symptoms; if none, then symptomatic therapy (E-I).

Pediatric and Pregnancy Considerations
- Doxycycline should be avoided.
- Transplacental transmission of disease has been reported in a few patients (rare).

ADDITIONAL TREATMENT
General Measures
- Carditis: Temporary pacing may be necessary.
- Arthritis: Symptomatic therapy includes nonsteroidal anti-inflammatory agents, intra-articular injections of corticosteroids, or disease-modifying antirheumatic drugs, such as hydroxychloroquine. Arthroscopic synovectomy for persistent synovitis.

IN-PATIENT CONSIDERATIONS
Admission Criteria
- Carditis: Hospitalize patients who are symptomatic (syncope, dyspnea, or chest pain), or those with PR prolongation ≥30 msec, second- or third-degree AV block.
- Meningitis or radiculopathy in early disease.
- Central or peripheral nervous system disease in late disease.

 ONGOING CARE
COMPLICATIONS
Arthritis unresponsive to antibiotics, especially in patients who are HLA-DR4-positive.

REFERENCES
1. Bacon RM, Kugeler KJ, Mead PS. Surveillance for Lyme disease–United States, 1992–2006. *MMWR Surveill Summ* 2008;57:1–9.
2. Wormser GP, Ramanathan R, Nowakowski J, et al. Duration of antibiotic therapy for early Lyme disease. A randomized, double-blind, placebo-controlled trial. *Annals Intern Med* 2003;138: 697–704.
3. Borg R, Dotevall L, Hagberg L, et al. Intravenous ceftriaxone compared with oral doxycycline for the treatment of Lyme neuroborreliosis. *Scand J Infect Dis* 2005;37:449–454.
4. Dattwyler RJ, Wormser GP, Rush TJ, et al. A comparison of two treatment regimens of ceftriaxone in late Lyme disease. *Wien klin Wochenschr* 2005;117(11–12):393–397.

ADDITIONAL READING
- Feder HM Jr, Johnson BJ, O'Connell S, et al. A critical appraisal of "chronic Lyme disease". *N Engl J Med* 2007;357(14):1422–1430.
- Wormser GP, Dattwyler RJ, Shapiro ED, et al. The clinical assessment, treatment, and prevention of Lyme disease, human granulocytic anaplasmosis, and babesiosis: Clinical practice guidelines by the Infectious Diseases Society of America. *Clin Infect Dis* 2006;43:1089–1134.

 CODES
ICD9
088.81 Lyme disease

CLINICAL PEARLS
- Most patients with erythema migrans do not recall a tick bite. Presence of EM allows clinical diagnosis in the absence of laboratory confirmation.
- A two-test approach is recommended for the laboratory diagnosis of Lyme disease. PCR can be used in CSF or synovial fluid.
- Consider coinfection with *B. microti* or *A. phagocytophilum* in endemic areas.

L

LYMPHANGITIS

Wei Lu
Petros I. Rafailidis
Matthew E. Falagas

 BASICS

DESCRIPTION
Lymphangitis is defined as an inflammation of the lymphatic channels that occurs as a result of infection at a site distal to the channel.

EPIDEMIOLOGY
No specific data are available.

RISK FACTORS
- Lymphedema
- Trauma
- Bites, insect stings (1)
- Fungal disease (i.e., tinea pedis)

PATHOPHYSIOLOGY
- Pathogenic organisms enter the lymphatic channels directly through an abrasion or wound or as a complication of infection.
- After the organisms enter the channels, local inflammation and subsequent infection ensue, manifesting as red streaks on the skin.
- The inflammation or infection then extends proximally toward regional lymph nodes.

ETIOLOGY
- In individuals with normal host defenses, group A beta-hemolytic streptococcal (GABHS) species are the most common causes of lymphangitis.
- Lymphangitis is more likely to occur in patients with cellulitis due to GABHS than in patients with cellulitis caused by *Staphylococcus aureus*.
- Other organisms include S. aureus and *Pseudomonas* species. *Streptococcus pneumoniae* is a relatively uncommon cause of lymphangitis.
- *Pasteurella multocida*, associated with dog and cat bites, can cause cellulitis and lymphangitis.
- In immunocompromised hosts, gram-negative rods, gram-negative bacilli, and fungi may cause cellulitis and resultant lymphangitis.
- Wounds that occur in freshwater can become contaminated with *Aeromonas hydrophila*.
- Worldwide, *Wuchereria bancrofti* is a major cause of acute lymphangitis. Signs and symptoms of lymphangitis caused by W. *bancrofti* are indistinguishable from those of lymphangitis caused by bacteria.

- Children with diabetes, immunodeficiency, varicella, chronic steroid use (2), or other systemic illnesses have increased risk of developing serious or rapidly spreading lymphangitis.
- Nodular lymphangitis (with a sporotrichoid distribution) is usually due to Sporothrix schenckii, Mycobacterium marinum, Nocardia brasiliensis, Leishmania braziliensis (3). Other pathogens involved are the following: *Streptococcus pyogenes*, *S. aureus, Bacillus anthracis, Francisella tularensis, Pseudomonas pseudomallei*, atypical mycobacteria, Fungi (*Blastomyces dermatitidis, Coccidioides immitis, Cryptococcus neoformans, Histoplasma capsulatum*) (4).
- Bite from venomous snake
- *Rickettsia sibirica* mongolotimonae (5)
- Erysipelas is associated with lymphangitis (6)
- Carcinomatous lymphangitis (7)

 DIAGNOSIS

HISTORY
- A history of trauma (either minor or major) to an area of skin distal to the site of infection is often elicited in patients with lymphangitis.
- Children with lymphangitis often have fever, chills, and malaise.
- Some children may report a headache, loss of appetite, and muscle aches.
- Patients often have a history of a recent cut or abrasion or of an area of skin that appears infected and spreading.
- Lymphangitis can progress rapidly to bacteremia and disseminated infection and sepsis, particularly when caused by group A streptococci.

PHYSICAL EXAM
- Erythematous and irregular linear streaks extend from the primary infection site toward draining regional nodes.
- These streaks may be tender and warm.
- The primary site may be an abscess, an infected wound, or an area of cellulitis.
- Blistering of the affected skin may occur.
- Lymph nodes associated with the infected lymphatic channels are often swollen and tender.
- Children may be febrile and tachycardic.

DIAGNOSTIC TESTS & INTERPRETATION
Lab
- A CBC count and blood culture should be obtained. In addition, a leading-edge culture or aspiration of pus should be considered.
- The CBC and differential counts often reveal marked leukocytosis.
- Blood cultures may reveal that infection has spread to the bloodstream; however, results are rarely positive.
- Culture and Gram staining of aspirate from the primary site of infection may help in identifying the infectious organism and aid in choosing antimicrobials.
- Aspiration of the leading edge of maximal inflammation is recommended as it is thought to be helpful in the acute management of cases of acute lymphangitis.

Imaging
Plain radiography is unnecessary in routine cases.

Diagnostic Procedures/Other
- Abscessed areas may require incision and drainage.
- Cultures and Gram staining of fluid may help identify the causative organism and help select appropriate antimicrobial agents.
- Cultures for fungi or mycobacteria if nodular lymphangitis is present.
- Histopathological examination may be necessary (3,4).

DIFFERENTIAL DIAGNOSIS
- Contact dermatitis
- Cellulitis
- Septic thrombophlebitis
- Superficial thrombophlebitis
- Necrotizing fasciitis
- Myositis
- Sporotrichosis

TREATMENT

MEDICATION

- Treat patients with lymphangitis with an appropriate antimicrobial agent.
- Provide empiric coverage for group A *streptococcal* species and *S. aureus* (8).
- Acceptable outpatient regimens include penicillinase-resistant synthetic penicillin or a first-generation cephalosporin (9).
- Acceptable inpatient regimens include a second- or third-generation cephalosporin (e.g., cefuroxime, ceftriaxone) or a penicillinase-resistant synthetic penicillin. In certain geographical areas of the country with high rates of methicillin-resistant *S. aureus* (MRSA), alternative antimicrobial agents such as clindamycin or trimethoprim-sulfamethoxazole (TMP-SMZ) should be considered (10).
- Children in stable social situations who appear non-toxemic and who are older than 3 years, afebrile, and well hydrated may be treated initially with oral (PO) antibiotics on an outpatient basis. Ensure close follow-up.
- Parenteral antibiotics may be required for a patient with signs of systemic illness (e.g., fever, chills and myalgia, lymphangitis).
- Aggressively treat suspected cases of GABHS; these cases can progress rapidly and have been associated with serious complications.
- Analgesics can be used to control pain, and anti-inflammatory medications can help reduce inflammation and swelling. Hot, moist compresses also help reduce inflammation and pain.

ADDITIONAL TREATMENT
General Measures
- Some patients with lymphangitis may require admission for intravenous (IV) antimicrobial therapy, esp. for children younger than 3 years or children who are febrile and who appear toxic.
- Children who have not improved clinically after 48 hours of appropriate PO antimicrobial therapy should receive IV anti-staphylococcal and antistreptococcal therapy.
- When erythema, warmth, and edema are markedly reduced, antibiotics can be changed to the oral (PO) route.
- Foot care is important in terms of providing protection against trauma or treatment with antifungals of tinea pedis.

 ONGOING CARE

PROGNOSIS
- The prognosis for patients with uncomplicated lymphangitis is good.
- Antimicrobial regimens are effective in more than 90% of cases.

COMPLICATIONS
- Lymphangitis may spread within hours.
- Bacteremia and sepsis can occur.
- Without appropriate antimicrobial therapy, cellulitis may develop or extend along the channels; necrosis and ulceration may occur.
- Lymphangitis caused by GABHS can progress rapidly, leading to bacteremia, sepsis, and death.
- Guidelines to prevent transmission of methicillin-resistant *S. aureus* have been established.

REFERENCES

1. Abraham S, Tschanz C, Krischer J, et al. Lymphangitis due to insect sting. *Dermatology* 2007;215:260–261.
2. Boughrara Z, Ingen-Housz-Oro S, Legrand P, et al. Cutaneous infections in bullous pemphigoid patients treated with topical corticosteroids. *Ann Dermatol Venereol* 2010;137:345–351.
3. Tobin EH, Jih WW. Sporotrichoid lymphocutaneous infections: Etiology, diagnosis and therapy. *Am Fam Physician* 2001;63: 326–332.
4. Kostman JR, DiNubile MJ. Nodular lymphangitis: A distinctive but often unrecognized syndrome. *Ann Intern Med* 1993;118:883–888.
5. Fournier PE, Gouriet F, Brouqui P, et al. Lymphangitis-associated rickettsiosis, a new rickettsiosis caused by Rickettsia sibirica mongolotimonae: Seven new cases and review of the literature. *Clin Infect Dis* 2005;40:1435–1444.
6. Bonnetblanc JM, Bédane C. Erysipelas: Recognition and management. *Am J Clin Dermatol* 2003;4:157–163.
7. Damstra RJ, Jagtman EA, Steijlen PM.Cancer-related secondary lymphoedema due to cutaneous lymphangitis carcinomatosa: Clinical presentations and review of literature. *Eur J Cancer Care (Engl)* 2010;19:669–675.
8. Hirschmann JV. Antimicrobial therapy for skin infections. *Cutis* 2007;79:26–36.
9. Badger C, Seers K, Preston N, et al. Antibiotics/anti-inflammatories for reducing acute inflammatory episodes in lymphoedema of the limbs. *Cochrane Database Syst Rev* 2004: CD003143.
10. Calfee DP, Salgado CD, Classen D, et al. Strategies to prevent transmission of methicillin-resistant Staphylococcus aureus in acute care hospitals. *Infect Control Hosp Epidemiol* 2008;29(Suppl 1): S62–S80.

 CODES

ICD9
457.2 Lymphangitis

CLINICAL PEARLS

- Consider local data regarding MRSA prevalence when prescribing anti-staphylococcal treatment.
- Try to discern whether nodular lymphangitis is present, which, according to its cause, may necessitate more specific treatment.
- Be meticulous in identifying even minor trauma on physical examination.
- Consider carcinomatous lymphangitis in difficult-to-treat cases.

L

LYMPHOGRANULOMA VENEREUM

Paschalis I. Vergidis
Matthew E. Falagas

BASICS

DESCRIPTION
Lymphogranuloma venereum (LGV) is a sexually transmitted infection manifested as one or more lesions at the site of inoculation.

EPIDEMIOLOGY
Prevalence
- Endemic in Africa, South America, and parts of Asia.
- Rare in North America, Europe, Australia, but outbreaks have been reported in men who have sex with men.
- 6–10 times more common in men than in women.

RISK FACTORS
- Geographic location in endemic areas: Residence, travel, and work.
- Inconsistent use of barrier contraceptives.
- HIV seropositivity.

GENERAL PREVENTION
Safe sex; use of barrier contraceptives.

ETIOLOGY
Chlamydia trachomatis serovars L1, L2, L3

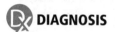

DIAGNOSIS

HISTORY
Incubation period: 5–21 days

PHYSICAL EXAM
- Primary stage:
  - Small herpetiform or papular genital lesion. This is self-limited. By the time the patient seeks care, the lesion may have resolved.
  - Cervicitis may occur in women.
- Secondary stage:
  - Tender inguinal and/or femoral lymphadenopathy ("groove" sign) that is typically unilateral. Bilateral lymphadenopathy occurs in 30%; it can be extensive.

- If untreated, the lymph nodes can ulcerate and drain. This occurs in one-third of patients. This is more commonly seen in chancroid.
  - Anorectal diseases in women and in men who have sex with men: Anal pruritus, mucus, mucopurulent rectal discharge, rectal pain, and tenesmus. Systemic symptoms, such as fever, may be prominent.
- Late stage:
  - Fibrosis and strictures in the anogenital tract.
  - Lymphatic obstruction causes genital elephantiasis.
- History and physical examination alone often lead to an inaccurate diagnosis.

DIAGNOSTIC TESTS & INTERPRETATION
Lab
- Genital and lymph node specimens (i.e., lesion swab or bubo aspirate) may be tested for *C. trachomatis* by culture, direct immunofluorescence, or nucleic acid detection.
- Nucleic acid amplification tests for *C. trachomatis* are not FDA-cleared for testing rectal specimens.
- Serologic tests support the diagnosis in the appropriate setting. These tests are not standardized.
- Complement fixation (titers >1:64).
- Microimmunofluorescence test
- Isolation of LGV Chlamydia serovars
- In patients with suspected proctocolitis (1), empiric treatment should be given pending the results of laboratory tests.

Diagnostic Procedures/Other
- Gently abrade the lesion with a sterile gauze pad to provoke oozing, but not gross bleeding.
- Squeeze the lesion between a gloved thumb and forefinger to increase exudate from the lesion.
- Apply the exudate directly onto a microscope slide if used for dark-field and direct immunofluorescence tests.

Pathological Findings
- Biopsy of lymph nodes shows areas of necrosis, which may enlarge to form stellate abscesses.
- Anorectal disease is characterized by granular or ulcerative proctitis.

DIFFERENTIAL DIAGNOSIS
- Urethritis
- Mucopurulent cervicitis
- Pelvic inflammatory disease
- Proctitis
- Proctocolitis

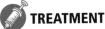 TREATMENT

MEDICATION

First Line
- Doxycycline 100 mg PO 2 times per day for 21 days (2).
- HIV-infected patients may need longer treatment.

Second Line
- Erythromycin base 500 mg PO 4 times per day for 21 days.
- Azithromycin 1 g orally once weekly for 3 weeks is probably effective, although clinical data are lacking.
- Sulfonamide treatment may not sterilize LGV lesions, and treatment failures have occurred.

Pregnancy Considerations
- Doxycycline is contraindicated.
- Treatment of choice is erythromycin.
- Azithromycin may prove a safe alternative.

SURGERY/OTHER PROCEDURES
Fluctuant inguinal lymph nodes may require aspiration or incision and drainage through intact skin.

 ONGOING CARE

FOLLOW-UP RECOMMENDATIONS
- Examination, serologic testing, and presumptive treatment of sexual partners.
- Persons who have had sexual contact with an LGV patient within 60 days before onset of the patient's symptoms should be examined and tested for urethral or cervical *Chlamydia* infection, and treated with a standard *Chlamydia* regimen (Azithromycin 1 g orally once or doxycycline 100 mg orally twice a day for 7 days).

COMPLICATIONS
- If left untreated, LGV leads to fibrosis of lymph nodes, fistulas, strictures, frozen pelvis, and infertility.
- Secondary bacterial superinfection.

REFERENCES

1. van der Bij AK, Spaargaren J, Morre SA, et al. Diagnostic and clinical implications of anorectal lymphogranuloma venereum in men who have sex with men: A retrospective case-control study. *Clin Infect Dis* 2006;42:186–194.
2. McLean CA, Stoner BP, Workowski KA. Treatment of lymphogranuloma venereum. *Clin Infect Dis* 2007;44(Suppl 3):S147–S152.

ADDITIONAL READING

- Mabey D, Peeling RW. Lymphogranuloma venereum. *Sex Transm Inf* 2002;78(2):90–2.
- Workowski KA, Berman SM. Sexually transmitted diseases treatment guidelines, 2010. *MMWR Recomm Rep* 2010;59(RR-12):1–110.

 CODES

ICD9
099.1 Lymphogranuloma venereum

CLINICAL PEARLS
- LGV, caused by *C. trachomatis* serovars L1, L2, L3, may lead to severe inflammation, in contrast to infection due to *C. trachomatis* serovars A through K.
- Serologic tests for LGV are not standardized and should be interpreted in the appropriate clinical context.
- Empiric therapy should be started in suspected proctocolitis, pending the results of laboratory tests.

L

MALARIA

Padma Srikanth
Paschalis Vergidis
Matthew E. Falagas

 BASICS

DESCRIPTION
Malaria is a vector-borne disease transmitted by the female *Anopheles* mosquito and is caused by a protozoan parasite.

EPIDEMIOLOGY
Incidence
- Every year 300–500 million people suffer from this disease and 1.5–3 million die (mostly children).
- *P. falciparum* occurs in Africa, Papua New Guinea, Haiti, and East Asia.
- *P. vivax* occurs in Central and South America, India, North Africa, and East Asia.
- *P. ovale* occurs in West Africa.
- *P. malariae* is present worldwide, but it is found mostly in Africa.

Prevalence
Malaria affects more than 2,400 million people, over 40% of the world's population, in more than 100 countries in the tropics.

RISK FACTORS
- Travel to endemic areas
- Rarely blood transfusion, mother to fetus transmission

Genetics
- Presence of HLA antigen Bw53 may protect against severe disease among children.
- *P. vivax* requires red cell antigens (Duffy factor) to invade red blood cells (RBCs). *P. vivax* infection is uncommon in blacks because their RBCs lack the Duffy factor.
- Sickle cell trait confers a survival advantage.

GENERAL PREVENTION
- Reducing vector–human contact with use of insecticide-impregnated bed nets or insect repellants containing DEET
- For chloroquine-susceptible malaria:
  – Chloroquine 300 mg base PO once weekly starting 1 week prior to exposure, during exposure, and for 4 weeks following exposure
- For chloroquine-resistant and chloroquine-susceptible malaria:
  – Atovaquone-proguanil daily beginning 2 days prior to exposure, during exposure, and for 1 week following exposure
  – Mefloquine 250 mg PO weekly beginning 2 weeks prior to exposure, during exposure, and for 4 weeks following exposure.
  – Doxycycline 100 mg PO daily beginning 2 days prior to exposure, during exposure, and daily for 4 weeks following exposure.
- Individuals born in endemic areas, who have emigrated outside these areas, are at risk of disease upon return due to waning immunity.

PATHOPHYSIOLOGY
- During a blood meal, a malaria-infected mosquito inoculates sporozoites into the human host. Sporozoites infect liver cells and mature into schizonts, which rupture and release merozoites.
- The time from insect bite to the release of merozoites into the bloodstream varies:
  – *P. falciparum*: between 5–15 days
  – *P. vivax*: 13.4 days
  – *P. ovale*: 14.1 days
  – *P. malariae*: 34.7 days
- Malaria causes hemolysis of parasitized RBCs that activates cytokines.
- *P. falciparum* infections are more severe due to the phenomenon of cyto-adherence. Characteristic knobs on the surface of parasitized RBCs enable cyto-adherence to endothelial cells in capillaries and post-capillary venules, and their sequestration in affected organs.
- Sequestration of *P. falciparum* parasitized red cells contributes to low oxygen tension, which increases sickling of parasitized HbAS cells.
- Sickle-hemoglobin protects against severe falciparum malaria, but does not protect against parasites that do not sequestrate (*P. vivax*, *P. malariae*, and *P. ovale*).

ETIOLOGY
- *P. falciparum* and *P. vivax* account for 95% of the infections
- *P. falciparum* can invade erythrocytes at all stages of maturation, is responsible for severe disease, and is often drug resistant. Because of the lack of a dormant live stage, *P. falciparum* does not cause relapses.
- *P. vivax* and *P. ovale* cause acute illness, and late relapse over 6–11 months after acute infection
- *P. malariae* infections may persist for decades within the bloodstream, but relapse does not occur, except under rare circumstances, such as trauma or surgery
- *P. knowlesi* has been recently recognized in Southeast Asia

COMMONLY ASSOCIATED CONDITIONS
Gram-negative bacteremia, sepsis

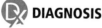 **DIAGNOSIS**

HISTORY
- History of travel to endemic area
- Cyclical fever (Periodicity not a reliable clue to diagnosis)
  – Tertian (every 48 hours) for *P. falciparum*, *P. vivax*, and *P. ovale*
  – Quartan (every 72 hours) for *P. malariae*
- Malaise, fatigue
- Myalgias
- Headache
- Back pain
- Flu-like symptoms, cough
- Vomiting, diarrhea, abdominal cramping

PHYSICAL EXAM
- The malarial paroxysm is characterized by 3 stages:
  – "Cold or chilling stage" that lasts 15 minutes to several hours
  – "Hot stage" lasts for several hours (this coincides with schizont rupture), temperature $\geq 40\,^{\circ}$C. Risk of convulsions, hyperthermia, and brain damage
  – "Sweating stage" (after 2–6 hours) characterized by resolution of fever and intense fatigue.
- Tachycardia
- Hypertension
- Splenomegaly

DIAGNOSTIC TESTS & INTERPRETATION
Lab
Initial lab tests
- Anemia
- Thrombocytopenia
- Decreased haptoglobin, increased lactate dehydrogenase and reticulocytes
- Microscopic examination of thin and thick smear for diagnosis and species identification. Sensitivity and specificity depends on the skill of the performer.
- Rapid detection tests targeting malarial antigens.
  – Targets conserved across all human malarias include: Plasmodium lactate dehydrogenase and aldolase enzymes
  – Diagnostic targets specific for *P. falciparum* include: Histidine-rich protein-2 (HRP-2) and *P. falciparum* lactate dehydrogenase
- BinaxNOW Malaria test is FDA-approved and targets HRP-2 and aldolase. Sensitivity and specificity for *P. falciparum* are >95% (1). Sensitivity is lower for other malaria species.
- Polymerase chain reaction (PCR) and other molecular techniques. Used for diagnosis but not widely available. Also used to confirm species.

Follow-Up & Special Considerations
- Monitor for acute renal failure (proteinuria, hemoglobinuria, and increased serum creatinine).
- Monitor peripheral smears to determine response to therapy.

Imaging
Generally not helpful except in cerebral malaria where CT/MRI may be indicated.

Pathological Findings
- Multiorgan failure occurs due to:
  – Diffuse microvascular disease resulting from large numbers of adherent parasitized red cells that cause a functional obstruction to flow
  – Damage following hypoxia and hypoglycemia.
- Tissue damage in the brain characterized by scattered ring hemorrhages and mild perivascular inflammation

DIFFERENTIAL DIAGNOSIS
- Influenza
- Typhoid fever
- Bacteremia
- Dengue fever
- Yellow fever
- Acute schistosomiasis
- East African trypanosomiasis
- Leptospirosis

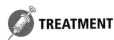 TREATMENT

MEDICATION
Uncomplicated malaria, chloroquine-susceptible
- Chloroquine phosphate 600 mg base orally, followed by 300 mg base at 6 hours, and on day 2 and day 3
- Eradication of persistent hypnozoites in *P. vivax* or *P. ovale* infection by primaquine 30 mg base once daily for 14 days.
  - Primaquine is contraindicated in persons with severe G6PD deficiency

Uncomplicated malaria, chloroquine-resistant
- Quinine sulfate 650 mg salt every 8 hours for 3–7 days plus doxycycline 100 mg PO b.i.d for 7 days (Instead of doxycycline, can use tetracycline or clindamycin for 7 days)
  - Note: For infections acquired in Southeast Asia, quinine treatment should continue for 7 days. For infections acquired elsewhere, quinine treatment should continue for 3 days.
- Atovaquone-proguanil (250 mg atovaquone/ 100 mg proguanil) 4 tablets PO daily for 3 days
- Artemether-lumefantrine (20 mg artemether/ 120 mg lumefantrine) 1st day: 4 tabs initially, followed by 4 tabs after 8 hours 2nd day: 4 tabs twice daily, 3rd day: 4 tabs twice daily.
- Mefloquine 750 mg salt orally, followed by 500 mg after 6–12 hours. Not recommended in persons who have acquired infections in Southeast Asia (due to drug resistance)

Severe *P. falciparum* malaria or severe *P. knowlesi* malaria
- Quinidine 10 mg salt/kg IV loading dose in normal saline over 2 hours, followed by 0.02 mg/kg/min until oral therapy can be started. Complete therapy with quinine plus doxycycline regimen to complete a 7-day total course of therapy.
  - Monitor for QT prolongation while on quinidine treatment
- Quinine dihydrochloride 20 mg/kg IV loading dose in 5% dextrose infused slowly at a constant rate over 4 hours, followed by maintenance dose 10 mg/kg over 3–4 hours at 8-hour intervals until oral therapy can be started. Complete treatment with oral quinine.

- Artesunate (2) 2.4 mg/kg IV as first dose, followed by 2.4 mg/kg at 12 and 24 hours, followed by 2.4 mg/kg once daily. Usually given for a total of 3 days
- Artemether 3.2 mg/kg IM on first day, followed by 1.6 mg/kg daily for 4 days.
  - After artemisin derivative treatment, complete therapy with a standard dose of atovaquone-proguanil, mefloquine, doxycycline, or clindamycin.

ADDITIONAL TREATMENT
General Measures
Supportive measures in the intensive care unit for severe malaria

Additional Therapies
Exchange blood transfusions are used adjunctively in hyperparasitemia.

IN-PATIENT CONSIDERATIONS
Initial Stabilization
- Intense care for all patients with signs of severe illness
- Monitoring for hypoglycemia and hyponatremia

Admission Criteria
- *P. falciparum* malaria in a nonimmune individual (Increased risk for complications, even if they appear well on presentation)
- Persistent fever
- Hypoglycemia
- Complications of *P. falciparum* malaria

IV Fluids
Isotonic saline (1000–3000 mL during the first 24 hours of hospital admission)

Discharge Criteria
Clinical improvement, ability to take oral medications, documented decreasing parasitemia levels

 ONGOING CARE

FOLLOW-UP RECOMMENDATIONS
- Further inpatient care:
  - Perform thick and thin blood smears every 6–12 hours until parasitemia falls below 1% to monitor response. If parasitemia does not fall by 75% within 48 hours or if the blood is not cleared of parasites after 7 days, initiate a different therapeutic regimen immediately.
- Further outpatient care: Obtain thick and thin blood smears weekly for 1 month post commencement of treatment.

PATIENT EDUCATION
- Inform travelers about the prevention of malaria
- Advise treated patients about the risk of relapse

PROGNOSIS
- Patients with uncomplicated malaria show marked improvement within 48 hours after the initiation of treatment and are afebrile after 96 hours
- *P. falciparum* infection carries a poor prognosis with a high mortality rate if untreated. However, if diagnosed early and treated appropriately, prognosis is good.

COMPLICATIONS
- Cerebral malaria: More common with *P. falciparum* due to microvascular obstruction
- Convulsions and coma – more common in children
- Hypoglycemia
- Lactic acidosis
- Hyperthermia
- Acute renal failure – more common in nonimmune individuals, usually oliguric with severe *P. falciparum* infection
- Blackwater fever (hemoglobinuria and malarial pigment in the urine)
- Pulmonary edema – uncommon
- Gastroenteritis – common in young children
- Anemia

REFERENCES
1. Stauffer WM, Cartwright CP, Olson DA, et al. Diagnostic performance of rapid diagnostic tests versus blood smears for malaria in US clinical practice. *Clin Infect Dis* 2009;49(6):908–913.
2. Dondorp A, Nosten F, Stepniewska K, et al. Artesunate versus quinine for treatment of severe falciparum malaria: A randomised trial. *Lancet* 2005;366(9487):717–725.

ADDITIONAL READING
- WHO – Guidelines for the treatment of malaria http://www.who.int/malaria/publications/atoz/ 9789241547925/en/index.html.
- CDC – Treatment of Malaria: Guidelines for Clinicians http://www.cdc.gov/malaria/diagnosis_ treatment/index.html.

 CODES

ICD9
- 084.0 Falciparum malaria (malignant tertian)
- 084.1 Vivax malaria (benign tertian)
- 084.6 Malaria, unspecified

CLINICAL PEARLS
- Rapid diagnostic tests are useful in determining if the patient has *P. falciparum* malaria.
- Artemisinin and its derivatives should not be used as monotherapy.
- Nonimmune individuals with *P. falciparum* malaria are at risk for severe disease and must be hospitalized.

M

MASTITIS

Stavros S. Athanasiou
Petros I. Rafailidis
Matthew E. Falagas

 BASICS

DESCRIPTION
- Mastitis is an infectious inflammation of the breast.
- Most commonly affects breast-feeding women (puerperial mastitis).

EPIDEMIOLOGY
Incidence
- The incidence of mastitis in women who were breastfeeding is 20% in the 6 months after delivery (1).
- Peak incidence occurs within the first 2 months after delivery (1).

RISK FACTORS
- Nipple damage
- Plugged ducts
- Local milk stasis
- Engorgement
- Infant attachment difficulties
- Cleft lip or palate
- History of mastitis with a previous child (2)
- Using a manual breast pump (2)
- Using only 1 position to breast-feed
- Published evidence suggests that supplementation of HIV-infected women with vitamins increased the risk of subclinical mastitis (3).
- No association has been established between maternal nasal carriage of *Staphylococcus aureus* and mastitis. However, published evidence suggests that nasal carriage in the infant may be associated with mastitis (4).

GENERAL PREVENTION
- Prompt attention to any signs of milk stasis
- Care should be taken when cracked nipples occur.
- Optimizing breastfeeding techniques to avoid milk stasis
- Published evidence suggests that bedside hand disinfection by breastfeeding mothers in the postpartum unit may lead to a reduction of the incidence of mastitis (5).
- Insufficient evidence to show effectiveness of interventions such as breastfeeding education, pharmacological treatments, and alternative therapies, with regard to the occurrence of mastitis (6).

PATHOPHYSIOLOGY
Insertion of bacteria from the infant's mouth and/or from the skin through cracked nipples, along with milk stasis and milk overproduction.

ETIOLOGY
- Usually, *Staphylococcus* spp. and *Streptococcus* spp. are isolated from the breast.
- *Methicillin-resistant S. aureus* (MRSA) has emerged in patients with puerperal mastitis during the past decade (7,8).
- *Mycobacterium tuberculosis* (may be associated with tuberculous tonsillitis in the infant.)
- *Escherichia coli*
- *Candida* spp.

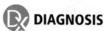 **DIAGNOSIS**

HISTORY
Diagnosis is mainly clinical.

PHYSICAL EXAM
- The spectrum of disease is from a small nodule to a large abscess.
- Breast tenderness and erythema
- Usually accompanied with fever, malaise, and fatigue
- Disease is unilateral, often in the upper and outer quadrants.
- Tender axillary lymph nodes may occur.
- Checking for possible extra-mammary tuberculosis infection.

DIAGNOSTIC TESTS & INTERPRETATION
Lab
- Cultures of milk, nipple drainage, or aspirated material.
- Blood culture in cases when the patient looks septic.

Imaging
- Ultrasonogram for identification of an underlying abscess, or for direction of needle-aspiration damage.
- Biopsy for identification of tissue infection, tuberculosis, and possible malignancy.

Diagnostic Procedures/Other
- Incision and drainage is needed if an abscess is present.
- In cases of recurrences in the same area, further evaluation (including ultrasonogram followed mammography in case of ambiguous results) is warranted to exclude an underlying breast mass.

DIFFERENTIAL DIAGNOSIS
- Idiopathic granulomatous mastitis
- Skin infections (e.g., streptococcal necrotizing fasciitis) may masquerade as mastitis (9).
- Carcinoma of the breast
- Engorgement of the breast from milk stasis (often bilateral and without fever/erythema)

 TREATMENT

MEDICATION
First Line
- Antibiotics such as dicloxacillin (125–500 mg 6 hourly), or cephalexin (250–500 mg 6 hourly) are recommended.
- In case of mastitis due to MRSA: Vancomycin, trimethoprim-sulfamethoxazole, clindamycin. Avoid continuation of breastfeeding in infants <2 months old or premature or ill or having increased levels of serum bilirubin, if prescribing trimethoprim-sulphamethoxazole. Glucose-6 dehydrogenase deficiency in the infant is also a contraindication to the use of trimethoprim-sulphomethoxazole.
- The recommended duration of antibiotic treatment is 10–14 days (10).
- Analgesics, anti-inflammatory agents
- Lactation should not be stopped during an episode of mastitis to avoid milk stasis!
- Concurrent treatment of the neonate may be considered, especially if streptococcal infection is involved

ADDITIONAL TREATMENT
General Measures
- Frequent breast drainage to avoid milk stasis (continuing breastfeeding – pumping – hand expression)
- Moist heat (hot compresses) is applied to the breast.
- Bed rest and avoidance of wearing a constricting bra are recommended.

COMPLEMENTARY & ALTERNATIVE THERAPIES
- Supportive counseling is very important.
- A recent randomized controlled trial (RCT) suggested that orally administered probiotics (specifically, *L. fermentum* CECT5716 or *L. salivarius* CECT5713) may potentially be a useful alternative to antibiotics treatment option for mastitis (11)
- The evidence are insufficient to support a beneficial effect of homeopathic remedies including chamomilla and sulfur (12)

SURGERY/OTHER PROCEDURES
- In case of breast abscess: Incision and drainage or ultrasound-guided needle aspiration, parenteral antibiotics may also be required
- Surgery may be required in some patients who have developed mastitis in previously reconstructed breasts. A plastic surgeon should be consulted.

IN-PATIENT CONSIDERATIONS
Admission Criteria
Community-acquired MRSA seems to be associated with the development of breast abscess that requires incision and drainage and results in discontinuation of breastfeeding (7,8).

ONGOING CARE

FOLLOW-UP RECOMMENDATIONS
- Supportive counseling is very important.
- Optimizing breastfeeding techniques to avoid milk stasis
- In cases of recurrences in the same area, further evaluation is warranted to exclude an underlying breast mass.

PROGNOSIS
Mastitis usually resolves with treatment.

COMPLICATIONS
- Recurrent mastitis
- Breast abscess
- Sepsis and septic shock

REFERENCES
1. Kinlay JR, O'Connell DL, Kinlay S. Incidence of mastitis in breastfeeding women during the six months after delivery: A prospective cohort study. *Med J Aust* 1998;21;169(6):310–312.
2. Foxman B, D'Arcy H, Gillespie B, et al. Lactation mastitis: Occurrence and medical management among 946 breastfeeding women in the United States. *Am J Epidemiol* 2002;155(2):103–114.
3. Arsenault JE, Aboud S, Manji KP, et al. Vitamin supplementation increases risk of subclinical mastitis in HIV-infected women. *J Nutr* 2010; 140(10):1788–1792.
4. Amir LH, Garland SM, Lumley J. A case-control study of mastitis: Nasal carriage of Staphylococcus aureus. *BMC Fam Pract* 2006;7:57.
5. Peters F, Flick-Filliés D. Hand disinfection to prevent puerperial mastitis. *Lancet* 1991; 338(8770):831.
6. Crepinsek MA, Crowe L, Michener K, et al. Interventions for preventing mastitis after childbirth. *Cochrane Database Syst Rev* 2010; (8):CD007239.
7. Lee IW, Kang L, Hsu HP, Kuo PL, Chang CM. Puerperal mastitis requiring hospitalization during a nine-year period. *Am J Obstet Gynecol* 2010; 203(4):332.e1–332.e6.
8. Stafford I, Hernandez J, Laibl V, Sheffield J, Roberts S, Wendel G Jr. Community-acquired methicillin-resistant Staphylococcus aureus among patients with puerperal mastitis requiring hospitalization. *Obstet Gynecol* 2008;112(3): 533–537.
9. Tillett RL, Saxby PJ, Stone CA, et al. Group A streptococcal necrotising fasciitis masquerading as mastitis. *Lancet* 2006;368(9530):174.
10. World Health Organization, Geneva 2002, Mastitis, Causes and Management.
11. Arroyo R, Martín V, Maldonado A, et al. Treatment of infectious mastitis during lactation: Antibiotics versus oral administration of Lactobacilli isolated from breast milk. *Clin Infect Dis* 2010;50(12):1551–1558.
12. Fetherston C. Management of lactation mastitis in a Western Australian cohort. *Breastfeed Rev* 1997;5(2):13–19.

ADDITIONAL READING
- Han BK, Choe YH, Park JM, et al. Granulomatous mastitis: Mammographic and sonographic appearances. *AJR* 1999;173(2):317–320.
- O'Hara RJ, Dexter SP, Fox JN. Conservative management of infective mastitis and breast abscesses after ultrasonographic assessment. *Br J Surg* 1996;83(10):1413–1414.
- Schoenfeld EM, McKay MP. Mastitis and methicillin-resistant Staphylococcus aureus (MRSA): The calm before the storm? *J Emerg Med* 2010; 38(4):e31–e34.
- Vogel A, Hutchison BL, Mitchell EA. Mastitis in the first year postpartum. *Birth* 1999;26(4):218–225.

 CODES

ICD9
- 611.0 Inflammatory disease of breast
- 675.20 Nonpurulent mastitis associated with childbirth, unspecified as to episode of care

CLINICAL PEARLS
- Breastfeeding should be continued to avoid milk stasis
- Community-acquired MRSA should be considered in diagnosis
- Recurrent episodes warrant further investigation to exclude an underlying breast mass.

M

MASTOIDITIS

Petros I. Rafailidis
Matthew E. Falagas

 BASICS

DESCRIPTION
- Mastoiditis is the inflammation of the mastoid air cells, classified as acute or chronic, depending on the duration of infection.
- Specifically, painless otorrhea with duration >3 weeks, in conjunction with a perforated tympanic membrane (either due to the disease or through iatrogenic tube insertion) is the hallmark of chronic mastoiditis.

EPIDEMIOLOGY
Incidence
- The incidence of mastoiditis has decreased significantly in the antibiotic era because of prompt treatment of otitis media with antimicrobial agents.
- However, since a watchful waiting approach has been adopted for the treatment of acute otitis media, the incidence has increased in some countries during the last decade (1) but not in other (2).
- The incidence is 1.2–2/100000 patient years in the US and Canada, while the incidence may reach 3.8/100000 patient years in European countries (3).
- Furthermore, the increasing resistance of microbes to antimicrobial agents during recent years has been associated with increasing rates of mastoiditis (4).

RISK FACTORS
- Inadequate treatment of otitis media.
- Non-vaccination against *Streptococcus pneumoniae* (*S. pneumoniae*) and *Haemophilus influenzae* (*H. influenzae*).
- Presence of cochlear implants.

GENERAL PREVENTION
- Early treatment of acute otitis media with effective antibiotics.
- Vaccination against *S. pneumoniae* and *H. influenzae*.
- Testing with audiogram in case history of recurrent acute otitis media and hearing problem.

ETIOLOGY
- Infection of the mastoid air cells usually follows middle ear infection.
- In acute mastoiditis, the involved bacteria are similar to those implicated in acute otitis media (usually *S. pneumoniae* and *H. influenzae*), except for *Moraxella catarrhalis* (5).
- Serotypes not included in the current vaccines against *S. pneumoniae* and *H. influenzae* are responsible for the majority of cases.
- *Pseudomonas aeruginosa* and *Streptococcus pyogenes* are significant causes of acute mastoiditis (6).
- *Staphylococcus aureus* is responsible for a small minority of cases of acute mastoiditis.

- In cases of chronic mastoiditis, *P. aeruginosa*, *Staphylococcus aureus*, gram-negative bacilli, and anaerobes are frequently involved. Polymicrobial causes are usual.
- Tuberculosis and atypical mycobacterial infections are rare causes of chronic mastoiditis.
- Rarely, fungi (mainly *Aspergillus*) can cause mastoiditis in immunosuppressed persons.

COMMONLY ASSOCIATED CONDITIONS
Acute otitis media

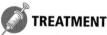 **DIAGNOSIS**

HISTORY
Acute otitis media (fever, ear pain, and impaired hearing).

PHYSICAL EXAM
- Erythematous tympanic membrane.
- Otorrhea ear discharge.
- Postauricular pain, tenderness, swelling, and fluctuance over the mastoid bone.
- The pinna is often displaced outward and downward.
- Vestibular signs (vertigo)
- Cervical signs (mass, edema)
- Chronic mastoiditis may be manifested by hearing loss, persistent ear discharge, and/or ear pain (although the latter may be lacking).

DIAGNOSTIC TESTS & INTERPRETATION
Lab
Usually involve increased white blood cell count, C-reactive protein, and erythrocyte sedimentation rate. Interestingly, a higher number of WBC and CRP are reported to differentiate among children with simple versus complicated mastoiditis (7).

Imaging
Initial approach
- Radiography reveals coalescence of the mastoid air cells due to destruction of their bony septa. Also, it may show haziness of the mastoid air cells due to the presence of fluid.
- CT scan or MRI is very helpful in evaluating the extension of the disease.

Follow-Up & Special Considerations
- Clinical follow-up, especially in regard to the presence of neurological signs (focal or diffuse), nonresponse to conservative treatment is of paramount importance and should not be deemed inferior to radiological imaging.

Diagnostic Procedures/Other
Cultures of ear discharge should be taken (if the tympanic membrane is not perforated, tympanocentesis should be performed).

Pathological Findings
Evidence of acute or subacute infection in cases of acute mastoiditis (8). An infiltrate consisting of lymphocytes, macrophages, and plasmacytes is present in chronic mastoiditis. A cholesteatoma is commonly an associated finding in chronic mastoiditis (9).

DIFFERENTIAL DIAGNOSIS
- Postauricular cellulitis
- Postauricular lymphadenopathy
- Parotitis
  - Tumors in the mastoid air cells.
  - Luc's abscess: Subperiosteal temporal collection without evidence of mastoid involvement.
  - Congenital cholesteatoma.
  - Histiocytosis X.

TREATMENT

MEDICATION
First Line

- In acute infection, therapy should be guided by results of the cultures of middle ear fluid. If there is no drainage of middle ear fluid, a myringotomy should be performed (10,11 [A]).
- Intravenous antimicrobial treatment is preferred for the initial management because mastoiditis is associated with a high probability of complications (12 [A]).

- An appropriate regimen for acute mastoiditis would therefore include a third or fourth generation cephalosporin (cefotaxime, ceftazidime, or cefepime), piperacillin/tazobactam, ticarcillin/clavulanate, or ciprofloxacin (not for children) for *P. aeruginosa*, or penicillin G for *S. pneumoniae* (or ceftriaxone/vancomycin for more resistant strains), or ampicillin/sulbactam (alternatively amoxicillin/clavulanate) for *H. influenzae*.
- Although the majority of data point to the fact that *S. pneumoniae* remain susceptible to penicillin in the vast majority, some data report increased resistance to ceftriaxone (13).
- An empirical combination regimen consisting of clindamycin (against gram-positives) plus aztreonam would cover potential culprits of acute mastoiditis.
- The recommended duration of treatment is 3–4 weeks. Oral antibiotics can be used after the initial successful management with intravenous antibiotics.
- A low threshold for ENT or neurosurgical consultation should exist, in case of doubt.

- In chronic mastoiditis the infection is usually polymicrobial. Treatment options against *P. aeruginosa* are those described above for acute mastoiditis. The role of treatment against *S. aureus* has to be pointed out.
- Aural toilet performed daily is an essential part of the initial conservative treatment of chronic mastoiditis.
- Local antibiotics (ofloxacin solution for aural use) may be attempted prior to or in addition to parenteral antibiotic treatment in patients with chronic mastoiditis.

ADDITIONAL TREATMENT
Issues for Referral
Neurological signs, presence of a postauricular abscess, coalescence of air cells, or erosion of the mastoid bone should lead to a referral to an ENT surgeon or neurosurgeon.

SURGERY/OTHER PROCEDURES
- Mastoidectomy (radical or canal wall up) (14–16[A]) should be performed when there is evidence of osteomyelitis (by CT scan or MRI), spread to the central nervous system, or failure of medical treatment.
- Surgery is also needed in cases of chronic mastoiditis that do not respond to antibiotic treatment. The empirical broad-spectrum perioperative antimicrobial therapy should be adjusted on the basis of culture results.
- A more conservative approach with retroauricular puncture and grommet tube (ventilation tube) insertion may be attempted when no intracranial complications are present and when the causative pathogen is not *Fusobacterium necrophorum* (11).
- In mastoiditis associated with cochlear implants, a more conservative approach with intravenous antibiotics and aspiration of the abscess has also been proposed (17).

IN-PATIENT CONSIDERATIONS
Admission Criteria
All children with mastoiditis should be admitted.

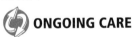 ONGOING CARE

FOLLOW-UP RECOMMENDATIONS
Follow-up audiograms are needed to check for hearing loss.

PROGNOSIS
Very good if diagnosis established early.

COMPLICATIONS
- Subperiosteal abscess of the temporal bone.
- Neck abscess deep to the sternocleidomastoid muscle (Bezold's abscess).
- Cellulitis
- Facial nerve paralysis

- Intracranial complications (epidural abscess, dural venous thrombophlebitis, meningitis, and brain abscess).
- Gradenigo syndrome: Ipsilateral paralysis of the 6th cranial nerve (abducens nerve), infliction of the 1st branch of the 5th cranial nerve (increased lacrimation, pain in the ipsilateral retro-orbital area, and reduced corneal sensation).
- Chronic mastoiditis may cause irreversible hearing loss.

REFERENCES
1. Van Zuijlen DA, Schilder AG, Van Balen FA, et al. National differences in incidence of acute mastoiditis: Relationship to prescribing patterns of antibiotics for acute otitis media? *Pediatr Infect Dis J* 2001;20:140–144.
2. Thorne MC, Chewaproug L, Elden LM. Suppurative complications of acute otitis media: Changes in frequency over time. *Arch Otolaryngol Head Neck Surg* 2009;135:638–641.
3. Stenfeldt K, Hermansson A. Acute mastoiditis in southern Sweden: A study of occurrence and clinical course of acute mastoiditis before and after introduction of new treatment recommendations for AOM. *Eur Arch Otorhinolaryngol* 2010;267(12):1855–1861.
4. Antonelli PJ, Dhanani N, Giannoni CM, et al. Impact of resistant pneumococcus on rates of acute mastoiditis. *Otolaryngol Head Neck Surg* 1999;121:190–194.
5. Broides A, Dagan R, Greenberg D, et al. Acute otitis media caused by Moraxella catarrhalis: Epidemiologic and clinical characteristics. *Clin Infect Dis* 2009;49:1641–1647.
6. Butbul-Aviel Y, Miron D, Halevy R, et al. Acute mastoiditis in children: Pseudomonas aeruginosa as a leading pathogen. *Int J Pediatr Otorhinolaryngol* 2003;67:277–281.
7. Bilavsky E, Yarden-Bilavsky H, Samra Z, et al. Clinical, laboratory, and microbiological differences between children with simple or complicated mastoiditis. *Int J Pediatr Otorhinolaryngol* 2009;73:1270–1273.
8. Stähelin-Massik J, Podvinec M, Jakscha J, et al. Mastoiditis in children: A prospective, observational study comparing clinical presentation, microbiology, computed tomography, surgical findings and histology. *Eur J Pediatr* 2008;167:541–548.
9. Popescu C, Ioni E, Mogoant CA, et al. Clinical and histopathological aspects in otomastoiditis. *Rom J Morphol Embryol* 2009;50:453–460.
10. Khafif A, Halperin D, Hochman I, et al. Acute mastoiditis: A 10-year review. *Am J Otolaryngol* 1998;19:170–173.
11. Trijolet JP, Bakhos D, Lanotte P, Pondaven S, et al. Acute mastoiditis in children: Can mastoidectomy be avoided? *Ann Otolaryngol Chir Cervicofac* 2009;126:169–174.

12. Katz A, Leibovitz E, Greenberg D, et al. Acute mastoiditis in Southern Israel: A twelve year retrospective study (1990 through 2001). *Pediatr Infect Dis J* 2003;22:878–882.
13. Roddy MG, Glazier SS, Agrawal D. Pediatric mastoiditis in the pneumococcal conjugate vaccine era: Symptom duration guides empiric antimicrobial therapy. *Pediatr Emerg Care* 2007;23:779–784.
14. Isaacson B, Mirabal C, Kutz JW Jr, et al. Pediatric otogenic intracranial abscesses. *Otolaryngol Head Neck Surg* 2010;142:434–437.
15. Taylor MF, Berkowitz RG. Indications for mastoidectomy in acute mastoiditis in children. *Ann Otol Rhinol Laryngol* 2004;113:69–72.
16. Zanetti D, Nassif N. Indications for surgery in acute mastoiditis and their complications in children. *Int J Pediatr Otorhinolaryngol* 2006;70:1175–1182.
17. Rodríguez V, Cavallé L, De Paula C, et al. Treatment of acute mastoiditis in children with cochlear implants. *Acta Otorrinolaringol Esp* 2010;61:180–183.

ADDITIONAL READING
- Lin HW, Shargorodsky J, Gopen Q. Clinical strategies for the management of acute mastoiditis in the pediatric population. *Clin Pediatr (Phila)* 2010; 49:110–115.
- Tamir S, Shwartz Y, Peleg U, et al. Shifting trends: Mastoiditis from a surgical to a medical disease. *Am J Otolaryngol* 2010;31:467–471.

CODES

ICD9
- 383.00 Acute mastoiditis without complications
- 383.1 Chronic mastoiditis
- 383.9 Unspecified mastoiditis

CLINICAL PEARLS
- Always examine the postauricular area for signs of infection.
- *S. pneumoniae* is still the commonest cause of acute mastoiditis despite vaccination.
- The physician has to think of specific treatment against *P. aeruginosa* and *S. aureus* in acute as well as chronic mastoiditis. As these are not common causes of acute otitis media (the usual precursor of mastoiditis), attention has to be paid.
- Loss of hearing may be a subtle finding during the initial stage of the disease and has to be specifically searched for.

M

MEASLES

Murat Akova
Matthew E. Falagas

BASICS

DESCRIPTION
- The disease is characterized by fever and a maculopapular rush starting from the head and spreading to trunk and extremities. The rash is preceded by coryza, conjunctivitis, and a characteristic enanthem namely Koplik's spots.
- Although the disease is usually benign in unvaccinated, immunocompetent children, it causes significant morbidity and mortality especially in malnourished children in the developing world and in those with immunosuppression.

EPIDEMIOLOGY
Incidence
- More than 20 million people are estimated to be affected by measles each year.
- 222,408 cases were reported by WHO from 193 countries worldwide, in 2009. Highest numbers were from Burkina Faso (54,118), China (52,461), Indonesia (20,818) and, Iraq (30,328).
- 82% of the susceptible population worldwide were estimated to be covered by measles vaccine.
- 60% of countries reached >90% vaccine coverage.
- Despite of these figures, there were 164,000 estimated deaths due to measles, in 2008 (1).

RISK FACTORS
- Any person without previous immunization. Young nonimmune healthcare workers are at risk and may themselves transmit disease to nonimmune or immunocompromised patients.
- Travel to countries where measles is endemic.
- Immunocompromised patients, pregnant women, persons with vitamin A deficiency (2) or poor nutritional status, and individuals at the extremes of age are at increased risk of complications.
- Outbreaks can cause significant mortality in areas during and after natural disasters and conflicts.
- 95% of measles deaths occur in low income countries.

GENERAL PREVENTION
- Measles can be prevented by vaccination (2).
- Routine vaccination (usually in combination with mumps and rubella (MMR) vaccine) with attenuated live vaccine at age 12–15 months, followed by a booster at ages 4–6 years (or any time >4 weeks after the 1st dose).
- In areas with high prevalence, the first dose can be administered at age 9 months.
- Asymptomatic and non-severely immunosuppressed AIDS/HIV patients can be vaccinated.
- The vaccine should be used with caution in severely immunocompromised for any reason.
- Adverse reactions to vaccine include:
  - Transient fever (5–15%) occurring 1–2 weeks after vaccination
  - Transient rash (5%)
  - Thrombocytopenia 1 per 25,000–40,000 doses
  - No evidence for any link between autism and measles vaccination
- Contraindications:
  - Pregnancy
  - Allergy against gelation or neomycin
  - Egg anaphylaxis is not a contraindication

PATHOPHYSIOLOGY
- It is spread by respiratory droplets.
- Invading respiratory mucosa the virus spreads to local lymph nodes, reticuloendothelial system, epithelial and endothelial cells including conjunctiva, lungs, intestines, and skin.
- Appearance of rash coincides with emerging serum antibody and termination of transmissibility of the disease.

ETIOLOGY
Measles is a viral disease caused by rubeola which is an RNA virus and a member of the family Paramyxoviridae, genus *Morbillivirus*.

COMMONLY ASSOCIATED CONDITIONS
- Respiratory symptoms and conjunctivitis precedes rash.
- Fever

DIAGNOSIS

HISTORY
History taking about incomplete or absence of vaccination, immunosuppression, and contact with infected person.

PHYSICAL EXAM
- Initial prodromal phase:
  - Fever
  - Cough
  - Conjunctivitis
  - Coryza
- Koplik's spots: 1 mm spots or grains along the buccal mucosa during the initial phase. Following this, patients develop a red maculopapular and sometimes confluent rash, initially occurring behind the ears and on the forehead, then proceeding down the body to the extremities.
- Patients have high fever during the time the rash is developing. In each location on the body, the rash usually takes 5 days to begin to clear.
- Desquamation of the hands and feet occurs in some cases.
- In adolescents or young adults who had received the live virus vaccination in early childhood but no booster, a mild, atypical infection can occur as immunity has waned. Cough; a mild, evanescent rash; and a pulmonary infiltrate are most common (3).

DIAGNOSTIC TESTS & INTERPRETATION
Lab
Initial lab tests
Leukopenia is frequent. T-cell cytopenia and thrombocytopenia may be observed

Follow-Up & Special Considerations
Serologic response may be sought in atypical cases and for documenting previous immunity.

Imaging
Initial approach
Chest x-ray may indicate interstitial pneumonitis.

Diagnostic Procedures/Other
- Measles antigen can be searched by immunofluorescent examination of cells from nasal secretions or urinary sediment.
- High measles antibody titers in serum and CSF may be diagnostic for subacute sclerosing panencephalitis (SSPE).

Pathological Findings
Virus isolation or searching viral RNA in infected tissues is difficult, but may be useful in patients with fatal pneumonia and in those with immunosuppression.

DIFFERENTIAL DIAGNOSIS
- Rubella
- Kawasaki syndrome
- Roseola
- Scarlet fever
- HHV-6 infection
- Infectious mononucleosis
- Rickettsial, enteroviral and adenoviral infections
- Dengue fever
- *Mycoplasma pneumoniae*

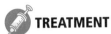 TREATMENT

MEDICATION
First Line
No approved antiviral therapy.

Second Line
- WHO recommends that 2 doses of vitamin A supplements be given 24 hours apart to all children with measles in developing countries.
- Immunosuppressed patients with severe measles may be treated with ribavirin (not approved by FDA).
- Antibiotics are reserved for secondary bacterial infections.

ADDITIONAL TREATMENT
Additional Therapies
Immune serum globulin (ISG), given within 6 days of exposure to a susceptible person may prevent or modify disease.

IN-PATIENT CONSIDERATIONS
- Respiratory isolation is required for admitted patients.
- Susceptible health care workers should not enter the patient's room.

 ONGOING CARE

FOLLOW-UP RECOMMENDATIONS
- Patients are advised to call their doctor if they develop any of the following while being affected by measles:
  – Difficulty breathing or noisy breathing
  – Changes in vision
  – Changes in behavior, confusion
  – Chest or abdominal pain

DIET
Ensure adequate diet, especially regarding vitamin A intake.

PATIENT EDUCATION
Regarding secondary complications

PROGNOSIS
- Recovery from measles gives lifelong immunity
- Complications are more common in <5 and >20 years of age
- Mortality can be up to 10% among malnourished children

COMPLICATIONS
- Bacterial pneumonia
- Bronchitis
- Sinusitis
- Encephalitis
- Blindness
- Severe diarrhea
- Otitis media
- Myocarditis and pericarditis
- Respiratory failure in immunocompromised and the pregnant
- SSPE is a fatal, progressive degenerative disease of CNS and may occur in 8.5 cases per 1 million of measles cases after 7–10 years of natural infection.

ADDITIONAL READING
- Botelho-Nevers E, Cassir N, Minodier P, et al. Measles among healthcare workers: A potential for nosocomial outbreaks. *Eurosurveillance* 2011;16: 19764.
- Centers for Disease Control and Prevention (CDC). Global measles mortality 2000–2008. *MMWR* 2009;58:1321–1326.
- Kelly H, Riddell M, Heywood A, Lambert S. WHO criteria for measles elimination: A critique with reference to criteria for polio elimination. *Euro Surveill* 2009;14:19445.
- Sabella C. Measles: Not just a childhood rash. *Cleve Clin J Med* 2010;77(3):207–213.
- Sudfeld CR, Navar AM, Halsey NA. Effectiveness of measles vaccination and vitamin A treatment. *Int J Epidemiol* 2010;39 (Suppl 1):i48–i55.

 CODES

ICD9
- 055.8 Measles with unspecified complication
- 055.9 Measles without mention of complication

CLINICAL PEARLS
- Measles is a highly communicable viral disease whose natural transmission has been halted in the developed world by mass immunization.
- Significant morbidity and mortality occurs in malnourished children in the developing world and in those with immunosuppression.
- Immunization requires 2 doses: 1 at 12–15 months of age and 1 at school age (4–6 years of age).
- Presentation includes a prodrome of fever, cough, coryza, and conjunctivitis, followed by a descending maculopapular rash.
- Measles-associated pneumonia is the most common cause of mortality.

M

MEDIASTINITIS

Jiayi Xu
Jieming Qu
Paschalis Vergidis
Matthew E. Falagas

 BASICS

DESCRIPTION
- Mediastinitis is an infection involving the mediastinum and may be acute or chronic.
- Acute mediastinal infections can result from esophageal perforation, cardiothoracic procedures, penetrating trauma, pneumonia, empyema, foreign body aspiration, and head and neck infections.
- One of the most serious and often lethal forms of mediastinitis is descending necrotizing mediastinitis, which includes mediastinitis secondary to head and neck infections and odontogenic diseases.
- Chronic mediastinitis may follow acute mediastinitis or may be secondary to granulomatous processes, including infections such as histoplasmosis, syphilis, tuberculosis, and coccidiomycosis. It has been also associated with immunologic abnormalities. Foreign bodies that have not been removed may lead to chronic mediastinitis.

EPIDEMIOLOGY
Incidence
- Most cases now are seen in post-cardiac surgery patients. The risk of infection after sternotomy is between 0.4–5%.
- Recent progress in cardiac surgery has led to an increasing number of elderly and immunocompromised patients with multiple risk factors treated surgically. Therefore, despite in-hospital infection control and antibiotic treatment, the incidence of mediastinitis has remained constant over the years.

Prevalence
- Currently most cases of mediastinitis are found to occur after cardiovascular surgery.
- Mediastinitis due to extension of infections from adjacent structures are now less frequent due to the increased use of antibiotics.

RISK FACTORS
- Reoperation
- Diabetes mellitus
- Obesity
- Chronic obstructive pulmonary disease
- Coexistence of peripheral vascular disease
- Bilateral use of internal mammary artery
- Lengthy surgical procedures of the thoracic area

GENERAL PREVENTION
- Perioperative antibiotic prophylaxis: Cefazolin or cefuroxime. Use vancomycin if penicillin allergy or history of methicillin-resistant *Staphylococcus aureus* (MRSA) colonization/infection.
- Early treatment of head and neck infection
- Observing aseptic techniques to minimize postoperative infections
- Postoperative incision care.

PATHOPHYSIOLOGY
- Inflammatory response due to invasion of the mediastinum by bacterial pathogens.
- Multiplication of pathogens and fibrin formation.
- Mediastinal structures become immobile.
- Dissemination of infection throughout mediastinum by sinus tracts.
- Increased area of dead space beneath sternum.

ETIOLOGY
- Patients with mediastinitis secondary to median sternotomy often have infection due to gram-positive organisms such as *Staphylococcus aureus*, *Staphylococcus epidermidis*, or *Enterococcus*.
- Infections resulting from esophageal perforation or secondary to spread from head and neck infections might be caused by gram-negative aerobic and anaerobic organisms. The most common anaerobic organisms are anaerobic streptococci and *Bacteroides* spp.
- Usually, in acute mediastinitis, infections are polymicrobial. Particular attention should be given to the usual oral pharyngeal flora, as well as *Candida* and *Aspergillus* spp. in the deteriorating or debilitated patient.
- Mediastinitis secondary to rib or vertebral osteomyelitis is extremely rare, but has been described in cases of tuberculosis or fungal infections.

COMMONLY ASSOCIATED CONDITIONS
- Acute mediastinitis
  - Esophageal perforation
  - Infection following a transsternal cardiac procedure (anterior mediastinitis)
  - Penetrating trauma
  - Oropharyngeal abscesses caused by odontogenic, peritonsillar infections
  - Pneumonia
  - Empyema
- Chronic mediastinitis
  - Granulomatous processes (histoplasmosis, syphilis, tuberculosis)
  - Noninfectious granulomatous processes (sarcoidosis)

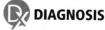 **DIAGNOSIS**

HISTORY
- Acute mediastinitis
  - Fever with no discernible source
  - Chest pain
  - Dysphagia
  - Respiratory distress
  - Epigastric pain (patients with esophageal perforation)
  - Cervical swelling and cervical pain
- Chronic mediastinitis
  - Usually asymptomatic in the early stage.
  - Symptoms usually arise secondary to compression or obstruction of major airways and vascular structures. They are nonspecific and include cough, dyspnea, wheezing, chest pain, dysphagia, and hemoptysis.

PHYSICAL EXAM
- Sternal click with instability
- Hamman's sign (a crunching sound audible over the precordium) noted in patients with head and neck infections and esophageal perforation
- Crepitus (especially in the neck or anterior chest wall)
- Swelling and edema of the pharynx/larynx
- Patients with chronic mediastinitis develop superior vena cava syndrome.

DIAGNOSTIC TESTS & INTERPRETATION
Lab
Initial lab tests
- Patients often exhibit an elevated white blood cell count with neutrophilic predominance.
- C-reactive protein is usually elevated.
- Blood culture can often be positive in patients with head and neck infections.
- Blood must be sent for bacterial and fungal cultures in deteriorating or debilitated patients or in patients with osteomyelitis and in patients with recent cardiothoracic surgery.
- In mediastinitis secondary to rib or vertebral osteomyelitis, acid-fast bacilli stain and mycobacterial culture must be done.

Imaging
Initial approach
- Chest radiographs may demonstrate diffuse mediastinal widening and findings associated with mediastinal abscess, including gas bubbles or an air–fluid level.
- CT scan is useful in determining the extent of mediastinal involvement. Mediastinal fluid collection, extraluminal gas, pericardial and pleural effusions, and soft tissue edema may be seen.

Follow-Up & Special Considerations
- CT scan can help in excluding other conditions.
- Head and neck CT scans are useful when descending necrotizing mediastinitis is considered.

Diagnostic Procedures/Other
- CT-guided transthoracic needle aspiration for microbiological testing
- Thoracoscopy or mediastinoscopy
- Exploratory thoracotomy

Pathological Findings
- Abscess formation
- Effusion/Empyema
- Granuloma and fibrosis (seen in chronic mediastinitis)

DIFFERENTIAL DIAGNOSIS
- Infectious: Pneumonia and complications, parasitic lung infections
- Lung cancer
- Mediastinal mass
- Lymphoma

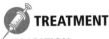# TREATMENT

MEDICATION
- Broad-spectrum or combination antibiotics should be initiated. Modification following culture results is advocated.
- Prolonged course of treatment is recommended (several weeks)

First Line
- Cefepime IV q12h or ceftazidime 2g IV q8h plus: Metronidazole 500 mg IV q8h or clindamycin 600 mg IV q8h
- Piperacillin-tazobactam 3.375 g IV q6h
- For MRSA infections: Vancomycin 15 mg/kg IV q12h or linezolid 600 mg IV q12h or daptomycin 6 mg/kg IV q12h.

Second Line
- Carbapenems, such as imipenem
- Quinolones

ADDITIONAL TREATMENT
General Measures
- Adequate nutrition
- Appropriate intravenous fluids

SURGERY/OTHER PROCEDURES
- Surgical drainage remains the gold standard.
- Debridement of necrotic tissue is essential.
- Controversies still exist on the surgical approach of choice: Cervical drainage alone or cervical drainage along with thoracotomy or thoracoscopy.
- Video-assisted thoracic surgery
- Negative pressure wound therapy, also called vacuum-assisted wound closure, for open wounds
- Irrigation through drainage tubes after closure of sternal wound

IN-PATIENT CONSIDERATIONS
Initial Stabilization
- Evaluation and management of patient's vital signs.
- Protection of airway in those with airway compromise.
- Oxygen supplementation
- Analgesia

Admission Criteria
- Need for administration of intravenous antibiotics
- Need for surgical drainage and debridement

Nursing
- Monitor patency of airway
- Care of surgical drains

Discharge Criteria
- Symptom alleviation or disappearance

ONGOING CARE

FOLLOW-UP RECOMMENDATIONS
- Decrease in fever expected 3–5 days after starting antibiotics.
- For patients with poor response to antibiotic therapy, infection with resistant bacteria, mycobacteria, fungi, or inappropriate drainage of the mediastinum should be considered.

Patient Monitoring
- Serial radiographs or CT scans are useful in identifying any progression of the infection.
- Monitoring vital signs, symptoms, and urine volume.

DIET
High energy and adequate nutrition

PATIENT EDUCATION
- Eliminate and control the risk factors (including losing weight, controlling blood glucose)
- Treat the initial infective diseases (head and neck infections, pneumonia) in time.

PROGNOSIS
- Mortality rates of up to 50%.
- Delayed diagnosis and inappropriate drainage are associated with worse prognosis.

COMPLICATIONS
- Pleural effusion or pleural empyema
- Sternal osteomyelitis
- Severe sepsis or septic shock
- Thrombosis
- Acute respiratory distress syndrome
- Graft destruction
- Infection of pacemakers or cardiac prosthetic valves in situ
- Superior vena cava syndrome

ADDITIONAL READING
- Kalliopi A. Athanassiadi. Infections of the mediastinum. *Thorac Surg Clin* 2009;19(1): 37–45, vi.
- Misthos P, Katsaragakis S, Kakaris S, et al. Descending necrotizing anterior mediastinitis: Analysis of survival and surgical treatment modalities. *J Oral Maxillofac Surg* 2007;65: 635–639.
- Passet E, Rossi P, Nadalin J, et al. Ten years of descending necrotizing mediastinitis: Management of 23 cases. *J Oral Maxillofac Surg* 2007;65: 1716–1724.
- Ridder GJ, Maier W, Kinzer S, et al. Descending necrotizing mediastinitis: Contemporary trends in etiology, diagnosis, management, and outcome. *Ann Surg* 2010;251(3):528–534.
- Singhal P, Kejriwal N, Lin Z, et al. Optimal surgical management of descending necrotising mediastinitis: Our experience and review of literature. *Heart Lung Circ* 2008;17:124–128.
- Tanaka Y, Maniwa Y, Yoshimura M, et al. Successful treatment of descending necrotizing mediastinitis. *Gen Thorac Cardiovasc Surg* 2007;55:366–369.

CODES

ICD9
519.2 Mediastinitis

CLINICAL PEARLS
- Acute mediastinitis is a severe infection that necessitates early diagnosis and treatment.
- Prolonged antibiotic treatment is needed.
- Descending necrotizing mediastinitis is caused by head and neck infections that spread to the mediastinum.

M

MENINGITIS, ACUTE

Souha S. Kanj
Paschalis Vergidis
Matthew E. Falagas

 BASICS

DESCRIPTION
Acute meningitis typically develops over a period of hours and resolves rapidly either by itself, when a viral etiology is implicated, or if treated appropriately when a bacterial etiology is found.

EPIDEMIOLOGY
- Meningitis occurs worldwide and can occur at any age and in previously healthy individuals.
- Meningococcus is the only bacterial pathogen that can lead to epidemics.
- Decrease in *H. influenzae* type B meningitis has been reported in countries giving the vaccine.

Incidence
- The overall incidence of meningitis is about 2–10 cases/100,000 population/year in the US
- Attack rate in neonates: 400 per 100,000, compared with 1–2 per 100,000 in adults and 20 per 100,000 in those ≤2 years old.
- The rates of meningitis in 1995 were (1):
  – Pneumococcal meningitis: 1.1 case per 100,000
  – Meningococcal meningitis: 0.6 case per 100,000
  – *H. influenzae* meningitis: 0.2 case per 100,000

RISK FACTORS
- Extremes of age
- Living in crowded conditions
- Household contact with meningitis cases
- Bacterial endocarditis
- Intravenous drug abuse
- Dural defect
- Head trauma
- Ventriculoperitoneal shunts and cochlear implants
- Asplenic patients have a higher incidence of infections with pneumococcus, meningococcus, and *H. influenzae*.
- Patients with complement deficiency have a higher risk for meningococcal meningitis.
- Patients with cerebrospinal fluid (CSF) rhinorrhea, head trauma, otitis media, mastoiditis, and alcoholism have a higher risk of pneumococcal meningitis.
- Unprotected sex increases risk of HIV meningitis and primary syphilis with invasion of the central nervous system (CNS).
- *Ixodes* tick bites in endemic areas are a risk factor for Lyme meningitis.

GENERAL PREVENTION
- Meningococcus polysaccharide vaccine confers immunity against serogroups A, C, W-135, and Y. No vaccine against serogroup B.
- Indicated in military recruits, travel to areas of high incidence, patients with asplenia and terminal complement disorders.
- *H. influenzae* type B vaccine, given at age 2, 3, and 6 months.
- A 23-polysaccharide pneumococcal vaccine should be given to children and adults with chronic CSF leak, splenectomy and to elderly and debilitated patients.
- A heptavalent conjugated pneumococcal vaccine has been recommended in children with 90% protection against the included serotypes.
- Chemoprophylaxis for meningococcus
  – Given to close contacts of index cases, such as housemates, daycare contacts, and hospital personnel (2):
    ○ Ciprofloxacin 500 mg orally, single dose (adults)
    ○ Rifampin 600 mg (or 10 mg/kg for children) every 12 hours for 2 days
    ○ Ceftriaxone 250 mg IM, single dose (125 mg for children)
    ○ Chemoprophylaxis for *H. influenzae*
- Rifampin 600 mg oral (20 mg/kg) once daily for 4 days for children.

PATHOPHYSIOLOGY
- Pathogens colonize the upper respiratory tract by attaching to the nasopharynx and can then evade the host's immune system and cross the blood–brain barrier to enter the CSF where they proliferate.
- Pathogens enter the CNS by hematogenous spread or by direct extension from a contiguous site.

ETIOLOGY
- Viral infections account for most cases.
- Enteroviral infection is the leading cause, especially in the late summer and early fall.
- HIV (acute retroviral syndrome), arboviruses, herpes viruses, mumps virus, adenovirus
- Most common bacterial causes [2]:
  – Pneumococcus
  – *Neisseria meningitides*
  – Group B *Streptococcus*
  – *Listeria monocytogenes*
  – *Haemophilus influenzae* type B
- *Treponema pallidum* and *Borrelia burgdorferi*
- Group B *Streptococcus* in neonates.
- Gram-negative organisms and *Staphylococcus aureus* in the postoperative setting or endocarditis.

COMMONLY ASSOCIATED CONDITIONS
- Malignancy
- Immunosuppression
- Hematologic disorders (sickle cell disease, thalassemia)
- Diabetes mellitus
- Cirrhosis
- HIV infection
- Immunoglobulin deficiency
- Contiguous infections, such as sinusitis
- Pneumonia or otitis media would suggest pneumococcal meningitis.
- Associated manifestations due to specific viral infections should be sought:
  – Mumps with parotitis or orchitis
  – Herpangina with Coxsackie virus A
  – Vesicles on genitalia with HSV-2
  – Vesicular rash with varicella

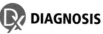 **DIAGNOSIS**

HISTORY
- Symptoms and signs often differ depending on many variables and are usually present in only half of adult patients.
- Certain patients have a subtle presentation
- Fevers with headache and vomiting initially
- Rapid progression to confusion and coma
- Cranial nerve abnormalities can be seen especially with Lyme disease.
- Focal neurologic abnormalities with infarction.
- Seizures occur in 5–28% of adults who have meningitis (3).

PHYSICAL EXAM
- Nuchal rigidity, Brudzinski, and Kernig signs
- Skin rash that ranges from petechiae to diffuse ecchymosis would suggest meningococcal disease, although it may be present with any bacterial meningitis (4).

Geriatric Considerations
- Numerous chronic illnesses, comorbid conditions predispose to infections.
- *S. pneumoniae*, less often *L. monocytogenes*
- Classical signs are often absent.

Pediatric Considerations
- In neonates (younger than 1 month) meningitis is caused by the same organisms that cause bacteremia and sepsis: Group B β-hemolytic streptococci, gram-negative enteric bacteria, and *L. monocytogenes*.
- Risk factors: Prematurity, low birth weight, maternal urinary tract infection, prolonged rupture of the membranes, endometritis/chorioamnionitis.

DIAGNOSTIC TESTS & INTERPRETATION
Lab
Initial lab tests
- CBC, glucose, electrolytes, BUN, creatinine, and blood cultures.
- Lumbar puncture (LP) with CSF determination of cell count/differential, glucose, protein, Gram stain and culture
- Gram stain for bacterial pathogens is positive in 50–90% of cases.
- CSF polymerase chain reaction (PCR) can help with the diagnosis of bacterial and viral pathogens.

Follow-Up & Special Considerations
- CSF Profiles
  - Bacterial meningitis
    - Often show 1,000–5,000 WBCs, with 90% or higher neutrophils
    - CSF glucose is often <40% of the serum glucose
    - CSF protein is elevated.
  - Viral meningitis
    - Generally <1,000 WBC cells.
    - Initially, neutrophils; however, over time, lymphocytes predominate.
    - Glucose is normal, except for mumps.
    - CSF protein is often mildly elevated.
- Bacterial antigen tests on CSF studies may be useful in patients who have partially treated meningitis.

Imaging
- Head CT may show mastoiditis, cerebral edema, ventriculitis, hydrocephalus, infarcts, or abscess.
- A head CT scan prior to the LP is indicated if (5):
  - Head trauma
  - Immunocompromised state
  - Seizure (within the last 7 days)
  - Altered level of consciousness
  - Focal weakness, abnormal speech, abnormal visual fields, or gaze paresis
  - History of mass lesions, focal infection, or stroke

DIFFERENTIAL DIAGNOSIS
- Encephalitis
- Meningitis due to drugs (NSAIDs, trimethoprim-sulfamethoxazole)
- Brain abscess
- Subarachnoid hemorrhage
- Cerebral vasculitis

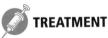 TREATMENT

MEDICATION
- Rapid administration of appropriate bactericidal antibiotics with rapid entry into the CSF. Empiric broad-spectrum antibiotic treatment is initially necessary.
- Empiric antibiotic therapy
  - Regimens include a third- or fourth-generation cephalosporin plus vancomycin
  - Meropenem is an alternative to cephalosporins.
  - Ampicillin is added when *Listeria* meningitis is suspected
  - Trimethoprim/sulfamethoxazole is an alternative for ampicillin (excluding newborns).

- Community-acquired bacterial meningitis
  - Ceftriaxone 2 g IV every 12 hours or cefotaxime 2 g IV every 4–6 hours
  - Add vancomycin until penicillin-resistant pneumococcus has been ruled out.
  - *Listeria* meningitis: Ampicillin 2 g every 4 hours plus gentamicin 1 mg/kg every 8 hours
  - For gram-negative bacteria: Ceftazidime 2 g IV every 8 hours with gentamicin 1 mg/kg every 8 hours
  - Meningococcal and *H. influenza* meningitis is treated for 7 days.
  - Pneumococcal meningitis is treated for 10 days.
  - *Listeria* meningitis is treated for 21 days.

ADDITIONAL TREATMENT
Additional Therapies
- Adjunctive corticosteroid therapy remains controversial.
- Contraindicated in neonates.
- Recommended in infants/children ≥6 weeks and adults with pneumococcal meningitis.
- Dose is 0.15 mg/kg per dose IV every 6 hours for 2–4 days, first dose given with the first dose of antibiotics.
- Might affect CNS concentration of antibiotics

SURGERY/OTHER PROCEDURES
A shunt might be indicated if hydrocephalus

IN-PATIENT CONSIDERATIONS
Admission Criteria
All patients with acute meningitis should be admitted for close monitoring.

Discharge Criteria
Upon completion of IV antibiotics or in those deemed to have self-limited viral infection.

 ONGOING CARE

FOLLOW-UP RECOMMENDATIONS
Patients who survive may need rehabilitation and close neurologic follow-up.

Patient Monitoring
Repeat LP is indicated if the patient is not improving on appropriate antibiotics.

PROGNOSIS
- Depends on age (6), comorbidities, pathogen, and severity at presentation.
- Mortality rate increases if:
  - Decreased level of consciousness at admission
  - Signs of increased intracranial pressure
  - Seizures within 24 hours of admission
  - Age >50 years or infancy
  - Comorbidity
  - Need for mechanical ventilation
  - Delay in initiation of treatment

COMPLICATIONS
- Altered mental status/coma
- Shock and disseminated intravascular coagulation
- Apnea and respiratory failure
- Seizures
- Hydrocephalus
- Inappropriate antidiuretic hormone secretion
- Subdural effusions or subdural empyema
- Brain abscess
- Cerebral infarct
- Impaired intellectual functioning and cognition, personality changes
- Cranial nerve abnormalities
- Sensorineural hearing loss
- Blindness
- Paralysis

REFERENCES

1. Schuchat A, Robinson K, Wenger JD, et al. Bacterial meningitis in the United States in 1995. Active Surveillance Team. *N Engl J Med* 1997;337(14): 970–976.
2. Mace SE. Acute bacterial meningitis. *Emerg Med Clin North Am* 2008;26(2):281–317, viii.
3. Hussein AS, Shafran SD. Acute bacterial meningitis in adults. A 12-year review. *Medicine (Baltimore)* 2000;79(6):360–368.
4. Chavez-Bueno S, McCracken GH Jr. Bacterial meningitis in children. *Pediatr Clin North Am* 2005;52(3):795–810, vii.
5. Hasbun R, Abrahams J, Jekel J, et al. Computed tomography of the head before lumbar puncture in adults with suspected meningitis. *N Engl J Med* 2001;345(24):1727–1733.
6. Miller LG, Choi C. Meningitis in older patients: How to diagnose and treat a deadly infection. *Geriatrics* 1997;52(8):43–44, 47–50, 55.

ADDITIONAL READING

- Brouwer MC, McIntyre P, de Gans J, et al. Corticosteroids for acute bacterial meningitis. *Cochrane Database Syst Rev* 2010;(9):CD004405.
- Hughes DC, Raghavan A, Mordekar SR, et al. Role of imaging in the diagnosis of acute bacterial meningitis and its complications. *Postgrad Med J* 2010;86(1018):478–485.
- Nudelman Y, Tunkel AR. Bacterial meningitis: Epidemiology, pathogenesis and management update. *Drugs* 2009;69(18):2577–2596.

 CODES

ICD9
- 047.9 Unspecified viral meningitis
- 320.9 Meningitis due to unspecified bacterium
- 322.9 Meningitis, unspecified

M

MENINGITIS, CHRONIC

Souha S. Kanj
Paschalis Vergidis
Matthew E. Falagas

 BASICS

DESCRIPTION
Chronic meningitis is an inflammation of the meninges with subacute onset and persistence of clinical symptoms and signs of meningitis for more than 4 weeks.

EPIDEMIOLOGY
Incidence
- Chronic meningitis is rare. Precise incidence rates are not available.
- The incidence and the cause of the disease have significant geographic variability.

RISK FACTORS
- Risk factors for chronic meningitis depend on the etiologic agent.
  - For tuberculous meningitis:
    - People from developing countries
    - History of alcoholism
    - HIV/AIDS
  - For *Brucella* meningitis: Close contact with farm animals in endemic areas
  - For fungal infections: Immunosuppression

GENERAL PREVENTION
- Early diagnosis and prompt treatment of certain infections (such as tuberculosis) will prevent the occurrence of chronic meningitis with these organisms.
- Except for BCG vaccination that might prevent tuberculous meningitis in infants there are no effective vaccines for any of the other causative agents.
- Initiation of Highly Active Antiretroviral Therapy in HIV-infected patients may prevent chronic meningitis (such as cryptococcal meningitis).

PATHOPHYSIOLOGY
- Infectious agents can invade directly the meninges, perivascular space, or the brain parenchyma.
- Some pathogens can trigger an immunologic process leading to an inflammatory reaction. Others cause granulomas in the meninges or the brain parenchyma

ETIOLOGY
- Chronic meningitis can be due to infectious or noninfectious causes.
- No etiology can be identified in one-third of patients (idiopathic chronic meningitis)
- Bacterial causes
  - Partially treated pyogenic meningitis.
  - Tuberculous meningitis (1): Leading cause of chronic meningitis worldwide (causes 40% of the chronic meningitis cases)
  - Syphilitic meningitis

- Lyme disease
- *Brucella* meningitis (Endemic areas: Middle East, Mediterranean countries, Mexico)
- *Nocardia* may cause focal cerebral disease and is a rare cause of chronic meningitis.
- Actinomyces (rare)
- Nontuberculous mycobacteria (rarely cause, usually in AIDS patients)
- Leptospirosis
- Relapsing fever
- *Listeria* (rare)
- *Francisella tularensis*
- *Tropheryma whipplei* (Whipple's disease)
- Fungal meningitis
  - Cryptococcal meningitis: Causes 7% of chronic meningitis cases.
  - Coccidioidomycosis (endemic in the deserted southwestern US).
  - Histoplasmosis
  - Candidiasis
  - Blastomycosis
  - Sporotrichosis (exposure to the thorns of rose plants)
  - Aspergillosis
- Viruses
  - HIV can lead to chronic meningitis, especially early in the course of illness.
  - Cytomegalovirus
  - Lymphocytic choriomeningitis
  - Enterovirus
  - Herpes simplex virus (recurrent meningitis)
  - Mumps virus
- Parasitic causes
  - Toxoplasmosis
  - Cysticercosis
  - *Angiostrongylus cantonensis*
  - *Baylisascaris procyonis* (raccoon parasite)
  - *Gnathostoma spinigerum* (endemic in Southeast Asia)
  - *Acanthamoeba* (rare)
- Other causes
  - Sarcoidosis
  - Systemic lupus erythematosus
  - Behçet's disease
  - Vasculitis
  - Diffuse gliomatosis
  - Metastatic malignancy
  - Drugs (intrathecal, systemic)

COMMONLY ASSOCIATED CONDITIONS
- In tuberculous meningitis, it is not uncommon for other signs of disease to be present (such as cough, hemoptysis, fevers, and weight loss).
- In *Brucella* meningitis, other foci of infection such as vertebral osteomyelitis might be present at the same time.

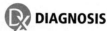 **DIAGNOSIS**

HISTORY
- Patients usually complain of insidious onset of headaches, mild neck stiffness, and low-grade fevers.
- Patients can present with focal neurological signs, chronic meningismus, nausea, vomiting, and confusion.
- Symptoms persist for at least 1 month if untreated.
- *Coccidioides* meningitis often leads to hydrocephalus, and patients may present with headache, confusion progressing to stupor, and coma.

PHYSICAL EXAM
- Evidence of lymphadenopathy, vasculitic rashes, and thrush should be sought.
- Tuberculous meningitis with basilar involvement may cause cranial nerve abnormalities, especially VI nerve palsy.
- Skin nodules support the diagnosis of disseminated coccidioidomycosis.

DIAGNOSTIC TESTS & INTERPRETATION
Lab
Initial lab tests
- Initial lab tests include complete blood count, routine chemistry, erythrocyte sedimentation rate, C-reactive protein, blood cultures, serology for HIV, syphilis, and Lyme.
- Other tests: Cryptococcal antigen, *Coccidioides* serology, *Histoplasma* antigen, *Blastomyces* antigen, and *Aspergillus* galactomannan
- Tuberculin skin test or Quantiferon for suspected tuberculous meningitis
- In areas of *Brucella* endemicity: Serology for brucella (direct, indirect), cerebrospinal fluid (CSF) culture
- Antinuclear antibody, rheumatoid factor, extractable nuclear antigens, anti-neutrophil cytoplasmic antibody and angiotensin-converting enzyme depending on clinical suspicion.
- CSF studies
  - Microscopy for cell count, organisms (Gram stain, acid-fast bacilli, India ink).
  - Culture for bacteria, mycobacteria, and fungi
  - Protein concentration
  - Glucose concentration: <40 mg/dL in fungal, tuberculous chronic meningitis
  - Syphilis serology (RPR)
  - Cryptococcal antigen
  - *Histoplasma* antigen
  - Bacterial antigens (in partially treated bacterial meningitis)
  - Polymerase chain reaction, particularly for tuberculosis, herpes simplex virus
  - Electrophoresis for oligoclonal bands
  - Angiotensin-converting enzyme
  - Cytology

Follow-Up & Special Considerations
- Tuberculous Meningitis
  - CSF often shows 100–500 cells, with a lymphocytic profile.
  - Up to 85% of patients have a decreased glucose in the CSF.
  - Acid-fast bacilli detected in CSF in 10–40% of cases.
  - CSF cultures are positive in 38–88% of cases.
  - Sputum cultures are positive for tuberculosis in 14–50% of cases.
  - Skin tests for tuberculosis (PPD) may be negative in over 50% of patients with tuberculosis meningitis. In AIDS patients, the percentage is higher.
- Cryptococcal Meningitis
  - The CSF often shows 40–400 cells, with a lymphocytic profile.
  - AIDS patients may have fewer than 10 cells.
  - CSF glucose is decreased in 55% of patients.
  - India-ink evaluation is positive in 50% of patients
  - Combination of a positive serum and CSF cryptococcal antigen (>1:8 in the CSF) is diagnostic.
  - Cultures are positive.
- Other
  - Diagnosis of coccidioidomycosis can be based on CSF culture or high titers of antibodies in both serum and CSF.
  - Parasitic infections can cause eosinophilic meningitis: Angiostrongylus cantonensis, Gnathostomiasis, and Baylisascariasis

Imaging
- Chest x-ray
- Brain imaging by CT or ideally MRI (with gadolinium)
- Spinal MRI
- Tuberculous meningitis
  - Chest x-ray may reveal changes consistent with old tuberculosis or a miliary pattern.
  - In 50% of all patients, the chest x-ray is normal.

Diagnostic Procedures/Other
Meningeal biopsy is indicated in certain cases (2).

Pathological Findings
- Granulomas with positive AFB smear in tuberculous meningitis.
- Special stains might reveal the causative fungal agents in some cases.
- Inflammatory changes can be seen in cases of vasculitis.

DIFFERENTIAL DIAGNOSIS
- Encephalitis
- Brain abscess
- Chronic parameningeal infection
- Stroke
- Brain tumor
- Intracranial epidermoid cyst with leakage of contents into the subarachnoid space

 # TREATMENT

MEDICATION
First Line
- Tuberculous Meningitis: Isoniazid, rifampin, pyrazinamide, and ethambutol should be used unless known resistance.
- *Brucella* meningitis: Streptomycin, doxycycline, rifampin, ceftriaxone (2 or preferably 3 drugs at the same time)
- Cryptococcal meningitis
  - Induction: Amphotericin B with flucytosine
  - Consolidation and maintenance: Fluconazole

Second Line
- Tuberculous meningitis: Streptomycin, fluoroquinolones can be used for resistant tuberculous
- *Brucella* meningitis: Fluoroquinolones, TMP/SMX

ADDITIONAL TREATMENT
Additional Therapies
- Dexamethasone is given in most cases of tuberculous meningitis for the first month of treatment.
- Treatment of increased intracranial pressure, osmotic therapy and anti-inflammatory treatment in cases of autoimmune diseases might be necessary.

SURGERY/OTHER PROCEDURES
Shunt placement may be indicated in cases of hydrocephalus.

IN-PATIENT CONSIDERATIONS
Admission Criteria
Admit to neuro-ICU for close monitoring if the patient presents acute neurologic deterioration.

Discharge Criteria
The patient can be discharged once stabilized, a diagnosis has been reached, and proper therapy has been initiated.

 # ONGOING CARE

FOLLOW-UP RECOMMENDATIONS
Patients who survive an episode of meningitis may need rehabilitation and close neurologic follow-up.

Patient Monitoring
- Depending on the condition, repeated lumbar puncture for CSF analysis may be needed to determine appropriate response to therapy.
- In cryptococcal meningitis, check serum of CSF cryptococcal antigen to assess response to treatment.
- In patients receiving antituberculous drugs, check liver enzymes within 2 weeks from treatment initiation.
- In some cases (such as coccidiomycosis and cryptococcal meningitis in AIDS) lifelong treatment may be required.

DIET
In patients with normal level of consciousness: No diet restriction. Otherwise follow aspiration precautions.

PROGNOSIS
- Idiopathic chronic meningitis has a good outcome
- Mortality rates for tuberculous meningitis are up to 30%.
- The outcome of tuberculous meningitis is mainly determined by the clinical stage at admission and the delay in starting treatment (3).
- Marked morbidity with cranial nerve palsies, seizures, and cerebral infarcts can be permanent.

COMPLICATIONS
- Seizures
- Mental retardation
- Cerebral infarct
- Chronic meningitis due to *Coccidioides* can lead to hydrocephalus.

REFERENCES
1. Katrak SM, Shembalkar PK, Bijwe SR, et al. The clinical, radiological and pathological profile of tuberculous meningitis in patients with and without human immunodeficiency virus infection. *J Neurol Sci* 2000;181(1–2):118–126.
2. Cheng TM, O'Neill BP, Scheithauer BW, et al. Chronic meningitis: The role of meningeal or cortical biopsy. *Neurosurgery* 1994;34(4): 590–595; discussion 596.
3. Verdon R, Chevret S, Laissy JP, et al. Tuberculous meningitis in adults: Review of 48 cases. *Clin Infect Dis* 1996;22(6):982–988.

ADDITIONAL READING
- Ginsberg L, Kidd D. Chronic and recurrent meningitis. *Pract Neurol* 2008;8(6):348–361.
- Helbok R, Broessner G, Pfausler B, et al. Chronic meningitis. *J Neurol* 2009;256(2):168–175.

CODES

ICD9
322.2 Chronic meningitis

M

MESENTERIC ADENITIS

Francisco Nacinovich
Martin E. Stryjewski
Matthew E. Falagas

 BASICS

DESCRIPTION
- Acute inflammation of the mesenteric lymph nodes often mimicking appendicitis. It can be preceded or accompanied by enterocolitis.
- Mesenteric adenitis is either primary or secondary to other causes.
- Secondary mesenteric adenitis occurs in the setting of Crohn's disease, infectious colitis, appendicitis, colonic diverticulitis, and systemic lupus erythematosus (1).

EPIDEMIOLOGY
Incidence
Up to 8% of patients are admitted with diagnosis of appendicitis (2).

Prevalence
- Seroprevalence of antibodies against *Yersinia enterocolitica* and *Yersinia pseudotuberculosis* in healthy Austrians has been estimated at 29.7%. However, the number of reported cases is far smaller and hence the vast majority of these infections is concluded to be subclinical or mild (3).
- Most common in children between 5–14 years of age.
- Cases can be sporadic or in outbreaks.

RISK FACTORS
- Outbreaks associated with consumption of raw or undercooked pork, chitterlings, unpasteurized or chocolate milk, and carrots (4,5).
- Intrafamilial outbreaks described.
- Blood transfusion (6)

GENERAL PREVENTION
- Avoid incompletely cooked pork, chitterlings, and unpasteurized milk.
- Adequate hand washing; avoid contamination with stools.

PATHOPHYSIOLOGY
- Gastrointestinal infection usually due to bacterial agents, affecting Peyer's patches and spreading to mesenteric lymph nodes. It can be also associated with terminal ileitis and colonic ulcerations.
- TLR-2 receptors seem to be critical inducing c-type lectin Reg3β to contain Yersinial infection at Peyer's patches (7).
- Invasin is the major factor of adhesion and invasion of *Yersinia enterocolitica* (8)

ETIOLOGY
- Most common cause: *Yersinia enterocolitica*
  – Other causes: *Yersinia pseudotuberculosis*, *Salmonella*, *Mycobacterium tuberculosis*.
  – Rare: Viruses (EBV, Adenovirus), *Bacillus anthracis*. In patients with HIV: *Mycobacterium Avium* intracellulare in adults
- Acute enterocolitis due to *Yersinia enterocolitica* is more common in Europe (e.g., Belgium) than in the USA. This is probably related to pork consumption. *Yersinia* pseudotuberculosis that frequently infects animal is an uncommon cause of human disease; it does produce mesenteric adenitis but not enterocolitis.

 DIAGNOSIS

HISTORY
- Abdominal pain (commonly in right lower quadrant [RLQ]) and fever frequently mimicking appendicitis.
- Diarrhea and nausea are common
  – Vomiting is less common
- Consumption of suspected food (e.g., undercooked pork) within 1–2 weeks prior to onset of symptoms is frequent

PHYSICAL EXAM
- Acutely ill patient
- Fever and abdominal tenderness usually in the RLQ
- Rebound tenderness in RLQ but less common than in acute appendicitis
- Less frequent: Immunologic phenomena such as erythema nodosum or reactive arthritis (in patients carrying HLA-B27).

DIAGNOSTIC TESTS & INTERPRETATION
Lab
Initial lab tests
- Increased white blood cells (WBC)
  – WBCs in stool if diarrhea

Follow-Up & Special Considerations
- Stool samples for bacterial culture including Yersinia. Culturing Yersinia from feces requires enrichment techniques (e.g., cold enrichment).
- Serologic tests (ELISA and agglutination) for Yersinia are useful to investigate outbreaks. Immunoblot is also available
- 16s rRNA sequencing may also employed.

Imaging
Initial approach
- Abdominal ultrasound has proven to be very useful in children. Normal appendix and enlarged mesenteric lymph nodes (usually at the ileocolonic junction) are found (9).
- Abdominal x-ray to rule out intestinal obstruction or perforation.
- CT scan useful in adults (although radiation should be considered). Clustered and enlarged mesenteric lymph nodes with normal appendix are found.

Follow-Up & Special Considerations
Follow-up is clinically guided as dictated by the abdominal pain, fever, and white blood cells.

Diagnostic Procedures/Other
Laparoscopy when appendicitis is suspected.

Pathological Findings
- Inflamed mesenteric lymph nodes with normal appendix.
  – Terminal ileitis and colonic ulcerations can be found.

DIFFERENTIAL DIAGNOSIS
- Acute appendicitis
- Inflammatory bowel disease (e.g., Crohn's disease)
- Tuberculosis
- Lymphoma
- Solid tumor (breast, lung, and gastrointestinal, pancreas) may lead to enlarged mesenteric lymph nodes
- Typhoid fever
- Paratyphoid fever

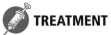 TREATMENT

MEDICATION

- Symptomatic – Self-limited disease; antibiotic therapy usually not needed for enterocolitis or mesenteric adenitis.
- In patients with diarrhea, fever, and stool culture positive for Yersinia, trimethoprim-sulphamethoxazole (TMP-SMX) can be used in children and TMP-SMX or ciprofloxacin in adults.
- Other antibiotics that can be considered: Tetracycline or doxycycline or ampicillin or/and an aminoglycoside (gentamicin or tobramycin)

ADDITIONAL TREATMENT
General Measures
Adequate hydration and diet in patients with diarrhea and/or vomiting.

Issues for Referral
Consult surgery in patients with fever and rebound tenderness in the abdomen

SURGERY/OTHER PROCEDURES
Laparoscopy if appendicitis is suspected

IN-PATIENT CONSIDERATIONS
Admission Criteria
- Fever, acute abdominal pain, and rebound tenderness in the RLQ
  – Hypotension

IV Fluids
In patients with hypotension, those who cannot tolerate diet and/or patients undergoing or being considered for surgery

Nursing
No specific indications

Discharge Criteria
When abdominal pain improves and fever resolves

 ONGOING CARE

COMPLICATIONS
- Mesenteric adenitis usually has a benign course. Complications are uncommon.
- Bacteremia, septic shock, and/or metastatic foci (e.g., liver) can be seen in immunosuppressed patients or in those with iron chelating therapies (e.g., deferoxamine).
- Lower gastrointestinal bleeding
- Intestinal necrosis with subsequent rupture and peritonitis
- Intestinal intussusception
- After *Yersinia enterocolitica or Yersinia pseudotuberculosis* infection the following may appear: erythema nodosum, reactive arthritis, uveitis, nephritis (10)
- Interestingly, there seems to be a decreased risk of subsequent ulcerative colitis data from a large cohort study (11).

REFERENCES

1. Macari M, Hines J, Balthazar E, et al. Mesenteric adenitis: CT diagnosis of primary versus secondary causes, incidence, and clinical significance in pediatric and adult patients. *Am J Roentgenol* 2002:178;853–858.
2. Rao PM, Rhea JT, Novelline RA. CT diagnosis of mesenteric adenitis. *Radiology* 1997:202; 145–149.
3. Tomaso H, Mooseder G, Dahouk SA, et al. Seroprevalence of anti-Yersinia antibodies in healthy Austrians. *Eur J Epidemiol* 2006:21; 77–81.
4. Black RE, Jackson RJ, Tsai T, et al. Epidemic Yersinia enterocolitica infection due to contaminated chocolate milk. *N Engl J Med* 1978:298;76–79
5. Jalava K, Hakkinen M, Valkonen M, et al. An outbreak of gastrointestinal illness and erythema nodosum from grated carrots contaminated with Yersinia pseudotuberculosis. *J Infect Dis* 2006:194;1209-1216.
6. Tipple MA, Bland LA, Murphy JJ, et al. Sepsis associated with transfusion of red cells contaminated with Yersinia enterocolitica. *Transfusion* 1990:30:207–213.
7. Dessein R, Gironella M, Vignal C, et al. Toll-like receptor 2 is critical for induction of Reg3 beta expression and intestinal clearance of Yersinia pseudotuberculosis. *Gut* 2009:58:771–776.
8. Gaus K, Hentschke M, Czymmeck N, et al. Destabilization of YopE by the ubiquitin-proteasome pathway fine-tunes Yop delivery into host cells and facilitates systemic spread of Yersinia enterocolitica in the host lymphoid tissue. *Infect Immun* 2011:79: 1166–1175.
9. Karmazyn B, Werner EA, Rejaie B, Applegate KE. Mesenteric lymph nodes in children: What is normal? *Pediatr Radiol* 2005:35:774–777.
10. Press N, Fyfe M, Bowie W, et al. Clinical and microbiological follow-up of an outbreak of Yersinia pseudotuberculosis serotype Ib. *Scand J Infect Dis* 2001:33:523–526.
11. Frisch M, Pedersen BV, Andersson RE. Appendicitis, mesenteric lymphadenitis, and subsequent risk of ulcerative colitis: Cohort studies in Sweden and Denmark. *BMJ* 2009:338:b716.

 CODES

ICD9
- 008.44 : *Intestinal infection due to yersinia enterocolitica*
- 289.2 Nonspecific mesenteric lymphadenitis

CLINICAL PEARLS

- Mesenteric lymphadenitis can mimic acute appendicitis
- In a child with fever and abdominal pain, an ultrasound revealing normal appendix and enlarged mesenteric lymph nodes is suggestive of mesenteric adenitis.
- *Yersinia enterocolitica* is the most common cause of the disease and can be isolated from the stool culture. However, don't assume that mesenteric adenitis is synonymous with *Yersinia enterocolitica* infection, as other bacteria may cause mesenteric adenitis as part of their clinical manifestation.
- Mesenteric lymph nodes may be enlarged without necessarily other accompanying symptoms such as pain.

M

MITES (INCLUDING CHIGGERS)

Abdul Ghafur
Vasant Nagvekar
Petros I. Rafailidis
Matthew E. Falagas

BASICS

DESCRIPTION
- Mites and chiggers (1) are arthropods with 4 pairs of legs that can parasitize humans and produce localized skin disease or spread diseases such as typhus or plague. *Sarcoptes scabiei* causes scabies (2) in humans (please see also the Scabies chapter) and mange in animals.
- Scrub typhus is transmitted by the bite of chiggers, which are larval forms of the Trombiculid mite *Leptotrombidium*. Scrub typhus is a rickettsiosis caused by *Orientia tsutsugamushi* and is more of a rural disease.

EPIDEMIOLOGY
Incidence
- Scabies has a worldwide distribution, but is seen most commonly in tropical areas. Worldwide estimation of disease is 300 million cases a year.
- Scabies is more common in poorer communities worldwide. The organism can be transmitted by fomites or sexual contact with an infected person. The number of organisms on fomites is generally low. Secondary household cases can be as high as 38% for all cases of scabies. In patients with a variant called Norwegian scabies, the organisms are abundant and the spread is common.
- Scrub typhus is widespread in India, Thailand, and Malaysia. Endemic in the "tsutsugamushi triangle," a triangle extending between northern Japan, northern Australia, and Afghanistan.

Prevalence
Exact prevalence not known but highly underreported.

RISK FACTORS
Scrub typhus: People working in forest areas and farmers.

Genetics
No genetic predisposition.

GENERAL PREVENTION
- Scabies can be prevented in a hospitalized setting by use of contact precautions and frequent, thorough hand washing.
- Norwegian scabies requires persons to be in contact with patients and their clothing and bed linens; wear long-sleeved gowns and shoe covers.
- Laundry workers have been infected; linens should be held in bags for 10 days before laundering.
- Anyone in contact with a patient should be treated empirically, following the regimen for a patient.
- Scrub typhus can be prevented by protective clothing and insect repellents when walking in terrain of endemic areas.

PATHOPHYSIOLOGY
Scrub typhus: Perivasculitis of small blood vessels due to intracellular pathogen.

ETIOLOGY
- Mites that infest humans
  - *S. scabiei* var. hominis causes scabies.
  - The mite resides within the skin and lays its eggs.
  - Localized inflammation within the burrow, caused by a reaction to the mite, the eggs, and feces, leads to pruritus.
  - The mite is not a vector for other infections.
  - The life cycle from egg to egg takes less than 2 weeks.
- Mites that infest animals
  - Various species, including *S. scabiei* var. canis
  - These normally infest dogs, but, upon contact with an infected dog, may cause disease in humans.
- Chiggers
  - These arthropods live in the warm climates; the larval form bites humans (2).
  - Chigger bite leads to intense inflammation and red papules.
  - Wheals develop approximately 3–6 hours after exposure.
  - Chiggers have been known to transmit scrub typhus.
- Scrub typhus
  - Is caused by *Orientia tsutsugamushi*, a rickettsial organism.

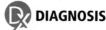

DIAGNOSIS

HISTORY
- Chiggers: Intensely pruritic lesions after walking outdoors (over grass) or sleeping in hotels
- Scrub typhus: Fever, headache, cough, and gastrointestinal symptoms. If untreated, can develop symptoms due to acute respiratory distress syndrome (ARDS), renal failure, or hepatic failure.

PHYSICAL EXAM
- Scabies produces linear burrows (3–15 mm) and erythematous papular lesions.
  - They may be on the hands or penis initially.
  - Lesions on the hands may be in the web spaces. At times, they can become nodular, especially with Norwegian scabies.
- Norwegian scabies occurs in immunocompromised patients, including AIDS patients.
  - The patient often has widespread nodular, crusty lesions.
  - At times, the lesions are less distinct and resemble psoriasis.
  - The lesions may not be pruritic, leading to confusion and delay in diagnosis. These lesions may become superinfected.
- Chiggers: Papule or pustule that may be hemorrhagic in the legs (usually ankles) or waistline
- Scrub typhus: An eschar, firm adherent scab, black in color 3–6mm in diameter. Eschar is usually seen in the groin, waist, or below breasts in females where the clothing is tight.

DIAGNOSTIC TESTS & INTERPRETATION
Lab
Initial lab tests
Scrub typhus: Serology IgM for by Elisa. Lymphopenia, then lymphocytosis thrombocytopenia. Increased transaminases.

Follow-Up & Special Considerations
Monitor platelets and creatinine levels.

Imaging
Scrub typhus: Chest x-ray to rule out early ARDS.

DIFFERENTIAL DIAGNOSIS
- Regarding chiggers (3)
  - Scabies
  - Cutaneous leishmaniasis
  - Cutaneous myiasis
  - Furunculosis
- Regarding scrub typhus
  - Leptospirosis,
  - Malaria
  - Enteric fever
  - Dengue fever
  - Hantavirus infection

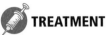 ## TREATMENT
MEDICATION
First Line
- Scabies
  - Cure rates with permethrin are much higher than with lindane, and the toxicity is much less with permethrin.
  - Permethrin 5% cream over the entire body (below chin) for 8–10 hours. Repeat in 1 week.
  - Lindane 1% lotion over the entire body (below chin) for 8–10 hours. Repeat in 1 week.
  - Ivermectin 200 μg/kg orally
  - Antihistamines to relieve patient's itching
- NORWEGIAN SCABIES
  - Permethrin or lindane following bathing, repeated in 12 hours. The second dose should be washed off after being on for 12 hours. Repeat in 1 week.
  - Alternately, treat with permethrin on the first day and with sulfur 6% in petrolatum on days 2 through 7, repeating the cycle until the condition is clear.
  - Lindane is contraindicated in young children and pregnant women due to its neurotoxicity.
- CHIGGERS
  - Symptomatic treatment of itching with local or systemic antihistamine medications or local steroids
- Scrub Typhuss
  - Doxycycline 100 mg b.i.d for 7–10 days.

Second Line
Azithromycin 500 mg once daily for 7 days in children and pregnant ladies.

ADDITIONAL TREATMENT
Issues for Referral
Regarding scrub typhus: Features of ARDS or renal failure.

IN-PATIENT CONSIDERATIONS
Admission Criteria
Regarding scrub typhus: Oliguria, breathlessness, or severe thrombocytopenia.

Discharge Criteria
Afebrile with no breathlessness and recovery of thrombocytopenia.

 ## ONGOING CARE
FOLLOW-UP RECOMMENDATIONS
No follow-up is needed if the patient is fully treated.

PATIENT EDUCATION
Use protective clothing and insect repellents if traveling to high risk areas to avoid scrub typhus infection.

PROGNOSIS
Regarding scrub typhus: Good prognosis if treated early. Delay in treatment leads to more complications (threefold risk) (4). 3–30% mortality if untreated.

COMPLICATIONS
- Superinfection may occur with staphylococcal or streptococcal organisms.
- Regarding scrub typhus, the following complications may arise (5):
  - ARDS
  - Acute renal failure
  - Acute hepatitis/granulomatous hepatitis
  - Myocarditis
  - Disseminated intravascular coagulation
  - Acute hearing loss
  - Meningoencephalitis
  - Hemophagocytic syndrome (6)

REFERENCES
1. Elston DM. What's eating you? Chiggers. *Cutis* 2006;77:350–352.
2. Chosidow O. Clinical practices. Scabies. *N Engl J Med* 2006;354:1718–1727.
3. Porter A, Lang P, Huff R. Persistent pruritic papules. *Am Fam Physician* 2004;69:2640–2642.
4. Yasunaga H, Horiguchi H, Kuwabara K, et al. Delay in tetracycline treatment increases the risk of complications in Tsutsugamushi disease: Data from the Japanese Diagnosis Procedure Combination database. *Intern Med* 2011;50:37–42.
5. Kim DM, Kim SW, Choi SH, et al. Clinical and laboratory findings associated with severe scrub typhus. *BMC Infect Dis* 2010;10:108.
6. Valsalan R, Kosaraju K, Sohanlal T, et al. Hemophagocytosis in scrub typhus. *J Postgrad Med* 2010;56:301–302.

ADDITIONAL READING
- Frequently asked questions. Scrub Typhus. WHO Regional Office for South-East Asia. (accessed December 2010 http://www.searo.who.int/LinkFiles/CDS_faq_Scrub_Typhus.pdf)

CODES
ICD9
- 081.2 Scrub typhus
- 133.0 Scabies
- 133.9 Acariasis, unspecified

CLINICAL PEARLS
- Chigger bites in North America do not transmit any disease but cause highly itchy lesions known as chigger hives.
- Chigger bites in Asia Pacific cause Scrub typhus. Search for eschar or you will miss it.

M

MUCORMYCOSIS

Paschalis I. Vergidis
Matthew E. Falagas

 BASICS

DESCRIPTION
Mucormycosis is a life-threatening opportunistic fungal infection characterized by extensive vascular occlusion and tissue necrosis, primarily seen in immunosuppressed individuals.

EPIDEMIOLOGY
Incidence
- There are no good available data for the incidence of mucormycosis.
- Estimated annual incidence in the US is 1.7 cases per million people (about 500 cases per year).
- 1-year cumulative incidence rates for mucormycosis are 3.8 per 1000 in stem cell transplantations and 0.6 per 1000 solid organ transplantations.
- Breakthrough infections noted in patients on prophylaxis/treatment for aspergillosis, but not mucormycosis (i.e., voriconazole, echinocandins)

Prevalence
Geographic distribution of this infection is worldwide.

RISK FACTORS
- Uncontrolled diabetes mellitus, particularly patients with ketoacidosis (and other forms of metabolic acidosis)
- Hematologic malignancies (risk increases with neutropenia and prolonged antibiotic use)
- Solid-organ or bone marrow transplantation.
- Deferoxamine therapy for iron and aluminium overload (patients in multiple transfusion programs and in hemodialysis)
- Burns and complicated wounds
- Intravenous drug use
- Protein–energy malnutrition
- Chronic steroid use
- HIV infection, mostly due to defective neutrophil numbers and function
- Nosocomial outbreaks in leukemic patients have been described. In one outbreak, cutaneous infection cases were attributed to contaminated dressings.

GENERAL PREVENTION
- Oral and trauma hygiene precautions (especially for diabetics and bone marrow transplant/neutropenic patients)
- In neutropenic and bone marrow transplant patients: HEPA filtered air/laminar air flow for primary prophylaxis. In patients with graft-versus-host disease (GVHD), posaconazole has been reported to prevent invasive mold infections (BI) (1). The optimal duration of prophylaxis is not defined.
- Secondary prophylaxis: Posaconazole (800 mg PO daily), intermittent infusions of liposomal amphotericin B (5–10 mg/kg per day 1 or 2 times per week).
- Emphasis should be given to prevention of diabetic ketoacidosis.

PATHOPHYSIOLOGY
- Most commonly, inhalation of the spores leads to infection of the lungs and paranasal sinuses; ingestion leads to gastrointestinal infection; traumatic inoculation leads to skin and soft-tissue infections.
- In intravenous drug users, inoculation of the organism occurs by venipuncture and leads to local or distant abscesses formation.
- Mucorales, after inoculation, invades the blood vessels, causing thrombosis, infarction, and tissue necrosis. Adjacent tissue and bone infection follows.
- Dissemination occurs by the hematogenous or lymphatic route.

ETIOLOGY
- Molds belonging to the family Mucorales (genera: *Rhizopus, Mucor, Rhizomucor, Absidia, Cunninghamella,* and *Saksenaea*).
- There is no animal reservoir for Mucorales.
- Mucorales organisms are ubiquitous in nature, and are found in abundance in soil and decomposing organic material.

DIAGNOSIS

HISTORY
- Symptoms and signs depend on the system affected; clinical course is related to the underlying conditions.
- Rapid onset of fever and tissue necrosis is common to all forms of the disease.

PHYSICAL EXAM
Rhinocerebral/Craniofacial
- This type is most frequently seen in diabetics and patients with hematologic malignancies.
- Infection begins in the paranasal sinuses and rapidly spreads to the orbit, face, palate, and/or brain.
- Unilateral headache, nasal or sinus congestion or pain, and serosanguineous nasal discharge occur.
- Due to CNS involvement, two-thirds of the patients are comatose by the time of the first clinical examination.
- Orbital edema, induration, and discoloration.
- Ptosis, proptosis of the eyeball, dilatation and fixation of the pupil, and loss of vision, accompanied by drainage of black pus from the eye.
- Violaceous discoloration and/or black necrotic lesion on the hard palate, turbinates; nasal septum or palatal perforation.
- In comatose diabetic patients, never forget to remove the dentures and examine the palate area.
- Diabetics who have persistence of mental status changes longer than 1–2 days after beginning appropriate treatment and resolution of metabolic abnormalities need further exploration, as the probability of mucormycosis is high.

Pulmonary
- Most cases are seen in leukemic patients undergoing intensive chemotherapy.
- Unexplained fever and progressive development of lung infiltrates, despite broad-spectrum antibiotics.
- Unilateral involvement of one anatomic segment and rapid progress to involve the whole lung.
- Pleural effusion, hemoptysis, and pleuritic chest pain are uncommon.

Gastrointestinal
- Most cases occur in malnourished infants and children.
- Lesions are most commonly found in the stomach, colon, and ileum.
- Nonspecific symptoms (abdominal pain, hematemesis)
- Peritonitis (if bowel perforation or infarction occurs)

Cutaneous
- Most cases occur in patients with burns, open fractures, and crush injuries or after applying contaminated surgical dressings to the skin.
- Also at insulin injection sites, catheter insertion sites
- Fever, persistent swelling, conversion from partial to full-thickness burn, ulceration, induration, tenderness, early separation of eschar, and muscle necrosis
- Lesions resembling erythema gangrenosum may develop following hematogenous dissemination.
- They begin as erythematous, indurated, painful lesions that subsequently ulcerate; a black eschar is present.

Disseminated Infection
- Usually follows pulmonary infection
- The most common site of spread is the brain, but other sites, such as the spleen, liver, and heart, can be involved.
- Cerebral infection distinct from the rhinocerebral form results in abscess formation and infarction.

Unusual Focal Forms
- Mainly seen in intravenous drug users
- Endocarditis, osteomyelitis, and pyelonephritis

DIAGNOSTIC TESTS & INTERPRETATION
Lab
Initial lab tests
- Fungal hyphae (wide, disorganized, with random branching and no septa) can be seen in tissue/fluid KOH preparations.
- Sources of culture: Nasal or sinus tissue, aspirates or biopsies of the lung or other sites
- Recovery from tissue can be improved by mincing (not homogenizing) tissue.
- Growth on fungal media, such as Sabouraud dextrose agar, incubated at 25°–30°C.

- Identification of genera is made by the level of development of the rhizoids, the shape of the sporangium, and the location of the sporangiospores. Polymerase chain reaction-based methods are increasingly used in identification.
- Mucorales organisms are ubiquitously found and may be colonizing the sinuses or airways. Nonetheless, identification of mold in immunocompromised patients may be indicative of infection. Histopathological evidence of fungal invasion confirms true infection.
- Antigen tests for β-d-glucan are not useful for mucormycosis.
- Cerebrospinal fluid (CSF) findings are nonspecific. CSF protein may be slightly elevated, but glucose is normal. There may be modest mononuclear pleocytosis. CSF cultures are usually sterile.

Follow-Up & Special Considerations
Antifungal susceptibility testing is performed only in reference or research laboratories.

Imaging
- Findings are nonspecific
- Plain x-rays: Sinus opacification and bone destruction in rhinocerebral/craniofacial disease
- In lung involvement, focal or diffuse infiltrates progressing to consolidation or cavitation
- Unilateral, segmental involvement in the beginning
- Wedge-shaped peripheral lesions, representing hemorrhagic infarction
- CT scans and MRIs: Space-occupying lesions and bone destruction findings in rhinocerebral and CNS disease
- Useful in delineating the disease extent and planning surgical intervention.

Diagnostic Procedures/Other
- Endoscopic examination of nasal turbinates
- Bronchoscopy with bronchoalveolar lavage
- Skin biopsy
- Biopsy at other sites (such as brain)

Pathological Findings
- Neutrophil infiltration of tissues, necrosis, thrombosis and hemorrhage, inflammatory vasculitis (arteries and veins)
- Broad (3–25 μm in diameter), empty, thin-wall, mostly aseptate fungal hyphae are present.

DIFFERENTIAL DIAGNOSIS
Rhinocerebral/Craniofacial
- Cavernous sinus thrombosis due to extension of bacterial facial infection
- Bacterial orbital cellulitis
- Rhinocerebral aspergillosis
- Pseudallescheriasis
- Rapidly growing orbital tumor

Pulmonary
- Bacterial pneumonia
- Aspergillosis
- Pseudallescheriasis
- Pulmonary embolism

Cutaneous
- Ecthyma gangrenosum (in leukemic patients)
- Anthrax

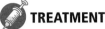 TREATMENT
MEDICATION
First Line
- Amphotericin B deoxycholate 1.0–1.5 mg/kg IV daily
- Liposomal amphotericin B 5–10 mg/kg IV daily (2)
- Amphotericin B lipid complex 5 mg/kg IV daily (3)
- Duration of treatment depends on resolution of clinical symptoms, radiographic findings, negative cultures, and recovery from immunosuppression.

Second Line
- Posaconazole 800 mg PO daily, in 4 divided doses. Administer along with high-fat diet. Absorption may be erratic in patients with mucositis.
- Posaconazole has been used as salvage therapy (4). Steady state concentrations are achieved 1 week after therapy.
- Combinations of amphotericin B with posaconazole, caspofungin, rifampin, or terbinafine have been used with variable results.

ADDITIONAL TREATMENT
Additional Therapies
- Treatment of hyperglycemia, ketoacidosis
- Decrease in immunosuppression
- Granulocyte transfusions in neutropenic patients
- Granulocyte colony-stimulating factor, granulocyte-macrophage colony-stimulating factor, or interferon-γ
- Hyperbaric oxygen therapy, particularly for diabetic patients (5)
- Iron chelators without xenosiderophore activity in Mucorales (deferiprone and deferasirox)

SURGERY/OTHER PROCEDURES
- Surgical debridement of infected tissues with removal of necrotic tissue is crucial in the treatment of rhino-orbital mucormycosis.
- Orbit exenteration in life-threatening infections.
- Lobectomy or pneumonectomy may be necessary in pulmonary disease.

 ONGOING CARE
FOLLOW-UP RECOMMENDATIONS
Patient Monitoring
- Target trough posaconazole concentrations:
  - Prophylaxis ≥0.5 μg/mL
  - Treatment ≥0.7 μg/mL

PROGNOSIS
- If untreated, rhinocerebral/craniofacial mucormycosis is fatal, usually within a week of onset.
- After appropriate treatment, the survival rate in diabetics with rhinocerebral mucormycosis is 50%.
- The prognosis in other high-risk groups and for other system involvement is very poor.
- Diagnosis of lung and gastrointestinal forms of the disease is usually made postmortem.

COMPLICATIONS
- Rhinocerebral/craniofacial: Cavernous sinus and internal carotid artery thrombosis, brain abscesses
- Lung: If untreated, dissemination follows with brain abscess formation and death within 2–3 weeks of onset.
- Gastrointestinal: Bowel infarction/perforation, sepsis, gastrointestinal bleed, and hemorrhagic shock, death within weeks.
- Cutaneous: Extensive local destruction, dissemination with distant abscess formation.

REFERENCES
1. Ullmann AJ, Lipton JH, Vesole DH, et al. Posaconazole or fluconazole for prophylaxis in severe graft-versus-host disease. *N Engl J Med* 2007;356:335–347.
2. Cornely OA, Maertens J, Bresnik M, et al. Liposomal amphotericin B as initial therapy for invasive mold infection: A randomized trial comparing a high-loading dose regimen with standard dosing (AmBiLoad trial). *Clin Infect Dis* 2007;44:1289–1297.
3. Larkin JA, Montero JA. Efficacy and safety of amphotericin B lipid complex for zygomycosis. *Infect Med* 2003;20:201–206.
4. Greenberg RN, Mullane K, van Burik JA, et al. Posaconazole as salvage therapy for zygomycosis. *Antimicrob Agents Chemother* 2006;50:126–133.
5. John BV, Chamilos G, Kontoyiannis DP. Hyperbaric oxygen as an adjunctive treatment for zygomycosis. *Clin Microbiol Infect* 2005;11:515–517.

 CODES

ICD9
117.7 Zygomycosis (phycomycosis or mucormycosis)

CLINICAL PEARLS
- Rhino-orbital mucormycosis is most commonly seen in diabetics and patients with hematologic malignancies
- Amphotericin B is the treatment of choice. Posaconazole has been used as salvage therapy.

M

MUMPS

Georgia Georgantzi
Petros I. Rafailidis
Matthew E. Falagas

 BASICS

DESCRIPTION
Mumps is a benign viral infection of childhood, manifested by swelling of the parotid glands. In adults and, rarely, in children, the disease can cause orchitis, pancreatitis, and aseptic meningitis.

EPIDEMIOLOGY
Incidence
- Mumps is found worldwide and is only present in humans.
- It is most common in children aged 5–9 years. About one-third of those infected are above the age of 15 years.

Prevalence
- In the US, vaccination programs have reduced the number of cases to fewer than 350 per year between years 2000–2005 (1).
- There was a large outbreak of mumps in college campuses in 9 Midwestern states in 2006 despite the high rate of vaccinated students (2).

GENERAL PREVENTION
- Isolation of both suspected and proven cases for 5 days after the onset of parotitis is warranted (3).
- Vaccination with attenuated virus at ages 12–15 months and at 4–6 years. The second dose may be administered before age 4 with at least 28 days between doses (4).
- Adults who have not been immunized should be immunized. Administer 2 doses with at least 28 days between doses, if not previously vaccinated, or the second dose, if vaccinated, with only 1 dose (4).
- The mumps vaccine is part of the combined measles—mumps–rubella vaccine and the combined measles—mumps—rubella–varicella vaccine.

ETIOLOGY
Mumps is an enveloped RNA virus of the family *Paramyxoviridae* and genus *Rubulavirus*. It is contracted by direct contact with secretions of infected individuals.

DIAGNOSIS

HISTORY
- Incubation is between 14–21 days.
- Asymptomatic in 30–40% of cases.
- Fever
- Malaise
- Headache
- Painful swelling of the parotid gland develops in the first 2 days.
- Bilateral swelling (70%) may occur after another 2 days.
- Consumption of sour foods may be painful.
- Less commonly swelling of other salivary glands.
- Resolution of pain, swelling, and fevers occurs within 1 week.
- Testicular pain.

PHYSICAL EXAM
- The mandibular angle is obliterated, while the ear is dislocated upward and outward.
- Signs of meningitis can occur at any time during mumps infection; aseptic meningitis is self-limited and resolves in less than 1 week.
- Epididymo-orchitis is common in adults with mumps, occurring in as many as 30% of post pubertal males. Patients present with testicular pain, marked swelling, and high fevers; resolution occurs in less than 1 week.
- In post pubertal females, mumps can cause oophoritis and mastitis.
- Mumps can commonly cause transient hearing loss, usually unilateral.
- Mumps can cause transient pancreatitis.

DIAGNOSTIC TESTS & INTERPRETATION
Lab
- Diagnosis is made on clinical grounds.
- Leukopenia may occur.
- Serum amylase are elevated with parotitis.
- Lipase and amylase isoenzymes are required to identify the involvement of pancreas.
- Serology can be done to confirm the diagnosis.
- IgG and IgM ELISA antibody may be present in serum specimens.
- Virus detection with PCR.
- Viral isolation from the saliva, cerebrospinal fluid, or urine can be obtained in some laboratories (viral culture).
- Lumbar puncture: CSF: 1000cells/μL (lymphocytes), mildly elevated protein, slightly decreased or normal glucose.

DIFFERENTIAL DIAGNOSIS
- Influenza A
- Coxsackievirus
- Parainfluenza 3
- HIV
- Suppurative parotitis

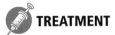 **TREATMENT**

MEDICATION

There is no specific treatment for mumps.

ADDITIONAL TREATMENT

General Measures
- Supportive care, fluids, and analgesics are recommended.
- In orchitis, bed rest, elevation of the scrotum, local cooling, and NSAIDs are recommended (5).

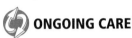 **ONGOING CARE**

PATIENT EDUCATION
- A vaccinated subject should not be in contact with a pregnant woman for 3 months and should not use aspirin for 6 weeks after the vaccination.
- Vaccination should not be performed during pregnancy.

PROGNOSIS
- It is mild and self-limited in general.
- It produces lifelong immunity.

COMPLICATIONS
- Hearing loss is transient and permanent damage is uncommon (2).
- Atrophy of the testes is a complication of severe disease, but sterility is rare, even after bilateral disease (5).
- Low or absent sperm counts.
- Another rare complication is encephalitis with permanent neurologic damage (2).
- Mumps during pregnancy is associated with congenital malformations, low birth weight, and fetal demise.
- Mumps infection also has been associated with the onset of juvenile diabetes mellitus (type I).

REFERENCES

1. Quinlisk MP. Mumps Control Today. *J Infect Dis* 2010;202:655–656.
2. Anderson LJ, Seward JF. Mumps epidemiology and immunity: The anatomy of a modern epidemic. *Pediatr Infect Dis J* 2008;27:S75–S79.
3. Kutty PK, Kyaw MH, Dayan GH, et al. Guidance for isolation precautions for mumps in the United States: A review of the scientific basis for policy change. *Clin Infect Dis* 2010;50:1619–1628.
4. American Academy of Pediatrics, Immunization schedule USA 2010, www.aap.org/healthtopics/immunizations.cfm. Accessed October 18, 2010.
5. Ternavasio-de la Vega HG, Boronat M, Ojeda A, et al. Mumps orchitis in the post-vaccine era (1967–2009): A single-center series of 67 patients and review of clinical outcome and trends. *Medicine (Baltimore)* 2010;89:96–116.

ADDITIONAL READING

- Kutty PK, Kruszon-Moran DM, Dayan GH, et al. Seroprevalence of antibody to mumps virus in the US population, 1999–2004. *J Infect Dis* 2010;202:667–674.

- Marin M, Broder KR, Temte JL, et al. Use of combination measles, mumps, rubella, and varicella vaccine: Recommendations of the Advisory Committee on Immunization Practices (ACIP). *MMWR Recomm Rep* 2010;59:1–12.
- Smallman-Raynor MR, Cliff AD, Ord JK. Common acute childhood infections and appendicitis: A historical study of statistical association in 27 English public boarding schools, 1930–1934. *Epidemiol Infect* 2010;138:1155–1165.

 CODES

ICD9
- 072.0 Mumps orchitis
- 072.1 Mumps meningitis
- 072.2 Mumps encephalitis

CLINICAL PEARLS
- It produces lifelong immunity.
- Isolation should be practiced during the period of maximum infectiousness (3 days before onset of symptoms until 5 days after onset) (2).
- Children should be routinely vaccinated with 2 doses of the vaccine. Adults unvaccinated or vaccinated with 1 dose should also be vaccinated (4).

M

MYCOTIC ANEURYSMS

Francisco Nacinovich
Martin E. Stryjewski
Matthew E. Falagas

BASICS

DESCRIPTION
- An aneurysm that develops in a vessel as part of an infectious process, such as infective endocarditis. The term "mycotic" refers to the shape of the dilation which resembles a fungus and not to the etiology, which is most commonly bacterial.
- Mycotic aneurysms (MA) are described as intracranial or extracranial (1). The term MA is also commonly used in patients with infections of preexisting aneurysms.
- However, one must acknowledge that there is no consensus regarding the terminology (2). Indeed, terms proposed by Wilson (3) seem the most appropriate: Mycotic aneurysms are endocarditis-related infected aneurysms, infection of existing aneurysms or microbial arteritis are bacteremia-related infected aneurysms, and the last category are posttraumatic infected false aneurysms.

EPIDEMIOLOGY
Incidence
- Around 2–4% of patients with IE develop intracranial MA. The incidence is underestimated because of the asymptomatic cases.
- In studies from the 1970s, up to 15% of patients with IE developed MA.

Prevalence
- Prevalence of MA in the general population is unknown. Most probably it decreased in the post antibiotic era.
- Annual prevalence of MA among injection drug users is 0.03%.
- <1% of aortic aneurysms are MA.

RISK FACTORS
- Infective endocarditis
- Other: Deep infections contiguous to a blood vessel, impaired immunity, arterial trauma, and older age
- Intravenous drug abuse

GENERAL PREVENTION
Early recognition, diagnosis, and prompt initiation of antibiotic therapy in patients with IE.

PATHOPHYSIOLOGY
- *Staphylococcus aureus*, *Salmonella* spp. and *Treponema pallidum* are the organisms with greatest affinity for the arterial wall.
- MAs can occur through different mechanisms:
  - Septic emboli from valvular vegetations in IE to the vasa vasorum or the intraluminal space (1)
  - Bacteremic seeding on a previous intimal injury (e.g., atherosclerotic plaque)
  - Spread of infection through a contiguous foci (e.g., osteomyelitis, deep abscesses).
  - Arterial trauma with direct inoculation of microorganisms (e.g., penetrating injury, intravenous drug abuse) or surgery (e.g., percutaneous angiography).

ETIOLOGY
- *S. aureus* is the most common cause (up to70%), followed by *Salmonella* spp. (up to 24%); *T. pallidum* is now rare. Non-typhi Salmonella bacteremia can result in aortitis or MA especially in the elderly with atheromatous lesions.
- MAs associated with *Salmonella* spp. almost always occur below the renal arteries and usually develop in preexisting vascular lesions (e.g., atherosclerosis plaques).
- Other pathogens: *S. viridans*, *S. pneumoniae*, gram-negative bacilli (e.g., *Brucella*, *Pseudomonas*, *Klebsiella*), *Mycobacterium tuberculosis*, fungi (Candida, Zygomycosis, Cryptococcus, and Aspergillus).
- Take into consideration local epidemiology, that is, in Thailand, *Burkholderia pseudomallei* is the most frequent pathogen associated with mycotic aneurysms (4).

COMMONLY ASSOCIATED CONDITIONS
- Infective endocarditis. Mycotic aneurysm constitutes a minor criterion according to the modified Duke endocarditis criteria (1)
- Persistent bacteremia in patients with previous arterial lesions

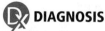

DIAGNOSIS

HISTORY
- MAs are usually asymptomatic unless there is an arterial leak or rupture. Symptoms are dictated by the anatomic region of the vessel.
- Stroke like syndromes with fever, headache, and/or seizures are common in patients with symptomatic intracranial MAs.
- Fever and abdominal or low pain can be seen in patients with MA in the aorta. Secondary infection of preexisting aneurisms is most common in the abdominal aorta.
- In patients with IE, premonitory signs and symptoms can precede the rupture of MA with a median of 6 days (up to 1 month).

PHYSICAL EXAM
- Leak or rupture of intracranial MA (ICMA) can produce meningeal irritation, focal neurologic signs, hemianopsia, and/or coma. Meningeal irritation can be the only finding.
- Intra-abdominal MAs can present with peritoneal signs, back pain, gastrointestinal bleeding, or shock.

DIAGNOSTIC TESTS & INTERPRETATION
Lab
Initial lab tests
- Increased WBCs (65–70%) and anemia (50%) are often present
- Blood cultures are positive in most patients (50–85%)

Follow-Up & Special Considerations
Culture of tissue (affected vessel) is positive in approximately 80% of cases

Imaging
Several procedures are available; suspecting the localization of the MA is the key in selecting the initial procedure.

Initial approach
- Conventional angiography is the gold standard in all cases of MA
- Doppler ultrasound (US) is useful as a first step in extremities or abdominal aorta
- Contrast enhanced CT can detect blood vessel rupture or aneurysmal dilatation in the CNS and in the aorta; normal brain CT scan makes intracranial MA unlikely.

- Transesophageal Doppler US is useful to evaluate heart abnormalities (e.g., valves).
- MRI and also digital subtraction angiography are sensitive for intracranial aneurysms. False–positive results may occur.

Follow-Up & Special Considerations
Compromise of multiple vessels could be found in up to 25% of patients.

Diagnostic Procedures/Other
- Radionuclide scintigraphy (e.g., Tc_{99}) may help to differentiate infectious from noninfectious processes; false–positive results occur.
- Although experience is still limited, PET is a promising diagnostic tool in patients with vascular infections.

Pathological Findings
Destruction of the normal arterial wall architecture with acute and chronic inflammation starting from vasa vasorum and progressively compromising the adventitial surface, the adjacent muscular layer, and then the internal elastic membrane allowing dilation and rupture. The intima can be intact. MAs usually occur at branching sites.

DIFFERENTIAL DIAGNOSIS
- Stroke
- Polyarteritis nodosa
- Congenital aneurysm
- Ruptured viscus

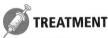 **TREATMENT**

MEDICATION
- Most patients with intracranial aneurysms have resolution with antibiotics alone. Parenteral antibiotics should be directed to the isolated microorganism for at least 6–8 weeks (regardless of surgical resection).
- Some experts recommend a longer duration of treatment if biochemical markers (such as white blood cell count, erythrocyte sedimentation rate, and C-reactive protein) do not return to normal values.
- Long-term oral suppressive therapy following parenteral antimicrobials should be considered for difficult to treat microorganisms.

ADDITIONAL TREATMENT
General Measures
According to the clinical status

Issues for Referral
Consult vascular surgery and or neurosurgery according to the affected vessels.

SURGERY/OTHER PROCEDURES
- Surgical treatment depends on the anatomic location and it is usually reserved for those patients with bleeding or enlarging aneurysms despite adequate antibiotic treatment (5).
- Endovascular surgical treatment is a valid alternative to open surgery for the treatment of mycotic aneurysms (6)
- Cryopreserved aortic allografts have also been used for the treatment of mycotic aneurysms of the aorta (7)

IN-PATIENT CONSIDERATIONS
Admission Criteria
Clinical signs due to MA (e.g., compression, rupture, and leak) in a patient with risk factors (e.g., IE).

IV Fluids
According to the clinical scenario

Nursing
No specific recommendation.

Discharge Criteria
When clinical status improves, patient is afebrile, and complications have resolved or have been adequately managed. Aneurysm should be stabilized or resolving.

 ONGOING CARE

FOLLOW-UP RECOMMENDATIONS
- Intracranial bleeding due to a ruptured MA usually occurs early in the course of the IE. The first weeks of treatment are critical for follow-up.
- Rupture occurring months or even 2 years after the treatment have been described.

Patient Monitoring
- Patient should be clinically followed with inflammatory markers such as WBC, sedimentation rate, and CRP
- Blood cultures should be obtained (before, during, and after treatment)
- Images (noninvasive procedures or angiogram) should be obtained to ensure the MA is getting smaller (expert opinion)

DIET
Rich in fiber to avoid constipation and excessive Valsalva (expert opinion)

PATIENT EDUCATION
Patients should be aware of fever and symptoms that can be associated with their MA (e.g., headache, vision loss).

PROGNOSIS
The mortality of MA is high and depends on the rupture. In patients with intracranial MA associated with IE, the overall mortality is around 50%; mortality in those who had a ruptured MA is 80%, and in those with intact MA is 30%, respectively.

COMPLICATIONS
- Rupture and bleeding, embolization, and vascular insufficiency are the most common complications of MAs.
- Subarachnoid hemorrhage from a MA occurs in <2% of cases of IE.

REFERENCES
1. Baddour LM, Wilson WR, Bayer AS, et al. Infective endocarditis: Diagnosis, antimicrobial therapy, and management of complications. *Circulation* 2005;111:e394–e434.
2. Wilson SE, Van Wagenen P, Passaro E Jr. Arterial infection. *Curr Probl Surg* 1978;15:1–89.
3. Bisdas T, Teebken OE. Mycotic or infected aneurysm? Time to change the term. *Eur J Vasc Endovasc Surg* 2011;41:570.
4. Anunnatsiri S, Chetchotisakd P, Kularbkaew C. Mycotic aneurysm in Northeast Thailand: The importance of Burkholderia pseudomallei as a causative pathogen. *Clin Infect Dis* 2008;47: 1436–1439.
5. Peters PJ, Harrison T, Lennox JL. A dangerous dilemma: Management of infectious intracranial aneurysms complicating endocarditis. *Lancet Infect Dis* 2006;6:742.
6. Silverberg D, Halak M, Yakubovitch D, et al. Endovascular management of mycotic aortic aneurysms. *Vasc Endovascular Surg* 2010;44: 693–696.
7. Bisdas T, Bredt M, Pichlmaier M, et al. Eight-year experience with cryopreserved arterial homografts for the in situ reconstruction of abdominal aortic infections. *J Vasc Surg* 2010;52:323–330.

ADDITIONAL READING
- Soravia-Dunand VA, Loo VG, Salit IE. Aortitis due to Salmonella: Report of 10 cases and comprehensive review of the literature. *Clin Infect Dis* 1999;29:862.
- Tsao JW, Marder SR, Goldstone J, et al. Presentation, diagnosis, and management of arterial mycotic pseudoaneurysms in injection drug users. *Ann Vasc Surg* 2002;16:652–662.

CODES

ICD9
- 421.0 Acute and subacute bacterial endocarditis
- 442.9 Other aneurysm of unspecified site

CLINICAL PEARLS
- MAs are usually seen in patients with IE and they are most commonly asymptomatic.
- *S. aureus* is the most common pathogen

M

MYELITIS

Paschalis I. Vergidis
Matthew E. Falagas

BASICS

DESCRIPTION
Myelitis is a disease involving infection of the spinal cord or the adjacent tissues, leading to alteration of cord function.

EPIDEMIOLOGY
Much depends on the specific etiology of this diverse group of infections. See individual topics for more detail.

RISK FACTORS
Immunocompromised status.

GENERAL PREVENTION
Vaccines are available for poliomyelitis and varicella zoster virus.

PATHOPHYSIOLOGY
- Inflammation can occur throughout the cross-section of the cord at one or at multiple levels, leading to a focal myelitis or a transverse myelitis.
- Infection of the nerve roots is termed radiculomyelitis.

ETIOLOGY
- Herpes viruses (HSV, EBV, VZV, CMV, HHV-6) have been implicated in causing transverse myelitis, especially in immunocompromised patients (1).
- HIV can lead to a diffuse vacuolar myelopathy with myelitis and cord dysfunction.
- HTLV-1 leads to tropical spastic paraparesis, a meningomyelitis.
- Influenza virus can cause myelitis.
- Infectious agents have various tropisms for compartments within the spinal cord.

- Poliomyelitis is most commonly found in the anterior horn cells.
- Enteroviruses such as coxsackievirus, echovirus, and enterovirus types 70 and 71, and flaviviruses such as West Nile virus, also affect the anterior horns.
- Posterior column disease is seen with syphilis, as in tabes dorsalis.
- Dorsal root ganglia are affected in varicella zoster infection. During infection, inflammation of the associated spinal cord segment occurs.
- Tuberculous spondylitis and spinal cord tuberculomas can cause myelopathic symptoms.
- Infection caused by *Mycoplasma pneumoniae*, Lyme borreliosis, and leptospirosis, are other causes of myelitis.
- *Aspergillus, Coccidioides, and Blastomyces* may invade the spinal epidural space.
- Schistosomiasis and neurocysticercosis can also cause myelitis.
- Epidural abscess can lead to cord compression.

DIAGNOSIS

HISTORY
- Myelopathies are characterized by motor weakness, sensory abnormalities referable to the spinal cord, and bladder or bowel dysfunction.
- Symptoms and signs evolve over the course of hours to days and are usually bilateral.
- Neuropathic pain can occur in the midline (back pain), or in a dermatomal distribution.

PHYSICAL EXAM
Transverse Myelitis
- Characterized by a well-defined truncal sensory level, below which the sensation of pain and temperature is altered or lost.
- Loss of motor and sensory function depending on the level of myelitis.
- Reflexes are initially lost, but then become hyperactive below the lesion.

Poliomyelitis
- Patients in the paralytic stage note asymmetric weakness in the arms and legs.
- Examination reveals fasciculations, atrophy, and loss of reflexes—the picture of lower motor neuron involvement.
- Bulbar paralysis may lead to dysphagia and respiratory failure.

Zoster Myelitis
- Patients may have inflammation of the dorsal root ganglion and posterior horn.
- Symptoms are ipsilateral to the rash.
- Dysesthesias give way to radicular pain in dermatomal distribution.
- Sensory loss is common, but motor impairment occurs in fewer than 5% of patients.

DIAGNOSTIC TESTS & INTERPRETATION
Lab
- Cerebrospinal fluid (CSF) can be obtained and sent for cell counts, glucose, protein, cultures, HSV/CMV/VZV polymerase chain reaction, West Nile virus IgM, and VDRL.
- Serology is used to detect possible HIV, enterovirus, syphilis, or Lyme borreliosis (2).
- In viral etiologies, CSF glucose is often normal. The protein can be elevated.
- With poliomyelitis, CSF lymphocytosis is noted.
- In herpes virus infections, polymorphonuclear cells may predominate at an initial stage.

Imaging
Magnetic resonance imaging demonstrates a focal enhancing lesion of the cord.

Pathological Findings
Lymphocytic and monocytic infiltration with varying degrees of demyelination, axonal injury, and gliosis.

DIFFERENTIAL DIAGNOSIS
Noninfectious Etiologies
- Multiple sclerosis and other demyelinating diseases
- Vitamin B12 deficiency
- Autoimmune diseases such as systemic lupus erythematosus (3)
- Neurosarcoidosis
- Paraneoplastic syndrome (small cell lung carcinoma, breast carcinoma)

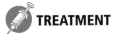 TREATMENT

MEDICATION
First Line
- Treatment of the viral infection likely to be causing the myelitis is necessary:
  – Herpes should be treated with acyclovir
  – Cytomegalovirus should be treated with ganciclovir or foscarnet.
  – HIV requires highly active antiretroviral therapy.
- Treatment of other infectious causes based on specific etiology.

ADDITIONAL TREATMENT
Additional Therapies
Steroids have been used mainly in the form of intravenous methylprednisolone for transverse myelitis associated with infectious causes. However, there is no consensus regarding their clinical role despite their use (2,4).

SURGERY/OTHER PROCEDURES
Emergency surgical decompression is indicated when the cord is compromised by epidural abscess.

 ONGOING CARE

FOLLOW-UP RECOMMENDATIONS
- Patients often require rehabilitation and close follow-up with neurologists (5).
- Relapses may occur (6).

COMPLICATIONS
- Chronic pain
- Partial or total paralysis

REFERENCES

1. Fux CA, Pfister S, Nohl F, et al. Cytomegalovirus-associated acute transverse myelitis in immunocompetent adults. *Clin Microbiol Infect* 2003;9:1187–1190.
2. Frohman EM, Wingerchuk DM. Clinical practice. Transverse myelitis. *N Engl J Med* 2010;363: 564–572.
3. Birnbaum J, Petri M, Thompson R, et al. Distinct subtypes of myelitis in systemic lupus erythematosus. *Arthritis Rheum* 2009;60: 3378–3387.
4. Hammerstedt HS, Edlow JA, Cusick S. Emergency department presentations of transverse myelitis: Two case reports. *Ann Emerg Med* 2005;46: 256–259.
5. Pidcock FS, Krishnan C, Crawford TO, et al. Acute transverse myelitis in childhood: Center-based analysis of 47 cases. *Neurology* 2007;68:1474–1480.
6. Seifert T, Enzinger C, Ropele S, et al. Relapsing acute transverse myelitis: A specific entity. *Eur J Neurol* 2005;12:681–684.

ADDITIONAL READING
- Transverse Myelitis Consortium Working Group. Proposed diagnostic criteria and nosology of acute transverse myelitis. *Neurology* 2002;59:499–505.

 CODES

ICD9
- 323.9 Unspecified cause of encephalitis, myelitis, and encephalomyelitis
- 341.20 Acute (transverse) myelitis NOS

CLINICAL PEARLS
- Transverse myelitis may be caused by various bacterial, fungal, viral, or parasitic infections.
- Symptoms are typically rapid in onset, acute, and bilateral.
- Exclude spinal cord compression!
- MRI is the imaging modality of choice.

M

MYOCARDITIS

Wei Lu
Paschalis Vergidis
Matthew E. Falagas

 BASICS

DESCRIPTION
- An inflammatory disease of the myocardium due to a wide variety of infectious organisms, autoimmune disorders, and exogenous agents
- Myocarditis may be due to infection of the heart or due to cross-reacting antibodies to the myocardium.

EPIDEMIOLOGY
Incidence
- Usually estimated at 1–10 cases per 100,000 persons, similar between males and females, although young males are particularly susceptible.
- This rare disease continues to be implicated in as many as 12% of sudden cardiac deaths among adolescents and young adults.

Prevalence
- Difficult to ascertain, owing to the wide variation of clinical presentation.
- Up to 5% of all cases of Coxsackie B virus infection are associated with myocarditis.
- Up to 40% of cases of *T. cruzi* infection are associated with myocarditis.

RISK FACTORS
HIV infection increases the risk of myocarditis from a wide variety of organisms, including cytomegalovirus, herpes simplex virus, *Toxoplasma gondii,* and, at times, *Cryptococcus*.

GENERAL PREVENTION
Vaccination against viral causes of myocarditis

PATHOPHYSIOLOGY
- Direct cytotoxic effect
- Secondary immune response
- Cytokine expression in the myocardium (e.g., tumor necrosis factor-alpha, nitric oxide synthase)
- Aberrant induction of apoptosis

ETIOLOGY
- Viral – Enterovirus (Coxsackie A, Coxsackie B, echovirus, and poliovirus), adenovirus, influenza and parainfluenza virus, cytomegalovirus, Epstein-Barr virus, HIV, viral hepatitis, mumps, rubeola, varicella, variola/vaccinia, arbovirus, respiratory syncytial virus, herpes simplex virus, dengue, yellow fever virus, rabies, and parvovirus
- Rickettsial – Scrub typhus, Rocky Mountain spotted fever, and Q fever

- Bacterial – Diphtheria, tuberculosis, streptococci, meningococci, brucellosis, clostridia, staphylococci, melioidosis, *Mycoplasma pneumoniae*, psittacosis. Bacteria can cause pericarditis with extension to the myocardium.
- Spirochetal – Syphilis, leptospirosis, relapsing fever/Borrelia, and Lyme disease
- Fungal – Candidiasis, aspergillosis, cryptococcosis, histoplasmosis, actinomycosis, blastomycosis, coccidioidomycosis, and mucormycosis
- Protozoal – Chagas disease, toxoplasmosis, trypanosomiasis, malaria, leishmaniasis, balantidiasis, sarcosporidiosis
- Helminthic – Trichinosis, echinococcosis, schistosomiasis, heterophyiasis, cysticercosis, visceral larva migrans, and filariasis
- Bites/stings – Scorpion venom, snake venom, black widow spider venom, wasp venom, and tick paralysis
- Acute rheumatic fever
- Kawasaki disease causes myocarditis and coronary artery aneurysm; the mechanism is uncertain.

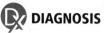 **DIAGNOSIS**

HISTORY
- A history of recent (within 1–2 weeks) flu-like syndrome of fevers, arthralgias, and malaise or pharyngitis, tonsillitis, or upper respiratory tract infections
- Chest pain is usually associated with pericarditis. Can mimic myocardial ischemia
- Symptoms of palpitations, syncope, or even sudden cardiac death, due to underlying ventricular arrhythmias or atrioventricular block
- Adults may present with heart failure years after initial index event of myocarditis (as many as 12.8% of patients with idiopathic dilated cardiomyopathy had presumed prior myocarditis in 1 case series).

PHYSICAL EXAM
- Patients often have typical upper respiratory tract viral symptoms.
- Over time, fevers, palpitations, shortness of breath, and malaise develop.
- Chest pain, pleuritic in nature, occurs.
- Examination often reveals tachycardia.
- S3 and signs of failure may develop.
- Arrhythmias
- Acute rheumatic fever (usually affects heart in 50–90%) – associated signs such as erythema marginatum, polyarthralgia, chorea, and subcutaneous nodules (Jones criteria)

DIAGNOSTIC TESTS & INTERPRETATION
Lab
- Complete blood count – leukocytosis (may demonstrate eosinophilia)
- Elevated erythrocyte sedimentation rate (and other acute phase reactants such as C-reactive protein)
- Elevated cardiac enzymes are seen in some but not all patients with myocarditis. Cardiac troponin elevation may be more common than creatine kinase-MB isoenzyme.
- Serum viral antibody titers for viral myocarditis including Coxsackie virus group B, HIV, cytomegalovirus, Epstein-Barr virus, hepatitis virus family, and influenza viruses.
- Rheumatologic screening – to rule out systemic inflammatory diseases

Imaging
- Chest x-ray: Cardiomegaly with or without vascular congestion
- Echocardiography: To exclude other causes of heart failure and evaluate the degree of cardiac dysfunction (usually diffuse hypokinesis and diastolic dysfunction); to allow gross localization of the extent of inflammation (i.e., wall motion abnormalities, wall thickening, and pericardial effusion).
- Cardiac angiography: To rule out coronary ischemia as a cause of new-onset heart failure, especially when clinical presentation mimics acute myocardial infarction. It usually shows high filling pressures and reduced cardiac outputs.
- Gadolinium-enhanced magnetic resonance imaging (MRI): To assess the extent of inflammation and cellular edema, although it is still nonspecific.
- Nuclear imaging: Antimyosin scintigraphy (using antimyosin antibody injections) can identify myocardial inflammation with high sensitivity (91–100%) and negative predictive power (93–100%) but has low specificity (31–44%) and low positive predictive power (28–33%). Positron emission tomography (PET) scanning has been used in selected cases (e.g., sarcoidosis) to assess the degree and location of inflammation.

Diagnostic Procedures/Other

- Electrocardiogram shows nonspecific ST/T-wave changes, AV block, or bundle branch blocks.
- Endomyocardial biopsy is the criterion standard for diagnosis of myocarditis; sensitivity may increase with multiple biopsies (50% for 1 biopsy, 90% for 7 biopsies). The standard is to obtain at least 4 or 5 biopsies, although false-negative rates still may be as high as 55%.
- The risk of adverse events approaches 6% (including complications with 2.7% on sheath insertion and 3.3% on the biopsy procedure), including 0.5% probability of perforation.

Pathological Findings

Endomyocardial biopsy specimens reveal an inflammatory infiltrate of the myocardium with necrosis and/or degeneration of adjacent myocytes.

DIFFERENTIAL DIAGNOSIS

- Acute myocardial infarction
- Sarcoidosis
- Peripartum cardiomyopathy
- Hyper- and hypothyroidism
- Drugs such as alcohol, cocaine, doxorubicin, trastuzumab, interleukin-2, and methyldopa
- Antibiotics such as tetracycline and sulfonamides
- Rheumatoid disorders such as lupus, rheumatoid arthritis, and scleroderma

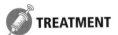 TREATMENT

MEDICATION

- Supportive therapy for symptoms of acute heart failure with the use of diuretics, nitroglycerin/nitroprusside, and angiotensin-converting enzyme (ACE) inhibitors
- Long-term treatment follows the same medical regimen, including ACE inhibitors, beta blockers, and aldosterone receptor antagonists. However, in some instances, some of these drugs cannot be implemented initially because of hemodynamic instability.
- Intravenous immunoglobulin (IVIG) and immunosuppressive therapies are possible adjunctive therapies

SURGERY/OTHER PROCEDURES

- Left ventricular assistive devices (LVADs) and extracorporeal membrane oxygenation may be indicated for short-term circulatory support for cardiogenic shock.
- Cardiac transplantation

 ONGOING CARE

FOLLOW-UP RECOMMENDATIONS

- Consists of largely supportive care, with slow rehabilitation and implementation of evidence-based medical therapy.
- Repeat assessment with echocardiography may be helpful to determine the persistency of cardiac dysfunction
- Patients with a history of myocarditis should be monitored at intervals of 1–3 months initially, with gradual return of physical activity.
- Any evidence of residual cardiac dysfunction or remodeling should be treated in the same manner as chronic heart failure.

DIET

Low-sodium diet similar to that of heart failure management

PROGNOSIS

- Sudden cardiac death accounts for 5–15% of people with undiagnosed and untreated myocarditis.
- Patients who have survived fulminant myocarditis have a good prognosis.

COMPLICATIONS

- Cardiogenic shock may occur in fulminant cases of myocarditis.
- Viral myocarditis may lead to dilated cardiomyopathy.
- Severe heart block requiring permanent pacemaker placement occurred in 1% of patients in the Myocarditis Treatment trial.

ADDITIONAL READING

- Ellis CR, Di Salvo T. Myocarditis: Basic and clinical aspects. *Cardiol Rev* 2007;15(4):170–177.
- Feldman AM, McNamara D. Myocarditis. *N Engl J Med* 2000;343(19):1388–1398.
- Frishman WH, Zeidner J, Naseer N. Diagnosis and management of viral myocarditis. *Curr Treat Options Cardiovasc Med* 2007;9(6):450–464.
- Maria CL, Darren K, Stephen JT. Update on myocarditis in children. *Curr Opin Pediatr* 2010;22:278–283.

 CODES

ICD9

- 074.23 Coxsackie myocarditis
- 422.90 Acute myocarditis, unspecified
- 429.0 Myocarditis, unspecified

CLINICAL PEARLS

- Most common causes of viral myocarditis are enterovirus and adenovirus.
- Suspect myocarditis if new onset cardiac abnormalities (arrhythmias, heart failure) and a viral prodromal illness.
- Supportive therapy is required for symptoms of acute heart failure. IVIG and immunosuppressive therapies are possible adjunctive therapies.

M

MYOSITIS

Petros I. Rafailidis
Matthew E. Falagas

 BASICS

DESCRIPTION
- Myositis is an inflammation of the muscles and can be either infectious (i.e., bacteria, fungi, parasites, viruses, and mycobacteria) or noninfectious (1).
- Pyomyositis is an infection of the muscle that is the result of hematogenous result only, and complicated often by abscess formation (2).
- Acute bacterial myositis, on the other hand, is defined as diffuse muscle infection without abscess formation (1).

EPIDEMIOLOGY
Incidence
The incidence of myositis is correlated with the incidence of the infectious agent involved.

Prevalence
- Pyomyositis is a rare disease in nontropical regions of the world.
- It is often associated with trauma or a foreign body in the muscles or in patients who are intravenous drug users.
- In tropical regions, pyomyositis may account for as many as 4% of hospital admissions.

Bacterial myositis is rare. When it occurs, it may be due to local extension from the skin (decubitus ulcer) or from an underlying source (osteomyelitis). On occasion, it may be secondary to hematogenous spread.

RISK FACTORS
- HIV
- Alcoholism
- Malignancy (i.e., colon cancer, hematologic (3))
- Residing in a tropical country
- Wound
- Surgical operation of the gastrointestinal tract
- Peripheral vascular disease
- Diabetes mellitus
- Obesity

GENERAL PREVENTION
- There is no way to prevent pyomyositis.

PATHOPHYSIOLOGY
- Blunt trauma to the muscles may precede the development of pyomyositis, presumably due to an area of infarct or hemorrhage.

ETIOLOGY
Viral
- Viral myositis is associated with the following:
  – HIV and HTLV-1
  – Influenza A virus
  – Adenovirus
  – Coxsackievirus
  – Epstein-Barr virus
  – Cytomegalovirus
  – Herpes simplex virus
  – Parainfluenza virus

Parasitic
- *Trichinella spiralis* can grow within muscle fibers.
- *Toxocara canis* and *Toxocara cati* also enter the muscle compartment as part of visceral larvae migrans syndrome.
- Cysts from *Cysticercus cellulosae* commonly infect muscle tissue, which leads to calcification over time.
- Hydatid disease caused by *Echinococcus granulosus* or *Echinococcus multilocularis* commonly infects muscles. *Toxoplasma gondii* may also encyst within muscles.

Bacterial
- Pyomyositis: *Staphylococcus aureus* is the pathogen in 95% of patients. Rare causes of pyomyositis include streptococci or coliforms.
  Often seen in tropical areas. Also in HIV-positive patients
- Acute Bacterial myositis (1): The following pathogens are culprits
  – Group A, group B, and group C Streptococci (can lead to both a fasciitis and a myositis)
  – Clostridium species (*C. perfringens*, *C. septicum*, *C. sordellii*): Gas gangrene
  – Non-clostridial myositis is either due to aerobic and anaerobic Streptococci plus *S. aureus* or due to mixed organisms (aerobic and anaerobic Streptococci plus anaerobic gram-negative (Bacteroides) and aerobic gram-negative (Enterobacteriaceae)
- A specific subtype of infectious muscle involvement is the psoas muscle abscess that can be due to extension of a vertebral focus of infection. *S. aureus* and tuberculosis are most commonly implicated. Gravity may lead the bacterial infection downward causing differential diagnosis challenges.
  – Bacterial myositis associated with aquatic environment (1)
- *Aeromonas hydrophila* (Freshwater exposure)
- *Vibrio vulnificus* (salt water exposure)

Fungal Myositis
Various fungi have been reported to be associated with myositis: Candida spp., *Cryptococcus neoformans*, and Aspergillus spp.

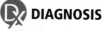 DIAGNOSIS

HISTORY
- The onset of symptoms may be insidious.
- Pain associated with fevers may be the only initial symptom or sign.

PHYSICAL EXAM
- Swelling depends on the depth of infection within the muscle.
  Search for crepitus.
- Over time, the area becomes indurated and woody, and extreme tenderness is noted on palpation.
- Skin changes may not occur if the infection is within a deep muscle group.
  Malodorous discharge
  Hemorrhagic bullae
- Sepsis may be a late manifestation.

DIAGNOSTIC TESTS & INTERPRETATION
Lab
Initial lab tests
- Leukocytosis with a left shift occurs.
- Creatine phosphokinase levels and lactic dehydrogenase may be increased
- Aldolase levels are often within normal limits.
- Gram stain and cultures of discharge are mandatory. However, keep in mind that bacterial myositis remains a spectrum of diseases with high mortality and thus do not completely rely on initial data. Culture received from deeper tissues is more revealing.
- Blood cultures may be positive in 5–35% of patients.
- Hemolytic anemia points to clostridial etiology.

Follow-Up & Special Considerations
Stains for parasites, fungi, and mycobacteria is warranted in the appropriate setting.

Imaging
Initial approach
- A CT or MRI is needed to define the extent of muscles affected.
- An ultrasound is helpful in the emergency setting and to detect abscesses.

Follow-Up & Special Considerations
- Needle aspiration should reveal the organism on Gram stain or culture.

Diagnostic Procedures/Other
- Bone films may show infection secondary to extension of osteomyelitis.

DIFFERENTIAL DIAGNOSIS
- Deep vein thrombosis
- Osteomyelitis
- Gas gangrene
- Fasciitis
  Disseminated intravascular coagulation
- Affected muscles over the abdomen may suggest an underlying abdominal process.
- Affected intercostal muscles may suggest ischemic cardiac pain.

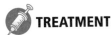

TREATMENT
MEDICATION
First Line
- A combined medical and surgical approach (4) is needed for the vast majority of bacterial myositis.
- When an abscess is visualized by CT or ultrasound, it should be drained, preferably by a guided needle aspiration.
- β-Lactamase penicillin (nafcillin 2 g IV every 4 hours) or a first-generation cephalosporin (cefazolin 2 g IV every 6 hours) is initiated for infection due to methicillin-susceptible S. aureus.
- Vancomycin intravenously is indicated for methicillin-resistant S. aureus.
- For bacterial myositis due to Streptococci group A or B and for clostridial myonecrosis (1,5)
  – Immediate surgical debridement of infected tissue plus a combination of high dose of penicillin (24 million units of penicillin divided in 6 doses [i.e., q4h]) plus clindamycin (900 mg IV q8h). Regarding clostridial myonecrosis and synergistic non-clostridial myositis in addition to penicillin and clindamycin, also add an antibiotic against gram-negative bacteria (i.e., ciprofloxacin).
- Treatment of parasitic myositis depends on the specific infectious agent (i.e., albendazole plus prednisone for Trichinosis).
- Treatment of viral myositis is generally supportive.
- HIV and immunocompromised patients need coverage for S. aureus and gram-negative bacteria.
- Treatment for aquatic environment related myositis (A. hydrophila and V. vulnificus) should include ceftazidime or a fluoroquinolone.

ADDITIONAL TREATMENT
General Measures
- Wound care

Additional Therapies
- Hyperbaric oxygen for the treatment of clostridial myositis.
- Patients should have physical therapy for joint involvement following medical treatment.
- Immunoglobulin for streptococcal toxic shock

IN-PATIENT CONSIDERATIONS
Initial Stabilization
- Mandatory for many cases of bacterial myositis.

Admission Criteria
- Patients with myositis due to bacterial or parasitic causes should generally be admitted.

Discharge Criteria
In case of bacterial myositis when no clinical symptoms and signs are present, and when laboratory/radiological findings are compatible with patient improvement. It has to be noted that clinical picture may at times be trivial and thus lead to underestimation.

ONGOING CARE
PROGNOSIS
Mortality in bacterial myositis due to Streptococci or Clostridia despite aggressive surgical and medical management remains high at levels of 25% and 85% respectively (1).

COMPLICATIONS
- Bacteremia
- Septic shock
- Limb necrosis
- Streptococcal toxic shock
- Death

REFERENCES
1. Crum-Cianflone NF. Bacterial, fungal, parasitic, and viral myositis. *Clin Microbiol Rev* 2008;21: 473–494.
2. Crum NF. Bacterial pyomyositis in the United States. *Am J Med* 2004;117:420–428.
3. Falagas ME, Rafailidis PI, Kapaskelis A, et al. Pyomyositis associated with hematological malignancy: Case report and review of the literature. *Int J Infect Dis* 2008;12:120–125.
4. Mills MK, Faraklas I, Davis C, et al. Outcomes from treatment of necrotizing soft-tissue infections: Results from the National Surgical Quality Improvement Program database. *Am J Surg* 2010;200:790–796.
5. Bryant AE, Stevens DL. Clostridial myonecrosis: New insights in pathogenesis and management. *Curr Infect Dis Rep* 2010;12:383–391.

ADDITIONAL READING
- Vigil KJ, Johnson JR, Johnston BD, et al. *Escherichia coli* Pyomyositis: An emerging infectious disease among patients with hematologic malignancies. *Clin Infect Dis* 2010;50:374–380.
- Crum NF, Lee RU, Thornton SA, et al. Fifteen-year study of the changing epidemiology of methicillin-resistant *Staphylococcus aureus*. *Am J Med* 2006; 119:943–951.

CODES
ICD9
- 728.0 Infective myositis
- 729.1 Myalgia and myositis, unspecified

CLINICAL PEARLS
- Do not underestimate bacterial myositis. The disease may be fulminant.
- Consider sending creatine phosphokinase serum levels when in doubt of whether there is only skin and subcutaneous tissue infection.
- Discordant severe skin sensitivity when other signs of infection are trivial, may signify severe muscle involvement
- Community acquired methicillin-resistant Staphylococcus is more frequent that in the past and thus antibiotics against it should be appropriate.
- If the pathogen of gas gangrene is C. septicum and no trauma has preceded it, suggest colonoscopy to detect possible colon cancer.
- Hemolytic anemia may be due to clostridia but also consider penicillin as a potential cause of hemolysis.

M

NECROTIZING SOFT-TISSUE INFECTIONS

Michael N. Mavros
Petros I. Rafailidis
Matthew E. Falagas

 BASICS

DESCRIPTION
- Severe invasive infections progressing rapidly from the superficial fascia to muscle compartments, causing tissue destruction.
- Usually secondary to a break in the skin from trauma, surgery, or insect bite.
- Depending on the site involved, the disease can manifest as:
  - Necrotizing cellulitis
  - Necrotizing fasciitis
  - Pyomyositis
- Highly lethal, uncommon disease: Mortality >20% in most series (pooled mortality ~34%) (1,2).

EPIDEMIOLOGY
Incidence
- Increasing incidence in the US, currently 0.04 cases per 1000 person-years (3).
- It is estimated that any physician will encounter at least one case of NSTI during practice (1).

RISK FACTORS
- Comorbidities (2–4):
  - Immunocompromised patients, particularly those with diabetes mellitus and peripheral vascular disease.
  - Other: Obesity, chronic liver failure, chronic renal failure, HIV, intravenous drug use, age >50, frequent hospitalizations.
  - Specifically for community-associated methicillin-resistant *Staphyolococcus aureus* (CA-MRSA): Athletes, institutionalized, intravenous drug users.
- Common inciting events (3,4):
  - Trauma, insect bites, iatrogenic interventions (catheters, surgery), chickenpox.
  - No inciting event identified in 20–50% of cases.

Genetics
Certain HLA-II haplotypes seem protective, while others appear to be predisposed to invasive streptococcal infection (4).

GENERAL PREVENTION
- Optimal initial wound care of traumatic injuries
- Prompt treatment of comorbidities

PATHOPHYSIOLOGY
- Bacteria invade subcutaneous tissues after trauma or internal injury.
- Bacterial production of endo- and exotoxins can cause local ischemia, tissue necrosis, and often systemic symptoms.
- Impaired local perfusion and immune response cannot withhold infection from spreading rapidly through the fascial planes, with progressive tissue necrosis.

ETIOLOGY
- 2/3 of cases are polymicrobial (Type 1 NSTI) (2,3):
  - Average of 4 different microorganisms per wound (Gram-positive cocci, Gram-negative rods, and/or anaerobes).
  - Main causative pathogen is *S. aureus*.
- 1/3 of cases are monomicrobial (Types 2 & 3) (2,3):
  - Usually due to GAS (Group A *Streptococcus*), *S. aureus*, and *Clostridium* spp.
- Alarming increase in incidence of CA-MRSA (2,3).

 DIAGNOSIS

HISTORY
- Possible traumatic injury or insect/animal bite
- Patient's comorbidities

PHYSICAL EXAM
- The clinical presentation remains the cornerstone of diagnosis.
  - If in doubt, surgical exploration is recommended.
- Initially (1–4): Local edema, erythema, pain, and tachycardia.
- Progression of infection (1–4):
  - Local signs: Diffuse edema, discoloration, pain disproportionate to appearance or anesthesia, bullae, crepitus, induration, subcutaneous gas.
  - Systemic manifestations: Fever, tachycardia, hypotension, shock.
- May rapidly progress to sepsis and multi-organ failure (2,3).

DIAGNOSTIC TESTS & INTERPRETATION
Lab
Initial lab tests
- Complete Blood Count (CBC), Basic Metabolic Panel (BMP), C-Reactive Protein (CRP)
- Laboratory Risk Indicator for NECrotizing fasciitis score (LRINEC) (5):
  - CRP: If >150 mg/dL: 4 points
  - WBC: If 15–25 cells/mm^3: 1 point, if >25 cells/mm^3: 2 points
  - Hb: If 11–13.5 g/dL: 1 point, if <11 g/dL: 2 points
  - Serum sodium: If <135 mmol/L: 2 points
  - Serum creatinine: If >1.6 mg/dL: 2 points
  - Serum glucose: If >180 mg/dL: 1 point
  - A score ≥6 has high accuracy for NSTI.
  - Although LRINEC may be useful as a screening test, diagnosis relies on surgical exploration (1–3).
- Wound and blood cultures (2,4):
  - Usually don't yield causative microorganism.
  - Primarily used for antibiotic susceptibility testing to guide further treatment.

Follow-Up & Special Considerations
- Sequential CBCs q6h (1).
- A further increase in WBC after surgical debridement may indicate need for further surgical exploration (1).

Imaging
- X-ray may show subcutaneous gas (high specificity, low sensitivity for NSTI) (1–4).
- CT or MRI may show signs of inflammation (e.g., thickened fascia), abscess, or gas formation (1–4,6).
- A delay pending imaging procedures may prove detrimental for the patient with NSTI (2–4).

Diagnostic Procedures/Other
- Gold standard for diagnosis of NSTI is surgical exploration (1–5).
  - Findings include gray necrotic tissue, lack of bleeding, pus, and noncontracting muscle.
- Although often deemed impractical, tissue biopsy or percutaneous needle aspiration may aid in early diagnosis (1–3).
- Measurement of affected tissue oxygen saturation by near-infrared spectroscopy has shown promising results (low oxygen saturation may be indicative of NSTI).

DIFFERENTIAL DIAGNOSIS
- Superficial skin and soft-tissue infections (3):
  - Erysipelas
  - Non-necrotizing cellulitis
- Noninfectious (3):
  - Myositis
  - Lymphedema
  - Eosinophilic fasciitis
  - Phlegmasia cerulea dolens
  - Myxedema
  - Iatrogenic subcutaneous emphysema (e.g., thoracentesis, chest-tube insertion)

 TREATMENT

MEDICATION
First Line
- Surgical treatment along with intravenous antibiotics is necessary (1–4).
- Mixed infection (1–4):
  - Ampicillin-sulbactam or piperacillin-tazobactam + clindamycin + ciprofloxacin
  - Imipenem-cilastatin, meropenem, or ertapenem
  - Cefotaxime + metronidazole or clindamycin
  - Clindamycin or metronidazole + aminoglycoside or fluoroquinolone
- *S. aureus* infection (1–4):
  - Empirical: Vancomycin
  - If methicillin-sensitive *S. aureus*: Nafcillin, oxacillin, or cefazolin

- *Streptococcus* infection (1–4):
  – Penicillin + clindamycin
- *Clostridium* infection (1–3):
  – Penicillin + clindamycin
- Duration of intravenous antibiotic therapy: Until no additional surgical exploration is needed, and patient has had no systemic signs for 48–72 hours (usually >10 days) (1,3).
- Available evidence on antibiotic treatment is limited since patients with NSTIs are typically excluded from RCTs.

Second Line
- *S. aureus* infection:
  – Empirical: Linezolid, daptomycin, tigecycline, or quinupristin-dalfopristin
  – If MSSA: Clindamycin
- *Streptococcus* infection:
  – Vancomycin, linezolid, daptomycin, or quinupristin-dalfopristin

ADDITIONAL TREATMENT
General Measures
- Aggressive early surgical debridement of the compromised area (1–4).
- ICU admission postoperatively (1–4).

Additional Therapies
- Hyperbaric oxygen (HBO) (1–4)
  – May be a useful adjunct, but is generally impractical.
  – Evidence is insufficient to issue a recommendation.
- IV immune globulin (IVIg) (1–4)
  – May be useful in critically ill patients with streptococcal or staphylococcal NSTI.
  – Evidence is insufficient to issue a recommendation.

SURGERY/OTHER PROCEDURES
- Early and aggressive surgical debridement reduces mortality (1–4).
  – Generous initial incision.
  – Tissue should be debrided up to the areas with moderate digital probing and bleeding.
  – Occasionally, amputation may be necessary.
- Fluid and tissue samples should be sent for Gram stain and culture (4).
- Vacuum-assisted closure (VAC) appears beneficial, particularly in patients with large wounds (2–4).
- Transfer to the ICU postoperatively (1–4).
- Re-exploration within 4–48 hours to ensure lack of progression is recommended (1–4).
  – Usually 3–5 procedures per patient are needed.
- Meticulous postoperative wound care (1–4).

IN-PATIENT CONSIDERATIONS
Initial Stabilization
- Close monitoring in ICU setting postoperatively.
- Appropriate early nutritional support (enterically if possible). Indirect calorimetry is preferred (4).
- Aggressive fluid resuscitation and blood component therapy may be required (1,2).
- Control of glucose, sepsis (1,2).
- Derangement in the physiology of the patient or an increase in WBC postoperatively may prompt surgical re-exploration (1).

Admission Criteria
Any patient with the slightest suspicion of a NSTI should be admitted immediately.

 ONGOING CARE

FOLLOW-UP RECOMMENDATIONS
- Particular focus on the prevention of infections (e.g., influenza and streptococcal vaccinations).
- Aggressive treatment of comorbidities:
  – Obesity
  – Diabetes mellitus
  – Smoking
  – Atherosclerosis

PROGNOSIS
- Mortality >20%, lately decreasing through timely diagnosis and aggressive surgical and antimicrobial treatment (1–4).
- Survivors are still at risk for premature death (often due to infectious causes) (3).

COMPLICATIONS
- Nosocomial infections (3):
  – Pneumonia
  – Cholecystitis
  – Urinary tract infections
  – Sepsis
- Adult respiratory distress syndrome (ARDS) (1,3)
- Acute renal failure (1–3)
- Seizures, stroke, or heart failure can sometimes occur (3).
- Amputation in ~15–20% of cases (1–3).

REFERENCES
1. Anaya DA, Dellinger EP. Necrotizing soft-tissue infection: Diagnosis and management. *Clin Infect Dis* 2007;44:705–710.
2. Phan HH, Cocanour CS. Necrotizing soft tissue infections in the intensive care unit. *Crit Care Med* 2010;38:S460–S468.
3. Sarani B, Strong M, Pascual J, et al. Necrotizing fasciitis: Current concepts and review of the literature. *J Am Coll Surg* 2009;208:279–288.
4. Endorf FW, Cancio LC, Klein MB. Necrotizing soft-tissue infections: Clinical guidelines. *J Burn Care Res* 2009;30:769–775.
5. Wong CH, Khin LW, Heng KS, et al. The LRINEC (Laboratory Risk Indicator for Necrotizing Fasciitis) score: A tool for distinguishing necrotizing fasciitis from other soft tissue infections. *Crit Care Med* 2004;32:1535–1541.
6. Zacharias N, Velmahos GC, Salama A, et al. Diagnosis of necrotizing soft tissue infections by computed tomography. *Arch Surg* 2010;145:452–455.

ADDITIONAL READING
- Stevens DL, Bisno AL, Chambers HF, et al. Practice guidelines for the diagnosis and management of skin and soft-tissue infections. *Clin Infect Dis* 2005;41:1373–1406.

 CODES

ICD9
- 728.0 Infective myositis
- 728.86 Necrotizing fasciitis

CLINICAL PEARLS
- Although rare, every physician is estimated to encounter at least one patient with a NSTI.
- Diagnosis is based on clinical manifestations. High index of suspicion is needed.
- Most important determinant of mortality is time to operative intervention.

N

NEUROPATHIES, INFECTIOUS

Paschalis Vergidis
Matthew E. Falagas

 BASICS

DESCRIPTION
- Infectious neuropathy is an inflammation of nerves, which can be caused by viruses, bacteria, parasites, or toxins.
- Acute inflammatory demyelinating polyneuritis or the Guillain-Barré syndrome (GBS) is an immune-mediated disease that has been associated with diverse infections.

EPIDEMIOLOGY
Incidence
- The incidence of GBS is 1.2–3.0 cases per 100,000 people.
- GBS occurs at all ages. There is a bimodal distribution with peaks in young persons (15–35 years) and in older adults (50–75 years).

RISK FACTORS
- Herpes virus may reactivate in immunosuppressed individuals.
- Individuals older than 60 years are at higher risk for post-herpetic neuralgia.
- Cytomegalovirus (CMV) radiculomyelopathy usually in AIDS with CD4 <50/mm^3.
- Advanced AIDS was a risk factor for HIV-associated peripheral neuropathy in the pre-HAART era. In the post-HAART era, most studies have not shown an association between the degree of immunosuppression and risk of disease.
- Living or traveling to endemic areas is a risk factor for Lyme disease, leprosy and American trypanosomiasis.

GENERAL PREVENTION
- Vaccination (zoster, rabies, tetanus, diphtheria)
- Prophylaxis for Lyme disease after tick bite: Doxycycline 200 mg (single dose). Use if local rate of infection of ticks >20%.
- There is no way to prevent either the postinfectious or the idiopathic form of Guillain-Barré syndrome.

PATHOPHYSIOLOGY
- GBS: An antecedent event (such as infection) evokes an immune response which cross-reacts with peripheral nerve components causing an acute neuropathy.
  - Immune reactions against epitopes in Schwann cells or myelin cause acute inflammatory demyelinating neuropathy (85% of cases).
  - Immune reactions against epitopes in the axonal membrane cause axonal forms of GBS (15% of cases).

ETIOLOGY
- Viral
  - Herpes simplex virus (HSV) and varicella zoster virus (VZV) reside within the sensory ganglia and cause neuropathy when reactivated.
  - CMV can lead to a radicular neuropathy in patients with AIDS.
  - HIV-associated neuropathies:
    - Distal sensory polyneuropathy (most common)
    - Inflammatory demyelinating polyneuropathy
    - Mononeuritis multiplex
    - Nucleoside neuropathy (Toxic neuropathy due to didanosine or stavudine)
  - Rabies virus can spread into the central nervous system by peripheral nerves.
- Bacterial
  - Lyme disease (caused by *Borrelia burgdorferi*) may present with neurologic symptoms.
  - Leprosy (caused by *Mycobacterium leprae*) leads to neuronal destruction with anesthesia of the skin.
- Parasitic
  - Chagas' disease (caused by *Trypanosoma cruzi*) has the ability to invade peripheral nerves, leading to neuropathy (mainly autonomic dysfunction).
- Toxin-mediated
  - Toxin produced by *Corynebacterium diphtheriae* can cause injury to Schwann cells and neuronal degeneration, especially of the cranial nerves.
  - *Clostridium botulinum* produces a toxin that can lead to ophthalmoplegia along with a descending motor paralysis.
  - *Clostridium tetani* produces a toxin that acts at the level of the neuromuscular junction and causes the characteristic muscle spasm.
- Immune-mediated
  - GBS is triggered by an antecedent event (infection, immunization, trauma, surgery, bone marrow transplantation).
  - GBS occurs within 2–4 weeks after the antecedent event.
  - Two-thirds of patients have a gastrointestinal or respiratory tract infection.
  - Infectious causes:
    - *Campylobacter jejuni* (1) (20–30% of cases)
    - HIV
    - Herpesvirus: EBV, CMV, HSV, VZV
    - Hepatitis C
    - Mycoplasma
    - Influenza

- Systemic disease:
  - Hodgkin's lymphoma
  - Systemic lupus erythematosus
  - Sarcoidosis
- Other causes:
  - Immunization (influenza, meningococcal vaccination)
  - Trauma
  - Surgery
  - Bone marrow transplantation

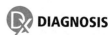 **DIAGNOSIS**

HISTORY
- Viral
  - Pain is the most common symptom of zoster and is caused by acute neuritis. In the absence of vesicular rash ("zoster sine herpete"), the disease may be difficult to diagnose.
  - Post-herpetic neuralgia: Pain persisting longer than 4 months from rash onset.
  - CMV radiculopathy: Insidious onset of paresthesias and distal weakness.
- Bacterial
  - Lyme: Living/traveling in endemic area. Recall of tick bite cannot always be elicited.
  - Leprosy: Epidemiologic history
- Toxin-mediated
  - Botulism: Congestion of contaminated food.
  - Tetanus: History of penetrating injury
- Immune-mediated
  - GBS starts with weakness of the lower legs, which, over days to weeks, ascends to the entire body, including the respiratory muscles.
  - Patients may note mild sensory changes, often paresthesias.
  - Autonomic dysfunction also occurs.
  - Maximal symptoms occur usually within 1 month.
  - Following the paralysis, the patients slowly recover, usually within 1 year of onset.
  - One-third of patients are left with mild residual neurologic dysfunction.
  - Note: GBS in HIV has a rapid onset and progression. GBS develops during seroconversion or early in HIV infection.

PHYSICAL EXAM
- Viral
  - HSV infection: Vesicular rash and pain in dermatomal distribution.
  - Primary genital HSV infection: Urinary retention, constipation, poor rectal tone, and hyperesthesia or anesthesia of the perineum, lower back, or sacral regions.
  - Vesicular rash in herpes zoster. Dermatomal distribution of pain. In 3% of patients, segmental motor paresis due to spread of infection to the anterior horn.
  - CMV infection
    - Polyradiculopathy: Lower extremity weakness, decreased or absent reflexes, cauda equina syndrome, urinary retention
    - Peripheral neuropathy: Multifocal or asymmetric sensory and motor deficits in the distribution of major peripheral or cranial nerves

- HIV infection: Distal symmetric neuropathy. Both feet are affected simultaneously by painful sensation of the burning type and allodynia. Usually no motor involvement. Ankle reflexes are absent or decreased.
- Paralytic rabies: Quadriparesis with sphincter involvement
- Atypical rabies (usually after bat exposure): Neuropathic pain, sensory or motor deficits, choreiform movements of the bitten limb, cranial nerve palsies
- Bacterial
  - Lyme disease
    ○ Erythema migrans followed weeks or months later by neurologic symptoms
    ○ Meningitis
    ○ Cranial neuropathy, especially involving the facial or optic nerve (unilaterally or bilaterally)
    ○ Radiculopathy: Radicular back pain, at times with focal weakness
  - Leprosy
    ○ Sensory loss varies in distribution (small skin patch to most of the body surface)
    ○ Nerve hypertrophy
    ○ Cutaneous lesions, such as maculae or leproma, especially in polybacillary-lepromatous type.
- Toxin-mediated
  - Diphtheria
    ○ Cranial polyneuropathy (2–3 weeks after primary infection) causing dysphagia, paralysis of accommodation of pupils
    ○ Sensory-motor polyneuropathy (8–12 weeks later)
  - Botulism
    ○ Prodrome: Nausea, vomiting, abdominal pain, diarrhea
    ○ Cranial nerve involvement: Blurred vision, diplopia, dysarthria, dysphagia
    ○ Descending motor paralysis
- Immune-mediated
  - Symmetric muscle weakness (from mild difficulty with walking to nearly complete paralysis)
  - Absent or depressed deep tendon reflexes.

DIAGNOSTIC TESTS & INTERPRETATION
Lab
- Viral
  - Detection of CMV DNA in cerebrospinal fluid (CSF).
  - Rabies: Detection of virus RNA/antigen in saliva, skin biopsy. Detection of antibody in serum and CSF.
- Bacterial
  - Lyme serology
- Toxin-mediated
  - Diphtheria: Special culture media (Loeffler's, Tindale's). Testing for toxin production.
  - Botulism: Detection of toxin in serum (performed in specialized laboratories).
- Immune-mediated
  - Diagnosis of GBS is often made on clinical grounds.
  - CSF cell count is typically normal (<5 cells/mm^3).
  - Elevated CSF protein
  - A minority of patients have mildly elevated cell counts. Elevated cell count is more common in HIV-infected patients.

Imaging
- MRI or contrast CT scan of the spinal cord show nerve root thickening in CMV radiculopathy.
- MRI may show enhancement of the nerve roots in GBS.

Diagnostic Procedures/Other
- Nerve conduction studies for HIV-associated sensory neuropathy: Low-amplitude or absent sural nerve action potentials.
- Histopathology or skin slit smears for leprosy.

Pathological Findings
Nerve biopsy in HIV-associated peripheral neuropathy demonstrates axonal loss with frequent foci of inflammation in the endoneurium or around perineurial blood vessels.

 ## TREATMENT
MEDICATION
First Line
- Viral
  - HSV, VZV infection: Acyclovir. Use foscarnet for AIDS patients with acyclovir-resistant virus.
  - CMV neurologic disease: IV ganciclovir or foscarnet or both for 3–6 weeks.
  - The effect of HAART on HIV-associated neuropathy is unclear.
  - Withdraw didanosine, stavudine in toxic neuropathy.
- Bacterial
  - Lyme disease
    ○ Isolated cranial neuropathy: Doxycycline 100 mg PO twice daily for 14–28 days.
    ○ Meningitis, radiculopathy: Ceftriaxone 2 g IV daily for 28 days.
- Toxin-mediated
  - Diphtheria: Erythromycin or penicillin, diphtheria antitoxin
  - Botulism:
    ○ Equine serum heptavalent botulin antitoxin for adults and children older than 1 year
    ○ Botulism immune globulin for infants less than 1 year
  - Tetanus: Penicillin G, tetanus immune globulin
- Immune-mediated
  - Treatment of GBS includes either plasmapheresis for 4–6 treatments (over 8–10 days) (2), or intravenous immune globulin (0.4 g/kg/d) for 3–6 days (3).
  - Initiation of these interventions should be done as early as possible.

ADDITIONAL TREATMENT
General Measures
- Close observation for respiratory muscle weakness. Early endotracheal intubation if needed.
- Blood pressure control and control of cardiac arrhythmias
- Bowel, bladder care

Issues for Referral
Close observation by a neurologist is needed.

Additional Therapies
- Physical therapy is often required.
- Glucocorticoids have not been shown to be beneficial for GBS.

 ## ONGOING CARE
COMPLICATIONS
- Residual neurologic damage occurs commonly with GBS.
- Recurrent disease has also been described.

REFERENCES
1. McCarthy N, Giesecke J. Incidence of Guillain-Barre syndrome following infection with *Campylobacter jejuni. Am J Epidemiol* 2001;153(6):610–614.
2. Raphael JC, Chevret S, Hughes RA, et al. Plasma exchange for Guillain-Barre syndrome. *Cochrane Database Syst Rev* 2002(2):CD001798.
3. Hughes RA, Swan AV, Raphael JC, et al. Immunotherapy for Guillain-Barre syndrome: A systematic review. *Brain* 2007;130(Pt 9): 2245–2257.

ADDITIONAL READING
- Said G. Infectious neuropathies. *Neurol Clin* 2007;25(1):115–137.
- Wulff EA, Wang AK, Simpson DM. HIV-associated peripheral neuropathy: Epidemiology, pathophysiology and treatment. *Drugs* 2000;59(6): 1251–1260.

 ## CODES

ICD9
- 354.5 Mononeuritis multiplex
- 357.0 Acute infective polyneuritis

CLINICAL PEARLS
- Guillain-Barré syndrome is an immune-mediated polyneuropathy characterized by symmetric muscle weakness and areflexia.
- Most common antecedent event is infection with *Campylobacter jejuni.*
- CSF analysis typically shows albumin-cytological dissociation (elevated protein with normal cell count).

N

NOCARDIOSIS

Paschalis Vergidis
Matthew E. Falagas

 BASICS

DESCRIPTION
- Invasive disease associated with *Nocardia* species, first described by Nocard in 1889.
- *Nocardia* species belong to higher bacteria – Family: Nocardiaceae; order: Actinomycetales; Gram-positive filamentous growth with true branching; aerobic.
- Localized or disseminated infection
  – Pulmonary disease (transient or subclinical, acute or chronic)
  – Disseminated (hematogenous spread, particularly in the nervous system)
  – Cellulitis, lymphocutaneous syndrome, actinomycetoma
  – Keratitis
- Systems affected: Lungs, central nervous system (CNS), heart (endocardium, pericardium), genitourinary (kidneys, prostate, testis, epididymis), thyroid, adrenal glands, liver, spleen, peritoneum, soft tissues, and bones. Dissemination to nearly every organ has been reported.

EPIDEMIOLOGY
Incidence
PATHOPHYSIOLOGY
- The aerosol route is the major portal of entry; the lung is the most common site of infection. The gastrointestinal system is an alternative route, through breaks of mucosa. Traumatic inoculation through the skin or eye occurs rarely.
- Frequent contact with soil or vegetate matter.
- No clear evidence for person-to-person transmission.
- Approximately 1000 cases are diagnosed every year in the US (85% pulmonary and/or systematic). Outbreaks are rare.
- Actinomycetoma occurs mainly in tropical/subtropical regions (Mexico, Central and South America, Africa, India). Mainly caused by *N. brasiliensis*.
- Predominant age: All ages (even neonates); more common among adults.
- Predominant sex: The male–female ratio is 3:1.
- Age-related factors: Infection in childhood may present as cervicofacial syndrome and cause cervical adenitis.

RISK FACTORS
- Malignancy
- AIDS
- Treatment with corticosteroids or TNF-alpha blockers
- Cushing's syndrome
- Organ transplantation
- Pulmonary alveolar proteinosis
- Chronic granulomatous disease of childhood
- Congenital immunodeficiency diseases
- Every disease/situation that causes deficient cell-mediated immunity
- Approximately one-third of patients are immunocompetent

GENERAL PREVENTION
Avoidance of direct contact with soil or vegetable matter (patients with immunosuppression)

ETIOLOGY
- *Nocardia* species are neither human nor animal commensals. Other mammals can be infected, too.
- *N. asteroides* is the prominent human pathogen (causes at least 50% of invasive disease). *N. abscessus*, *N. brasiliensis*, *N. otitidiscaviarum*, *N. farcinica*, *N. nova*, *N. transvalensis*, and *N. pseudobrasiliensis* are also associated with human disease (1).

 DIAGNOSIS

HISTORY
- Clinical manifestations are nonspecific.
- Cough is prominent and productive (small amounts of thick, purulent, nonmalodorous sputum).
- Fever, anorexia, weight loss, and malaise are common.
- Dyspnea, pleuritic pain, and hemoptysis are less common.
- Tracheitis and bronchitis are uncommon.
- Remissions over periods of several weeks are frequent.
- Metastatic brain foci may be silent early on. Symptoms and signs depend on location; these are more indolent than abscesses due to other bacteria.
- Meningitis without apparent brain abscess is rare.
- Epididymo-orchitis

PHYSICAL EXAM
- Symptoms and signs from abscesses of skin and supporting structures, bone (rarely), muscles, sinuses, kidneys, thyroid, adrenal glands, and so on.
- Keratoconjunctivitis (traumatic inoculation), endophthalmitis (hematogenous spread).
- Cellulitis (1–3 weeks after breach of skin): Pain, swelling, erythema, warmth; firm, not fluctuant, lesions. It may progress to involve underlying tissues. Dissemination is rare.
- Lymphocutaneous syndrome: Pyodermatous lesion at site of inoculation, central ulceration, purulent or honey-colored drainage; subcutaneous nodules along local-draining lymphatics.
- Actinomycetoma: Nodular swelling, typically feet or hands, but also posterior part of neck, upper back, head, and other sites. A fistula appears when the nodule breaks down, and is soon accompanied by others that come and go. There is extensive deformation of affected areas over a period of months to years.

DIAGNOSTIC TESTS & INTERPRETATION
Lab
- Examination of sputum or pus for crooked, branching, beaded Gram-positive filaments. Modified acid-fast or silver stain is needed.
- These organisms grow relatively slowly; culture plates should be held 7–10 days. (Sometimes colonies take 2 weeks to appear and 4 weeks to take the characteristic appearance.) Colonies are chalky, raised, pink to orange, and crumbly, with a characteristic "mildew" odor. Notify the laboratory when *Nocardia* is suspected.
- Antimicrobial susceptibility testing should be performed in invasive disease.
- *Nocardia* species are rarely skin contaminants or respiratory tract saprophytes. Even in the immunocompetent host, isolation of the organism usually reflects disease (and not only colonization).
- Cerebrospinal fluid or urine specimens should be concentrated and cultured if clinically indicated, but they are rarely positive.
- Polymerase chain reaction may aid in diagnosis.

Imaging
Initial approach
- Chest X-ray: No pathognomonic radiographic picture. Infiltrates vary in size, usually of moderate or greater density. Nodules and cavitation are common. Empyema is evident in one-third of cases. Calcification is rare. Miliary lesions have been reported.
- CT or MRI of head (with or without contrast material) if brain involvement suspected.
- Ultrasound examination of soft tissues (to estimate the presence and size of lesions).

Follow-Up & Special Considerations
Neuroimaging to document resolution of brain abscess

Diagnostic Procedures/Other
Aspiration of brain lesion when diagnosis in doubt

Pathological Findings
- Neutrophils and phagocytes limit organism growth, but do not kill them efficiently.
- Cell-mediated immunity is important for definite control and elimination of organism.
- Suppurative necrosis and abscess formation are typical.
- Granulation tissue usually surrounds the lesion; extensive fibrosis or encapsulation is uncommon.
- Pulmonary lesions: Multiple, confluent abscesses and daughter abscesses are common; peribronchial lymphadenitis may be present.
- There may be extension to the pleura of chest wall.
- In mycetoma and lymphocutaneous syndromes: Sulfur granules appear (absent in visceral nocardiosis).
- Brain abscesses: Any part of brain, usually multiloculated; satellite extensions common.

DIFFERENTIAL DIAGNOSIS
- Tuberculosis
- Bronchogenic carcinoma
- Lung abscess
- Brain tumor
- Brain abscess
- Sarcoidosis
- Actinomycosis
- Fungal disease
- Acute pulmonary infections due to common pathogens
- *Mycobacterium fortuitum* (presenting with postsurgical or skin lesions)
- *Rhodococcus bronchialis* (postsurgical sternotomy infections)
- *Rhodococcus equi* (pulmonary infections)

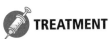 TREATMENT
MEDICATION
First Line
- Sulfonamides: The most effective and best-studied drugs, even though no prospective randomized trials. Sulfamethoxazole-trimethoprim (15–20 mg/kg/d based on trimethoprim, divided in 3–4 doses). Sulfadiazine (1.5–2.0 g q6h) or sulfisoxazole
- Amikacin: The best-established drug for parenteral use (5.0–7.5 mg/kg q12h)
- Imipenem 500 mg i.v. q6h, meropenem 1 g q8h
- Ceftriaxone 2 g i.v. q12h, cefotaxime 2 g i.v. q8h
- Minocycline: The best-established alternative oral drug for use against all *Nocardia* species (100–200 mg q12h)
- Combined therapy: Some advocate the use of two drugs awaiting susceptibility testing. Sulfamethoxazole-trimethoprim plus amikacin, imipenem plus TMP/SMX, imipenem plus amikacin, imipenem plus cefotaxime
- Duration of therapy
  - In the immunocompetent with pulmonary or systemic nocardiosis (outside the CNS) 6–12 months
  - In the immunocompetent with CNS nocardiosis: 12 months. (If all apparent lesions excised, 6 months of therapy may be reasonable.)
  - In the immunosuppressed, pulmonary or systemic: 12 months
  - If only soft tissues: 2 months
  - If soft tissues and bone are involved or a slow response of soft lesions: 4 months
  - If unusually extensive soft-tissue lesion or immunosuppressed: Longer treatment duration needed
  - In actinomycetoma: 6–12 months after clinical cure
  - In keratitis: Oral and topical use of sulfonamides until apparent cure and then oral alone for 2–4 months

Second Line
- Linezolid 600 mg p.o. twice daily (2). Long-term use associated with hematologic toxicity
- Extended spectrum fluoroquinolones (e.g., moxifloxacin 400 mg daily)
- Amoxicillin/clavulanate for cutaneous disease, or for chronic suppression

SURGERY/OTHER PROCEDURES
- Large, accessible abscesses should be aspirated or drained. Smaller abscesses can be treated with antimicrobials only (3).
- For deep or extensive disease due to actinomycetoma, excision can be considered.

 ONGOING CARE
FOLLOW-UP RECOMMENDATIONS
- All patients with cutaneous nocardiosis should initially be evaluated for disseminated disease. Cutaneous lesions are not always due to inoculation. Occasionally, disseminated disease results in secondary seeding of the skin.
- Investigate any evidence of complication or recurrence until several months after apparent cure, because there is a tendency for relapse or appearance of metastatic abscesses during or after effective therapy (at least 6 months after therapy has ended).
- If there is a poor response or development of a new pulmonary or extrapulmonary lesion, investigate for a second pathogen (*Pneumocystis jirovecii*, *Aspergillus*, *Cryptococcus*, *Mycobacterium tuberculosis*)
  - Any child with nocardiosis and no known cause of immunosuppression should undergo tests to determine the adequacy of the phagocytic respiratory burst.

Patient Monitoring
Sulfonamide levels should be monitored in patients with severe disease and those who fail treatment. Goal trough: 100–150 mcg/mL.

PROGNOSIS
- Death is due to sepsis, brain abscess, and overwhelming pneumonia.
- Mortality is increased in patients:
  - With acute infection
  - Being treated with corticosteroid or antineoplastic agents
  - With Cushing's disease
  - With dissemination of infection in multiple organs or the CNS
- Mortality is 15% in otherwise healthy patients with pulmonary nocardiosis.
- Dissemination occurs equally in all categories of patients.

COMPLICATIONS
- Brain abscesses could drain into ventricles or out into the subarachnoid space.
- Epidural spinal cord compression from vertebral osteomyelitis
- Pleuropulmonary fistula
- Iliopsoas, ischiorectal, perirectal abscess
- Pericarditis, endocarditis (natural and prosthetic values), aortitis
- Mediastinitis with superior vena cava obstruction
- Empyema
- Obstructive bronchial masses
- Peritonitis (in chronic peritoneal dialysis)
- Septic arthritis and bursitis
- Diffuse organ abscesses

REFERENCES
1. Brown-Elliott BA, Brown JM, Conville PS, et al. Clinical and laboratory features of the *Nocardia* spp. based on current molecular taxonomy. *Clin Microbiol Rev* 2006;19(2):259–282.
2. Moylett EH, Pacheco SE, Brown-Elliott BA, et al. Clinical experience with linezolid for the treatment of *Nocardia* infection. *Clin Infect Dis* 2003;36: 313–318.
3. Lee GY, Daniel RT, Brophy BP, et al. Surgical treatment of nocardia brain abscesses. *Neurosurgery* 2002;51:668–671; discussion 671–672.

ADDITIONAL READING
- Peleg AY, Husain S, Qureshi ZA, et al. Risk factors, clinical characteristics, and outcome of *Nocardia* infection in organ transplant recipients: A matched case-control study. *Clin Infect Dis* 2007;44: 1307–1314.
- Lederman ER, Crum NF. A case series and focused review of nocardiosis: Clinical and microbiologic aspects. *Medicine* 2004;83:300–313.

 CODES

ICD9
- 039.1 Pulmonary actinomycotic infection
- 039.8 Actinomycotic infection of other specified sites
- 039.9 Actinomycotic infection of unspecified site

CLINICAL PEARLS
- *Nocardia* can cause localized pulmonary or cutaneous disease, but may also disseminate. Neuroimaging to exclude CNS involvement should be performed in all immunocompromised hosts.
- If suspicion for *Nocardia*, notify the microbiology lab to ensure adequate incubation time.
- Sulfonamides are the drugs of choice. After initial intravenous induction, therapy may be stepped-down to oral.

N

NON-TYPHOIDAL *SALMONELLA* INFECTIONS

Abiola C. Senok
Atef M. Shibl
Paschalis Vergidis
Matthew E. Falagas

 BASICS

DESCRIPTION
Infections caused by *Salmonella* spp. causing self-limiting diarrhea, bacteremia, and occasionally extra-intestinal focal disease in humans

EPIDEMIOLOGY
Incidence
- Important cause of reportable food-borne infection in developed and developing countries
- Estimates of 1–3 million cases annually in the US

Prevalence
Chronic carrier state is uncommon, occurring in only 0.5% of cases.

RISK FACTORS
- Ingestion of contaminated eggs, poultry, dairy products, and meat.
- Pet animals including reptiles and birds have been implicated as sources of infection.
- Nosocomial spread has been documented.
- Risk factors for severe infections are extremes of age and immunocompromised status.
- Growing antibiotic resistance is a major concern.

GENERAL PREVENTION
- Eggs should be well cooked.
- Meat and poultry should be washed prior to cooking and be well cooked.
- Good hand washing after contact with pets is recommended.
- Pets, such as reptiles, should be avoided in families with young children or immunocompromised individuals.
- Outbreaks should be reported to public health authorities for investigation.

PATHOPHYSIOLOGY
- Infectious dose of 103–106 colony-forming units.
- Infection affects the lining of the terminal ileum and large bowel.
- Spread beyond the gastrointestinal mucosa leads to bacteremia and metastatic focal infection.
- Nontyphoidal *Salmonella* spp. have the ability to live within macrophages.
- Fecal shedding persists for approximately 4 weeks in adults and 7 weeks in young children.

ETIOLOGY
- Gram-negative facultative anaerobic rods belonging to the Enterobacteriaceae family

 DIAGNOSIS

HISTORY
- Acute diarrhea with non-bloody stools of moderate volume.
- Associated fever, chills, nausea, vomiting and abdominal cramps frequently occur.
- Dysentery or cholera-like symptoms are uncommon.
- Gastroenteritis is usually self-limiting. Fevers resolve after 2–3 days and diarrhea within the first week.

DIAGNOSTIC TESTS & INTERPRETATION
Lab
- Freshly passed stool cultures for identification of the organism
- Blood cultures
- Leukocytosis is common
- High erythrocyte sedimentation rate suggests osteomyelitis or abscess formation
- Culture other body fluids when metastatic disease is suspected

Imaging
- Abdominal CT scan shows slight symmetrical thickening of the wall of the terminal ileum and mild thickening of the colon.
- For suspected endovascular foci, imaging investigations are required, e.g., CT scanning.

DIFFERENTIAL DIAGNOSIS
- Other causes of enteritis:
  - *Escherichia coli*
  - *Campylobacter*
  - *Yersinia*
  - *Shigella*
  - *Clostridium difficile*

 TREATMENT

MEDICATION
First Line
- No antibiotics for immunocompetent patients with uncomplicated salmonellosis.
- Severe diarrhea can be treated with ciprofloxacin 500 mg p.o. b.i.d. for 3–5 days.
- For patients at risk of bacteremia, give oral or i.v. ciprofloxacin until afebrile.
- For bacteremia, give ceftriaxone 2 g i.v. daily plus ciprofloxacin 400 mg i.v. q12 until susceptibility testing is available, then de-escalate to single agent for 14 days.
- Endovascular infection should be treated for at least 6 weeks.
- HIV-positive patients may require long-term ciprofloxacin suppressive therapy.

Second Line
For severe diarrhea: 1 double-strength tablet of trimethoprim–sulfamethoxazole p.o. b.i.d. for 3–5 days

ADDITIONAL TREATMENT
General Measures
Rehydration and electrolyte replacement

SURGERY/OTHER PROCEDURES
Surgical intervention may be indicated for some focal infections

IN-PATIENT CONSIDERATIONS
Admission Criteria
Patients with severe diarrhea, systemic infection should be admitted

IV Fluids
For rehydration and electrolyte replacement

Nursing
- Adherence to strict hand washing
- Proper disposal of fecal material

 ONGOING CARE

FOLLOW-UP RECOMMENDATIONS
- Routine follow-up cultures not recommended after uncomplicated *Salmonella* gastroenteritis in immunocompetent patients.
- For infected health care workers or food handlers, 1 or 2 negative stool cultures obtained at least 48 hours after cessation of antibiotics is required before return to work.
- Treatment of chronic asymptomatic carriers is controversial.

PATIENT EDUCATION
Understand general preventive measures

PROGNOSIS
- Morbidity and mortality is highest in the extremes of age and in immunocompromised patients
- Central nervous system infection is fatal in approximately 50% of cases

COMPLICATIONS
- Bacteremia occurs in about 4% of immunocompetent patients
- Higher risk of bacteremia is seen in immunocompromised patients (especially HIV-infected patients), patients in extremes of age, and those with comorbidities, e.g., prostheses, valvular heart disease, and diabetes
- Metastatic spread of infection to vascular grafts, bone, joints, kidney, liver, and spleen has been well documented in bacteremic patients
- Infectious endarteritis, especially involving the abdominal aorta and endocarditis
- Osteomyelitis has been described in patients with sickle cell anemia and *Salmonella* bacteremia

ADDITIONAL READING
- Crum-Cianflone NF. Salmonellosis and the gastrointestinal tract: More than just peanut butter. *Curr Gastroenterol Rep* 2008;10:424–431.
- Hohmann EL. Nontyphoidal salmonellosis. *Clin Infect Dis* 2001;32:263–269.
- Majowicz SE, Musto J, Scallan E, et al. The global burden of nontyphoidal *Salmonella* gastroenteritis. *Clin Infect Dis* 2010;50:882–889.
- Mead P, Slutsker L, Dietz V, et al. Food-related illness and death in the United States. *Emerg Infect Dis* 1999;5:607–625.

 CODES

ICD9
- 003.0 *Salmonella* gastroenteritis
- 003.9 *Salmonella* infection, unspecified

CLINICAL PEARLS
- Non-typhoidal *Salmonella* infection is an important cause of food-borne gastroenteritis acquired via ingestion of contaminated eggs, poultry, and meat.
- Bacteremia and metastatic focal infection occur in at-risk patient groups, e.g. very young, elderly, immunocompromised.
- Stool and blood cultures are diagnostic.
- Antibiotic treatment is generally not indicated except for severe complicated infections.

N

ODONTOGENIC INFECTIONS

Ata Nevzat Yalcin
Paschalis Vergidis
Matthew E. Falagas

BASICS

DESCRIPTION
- Odontogenic infections originate within the mouth and are associated with the teeth and surrounding structures. These infections can range from small apical abscesses to large soft-tissue infections extending to the neck and beyond.
- Odontogenic orofacial infections include dental caries, pulpitis, periapical abscess, gingivitis, periodontal disease, peri-implantitis, and infections in the deep fascia.

EPIDEMIOLOGY
Prevalence
- Odontogenic infections are prevalent worldwide and are the principal reason for seeking dental care.
- Periapical abscess, pericoronitis, and periodontal abscess are the most common emergency odontogenic infections.

RISK FACTORS
- Old age
- Pregnancy
- Diabetes
- Immunodeficiency
- Malnutrition
- Eruption of deciduous dentition
- Poor oral hygiene
- Smoking
- Disorders of salivation
- Hospitalization

GENERAL PREVENTION
- Good oral hygiene to prevent plaque build-up.
- Fluoride promotes remineralization of the teeth and can prevent caries.
- Chlorhexidine can reduce the amount of plaque formation and prevent disease

PATHOPHYSIOLOGY
- The dental biofilm is the etiological agent of odontogenic infections. It is defined as a proliferative bacterial, enzyme-active ecosystem.
- Perturbation of the colonizing microflora can lead to the development of disease within the mouth.
- Patients with poor oral hygiene have higher colony counts of mouth flora.
- Hospitalized patients have higher numbers of Gram-negative facultative rods (e.g. *Escherichia coli*, *Klebsiella* spp.).
- Disorders of salivation are associated with greater numbers of organisms.
- Disorders of cell-mediated immunity, deficiency of IgA, and reduction in neutrophils are all risk factors for the development of oral infections.

ETIOLOGY
- Odontogenic infection is polymicrobial and mixed.
- Most frequent pathogens isolated from odontogenic infections are
  - *Streptococcus* spp. (*S. mutans* group, *S. anguis*, *S. mitis*, *S. salivarius*)
  - *Lactobacillus*
  - *Peptostreptococcus* spp.
  - *Actinomyces* spp.
  - *Fusobacterium* spp.
  - *Veillonella*
- *S. mutans* is the only microorganism consistently isolated from all decayed dental fissures and caries cases.
- Periodontal infections are generally polymicrobial: Gram-positive aerobes, primarily streptococci, predominate in gingivitis, and the Gram-negative anaerobic rods predominate in bone-destroying periodontitis.

COMMONLY ASSOCIATED CONDITIONS
Necrotizing ulcerative periodontitis involves severe loss of periodontal attachment and alveolar bone. This entity may be associated with HIV infection.

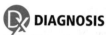

DIAGNOSIS

HISTORY
- Diagnosing the origin of odontogenic infection is important in order to manage the disease appropriately.
- Clinical manifestations may be useful when they are referred to a specific tooth.
- Periapical abscess and pulpitis
  - Patients complain initially of hot and cold sensitivity of the tooth; this may develop into a throbbing sensation that is worsened with eating.
  - Eventually, the tooth generates continuous pain.
- Gingivitis
  - Inflammation of the gums may lead to halitosis and bleeding after brushing.
- Periodontitis
  - Periodontal disease is often associated with localized pain along with hot and cold sensitivity.

PHYSICAL EXAM
- Pulpitis
  - Mild inflammation in early disease. Occlusion of blood vessels and necrosis of the pulp tissue in advanced disease.
- Gingivitis
  - The gums are hyperemic.
  - In acute necrotizing ulcerative gingivitis (Vincent's angina or trench mouth) the gingival surface becomes necrotic. Fever may be present.
- Periodontitis
  - Gingivitis may be present. Loss of the supporting structure may lead to motion of the tooth, and pressure on the tooth leads to formation of pus around the tooth.

DIAGNOSTIC TESTS & INTERPRETATION
Lab
- Microbiological testing can help to identify the cause, although all odontogenic infections are the result of biofilm evolution with marked similarities in the bacterial composition.
- Odontological microbiological studies are complex because of potential contamination.
- Bacterial culture is the traditional method of identification and also allows susceptibility testing.
- Immunofluorescent techniques and DNA hybridization are also useful.

Imaging
- X-rays provide essential information, but certain limitations should be considered.
- Radiographs can detect bone loss, areas of abscess formation, and loss of dentin and enamel.
- With deep extension of infection, CT or MRI scanning is most helpful.

 TREATMENT

- The objective of treatment is to control the infective bacterial load by combining mechanical debridement, surgery, and/or systemic antibiotic treatment, where appropriate.
- Indications for antibiotic therapy
  - Acute-onset fascial or oral swelling
  - Swelling inferior to the mandible
  - Trismus
  - Dysphagia
  - Lymphadenopathy
  - Fever ($>38.3°C$)
  - Pericoronitis
  - Osteomyelitis

MEDICATION
First Line
- Outpatient treatment: Penicillin G, clindamycin, azithromycin
- Inpatient treatment: Clindamycin, ampicillin plus metronidazole, ampicillin/sulbactam, amoxicillin/clavulanate
- Early-onset aggressive or localized juvenile periodontitis: Doxycycline, metronidazole

Second Line
- Out-patient treatment (penicillin allergy): Clindamycin, azithromycin
- In-patient treatment (penicillin allergy): Clindamycin, third-generation cephalosporins

SURGERY/OTHER PROCEDURES
- All abscesses need to be drained. There are many intraoral routes for drainage.
- At times, the crown of the tooth needs to be removed or the tooth extracted.

 ONGOING CARE

FOLLOW-UP RECOMMENDATIONS
- Frequent periodontal scaling can avert plaque formation and periodontitis.
- Frequent follow-up with a dentist, at least every 6 months, is mandatory.

COMPLICATIONS
- Fascial space infections (e.g., osteomyelitis of the jaw)
- Necrotizing fasciitis
- Odontogenic sinusitis
- Buccal and periorbital cellulitis
- Ludwig's angina: Bilateral infection that causes elevation of the tongue and floor of the mouth
- Lateral pharyngeal space infections are rarely caused by an odontogenic source
- Suppurative jugular thrombophlebitis (Lemierre's syndrome)
- Orbital and intracranial complications:
  - Orbital and intracranial abscess
  - Septic cavernous sinus thrombosis
  - Brain abscess and subdural empyema

ADDITIONAL READING
- Levi ME, Eusterman VD. Oral infections and antibiotic therapy. *Otolaryngol Clin North Am* 2011;44(1):57–78.
- Lopez-Piriz R, Aguilar L, Gimenez MJ. Management of odontogenic infections. *Med Oral Patol Oral Cir Bucal* 2007;12:E154–E159.

 CODES

ICD9
- 521.00 Dental caries, unspecified
- 522.0 Pulpitis
- 522.4 Acute apical periodontitis of pulpal origin

O

ORCHITIS

Renato Finkelstein
Matthew E. Falagas

 BASICS

DESCRIPTION
Inflammation of testes—generally due to infectious causes. Orchitis frequently occurs in patients with concurrent epididymitis, and in this situation the causative pathogens of both conditions are similar. In contrast to infections occurring in other genitourinary sites, viruses, particularly mumps, are important causes of orchitis.

EPIDEMIOLOGY
Incidence
- Not well known, but less common than other causes of lower UTI in men (e.g. prostatitis and epididymitis).
- Commonly seen in the outpatient setting.
- Epididymitis and orchitis accounts for 1 in 144 outpatient visits (0.69%) in men 18–50 years of age (1).
- Orchitis is found in association with acute epididymitis in 20–40% of cases.

RISK FACTORS
- Urethral catheterization (2,3)
- Epididymitis

GENERAL PREVENTION
- Preventing the most common causes of sexually transmitted diseases (STDs) causing urethritis and epididymitis, i.e., *Neisseria gonorrhoeae* or *Chlamydia trachomatis* infection. The most reliable way to avoid transmission of STDs is to abstain from sex or to be in a long-term, mutually monogamous relationship with an uninfected partner.
- Immunization against mumps

PATHOPHYSIOLOGY
- Contiguous spread from an inflammatory process in the epididymitis (epididymo-orchitis)
- Blood-borne dissemination is the major route of infection of isolated testicular infection

ETIOLOGY
- Bacterial: Usually in patients in epididymitis and caused by the same organisms
  - Common causes:
    - Age 14–35 years: *N. gonorrhoeae* or *C. trachomatis* (2)
    - Other ages: *Escherichia coli, Klebsiella pneumoniae, Proteus mirabilis, Pseudomonas aeruginosa*.
    - Less common: *Ureaplasma urealyticum*, staphylococci and streptococci.
    - Rare: *Brucella* spp. (endemic areas) (4), *Mycobacterium tuberculosis* (5), *Nocardia* spp. (6) (immunosuppression), *Haemophilus influenzae* (AIDS)

- Viral: The most common cause of primary testicular infection: Mumps (20–30% of post pubertal mumps infection)
  - Rare: Coxsackie B virus, lymphocytic choriomeningitis virus.
- Fungal: Few cases reported in disseminated histoplasmosis (7).
- Noninfectious causes
  - Xanthogranulomatous orchitis: A very rare disease characterized by replacement of testicular tissue by lipid-laden macrophages.

COMMONLY ASSOCIATED CONDITIONS
Epididymitis

 DIAGNOSIS

HISTORY
- Testicular pain and swelling
- Abrupt onset when caused by viruses
- Nausea, vomiting, prostration, high fever, and constitutional symptoms may be present
- In mumps, manifestations appear generally 4–8 days after parotitis; intervals of up to 6 weeks have been reported, progress for 2–3 days and resolve within a week or 2. Residual testicular tenderness can persist for weeks. Bilateral in 15–30% of cases.

PHYSICAL EXAM
- Testicular swelling and tenderness.
- Normal cremasteric reflex (i.e., ipsilateral cremasteric muscle contraction producing unilateral testis elevation).
- Concomitant signs of inflammation of the spermatic cord may and may not be noted.
- Reactive hydrocele and scrotal wall erythema may mimic testicular torsion.

DIAGNOSTIC TESTS & INTERPRETATION
Lab
Initial lab tests
- If urethritis is suspected, gram stain and culture of swabbed urethral discharge may detect urethritis, even if asymptomatic. In addition, the patient should be also evaluated for other STDs.
- Urinalysis and urine culture, preferably on first-void urine samples.
- C-reactive protein (CRP) levels and erythrocyte sedimentation rate are useful in differentiating from testicular torsion
- Blood culture may be diagnostic when epididymitis is associated with urosepsis.
- Brucellar orchitis is diagnosed by blood cultures and serologic tests.

- In mumps, serum amylase concentrations are raised. In most cases white blood cell and differential counts are normal, although leukocytosis has been reported. The virus can be readily isolated from saliva, CSF, urine, or seminal fluid within the first week. The virus has been rarely been isolated from blood and only during the first 2 days of illness. Viral detection using RT-PCR is more rapid, sensitive and specific and is done directly on the clinical specimens. In most cases clinical diagnosis is confirmed by serological means which is typically based on detection of virus-specific IgM antibody, measured by direct or indirect ELISA.

Follow-Up & Special Considerations
- Polymerase chain reaction (PCR) assays for *C. trachomatis* and *N. gonorrhoeae* should be performed on urethral swab or urine specimens.
- In case of positive testing for either *Chlamydiae* or *N. gonorrhoeae*, consider, after discussion with the patient, testing also for other sexually transmitted diseases.

Imaging
Initial approach
Color Doppler ultrasonography, particularly to rule out testicular torsion.

Follow-Up & Special Considerations
- Cultures, histopathologic examination, and PCR assays (if available) should be performed in all surgically removed tissue specimens.
- If tuberculosis is considered, chest x-rays and appropriate urine cultures should be performed. Scrotal draining sinuses, if present, should also be cultured.

Diagnostic Procedures/Other
If the diagnosis remains unclear, and testicular torsion is suspected, surgical exploration of the scrotum is warranted.

DIFFERENTIAL DIAGNOSIS
- Testicular torsion is the most important differential diagnosis
- Indirect inguinal hernia
- Tumors
- Trauma/testicular hematoma
- Polyarteritis nodosa
- Henoch–Schönlein purpura
- Testicular infarction
- Adamantiades–Behçet syndrome
- Fournier's gangrene

TREATMENT

MEDICATION

- Bacterial orchitis is in general associated with epididymitis and treated according to the specific causes for this entity (see also epididymitis).
- Gonorrhea should be treated with 1 dose of ceftriaxone 250 mg intramuscularly (8)[A].
- *Chlamydiae* spp. should be treated with doxycycline 100 mg p.o. b.i.d. for 10 days (8)[A]. Azithromycin 1 g once only is an alternative option for the treatment of *Chlamydiae* spp. While *N. gonorrhoeae* may be susceptible to azithromycin 2 g once only, do not use azithromycin to treat coinfection of gonorrhea and chlamydial infection because of fears regarding emergence of resistance of gonococci to azithromycin.
- Treat presumptively for both gonorrhea and chlamydial infection even if only 1 of them is detected since coinfection rates are high (8).
- Quinolones cannot be suggested for the treatment of *N. gonorrhoeae* due to the emergence of resistance to them (8). However, in a setting of less than 5% of the *N. gonorrhoeae* strains showing resistance to quinolones, the physician may consider them (8) i.e., ofloxacin 300 mg postprandial b.i.d. for 10 days.
- Pyogenic orchitis due to coliforms should be treated with β-lactam/β-lactamase inhibitor or a third-generation cephalosporin or ciprofloxacin. Duration of treatment should be 7–10 days.
- No specific treatment is available for the treatment of viral orchitis.
- Specific treatments are required for uncommon causes such as tuberculosis and brucellosis.

ADDITIONAL TREATMENT

General Measures
Includes bed rest and the use of cold packs for pain.

Issues for Referral
To an urologist if surgery needed.

SURGERY/OTHER PROCEDURES
Surgery is usually required for treatment of complications such as testicular abscess and pyocele

IN-PATIENT CONSIDERATIONS

Initial Stabilization
Necessary if septic.

Admission Criteria
- If infectious cause is not clear, especially if considerations like brucella or tuberculosis are possible.
- If septic or abscess is present
- If non-infectious cause is likely
- If testicular torsion has not been ruled out.

IV Fluids
In a septic patient with hypoalbuminemia, monitor fluid intake, by examining also the testes for edema.

Nursing
Scrotal elevation is necessary.

Discharge Criteria
When afebrile, without pain and without evidence of abscess. Compliance is necessary.

ONGOING CARE

FOLLOW-UP RECOMMENDATIONS
If symptoms persist or noncompliance suspected, follow-up in 3–4 weeks time (8). Otherwise, retest men in 3–6 months (8).

Patient Monitoring
Persistence of pain or fever, worsening of the swelling in conjunction with hardness and fluctuance will make a urological consultation obligatory.

PATIENT EDUCATION
Discuss with the patient regarding the value of testing for other sexually transmitted diseases and also for testing in sexual partner.

PROGNOSIS
Despite the anxiety about the potential consequences of mumps orchitis on fertility, it appears that mumps orchitis seldom results in infertility (9). Some degree of reduced testicular size can be seen in up to half of affected patients and abnormalities of spermatograms (in terms of sperm count, morphology, or motility) arise in up to 25% of patients (10).

COMPLICATIONS
- Complications of pyogenic bacterial orchitis include testicular infarction, abscess formation, and pyocele of the scrotum.
- Infertility

REFERENCES

1. National Center for Health Statistics. National Ambulatory Medical Care Survey, 2002. http://www.cdc.gov/nchs/about/major/ahcd/ahcd1.htm. Accessed January 23, 2009.
2. Ku JH, Jung TY, Lee JK, et al. Influence of bladder management on epididymo-orchitis in patients with spinal cord injury: Clean intermittent catheterization is a risk factor for epididymo-orchitis. *Spinal Cord* 2006;44:165–169.
3. Mirsadraee S, Mahdavi R, Moghadam HV, et al. Epididymo-orchitis risk factors in traumatic spinal cord injured patients. *Spinal Cord* 2003;41:516–520.
4. Roushan MR, Javanian M, Kasaeian AA. Brucellar epididymo-orchitis: Review of 53 cases in Babol, northern Iran. *Scand J Infect Dis* 2009;41(6–7):440–444.
5. Tsili AC, Tsampoulas C, Giannalis D, et al. Tuberculous epididymo-orchitis: MRI findings. *Br J Radiol* 2008;81:e166–e169.
6. Routh JC, Lischer GH, Leibovich BC. Epididymo-orchitis and testicular abscess due to *Nocardia asteroides* complex. *Urology* 2005;65:591.
7. Tichindelean C, East JW, Sarria JC. Disseminated histoplasmosis presenting as granulomatous epididymo-orchitis. *Am J Med Sci* 2009;338:238–240.
8. Sexually transmitted diseases treatment guidelines, 2010: Fluoroquinolones no longer recommended for treatment of gonococcal infections. *MMWR Recomm Rep* 2010;59:RR-12.
9. Beard CM, Benson RC Jr, Kelalis PP, et al. The incidence and outcome of mumps orchitis in Rochester, Minnesota, 1935 to 1974. *Mayo Clin Proc* 1977;52:3–7.
10. Barták V. Sperm count, morphology and motility after unilateral mumps orchitis. *J Reprod Fertil* 1973;32:491–494.

ADDITIONAL READING

- Trojiant TH, Lishnakt TS, Heiman D. Epididymitis and orchitis: An overview. *Am Fam Physician* 2009;79:583–587.

CODES

ICD9
- 072.0 Mumps orchitis
- 604.90 Orchitis and epididymitis, unspecified

CLINICAL PEARLS
- Orchitis usually occurs in patients with concurrent epididymitis, and the causative pathogens of both conditions are similar.
- Blood-borne dissemination is the major route of isolated testicular infection.

OSTEOMYELITIS

Petros I. Rafailidis
Matthew E. Falagas

 BASICS

DESCRIPTION
Osteomyelitis is an infection of bone, usually bacterial and rarely fungal in nature (1). It is acute (developing over days or weeks) or chronic (over months or years associated with dead bone [sequestrum]).

EPIDEMIOLOGY
Incidence
10–100 per 100,000 general population

RISK FACTORS
- Although *Staphylococcus aureus* is more common, patients with sickle cell anemia account for most of the bone infections with *Salmonella*.
- Diabetics have increased risk for osteomyelitis caused by *S. aureus*. Diabetic foot ulcers predispose to bone infections.
- Intravenous drug users
- Patients with peripheral vascular disease or peripheral neuropathy
- Osteopetrosis
- Radiotherapy
- Immunosuppression (AIDS, chronic granulomatous disease)
- Cat scratch
- Trauma
- Risk factors for tuberculosis

GENERAL PREVENTION
- Diabetic patients with neuropathy should always be made aware of the risk of developing ulcers on their feet.
- Every effort should be made to provide a sterile operating room environment for patients receiving prosthetic joints (2).

ETIOLOGY
Infection can occur via the following:
- Hematogenous spread.
  - In adults, hematogenous spread to bone often occurs with *S. aureus*.
  - *Mycobacterium tuberculosis* may be isolated, often in the thoracic spine. It spreads from the intervertebral disks to involve bone above and below the disk and is the result of hematogenous spread in most instances.
- Direct inoculation during trauma or surgery.
- Spread from contiguous sites, such as joints or soft-tissue infections.
  - Infection contiguous to a prosthetic device may lead to persistent infection despite adequate antibiotic therapy.
- Infection is often subacute in nature.
- All areas of the bone, including the cortex, medullary cavity, and periosteum, can be affected. Necrotic bone is termed the sequestrum.
- Osteomyelitis in children often is present in the metaphysis of long bones.

- *Pseudomonas aeruginosa* is often isolated in osteomyelitis in intravenous drug users and in diabetics with foot infections. Also, it can inoculate bone when a sharp object, such as a nail, penetrates a wet sneaker.
- *Staphylococcus epidermidis* can infect bone contiguous to an infected prosthetic device, such as a rod or total knee replacement.
- Enterobacteriaceae can cause vertebral osteomyelitis. They often spread from Batson's plexus in patients with bladder or prostate infections to the vertebral column. These organisms also may be present in the bones of the foot in patients with diabetes or vascular insufficiency.
- Atypical mycobacterial infection with *Mycobacterium avium*-intracellulare is seen within the bone marrow of patients with AIDS. Cases with bony destruction are seen during a reconstitution syndrome in patients starting highly active antiretroviral therapy.
- Fungal osteomyelitis is seen with coccidioidomycosis and blastomycosis.
- Infections with *Candida* are seen in patients with chronic indwelling catheters and in intravenous drug users.
- *Brucella* spp. which has a worldwide burden should be considered in the differential.
- Consider melioidosis when a history of travel to Southeast Asia is present.

COMMONLY ASSOCIATED CONDITIONS
- Septic arthritis
- Cellulitis

 DIAGNOSIS

HISTORY
- There is a wide range of clinical presentations in patients with osteomyelitis.
- Much depends on the acuity of the infection, the location of the involved bones, and the organism isolated.
- In general, patients present with fever and pain over the affected bone.
- Ask for a history of cat scratch.
- Travel (brucellosis or melioidosis).

PHYSICAL EXAM
- Swelling may be present.
- Increased temperature may be present over the affected bone.
- When the infection is chronic, sinus drainage may occur.
- Overlying cellulitis is common. Recurrent cellulitis should alert the clinician to the possibility of an underlying osteomyelitis.
- The diagnosis of osteomyelitis should be considered in any patient who presents with bone pain or swelling that is not associated with trauma.

DIAGNOSTIC TESTS & INTERPRETATION
Lab
Initial lab tests
- The organism responsible for osteomyelitis can be recovered via positive blood cultures in 40% of cases of acute osteomyelitis.
- Sinus tract cultures, if positive for *S. aureus*, may be accurate; however, other organisms found in the tract may not reflect the infection in the bone, especially when overlying cellulitis is present.
- Bone biopsy obtained through surgery or CT-guided fine-needle aspiration (send for culture and histology), while the patient is not on antibiotics, is the only reliable way to recover the organism causing osteomyelitis.
- An elevated erythrocyte sedimentation rate (ESR) is helpful in making the diagnosis and in following treatment of the disease.
- A Wright agglutination test as well as specific antibodies against *Brucella* spp. or PCR for brucellar DNA may help establish the diagnosis (3).
- Sonication of removed prostheses.
- Protracted time for culture up to 2 weeks.

Follow-Up & Special Considerations
Multiplex real time PCR is a helpful tool to expedite diagnosis.

Imaging
Initial approach
- X-rays are important in making the diagnosis; however, the radiographs may be normal in the early stages of illness.
- CT scans may reveal subtle cortical changes and soft-tissue changes before they are seen on plain x-rays.
- MRI is very useful for evaluation of the spine in suspected osteomyelitis (4).
- Radionuclide scanning is the best means of making an early diagnosis. The entire body can be scanned and occult sites of metastatic infection can be detected. Various tracers include ciprofloxacin, technetium-99m (Tc-99m) methylene diphosphonate, gallium, indium-labeled leukocytes, Tc-99m-labelled antileukocyte fragment Fab' or Tc-99m-hexamethylpropyleneamine oxime.
- Ultrasound of the affected bone and adjacent soft tissue to detect a collection.

Follow-Up & Special Considerations
Bone erosion, periosteal reaction, fat fluid level, and Brodie's abscess are potential findings on x-rays or MRI.

Diagnostic Procedures/Other
A positron emission tomography scan may be necessary in cases of possible chronic osteomyelitis.

Pathological Findings
- Polymorphonuclear infiltrate of the metaphysis that may extend either in the bone marrow or towards the bone cortex forming an abscess.
- When a more indolent course is present, a Brodie's abscess may be present.

DIFFERENTIAL DIAGNOSIS
- Tumors of the bone
- SAPHO syndrome: Synovitis, acne, pustulosis, hyperostosis
- Cellulitis
- Eosinophilic granuloma (in children)
- Metastasis (rule out when involvement of fingers or toes is there)

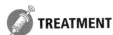 TREATMENT

MEDICATION
First Line
- Long-term antibiotic therapy can work only if necrotic tissue and bone are surgically debrided. In early disease, it is not always necessary to debride.
- At times, revascularization is necessary for adequate treatment.
- It is best to treat for specific causes.
- Methicillin-susceptible *S. aureus* should be treated with nafcillin (1.5 g every 4–6 hours) or oxacillin for 6 weeks (1,2).
- Methicillin-resistant *S. aureus* treatment depends on whether *S. aureus* infection is community-acquired or hospital-associated.
- Vancomycin 1 g every 12 hours i.v. (plus rifampin 600–900 mg i.v. daily if the presence of foreign body (infected prosthesis) is appropriate for *S. aureus* osteomyelitis for hospital-associated MRSA. Pay attention to guidelines regarding vancomycin use. Teicoplanin for i.v. use (10 mg/kg daily) is available in Europe as an alternative to vancomycin. For community-acquired MRSA, treatment may include trimethoprim–sulfamethoxazole or clindamycin or ciprofloxacin ± rifampicin depending on antimicrobial susceptibility testing.
- The same principles regarding *S. aureus* apply to coagulase-negative *Staphylococcus*.
- Susceptible gram-negative rods should be treated with ciprofloxacin (400 b.i.d. i.v. or 750 mg p.o. b.i.d.) or a third-generation cephalosporin such as ceftriaxone 2 g once daily i.v.
- Treat *P. aeruginosa* osteomyelitis with i.v. ceftazidime 2 g every 8 hour or cefepime 2 g every 12 hour (consider a combination regimen with a once-daily aminoglycoside) or piperacillin/tazobactam 4/0.5 g every 6 hour for 2–4 weeks. Continue with ciprofloxacin 750 mg q12h p.o. (1,2).

- Treatment of diabetic foot osteomyelitis should be geared towards the culprit. The most common of them is MRSA. Streptococci, anaerobes, *Pseudomonas aeruginosa* and Enterobacteriaceae play also an important pathogenetic role. Empirical treatment may include clindamycin plus ciprofloxacin (or levofloxacin), or vancomycin plus ceftazidime. Once culture results and susceptibility data are available modify accordingly (5).

Second Line
Consideration of linezolid or daptomycin if difficulty is encountered to treat *Staphylococcal* infections.

ADDITIONAL TREATMENT
Issues for Referral
- Foreign bodies, if infected, should be removed, if possible.
- Presence of sinus tract points to necessity for surgery.

Additional Therapies
Hyperbaric oxygen

SURGERY/OTHER PROCEDURES
- Surgical debridement of necrotic tissue
- After debridement, dead space management includes: Insertion of polymethylacrylate cement mixed with an antibiotic before reconstruction or
- Use of muscle flaps and skin with or without bone revascularization or microvascular transfer of flaps (including myocutaneous, muscle, osteocutaneous, osseous)
- The Ilizarov technique has been employed at times as a therapeutic tool for osteomyelitis
- Consider amputation when there is no satisfactory response to medical and surgical treatment

IN-PATIENT CONSIDERATIONS
Initial Stabilization
Required when generalized sepsis is present

Admission Criteria
Necessary initially for all cases of acute osteomyelitis (exclude concurrent bacteremia) and provide intravenous treatment

 ONGOING CARE

FOLLOW-UP RECOMMENDATIONS
- Osteomyelitis may recur, and close follow-up is always needed.
- Follow-up x-rays may not indicate whether the infection is eradicated. Bone is often in the process of remodeling, and the findings on x-ray may be hard to evaluate.
- Following ESRs every month for the first 2 months and then every 4 months is suggested for the first year following treatment. Follow-up for 2 years in case of foreign body.

Patient Monitoring
Liver/renal function tests (1–2 times/month).

PATIENT EDUCATION
Persuading a patient for the continuation of treatment while one has improved is a challenge for the physician.

PROGNOSIS
- Good for acute osteomyelitis
- Guarded for chronic osteomyelitis

COMPLICATIONS
- Bony destruction may lead to loss of function of the bone or limb.
- Vertebral osteomyelitis may produce an epidural abscess and cord compression and myelitis. Spread to the paravertebral area may lead to a psoas abscess.
- Osteomyelitis of the base of the skull may lead to cranial neuropathies.
- Amyloidosis after chronic osteomyelitis
- Marjolin's ulcer (cancer) (6)
- Chronic multifocal osteomyelitis

REFERENCES
1. Lew DP, Waldvogel FA. Osteomyelitis. *Lancet* 2004;364:369–379.
2. Zimmerli W, Trampuz A, Ochsner PE. Prosthetic-joint infections. *N Engl J Med* 2004;351: 1645–1654.
3. Colmenero JD, Morata P, Ruiz-Mesa JD, et al. Multiplex real-time polymerase chain reaction: A practical approach for rapid diagnosis of tuberculous and brucellar vertebral osteomyelitis. *Spine (Phila Pa 1976)* 2010;35:E1392–E1396.
4. Hui CL, Naidoo P. Extramedullary fat fluid level on MRI as a specific sign for osteomyelitis. *Australas Radiol* 2003;47:443–446.
5. Lipsky BA, Berendt AR, Deery HG, et al. Infectious Diseases Society of America. Diagnosis and treatment of diabetic foot infections. *Clin Infect Dis* 2004;39:885–910.
6. Samaras V, Rafailidis PI, Mourtzoukou EG, Peppas G, Falagas ME. Chronic bacterial and parasitic infections and cancer: a review. *J Infect Dev Ctries* 2010;4:267–281.

ADDITIONAL READING
- Schade VL, Roukis TS. The role of polymethyl-methacrylate antibiotic-loaded cement in addition to debridement for the treatment of soft tissue and osseous infections of the foot and ankle. *J Foot Ankle Surg* 2010;49:55–62.

 CODES

ICD9
- 730.00 Acute osteomyelitis, site unspecified
- 730.10 Chronic osteomyelitis, site unspecified
- 730.20 Unspecified osteomyelitis, site unspecified

CLINICAL PEARLS
Deep tissue culture rather than superficial or sinus tract culture reveals the true pathogen

OTITIS EXTERNA

Petros I. Rafailidis
Matthew E. Falagas

BASICS

DESCRIPTION
Infection of the external auditory canal; subdivided into 4 categories:
- Acute localized otitis externa
- Acute diffuse otitis externa (swimmer's ear)
- Chronic otitis externa (more than 6 weeks)
- Invasive (malignant or necrotizing) otitis externa: Spread beyond the external auditory canal to soft tissue and bone, often with associated necrosis

EPIDEMIOLOGY
Incidence
All forms of otitis externa (except the invasive form) are common. ~4 per 1000 of the general population (1).

RISK FACTORS
- Hot, humid weather, water exposure, and mechanical trauma are risk factors for acute diffuse otitis externa.
- Diabetic, elderly, immunocompromised, and debilitated patients are at particular risk for invasive (malignant) otitis externa.

GENERAL PREVENTION
- Good management of diabetes mellitus may decrease the risk of invasive otitis externa.
- Avoid trauma.

PATHOPHYSIOLOGY
There is some evidence regarding a potential role of the decreased amount of lysozyme, immunoglobulins IgA and IgG in wax and otitis externa (2). Microbial factors are very important. Specifically, transcription levels of exotoxin, a gene of *Pseudomonas aeruginosa*, are increased in patients with external otitis (3).

ETIOLOGY
- Acute localized otitis externa: Pustule or furuncle associated with hair follicles; usually due to *Staphylococcus aureus*.
- Acute diffuse otitis externa (swimmer's ear): Occurs mostly in hot, humid weather and may be due to a decrease in canal acidity. The most common pathogens are *P. aeruginosa*, other gram-negative bacilli, *S. aureus*, and fungi (e.g., *Aspergillus* spp.).
- Chronic otitis externa: Due to irritation of the external auditory canal from drainage of a chronic middle-ear infection. Rare causes include tuberculosis, syphilis, yaws, and leprosy.

- Invasive (malignant) otitis externa: Severe, necrotizing infection that slowly invades from the squamous epithelium of the ear canal into adjacent soft tissues, blood vessels, cartilage, and bone. *P. aeruginosa* is the pathogen involved in more than 95% of cases; in the remaining cases, the pathogens include *S. aureus*, *Staphylococcus epidermis*, *Aspergillus* spp., *Fusobacterium*, and *Actinomyces* (4).

COMMONLY ASSOCIATED CONDITIONS
Chronic otitis externa is associated with chronic suppurative otitis media

DIAGNOSIS

HISTORY
- Acute localized otitis externa
  - Presentation of pustule or furuncle
- Acute diffuse otitis externa (swimmer's ear)
  - Otalgia, pruritus
- Chronic otitis externa: Causes pruritus rather than ear pain
- Invasive (malignant) otitis externa
  - Severe pain and tenderness from the tissues around the ear
  - Drainage of pus from the canal

PHYSICAL EXAM
- Otoscopy is essential
- Acute diffuse otitis externa
  - Manipulation of the auricle often elicits pain.
  - Often purulent discharge
  - Erythema and edema of the ear canal skin
  - Erythematous tympanic membrane: In contrast to acute otitis media, however, it moves normally with pneumatic otoscopy
- Invasive otitis externa
  - Drainage of pus from the canal
  - Edematous canal with granulation tissue, usually in the posterior wall
  - Permanent facial paralysis is frequent (cranial nerves VI, IX, X, XI, or XII also may be affected).
  - Fever is rare and of low grade

DIAGNOSTIC TESTS & INTERPRETATION
Lab
- In invasive (malignant) otitis externa: Laboratory studies usually reveal a normal WBC but an increased erythrocyte sedimentation rate.
- Cultures of discharge from the external canal are unreliable. A deep-tissue specimen should be obtained for culture and pathologic examination.
- In malignant otitis, diagnostic tests for underlying disease should be performed especially to exclude diabetes mellitus, hematologic malignancy, and AIDS. In addition, one should know that immunosuppressive treatment predisposes to malignant otitis externa.

Imaging
Initial approach
- CT and MRI are helpful for defining the extent of bone (CT better) and soft-tissue involvement (MRI better).
- Scintigraphy with technetium 99 (very sensitive for diagnosis of bone involvement, but remains positive even after treatment) (5).

Follow-Up & Special Considerations
- Repeat CT or MRI
- Scintigraphy with gallium 67 citrate (becomes normal after treatment) provides additional help

Diagnostic Procedures/Other
Biopsy of tissue of the external auditory canal to reveal pathogen or other diagnosis (neoplasm)

Pathological Findings
Malignant otitis externa
- Suppuration and continuous formation of granulation tissue and possible extension to the soft tissues beneath the temporal bone
- If untreated, spreads mainly through vascular and fascial planes to osteomyelitis of the base of the skull, sigmoid sinus thrombosis, and cranial nerve palsies (6)

DIFFERENTIAL DIAGNOSIS
- Herpes zoster (oticus), bullous myringitis, foreign body, neoplasm, cholesteatoma/keratosis obturans
- The involvement of the pinna should point to other diagnostic thoughts such as relapsing polychondritis, bacterial perichondritis, and eczema

TREATMENT

MEDICATION
First Line
- Acute localized otitis externa
  - Otic drops containing antibiotics with antistaphylococcal action are usually effective
  - Antibiotics by mouth (e.g., dicloxacillin 500 mg q6h or amoxicillin/clavulanic acid 500/125 mg q8h for 7 days if local antibiotic treatment is not effective)
- Acute diffuse otitis externa (swimmer's ear)
  - Protection of the ear from additional moisture and avoidance of further mechanical injury by scratching
  - Gentle removal of debris and cleaning with mixture of alcohol, acetic acid, and distilled water
  - Otic drops containing a mixture of antibiotic and corticosteroid in an acid vehicle (e.g., neomycin–polymyxin and hydrocortisone or quinolone plus dexamethasone) are very effective (7–9) [A]
  - An ear wick or a gauze to which the medication is instilled may be necessary occasionally

- Chronic otitis externa: Treatment for chronic otitis media will also treat this condition
- Invasive (malignant) otitis externa
  - Intravenous antibiotic treatment active against *P. aeruginosa* should be used for 6–8 weeks (9,10). Use 1 of the following:
  - Imipenem 0.5–1 g q6h
  - Meropenem 1–2 g q8h
  - Ciprofloxacin 400–600 mg q12h
  - Ceftazidime 2 g q8h
  - Cefepime 2 g q12h
  - Piperacillin 4–6 g q4–6h plus tazobactam 0.5 g q4–6h [or an antipseudomonal aminoglycoside i.e. gentamicin]
  - Ticarcillin 3 g plus 0.375 g clavulanate q4h [or an antipseudomonal aminoglycoside]
  - In early cases, oral ciprofloxacin alone (750 mg q12h) may follow the initial 2 weeks of intravenous therapy if cultures reveal a *P. aeruginosa* strain sensitive to this drug
  - Cleansing of the canal and removing of the devitalized tissue
  - Treatment against other less-frequent pathogens such as *Aspergillus* includes antifungal treatment with itraconazole (400–800 mg/day) or voriconazole (400–600 mg/day) or amphotericin B (median total dose of 2 g). The duration of treatment with the oral antifungals reaches usually many weeks (10)

ADDITIONAL TREATMENT
General Measures
Avoid water exposure and trauma (including insertion of finger or foreign body into the external auditory canal)

Issues for Referral
To ENT surgeon when inadequate response to medical treatment is there.

Additional Therapies
Hyperbaric oxygen is reserved for recalcitrant cases; more data needed to assess effectiveness (5).

SURGERY/OTHER PROCEDURES
Surgical debridement of the infected bone is reserved for cases of deterioration despite medical therapy in malignant otitis externa.

IN-PATIENT CONSIDERATIONS
Admission Criteria
Invasive (malignant) otitis

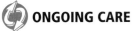 **ONGOING CARE**

FOLLOW-UP RECOMMENDATIONS
Otoscopy in a follow-up appointment

Patient Monitoring
- Monitoring of hearing with audiogram
- Monitoring of erythrocyte sedimentation rate to assess duration of antimicrobial treatment

PATIENT EDUCATION
- Instruct the patient not to use vigorous cleaning methods and to avoid moisture
- Explain to the patient that the term "malignant" does not refer to cancer and that the prognosis is much better today

PROGNOSIS
- Regarding the malignant form, the involvement of the facial nerve, or any other nerve, the presence of *Aspergillus*, bilateral involvement, and the presence of granulation tissue all affect negatively the prognosis (11). Presence of immune deficiency is also associated with worse outcome (12).
- Up to 95% of patients with malignant otitis externa may be cured (9), and this contrasts sharply with the much higher mortality reported decades ago.

COMPLICATIONS
In invasive (malignant) otitis externa, the infection may spread to the temporal bone, sigmoid sinus, jugular bulb, base of the skull, cranial nerves, meninges, and brain.

REFERENCES
1. Holten KB, Gick J. Management of the patient with otitis externa. *J Fam Pract* 2001;50:353–360.
2. Petrakis NL, Doherty M, Lee RE, et al. Demonstration and implications of lysozyme and immunoglobulins in human ear wax. *Nature* 1971;229:119–120.
3. Matar GM, Ramlawi F, Hijazi N, et al. Transcription levels of *Pseudomonas aeruginosa* exotoxin a gene and severity of symptoms in patients with otitis externa. *Curr Microbiol* 2002;45:350–354.
4. Franco-Vidal V, Blanchet H, Bebear C, et al. Necrotizing external otitis: A report of 46 cases. *Otol Neurotol* 2007;28:771–773.
5. Carfrae MJ, Kesser BW. Malignant otitis externa. *Otolaryngol Clin North Am* 2008;41:537–549
6. Chandler JR. Malignant external otitis: Further considerations. *Ann Otol Rhinol Laryngol* 1977;86:417–428.
7. Abelardo E, Pope L, Rajkumar K, et al. A double-blind randomised clinical trial of the treatment of otitis externa using topical steroid alone versus topical steroid-antibiotic therapy. *Eur Arch Otorhinolaryngol* 2009;266:41–45.
8. Mösges R, Schröder T, Baues CM, et al. Dexamethasone phosphate in antibiotic ear drops for the treatment of acute bacterial otitis externa. *Curr Med Res Opin* 2008;24:2339–2347.
9. Rahman A, Rizwan S, Waycaster C, et al. Pooled analysis of two clinical trials comparing the clinical outcomes of topical ciprofloxacin/dexamethasone otic suspension and polymyxin B/neomycin/hydrocortisone otic suspension for the treatment of acute otitis externa in adults and children. *Clin Ther* 2007;29:1950–1956.
10. Parize P, Chandesris MO, Lanternier F, et al. Antifungal therapy of *Aspergillus* invasive otitis externa: Efficacy of voriconazole and review. *Antimicrob Agents Chemother* 2009;53:1048–1053.
11. Eveleigh MO, Hall CE, Baldwin DL. Prognostic scoring in necrotising otitis externa. *J Laryngol Otol* 2009;123:1097–1102.
12. Joshua BZ, Sulkes J, Raveh E, et al. Predicting outcome of malignant external otitis. *Otol Neurotol* 2008;29:339–343.

ADDITIONAL READING
- Rosenfeld RM, Brown L, Cannon RC, et al. Clinical practice guideline: Acute otitis externa. *Otolaryngol Head Neck Surg* 2006;134:S4–S23.

 CODES

ICD9
- 380.10 Infective otitis externa, unspecified
- 380.14 Malignant otitis externa
- 380.23 Other chronic otitis externa

CLINICAL PEARLS
- Don't use ototoxic ear drops (aminoglycoside either in suspension or solution or acetic acid) when the tympanic membrane is perforated.
- Don't use local treatment (drops) for the malignant form as an initial treatment.
- When the clinical response to treatment is not the expected one, consider the following:
  - Is access to the area optimal (lack of debris, dependent posture [ear with disease is higher than healthy one])?
  - Microbiological data are mandatory at this stage, i.e., culture and susceptibility pattern to identify the pathogen
  - Has resistance to a topical agent emerged?
  - Is surgical treatment needed (if diagnosis is correct) or do you need to broaden your differential diagnosis (i.e. presence of neoplasm)? Consider biopsy.

OTITIS MEDIA

Petros I. Rafailidis
Matthew E. Falagas

 BASICS

DESCRIPTION

- Inflammation of the mucosa of periosteum of the middle ear
- Acute otitis media: Presence of fluid in the middle ear, with signs or symptoms of acute illness
- Recurrent acute otitis media: 3 or more episodes in 6 months, 4 or more in 1 year, or 2 or more episodes in the first year of life
- Otitis media with effusion or serous otitis media: Persistence of middle-ear fluid for several months without other signs of infection
- Chronic suppurative otitis media: Chronic purulent drainage from the affected ear through perforated tympanic membrane with or without cholesteatoma

EPIDEMIOLOGY
Incidence
- More than two-thirds of children under age 3 have at least 1 episode of acute otitis media and one-third have 3 or more; the prevalence among adults is only 0.25%. 2300 outpatient visits for acute otitis media per 1000 child-years (1).
- The peak incidence is at ages 6–24 months (with a second smaller peak between 5 and 6 years, the time of school entrance); incidence declines after age of 6 years and is infrequent in adults. The vaccination against pneumococci has decreased the incidence of the disease.
- Acute otitis media occurs more often in males.

RISK FACTORS
- Anatomic changes (cleft palate, cleft uvula)
- Alteration of normal physiologic defenses (patulous eustachian tube), i.e., viral infection of the upper respiratory tract or allergy
- Congenital or acquired immunologic deficiencies
- Daycare attendance
- Passive smoking
- Family history
- Being of young age at the time of the first episode is a risk factor of recurrent middle-ear infections.
- Risk factors for developmental delay (i.e. Down's syndrome, cleft palate) put patients with otitis media with effusion at increased risk for hearing loss

GENERAL PREVENTION
- Vaccination against Pneumococci and *Haemophilus influenzae*
- Immunoprophylaxis with killed and live vaccine against influenza
- Breastfeeding for 6 months
- Appropriate antimicrobial treatment of patients with acute otitis media decreases the probability of recurrence.

PATHOPHYSIOLOGY
Anatomic or physiologic dysfunction of the eustachian tube appears to lead to fluid collection in the middle-ear and mastoid cavities, providing a culture medium for any bacterium present. Viral upper respiratory infections, which can cause congestion of the mucosa of the eustachian tube, often precede episodes of acute otitis media.

ETIOLOGY
- Acute otitis media
  - In children (non-neonates)
  - *Streptococcus pneumoniae*: 35%; the most common types in order of decreasing frequency are 19, 23, 6, 14, 3, and 18.
  - *H. influenzae*: Approximately 25%; about 90% of *H. influenzae* infections are due to nontypable strains; bacteremia or meningitis may accompany infections due to type b *H. influenzae* (20% of strains produce beta lactamases).
  - *Moraxella catarrhalis*: Approximately 15% (90% of *M. catarrhalis* strains produce beta-lactamases)
  - Group A streptococci: 12%
  - *Staphylococcus aureus*: 12%
  - Sterile (no pathogen grown in cultures of middle-ear fluid): Up to 30% in some studies
  - In neonates: Group B streptococci and gram-negative bacilli are important causes. Also, *Chlamydia trachomatis* infection may be a pathogen
  - In adults: *H. influenza* (26%) and *S. pneumoniae* (21%) are the most common pathogens.
- Recurrent acute otitis media
  - Most cases are due to the same pathogens that cause acute otitis media. Most cases of early recurrence (75%) are not due to relapse (of the same strain) but due to new infections (organisms different from those that caused the initial episode).
- Otitis media with effusion
  - Cultures of middle-ear fluid are frequently negative.
- Chronic suppurative otitis media
  - Aerobic cultures of draining fluid reveal a high percentage of *S. aureus*, *Pseudomonas aeruginosa*, and enteric gram-negative bacilli (*Klebsiella*, *Escherichia coli*, *Proteus*)
  - Anaerobes, including *Prevotella*, *Fusobacterium*, *Porphyromonas*, and some *Bacteroides* species, are found in 50% of cases, usually in mixed culture with aerobes.
  - Tuberculous otitis media is a rare cause. It is characterized by a tympanic membrane with multiple perforations, extensive granulation tissue, and severe hearing loss.

COMMONLY ASSOCIATED CONDITIONS
Chronic otitis media may coexist with chronic otitis externa

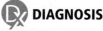 **DIAGNOSIS**

HISTORY
- Acute otitis media
  - Earache
  - Fever (may be absent)
  - Decreased hearing
- Acute otitis media in infants
  - May cause no symptoms or cause septic profile
  - Often irritability, anorexia, nausea, vomiting, and diarrhea
- Otitis media with effusion
  - Usually asymptomatic
  - Sense of fullness in the affected ear
  - Vertigo or tinnitus may occur
  - Associated with an approximate 25-dB hearing loss of the affected ear
- Chronic suppurative otitis media is divided into 2 groups: With or without cholesteatoma
  - Chronic purulent drainage from the affected ear
  - Hearing loss
  - Perforation of the tympanic membrane
  - May be accompanied by mucosal changes, such as polypoid degeneration and granulation tissue, and osseous changes, such as osteitis and sclerosis

PHYSICAL EXAM
- Acute otitis media
  - Ear drainage if eardrum is perforated
  - Vertigo, nystagmus, and tinnitus may occur
  - Decreased eardrum mobility (as observed by pneumatic otoscopy)
  - The eardrum is usually red, opaque, and bulging. Redness is an early sign of acute otitis media, but erythema alone is not diagnostic of middle-ear infection
- Otitis media with effusion
  - The eardrum is often dull but not bulging and is hypomobile

DIAGNOSTIC TESTS & INTERPRETATION
Lab
Initial lab tests
- White blood cells may be increased; a polymorphonuclear type points to a bacterial pathogen
- Culture obtained by tympanocentesis to define the microbiology (cause of infection) should be considered in the following:
  - The patient who is critically ill at the onset
  - The patient with altered host defenses, including the newborn infant
- Blood cultures when toxic appearance is there

Follow-Up & Special Considerations
Tympanocentesis for the patient who has not responded to initial antimicrobial therapy in 48–72 hours

Imaging
In patients with chronic suppurative otitis media, a CT scan should be used to rule out a surgically treatable nidus of infection, such as an infected cholesteatoma or mastoid sequestrum.

Diagnostic Procedures/Other
- Tympanometry, acoustic reflex measurement, or acoustic reflectometry: To document the presence of middle-ear fluid
- Hearing testing ± language testing if acute otitis media with effusion with a duration of over 3 months is present

DIFFERENTIAL DIAGNOSIS
- Earache due to referred pain from the jaw or teeth (otoscopic examination is normal).
- In an adult with persistent unilateral serous otitis media, nasopharyngeal carcinoma must be excluded.

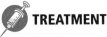

TREATMENT
MEDICATION
First Line
- In children (non-neonates) and adults
  – Drug of choice: Amoxicillin 80–90 mg/kg/d divided q8h (2) [maximum daily dose 1.5 g according to two-thirds of the committee releasing the guidelines] or 500 mg t.i.d. in adults for 10 days
  – Alternative drugs are indicated for the following cases: Persistent symptoms after 48–72 hours of amoxicillin treatment and in immunocompromised hosts
  – Amoxicillin–clavulanate: 80–90 mg/kg/d for amoxicillin component divided q8h or 625 mg t.i.d. in adults for 10 days
  – Cefuroxime axetil: 30 mg/kg/d divided q12h or 250 mg b.i.d. in adults for 10 days
  – Cefprozil: 30 mg/kg/d divided q12h or 500 mg b.i.d. in adults for 10 days
  – Cefpodoxime proxetil: 10 mg/kg/d divided q12h or 100 mg b.i.d. in adults for 10 days
  – Ceftriaxone: 50 mg/kg i.m. single dose
- Patients with penicillin allergy
  – Clarithromycin: 15 mg/kg/d divided q12h or 250 mg b.i.d. in adults for 10 days
  – Azithromycin: 10 mg/kg q.d. on day 1 and then 5 mg/kg q.d. on days 2–5; in adults, 500 mg q.d. on day 1 and then 250 mg q.d. on days 2–5
  – Erythromycin–sulfisoxazole: 40 mg/kg/d for erythromycin component divided q6h
  – Trimethoprim–sulfamethoxazole (TMP/SMX): 8 mg TMP/kg/d divided q12h or 160 mg TMP/800 mg SMX b.i.d. in adults for 10 days
- In neonates: Initially, intravenous antimicrobial chemotherapy is needed (ampicillin plus cephalosporin of third generation)
  – A watchful waiting approach has been adopted in recent years provided that the child is older than 6 months and the patient's carer fully understands the paramount importance of a follow-up visit in the 2–3 next days and no deterioration of the child's health happens in the meantime. This approach is not suitable when there is presence of grommets.

Second Line
Recurrent Acute Otitis Media
- Chemoprophylaxis for 3–6 months with antibiotics provides has been reported by some to provide a minor benefit and has not been recommended as a general measure; it has to be individualized.

Otitis Media with Effusion
- Antihistamines and decongestants are usually ineffective (3)
- A short course of oral antibiotics or steroids or a combination of the 2 provides only little lasting benefit (3).

Chronic Suppurative Otitis Media
- Surgical drainage of infected areas of the middle ear, followed by a prolonged course of topical antibiotic drops
- Surgical management of cholesteatoma
- In exacerbations: Culture of the drainage and oral antimicrobial based on antibiogram

ADDITIONAL TREATMENT
General Measures
Pain has to be managed with analgesics independently of the decision regarding antibiotic treatment.

SURGERY/OTHER PROCEDURES
- Referral for surgery if the patient with otitis media with effusion has the following: More than 4–6 months of bilateral otitis media with effusion, more than 6 months of unilateral otitis media with effusion and/or hearing loss greater than 40 dB (individualize if 21–39 dB), developmental delay risk factors. Surgery includes initially the use of tympanostomy tubes and, if repeat surgery necessary, then the combination of adenoidectomy plus myringotomy (± tube insertion).
- Recurrent acute otitis media: Individualization is required; the risk of grommet insertion has to be considered.

IN-PATIENT CONSIDERATIONS
Admission Criteria
Neonate or indication for surgery

 ONGOING CARE
FOLLOW-UP RECOMMENDATIONS
- Not necessary if symptoms of acute otitis media clearly disappear with appropriate treatment.
- Regarding otitis media with effusion, watchful waiting for 3 months is suggested if no risk factors for developmental difficulties exist. Follow-up at 3- to 6-month intervals is suggested thereafter until effusion is not present, hearing loss is identified, or structural abnormalities are suspected (i.e., ossicular erosion).

PROGNOSIS
Acute: Excellent usually. When effusion is present depends on good follow-up.

COMPLICATIONS
- Acute and chronic mastoiditis, hearing loss
- Labyrinthitis
- Facial nerve paralysis
- Petrous apicitis, Gradenigo's syndrome
- Otogenic skull base osteomyelitis
- Sigmoid sinus thrombosis
- CNS infection (meningitis, epidural abscess, subdural abscess, brain abscess)

REFERENCES
1. Daly KA, Hoffman HJ, Kvaerner KJ, et al. Epidemiology, natural history, and risk factors: Panel report from the Ninth International Research Conference on Otitis Media. *Int J Pediatr Otorhinolaryngol* 2010;74:231–240.
2. Christian-Kopp S, Sinha M, Rosenberg DI, et al. Antibiotic dosing for acute otitis media in children: A weighty issue. *Pediatr Emerg Care* 2010;26: 19–25.
3. American Academy of Family Physicians; American Academy of Otolaryngology-Head and Neck Surgery; American Academy of Pediatrics Subcommittee on otitis media with effusion. Otitis media with effusion. *Pediatrics* 2004;113: 1412–1429.

CODES

ICD9
- 381.4 Nonsuppurative otitis media, not specified as acute or chronic
- 382.3 Unspecified chronic suppurative otitis media
- 382.9 Unspecified otitis media

CLINICAL PEARLS
- Don't abandon follow-up when a middle-ear effusion is present beyond 3 months

O

PARVOVIRUS INFECTION

Paschalis Vergidis
Matthew E. Falagas

 BASICS

DESCRIPTION

- Parvovirus B19 has been associated with erythema infectiosum (fifth disease), transient aplastic crisis in chronic hemolytic anemia patients, chronic anemia in immunocompromised (including HIV-infected) patients, and fetal infection (hydrops fetalis and fetal death).
- Parvovirus B19 is responsible for most transient aplastic anemia episodes in patients with chronic hemolytic disorders (i.e., 80–92% of transient pure red-cell aplasia crises in sickle cell disease).

EPIDEMIOLOGY

Prevalence

- Global distribution: Humans are the principal infection reservoir.
- Seroprevalence rates rise rapidly between the ages of 5–18, and reach 30–60% in adults.
- Erythema infectiosum is a childhood illness and occurs in outbreaks in schools, mostly during late winter and early spring, but it can affect any age. Secondary attack rates rise up to 50%.
- Although there is no sex predominance for most manifestations of parvovirus infection, arthritis most commonly affects women.
- Failure to clear parvovirus B19 viremia seems to be a common causative factor for chronic anemia in immunocompromised patients.

RISK FACTORS

- Seronegative pregnant women
- Patients with chronic hemolytic anemias (thalassemia, sickle cell disease, etc.)
- HIV-infected individuals
- Bone marrow and solid organ transplant recipients (1)
- Patients with other forms of cell-mediated immunity suppression

GENERAL PREVENTION

- Prevention by vaccine is not available. Study of the vaccine has been suspended due to adverse events.
- As the patients are infectious before the appearance of any signs and symptoms, prevention by exclusion from school or the workplace is of no help. Exclusion should be individualized (i.e., exclusion of a high-risk individual during an outbreak).
- Hand washing in the case of direct contact
- Separation of admitted patients from those in high-risk groups (including seronegative pregnant hospital workers)
- When treating viremic patients, hospital staff should wear gowns, gloves, and masks to avoid hospital outbreaks.

PATHOPHYSIOLOGY

- Transmission may occur by the respiratory route and close person-to-person contact. The virus is present in oral and/or respiratory secretions.
- Parenteral transmission by blood and blood products has also been documented. Risk by single blood donation is 1:50,000, but this increases with the use of concentrated coagulation factors.
- Vertical transmission also occurs and may lead to hydrops fetalis and fetal death.
- Nosocomial and laboratory transmission has been documented.
- Viremic patients with aplastic crises are highly infective for other patients belonging to the high-risk groups.
- Infection may be asymptomatic.
- Incubation lasts about a week and is followed by viremia of 1 week duration. During the viremic period, the virus can be detected in oral and/or respiratory secretions.
- About the tenth day, pure red-cell aplasia in bone marrow has been established, due to infection and lysis of the red-cell precursors.
- Rash appears after resolution of viremia (more than 2 weeks after challenge) and lasts for 2–3 days. Joint involvement may persist several days after the rash resolution. Both phenomena seem to be immune-mediated reactions.
- IgM–parvovirus B19 complexes can be detected on about day 10, and IgG about 1 week later.
- Resolution of anemia and recovery from viremia correlate with virus-specific IgM and IgG antibodies. The latter may persist lifelong.
- Failure to form a proper antibody response results in chronic infection in the immunocompromised patient.
- Failure to effectively overcome the pure red-cell aplasia in hemolytic anemia patients results in transient aplastic crisis.

Pregnancy Considerations

Infection of the fetus may lead to severe anemia, resulting in cardiac failure, hydrops fetalis, and endometrial death.

ETIOLOGY

Parvovirus B19 is a small, non-enveloped, single-stranded DNA virus, the only human-specific member of the family *Parvoviridae*. It has been named after the code number of the human serum where it was discovered in the early 1970s.

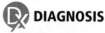 DIAGNOSIS

HISTORY

- The appearance of the rash is preceded by mild symptoms (fever, malaise, myalgias, headache, and pruritus).
- There may be sore throat and respiratory and abdominal symptoms.
- Joint symptoms (stiffness, pain) begin about 1 day after rash resolution, mostly affecting women. Hands, knees, and wrists are usually involved. Peripheral polyarthropathy is symmetric and improves in about 2 weeks.
- Symptoms of severe anemia predominate in aplastic crises and in hemolytic anemia patients.

PHYSICAL EXAM

- Erythema infectiosum appears about the tenth day of illness, presenting as a fine, reticular, maculopapular, bright-red facial rash (slapped cheek). It spares the region around the mouth, but may involve the extremities and, less often, the trunk, the palms, and the soles. It usually resolves within 1 week but can recur for several weeks after exposure to heat, cold, exercise, or stress.
- Swelling of the affected joints and fluid formation can be present.
- Signs of severe anemia predominate in aplastic crises and in hemolytic anemia patients. Rash may be absent.

DIAGNOSTIC TESTS & INTERPRETATION

Lab

- Diagnosis of erythema infectiosum in children is clinical.
- Detection of viral IgM (RIA, ELISA) can be achieved within 3 days of onset of symptoms of viremia. The IgM level decreases after 1 month but remains detectable by 2–3 months.
- A fourfold or larger increase of viral IgG (RIA, ELISA) between acute phase and convalescent serum samples confirms the diagnosis.
- Antibodies might be of no help in immunocompromised individuals, as the titer's rise might be transient or absent. In these patients, detection of parvovirus B19 DNA by hybridization or PCR in serum, respiratory secretions, bone marrow, spleen, and tissue specimens is recommended.
- Parvovirus-related aplastic episodes in the setting of hemolytic anemia are suspected when the degree of anemia is high (Hb <2 g/dL below baseline, reticulocytes <0.2%), and bone marrow is hypoplastic, with characteristic giant pronormoblasts present.

Pregnancy Considerations
- When hydrops fetalis develops, maternal IgM is usually no longer present.
- Amniotic fluid and cord blood PCR are recommended for diagnosis.
- Maternal α-fetoprotein and ultrasound of the fetus are used to detect hydrops.

DIFFERENTIAL DIAGNOSIS
- Rubella
- Scarlet fever
- Facial erysipelas
- Roseola
- Infectious mononucleosis
- Echovirus infection
- Toxic shock syndrome
- Rickettsioses
- Meningococcemia
- Lyme disease
- Vasculitic disease
- Allergic and drug reactions

 TREATMENT

MEDICATION
- Parvovirus B19 infection in the immunocompetent host is self-limited and does not need specific treatment.
- Symptomatic relief with anti-inflammatory drugs may be necessary in cases of arthritis.
- Transient aplastic crisis and chronic anemia:
  - Supportive blood transfusions as anemia is usually severe
  - Intravenous immunoglobulin (IVIG) infusions for patients with chronic anemia
  - Recurrence of aplastic anemia and chronic anemia responds to retreatment with IVIG.
- If feasible, reduction of immunosuppression in the immunocompromised host is recommended. Dose and duration of IVIG treatment are not standardized.

ADDITIONAL TREATMENT
General Measures
Counseling parents in the case of infection during pregnancy. Therapeutic abortion is not indicated. Intrauterine transfusions may be necessary in the case of hydrops fetalis.

 ONGOING CARE

FOLLOW-UP RECOMMENDATIONS
- Complete blood count and reticulocytes in hemolytic anemia and immunocompromised (including HIV-positive) patients.
- Maternal α-fetoprotein, ultrasound of the fetus to detect hydrops, in the case of maternal infection during pregnancy.

COMPLICATIONS
- There are no major complications in the immunocompetent host.
- Erythema infectiosum and related arthritis are benign, self-limited conditions.
- In the case of infection during pregnancy, risk of fetal infection is 33%. The risk of fetal death is 11% for infection that occurs within the first 20 weeks of pregnancy, and <1% after 20 weeks (2,3). Parvovirus B19 rarely causes congenital anomalies.
- Hemophagocytic syndrome (4).
- Transient aplastic episodes in hemolytic anemia patients may be fatal if not readily managed.
- Chronic anemia in immunocompromised patients has a high recurrence rate but responds to IVIG retreatment.
- Papular purpuric glove and socks syndrome.
- Hepatitis: Acute (including fatal liver failure) or chronic (5,6).
- Antiphospholipid antibodies (7).
- Presence of parvovirus is frequently detected by PCR in myocardial tissue. However, patients with the presence of parvovirus do not have more inflammatory infiltrates than those without detectable virus. Of note, the clinical presentation of 12 patients with detectable virus among a cohort of 100 patients presenting for cardiomyopathy workup included a variety of presentation ranging from acute heart failure to chronic heart failure and also patients with ischemic cardiomyopathy (8).
- Acute meningoencephalitis (9).
- Chronic allograft dysfunction (10).

REFERENCES
1. Eid AJ, Brown RA, Patel R, et al. Parvovirus B19 infection after transplantation: A review of 98 cases. *Clin Infect Dis* 2006;43:40–48.
2. Enders M, Weidner A, Zoellner I, et al. Fetal morbidity and mortality after acute human parvovirus B19 infection in pregnancy: Prospective evaluation of 1018 cases. *Prenatal diagnosis* 2004;24:513–518.
3. Schiesser M, Sergi C, Enders M, et al. Discordant outcomes in a case of parvovirus B19 transmission into both dichorionic twins. *Twin Res Hum Genet* 2009;12:175–179.
4. Rouphael NG, Talati NJ, Vaughan C, et al. Infections associated with haemophagocytic syndrome. *Lancet Infect Dis* 2007;7:814–822.
5. Hillingsø JG, Jensen IP, Tom-Petersen L. Parvovirus B19 and acute hepatitis in adults. *Lancet* 1998; 351:955–956.

6. Mogensen TH, Jensen JM, Hamilton-Dutoit S, et al. Chronic hepatitis caused by persistent parvovirus B19 infection. *BMC Infect Dis* 2010;10:246.
7. von Landenberg P, Lehmann HW, Modrow S. Human parvovirus B19 infection and antiphospholipid antibodies. *Autoimmun Rev* 2007;6:278–285.
8. Stewart GC, Lopez-Molina J, Gottumukkala RV, et al. Myocardial Parvovirus B19 persistence: Lack of association with clinicopathologic phenotype in adults with heart failure. *Circ Heart Fail* 2011; 4: 71–78.
9. Barah F, Vallely PJ, Chiswick ML, et al. Association of human parvovirus B19 infection with acute meningoencephalitis. *Lancet* 2001;358:729–730.
10. Waldman M, Kopp JB. Parvovirus B19 and the kidney. *Clin J Am Soc Nephrol* 2007;2:S47–S56.

ADDITIONAL READING
- Frickhofen N, Abkowitz JL, Safford M, et al. Persistent B19 parvovirus infection in patients infected with human immunodeficiency virus type 1 (HIV-1): A treatable cause of anemia in AIDS. *Ann Intern Med* 1990;113:926–933.
- Kurtzman G, Frickhofen N, Kimball J, et al. Pure red-cell aplasia of 10 years' duration due to persistent parvovirus B19 infection and its cure with immunoglobulin therapy. *N Engl J Med* 1989;321:519–523.

 CODES

ICD9
- 057.0 Erythema infectiosum (fifth disease)
- 079.83 Parvovirus B19
- 647.63 Other antepartum viral diseases

CLINICAL PEARLS
- Parvovirus B19 is associated with transient aplastic crisis in chronic hemolytic anemia patients, and chronic anemia in immunocompromised patients (including those with HIV-infection).
- Treatment consists of supportive blood transfusions and IVIG infusions.
- Infection during pregnancy can lead to hydrops fetalis. Parvovirus B19 rarely causes congenital abnormalities.

PELVIC INFLAMMATORY DISEASE

Paschalis I. Vergidis
Matthew E. Falagas

 BASICS

DESCRIPTION
- Pelvic inflammatory disease (PID) covers a spectrum of inflammatory disorders of the upper female genital tract, manifesting with lower abdominal or pelvic pain, increased or changed vaginal discharge, dyspareunia, dysuria, metrorrhagia, or menorrhagia. Disorders include the following:
  - Endometritis
  - Salpingitis
  - Parametritis
  - Oophoritis
  - Tubo-ovarian abscess
  - Pelvic peritonitis

EPIDEMIOLOGY
Incidence
- Nearly 1 million cases are reported annually in the US (1).
- Although incidence rates have declined, PID remains a considerable cause of morbidity and the most frequent gynecologic emergency.
- Most prevalent in adolescent girls.

RISK FACTORS
- Multiple sex partners
- Unprotected sexual intercourse
- Intrauterine devices (IUDs), typically older models. The risk is mainly limited to the first 3 weeks after insertion.
- Previous episode of PID
- Bacterial vaginosis (BV) is more common among women with PID. However, BV is not thought to be responsible alone.

GENERAL PREVENTION
- Safe-sex practices:
  - Use condoms.
  - Limit the number of sex partners.
  - Treat infected partners.
- Avoid IUDs in women with multiple sex partners who are at risk of acquiring an STD.

ETIOLOGY
- Common organisms (50% of cases), either alone or in combination:
  - *Neisseria gonorrhoeae*
  - *Chlamydia trachomatis*
  - Anaerobes, such as *Bacteroides* and *Peptostreptococcus*
- Other organisms frequently isolated from inflamed tissue, but that may not be involved in pathogenesis:
  - *Gardnerella vaginalis*
  - Enteric gram-negative rods, such as *E. coli*
  - Streptococci, mainly *Streptococcus agalactiae* (group B Streptococcus)
  - *Mycoplasma hominis*
- Rarely, actinomycosis in women with an intrauterine device (IUD).
- In developing countries, *Mycobacterium tuberculosis* is a common cause.

 DIAGNOSIS

HISTORY
- Lower abdominal or pelvic pain, usually dull, bilateral, and subacute at onset.
- Increased or changed vaginal discharge.
- Metrorrhagia
- Menorrhagia
- Dyspareunia
- Dysuria

Less Common Symptoms and Signs
- Nausea and vomiting
- Pleuritic or right upper quadrant pain, caused by perihepatitis of Fitz-Hugh and Curtis syndrome.
- Symptoms of proctitis

PHYSICAL EXAM
- Cervical motion tenderness
- Uterine tenderness
- Adnexal tenderness or swelling
- Mucopurulent cervicitis
- Elevated temperature

DIAGNOSTIC TESTS & INTERPRETATION
Lab
Initial lab tests
- CBC count
- Pregnancy test
- Urinalysis
- Fecal occult blood test
- Erythrocyte sedimentation rate
- C-reactive protein
- Gram stain and microscopic examination of cervical discharge
- Gonococcal culture
- Nucleic acid amplification tests for *Chlamydia* and *N. gonorrhoeae*.

Follow-Up & Special Considerations
HIV screening is encouraged in women diagnosed with PID.

Imaging
If there is diagnostic uncertainty: Ultrasound (transvaginal) or CT or MRI examination of the pelvis. Thickened fluid-filled oviducts are supportive of the diagnosis.

Diagnostic Procedures/Other
Laparoscopy can be used to obtain a diagnosis of salpingitis when noninvasive tests are inconclusive.

DIFFERENTIAL DIAGNOSIS
- Acute appendicitis
- Ectopic pregnancy
- Endometriosis
- Ovarian tumor
- Uterine fibroids
- Mesenteric lymphadenitis
- Urinary tract infection
- Ruptured ovarian cyst
- Corpus luteum bleeding

TREATMENT

MEDICATION
Outpatient
First Line
- Ceftriaxone 250 mg IM or other parenteral third generation cephalosporin, for example, ceftizoxime or cefotaxime, plus doxycycline 100 mg orally twice daily for 14 days.
- Cefoxitin 2 g IM plus probenecid 1 g orally (PO) in a single concurrent dose plus doxycycline.
- Can add metronidazole 500 mg orally twice daily for 14 days to any of the above regimens.

Second Line
- Fluoroquinolone use may only be considered if parenteral cephalosporin use is not feasible, and community prevalence and individual risk of gonorrhea is low.
- Use levofloxacin 500 mg orally daily or ofloxacin 400 mg orally twice daily for 14 days with or without metronidazole 500 mg twice daily for 14 days.

Inpatient
First Line
- Cefoxitin 2 g IV every 6 hours plus doxycycline 100 mg IV or orally every 12 hours. Doxycycline should be administered orally when possible because of pain associated with infusion.
- Cefotetan 2 g IV every 12 hours plus doxycycline. Continue at least 24 hours after the patient demonstrates substantial clinical improvement.

- Clindamycin 900 mg IV every 8 hours plus gentamicin 2 mg/kg IV or IM as a loading dose, then gentamicin 1.5 mg/kg every 8 hours. The maintenance dose should be adjusted for renal dysfunction. Single daily aminoglycoside dosing may be substituted. Continue at least 24 hours after the patient demonstrates substantial clinical improvement, after which, doxycycline 100 mg orally twice daily or clindamycin 450 mg orally 4 times daily should be continued for a total of 14 days. Despite increasing resistance of anaerobes to clindamycin, there is no evidence of treatment failures in PID.

Second Line
- Ampicillin/sulbactam 3 g IV every 6 hours plus doxycycline (as above)
- Fluoroquinolones no longer recommended due to increased resistance to gonococci.

SURGERY/OTHER PROCEDURES
- Drainage of tubo-ovarian abscess that are large or do not respond to antimicrobial management
- There are conflicting data on the need to remove an IUD. Close clinical follow-up is required if the IUD remains in place.

IN-PATIENT CONSIDERATIONS
Admission Criteria
Hospitalize the patient if the following applies:
- Diagnosis is uncertain and surgical emergencies, such as appendicitis and ectopic pregnancy, cannot be excluded.
- Severe illness or nausea and vomiting preclude outpatient management.
- The patient is pregnant.
- The patient does not respond clinically to outpatient therapy within 72 hours of initiation of drug therapy
- A pelvic abscess is suspected.
- Clinical follow-up within 72 hours if starting antibiotics cannot be arranged.
- The patient is unable to follow or tolerate an outpatient regimen.

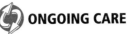 ONGOING CARE

FOLLOW-UP RECOMMENDATIONS
- 72 hours after initiation of drug therapy, the patient should show clear, marked improvement.
- 3–5 days from initiation of therapy for hospitalized patients, substantial clinical improvement should be evidenced by defervescence and reduction in abdominal, uterine, adnexal, and cervical motion tenderness.
- 7–10 days after completing drug therapy, all patients should have microbiologic examination.
- Sex partners:
  – Evaluate and treat for the likelihood of asymptomatic or symptomatic gonococcal and/or chlamydial infection. There is a high risk of reinfection of the patient if a partner is left untreated.
  – Empiric treatment for both gonococcal and chlamydial infection, regardless of microbiologic test results.

COMPLICATIONS
- Infertility may occur in 11% of women after 1 episode of PID, in 23% after 2 episodes, and in 54% after 3 episodes.
- Ectopic pregnancy occurs 7–10 times more frequently after PID.
- A syndrome of chronic abdominal pain attributed to pelvic adhesions may occur, mainly in infertile women with a history of multiple episodes of PID.
- Death occurs in about 6 per 100,000, usually caused by a ruptured tubo-ovarian abscess, with generalized peritonitis.
- Women with HIV infection respond to treatment similarly to those uninfected (2).

REFERENCES
1. Sutton MY, Sternberg M, Zaidi A, et al. Trends in pelvic inflammatory disease hospital discharges and ambulatory visits, United States, 1985–2001. *Sex Transm Dis* 2005;32:778–784.
2. Irwin KL, Moorman AC, O'Sullivan MJ, et al. Influence of human immunodeficiency virus infection on pelvic inflammatory disease. *Obstet Gynecol* 2000;95:525–534.

ADDITIONAL READING
- Ness RB, Soper DE, Holley RL, et al. Effectiveness of inpatient and outpatient treatment strategies for women with pelvic inflammatory disease: Results from the Pelvic Inflammatory Disease Evaluation and Clinical Health (PEACH) Randomized Trial. *Am J Obstet Gynecol* 2002;186:929–937.
- Walker CK, Wiesenfeld HC. Antibiotic therapy for acute pelvic inflammatory disease: The 2006 Centers for Disease Control and Prevention sexually transmitted diseases treatment guidelines. *Clin Infect Dis* 2007;44(Suppl 3):S111–S122.
- Workowski KA, Berman SM. Sexually transmitted diseases treatment guidelines, 2010. *MMWR Recomm Rep* 2010;59(RR-12):1–110.

 CODES

ICD9
- 614.3 Acute parametritis and pelvic cellulitis
- 614.4 Chronic or unspecified parametritis and pelvic cellulitis
- 614.9 Unspecified inflammatory disease of female pelvic organs and tissues

CLINICAL PEARLS
- PID covers a spectrum of inflammatory disorders of the upper female genital tract and manifests with lower abdominal or pelvic pain, usually dull, bilateral, and subacute at onset.
- Many women with PID have subtle symptoms.
- Surgical emergencies should be excluded in the evaluation of patients with suspected PID.

PERICARDITIS

Petros I. Rafailidis
Matthew E. Falagas

 BASICS

DESCRIPTION
Pericarditis is inflammation of the pericardium, and is caused by a wide assortment of infections, including viral, bacterial, fungal, and protozoal etiologies. Noninfectious etiologies also are common and must be ruled out.

EPIDEMIOLOGY
Incidence
- Is ~0.1% among hospitalized patients. The incidence among patients with chest pain attending emergency medicine departments is 5% (1).
- Bacterial pericarditis has an incidence of 5 per 100,000.

GENERAL PREVENTION
- There is no way to prevent idiopathic pericarditis.
- Early diagnosis and treatment may prevent the need for surgery.

PATHOPHYSIOLOGY
Depends on the particular pathogen. An autoimmune reaction seems to be the commonest scenario for the idiopathic variant. Directly infectious affliction of the pericardium occurs regarding bacterial pericarditis. CD4 lymphocytes and increased gamma interferon are present in tuberculous pericarditis in HIV negative patients (2).

ETIOLOGY
- Most cases of idiopathic pericarditis are never fully diagnosed, and thus are attributed to viral causes.
- Viral:
  - Coxsackievirus A and B are the most common infections, leading to pericarditis and myocarditis.
  - Herpes viruses (Epstein-Barr virus, varicella zoster virus, herpes simplex virus, and cytomegalovirus)
  - Hepatitis B virus
  - Adenovirus
  - Mumps
  - Echovirus
  - Influenza
  - Human immunodeficiency virus
- Bacterial:
  - Contiguous pulmonary processes such as pneumonia or empyema, caused by tuberculosis, Pneumococcus, Staphylococcus, and gram-negative organisms such as Klebsiella, Legionella, and Haemophilus influenzae
  - Part of a generalized infection of the mediastinum in patients who have had a median sternotomy as part of cardiac surgery
  - Nosocomial organisms, such as *Staphylococcus aureus*, or gram-negative organisms are often discovered.
  - *Coxiella burnetii*, *Bartonella quintana*, *Rickettsia conorii* and *Mycoplasma pneumoniae* are other culprits.

- Fungal:
  - Histoplasmosis
  - Coccidioides immitis
  - Candida
  - All are seen as part of a disseminated syndrome.
- Protozoal:
  - Disseminated toxoplasmosis
  - Spread of *Entamoeba histolytica* can occur from involvement of the liver, usually the left lobe, with extension through the diaphragm.

 DIAGNOSIS

HISTORY
- Retrosternal chest pain and fever are common. Patients get relief from the pain by sitting forward.
- Associated viral symptoms, such as upper respiratory tract infections in winter or the rash of chicken pox.
- In bacterial pericarditis, chest pain occurs in only one-third of patients with disease.
- Fevers
- Tachypnea and unexplained tachycardia; can lead to early tamponade.

PHYSICAL EXAM
- Physical examination may reveal a pulsus paradoxus, along with decreased pulse pressure.
- A three-component friction rub or decreased heart sounds may be noted.

DIAGNOSTIC TESTS & INTERPRETATION
Lab
- Serum should always be stored for acute and convalescent serology studies.
- A complete blood count may show increased (or decreased) WBC and an increase in polymorphonuclear leucocytes (or lymphocytes).
- Troponin levels may be elevated.
- Pericardiocentesis or surgical pericardial biopsy can help establish the diagnosis while relieving tamponade (window procedure).
- Various tests may be sent regarding the pericardial fluid such as protein amount, number and type of cells (including WBC), interferon γ, lactic dehydrogenase levels, adenine deaminase, lysozyme, as well as tests to rule out other conditions such as antinuclear antibodies, complement components C3 and C4, and cytology (3)
- Enteroviral isolation of the throat or stool should be attempted for cases in young healthy people who develop pericarditis.
- A PPD skin testing or a gamma interferon release assay (in blood) may provide help at times.

Imaging
Initial approach
Chest x-ray may provide some clues regarding the possible presence of pericardial fluid.
Follow-Up & Special Considerations
Computed tomography scans or magnetic resonance imaging can distinguish pulmonary processes and assess the thickness of the pericardium.

Diagnostic Procedures/Other
- An ECG often shows ST elevation in multiple leads, along with PR depression:
  - An ECG is the best diagnostic method.
  - Hemodynamic consequences can be seen.
  - An ECG shows evidence of constrictive pericarditis as is seen in cases of tuberculosis.
- T-wave inversions occur late.
- Electrical alternans and low voltage are seen with large pericardial effusions.
- Tamponade can be diagnosed by ECG or by catheterization of the right heart or pulmonary artery.

Pathological Findings
- In viral pericarditis, pathological findings are that of lymphocytic infiltrate of the pericardium, while leukocytic epicarditis is present in bacterial pericarditis.
- Caseous granulomas and fibrosis are at apparent in tuberculous pericarditis (1,4).

DIFFERENTIAL DIAGNOSIS
- Uremia
- Collagen-vascular diseases
- Post-myocardial infarct
- Hypothyroidism
- Sarcoidosis
- Neoplastic disease (solid tumor or hematological)
- Postradiation
- Familial Mediterranean fever
- Restrictive cardiomyopathy (NT pro-BNP may be higher while CRP is lower) (5)
- Rheumatic fever

TREATMENT

MEDICATION

First Line

- Nonsteroidal anti-inflammatory medications are used to treat pain and inflammation for up to 6 weeks: Aspirin 650 mg PO every 6–8 hours and then taper after 7 days or indomethacin 25–50 mg PO every 6–8 hours (1,4,6).
- Colchicine for up to 6 weeks (starting at 2–3 mg/day and then taper to 1 mg/day).
- In relapsing (recurrent) pericarditis colchicine for up to 1 year (1 mg/day) may be needed.
- Steroids are not given for most causes. Exception is constrictive pericarditis with tuberculosis, for which the use of steroids is recommended although more data are needed regarding their effectiveness.
- Antiviral agents are used when the viral diagnosis is evident:
  – Cytomegalovirus can be treated with ganciclovir 5 mg/kg twice a day in immunosupressed patients.
  – Herpes simplex virus can be treated with acyclovir 5 mg/kg q8h.
  – Influenza can be treated with rimantadine 100 mg PO b.i.d or oseltamivir 75 mg PO b.i.d.
  – Purulent pericarditis needs to be treated with appropriate antibiotics for at least 4–6 weeks.
  – Treatment for tuberculosis includes isoniazid plus rifampicin plus pyrazinamide plus ethambutol for 2 months, followed by isoniazid and rifampicin for 6 months.

ADDITIONAL TREATMENT

General Measures

- Bed rest is considered a mainstay of therapy.
- Provide gastric protection with misoprostol or omeprazole when prescribing NSAIDs.

Issues for Referral

- Tamponade
- Constrictive pericarditis

Additional Therapies

Interferon and immunoglobulins have been used mainly for viral perimyocarditis. Further evidence is necessary regarding their exact role.

SURGERY/OTHER PROCEDURES

- Pericardiotomy is often required in purulent pericarditis or when tamponade has occurred.
- Pericardiectomy is needed in constrictive pericarditis.
- Pericardiocentesis will be needed in cases of tamponade or need to establish a diagnosis (7).
- Intrapericardial administration of steroids after cardiac procedures has been used by some (8).

IN-PATIENT CONSIDERATIONS

Initial Stabilization

Needed as an emergency measure if cardiac tamponade is present.

Admission Criteria

These include: Severe pericardial effusion, fever >38°C, cardiac tamponade, trauma, anticoagulation, immunosuppression, failure of nonsteroidal anti-inflammatory agents (9).

IV Fluids

Cautious administration in constrictive pericarditis or presence of large pericardial effusion.

 ONGOING CARE

FOLLOW-UP RECOMMENDATIONS

Patients should have follow-up echocardiograms to rule out late fluid re-accumulation and tamponade.

Patient Monitoring

Monitoring of cardiac output, the amount of the pericardial effusion, and cardiac mechanics (diastolic collapse/mitral flow derangement) may be necessary in hospital.

PROGNOSIS

- Prognosis of idiopathic pericarditis is excellent in general for ~96.5% of the patients. However, cardiac tamponade may occur in 3.5% of patients.
- Predictors of poor outcome for acute pericarditis are the admission criteria mentioned above.
- Regarding tuberculous pericarditis with treatment, mortality up to 17% has been reported in HIV seronegative patients while mortality rates of 34% have been reported in HIV positive patients.
- Untreated bacterial and tuberculous pericarditis invariably leads to death.

COMPLICATIONS

- Recurrences may occur in idiopathic pericarditis
- Constrictive pericarditis probably complicates rarely idiopathic pericarditis
- Tamponade

REFERENCES

1. Khandaker MH, Espinosa RE, Nishimura RA, et al. Pericardial disease: Diagnosis and management. *Mayo Clin Proc* 2010;85:572–593.
2. Reuter H, Burgess LJ, Carstens ME, et al. Characterization of the immunological features of tuberculous pericardial effusions in HIV positive and HIV negative patients in contrast with non-tuberculous effusions. *Tuberculosis (Edinb)* 2006;86:125–133.
3. Mayosi BM, Burgess LJ, Doubell AF. Tuberculous pericarditis. *Circulation* 2005;112:3608–3616.
4. Maisch B, Seferović PM, Ristić AD, et al. Guidelines on the diagnosis and management of pericardial diseases executive summary of the European society of cardiology: The task force on the diagnosis and management of pericardial diseases. *Eur Heart J* 2004;25:587–610.
5. Leya FS, Arab D, Joyal D, et al. The efficacy of brain natriuretic peptide levels in differentiating constrictive pericarditis from restrictive cardiomyopathy. *J Am Coll Cardiol* 2005;45:1900–1902.
6. Lotrionte M, Biondi-Zoccai G, Imazio M, et al. International collaborative systematic review of controlled clinical trials on pharmacologic treatments for acute pericarditis and its recurrences. *Am Heart J* 2010;160:662–670.
7. Allen KB, Faber LP, Warren WH, et al. Pericardial effusion: subxiphoid pericardiostomy versus percutaneous catheter drainage. *Ann Thorac Surg* 1999;67:437–440.
8. Maxwell CB, Crouch MA. Intrapericardial triamcinolone for acute pericarditis after electrophysiologic procedures. *Am J Health Syst Pharm* 2010;67:269–273.
9. Imazio M, Demichelis B, Parrini I, et al. Day-hospital treatment of acute pericarditis: A management program for outpatient therapy. *J Am Coll Cardiol* 2004;43:1042–1026.

ADDITIONAL READING

- Levy PY, Corey R, Berger P, et al. Etiologic diagnosis of 204 pericardial effusions. *Medicine (Baltimore)* 2003;82:385–391.

 CODES

ICD9

- 420.91 Acute idiopathic pericarditis
- 420.99 Other acute pericarditis
- 423.9 Unspecified disease of pericardium

CLINICAL PEARLS

- Always consider the epidemiological setting, that is, in South Africa tuberculosis and HIV rank very high on the list of causes.
- When examining the patient's pulse, check whether it decreases/disappears during inspiration.

PERITONITIS (PRIMARY AND SECONDARY)

Petros I. Rafailidis
Matthew E. Falagas

 BASICS

DESCRIPTION
- Peritonitis is inflammation of the peritoneum, usually due to an infectious etiology. Peritonitis is classified as one of the following:
  - Primary (bacterial infection not associated with an intra-abdominal source)
  - Secondary (infection secondary to inflammation or perforation of a gastrointestinal or genitourinary source (1))
  - Tertiary (diffuse peritonitis, without a well-defined focus of infection) peritonitis is a persistent peritonitis after management of secondary peritonitis (2,3).
  - Related to peritoneal dialysis.

EPIDEMIOLOGY
Incidence
- Spontaneous bacterial peritonitis
  - Occurs in 25% of patients with cirrhosis of the liver
  - The most frequent infectious complication in patients with ascites
- Incidence of secondary peritonitis depends on the specific cause.
- Peritoneal dialysis infections
  - Occurs on an average of once a year in patients undergoing chronic peritoneal dialysis.

RISK FACTORS
- Severe liver disease with ascitic fluid albumin <1 g/dL
- Shock
- Gastrointestinal bleed
- Urinary tract infection
- Intestinal overgrowth
- Patients with the following conditions (1):
  - Nephrotic syndrome
  - Severe heart failure
  - Acute hepatitis
  - Metastatic cancer
  - Systemic lupus erythematosus

GENERAL PREVENTION
- Use of trimethoprim-sulfamethoxazole, double-stranded, every day for 5 days per week or norfloxacin 400 mg once daily has been shown to reduce the rate of spontaneous bacterial peritonitis (SBP) in patients with end-stage liver disease and a previous episode of SBP or a low (<1 g) albumin level in the ascitic fluid or presenting with variceal bleeding. In the latter setting, 1 g of ceftriaxone IV daily is a superior prophylactic option.
- The pneumococcal vaccine has led to a reduction of pneumococcal peritonitis; however, the disease is far from extinct and physicians should always bear in mind this notorious pathogen.

ETIOLOGY
- Primary peritonitis or spontaneous bacterial peritonitis
  - This occurs on rare occasions in healthy young children. More commonly, it occurs in children with the nephrotic syndrome. Often, the etiology is not known, but respiratory tract pathogens, including *Pneumococcus*, have commonly been isolated.
  - Most cases of spontaneous peritonitis occur in adult patients with advanced cirrhosis and ascites.
  - It is believed that the source of the infection is most likely the bloodstream, but transmural spread of bacteria across the bowel wall, lymphatics, or the fallopian tubes has been suggested as well.
  - In most cases, underlying cirrhosis leads to bypass of the reticuloendothelial system (liver and spleen).
  - Infections with gram-negative enteric organisms, such as *E. coli* and *Klebsiella*, account for 70% of cases.
  - Infections with gram-positive organisms, including *Streptococcus* species along with the *Pneumococcus*, account for 25% of cases.
  - *Staphylococcus aureus* accounts for only 2–4% of cases.
  - Isolation rates of anaerobes are low.
  - Tuberculosis peritonitis occurs infrequently in developed countries.
- Secondary peritonitis
  - Intra-abdominal source of infection
    - Includes diverticular abscess, ruptured appendicitis, cholecystitis, and penetrating abdominal trauma
  - Multiple aerobic and anaerobic organisms are isolated, derived from the bowel flora.
    - Candida may be isolated from perforations of the stomach and small bowel.
    - Enterococcus is isolated in as many as 20% of intra-abdominal infections; however, eradication has been noted despite antibiotic regimes not specific for the organism.
    - *Pseudomonas aeruginosa* can be isolated in 20% of cases in some hospitals, despite its not being a usual colonizer of the intestine.
- Tertiary peritonitis
  - Candida, Pseudomonas, and Enterococcus
  - 50% mortality, prolonged course
  - Multiple-organ failure

 DIAGNOSIS

HISTORY
- SPONTANEOUS BACTERIAL PERITONITIS
  - Ask for history of liver disease or nephrotic syndrome
  - Onset may be subclinical, with nothing more than a decompensation in fluid balance, low-grade fever, or mild encephalopathy.
  - Fevers occur in 50–80% of patients.
  - Abdominal pain occurs in 60% of patients.
  - Encephalopathy is noted in 50%, and this may be the only sign of infection.
  - Diarrhea occurs in 33% of patients.
  - Hypothermia occurs in 17% of patients.
  - Note: 10% of patients have no symptoms and signs.
- SECONDARY PERITONITIS
  - Symptoms are related to inflammation of the peritoneum adjacent to the organ affected.
  - Fevers and hypotension are often present.
  - Some pelvic infections may be occult and present with fevers and colonic irritation leading to diarrhea.
- TERTIARY PERITONITIS
  - Same as in secondary peritonitis
  - Chronic peritoneal drainage of purulent, culture-positive exudates
  - Hypotension, renal failure

PHYSICAL EXAM
- Regarding primary peritonitis, signs of cirrhosis may be present: Ascites, jaundice, spider angiomas, and asterixis
- Patients present with abdominal tenderness, rebound tenderness, which becomes diffuse and board-like, if the infection spreads.
- Specific signs may point to the diagnosis of secondary peritonitis at a time before full-blown peritonitis: Try to detect Murphy's sign (tenderness in the right upper quadrant) or McBurney's sign (right lower abdominal quadrant), Rovsing's sign (tenderness in the right lower abdominal quadrant on eliciting pressure on the lower left abdominal quadrant), iliopsoas sign, obturator sign, or tenderness in the left lower abdominal quadrant.
- Bowel sound frequency may be decreased.

DIAGNOSTIC TESTS & INTERPRETATION
Lab
Initial lab tests
- A complete blood count, serum creatinine, liver enzymes, serum albumin, blood glucose, serum electrolytes, prothrombin time and aPTT and cross match
- Pregnancy test
- If ascites is present, paracentesis should be performed (3).

- Ascitic fluid with >250 polys/mm³
- Ascitic protein <3.5 g/L
- Ascitic fluid pH <7.35 and lactate >25 mg/dL
- Positive blood cultures in 75% of patients with spontaneous bacterial peritonitis
- On rare occasion, patients will not have time following infection to mount a WBC response in the ascitic fluid. Cultures may be positive, with few WBCs present.
- Peritoneal fluid should be inoculated directly into blood culture bottles.
- Tuberculosis must be considered when routine cultures are negative. Peritoneal biopsy is often necessary to make this diagnosis.

Follow-Up & Special Considerations
Follow-up paracentesis (in primary peritonitis) should be performed to make sure the leukocyte counts in the ascitic fluid are falling. This should be done in 48 hours after the initial paracentesis, or sooner if the patient has not responded.

Imaging
Initial approach
- X-rays often help with the diagnosis of secondary peritonitis. Air under the diaphragm suggests disruption of the bowel or stomach wall.
- Abdominal CT scan or ultrasounds are needed to help diagnose/confirm the etiology of secondary peritonitis.

Follow-Up & Special Considerations
MRI may be necessary

Diagnostic Procedures/Other
Peritoneal lavage

DIFFERENTIAL DIAGNOSIS
- Aortic aneurysm rupture
- Dissecting aortic aneurysm
- Peritoneal carcinomatosis
- Acute pancreatitis
- Herpes zoster
- Acute porphyria
- Diabetic ketoacidosis
- Sickle cell crisis
- Familial Mediterranean fever

 TREATMENT

MEDICATION
First Line
- SPONTANEOUS BACTERIAL PERITONITIS
  – Aminoglycosides should be avoided.
  – Initial empiric treatment with cefotaxime 2 g IV every 8 hours (4)[A]
  – A β-lactam/β-lactamase inhibitor or carbapenem should be considered.
  – Treatment should be administered for 5 days (4).
  – The use of human albumin in association to antibiotics has decreased mortality more than antibiotic treatment alone (4)[A].

- SECONDARY PERITONITIS
  – A combined surgical – medical approach is beneficial.
  – Antibiotics should be directed against aerobes and anaerobes. Examples of regimens include a combination of gentamicin and clindamycin, second- or third-generation cephalosporins or quinolones with metronidazole, β-lactam/β-lactamase inhibitors, or carbapenems (5)[A].
- TERTIARY PERITONITIS
  – Various drainage procedures have been used.
  – Systemic antibiotics are used only for high fever and hypotension; local instillation of antibiotics is not effective.

ADDITIONAL TREATMENT
General Measures
Nil by mouth until convinced that no hollow organ rupture is present and in view of plan for surgical management.

Issues for Referral
To a general surgeon

COMPLEMENTARY & ALTERNATIVE THERAPIES
Contraindicated

SURGERY/OTHER PROCEDURES
Mandatory for the majority of causes of peritonitis.

IN-PATIENT CONSIDERATIONS
Initial Stabilization
Mandatory in the majority of cases and dependent on hemodynamic status of the patient.

Admission Criteria
All patients with primary and secondary peritonitis need admission to hospital.

IV Fluids
Mandatory for initial stabilization in secondary and tertiary peritonitis.

Discharge Criteria
Once clinical condition has improved (no pain, no fever, and no tenderness)

 ONGOING CARE

FOLLOW-UP RECOMMENDATIONS
Patient Monitoring
If prophylactic antibiotics are considered then monitoring for potential adverse events associated with antibiotic treatment may be necessary.

DIET
Nil by mouth if secondary peritonitis in view of surgical management.

PROGNOSIS
- In primary peritonitis, if there is underlying cirrhosis, mortality ranges from 10–30% with treatment.
- In secondary peritonitis mortality is decreased if swift control of the source is achieved.
- Tertiary peritonitis is associated with high mortality (~50%).

REFERENCES
1. Johnson CC, Baldesarre J, Levison ME. Peritonitis: Update on pathophysiology, clinical manifestations, and management. *Clin Infect Dis* 1997;24: 1035–1047.
2. Panhofer P, Izay B, Riedl M, et al. Age, microbiology and prognostic scores help to differentiate between secondary and tertiary peritonitis. *Langenbecks Arch Surg* 2009;394:265–271.
3. Chromik AM, Meiser A, Hölling J, et al. Identification of patients at risk for development of tertiary peritonitis on a surgical intensive care unit. *J Gastrointest Surg* 2009;13:1358–1367.
4. Runyon BA. AASLD Practice Guidelines Committee. Management of adult patients with ascites due to cirrhosis: An update. *Hepatology* 2009;49: 2087–2107.
5. Solomkin JS, Mazuski JE, Bradley JS, et al. Diagnosis and management of complicated intra-abdominal infection in adults and children: Guidelines by the Surgical Infection Society and the Infectious Diseases Society of America. *Clin Infect Dis* 2010;50:133–164.

ADDITIONAL READING
- Lamme B, Boermeester MA, Belt EJ, et al. Mortality and morbidity of planned relaparotomy versus relaparotomy on demand for secondary peritonitis. *Br J Surg* 2004;91:1046–1054.

 CODES

ICD9
- 567.9 Unspecified peritonitis
- 567.23 Spontaneous bacterial peritonitis
- 567.29 Other suppurative peritonitis

CLINICAL PEARLS
- In a patient with peritonitis rule out intrauterine pregnancy. However, a pregnant woman can still have peritonitis due to common causes. In this case classical signs may be altered. Admit patients with dubious signs for observation.

PERTUSSIS

Anastasios M. Kapaskelis
Petros I. Rafailidis
Matthew E. Falagas

 BASICS

DESCRIPTION
- Infection due to *Bordetella pertussis* and *Bordetella parapertussis*.
- Responsible for whooping cough.

EPIDEMIOLOGY
Incidence
- Pertussis is worldwide in distribution. The reported incidence of pertussis among vaccinated children is 31/100,000 person-years after 2 doses and 19/100,000 person-years after the third dose at 12 months of age (1).
- Although vaccination resulted in a substantial reduction in pertussis incidence among young children, considerably high infection rates are reported among older children and young adults.

Prevalence
- Pertussis causes outbreaks.
- Concerning adults, a prevalence of 12.4–26% has been reported in studies from US, Australia, and Germany (2).

RISK FACTORS
Older siblings and adults may transmit pertussis infection to unvaccinated infants and young children.

GENERAL PREVENTION
- Standard immunization: Pertussis acellular or whole-cell vaccine is given in conjunction with diphtheria and tetanus at ages 2, 4, 6, and 15–18 months and at ages 4–6 years.
- Booster adult vaccination: Consideration is being given to adding the acellular vaccine to tetanus and diphtheria for administration to adults.
- A potential association between pertussis infection and atopic disorders in pertussis vaccinated patients has been suggested (3). The issue of the association between pertussis vaccination during infancy and the development of childhood asthma is doubtful, since recent studies do not provide supportive evidence (3).
- A potential association between pertussis vaccination and the risk of seizures, encephalopathy, and sudden infant death syndrome (SIDS) has also been suggested (5,6).
- The rates of reported adverse events per 100,000 vaccinations is lower for the diphtheria and tetanus toxoids and acellular pertussis vaccine compared to the diphtheria and tetanus toxoids and whole-cell pertussis vaccine (7).
- Antibiotic prophylaxis of household contacts is needed, and should be started as soon as possible after the diagnosis is made. Erythromycin or TMP-SMX should be used for a full 14 days.

PATHOPHYSIOLOGY
- The Bps polysaccharide of *B. pertussis* contributes to its adherence to human nasal epithelia and also to the colonization and biofilm formation.
- The inflammatory peptide bradykinin may possibly account for the persistent, paroxysmal coughing observed during the initial phases of *B. pertussis* infection (8).

ETIOLOGY
- *B. pertussis* is a small, gram-negative coccobacillary organism.
- A number of toxins are produced, including the tracheal cytotoxin (a disaccharide-tetrapeptide) and the pertussis toxin (AB5-type exotoxin).

 DIAGNOSIS

HISTORY
- Incubation time is commonly 7–10 days (range of 4–21 days).
- Catarrhal phase: Lasts <2 weeks, associated with rhinorrhea, fever, and conjunctivitis.
- Paroxysmal phase: Lasts 2–4 weeks; the patient gradually develops a dry cough with episodes of coughing fits.
- Convalescent phase: Over the next 1–2 weeks, the episodes of coughing decrease and the patient returns to normal.

PHYSICAL EXAM
- The whoop (characteristic high-pitched sound) is the most common symptom in young unvaccinated children. It is associated with a paroxysm of coughing, followed by cyanosis and then by vomiting.
- In adults and previously vaccinated children the clinical manifestations may be atypical (prolonged cough), resulting in underdiagnoses.

DIAGNOSTIC TESTS & INTERPRETATION
Lab
Initial lab tests
- Culture of the organism by sputum or nasopharyngeal swab is positive within the first 2 weeks of illness. Cultures become negative after 5 days of antibiotic therapy.
- Lymphocytosis may be marked at the onset of the paroxysmal phase.
- Serology confirms the clinical diagnosis. Diagnosis can be made with a single high antibody titer to pertussis toxin or with a fourfold increase in antibodies titer over a 2-week period.

Follow-Up & Special Considerations
Triplex real-time PCR assay is also reported to be sensitive and specific for simultaneous identification and discrimination of *B. pertussis* and *B. parapertussis* (9).

Imaging
Chest radiography: May reveal perihilar infiltrates or edema, variable degrees of atelectasis. In cases of pertussis pneumonia and/or secondary bacterial infection, chest radiography may reveal consolidation.

DIFFERENTIAL DIAGNOSIS
- Pneumonia (bacterial or viral), adenoviral respiratory infection, respiratory syncytial virus infection, bronchitis, asthma.
- Particularly in infants: Foreign-body aspiration, gastroesophageal reflux.

TREATMENT

MEDICATION
First Line
- Supportive care is needed, especially in infants under the age of 1 year. Antibiotics do not reduce the duration of coughing if given initially in the paroxysmal phase.
- The aim of antibiotic treatment in pertussis is the eradication of the bacterium. However, antibiotics that act either through inhibition of protein synthesis (such as erythromycin), transcription (rifampin), or cell wall biosynthesis (including cefoperazone and piperacillin) and magnesium sulfate (inhibiting transcription of pertussis toxin, but not bacterial growth) did not prevent the release of preformed toxin (10):
  – Patients <1 month: Azithromycin (10–12 mg/kg/d per os for total of 5 days). Azithromycin is reported to be associated with lower risk for infantile hypertrophic pyloric stenosis-IHPS compared to erythromycin (11).
  – Patients ≥1 month: Macrolides: Erythromycin [40–50 mg/kg/d (stearate/base) per os divided 4 times daily; not to exceed 2 g/day], clarithromycin (15–20 mg/kg per os divided twice daily for 5–7 days; not to exceed 1 g/day), and azithromycin (10–12 mg/kg/d per os for 5 days).
  – Adults: Erythromycin 500 mg orally 4 times per day for 14 days, or trimethoprim-sulfamethoxazole (TMP-SMX), double-stranded, orally twice per day for 14 days.

Second Line
Patients ≥2 months with hypersensitivity to macrolides may be treated with trimethoprim-sulfamethoxazole

ADDITIONAL TREATMENT
Additional Therapies
The currently available evidence are insufficient to support the effectiveness of treatment strategies other than antibiotics and vaccines (including corticosteroids, beta 2-adrenergic agonists, pertussis-specific immunoglobulin, antihistamines, or leukotriene receptor antagonists) to suppress the cough in whooping cough (12).

IN-PATIENT CONSIDERATIONS
Admission Criteria
Patients that are at risk for severe disease (including infants <6 months old and unvaccinated children) may require hospitalization.

 ## ONGOING CARE

PATIENT EDUCATION
Patient and parent education are recommended after the establishment of pertussis diagnosis.

PROGNOSIS
- The prognosis following full recovery is excellent.
- Death and need for admission in the intensive care unit may occur in patients with risk factors for severe pertussis disease (such as comorbidity, elevated lymphocyte count, presentation with seizures/encephalopathy or shock) (13):
  – Increased mortality rates have been reported particularly for infants too young to be vaccinated (14).

COMPLICATIONS
- Major complications include secondary bacterial respiratory infections (such as pneumonia).
- Coughing paroxysms may result in eyelid ecchymosis, subconjunctival hemorrhage, dellen (peripheral corneal local thinning) (15).
- Coughing may lead to intracranial hemorrhage.
- Encephalopathy and meningoencephalitis.
- Seizures may occur in children and, less frequently, in adults.
- Barotrauma from coughing may cause pneumothorax.
- Specifically, regarding infants, complications such as weight loss, bronchitis, otitis media, apnea, cyanosis, inguinal hernia, and rectal prolapse may also be observed (16).
- Specifically, regarding adults, complications such as urinary incontinence, rib fracture, pneumothorax, inguinal hernia, aspiration, pneumonia, seizures, and otitis media may also be observed (17).

REFERENCES

1. Gustafsson L, Hessel L, Storsaeter J, et al. Long-term follow-up of Swedish children vaccinated with acellular pertussis vaccines at 3, 5, and 12 months of age indicates the need for a booster dose at 5 to 7 years of age. *Pediatrics* 2006;118:978–984.
2. Birkebaek NH. Bordetella pertussis in the aetiology of chronic cough in adults. Diagnostic methods and clinic. *Dan Med Bull* 2001;48:77–80.
3. Bernsen RM, Nagelkerke NJ, Thijs C, et al. Reported Pertussis infection and risk of atopy in 8- to 12-yr-old vaccinated and non-vaccinated children. *Pediatr Allergy Immunol* 2008;19: 46–52.
4. Spycher BD, Silverman M, Egger M, et al. Routine vaccination against pertussis and the risk of childhood asthma: A population-based cohort study. *Pediatrics* 2009;123:944–950.
5. Griffin MR, Ray WA, Mortimer EA, et al. Risk of seizures and encephalopathy after immunization with the diphtheria-tetanus-pertussis vaccine. *JAMA* 1990;263:1641–1645.
6. Baraff LJ, Ablon WJ, Weiss RC. Possible temporal association between diphtheria-tetanus toxoid-pertussis vaccination and sudden infant death syndrome. *Pediatr Infect Dis* 1983;2:7–11.
7. Rosenthal S, Chen R, Hadler S. The safety of acellular pertussis vaccine vs whole-cell pertussis vaccine. A postmarketing assessment. *Arch Pediatr Adolesc Med* 1996;150:457–460.
8. Hewitt M, Canning BJ. Coughing precipitated by Bordetella pertussis infection. *Lung* 2010; 188(Suppl 1):S73–S79.
9. Xu Y, Xu Y, Hou Q, et al. Triplex real-time PCR assay for detection and differentiation of Bordetella pertussis and Bordetella parapertussis. *APMIS* 2010;118:685–691.
10. Craig-Mylius KA, Weiss AA. Antibacterial agents and release of periplasmic pertussis toxin from Bordetella pertussis. *Antimicrob Agents Chemother* 2000;44:1383–1386.
11. Friedman DS, Curtis CR, Schauer SL, et al. Surveillance for transmission and antibiotic adverse events among neonates and adults exposed to a healthcare worker with pertussis. *Infect Control Hosp Epidemiol* 2004;25:967–973.
12. Bettiol S, Thompson MJ, Roberts NW, et al. Symptomatic treatment of the cough in whooping cough. *Cochrane Database Syst Rev* 2010;(1): CD003257.
13. Surridge J, Segedin ER, Grant CC. Pertussis requiring intensive care. *Arch Dis Child*. 2007;92:970–975.
14. Vitek CR, Pascual FB, Baughman AL, et al. Increase in deaths from pertussis among young infants in the United States in the 1990s. *Pediatr Infect Dis J* 2003;22:628–634.
15. Reisli I, Keles S, Kamis U, et al. Picture of the month: Coughing paroxysms associated with subconjunctival hemorrhage and dellen. *Arch Pediatr Adolesc Med* 2006;160:53–55.
16. Greenberg DP, von König CH, Heininger U. Health burden of pertussis in infants and children. *Pediatr Infect Dis J* 2005;24(5 Suppl):S39–S43.
17. Rothstein E, Edwards K. Health burden of pertussis in adolescents and adults. *Pediatr Infect Dis J* 2005;24(5 Suppl):S44–S47.

ADDITIONAL READING
- von König CH, Halperin S, Riffelmann M, et al. Pertussis of adults and infants. *Lancet Infect Dis* 2002;2:744–750.
- Kapaskelis AM, Vouloumanou EK, Rafailidis PI, et al. High prevalence of antibody titers against Bordetella pertussis in an adult population with prolonged cough. *Respir Med* 2008;102:1586–1591.

 ## CODES

ICD9
- 033.0 : *Whooping cough due to bordetella pertussis (b. pertussis)*
- 033.1 Whooping cough due to bordetella parapertussis (b. parapertussis)
- 033.9 : *Whooping cough, unspecified organism*

CLINICAL PEARLS
- Both natural and vaccine-induced immunity to pertussis wanes.
- Advise in favor of adherence to pertussis vaccination for children and recommend booster pertussis vaccination for adults to protect infants too young to be immunized and establish herd immunity.
- Consider pertussis diagnosis in an adult with prolonged cough of new origin in the absence of evidence of other respiratory tract infection.
- Young unvaccinated infants are at risk for severe pertussis disease and may require hospitalization.

PHARYNGITIS

Petros I. Rafailidis
Matthew E. Falagas

 BASICS

DESCRIPTION
Inflammation of the mucosa of the pharynx and tonsils.

EPIDEMIOLOGY
Incidence
- Most cases occur during the colder months of the year, with peak rates in late winter and early spring.
- It occurs in all age groups. Streptococcal pharyngitis is more frequent in children 5–10 years old (~15% of all cases).
- Incidence is equal in males and females.

Prevalence
Repeated Group A beta-hemolytic streptococci pharyngitis: 1% (children 4–15 years old) (1).

RISK FACTORS
- Age (the young are more susceptible)
- Close quarters, such as in new military recruits
- Smoking
- Excess alcohol consumption
- Oral sex (mainly for cases of gonococcal pharyngitis)
- Diabetes mellitus
- Recent illness
- Immunosuppression

GENERAL PREVENTION
Avoid contact with infected people. Patients are presumed to be noninfectious after 24 hours of antibiotic coverage.

ETIOLOGY
- Viral: Rhinovirus, coronavirus, adenovirus (types 3, 4, 7, 14, 21), herpes simplex virus (types 1, 2), parainfluenza virus (types 1–4), influenza virus (types A and B), coxsackievirus A (types 2, 4, 5, 6, 8, 9, 10, 21), coxsackievirus B (types 1–5), echovirus, enterovirus 71, Epstein-Barr virus, cytomegalovirus, human immunodeficiency virus, human herpes virus 6 (HHV-6), and others.
- Bacterial: Group A β-hemolytic Streptococcus; groups C, G, and β-hemolytic Streptococcus; *Neisseria gonorrhoeae*; *Haemophilus influenzae* type b; *Corynebacterium diphtheriae* (diphtheria); *Corynebacterium ulcerans*; *Arcanobacterium haemolyticum* (*Corynebacterium haemolyticum*); *Yersinia enterocolitica*; *Treponema pallidum*; and mixed anaerobic infection (2).
- Chlamydial: *Chlamydia pneumoniae*.
- Mycoplasmal: *Mycoplasma pneumoniae*, *Mycoplasma hominis* (type 1).
- In approximately 30% of patients with pharyngitis, the cause is unknown.

 DIAGNOSIS

Help for an etiologic diagnosis may come from the following:
- Patient's history
- Epidemiologic factors
- Patient's age

HISTORY AND PHYSICAL EXAM
- Streptococcal pharyngitis:
  - The severity of illness varies greatly.
  - Fever (>39°C in severe cases)
  - Pharyngeal pain, odynophagia
  - Headache, chills, malaise, and anorexia may occur.
  - Pharyngeal erythema, enlarged tonsils, and exudate that covers the posterior pharynx and tonsillar area
  - Edema of the uvula and soft palate petechiae
  - Cervical adenopathy
  - Absence of cough, hoarseness, or lower respiratory symptoms
  - In scarlet fever (strains of *Streptococcus pyogenes*, which produce erythrogenic toxin), there is a characteristic erythematous rash (punctate erythematous macules with reddened flexor creases and circumoral pallor) that involves the face, trunk, and skinfold and is followed by desquamation. The tongue is initially white and then red and the papillae are enlarged (white/red strawberry tongue respectively).
  - In cases of pharyngitis due to strains of group C or G β-hemolytic streptococci, the symptoms and signs are similar to those due to *S. pyogenes*.
- Pharyngitis in patients with influenza:
  - Sore throat
  - Fever
  - Myalgia, headache, malaise
  - Coryzal symptoms, hoarseness, possible cough
  - Edema and erythema of the pharyngeal mucosa
  - Pharyngeal exudates and adenopathy usually not present
- Pharyngoconjunctival fever (adenoviral pharyngitis):
  - Sore throat
  - Fever
  - Myalgia, headache, malaise
  - Pharyngeal erythema and exudate may be present, mimicking streptococcal pharyngitis.
  - In one-third to half of the cases, there is also conjunctivitis.
- Acute herpetic pharyngitis (due to herpes simplex virus, primary infection):
  - Vesicles and shallow ulcers of the palate are characteristic.
  - Often, there is an associated gingivostomatitis.

- Herpangina (caused by coxsackievirus A):
  - It is characterized by the presence of small vesicles (diameter, 1–2 mm) on the soft palate, uvula, and anterior tonsillar pillars. After rupture of these lesions, small white ulcers are present.
  - In some cases, there is abdominal pain mimicking acute appendicitis.
- Infectious mononucleosis (due to Epstein-Barr virus):
  - Exudative tonsillitis or pharyngitis occurs in approximately half of the cases (often membranous).
  - It is associated with fever, cervical or generalized adenopathy, persistent fatigue, and, often, splenomegaly.
- HIV infection:
  - Febrile pharyngitis (hyperemia; often mucosal ulcerations, but not exudate) associated with myalgia, arthralgia, adenopathy, and, often, maculopapular rash is a feature of primary infection with HIV.
- Pharyngitis associated with the "common cold":
  - It is characterized by soreness or irritation of the pharynx.
  - Mild edema and erythema may be present.
  - Fever is unusual (except in children).
  - Symptoms of acute upper respiratory illness are always present.
- Infection with *Corynebacterium diphtheriae*:
  - This still occurs in unvaccinated populations.
  - The characteristic tonsillar or pharyngeal membrane is gray and firmly adherent to the mucosa.
- Infection with *C. haemolyticum*:
  - It is clinically mimicking streptococcal pharyngitis.
  - It affects mainly children and young adults and is associated with a diffuse, erythematous, maculopapular skin rash on the extremities and trunk.
- Vincent's angina:
  - It is a mixed infection due to aerobic and anaerobic bacteria.
  - The most often isolated microorganism is *Fusobacterium necrophorum*.
  - It is characterized by a purulent exudate and a foul breath odor. It may be complicated with peritonsillar abscess and jugular vein septic phlebitis (Lemierre's disease)
- Gonococcal pharyngitis: *N. gonorrhoeae* may be a cause of mild pharyngitis.
- Yersinial pharyngitis: *Y. enterocolitica* may be a cause of exudative pharyngitis.
- Chlamydial pharyngitis: Isolated pharyngitis or in association with pneumonia or bronchitis.

- Mycoplasmal pharyngitis: Mild pharyngitis without distinguishing clinical features.
- Presence of pharyngeal exudate: Group A β-hemolytic *Streptococcus*; groups C and G β-hemolytic *Streptococcus*; *C. diphtheriae*; *C. haemolyticum*; *Y. enterocolitica*; anaerobic infection; adenovirus; herpes simplex virus; Epstein-Barr virus
- Presence of small vesicles or ulcers: Herpes simplex virus infection or herpangina.
- Presence of membranous exudates: Diphtheria, Vincent's angina, or Epstein-Barr virus. If it is pseudomembrane and firmly adhered, it suggests diphtheria.
- Presence of petechiae of the soft palate: Group A β-hemolytic *Streptococcus* or Epstein-Barr virus.
- Presence of skin rash: *S. pyogenes*, *C.* (Arcanobacterium) *haemolyticum*, HIV, and Epstein-Barr virus.
- Presence of conjunctivitis: Adenovirus and some types of enterovirus.
- Also helpful may be the presence of adenopathy (regional or generalized), splenomegaly, or other extrapharyngeal features.

DIAGNOSTIC TESTS & INTERPRETATION
Lab
- Leukocytosis suggests infection with bacteria.
- Group A β-hemolytic *Streptococcus*: Blood agar throat culture from swab, antigen agglutination test from throat swab, serologic tests (ASO titer) (rarely helpful).
- *N. gonorrhoeae*: may be detected on Thayer-Martin media from throat swab
- Vincent's angina: A crystal violet–stained smear of the pharyngeal exudate
- Diphtheria: Throat culture using Loeffler's medium
- Primary HIV infection: Detection of HIV antigen in serum or HIV RNA
- Epstein-Barr virus: Monospot test or specific serologic test
- Specific serologic tests are available for other etiologic agents.

DIFFERENTIAL DIAGNOSIS
Distinguish infectious pharyngitis from noninfectious pharyngitis, which may be associated with conditions such as systemic lupus erythematosus, Behçet's syndrome, Kawasaki syndrome, pemphigus, bullous pemphigoid, drug reactions, agranulocytosis, chemical irritation, and neoplasms, PFAPA syndrome (periodic fever, aphthous stomatitis, pharyngitis and cervical adenitis), temporal arteritis, adult onset Still's disease.

 TREATMENT
MEDICATION
- Streptococcal pharyngitis: The primary aim of treatment is the eradication of the microbe and prevention of acute rheumatic fever.
- Drug of choice:
  – Penicillin V 50,000 IU/kg/d divided q6h in children or 500,000 IU q.i.d in adults for 10 days, or
  – Benzathine penicillin G 25,000 IU/kg IM to a maximum of 1.2 million IU as a single dose or 1.2 million IU IM in adults.
  – In patients who are allergic to penicillin: Erythromycin 40 mg/kg/d divided q6h or 500 mg q8h in adults for 10 days.
- Alternative drugs: First-generation cephalosporins, newer macrolides.
- Recurrent pharyngitis associated with *S. pyogenes* and failure of the first-choice treatment: Amoxicillin-clavulanate, ampicillin-sulbactam, or clindamycin
- Asymptomatic carrier: No treatment required except when
  – Occurrence of rheumatic fever or nephritis in a population such as military recruits or school
  – Cases of streptococcal infection in families with a member who suffers from rheumatic fever or acute streptococcal toxic shock syndrome
- *C. diphtheriae*: Antitoxin plus erythromycin 40 mg/kg/d (divided in 4 doses) IV, or erythromycin 500 mg PO q6 h for 7–14 days. Strict isolation is necessary until at least 24 hours after initiation of appropriate treatment and 2 samples of pharyngeal secretions cultures are negative.
- Vincent's angina: Penicillin G 4 million IU q4h IV
- Gonococci: Ceftriaxone 250 mg IM as a single dose
- *A. haemolyticum*: Frequently nonsensitive to penicillin or other β-lactams. Doxycycline, vancomycin, or fluoroquinolones may be needed.
- Viral: Antiviral agents are not indicated, except for herpes simplex virus 1 or 2 infection (acyclovir 200 mg 5 times per day for 10 days) and HIV infection.

ADDITIONAL TREATMENT
General Measures
- Saltwater gargles, acetaminophen
- Corticosteroids act as analgesics in severe or exudative sore throat.

Issues for Referral
- To ENT for peritonsillar or retrotonsillar abscess drainage.
- Tonsillectomy reduces the incidence of throat infections in children who were severely affected with recurrent pharyngitis (3)[A].

IN-PATIENT CONSIDERATIONS
Admission Criteria
- Presence of complications, that is, mastoiditis, retropharyngeal abscess
- Vincent's angina and diphtheria

 ONGOING CARE
FOLLOW-UP RECOMMENDATIONS
Not necessary in appropriately managed cases with full recovery.

PROGNOSIS
Excellent in general, if uncomplicated.

COMPLICATIONS
- *S. pyogenes* pharyngitis:
  – Suppurative complications: Sinusitis, otitis media, mastoiditis, peritonsillar abscess, retropharyngeal abscess, bacteremia, and pneumonia
  – Nonsuppurative complications: Acute rheumatic fever, acute post-streptococcal glomerulonephritis, toxic shock syndrome, and scarlet fever
- Vincent's angina: Lemierre's disease

REFERENCES
1. St Sauver JL, Weaver AL, Orvidas LJ, et al. Population-based prevalence of repeated group A beta-hemolytic streptococcal pharyngitis episodes. *Mayo Clin Proc* 2006;81:1172–1176.
2. McMillan JA, Sandstrom C, Weiner LB, et al. Viral and bacterial organisms associated with acute pharyngitis in a school-aged population. *J Pediatr* 1986;109:747–752.
3. Paradise JL, Bluestone CD, Bachman RZ, et al. Efficacy of tonsillectomy for recurrent throat infection in severely affected children. Results of parallel randomized and nonrandomized clinical trials. *N Engl J Med* 1984;310:674.

ADDITIONAL READING
- Hayward G, Thompson M, Heneghan C, et al. Corticosteroids for pain relief in sore throat: Systematic review and meta-analysis. *BMJ* 2009;339:b2976.

 CODES

ICD9
- 034.0 Streptococcal sore throat
- 462 Acute pharyngitis

CLINICAL PEARLS
- The primary objectives in managing infectious pharyngitis are the following:
  – To detect and treat cases due to *S. pyogenes* (be aware of local macrolide resistance)
  – Identify the occasional case due to an unusual (infectious or noninfectious) cause for which treatment is available.

PILONIDAL ABSCESS

Michael N. Mavros
George Peppas
Paschalis Vergidis
Matthew E. Falagas

 ## BASICS

DESCRIPTION
Infection of a pilonidal (postanal) cyst

EPIDEMIOLOGY

Incidence
- Pilonidal disease is relatively common (1).
  - ~70,000 new cases in the US annually.
  - Male to female ratio 3:1.
  - Peak incidence is 18–30 years of age.
- More common in Mediterranean countries, rare in East Asia, Oceania, and sub-Saharan Africa (2).

RISK FACTORS
- Age between 18–30 years
- Male gender
- Hairiness
- Obesity
- Poor hygiene
- Deep natal cleft

GENERAL PREVENTION
- Generally cannot be prevented (1,2).
  - Good perianal hygiene and shaving may be beneficial.

PATHOPHYSIOLOGY
- Pilonidal disease is now considered an acquired, self-limited condition (2).
  - A hair follicle forms a skin pit, enlarges, fills with keratin and debris, and gets inflamed.
  - Folliculitis is deteriorated by the insertion and entrapment of hair within the pit, which trigger a foreign body reaction and infection in the subcutaneous fat (2,3).
  - The direction of the inserted hair likely determines the tract of the formed pilonidal sinus, in cases of chronic infection (3).

ETIOLOGY
- No clear causes identified.
  - Hair and local hygiene play a pivotal role.
  - Microbial pathogens usually include bowel and skin flora.

 ## DIAGNOSIS

HISTORY
- Patients may complain of a tender, warm, fluctuant mass (acute infection) or midline drainage (chronic infection).
  - Symptoms may wax and wane for weeks.

PHYSICAL EXAM
- Diagnosis is based on physical examination.
  - Characteristic midline gluteal cleft pits, approximately 5 cm post anus.
  - There may be an abscess (acute infection) or a single or multiple sinuses (chronic infection).
  - Inflammation may be minimal and sinus may be small.
  - Anorectal exam should be performed to rule out other diseases.

DIFFERENTIAL DIAGNOSIS
- Infectious diseases:
  - Perianal abscess
  - Hidradenitis suppurativa
  - Necrotizing fasciitis
  - Furunculosis
  - Herpes simplex virus, syphilis, tuberculosis, or actinomycosis
- Noninfectious diseases:
  - Anal fistula or fissures
  - Crohn's disease
  - Foreign body reaction
  - Radiation proctitis
  - Coccygodynia

 ## TREATMENT

MEDICATION

First Line
- Antibiotics have a limited role but may be beneficial when there is associated cellulitis, underlying immunosuppression, or concurrent systemic illness (1).
- Antibiotics may also be used pre- or perioperatively.
- Coverage should include anaerobes.

ADDITIONAL TREATMENT

General Measures
Meticulous local hygiene and shaving appears beneficial.

COMPLEMENTARY & ALTERNATIVE THERAPIES
- Injection of phenol or fibrin glue into the sinus (in conjunction with hair control and strict local hygiene) has been tried (1,2).
  - Intense pain may sometimes require hospitalization.
  - High success rates (without surgery) with acceptable morbidity.

SURGERY/OTHER PROCEDURES
- Mainstay of treatment for acute and chronic pilonidal disease (except minimally symptomatic cases) is surgery (1–3).
- An off-midline incision and excision of the skin pits (without wide excision of the abscess) seems adequate in most instances (2,3).
  - Simple day-case surgery, minimal care in the community, and rapid return to work.
  - Acceptable recurrence rates.
- Wide excision of the abscess with flattening of the natal cleft and off-midline skin closure can be performed for recurrent, extensive, or complicated disease (2).
  - Lower recurrence rates
  - High morbidity, potentially debilitating complications

 ONGOING CARE

FOLLOW-UP RECOMMENDATIONS
Strict local hygiene and hair control.

PROGNOSIS
- Recurrence is not uncommon.
  - May require more extensive surgery.
- Long-term prognosis is excellent.

COMPLICATIONS
- A large abscess may be associated with sepsis and shock.
- Carcinoma arising from a chronic, untreated pilonidal sinus is very rare (1).

REFERENCES

1. Humphries AE, Duncan JE. Evaluation and management of pilonidal disease. *Surg Clin N Am* 2010;90:113–124.
2. Thompson MR, Sepanati A, Kitchen P. Simple day-case surgery for pilonidal sinus disease. *Br J Surg* 2011;98:198–209.
3. Kitchen P. Pilonidal sinus – management in the primary care setting. *Aust Fam Physician* 2010;39:372–375.

 CODES

ICD9
685.0 Pilonidal cyst with abscess

CLINICAL PEARLS
- Simple day-case surgery is the preferred mode of treatment for pilonidal abscess.
- Antibiotics have a limited role but may be beneficial when there is associated cellulitis. Antibiotics may also be used perioperatively.
- Strict local hygiene and hair control is required after surgery to prevent recurrence.

PLAGUE

Sarah Taimur
Paschalis Vergidis
Matthew E. Falagas

 BASICS

DESCRIPTION
Plague is a zoonotic infection caused by *Yersinia pestis*. Of great historical significance, this organism caused the "Black Death" in the Middle Ages. The disease may be bubonic (lymph node involvement), septicemic, pneumonic, or meningeal.

EPIDEMIOLOGY
Incidence
- Plague has a worldwide distribution except in Australia and Antarctica.
- Between 1998 and 2003: 38,310 cases with 2845 deaths were reported in 25 countries.
- Most cases occur in poor, developing countries.
- In the US, 415 cases reported from 1970–2007. 80% in New Mexico, Arizona, and Colorado and 10% in California.
- Cases have been reported annually for the past 8 years from the US, Congo, Madagascar, Peru, Tanzania, China, and Vietnam.
- Recent major outbreaks (after silent periods of 30–50 years): India, Indonesia, Algeria, Congo, and Madagascar (1).

RISK FACTORS
- Travel or residence in endemic areas
- Poor rodent control
- Frequent rodent contact
- Rodent predator contact (endemic areas)
- Occupational exposure (veterinarians, researchers)
- Sleeping with pets (endemic areas)
- Poor animal flea control

GENERAL PREVENTION
- Vaccination is indicated for high risk individuals (laboratory workers, ecologists, field workers in high risk areas) (2). The vaccine is not commercially available in the US:
  – Primary vaccination series: 3 doses given at 0, 1–3 months and 5–6 month intervals.
  – Booster doses: Up to 3 doses at 6 month intervals depending on antibody response and continuing risk of exposure. Additional booster at 1–2 year intervals for continued risk may be given.
- Avoid direct handling of dead animal bodies.
- Avoid contact with persons with suspected pneumonic plague.
- Rodent and vector control measures.
- DEET application to skin and clothes.
- Post-exposure prophylaxis:
  – Adults:
    ○ Tetracycline 2 g/d orally divided in 2–4 doses for 7 days.
    ○ Doxycycline 100–200 mg orally every 12 hours for 7 days.
    ○ Trimethoprim-sulfamethoxazole (TMP-SMX) 160/800 mg every 12 hours for 7 days.

- For pneumonic plague: Isolation with respiratory droplet precautions.
- For bubonic plague: Standard hospital precautions.
- For clinical specimens: Biosafety level 2 procedures (level 3 might be indicated if activity is high risk for aerosol production)

PATHOPHYSIOLOGY
- Animal reservoir: Several mammalian species, including rodents, prairie dogs, ground squirrels, and domestic cats.
- Vector: Several species of fleas have been implicated in transmission of plague. The type of flea varies by geographic region.
- Humans are the accidental host and do not play a role in the maintenance of *Y. pestis* in ecosystem
- Transmission to human can occur as follows:
  – Bite from an infected rodent flea.
  – Direct contact with infected animals (scratches/bites, handling of carcasses).
  – Inhalation of aerosolized bacteria from animals, an infected human host with pneumonic plague, or laboratory specimens.
- Following exposure, incubation is generally between 2–8 days.
- The inoculated bacteria undergo intracellular multiplication followed by lysis of macrophages, bacterial release, and dissemination through lymphatics and bloodstream.
- Lymphatic spread to regional lymph nodes with inflammation and necrosis with creation of buboes.
- Hematogenous spread with sepsis and multiorgan disease.

ETIOLOGY
- *Yersinia pestis* is a gram-negative aerobic coccobacillus in the *Enterobacteriaceae* family
- Three biovars have been described: Antiqua, Medievalis, and Orientalis.

 DIAGNOSIS

HISTORY
Bubonic Plague
- Most common form of disease
- Sudden onset of fever, chills, headache, weakness.
- After 24 hours, patients note the onset of buboes, which are painful, massively enlarged lymph nodes.

Septicemic Plague
- May occur as primary disease or following bubonic/pneumonic plague.
- In 10% of cases, buboes are not present.
- Patients progress to multisystem disease:
  – Nausea, vomiting
  – Diarrhea
  – Abdominal pain
  – Severe prostration
  – Lethargy

Pneumonic Plague
- Primary pneumonic plague: Occurs following airborne transmission from an infected human or animal host.
- Secondary pneumonic plague: Develops as a complication of bubonic or septicemic plague.
- Cough productive of purulent to blood-tinged or grossly hemorrhagic sputum
- Pleuritic chest pain
- Rapidly progressing respiratory distress with hypoxia

Meningitic Plague
- Rare complication of usually untreated bubonic plague. It is caused by seeding of the central nervous system at the time of bacteremia.
- Fever
- Headache

Pharyngeal Plague
- Can occur following ingestion or inhalation of bacteria.
- Fever
- Sore throat

PHYSICAL EXAM
Bubonic Plague
- Formation of buboes within 24 hours proximal to the site of infected flea bite, most commonly in groin involving inguinal or femoral lymph nodes.
- Other common sites are axillary and cervical lymph nodes.
- Buboes are intensely inflamed lymph nodes which can be very large, firm to fluctuant, severely tender, and erythematous.
- Buboes eventually undergo ulceration.
- Small pustules or papules may be present in the area of the flea bite in 25% of patients.

Septicemic plague
- Toxic appearance
- Tachycardia, tachypnea
- Hypotension
- Buboes are uncommon
- Acral gangrene

Meningitic Plague
- Nuchal rigidity

Pharyngeal Plague
- Pharyngeal erythema
- Painful anterior cervical lymphadenitis

DIAGNOSTIC TESTS & INTERPRETATION
Lab
- Leukocytosis (can be severe depending on severity of illness)
- Thrombocytopenia
- Transaminitis
- Hyperbilirubinemia
- Elevated BUN and creatinine

- Disseminated intravascular coagulation (in severe cases of disease with sepsis)
- Blood cultures should be collected on all patients.
- Depending on clinical presentation, sputum, throat swabs, skin swabs, bubo aspirates or cerebrospinal fluid (CSF) can be collected and sent for Gram stain and culture.
- CSF analysis in meningeal plague: Pleocytosis with polymorphonuclear predominance. Gram stain may show gram-negative coccobacilli
- Special culture media: MacConkey agar, chocolate agar, brain-heart infusion broth, and sheep blood agar are recommended for culture of *Y. pestis*.
- Special stain: Wayson stain shows the characteristic "closed safety pin" appearance of *Y. pestis*. Bacilli stain light blue with darker blue staining at both poles.
- Plague bacilli express a unique diagnostic envelope glycoprotein called the Fraction 1 (F1) antigen.
- Serologic tests
  – Passive hemagglutination test:
    ○ Four-fold increase between acute and convalescent antibody titers can be used to make a diagnosis in culture negative cases.
  – ELISA based serological tests:
    ○ IgG and IgM antibodies to F1 antigen.
- Rapid antigen test is based on F1 antigen detection using monoclonal antibodies (3). The test can be used at the bedside.
- Polymerase chain reaction: Has been studied in respiratory specimens, but is not routinely available as a diagnostic tool (4).

Imaging
- Chest x-ray: Patchy or lobar pneumonia that progresses to cavitation.
- Pleural effusions
- Mediastinal or hilar lymphadenopathy
- Acute respiratory distress syndrome with diffuse opacities can be present

Diagnostic Procedures/Other
Injection of saline into the bubo is essential to obtain a good specimen.

DIFFERENTIAL DIAGNOSIS
- Streptococcal or staphylococcal lymphadenitis
- Other bacterial skin abscesses
- Cat scratch disease
- Incarcerated inguinal hernia
- Chancroid and lymphogranuloma venereum
- Streptococcal skin infection
- Anthrax
- Tularemia
- Hantavirus pulmonary syndrome

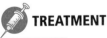 TREATMENT

MEDICATION
First Line
- Streptomycin 30 mg/kg/d IM in 2 divided doses:
  – Monitor for ototoxicity and nephrotoxicity.
  – Adjust dose in renal failure.
- Gentamicin 2.5 mg/kg IM every 12 hours (5). Equally effective as streptomycin.
- Duration of treatment is for 7 days.

Second Line
- Tetracycline 2–4 g/day in 4 divided doses. Loading dose of 2 g IV in severely ill patients.
- Doxycycline 100 mg IV or orally twice a day. Loading dose of 200 mg IV every 12 hours on day 1 in cases of severe illness.
- Chloramphenicol 25–30 mg/kg IV loading dose, followed by 50–60 mg/kg/d in 4 divided doses. Considered drug of choice in plague meningitis due to high tissue penetration.
- TMP-SMX 160/800 mg every 12 hours. Associated with higher failure rates. No ideal for monotherapy in severe disease.

ALERT
- Plague is a potential agent of bioterrorism due to high virulence and aerosol dissemination (6).
- Microbiology personnel should be notified of specimens potentially harboring the organism to take appropriate precautions.
- Emergence of multidrug resistant strains has been reported (7). Outbreaks due to multidrug resistant strains have not been reported.

ADDITIONAL TREATMENT
General Measures
- Intravenous fluid administration
- Symptom control (analgesic, antipyretics, and antiemetics)
- Intensive care unit care for critically ill patients.

SURGERY/OTHER PROCEDURES
Incision and drainage of buboes might be indicated if very large, painful, fluctuant with slow response to antimicrobials alone.

IN-PATIENT CONSIDERATIONS
Admission Criteria
- Careful clinical evaluation in a patient with suspected plague for respiratory distress and hypotension is needed to identify high-risk patients who may be in early sepsis and respiratory failure.
- If any of these findings are present, admission to the hospital should be advised.
- Other considerations for hospital admission are young children and older adults, and suspected pneumonic plague.

 ONGOING CARE

PROGNOSIS
- Mortality rates are as high as 50% for untreated disease.
- Pneumonic plague is an extremely fulminant condition with rapid progression to respiratory failure. Left untreated is almost always fatal.

COMPLICATIONS
- Superinfection of buboes with *Staphylococcus aureus* may occur at any time, and may require surgical drainage.
- Bubonic plague can be complicated by pneumonia, sepsis, and multiorgan failure.
- Unless diagnosed early, pneumonic plague may progress to respiratory failure.

REFERENCES
1. Human plague in 2002 and 2003. *Wkly Epidemiol Rec* 2004;79(33):301–306.
2. Prevention of plague: Recommendations of the Advisory Committee on Immunization Practices (ACIP). *MMWR Recomm Rep* 1996;45(RR-14):1–15.
3. Chanteau S, Rahalison L, Ralafiarisoa L, et al. Development and testing of a rapid diagnostic test for bubonic and pneumonic plague. *Lancet*. 2003;361(9353):211–216.
4. Loiez C, Herwegh S, Wallet F, et al. Detection of *Yersinia pestis* in sputum by real-time PCR. *J Clin Microbiol* 2003;41(10):4873–4875.
5. Mwengee W, Butler T, Mgema S, et al. Treatment of plague with gentamicin or doxycycline in a randomized clinical trial in Tanzania. *Clin Infect Dis* 2006;42(5):614–621.
6. Biological and chemical terrorism: Strategic plan for preparedness and response. Recommendations of the CDC Strategic Planning Workgroup. *MMWR Recomm Rep* 2000;49(RR-4):1–14.
7. Galimand M, Carniel E, Courvalin P. Resistance of *Yersinia pestis* to antimicrobial agents. *Antimicrob Agents Chemother* 2006;50(10):3233–3236.

 CODES

ICD9
- 020.0 Bubonic plague
- 020.5 Pneumonic plague, unspecified
- 020.9 Plague, unspecified

CLINICAL PEARLS
- Skin lesions due to flea bites distal to the buboes may help diagnosing plague.
- Wayson stain shows the characteristic bipolar staining ("closed safety pin" appearance).
- Treatment of choice is streptomycin, but manufacturing of the drug is limited. Gentamicin is equally effective.

PNEUMOCYSTIS JIROVECI (CARINII) INFECTION

Erica S. Shenoy (E. Mylonakis, Editor)

 BASICS

DESCRIPTION
Pneumocystis jiroveci is an opportunistic pathogen, the natural habitat of which is the lung. This unicellular fungus is an important cause of pneumonia in the immunocompromised host. It is most commonly known as Pneumocystis carinii pneumonia (PCP), though a recent change in the nomenclature has resulted in the organism formerly known as *Pneumocystis carinii* now identified as *Pneumocystis jiroveci*.

EPIDEMIOLOGY
- The incidence in immunocompromised (i.e., HIV/AIDS and transplant patients) has decreased with the use of prophylaxis, although it is still the most common opportunistic infection among HIV-infected patients.
- Pneumocystis pneumonia has been observed in patients on immune-modulating agents such as etanercept and infliximab.
- Extrapulmonary *P. jiroveci* infection is involved in fewer than 3% of cases.
- Internationally, the reported incidence of Pneumocystis pneumonia is "low"; this is thought to be the result of under-diagnosis.
- Pneumocystis pneumonia is found in approximately 80% of HIV-infected infants diagnosed with pneumonia.

RISK FACTORS
- HIV/AIDS, especially at CD4 counts <200.
- Malignancy (solid organ or hematologic)
- Patients on long-term immunosuppressive agents
- Patients with a primary immune deficiencies (i.e., hypogammaglobulinemia and severe combined immunodeficiency)
- Tobacco use
- Severe malnutrition

GENERAL PREVENTION
- Primary prophylaxis is indicated for HIV-infected patients at high risk of developing pneumocystosis—that is, those who have CD4+ cell counts of <200/mm^3 or in patients with oropharyngeal candidiasis, regardless of CD4 count. Clinicians should consider prophylaxis in patients with CD4 <15% as well. Primary prophylaxis can be discontinued if CD4 >200 for >3 months.
- Guidelines for the administration of primary prophylaxis to other immunocompromised hosts are less clear. Currently, in most centers, prophylaxis is given to patients in known risk groups, such as bone marrow transplant recipients and children with acute lymphoblastic leukemia.
- Secondary prophylaxis is indicated for all patients who have recovered from *P. jiroveci* pneumonia.

- The prophylactic regimen of choice is 1 double-strength tablet of trimethoprim-sulfamethoxazole (160 mg of trimethoprim) per day. Alternative regimens include the following:
  - Trimethoprim-sulfamethoxazole at a reduced dose or frequency (i.e., 1 single-strength tablet daily)
  - Dapsone (50 mg daily), pyrimethamine (50 mg once per week), and folinic acid (25 mg once per week)
  - Dapsone (100 mg daily)
  - Nebulized pentamidine (300 mg once per month through a Respirgard II nebulizer)
  - Pyrimethamine plus sulfadoxine for patients with hypersensitivity to sulfonamides. Patients taking this combination have a higher risk of Stevens–Johnson syndrome.

PATHOPHYSIOLOGY
- *P. jiroveci* is found in the lungs of healthy individuals. Infection occurs early in childhood and approximately two-thirds of children have been infected by age 4 years.
- In individuals with impaired immunity, the usually nonpathogenic organism may cause disease. For example, in patients with low CD4 counts, it is known that activated macrophages are not able to clear pneumocystis organisms. This results in increased alveolar-capillary permeability. This results in hypoxemia with increased alveolar-arterial oxygen gradient (PAO$_2$-PaO$_2$) and respiratory alkalosis.

ETIOLOGY
Pneumocystis pneumonia is caused by *P. jiroveci*.

COMMONLY ASSOCIATED CONDITIONS
As described in risk factors, HIV infection and other forms of immunosuppression put patients at risk for Pneumocystis pneumonia.

 DIAGNOSIS

HISTORY
- Symptoms are usually nonspecific and may include progressive exertional dyspnea, fever, chest pain, weight loss, chills, and hemoptysis.
- Among HIV-infected patients, the presentation is often subacute, as opposed to non-HIV infected patients who are otherwise immunocompromised.

PHYSICAL EXAM
- Physical findings may include tachypnea, fever, and tachycardia.
- Pulmonary examination may be normal in up to half of patients.
- Children with severe disease may have cyanosis, nasal flaring, and intercostal retractions.
- In the rare instances of extrapulmonary disease, involvement of CNS, bone marrow (necrosis leading to pancytopenia), lymphadenopathy, ocular involvement, thyroid involvement with enlarging mass, and GI tract involvement occur.

DIAGNOSTIC TESTS & INTERPRETATION
Lab
Initial lab tests
- Elevated serum concentrations of lactate dehydrogenase have been reported but are not specific to *P. jiroveci* infection.
- (1→3)β-D-glucan may be elevated in patients with Pneumocystis pneumonia, but is not diagnostic.
- The white blood cell (WBC) count is variable.
- Exercise-induced oxygen saturation is probably the most sensitive and specific noninvasive test for diagnosis of *P. jiroveci* pneumonia.
- Arterial blood gases usually demonstrate hypoxia, an increased alveolar-arterial oxygen gradient (PAO$_2$-PaO$_2$), and respiratory alkalosis.

Follow-Up & Special Considerations
- Disease severity is classified by alveolar-arterial gradients as follows:
  - Mild: <35 mm Hg
  - Moderate/Severe: 35–45 mm Hg
  - Severe: >45 mm Hg

Imaging
- The classic findings on chest radiography consist of bilateral diffuse infiltrates involving the perihilar regions.
- Early in the course of Pneumocystis, the chest radiograph may be normal.
- Patients who receive aerosolized pentamidine have an increased frequency of upper lobe infiltrates and pneumothorax.
- Obtain chest CT if x-ray is unrevealing.
- There may be increased uptake with nuclear imaging techniques (gallium scan), though such tests with high sensitivity, low specificity, and high cost make them less useful, except in cases of relapse, where bronchoalveolar lavage (BAL) may have lower yield.

Diagnostic Procedures/Other
- There is no reliable way to cultivate the organism in vitro.
- A definitive diagnosis is made by histopathologic staining (see below).
- The yield from different diagnostic procedures is higher in HIV-infected patients than in non-HIV-infected patients, probably because of the higher organism burden.
- Fiberoptic bronchoscopy with BAL remains the mainstay of *P. jiroveci* diagnosis.
- Expectorated sputum induction is a simple, noninvasive technique, but has very low sensitivity; should not be used in the diagnosis.
- Induced sputum, however, is used in the diagnosis of Pneumocystis pneumonia. Sensitivity and specificity vary.
- Transbronchial biopsy and open lung biopsy, which are the most invasive procedures, are reserved for situations in which a diagnosis cannot be made by BAL.
- Pulmonary function tests should be obtained as part of the work up in suspected Pneumocystis pneumonia.
- Pulse oximetry should be performed at rest and with exertion.

Pathological Findings
- Several stains are used to detect the trophozoite and cyst forms, including Cresyl violet, Giemsa, Romanowsky and Wright stains.
- The cell wall of the cysts can be stained using methenamine silver, toluidine blue, and Gram-Weigert stains.
- Direct immunofluorescence, using monoclonal antibodies to the organisms, is used as well.

DIFFERENTIAL DIAGNOSIS
- Includes other infectious causes of pneumonia such as:
  - Atypical presentation of pneumonococcal or fungal pneumonia
  - Legionnaires' disease
  - Tuberculosis
  - Viral pneumonia (i.e., influenza, RSV, etc)
  - CMV pneumonia
- Congestive heart failure
- Kaposi's sarcoma or lymphoma with pulmonary involvement
- Pulmonary embolism
- Lymphocytic interstitial pneumonia
- Acute respiratory distress syndrome (ARDS)

 ## TREATMENT

MEDICATION
First Line
- Trimethoprim-sulfamethoxazole (TMP-SMX) is the drug of choice; it should be dose-adjusted for renal function.
- Dosing for TMP/SMX is 20 mg of trimethoprim per day in 3–4 divided doses, administered IV or PO. In children >2 months, the dose is 15–20 mg/kg/d in 3 divided doses.
- Several studies have shown that the administration of glucocorticoids to HIV-infected patients with moderate to severe pneumocystosis (a PO_2 of 70 mm Hg or a PAO_2PaO_2 of 35 mm Hg) can improve the rate of survival. The recommended dosing is prednisone 40 mg PO twice a day for 5 days, then 40 mg/d for 5 days, then 20 mg per day for 11 days (administer 30 min before TMP-SMX). Steroids should be started immediately, and before 72 hours of starting anti-pneumocystis therapy.
- The use of steroids as adjunctive therapy in non-HIV adults with severe disease is also recommended.
- If steroids are used in the patients in their third trimester of pregnancy, glucose levels should be monitored closely.
- 10–45% HIV-infected patients experience serious adverse reactions, including fever, rash, neutropenia, thrombocytopenia, hepatitis, and hyperkalemia.
- Treatment of *P. jiroveci* pneumonia should be continued for 14 days in non-HIV-infected patients, and for 21 days in persons with HIV/AIDS.
- Clinicians should wait for a few days before concluding that therapy has failed. Most HIV infected patients should demonstrate clinical response within 4–5 days of treatment but if no improvement has been demonstrated at day 8, alternative treatments should be considered.
- Treatment for the extrapulmonary forms of pneumocystosis is the same as that for pneumonia.

Second Line
- Pentamidine is given as a single dose of 4 mg/kg/d by slow intravenous infusion. Its principal adverse effects are hypotension, cardiac arrhythmia, pancreatitis, dysglycemia, azotemia, electrolyte changes, and neutropenia.
- Other alternative treatments are clindamycin given intravenously (600–900 mg 4 times daily, based on severity) or by mouth (300–450 mg 4 times daily in mild–moderate disease) and primaquine by mouth (15–30 mg daily). Primaquine should be avoided in patients with glucose-6-phosphate dehydrogenase deficiency.
- Trimethoprim plus dapsone and atovaquone are less toxic oral regimens that are used in mild to moderate *P. jiroveci* pneumonia.

ADDITIONAL TREATMENT
General Measures
- Treatment failure occurs when the patient fails to respond to 4–8 days of treatment, as documented by lack of improvement or worsening of respiratory status or arterial blood gases.
- Failure can be related to intolerability of drug toxicity or lack of efficacy of TMP-SMX.
- If treatment failure has occurred, parenteral pentamidine or primaquine plus clindamycin is often an alternative therapeutic regimen. In mild disease, atovaquone can be used.

Issues for Referral
Infectious disease and pulmonary critical care expertise should be considered.

 ## ONGOING CARE

FOLLOW-UP RECOMMENDATIONS
Patients with a diagnosis of Pneumocystis pneumonia not on immunosuppressive agents should be tested for HIV as well as inherited immunodeficiencies.

Patient Monitoring
- Patients should be monitored closely for clinical response and treatment-related toxicity.
- Close monitoring of oxygenation.
- Close monitoring for pneumothorax or other complications.

PROGNOSIS
- Among patients with HIV, mortality rate is approximately 10–20%.
- In non-HIV infected patients, mortality rates of 30–50% have been observed, possibly the result of delayed diagnosis and treatment.

COMPLICATIONS
- In the typical case of untreated Pneumocystis pneumonia, progressive respiratory compromise leads to death.
- Therapy is most effective when instituted early in the course of the disease, before there is extensive alveolar damage.
- Concurrent pulmonary infections complicate management.

ADDITIONAL READING
- Bennett NJ, et al. Pneumocystis (carinii) jiroveci Pneumonia. *EMedicine Infectious Diseases*, 2009.

- Furrer H, Egger M, Opravil M, et al. Discontinuation of primary prophylaxis against Pneumocystis carinii pneumonia in HIV-1-infected adults treated with combination antiretroviral therapy. Swiss HIV Cohort Study. *N Engl J Med* 1999;340:1301–1306.
- Kaplan JE, et al. Guidelines for the prevention and treatment of opportunistic infections among HIV-infected adults and adolescents: Guidelines from the CDC, the National Institutes of Health and the HIV Medicine Association of the Infectious Diseases Society of America. *MMWR* 2009; 58(RR04);1–198.
- Masur H. Management of Opportunistic Infections Associated with Human Immunodeficiency Virus. Infection. In Principles and Practice of Infectious Diseases, 7th ed. Mandell, Douglas and Bennett, eds. 2009.
- Mofenson LM, et al. Guidelines for the prevention and treatment of opportunistic infections among HIV-exposed and HIV-infected children: Recommendations from the CDC, the National Institutes of Health, the Pediatric Infectious Diseases Society, and the American Academy of Pediatrics. *MMWR* 2009;58(RR11):1–166.
- Miller RF, Mitchell DM. AIDS and the lung: Update 1995. 1. Pneumocystis cariniipneumonia. *Thorax* 1995;50:191–200.
- O'Dowd EL. A Case of Pneumocystis Jirovecii Pneumonia in a Patient Treated with Etanercept for Rheumatoid Arthritis. American Journal of Respiratory and Critical Care Medicine 2010;181: A6180.
- Stringer JR, et al. A new name (Pneumocystis jiroveci) for ineumocystis in humans. *Emerg Infect Dis* 2002;8.
- Sepkowitz KA, Brown AE, Armstrong D. *Pneumocystis carinii* pneumonia without acquired immunodeficiency syndrome. More patients, same risk. *Arch Intern Med* 1995;155:1125–1128.
- Tai TL, et al. Pneumocystis carinii pneumonia following a second infusion of infliximab. *Rheumatology* 2002;41:951–952.
- Watanabe T, et al. Serum (1à3)beta-D-Glucan as a noninvasive adjunct marker for the diagnosis Pneumocystis pneumonia in patients with AIDS. *Clin Infect Dis* 2009;40:1128–1131.
- Weltzer PD. Pneumocystis carinii infection. In: Fauci AS, Braunwald E, Isselbacher KJ, et at., eds. *Harrison's principles of internal medicine*, 14th edition. New York, McGraw-Hill, 1998:1161–1163.

 ## CODES

ICD9
136.3 *Pneumocystis carinii*Pneumocystosis

CLINICAL PEARLS
- Pneumocystis pneumonia should be suspected in patients with epidemiological risk factors, even those who are on prophylaxis (especially if they are on TMP-SMX).
- Diagnosis is usually based on histological staining of induced sputum or BAL specimens.
- Early treatment with TMP-SMX (or alternative if needed) along with steroids, if indicated, leads to improved outcomes.

PNEUMONIA

Yinggang Zhu
Jieming Qu
Petros I. Rafailidis
Matthew E. Falagas

 BASICS

DESCRIPTION

- Pneumonia is defined as inflammation of the pulmonary parenchyma caused by an infectious agent. Inflammation of the lung is categorized by clinical setting as the following:
  - Community-acquired pneumonia (CAP): Typical (i.e., classic) pneumonia; Atypical pneumonia;
  - Nursing home: In nursing home residents
  - Nosocomial pneumonia: Hospital-associated pneumonia; ventilator-associated pneumonia
  - Pneumonia in immunocompromised hosts
  - Aspiration pneumonia

EPIDEMIOLOGY

Incidence

- 4 million patients with pneumonia annually in the US
- CAP: Affects 12 per 1,000 inhabitants annually in the US; the highest numbers being at the extremes of age
- Nosocomial: 0.5–1.5% of hospitalized patients

Prevalence

- CAP: More prevalent in children and individuals >60 years
- Nosocomial: Common among patients requiring mechanical ventilation, particularly among patients who remain ventilated for as long as 30 days

RISK FACTORS

- Alcoholism
- Aspiration
- Endotracheal intubation
- Immunosuppression
- Age >65 years
- Hospital or nursing home setting, especially the ICU
- Underlying disease (COPD, cystic fibrosis)

GENERAL PREVENTION

- Influenza and pneumococcal vaccine
- Avoid endotracheal intubation or at least minimize its duration

PATHOPHYSIOLOGY

- The host inflammatory response leads to release of inflammatory mediators and chemokines
- Inflammatory mediators released by macrophages and the recruited neutrophils create an alveolar capillary leak resulting in hemoptysis, infiltrates, rales.
- Alveolar filling leads to hypoxemia
- Decreased compliance due to capillary leak, hypoxemia, increased respiratory drive, increased secretions, and occasionally infection-related bronchospasm all contribute to dyspnea.

ETIOLOGY

- Community-acquired pneumonia
  - *Streptococcus pneumoniae* (20–65%)
  - *Mycoplasma pneumoniae* (~15%): Common in patients with "walking pneumonia"
  - *Haemophilus influenzae*
  - *Chlamydia pneumoniae*
  - *Staphylococcus aureus* (2–10%): More common with influenza; novel community-acquired strains of methicillin-resistant *S. aureus* (CA-MRSA) may contribute to necrotizing or cavitary pneumonia
  - Newly identified pathogens: Hantaviruses, metapneumoviruses, the coronavirus responsible for the severe acute respiratory syndrome (SARS)
  - Polymicrobial infections (10–15%): Including typical and atypical pathogens
  - *Coxiella burnetii* is an important cause

ALERT

Legionnaire's disease, SARS, psittacosis, avian influenza (H5N1), and possible agents of bioterrorism need to be reported.

- Nosocomial
  - Gram-negative bacilli (50–80%): Multidrug-resistant (MDR) *Pseudomonas*, *Xanthomonas*, *Klebsiella*, and *Acinetobacter* species have emerged
  - *S. aureus* (20–30%): MRSA
  - Anaerobic bacteria (<10%)
  - *Legionella* (~5%): May be found in epidemics associated with contaminated water supply
- Viral pathogens (Less common): Most frequently affects immunocompromised hosts
- Immunocompromised host
- Immunoglobulin and complement deficiencies
  - *S. pneumoniae*
  - *H. influenzae*
  - *S. aureus*
  - *Neisseria* spp.
- Granulocyte dysfunction or deficiency
  - Enteric gram-negative bacilli
  - *Aspergillus*
- Cellular and combined immune deficiencies
  - Fungal infections: *Pneumocystis jiroveci*, *Candida*, *Cryptococcus*
  - Parasitic infection: Toxoplasma, *Strongyloides stercoralis*
  - Mycobacteria: *M. tuberculosis*, *M. avium*, *M. kansasii*, etc.
  - Bacteria: *Listeria*, *S. pneumoniae*, *H. influenzae*, *S. aureus*, *P. aeruginosa*, *Legionella*
- Virus: Cytomegalovirus, herpes virus 6, herpes simplex virus, and Epstein-Barr virus

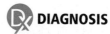 **DIAGNOSIS**

HISTORY

- Community-acquired Pneumonia
- Community-acquired pneumonia: Recent history of upper respiratory tract infection
- Nosocomial hospitalization for more than 48 h
- Symptoms may include fever with respiratory symptoms: Cough, sputum, pleurisy, dyspnea, etc. Other symptoms include chills, sweats, fatigue, headache, myalgias, and arthralgias. The elderly may initially display new-onset or worsening confusion.

PHYSICAL EXAM

- Tachypnea and tachycardia are common.
- Increased or decreased tactile fremitus
- Percussion notes vary from dull to flat, reflecting underlying consolidated lung and pleural fluid, respectively
- Crackles/bronchial breath sounds/a pleural friction rub
- Hypotension or evidence of organ failure may be found in severely ill patients.

DIAGNOSTIC TESTS & INTERPRETATION

Lab

Initial lab tests

- CBC
- Culture specimens uncontaminated by upper airway secretions
- Pulse oximetry/arterial blood gas measurements
- C-reactive protein (CRP)

Imaging

Initial approach

CXR

Follow-Up & Special Considerations

- If pneumonia is strongly suspected on clinical grounds and no opacity is seen on the initial chest radiograph, it is useful to repeat the radiograph in 24–48 h or to perform a CT of the chest.
- Pneumatoceles suggest infection with *S. aureus*, and an upper-lobe cavitating lesion suggests tuberculosis
- CT may be of value in a patient with suspected post-obstructive pneumonia caused by a tumor or foreign body.

Diagnostic Procedures/Other

In patients who are seriously ill or who present a diagnostic problem, invasive techniques should be considered for obtaining uncontaminated lower respiratory secretions or lung biopsies.

- Quantitative-culture approach
- Rapid urinary antigen tests for *S. pneumoniae* and *L. pneumophila*
- Polymerase chain reaction (PCR)
- Bronchoscopy with bronchoalveolar lavage
- Transbronchial biopsy
- Lung biopsy
- If suspected, rule out concurrent endocarditis or meningitis

Pathological Findings

Pattern for pneumococcal pneumonia: Edema, red hepatization, gray hepatization, and resolution. Viral and pneumocystis pneumonias represent alveolar rather than interstitial processes.

DIFFERENTIAL DIAGNOSIS

- **Infectious**: Bronchitis, acute exacerbations of chronic bronchitis, lung abscess, and empyema
- **Noninfectious:** Heart failure, pulmonary embolism, lung cancer, and lymphoma

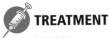 TREATMENT

MEDICATION

Empiric Antimicrobial Therapy for CAP

- Outpatients (2): 1. Previously healthy and no use of antibiotics in the preceding 3 months: Clarithromycin or azithromycin or doxycycline. 2. Having comorbidity or immunosuppression or received antibiotics in the last 3 months: a. Respiratory fluoroquinolone (moxifloxacin 400 mg OD PO or levofloxacin 750 mg OD PO) [if not used priorly] or b. β-lactam (e.g., high-dose (1 g t.i.d PO) amoxicillin or cefuroxime 500 mg b.i.d PO) plus macrolide. If locally a high rate of infection (>25%) is caused by highly macrolide resistant *S. pneumoniae* consider, even in previously healthy persons, the use of a respiratory fluoroquinolone or a beta lactam
- Inpatients, non-ICU (2)
  - Respiratory fluoroquinolone
  - β-lactam [cefotaxime or ceftriaxone or ampicillin or selected patients ertapenem] plus macrolide
- Inpatients, ICU (2)
- β-lactam (cefotaxime or ceftriaxone or ampicillin/sulbactam or amoxicillin/clavulanate) plus azithromycin or fluoroquinolone. Special concerns Pseudomonas: Antipseudomonal β-lactam plus either ciprofloxacin or levofloxacin
- CA-MRSA: Add linezolid
- Treatment duration for CAP: At least 5 days; the majority receive treatment for 7–10 days [A]. 14–21 days may be necessary for pneumonia due to *L. pneumophila* (if severe, consider adding rifampin), *Coxiella burnetii* (acute Q fever) and *S. aureus*.
- Use doxycycline for acute Q fever.
- Treatment must be tailored to microbiological/ serological data if available (i.e., penicillin G may suffice for *S. pneumoniae*).

Empiric Antimicrobial Therapy for Nosocomial Pneumonia

- Without risk factors for MDR pathogens
- Ceftriaxone or respiratory fluoroquinolone or
- or ampicillin/sulbactam or ertapenem
- With risk factors for MDR pathogens
  - β-lactam (e.g., ceftazidime or cefepime or piperacillin/tazobactam or imipenem or meropenem) plus aminoglycoside or fluoroquinolone plus (for hospital associated-MRSA) Linezolid or vancomycin
- Treatment duration for HAP: 8 days unless MDR *P. aeruginosa* or *A. baumannii* for which a 15 day regimen is appropriate 1[A].

ADDITIONAL TREATMENT

Issues for Referral

- To a cardiothoracic surgeon if presence of empyema
- To ICU if need for mechanical ventilation or Extra Corporeal Membrane Oxygenation

Additional Therapies

Corticosteroids or immunomodulatory therapy among patients with severe CAP

IN-PATIENT CONSIDERATIONS

Initial Stabilization

- Adequate hydration
- Oxygen therapy
- Initiation of empiric antibiotics within 4 h arrival to hospital
- Assisted ventilation if necessary

Admission Criteria

- CURB-65 severity score (Confusion, urea nitrogen levels >20mg/dL, increased respiratory rate >30/min, systolic pressure <90 mm Hg or diastolic pressure <60 mm Hg, age >65 years). Each parameter receives a score of 1 point. Admit if >2 (2).
- The pneumonia severity index (3) is another useful tool to decide admission or not. It is based on demographic factors, coexisting conditions (i.e., alcoholism), physical examination findings (i.e., altered mental status), laboratory and radiological findings (i.e., PaO$_2$ <60 mm Hg).
- Immunosuppressive therapy
- Chest x-ray indicating multiple lobe involvement or rapid spread

Nursing

Monitor oxygen saturation

Discharge Criteria

Clinically improved (no cardiorespiratory compromise), without fever over 72 h and oral administration of antibiotics possible

 ONGOING CARE

FOLLOW-UP RECOMMENDATIONS

Chest radiographic abnormalities may require 4–12 weeks to clear. If relapse or recurrence is documented, the possibility of an underlying neoplasm must be considered.

PROGNOSIS

- The overall mortality rate of CAP for the outpatient group is <1%. For patients requiring hospitalization, the overall mortality rate is estimated at 10%, with ~50% of the deaths directly attributable to pneumonia.
- VAP is associated with a reported 50–70% mortality, but the real issue is attributable mortality.

COMPLICATIONS

- Failure to respond to treatment as a result of the following: 1. Noninfectious conditions, 2. Drug resistant pathogen, 3. Inadequate dose of antibiotic, 4. Compromised or debilitated host, 5. Nosocomial superinfections
- Metastatic infection
- Complicated pleural effusion
- Lung abscess

REFERENCES

1. American Thoracic Society/Infectious Diseases Society of America. Guidelines for the management of adults with hospital-acquired, ventilator-associated, and healthcare-associated pneumonia. *Am J Respir Crit Care Med* 2005;171:388–416.
2. Mandell La, Wunderink RG, Anzueto A, et al. Infectious Diseases Society of America/American Thoracic Society consensus guidelines on the management of community-acquired pneumonia. *Clin Infect Dis* 2007;44(S2):S27–S72.
3. Fine MJ, Auble TE, Yealy DM, et al. A prediction rule to identify low-risk patients with community-acquired pneumonia. *N Engl J Med* 1997;336: 243–250.

 CODES

ICD9

- 482.30 Pneumonia due to Streptococcus, unspecified
- 486 Pneumonia, organism unspecified
- 507.0 Pneumonitis due to aspiration of food or vomitus

CLINICAL PEARLS

- Don't rely entirely on prognostic scores for admission to hospital, if hypoxemia or pneumonia complications or unreliable oral intake or underlying disease exacerbation are present (2).

POLIOMYELITIS

Girish Chinnaswamy
Balaji Veeraraghavan
Paschalis Vergidis
Matthew E. Falagas

BASICS

DESCRIPTION
- Poliomyelitis is an acute viral infection caused by a small RNA enterovirus.
- Most commonly the virus causes inapparent infection.
- In approximately 1% of cases, the central nervous system is affected. This can result in varying degrees of paralysis.

EPIDEMIOLOGY
Incidence
- No cases of wild-type poliovirus (WPV) infection have been reported in the US since 1979.
- Until 1998, an average of 8–10 vaccine-derived viruses were reported yearly.

Prevalence
- There are no chronic carriers and no animal source is documented.
- Wild-type polioviruses (WPV), live attenuated oral poliomyelitis vaccine (OPV) viruses, and virulent polioviruses derived from OPV strains (vaccine-derived polioviruses) (1) may circulate in different populations.
- By 2005, indigenous transmission of WPV types 1 and 3 had been eliminated from all but 4 countries (Afghanistan, India, Nigeria, and Pakistan) (2). WPV type 2 transmission has been globally interrupted.
- Outbreaks following WPV importations into previously poliomyelitis-free countries have been reported (3). There will be an ongoing risk until poliomyelitis is completely eradicated from all countries.

RISK FACTORS
- Overcrowding and poor sanitation provide opportunities for exposure to infection.
- Risk factors for paralysis:
  – B-cell immunodeficiency
  – Strenuous exercise within first 3 days of illness
  – Disease tends to localize in a limb where prior intramuscular injection was administered
  – Tonsillectomy

GENERAL PREVENTION
- 2 vaccines are available: Inactivated poliomyelitis vaccine (IPV) and attenuated oral poliomyelitis vaccine (OPV)
- In developed countries, IPV is administered parenterally.
  – Contains all 3 serotypes and has seroconversion rates equal to OPV.
  – Neutralizing antibodies are found in 100% of people after the third dose.
  – Recipients develop little or no secretory antibody and may develop natural asymptomatic infection and spread the virus to unvaccinated contacts.

- In the developing world, OPV is primarily used due to its lower cost and ease of administration.
  – OPV nonimmune recipients shed virus in feces up to 6 weeks.
  – OPV promotes antibody formation in the gut (providing local protection against viral entry) and boost herd immunity (Shortly after vaccination, children excrete virus that may be acquired by their contacts).
- A proportion of the population vaccinated with all the recommended doses of OPV may fail to seroconvert for all 3 serotypes. This is related to vaccine formulation. Concurrent acute diarrhea adversely affects seroconversion rates (4).
- The disadvantage of OPV is the rare occurrence of vaccine-derived paralytic poliomyelitis (1 person in every 2.6 million doses). Mainly occurs in immunocompromised individuals.
- To eliminate the risk of vaccine-derived disease, an all-IPV schedule is now recommended for routine childhood vaccination in the US and Europe. All children should receive 4 doses of IPV at 2 months, 4 months, 6–18 months, and 4–6 years.
- When IPV was used as a supplement to OPV immunization, markedly enhanced seroconversion rates were observed.

PATHOPHYSIOLOGY
- Humans are the only known reservoir of infection.
- The fecal–oral route is the main route of spread in developing countries.
- Droplet transmission through respiratory secretions is relatively more important in developed countries. It can occur in the acute phase when the virus is present in the throat. Close personal contact with an infected person facilitates droplet spread.
- Primary site of infection are the intestinal cells. From here it spreads and replicates in the local lymphatics, causing minor viremia. The infection is either terminated at this stage or reaches susceptible reticuloendothelial tissue through the bloodstream, resulting in major viremia.
- The central nervous system is infected by retrograde axonal transport from muscle to nerve to cord. Neurons throughout the grey matter are affected.
- The virus causes destruction of anterior horn cells and motor nuclei in the spinal cord, pons, and medulla. This leads to motor weakness or paralysis of the axial skeleton, the cranial nerves or the brainstem.

ETIOLOGY
- Poliovirus belongs to the family of *Picornaviridae*, genus *Enterovirus*,
- There are 3 serotypes 1, 2, and 3.
- Infection by one of the serotypes (1, 2, or 3) confers immunity only to that specific serotype, with little cross protection to others.
- Prior to vaccination, the majority of paralytic poliomyelitis was due to serotype-1 virus.

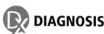

DIAGNOSIS

HISTORY
The incubation period from exposure to the viral prodrome is 9–12 days (minor illness) and from exposure to the onset of paralysis is 11–17 days (major illness).

PHYSICAL EXAM
- Inapparent (subclinical) infection
  – 95% of cases are asymptomatic. Disease can only be recognized by virus isolation or serology.
- Abortive polio or minor illness
  – This occurs in 4–8% of infected individuals.
  – Nonspecific upper respiratory tract illness, with sore throat and low-grade fevers.
  – There may be abdominal pain and diarrhea.
  – Self-limited disease
  – The patient recovers quickly.
- Nonparalytic poliomyelitis
  – This occurs in 1% of all infections.
  – Nonspecific respiratory illness with signs of meningeal irritation (Stiffness and pain in the neck and back)
  – Symptoms last for 2–10 days.
  – Recovery is rapid.
- Spinal paralytic poliomyelitis
  – Occurs in 0.1% of infection (major illness).
  – The patient notices the rapid onset of localized muscle pains 2–5 days following the "minor illness stage." Fasciculations are visible. Fevers return.
  – The predominant sign is asymmetrical flaccid paralysis with proximal muscle groups more involved than distal muscles.
  – Lower limb involvement is more common than upper limb weakness.
  – Sensory loss is rare.
  – Reflexes are lost.
  – Occasionally the disease progresses from weakness to quadriplegia and bulbar involvement.

- Bulbar paralytic poliomyelitis
  - Progression to bulbar involvement usually occurs over 2–3 days (but disease can progress even within hours).
  - Progression halts when the patient becomes afebrile.
  - Cranial nerves paralysis (IX and X are frequently involved) results in dysphagia, nasal speech, and dyspnea.
  - Occurs in 5%–35% of paralytic cases.
  - Mixed bulbar and spinal involvement is common
- Polioencephalitis
  - Rare form. Usually occurs in children.
  - May present with seizures.

DIAGNOSTIC TESTS & INTERPRETATION
Lab
- Cerebrospinal fluid (CSF) pleocytosis. CSF abnormalities are indistinguishable from those of other viral infections causing aseptic meningitis.
- Virus isolation – Poliovirus can be isolated from pharyngeal secretions during the first week of illness and from stool for several weeks. The virus is rarely isolated from the CSF.
- In sporadic cases, it is important to characterize the virus isolate as either wild-type or vaccine-derived by genotypic methods.
- The diagnosis can be established serologically by testing acute and convalescent sera by neutralization against antigens of the 3 serotypes.
  - Serology cannot distinguish between wild-type and vaccine-derived poliovirus infection

Imaging
Initial approach
- Neuroimaging (spinal or head CT/MRI) mainly to exclude other causes of paralytic disease.
- MRI shows T2-weighted hyperintensities involving bilateral anterior horn cells

Pathological Findings
Neuronal destruction and inflammatory lesions in the gray matter of the anterior horns of the spinal cord and in the motor nuclei of the pons and medulla.

DIFFERENTIAL DIAGNOSIS
- Other enteroviral infections
- Botulism
- West Nile virus infection
- Transverse myelitis
- Epidural mass lesion
- Tick paralysis
- Guillain-Barré syndrome (causes symmetrical, bilateral ascending paralysis)
- Neuropathy
- Stroke

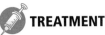 TREATMENT

MEDICATION
There is no specific antiviral therapy for poliovirus.

ADDITIONAL TREATMENT
General Measures
- Patients require hospitalization during the acute phase for supportive treatment.
- Bed rest is essential to prevent augmentation of paralysis.

Additional Therapies
Positive pressure ventilation is indicated when the vital capacity falls below 50%.

SURGERY/OTHER PROCEDURES
Total hip arthroplasty for patients with hip dysplasia due to paralytic poliomyelitis.

 ONGOING CARE

FOLLOW-UP RECOMMENDATIONS
Physical therapy should be prompt once progression of paralysis has ceased.

DIET
Use diet rich in fiber as patients may develop constipation.

PROGNOSIS
- Bulbar paralytic poliomyelitis has the highest rate of complications. Mortality is as high as 60%.
- Two-thirds of patients with paralytic disease have a degree of permanent weakness on recovery.
- Complete recovery is rare when acute paralysis is severe.
- Those who survive bulbar paralysis show significant improvement by 10 days.
- The eventual outcome can be estimated after a month, when most reversible damage has disappeared. Complete recovery from pharyngeal paralysis is usually seen.

COMPLICATIONS
- Complication of paralytic poliomyelitis:
  - Respiratory compromise
  - Gastrointestinal events such as gastric dilatation and paralytic ileus.
- Post-poliomyelitis syndrome:
  - 20–30% of patients who recover partially or completely from paralytic poliomyelitis have a gradual onset of muscle weakness, pain, muscle atrophy, and fatigue many years after the acute illness.
  - Usually occurs 25–35 years after initial infection
  - Typically involves the muscles that were affected initially.

REFERENCES
1. Centers for Disease Control and Prevention (CDC). Update on vaccine-derived polioviruses–worldwide, January 2008–June 2009. *MMWR Morb Mortal Wkly Rep* 2009;58(36):1002–1006.
2. Centers for Disease Control and Prevention (CDC). Progress toward interruption of wild poliovirus transmission – worldwide, 2009. *MMWR Morb Mortal Wkly Rep* 2010;59(18):545–550.
3. Centers for Disease Control and Prevention (CDC). Outbreaks following wild poliovirus importations—Europe, Africa, and Asia, January 2009-September 2010. *MMWR Morb Mortal Wkly Rep* 2010;59(43):1393–1399.
4. Myaux JA, Unicomb L, Besser RE, et al. Effect of diarrhea on the humoral response to oral polio vaccination. *Pediatr Infect Dis J* 1996;15(3):204–209.

 CODES

ICD9
- 045.10 Acute poliomyelitis with other paralysis, unspecified type of poliovirus
- 045.20 Acute nonparalytic poliomyelitis, unspecified type poliovirus

CLINICAL PEARLS
- Poliomyelitis typically causes asymmetrical flaccid paralysis with involvement of proximal muscle groups more than distal muscles.
- Two vaccines are available: Inactivated poliomyelitis vaccine (IPV) and attenuated oral poliomyelitis vaccine (OPV).
- To eliminate the risk of vaccine-derived paralytic poliomyelitis, an all-IPV schedule is now recommended for routine childhood vaccination in developed countries.

PROGRESSIVE MULTIFOCAL LEUKOENCEPHALOPATHY

Paschalis Vergidis
Mathew E. Falagas

 BASICS

DESCRIPTION
- Progressive multifocal leukoencephalopathy (PML) is a rare, subacute demyelinating disease of the brain white matter, caused either by primary infection or reactivation of JC virus (JCV).
- First identified as a clinical entity in 1958, it is primarily seen in patients with AIDS or other forms of cell-mediated immunity suppression, and is mainly characterized by rapidly deteriorating focal neurologic deficits, with a usually fatal outcome.
- PML is an AIDS-defining disease.

EPIDEMIOLOGY
Incidence
- Incidence in the US increased with the AIDS epidemic, but declined with the use of highly active antiretroviral therapy (HAART).
- Reported deaths due to PML in the pre-HIV era: 1.5 in 10 million persons in 1974.
- Reported deaths due to PML in 1987: 6.1 in 10 million persons.
- 1–4% of HIV-positive persons will develop PML if left untreated. In 1992, 2% of HIV-related deaths were due to PML.
- In a study from Denmark (1):
  - 1995–1996 (pre-HAART): 3.3 cases/1000 patient-years at risk (PYR)
  - 1997–1999 (early HAART): 1.8 cases/1000 PYR
  - 2000–2006 (late HAART): 1.3 cases/1000 PYR

Prevalence
- JCV seroprevalence in adults in the US and Europe is about 60–80%. A very small proportion of those show evidence of active viral replication, against about 33% among HIV-infected individuals.
- Antibody-based studies show that primary JCV infection occurs during childhood (10–14 years).
- Asymptomatic JCV and BKV viruria has been described in immunosuppressed patients, pregnant women, and the elderly.

RISK FACTORS
- AIDS, mainly advanced disease (CD4 count <100/mm³): More than 60% of cases of PML occur in this setting.
- Rare case reports of other forms of congenital or acquired immunosuppression (organ transplant recipients are at increased risk if the donor is seropositive for JCV), patients with hematologic malignancies, and patients in chronic steroid use (including patients with systemic lupus erythematosus, rheumatoid arthritis, or sarcoidosis).
- Isolated cases have been reported in the absence of any identifiable immunodeficiency.

ALERT
Rare cases of PML have been reported in patients with multiple sclerosis or Crohn's disease treated with natalizumab. Risk is increased with duration of therapy.

GENERAL PREVENTION
Proper antiretroviral treatment to avoid severe immunosuppression

PATHOPHYSIOLOGY
- Incubation period and mode of transmission are not known. Primary infection has been documented in renal transplant recipients from a seropositive donor.
- Demyelination results in rapid deterioration (over weeks) with multiple focal neurologic deficits, without signs of increased intracranial pressure. The disease is commonly fatal.
- PML may develop paradoxically after initiating HAART as an immune reconstitution syndrome (Inflammatory PML)

ETIOLOGY
- JCV, a DNA virus, belonging to the family Papovaviridae, genus *Polyomavirus*.
- The other known human polyomavirus, BK virus (BKV), does not cause PML.

 DIAGNOSIS

PHYSICAL EXAM
- No constitutional symptoms, such as fever.
- At presentation: Hemiparesis (42%), visual field deficits (32–45%), typically homonymous hemianopia, cognitive impairment (36%), aphasia (17%), ataxia (21%), and/or cranial nerve deficits (13%), sensory deficits (9%), seizures (accounts for 1% of seizures in HIV-positive patients), dementia, confusion, personality changes. Typically spares the spinal cord.
- Late in the course: Severe neurologic deficits (cortical blindness, quadriparesis, profound dementia, and coma; motor weakness in 75%)
- The clinical presentation can be much more impressive than the imaging and/or pathology findings.
- Clinical presentation in HIV-positive patients is similar to that in HIV-negative patients.

DIAGNOSTIC TESTS & INTERPRETATION
Lab
- Gold standard: Detection of JCV antigen or genomic DNA in brain tissue by immunocytochemistry, in situ hybridization, or PCR amplification, in association with the characteristic pathologic changes. Detection is not diagnostic unless accompanied by pathologic changes.
- Due to morbidity and mortality associated with brain biopsy, JCV PCR in cerebrospinal fluid (CSF) is the preferred diagnostic modality. PCR has a sensitivity of 72–92% and a specificity of 92–100%, if no HAART. The sensitivity decreases with use of HAART, probably due to a decrease in viral replication (2)
- CSF: nonspecific pleocytosis, increased IgG, and monoclonal bands have been described.
- Serum and CSF antibodies are not helpful.
- JCV grows slowly in culture (over weeks to months), and susceptible cells are not readily available.

Imaging
- CT scan: Hypodense, non-enhancing subcortical white matter lesions without edema or mass effect; usually periventricularly, in the centrum semiovale, in the parietal-occipital region, and in the cerebellum
- MRI scan: More sensitive than CT scan; shows multiple, asymmetric subcortical white matter lesions, with high signal on T2-weighted images
- Note: Inflammatory PML is characterized by contrast-enhancing lesions.

Diagnostic Procedures/Other
Electroencephalography (EEG) shows focal or diffuse slowing. Sometimes, EEG abnormalities precede CT changes.

Pathological Findings
- Demyelination occurs as a result of the direct infection of central nervous system (CNS) oligodendrocytes (myelin-producing cells) by JCV and the subsequent cytopathic effect, which leads to decreased myelin production.
- Multifocal areas of demyelination, varying greatly in size, scattered throughout the CNS, with minimal inflammation
- Reactive gliosis. Bizarre astrocytes with lobulated nuclei and lipid-laden macrophages.
- Cerebral hemispheres, cerebellum, and brainstem may all be involved. Spinal cord involvement is rare.
- Electron microscopy shows polyomavirus inclusions into enlarged nuclei of oligodendrocytes.

DIFFERENTIAL DIAGNOSIS
- HIV encephalopathy and leukoencephalomyelopathy
- Other opportunistic infections (cytomegalovirus, neurosyphilis, cryptococcosis, tuberculous meningitis, toxoplasmosis) and malignancies associated with HIV infection (primary CNS lymphoma, Kaposi's sarcoma)
- Acute multiple sclerosis
- Acute hemorrhagic leukoencephalitis
- Herpes simplex virus meningoencephalitis
- Multifocal varicella zoster virus leukoencephalitis
- Post-infectious or vaccinal immune-mediated encephalomyelitis
- Cyclosporin toxicity (encephalopathy, seizures) in transplant recipients

 ## TREATMENT

MEDICATION
First Line
- There is no available specific treatment for PML.
- For patient with AIDS, initiate aggressive antiretroviral treatment to reverse immunosuppression.
- Supervised drug administration may be necessary in patients with dementia.
- Decrease or discontinue immunosuppressants, if PML developed in the setting of immunosuppression.
- Intravenous or intrathecal cytarabine (cytosine arabinoside) for patients with hematologic malignancies may be of some benefit (3).
- No benefit from use of cidofovir (4).
- Corticosteroids may be beneficial for inflammatory PML (5).
- Treatment with plasma exchange (together with discontinuation of natalizumab) has been tried in natalizumab-associated PML.

 ## ONGOING CARE

FOLLOW-UP RECOMMENDATIONS
- Frequent clinical follow-up to check for recurrence of illness
- HIV infection monitoring

PROGNOSIS
Death occurs within about 6 months of the diagnosis, but spontaneous fluctuations over a period of 2–3 years have been described in HIV-positive patients, except if immunosuppression improves with aggressive management of HIV infection.

REFERENCES

1. Engsig FN, Hansen AB, Omland LH, et al. Incidence, clinical presentation, and outcome of progressive multifocal leukoencephalopathy in HIV-infected patients during the highly active antiretroviral therapy era: A nationwide cohort study. *J Infect Dis* 2009;199:77–83.
2. Marzocchetti A, Di Giambenedetto S, Cingolani A, et al. Reduced rate of diagnostic positive detection of JC virus DNA in cerebrospinal fluid in cases of suspected progressive multifocal leukoencephalopathy in the era of potent antiretroviral therapy. *J Clin Microbiol* 2005;43(8):4175–4177.
3. Aksamit AJ. Treatment of non-AIDS progressive multifocal leukoencephalopathy with cytosine arabinoside. *J Neurovirol* 2001;7:386–390.
4. De Luca A, Ammassari A, Pezzotti P, et al. Cidofovir in addition to antiretroviral treatment is not effective for AIDS-associated progressive multifocal leukoencephalopathy: A multicohort analysis. *AIDS (London, England)* 2008;22:1759–1767.
5. Tan K, Roda R, Ostrow L, et al. PML-IRIS in patients with HIV infection: Clinical manifestations and treatment with steroids. *Neurology* 2009;72: 1458–1464.

ADDITIONAL READING

- Kaplan JE, Benson C, Holmes KH, et al. Guidelines for prevention and treatment of opportunistic infections in HIV-infected adults and adolescents: Recommendations from CDC, the National Institutes of Health, and the HIV Medicine Association of the Infectious Diseases Society of America. *MMWR Recomm Rep* 2009;58(RR-4):1–207.

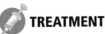 ## CODES

ICD9
- Irrelevant code
- 046.3 Progressive multifocal leukoencephalopathy

CLINICAL PEARLS
- PML is a rapidly progressing disease with focal neurologic deficits and usually fatal outcome
- Risk factors are: AIDS, immunosuppression after organ transplantation, hematologic malignancies, and natalizumab use.
- No specific treatment is available. Initiate HAART in AIDS. Decrease or discontinue immunosuppression, if PML developed in the setting of immunosuppression.

PROSTATITIS

Paschalis Vergidis
Matthew E. Falagas

 BASICS

DESCRIPTION
- The term prostatitis encompasses several infectious and noninfectious processes, including the following (1):
  - Acute bacterial prostatitis
  - Chronic bacterial prostatitis
  - Chronic prostatitis, Inflammatory subtype (formerly nonbacterial prostatitis)
  - Chronic prostatitis, noninflammatory subtype (formerly prostatodynia)
  - Asymptomatic inflammatory prostatitis
  - Granulomatous prostatitis
- The most common form is chronic prostatitis/chronic pelvic pain syndrome (90% of patients)

EPIDEMIOLOGY
Prevalence
The overall prevalence of prostatitis is 2–16%.

RISK FACTORS
Genitourinary procedures for acute bacterial prostatitis

GENERAL PREVENTION
Effective management of acute prostatitis cases will decrease the incidence of recurrent prostatitis or chronic bacterial prostatitis.

PATHOPHYSIOLOGY
- Bacterial prostatitis is associated with secretory dysfunction of the prostate.
- Prostatic secretions have an increased pH, which influences the local pharmacokinetic properties of several antibiotics.
- There is a reduced level of prostatic antibacterial factor, a zinc-containing polypeptide with antimicrobial properties found in prostatic secretions.

ETIOLOGY
- Acute bacterial prostatis is caused by the usual uropathogens, mainly:
  - *Escherichia coli*
  - Other Enterobacteriaceae
  - *Pseudomonas aeruginosa*
  - Enterococci
- Chronic bacterial prostatitis is usually caused by the same uropathogens.
- Chronic prostatitis, inflammatory subtype
  - Uncertain etiology
  - Leukocytes in the expressed prostatic secretions
  - Some cases caused by *Chlamydia* (2) or *Mycoplasma* species

- Chronic prostatitis, noninflammatory subtype:
  - Uncertain etiology
  - No evidence of an inflammatory response in prostatic secretions
  - In some cases, a voiding dysfunction is found by urodynamic testing, caused by dyssynergy between bladder detrusor and internal sphincter muscles.
- Granulomatous prostatitis. Rare condition.
  - Usually follows an episode of acute bacterial prostatitis
  - Other causes:
    - Tuberculosis
    - Nontuberculous mycobacteria
    - Fungi, mainly cryptococcosis, blastomycosis, coccidioidomycosis, or histoplasmosis
    - The prostate can be the focus of persistent cryptococcosis in patients with AIDS

 DIAGNOSIS

HISTORY
- ACUTE BACTERIAL PROSTATITIS
  - Prostatitis should be considered in every man with symptoms and/or signs consistent with urinary tract infection (UTI).
  - Perineal, pelvic, or lower back pain
  - Urinary frequency
  - Dysuria or urgency
  - Systemic symptoms such as fever with chills
- CHRONIC BACTERIAL PROSTATITIS
  - Can be the cause of persistence of bacteria in the urinary tract and leads to recurrent UTIs with the same pathogen.
  - Patients are usually asymptomatic in the periods between recurrent UTIs, although they sometimes complain of symptoms similar to those reported in chronic nonbacterial prostatitis.
- CHRONIC PROSTATITIS
  - Perineal, pelvic, lower back, scrotal, or inguinal pain or vague discomfort are common.
  - Symptoms are continuous or spasmodic.
  - Urinary frequency, dysuria, dribbling, hesitancy, and urgency are sometimes present.
  - Erectile dysfunction, ejaculatory complaints.
- ASYMPTOMATIC INFLAMMATORY PROSTATITIS
  - No history of genitourinary tract pain. Diagnosed during evaluation for other issues (elevated prostate-specific antigen, infertility, etc.)

PHYSICAL EXAM
- Acute bacterial prostatitis: A digital rectal examination, which should be done gently to avoid precipitating bacteremia, reveals an enlarged, tender prostate.
- Chronic prostatitis: Rectal examination reveals a normal prostate.
- Granulomatous prostatitis: Firm, indurated prostate.

DIAGNOSTIC TESTS & INTERPRETATION
Lab
- Specimens for urinalysis, urine culture, blood urea nitrogen, and creatinine should be taken before initiation of antimicrobial treatment.
- The differential diagnosis of prostatitis syndromes is based on the interpretation of segmented urine cultures (4-glass Meares-Stamey test).
  - For the appropriate collection of segmented urine cultures, the patient retracts the foreskin and cleans the glans penis.
  - The first 10 mL of voided urine is the urethral specimen and is labeled VB1 (voided bladder 1).
  - A midstream urine specimen is labeled VB2 (attention should be paid not to empty the bladder fully).
  - While the patient maintains foreskin retraction, the physician massages the prostate with continuous strokes for collection of the expressed prostatic secretions (EPS).
  - If there is no fluid, the patient milks the penis from the base toward the tip.
  - Finally, the first 10 mL of voided urine after the prostate massage is collected and labeled VB3. This specimen represents a mixture of prostatic secretions and urine.
- If VB2 is sterile or has $<10^3$ CFU/mL, the diagnosis of bacterial prostatitis is indicated by the higher colony counts of bacteria from the EPS or VB3 than from VB1, preferably by at least tenfold.
- If VB2 has $>10^3$ CFU/mL, a prostatic infection may be masked by a coexistent bladder infection. In this case, a 3-day regimen should be given with an antibiotic that will treat the bladder infection but will not penetrate well into the prostate (e.g., oral ampicillin 500 mg 4 times daily or oral nitrofurantoin 100 mg 3 times daily). The segmented urine cultures test should then be repeated.
- In the absence of urethral, bladder, and kidney infections, presence of 10 or more white blood cells per high-power microscopic field of the EPS or VB3 is indicative of prostatic inflammation.
- A more practical alternative to the Meares-Stamey test is to obtain pre-prostatic and post-prostatic massage urine culture (2-glass test) (3).

Imaging
Transrectal ultrasonography and CT imaging are useful in diagnosing prostatic stones and prostate abscess.

Diagnostic Procedures/Other
Elderly men with symptoms of chronic prostatitis without evidence of infection should have urine cytology, a bladder ultrasound examination, and, if necessary, cystoscopy to exclude the possibility of bladder cancer.

Pathological Findings
Granulomatous prostatitis: Granulomas containing lipid-laden histiocytes and plasma cells. Macrophages may fuse to form multinucleated giant cells.

DIFFERENTIAL DIAGNOSIS
- Prostate hyperplasia
- Bladder neck dysfunction
- Urethral stricture
- Prostatic calculi
- Prostate cancer

TREATMENT

MEDICATION

- ACUTE BACTERIAL PROSTATITIS
  - The severity of illness and the presence of nausea or vomiting dictate the route of treatment.
  - Mild illness, no nausea or vomiting
    - A fluoroquinolone (e.g., levofloxacin 500 mg once daily or ciprofloxacin 500 mg twice daily, orally), or
    - Trimethoprim-sulfamethoxazole (TMP-SMX), 1 double-strength tablet twice daily, orally
    - Drugs are given for 2 weeks. Some recommend 3–4 weeks of treatment.
  - Moderate or severe illness
    - Parenteral treatment (ampicillin and gentamicin, or ciprofloxacin, levofloxacin, or TMP-SMX) until fever resolves; then oral fluoroquinolones or TMP-SMX for a total of 4 weeks
  - Persistence of the pathogen would prompt retreatment for a 12-week course.
- CHRONIC BACTERIAL PROSTATITIS
  - Because many antimicrobial drugs do not penetrate well into the prostate that is not acutely inflamed, selection of an antibiotic based only on the segmented urine cultures results is not appropriate.
  - The preferred regimens for penetration into the prostate are an oral fluoroquinolone (e.g., levofloxacin 500 mg once daily, or ciprofloxacin 500 mg twice daily for 4 weeks), or oral TMP-SMX, 1 double-strength tablet (160 mg TMP, 800 mg SMX) twice daily for 6 weeks.
  - About one-third of patients with chronic bacterial prostatitis have a complete response, one-third have a partial response, and one-third have no response to this regimen.
  - For patients in the latter two categories, a 12-week course with the same or an alternative antibiotic is given.
  - When a cure is not achieved, continuous antimicrobial treatment with oral TMP-SMX, 1 single-strength tablet daily, is given for suppression of prostatic infection and prevention of recurrent UTIs.
- CHRONIC PROSTATITIS, INFLAMMATORY SUBTYPE
  - No good therapy for this syndrome because the etiology is uncertain.
  - A 2-week trial course of an antibiotic for the possibility of *Chlamydia* or *Mycoplasma* infection is reasonable.
  - The preferred agent is oral doxycycline 100 mg twice daily or an oral macrolide (erythromycin 500 mg 4 times daily)
  - If there is no clear improvement, additional antimicrobial treatment should not be given; if there is improvement, continue treatment for 2–4 more weeks.

- CHRONIC PROSTATITIS, NONINFLAMMATORY SUBTYPE
  - Patients with urodynamic dysfunction may benefit from therapy with an alpha-blocker [e.g., alfuzosin, tamsulosin, terazosin (4)].
- ASYMPTOMATIC INFLAMMATORY PROSTATITIS
  - Antibiotic therapy not indicated.

ADDITIONAL TREATMENT
Additional Therapies
- ACUTE BACTERIAL PROSTATITIS
  - Adjunctive treatment includes stool softeners, analgesics, and antipyretics.
  - Transurethral catheterization should be avoided to avoid obstructing drainage of prostatic secretions.
  - Acute urinary retention is managed by suprapubic catheterization.
- CHRONIC PROSTATITIS, INFLAMMATORY SUBTYPE
  - Reassurance about the benign nature of the illness and nonspecific therapy (hot sitz baths, anti-inflammatory agents such as ibuprofen) are helpful.
  - Prostatic massage, oral zinc, and vitamins have unproved efficacy. Sexual activity is encouraged.
- CHRONIC PROSTATITIS, NONINFLAMMATORY SUBTYPE
  - Some patients seem to have tension myalgia of the pelvic floor. Diathermy, special exercises, and diazepam have been helpful in these patients.

SURGERY/OTHER PROCEDURES
- CHRONIC BACTERIAL PROSTATITIS
  - In elderly men with considerable morbidity because of frequent recurrent UTIs despite suppressive antimicrobial treatment, transurethral or open prostatic resection should be considered.
  - Infected prostatic calculi can cause bacterial persistence in the prostate despite appropriate, prolonged therapy. Calculi may be another indication for resection.

ONGOING CARE

FOLLOW-UP RECOMMENDATIONS
A follow-up culture of urine should be performed 14 days after completing therapy in cases of acute bacterial prostatitis.

COMPLICATIONS
- ACUTE BACTERIAL PROSTATITIS
  - Prostatic abscess
  - Prostatic infarction
  - Bacteremia
  - Chronic bacterial prostatitis
  - Granulomatous prostatitis

REFERENCES

1. Krieger JN, Nyberg L Jr, Nickel JC. NIH consensus definition and classification of prostatitis. *JAMA* 1999;282(3):236–237.
2. Mazzoli S, Cai T, Rupealta V, et al. Interleukin 8 and anti-*Chlamydia trachomatis* mucosal IgA as urogenital immunologic markers in patients with *C. trachomatis* prostatic infection. *Eur Urol* 2007; 51(5):1385–1393.
3. Nickel JC, Shoskes D, Wang Y, et al. How does the pre-massage and post-massage 2-glass test compare to the Meares-Stamey 4-glass test in men with chronic prostatitis/chronic pelvic pain syndrome? *J Urol* 2006;176(1):119–124.
4. Cheah PY, Liong ML, Yuen KH, et al. Terazosin therapy for chronic prostatitis/chronic pelvic pain syndrome: A randomized, placebo controlled trial. *J Urol* 2003;169(2):592–596.

ADDITIONAL READING

- Nickel JC. Treatment of chronic prostatitis/chronic pelvic pain syndrome. *Int J Antimicrob Agents* 2008;31(Suppl 1):S112–S116.

 CODES

ICD9
- 601.0 Acute prostatitis
- 601.1 Chronic prostatitis
- 601.9 Prostatitis, unspecified

CLINICAL PEARLS

- Chronic prostatitis/chronic pelvic pain syndrome is the most common form of prostatitis. Etiology is uncertain.
- Obtaining pre- and post-prostatic massage urine culture is a more practical means of diagnosis prostatitis compared to the 4-glass Meares-Stamey test.
- A 2-week antibiotic trial is reasonable in chronic prostatitis. If symptoms improve, complete a 4-week course. If no improvement, discontinue antibiotics.

PSEUDOMONAS INFECTIONS, MELIOIDOSIS, AND GLANDERS

Erica S. Shenoy (E. Mylonakis, Editor)

BASICS

DESCRIPTION
- Members of the genus Pseudomonas that are motile, gram–negative, aerobic bacteria.
- *Burkholderia pseudomallei* (formerly *Pseudomonas pseudomallei*) causes a broad spectrum of disease processes called melioidosis. Melioidosis is also known as Whitmore's disease and Nightcliff gardener's disease.
- *Burkholderia mallei* (formerly *Pseudomonas mallei*) results in an infection termed glanders that occurs mainly in horses, mules, and donkeys though it is also able to infect humans, thereby making it a zoonotic agent.
- Both *B. pseudomallei* and *B. mallei* are considered possible bioterrorism agents.

EPIDEMIOLOGY
Incidence
- *Pseudomonas aeruginosa* is one of the most common causes of urinary tract infections, pneumonia, and bacteremia among hospitalized patients. It accounts for 10% of all hospital acquired infections and is the most common pathogen among patients hospitalized for greater than 1 week.
- *B. pseudomallei* and the infections it causes are found mainly in the tropics and are endemic in Southeast Asia. Person-to-person transmission is rare. In the US, there are approximately 0–5 cases per year.
- Glanders, a disease of equine animals that is occasionally transmitted to humans, is endemic in Africa, Asia, the Middle East, Central America, and South America.

RISK FACTORS
- Most *P. aeruginosa* infections are hospital acquired. Risk factors for *P. aeruginosa* infection include bypass of the normal barriers (e.g., endotracheal intubation, urinary bladder catheterization), immune compromise, and disruption of normal bacterial flora secondary to broad spectrum antibiotic therapy.
  - Risk factors for central nervous system infections include head and neck cancers, central nervous system (CNS) tumors, cerebrospinal fluid (CSF) leaks, indwelling hardware, lumbar puncture, neurosurgical procedures, bacteremia, parameningeal infection, penetrating head trauma, and spinal anesthesia.
  - Patients with cystic fibrosis can develop a chronic infection of the lower respiratory tract with *P. aeruginosa*.
  - *P. aeruginosa* is a major cause of ventilator-associated pneumonia (VAP).
  - *P. aeruginosa* is a common cause of bone and joint infection and can present with an indolent course.
  - Vertebral osteomyelitis is associated with complicated Pseudomonas urinary tract infections, genitourinary instrumentation, and intravenous drug abuse.
  - Bacteremia is associated with medical devices and the mortality rate exceeds 10%.
  - UTIs may be chronic or recurrent and usually result from instrumentation, obstruction, bacteremia, stones or other persistent foci, surgery, and urinary tract catheterization.

- Occasionally, *P. aeruginosa* leads to "malignant external otitis," an invasive process that is typically slow but destructive and is more common among diabetics and immunocompromised individuals and can extend to the CNS.
- *P. aeruginosa* infections of the symphysis pubis are associated with pelvic surgery and intravenous drug use.
- *P. aeruginosa* is often the cause of bacterial keratitis, scleral abscess, and endophthalmitis.
- Pseudomonas infections of the GI tract are observed, especially in neutropenic patients where it can result in necrotizing enterocolitis (NEC) and typhlitis.
- Pseudomonas infections are common in burn wounds.
- Risk factors for melioidosis include diabetes, thalassemia, kidney disease, occupational and environmental exposure history.

GENERAL PREVENTION
Minimization of risk factors is the only means of prevention of *Pseudomonas* infections. There is no vaccine.

PATHOPHYSIOLOGY
Pseudomonas species first attach and to and then colonize surfaces such as indwelling catheters and respirators, leading to local infection, and finally hematogenous spread and systemic disease.

ETIOLOGY
- *P. aeruginosa* is the most common human pathogen in this group. Others include:
  - *B. pseudomallei* (formerly *P. pseudomallei*), which causes melioidosis
  - *B. mallei* (formerly *P. mallei*), which causes glanders
  - *Burkholderia cepacia* (formerly *Pseudomonas cepacia*), which has been reported to cause bacteremia, burn-wound infections, chronic infections of the respiratory tract in patients with cystic fibrosis, endocarditis, meningitis, peritonitis, pneumonia, surgical wound infections, and urinary tract infections (UTIs).
  - *Burkholderia pickettii* (formerly *Pseudomonas pickettii*) has been the etiological outbreak in several documented nosocomial outbreaks.
  - *Comamonas acidovorans* (formerly Pseudomonas acidovorans) is a rare cause of endocarditis.
  - *Pseudomonas fluorescens* (mainly associated with infections related to the administration of contaminated stored blood products).
  - *Pseudomonas putida* is an opportunistic pathogen that can cause sepsis in neonates, neutropenic, and cancer patients and sometimes causes disease in immunocompetent hosts. There is evidence of emerging drug resistance in clinical isolates.
  - *Stenotrophomonas maltophilia* (formerly *Xanthomonas maltophilia*), which has been associated with pneumonia, bacteremia, cholangitis, endocarditis, meningitis, peritonitis, UTI, and wound infections.

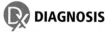

DIAGNOSIS

HISTORY
- Symptoms are in most cases related to the affected organ system. Documentation of risk factors may be helpful.
- Among patients with early cystic fibrosis, *P. aeruginosa* usually causes mild recurrent upper respiratory symptoms. As cystic fibrosis advances, episodes of pneumonia develop and can lead to chronic productive cough, generalized weakness, growth retardation, respiratory compromise, weight loss, and wheezing.
- The clinical features of bacteremia, meningitis, and UTIs due to *P. aeruginosa* are usually indistinguishable from those of other bacterial infections.
- Corneal ulcer due to *P. aeruginosa* may advance rapidly to involve the entire cornea.
- Patients with *P. aeruginosa* infections of the symphysis pubis present with pain. Fever is variable, and the duration of symptoms before diagnosis ranges from days to months.
- Patients presenting with Pseudomonas osteomyelitis of the foot may have history of penetrating injury of the foot.
- Patients with sternoclavicular septic arthritis may have history of IV drug use.
- Otalgia and otorrhea are common presenting symptoms of malignant external otitis.
- Manifestations of glanders are determined by the route of infection:
  - Chronic suppurative infection presents as multiple abscesses.
  - Mucous membrane infection results in the production of a mucopurulent discharge involving the eye, nose, or lips, with the subsequent development of granulomatous ulcers.
  - Pulmonary and systemic infection can present with fever, myalgia, headache, pleuritic chest pain, and diarrhea.
- Melioidosis most often involves the lungs and presents with fever, productive cough, and marked tachypnea. It can also cause acute or chronic suppurative infections involving the skin or internal organs.

PHYSICAL EXAM
- Physical findings are related to affected organ system.
- Pathognomonic skin lesions termed Ecthyma gangrenosum develop in a relatively small minority of patients with *P. aeruginosa* bacteremia. The lesions begin as small hemorrhagic vesicles surrounded by a rim of erythema and undergo central necrosis with subsequent ulceration.
- *P. aeruginosa* causes diffuse pruritic maculopapular and vesiculopustular rashes associated with exposure to contaminated hot tubs, spas, whirlpools, and swimming pools.
- In external otitis due to *P. aeruginosa*, there is a purulent discharge, and pain is elicited by pulling on the pinna. Physical examination in cases of malignant external otitis almost always reveals abnormalities of the external auditory canal, including swelling, erythema, purulent discharge, debris, and granulation tissue in the canal.
- In glanders, lymphadenopathy and splenomegaly may be documented.

DIAGNOSTIC TESTS & INTERPRETATION
Lab
In addition to basic laboratory tests, cultures (sputum, bronchial alveolar lavage (BAL), urine, blood, wound, etc) should be obtained and organisms isolated and tested for antibiotic susceptibility.

Imaging
- In malignant external otitis caused by Pseudomonas, computed tomography and magnetic resonance imaging (MRI) typically reveal bony erosions and new bone formation.
- In melioidosis, chest x-rays typically reveal upper lobe consolidation or thin-walled cavities. Progressive upper lobe disease can mimic tuberculosis.
- MRI is useful in the case of suspected osteomyelitis.
- Echocardiography is indicated in patients with Pseudomonas bacteremia in whom endocarditis is a consideration.

Diagnostic Procedures/Other
BAL or endotracheal aspirates in intubated patients should be obtained to confirm suspected cases of *P. aeruginosa*.

DIFFERENTIAL DIAGNOSIS
Differential diagnosis is broad and includes, in the case of Pseudomonas pneumonia, other causes of bacterial pneumonia, viral pneumonia, and pneumocystis jiroveci pneumonia (PJP) among other infections.

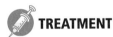 TREATMENT

MEDICATION
- Most types of *P. aeruginosa* disease are treated with one or two antibiotics to which the infecting organism is sensitive (usually a combination of an aminoglycoside or a quinolone and β-lactam).
- Antibiotics with antipseudomonal activity include aminoglycosides (gentamicin, tobramycin, etc.), carbapenems, certain extended-spectrum penicillins (e.g., ticarcillin, piperacillin), certain third-generation cephalosporins (e.g., ceftazidime, cefoperazone), fluoroquinolones (e.g., ciprofloxacin), and monobactams.
- Of note, there is increasing resistance to ciprofloxacin, hence care should be taken when considering as empiric therapy.

First Line
- *P. aeruginosa*:
  - Bacteremia: Treatment often consists of 2 agents, although no randomized control trial has been conducted to test single versus combination therapy. In general, ceftazidime, cefepime, meropenem, imipenem–cilastatin, piperacillin–tazobactam (high dose), and aztreonam (in the setting of β-lactam allergic patient). The addition of an aminoglycoside can be considered in settings where there are high levels of β-lactam resistance, and should be used in settings where susceptibility rates are <80%.
  - Pneumonia: Treatment is similar to that for bacteremia, though utility of parental aminoglycosides is doubtful. Inhaled tobramycin, however, is recommended at a dose of 300 mg daily. In the case of chronic respiratory tract infections, the clinician must distinguish between colonization and active infection.

- Osteomyelitis: Usually consists of an antipseudomonal β-lactam or fluoroquinolone at high doses for an extended period of time.
- CNS infections: Ceftazidime is the agent of choice, but cefepime and meropenem can be used as well. Imipenem should not be used because of rapid development of resistance and neurotoxicity. In cases of resistant organisms, an aminoglycoside, administered either intrathecally or intraventricularly may be used.
- Eye infections: Keratitis can be treated with topical or subconjunctival antibiotics; endophthalmitis is treated with systemic and intravitreal antibiotics.
- Ear infections: Malignant external otitis is treated with β-lactam antibiotics or ciprofloxacin; relapse can occur 1 year out from therapy.
- Urinary tract infections: Antipseudomonal β-lactams, ciprofloxacin, levofloxacin, and aminoglycosides can be used and achieve high concentrations in the urinary tract. 7–10 days are sufficient for UTIs, and 2 weeks for pyelonephritis.
- Burn wounds: Care should be taken to avoid imipenem, given the rapid development of resistance. Wound colonization can be treated with topical agents.
- Endovascular infections: Therapy often involves combination therapy with close monitoring for emergence of resistance.

- Melioidosis: Treatment is variable and depends on severity.
- Glanders: Can be treated initially with imipenem, ceftazidime, or meropenem in addition to ciprofloxacin and doxycycline. Initial treatment is followed by extended oral therapy to reduce likelihood of relapse.

ADDITIONAL TREATMENT
Issues for Referral
Involvement of infectious disease specialists should be considered, especially with melioidosis or glanders.

SURGERY/OTHER PROCEDURES
- Osteomyelitis usually requires surgical intervention in addition to antimicrobial therapy.
- Malignant otitis externa may require debridement.

 ONGOING CARE

FOLLOW-UP RECOMMENDATIONS
Very close follow-up is recommended, given the risk of resistance and relapse.

PROGNOSIS
In the case of *Pseudomonas* infections, prognosis depends on organ system affected, host factors, and treatment.

COMPLICATIONS
- Multidrug resistant *Pseudomonas* is being increasingly observed. Resistance mechanisms include chromosomal Bush group 1 β-lactamases and extended spectrum beta lactamases (EBSL).
- Other complications are specific to the site of infection. For example, in the case of *Pseudomonas* endocarditis, disseminated infection including brain abscess and septic emboli are possible.

- Septic shock and death as a consequence of bacteremia.
- Respiratory failure.
- Ear infections can result in involvement of cranial nerves; rarely, meningitis and brain abscesses are complications of this infection.

ADDITIONAL READING

- Pier GB, Ramphal R. Pseudomonas areuginosa. In: Mandell, Douglas, Bennett, eds, *Principles and Practice of Infectious Diseases,* 7th ed. 2009.
- Rega PP. Glanders and melioidosis. *EMedicine,* 2009.
- Qahar S et al. Pseudomonas aeruginosa Infections. *EMedicine* 2009.
- Han XY, RA Andrade. *Brevundimonas diminuta* infections and its resistance to fluoroquinolones. *J Antimicrob Chemother* 2005;55:853–859.
- Horowitz H, et al. Endocarditis Associated with Comamonas acidovorans. *J Clin Micro* 1990;28: 143–145.
- Horii T, Muramatsu H, Iinuma Y. Mechanisms of resistance to fluoroquinolones and carbapenems in *Pseudomonas putida. J Antimicrob Chemother* 2005;56:643–647.
- Pollack M. Infections due to *Pseudomonas* species and related organisms. In: Fauci AS, Braunwald E, Isselbacher KJ, et al., eds. *Harrison's principles of medicine,* 14th ed. New York: McGraw-Hill, 1998:943–950.
- Sanford JP. *Pseudomonas* species (including melioidosis and glanders). In: Mandell GL, Bennett JE, Dolin R, eds. *Principles and practice of infectious diseases,* 4th ed. 1995:2003–2009.
- Wilson R, Dowling RB. Lung infections. 3. *Pseudomonas aeruginosa* and other related species. *Thorax* 1998;53:213–219.

CODES

ICD9
- 024 Glanders
- 025 Melioidosis
- 041.7 Pseudomonas infection in conditions classified elsewhere and of unspecified site

CLINICAL PEARLS
- Treatment failure may occur given the propensity of the organism to develop resistance to first line antibiotics.

PSITTACOSIS
Rachel Simmons (E. Mylonakis, Editor)

 BASICS

DESCRIPTION
- Psittacosis is a systemic zoonotic infection caused by *Chlamydophila psittaci* (formerly *Chlamydia psittaci*).
- Psittacosis has a predilection for the lungs, causing an atypical pneumonia. The infection can be subclinical or can rarely cause severe sepsis.
- *C. psittaci* is transmitted from infected birds to humans.
- The name of the disease is derived from the Greek word for "parrot," psittakos; however, almost any bird may be a vector.
- Synonyms: Parrot fever and ornithosis.

EPIDEMIOLOGY
Incidence
- Since 2000, the annual number of reported cases of human psittacosis has ranged from 8 to 25 in the US. Psittacosis may be underdiagnosed and underreported due to mild, self-limited symptoms.
- The incidence is approximately 0.01 per 100,000 population in the US and is variable due to periodic outbreaks (2).
- *C. psittaci* is estimated to cause 0.5–1.5% of cases of community-acquired pneumonia.

Prevalence
Wild birds are variably infected with *C. psittaci* in different geographic regions.

RISK FACTORS
- Psittacosis is an occupational disease of pet shop owners, poultry workers, pigeon fanciers, taxidermists, veterinarians, workers at poultry-processing plants, and zoo attendants. Bird owners are also at risk.
- Almost any avian species can harbor *C. psittaci*. Psittacine birds (parrots, parakeets, cockatiels, cockatoos, and budgerigars) are most commonly infected, but human cases have been traced to contact with pigeons, ducks, turkeys, chickens, and many other birds.
- Infected birds are commonly asymptomatic though they can exhibit ruffled feathers, respiratory symptoms, conjunctivitis, or diarrhea. Shedding of *C. psittaci* increases in times of stress.
- Currently pet birds are considered to have low transmission risk for immunocompromised patients.

GENERAL PREVENTION
- Cases in the US have declined with the introduction of tetracycline-laced bird feed and the requirement of a 30-day quarantine period for imported birds.
- Infected birds should be treated by a licensed veterinarian.
- Employers should inform at-risk persons regarding the health risks of caring for birds or handling avian tissue or secretions.
- Workers should wear appropriate protective clothing such as gloves, eyewear, and an appropriately fitted respirator (N95 or higher rating) when handling potentially infected birds or bird tissue or when cleaning cages NASHPV compendium.

PATHOPHYSIOLOGY
- The agent is present in nasal secretions, excreta, tissues, and feathers of infected birds.
- Transmission to humans occurs through the respiratory route following exposure to feces, respiratory secretions, plumage, or tissue of infected birds.

ETIOLOGY
C. psittaci is a gram–negative, obligate intracellular bacterium. It has been divided into 8 serovars based on the major outer membrane protein.

 DIAGNOSIS

HISTORY
- The clinical manifestations of psittacosis are variable. Infection severity ranges from a subclinical illness to atypical pneumonia to a fatal systemic illness (1).
- Pulmonary, hepatic, CNS, cardiac, renal, rheumatic, gastrointestinal, dermatologic, and hematologic symptoms and signs have been described.
- After an incubation period of 5–21 days, symptoms typically begin abruptly with chills, fever, nonproductive cough, diaphoresis, headache, and myalgias.
- Respiratory symptoms can be mild or absent early in the illness.
- Diffuse, severe headache is a prominent symptom with up to one-third of patients undergoing lumbar puncture in case series.
- Meningoencephalitis with lethargy, mental depression, agitation, and disorientation has been described.
- Gastrointestinal problems such as abdominal pain, nausea, vomiting, and diarrhea can occur.
- *C. psittaci* is a rare cause of endocarditis, myocarditis, and pericarditis.
- Renal manifestations are rare and include interstitial nephritis and acute renal failure in severe infection.
- Fulminant psittacosis is rare, but potentially life-threatening with severe multisystem organ failure. Hypoxic respiratory failure, acute respiratory distress syndrome, septic shock, renal failure, hepatic failure, disseminated intravascular coagulation, and hemophagocytic syndrome have been reported.
- Psittacosis has also been associated with a chronic unilateral follicular conjunctivitis.
- Several studies of pathologic specimens have reported an association between ocular adnexal mucosa-associated lymphoid tissue (MALT) and psittacosis. This finding is controversial and warrants further study.

Pregnancy Considerations
Gestational psittacosis is rare and defined as severe infection including multisystem organ failure, placentitis, and fetal compromise. The fetal mortality rate is high (11 out of 14 cases).

PHYSICAL EXAM
- The most common findings on examination are fever, pharyngitis, hepatomegaly, and abnormal chest examination (fine rales, egophony, bronchial breath sounds, and rhonchi).
- Altered mental status, neck stiffness, and photophobia occur in 5–15% of patients.
- Splenomegaly occurs in up to 10% of patients.
- Other organ systems are variably affected, hence a detailed, complete physical exam should be performed.

DIAGNOSTIC TESTS & INTERPRETATION
Lab
Initial lab tests
- Psittacosis can present with multiple nonspecific lab findings; therefore, if suspected, complete blood count with differential, serum electrolytes, BUN, creatinine, liver function tests, coagulation studies, urinalysis, and blood cultures should be sent in addition to specific tests for psittacosis and other pathogens.
- The white blood cell count can be normal, moderately decreased, or increased without marked neutrophilia.
- The erythrocyte sedimentation rate (ESR) or C-reactive protein may be elevated.
- The results of liver function tests can be mildly elevated.
- The diagnosis of psittacosis can be made by culture, serology (most common), or polymerase chain reaction (PCR).
- Culture of *C. psittaci* is labor intensive and requires high level isolation facilities so is rarely performed.
- Serology is obtained in the acute and convalescent periods (at least 2–4 weeks apart).
- Fourfold or greater increase in IgG titers by complement fixation (CF) or microimmunofluorescence (MIF) is considered diagnostic. A single serology with an IgM titer ≥ 32 in a patient with an illness compatible with psittacosis also supports the diagnosis NASHPV compendium.
- Acute infections with *C. trachomatis* or *C. pneumoniae* can also produce titer rises in the antibody tests, hence positive serology should be interpreted with caution.
- Real-time PCR has been recently developed for the detection of *C. psittaci* genetic material in respiratory specimens. It has been validated in avian specimens and is undergoing further study in humans (3).

Follow-Up & Special Considerations
- Report all suspected and confirmed cases of psittacosis to the state health department.
- Obtain convalescent serology 2–4 weeks after acute-phase serologic tests.

Imaging
- In approximately 80% of patients, the chest radiograph is abnormal.
- Pulmonary findings include interstitial infiltrate, nodules, military pattern, or lobar consolidation.
- The radiographic findings are often more severe than physical examination would predict.
- Chest CT scan can also demonstrate a pulmonary process.

Diagnostic Procedures/Other
Bronchoscopy with bronchoalveolar lavage collection sent for *C. psittaci* PCR may aid in the diagnosis.

Pathological Findings
- Respiratory findings include tracheobronchitis with mononuclear cell infiltrate.
- In psittacosis, chlamydial organisms can be seen as inclusion bodies in the cytoplasm of pneumonocytes and inflammatory cells.

DIFFERENTIAL DIAGNOSIS
- The pulmonary diseases in the differential diagnosis include the following:
  - *Chlamydia pneumoniae* pneumonia
  - Common bacterial pneumonias
  - *Coxiella burnetii* pneumonia
  - *Legionella pneumophila* pneumonia
  - *Mycoplasma pneumoniae* pneumonia
  - Viral pneumonia (influenza A and B viruses, respiratory syncytial virus, adenovirus, and parainfluenza, avian influenza)
  - Histoplasmosis
  - Coccidioidomycosis
  - Carcinoma of the lung with bronchial obstruction
- In some studies, up to 25% of patients with psittacosis report no exposure to birds. Such patients may not have psittacosis because of serologic cross-reactivity between *C. psittaci* and *C. pneumoniae*, which has no particular relation to birds.

TREATMENT
MEDICATION
First Line
- Doxycycline is the first line therapy. Tetracycline may be used as an alternative agent (1).
- Fever and symptoms typically resolve within 24–48 hours after the institution of therapy.
- In mild to moderate cases, doxycycline 100 mg PO twice daily or tetracycline 500 mg PO 4 times daily can be used.
- Severe infections should be treated with intravenous doxycycline hyclate or intravenous tetracycline if doxycycline is not available.
- No cases of *C. psittaci* resistance to tetracyclines or macrolides have been reported.
- Duration of therapy is a minimum of 10 days or longer in severe infection. Therapy should be continued for 10–14 days after fever has resolved.

Second Line
- Macrolides (azithromycin or erythromycin) can be used in patients who are allergic to or intolerant of doxycycline and during pregnancy or childhood.
- Minocycline has been used with success.
- Tigecycline and some fluoroquinolones (ciprofloxacin, moxifloxacin, and levofloxacin) have in vitro activity against *C. psittaci* but very limited clinical data so these agents should be used with caution.

ADDITIONAL TREATMENT
General Measures
In severe cases, hospitalization and pulmonary intensive care may be indicated.

Issues for Referral
Psittacosis is a rare infection. Consultation with an infectious diseases specialist is recommended for suspected and confirmed cases.

IN-PATIENT CONSIDERATIONS
Initial Stabilization
- Assess and stabilize airway and respiratory system in psittacosis and other respiratory infections.
- Droplet transmission precautions in addition to standard infection control practices should be instituted.

Admission Criteria
- Alterations in mental status, hypoxemia, cardiac dysfunction, or renal impairment should prompt admission.
- Clinical prediction rules such as CURB-65 and the Pneumonia Severity Index can be used to determine if inpatient or outpatient care is more appropriate.
- In severe infection, patients may require mechanical ventilation and treatment in the intensive care unit.

Discharge Criteria
Patients may be discharged when fevers have abated for more than 24 hours, vital signs are normal, respiratory status has stabilized, and follow-up plans are in place.

 ## ONGOING CARE
FOLLOW-UP RECOMMENDATIONS
- Patients should remain on antimicrobial therapy until symptoms have resolved.
- The department of health will likely conduct an investigation of a potential source of transmission and other cases of psittacosis.

PATIENT EDUCATION
The signs and symptoms of psittacosis in both birds and humans, routes of transmission, and prevention strategies should be reviewed with patients.

PROGNOSIS
- Response to doxycycline is prompt.
- With appropriate treatment, psittacosis is rarely fatal.

COMPLICATIONS
- Fulminant psittacosis is rare, but potentially life-threatening with severe multisystem organ failure.
- Pancarditis, hepatitis, anemia, reactive arthritis, meningoencephalitis, keratoconjunctivitis, encephalitis, skin lesions, and, rarely, interstitial nephritis, glomerulonephritis, and acute renal failure are seen (1).
- Thrombophlebitis can occur during convalescence and may cause pulmonary infarction.

REFERENCES
1. Stewardson AJ, Grayson ML. Psittacosis. *Infect Dis Clin North Am* 2010;24(1):7–25.
2. Centers for Disease Control and Prevention. Summary of notifiable diseasesnited States, 2008. *MMWR* 2008;57(54):(14, 78, 80).
3. Mitchell SL, Wolff BJ, Thacker WL, et al. Genotyping of Chlamydophila psittaci by real-time PCR and high–resolution melt analysis. *J Clin Microbiol* 2009;47:175–181.

ADDITIONAL READING
- National association of State Public Health veterinarians. Compendium of measures to control Chlamydophila psittaci infection among human (psittacosis) and pet birds (avian chlamydiosis). *CDC* 2010. http://www.nasphv.org/documentsCompendiaPsittacosis.html.

 #### See Also (Topic, Algorithm, Electronic Media Element)
- Community acquired pneumonia
- Pneumonia severity index: http://pda.ahrq.gov/clinic/psi/psicalc.asp

 ## CODES
ICD9
- 073.0 Ornithosis with pneumonia
- 073.9 Ornithosis, unspecified
- 079.88 Other specified chlamydial infection

CLINICAL PEARLS
- Psittacosis is a zoonotic infection with protean manifestations. The respiratory manifestations are the most common signs and symptoms.
- *C. psittaci* is transmitted from infected birds to humans.
- Doxycycline or tetracycline is the treatment of choice.

PYELONEPHRITIS

Ioanna Zarkada
Petros I. Rafailidis
Matthew E. Falagas

 BASICS

DESCRIPTION
- Pyelonephritis is a common infection of the upper urinary tract, causing inflammation of the renal parenchyma, calyces, and pelvis. It is classified as acute uncomplicated, acute complicated (i.e. when it occurs in patients with anatomic abnormalities or patients with immunosuppression), chronic, and xanthogranulomatous.
- Chronic pyelonephritis is characterized macroscopically by uneven scarring of kidney and microscopically by chronic inflammatory changes, mainly in the renal interstitium and tubules of one or both kidneys.

EPIDEMIOLOGY
Incidence
- The annual incidence of outpatient pyelonephritis is 12–13 cases per 10,000 among females and 2–3 cases per 10,000 among males.
- The incidence is highest in young women followed by infants and the elderly (1).

Prevalence
In US, there are more than 250,000 cases each year (2).

RISK FACTORS
- Pregnancy
- Obstruction (prostate enlargement or inflammation; urethral obstruction)
- Stone formations
- Diabetes (emphysematous pyelonephritis)
- There is also high predisposition in young women with:
  - Frequency (≥3 times per week) of sexual intercourse in the previous 30 days.
  - Urinary tract infection (UTI) in the previous 12 months
  - Stress incontinence in the previous 30 days
  - New sex partner in the previous year
  - Recent spermicide use
  - UTI history in the patient's mother (3).

GENERAL PREVENTION
- Identification and treatment of predisposing clinical situations:
  - Reduction of spermicide use
  - Early identification and treatment of lower UTIs.

PATHOPHYSIOLOGY
- The infection of the renal parenchyma can be induced by:
  - Pathogens ascending through urethra to the bladder and then through ureters to the kidney.
  - Hematogenous spread to the kidney usually of gram–positive organisms (bacteremia) or fungemia (2).

ETIOLOGY
- Acute pyelonephritis:
  - *Escherichia coli* (80%)
  - Proteus spp.
  - Klebsiella spp.
  - Rare causes may be: *Pseudomonas aeruginosa*, *Enterococci*, and *Staphylococcus saprophyticus*.
  - A urine culture positive for *Staphylococcus aureus* usually indicates bacteremia.
- Emphysematous pyelonephritis (a gas-producing necrotizing infection of the renal parenchyma):
  - *E. coli*, Klebsiella spp., and Candida spp. (rare) (4).
- Chronic:
  - Infectious or noninfectious causes.

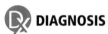 DIAGNOSIS

HISTORY
- Symptoms might be present for some hours or few days and may be:
  - Systemic (headache, nausea, vomiting, malaise, fever, chills)
  - Unilateral or bilateral flank pain or tenderness
  - Low back pain
  - Abdominal pain
- Symptoms of lower UTI are either concurrent or 1–2 days preceding symptoms of upper UTI (dysuria, urgency, hematuria):
- Elderly: There may be paucity of symptoms
- Children: Usually present with nonspecific symptoms for all UTIs.

PHYSICAL EXAM
- Fever (might be absent sometimes)
- Tachycardia (indicates fever, dehydration, or sepsis)
- Toxic appearance if patient is in sepsis
- Flank tenderness or pain

DIAGNOSTIC TESTS & INTERPRETATION
Lab
- Urinalysis to detect:
  - Pyuria
  - Bacteria in urine (absence does not exclude acute pyelonephritis)
- Pretreatment urine culture
- Blood urea nitrogen, and/or creatinine.
- A CBC may show increases in WBC with a shift to the left
- CRP levels and ESR may be increased
- A set of blood cultures may be of help

Imaging
Initial approach
- Imaging might be warranted in patients with:
  - Atypical features such as colicky pain and/or persistent hematuria
  - Slow or no improvement (symptoms persist longer than 72 hours with appropriate treatment)
  - Recurrent episodes
- A plain x-ray of kidneys, ureter, and bladder may locate radiopaque calculi and soft-tissue masses and detect gas in the kidneys in cases of emphysematous pyelonephritis.
- Ultrasonography is the preferred initial method in recurrent or atypical pyelonephritis.
- Computed tomography of the abdomen with the administration of intravenous contrast medium is used if further clarification of renal anatomy is required, such as in intrarenal and/or perinephric abscess or presence of obstruction.

Follow-Up & Special Considerations
Ultrasonography may need to be repeated in case of clinical deterioration despite initial response to treatment.

Diagnostic Procedures/Other
- Material from an obstructed region with obstruction should be examined by chemical analysis (in case of nephrolithiasis) and histologically (in case of neoplastic tissue). Microbiological testing may also be necessary.
- Intravenous pyelography
- Work up for nephrolithiasis may be needed

Pathological Findings
- Acute inflammation of the renal parenchyma and infiltration of the renal papillary tip by polymorphonuclear leukocytes with destruction of the urothelium (5).

DIFFERENTIAL DIAGNOSIS
- Cystitis
- Urethritis
- Vaginitis
- Appendicitis
- Pelvic inflammatory disease
- Tumor in bladder or kidney

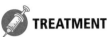 **TREATMENT**

MEDICATION
First Line
- For outpatients with acute uncomplicated pyelonephritis (it is imperative to know local susceptibility data):
  – Amoxicillin 500 mg every 8 hours orally for 10–14 days
  – Amoxicillin 500 mg plus clavulanate 125 mg every 8 hours
  – Trimethoprim-sulfamethoxazole (TMP-SMX) 160–800 mg orally every 12 hours for 10–14 days
  – Norfloxacin 400 mg every 12 hours orally for 10–14 days
  – Ciprofloxacin 500 mg every 12 hours orally for 10–14 days
  – Levofloxacin 750 mg every 24 hours orally for 5 days (6).
  – Cefpodoxime 200 mg every 12 hours orally for 10–14 days.
- For inpatients, parenterally:
  – Ciprofloxacin 400 mg every 12 hours
  – Levofloxacin 750 mg every 24 hours
  – Ceftriaxone 1–2 g every 24 hours
  – Gentamicin 1 mg/kg every 8 hours
  – Ampicillin 1 g every 6 hours.
  – Aztreonam 1 g every 8–12 hours
  – Imipenem/cilastatin 250–500 mg every 6–8 hours
  – Ertapenem (not active against *P. aeruginosa*): 1 g every 24 hours
  – Ticarcillin/clavulanic acid 3.2 g every 8 hours.
  – After fever resolves, an oral regimen should be administered to complete 10–14 days of treatment.

ADDITIONAL TREATMENT
General Measures
- Supportive treatment is essential:
  – Rest
  – Analgetics and antiemetics
  – Intravenous or oral fluids

Issues for Referral
- In case of obstruction or urogenital abnormality, a urologist should be consulted as further management may be needed to revoke the cause of obstruction (i.e. removal of stone or polyp)
- Consult an infectious diseases specialist if an unusual (*P. aeruginosa*) or resistant pathogen (i.e., extensive beta-lactamase producer) is isolated.

SURGERY/OTHER PROCEDURES
- Surgical management might be needed in:
  – Emphysematous pyelonephritis
  – Renal calculi
  – Renal/perinephric abscess
  – Xanthogranulomatous pyelonephritis

IN-PATIENT CONSIDERATIONS
Initial Stabilization
If the patient is hemodynamically unstable (sepsis), intravenous fluids are required.

Admission Criteria
- Severe illness (high fever, pain and debility)
- Dehydration
- Inability to take oral medications or concern about compliance.
- Pregnancy

Discharge Criteria
Defervescence and clinical improvement for 24–48 hours.

 ONGOING CARE

FOLLOW-UP RECOMMENDATIONS
- Posttreatment urine culture
- Patients with persistent symptoms on antibiotic therapy should be investigated with radiographic imaging and additional laboratory tests.

PATIENT EDUCATION
- Patients must receive drugs as prescribed.
- Advise patients to receive adequate fluids to prevent dehydration.

PROGNOSIS
- Acute uncomplicated pyelonephritis has very good prognosis.
- Overall in-hospital mortality is <1–2% (7).

COMPLICATIONS
- Bacteremia or/and septic shock
- Renal abscess
- Perinephric abscess
- Struvite urinary stones (ammonium magnesium phosphate) when infection by Proteus spp.

REFERENCES
1. Czaja, CA, Scholes, D, Hooton, et al. Population-based epidemiologic analysis of acute pyelonephritis. *Clin Infect Dis* 2007;45:273.
2. Scholes D, Hooton TM, Roberts PL, et al. Risk factors associated with acute pyelonephritis in healthy women. *Ann Intern Med* 2005;142:20.
3. Ramakrishan K, Scheid DC. Diagnosis and management of acute pyelonephritis in adults. *Am Fam Physician* 2005;71;933–942.
4. Grupper M, Kravtsov A, Potasman I, et al. Emphysematous cystitis: Illustrative case report and review of the literature. *Medicine (Baltimore)* 2007;86:47–53.
5. Craig WD, Wagner BJ, Travis MD. Pyelonephritis: Radiologic-pathologic review. *Radiographics* 2008;28:255–277.
6. Peterson J, Kaul S, Khashab M, et al. A double-blind, randomized comparison for levofloxacin 750 mg once-daily for five days with ciprofloxacin 400/500 mg twice-daily for 10 days for the treatment of complicated urinary tract infections and acute pyelonephritis. *Urology* 2008;71:17–22.
7. Foxman B, Klemstine KL, Brown PD. Acute pyelonephritis in US hospitals in 1997: hospitalization and in-hospital mortality. *Ann Epidemiol* 2003;13:144–150.

ADDITIONAL READING
- Vouloumanou EK, Rafailidis PI, Kazantzi MS, et al. Early switch to oral versus intravenous antimicrobial treatment for hospitalized patients with acute pyelonephritis: A systematic review of randomized controlled trials. *Curr Med Res Opin* 2008;24: 3423–3434.

 CODES

ICD9
- 590.00 Chronic pyelonephritis without lesion of renal medullary necrosis
- 590.10 Acute pyelonephritis without lesion of renal medullary necrosis
- 590.80 Pyelonephritis, unspecified

CLINICAL PEARLS
- *Escherichia coli* and *Klebsiella pneumoniae* have become notoriously resistant to many classes of antibiotics. Specifically, their extensive beta lactam producing capability linked occasionally to quinolone resistance is a true challenge for physicians. Carbapenems or fosfomycin disodium (available in Europe for systemic use) may be needed to treat such bacteria.
- The necessity to treat according to local susceptibility of uropathogens cannot be overemphasized.
- Avoid quinolones and sulfa derivatives in the treatment of pyelonephritis in pregnancy and in patients with glucose 6-phosphate dehydrogenase deficiency.

Q FEVER
Petros Karsaliakos (E. Mylonakis, Editor)

 BASICS

DESCRIPTION
Q fever is a globally distributed disease (Q for query, because the cause was unknown when the infection was first described in 1935), which is mainly presented as an acute and occasionally chronic infection caused by *Coxiella burnetii*.

EPIDEMIOLOGY
- Q fever is a zoonosis. The primary reservoirs of *C. burnetii* are cattle, sheep, and goats, but many other species, including rodents and cats, can be infected.
- In 1999 the disease was recognized as of epidemiologically important in the US.
- In many other countries the disease is underdiagnosed and underreported.
- The infection in animals is usually not clinically apparent, but *C. burnetii* may be excreted in milk, urine, feces, and amniotic fluid.
- *C. burnetii* is mostly contracted by inhaling infected aerosols; it has an incubation period of around 3 weeks.
- Blood transfusion is a rare route of transmission.
- The organism is particularly infectious (1–10 organisms are sufficient to infect humans) and is usually transmitted following contact with parturient ewes or cows, in which the organism is endemic in certain areas.
- In some series, up to 80% of the cases occurred between February and May.
- A high ratio of male to female patients (up to 1.0:3.5) has been noted.
- Reports of both sporadic cases and epidemics have been published.
- About 52 cases of Q fever are annually reported in the US.

GENERAL PREVENTION
- Consumption of only pasteurized milk.
- Aborted material from goats and sheep should be destroyed, and affected dams isolated.
- A vaccine is available in Australia for all workers in hazard of transmission.
- Vaccination requires pretest with skin testing and serology.

ETIOLOGY
- *C. burnetii* is a gram-negative coccobacillus with the capability of surviving inside host cell phagolysosomes.
- *C. burnetii* displays an antigenic-phase variation that is unique among the rickettsiae.
- In acute Q fever, antibodies to *C. burnetii* phase II antigens dominate the immune response, whereas in chronic Q fever, phase I antigen levels become elevated.
- It is not the strain of the pathogen that defines whether the disease will acquire an acute or chronic character.
- The immunologic reaction of the patient will determine the further clinical route.
- Interleukin-10 overproduction plays an important role for the intracellular survival of the microbe.
- Cellular immunity is responsible for the immunologic confrontation of *Coxiella*.
- T-cell activation participates the most in the killing of these bacteria.

DIAGNOSIS

Clinical Manifestations
Symptoms
- About 50% of patients with active Q fever infection present with no symptoms or signs.
- *C. burnetii* infection causes a variety of clinical syndromes. Most common are a self-limited febrile illness, a flulike syndrome, and a mild-to-moderate atypical pneumonia.
- Other symptoms include chills, sweats, nausea, vomiting, and diarrhea, which occur in 5–20% of patients.
- Pneumonia and hepatitis often coexist in the acute syndrome.
- Acute Q fever in pregnant women is of high severity and may lead to abortion or neonatal death.
- Headache is the most common neurologic manifestation of *C. burnetii* infection.

- Uncommon manifestations of acute Q fever include the following:
  - Epididymitis
  - Erythema nodosum
  - Extrapyramidal neurologic disease
  - Guillain-Barré syndrome
  - Hemolytic anemia
  - Inappropriate secretion of antidiuretic hormone
  - Mediastinal lymphadenopathy
  - Mesenteric panniculitis
  - Optic neuritis
  - Orchitis
  - Pancreatitis
  - Priapism
- Chronic Q fever is almost a synonym for *C. burnetii* endocarditis.
- Fever is absent or, if present, is of low grade.
- Q fever endocarditis more frequently predilects the aortic valve. Mitral valve infection is less common.
- In recent years the involvement of vascular grafts has been increased.
- Other manifestations of chronic Q fever include the following:
  - Hepatitis
  - Infection among immunocompromised hosts
  - Infection during pregnancy
  - Infection of aneurysms
  - Infection of vascular prostheses
  - Meningoencephalitis
  - Myocarditis
  - Osteomyelitis
  - Pericarditis
  - Prolonged fever
- Meningoencephalitis and abnormal cerebrospinal fluid findings are much less frequent in Q fever than in other rickettsial diseases.

Signs
- Hyperthermia is the main clinical feature in acute Q fever, with temperatures that can reach 40°C in up to 60% of the patients with pneumonia.
- The dissociation between pulse rate and temperature is found in one-third to half with Q fever.
- Hepatomegaly and splenomegaly can occur in certain cases.
- Rash is not prominent in acute Q fever as it is in the other Rickettsiosis.

DIAGNOSTIC TESTS & INTERPRETATION
Lab
- *C. burnetii* can be isolated from buffy-coat blood samples or tissue specimens by a shell-vial technique, but most clinical laboratories are not permitted to attempt the isolation of *C. burnetii*, because it is considered highly infectious.
- Polymerase chain reaction (PCR) can be used to amplify *C. burnetii* DNA from tissue or biopsy specimens. This technique also can be used on paraffin-embedded tissues.
- Serology is the most commonly used diagnostic tool. Three techniques are available:
  – Complement fixation
  – Indirect immunofluorescence (method of choice)
  – Enzyme-linked immunosorbent assay
- A fourfold rise in titer between acute- and convalescent-phase samples is seen in acute Q fever.
- A titer of IGM antibodies higher than 1:50 contributes to the diagnosis. Positive IGM antibodies may exist for about 2 years.
- Positive rheumatoid factor, high erythrocyte sedimentation rate, increased C-reactive protein level, augmented gamma globulin concentrations even if they are not specific , they often co-exist especially in chronic Q fever.
- The WBC count is usually normal, but monocytosis can occur with acute Q fever. Thrombocytopenia is present in about 25% of patients. Thrombocytosis is not rare with cases exceeding 1 million/mm³.
- Altered liver function, consisting more frequently in elevated alkaline phosphatase (70% of the cases) rather than transaminase, is found.

Imaging
- Pleurisy sometimes involves one-third of cases and might be large.
- Radiographic resolution may last even for 2 months.

DIFFERENTIAL DIAGNOSIS
- The differential diagnosis of *C. burnetii* pneumonia includes all other possible causes of atypical pneumonia, and *C. burnetii* should be considered in cases of culture-negative endocarditis (see also Section II chapter, "Pneumonia" and both chapters on endocarditis).
- Hepatitis due to *C. burnetii* can present as fever of unknown origin.
- CNS involvement may be presented with seizures and coma.

 TREATMENT
MEDICATION
- There are no adequate studies to support a specific treatment duration.
- The treatment should initiate early and is more successful in the first 3 days of clinical presentation.

First Line
- Treatment of acute Q fever with doxycycline (100 mg twice daily for 14 days) is usually successful.
- Doxycycline (100 mg twice daily) with hydroxychloroquine (200 mg t.i.d) is becoming the treatment of choice in *C. burnetii* endocarditis.
- The optimal duration of antibiotic therapy for chronic Q fever remains undetermined, but a minimum of 3–4 years of treatment is usually recommended. Therapy should be discontinued only if the phase I IgA antibody titer is ≤1:50 and the phase I IgG titer is ≤1:200.

COMPLEMENTARY & ALTERNATIVE THERAPIES
- The combination of rifampin (300 mg per day) and doxycycline (100 mg b.i.d) has been used with success for the treatment of chronic Q fever.
- Quinolones are also effective and can be used in the treatment of chronic Q fever, instead of rifampin.

 ONGOING CARE
FOLLOW-UP RECOMMENDATIONS
- Most acute Q fever infections resolve spontaneously.
- Measuring antibody titers every 6 months during endocarditis therapy is mandatory for the cessation of treatment.
- Chest radiographs return to normal in 80% of the patients within the first month.

COMPLICATIONS
- Acute Q fever shows a mortality of approximately 2%.
- Mortality due to *C. burnetii* endocarditis is up to 25–60%, and relapse is common.

ADDITIONAL READING
- Gikas A, Kokkini S, Tsioutis C. Q fever: Clinical manifestations and treatment. *Expert Rev Anti Infect Ther* 2010;8(5):529–539.
- Marrie TJ. Q fever pneumonia. *Infect Dis Clin North Am* 2010;24(1):27–41.
- Angelakis E, Raoult D. Q Fever. *Vet Microbiol* 2010;140(3–4):297–309.

CODES

ICD9
083.0 Q fever

CLINICAL PEARLS
- Processing culture specimens from patients with Q fever requires high yield of protection to avoid transmission to laboratory personnel.
- Transesophageal cardiac ultrasound might be negative in many instances of Q fever endocarditis.

RABIES

Vasant Nagvekar
Abdul Ghafur
Matthew E. Falagas

 BASICS

DESCRIPTION
Rabies is caused by a bullet-shaped single stranded RNA virus, belonging to the group Rhabdoviridae.

EPIDEMIOLOGY
Incidence
- 15,000,000 people receive postexposure prophylaxis every year (1).
- According to the WHO, many cases may be underreported and death toll may be >55,000 (1).

Prevalence
- More prevalent in developing countries.
- Seen all over the world except Antarctica and few island nations.
- Dog bite is the commonest mode of transmission in developing nations.
- A bite due to raccoons and bats is the mode of transmission in developed nations.

RISK FACTORS
- Scientists in rabies research laboratory and vaccine production.
- Veterinarians (exposure to wild dogs, skunks, raccoons, foxes, and bats).
- Wildlife officers, where rabies is common.
- Transmission can occur in caves, most likely from aerosolized bat excreta.

Genetics
No genetic predisposition.

GENERAL PREVENTION
- Mass vaccination of the animals is the key to the prevention of rabies in humans.
- Determination as to who does and does not need prophylaxis should be made on an individual basis.
- People at high risk may want to be immunized prior to any potential exposure.

- Travelers should be alerted to the risks when traveling to less-developed areas.
- In people who have high-risk professions or travel to high risk locations where animal contact is possible, preexposure vaccination is indicated. In this case, vaccine (1 mL IM) should be given at day 0, 7, and 21, or 28. Antibody titers should be determined at least every 6 months (laboratory staff) or every 2 years (wild life officers) (2). There should be neutralization at the 1:5 levels by the rapid fluorescent focus inhibition test.

PATHOPHYSIOLOGY
- Virus gain entry through broken skin or intact mucosa.
- Incubation period is in the range of 20–90 days.
- Virus spreads centripetally by axonal transport to CNS, where intracellular viral replication with formation of Negri bodies occurs.
- The virus then progresses centrifugally to many tissues including the salivary and lacrimal glands.

ETIOLOGY
- Human infection is through the bite of a rabid dog.
- Virus is present in high concentrations in the saliva and so apart from the bites, scratches or licks of a rabid animal can cause disease.

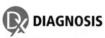 **DIAGNOSIS**

HISTORY
History of multiple bites through exposed skin and bites on the face are more likely to transmit the disease than single bite at extremities or through thick clothes which removes saliva from animal's teeth. Prodrome: Patients may note paresthesias at the site of the initial bite. Constitutional symptoms and signs, such as malaise and fevers, nausea, vomiting, and sore throat, may occur. The prodrome lasts 2–10 days.

PHYSICAL EXAM
After the prodrome, encephalitis is manifested:
- May be febrile
- Changes in personality and cognition
- Hyperactivity, agitation, biting, and hallucinations occur.
- Patients may also have hypertension, and spasms of the pharynx and larynx.
- In furious rabies hydrophobia (hydro: of water, phobia: fear: fear of water, i.e., spasms after visual stimulus of seeing water), aerophobia (fear of air, i.e., spasms after olfactory stimuli) and exaggerated irritant reflex of the respiratory tract with episodic hyperactivity.
- Seizures may occur also after tactile stimuli.
- The symptoms can wax and wane, and, between episodes of agitation, the patients are cooperative.
- On occasion, patients will have progressive confusion and clouding of consciousness, which progresses rapidly to coma. The patients complain of headache. Paralysis may occur at this stage.
- In the paralytic form patient will present with findings suggestive of Guillain Barré syndrome.

DIAGNOSTIC TESTS & INTERPRETATION
Lab
- History rather than any laboratory tests is the clue to the diagnosis.
- Direct fluorescent antibody (DFA) remains the standard laboratory test and is usually done on skin sample taken from the nape of neck.
  – RT-PCR of saliva, CSF or tissue are alternative options.

Imaging
- Brain imaging is usually normal in early stage.
- MRI – increased T2 signal in the hippocampi, hypothalamus, and brain stem may be seen.
- No imaging is pathognomonic of rabies.

Diagnostic Procedures/Other
- CSF may be normal or may show pleocytosis.
- RT-PCR in CSF may be positive (3).
- Biopsy of nape of neck above hair line for direct fluorescent antibody test, as virus tends to get localized in hair follicles.

Pathological Findings
- Presence of Negri bodies especially in the hippocampal pyramidal cells.
- Segmental demyelination in paralytic rabies similar to Guillain Barré syndrome.

DIFFERENTIAL DIAGNOSIS
- Tetanus and viral encephalitis may resemble furious forms of rabies.
- Acute demyelinating polyneuropathy, poliomyelitis, and acute disseminated encephalomyelitis can mimic paralytic rabies.

 TREATMENT

MEDICATION
- For unvaccinated persons: Human rabies immunoglobulin 20 units/kg body weight given once on day 0. If possible, infiltrate the majority of the dose around the wound and the rest in to the gluteal region.
- Do not inject immunoglobulin at the same site of vaccine administration.
- Immunoglobulin is not required for persons vaccinated prior to exposure to the virus.
- For unvaccinated persons: Human Diploid Cell Vaccine (HDVC), Rabies Vaccine Adsorbed (RVA) or Purified Chick Embryo Cell Vaccine (PCECV) preferably in deltoid region on day 0, 3, 7, 14, and 28.
- For vaccinated persons: Booster vaccine dose on days 0 and 3.

ADDITIONAL TREATMENT
General Measures
Thorough washing of the wound with 20% soap solution and irrigating the wound with iodine reduces the risk by 90%.

Issues for Referral
- Deep wounds, bleeding from the wound
- Altered behavior.

Additional Therapies
Immunocompromised patients may not respond to vaccination and measurement of antibodies at 2–4 weeks is recommended.

COMPLEMENTARY & ALTERNATIVE THERAPIES
Care of surgical wound

IN-PATIENT CONSIDERATIONS
Admission Criteria
- Deep and multiple bite wounds.
- Altered sensorium or behavior.

IV Fluids
Intravenous fluids are indicated only in furious and paralytic forms of rabies.

Nursing
Nursing care is very important especially in trying to avoid unnecessary exposure to stimuli that may provoke seizures.

 ONGOING CARE

FOLLOW-UP RECOMMENDATIONS
Observe the dog if possible for up to 10 days.

DIET
No need of any special diet for individuals bitten by a dog.

PATIENT EDUCATION
The dog must be observed for 10 days if located. If the animal dies, or is lost or killed within 10 days of exposure, it should be immediately reported.

PROGNOSIS
- 100% mortality in confirmed rabies in unvaccinated rabies.
- This contrasts sharply with the very good prognosis that persons who were vaccinated prior to their exposure and received an additional booster after the exposure.

COMPLICATIONS
- Encephalomyelitis
- Intractable seizures
- Guillain-Barré syndrome
- Myocarditis/arrhythmias
- Respiratory failure
- Vascular collapse
- Death

REFERENCES
1. WHO Technical report series 931. WHO Expert consultation on rabies. World Health Organization 2005. http://whqlibdoc.who.int/trs/WHO_TRS_931_eng.pdf. Accessed December 2010.
2. Warrell MJ, Warrell DA. Rabies and other lyssavirus diseases. *Lancet* 2004;363:959–969.
3. Dacheux L, Wacharapluesadee S, Hemachudha T, et al. More accurate insight into the incidence of human rabies in developing countries through validated laboratory techniques. *PLoS Negl Trop Dis* 2010;4(11):e765.

ADDITIONAL READING
- Wilson PJ, Oertli EH, Hunt PR, et al. Evaluation of a postexposure rabies prophylaxis protocol for domestic animals in Texas: 2000–2009. *J Am Vet Med Assoc* 2010;237:1395–1401.
- Bourhy H, Dautry-Varsat A, Hotez PJ, et al. Rabies, still neglected after 125 years of vaccination. *PLoS Negl Trop Dis* 2010;4:e839.

 CODES

ICD9
071 Rabies

CLINICAL PEARLS
- Rabies is a preventable disease.
- Always vaccinate pet dogs.

RELAPSING FEVER

Paschalis Vergidis
Matthew E. Falagas

 BASICS

DESCRIPTION
A spirochetal infection manifested with fever that lasts few days and subsequent recurrence(s) of fever after short period(s) of normal temperature. Occurs in 2 major forms: Louse-borne (or epidemic) and tick-borne (or endemic).

EPIDEMIOLOGY
Incidence
Louse Borne
- The incidence of relapsing fever due to *Borrelia recurrentis* (louse-borne epidemic relapsing fever) depends on socioeconomic and ecologic factors.
- Louse-borne relapsing fever usually occurs in epidemics related to catastrophic events, such as war, serious weather-related events, or famine because of easy dissemination of lice between humans due to overcrowding.
- There are a few areas of the world (highlands of Central and East Africa and the South America Andes) where louse-borne relapsing fever is still endemic.

Tick Borne
- The incidence of tick-borne relapsing fever is mainly influenced by environmental and social factors, which determine the probability of tick bites in humans.
- Tick-borne relapsing fever has a worldwide distribution but is especially endemic in tropical Africa.
- In the US, tick-borne disease usually occurs west of the Mississippi River. In the mountainous areas of California, Utah, Arizona, New Mexico, Colorado, Oregon, and Washington, infections are usually caused by *Borrelia hermsii*. In the non-mountainous regions of the Southwest, the usual agent of relapsing fever is *Borrelia turicatae*.

RISK FACTORS
- Overcrowding and homelessness are major risk factors for louse-borne relapsing fever.
- Recreational activities in areas where tick bites are more likely to occur increase the probability of tick-borne relapsing fever. *B. hermsii* is often acquired from exposure to cabins in pine forests. *B. turicatae* is often acquired by entering caves and crawling under houses.

GENERAL PREVENTION
- Control of lice and ticks
- In a high-risk environment, postexposure treatment for tick-borne relapsing fever with oral doxycycline (200 mg the first day and 100 mg per day for the next 4 days) is recommended (1).

PATHOPHYSIOLOGY
- When crushing lice, *B. recurrentis* is released and penetrates the skin (bite site, skin of the crushing fingers) or mucous membranes (conjunctivae after rubbing eyes).
- Tick-borne relapsing fever is transmitted during blood feeding, usually from tick saliva. Most people are not aware of the bite, as argasid ticks are night feeders, feed quickly (in <1 hour), and lack a painful bite.
- Fever occurs during bouts of spirochetemia. Spirochetes are sequestered in internal organs during afebrile periods. Under immune pressure, *Borrelia* undergoes antigenic modification and re-emerges in the bloodstream.

ETIOLOGY
- The pathogenic spirochetes causing relapsing fever are transmitted to humans by arthropods.
- The human body louse (*Pediculus humanus corporis*) transmits *B. recurrentis* to humans, causing epidemic relapsing fever.
- Argasid ticks (soft-bodied ticks), usually of the genus *Ornithodoros*, transmit over 15 species of *Borrelia* to humans, causing endemic relapsing fever.

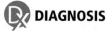 **DIAGNOSIS**

HISTORY
- The incubation period of relapsing fever is usually 8 days (range, 5–15 days).
- Acute onset of fever, accompanied by a combination of the following symptoms:
  - Chills
  - Rigors
  - Headache
  - Malaise
  - Arthralgias
  - Diffuse myalgias
  - Lethargy
  - Cough
  - Jaundice
  - Photophobia
- A petechial, macular, and/or papular rash may appear.
- Cardiac and/or central nervous system manifestations may complicate relapsing fever.
- The febrile episode terminates abruptly in 3–6 days.
- After 7–9 days with no fever, the patient has recurrence of the symptoms (relapsing fever).
- The number of relapses of fever is usually 1–2 in louse-borne relapsing fever, while multiple relapses of fever are common in tick-borne relapsing fever.

PHYSICAL EXAM
Common signs may include the following:
- Conjunctival injection and edema
- Hepatomegaly
- Splenomegaly
- Diffuse abdominal tenderness
- Abnormal respiratory sounds (rales and rhonchi)
- Lymphadenopathy
- Neurologic findings (more common in tick-borne than louse-borne relapsing fever)

DIAGNOSTIC TESTS & INTERPRETATION
Lab
- Demonstration of *Borrelia* in the peripheral blood of a febrile patient is the definitive test for the diagnosis of relapsing fever.
- Thick and thin smears of peripheral blood stained with Giemsa or Wright should be carefully checked.
- Organisms are rarely found during afebrile periods.
- Dark-field microscopy of peripheral blood may also prove the presence of *Borrelia*.
- Polymerase chain reaction can be performed on blood samples.
- Serology tests may be of help, but results should be interpreted with caution due to their limited sensitivity and specificity.

DIFFERENTIAL DIAGNOSIS
- The possibility of a coexisting epidemic of typhus should be entertained in cases of epidemic louse-borne relapsing fever.
- Malaria
- Leptospirosis
- Rat-bite fever
- Dengue
- Ehrlichiosis/Anaplasmosis
- Babesiosis
- Tularemia

TREATMENT
MEDICATION
First Line
- A single dose of tetracycline 500 mg or doxycycline 100 mg orally is the recommended treatment for louse-borne relapsing fever.
- Tetracycline (500 mg PO every 6 hours) or doxycycline (100 mg PO twice daily) for 7 days is the recommended treatment for tick-borne relapsing fever.
- Meningitis or encephalitis should be treated with parenteral antibiotics, such as penicillin G or ceftriaxone, for 10–14 days.

Second Line
- Eryrthromycin 500 mg single oral dose for louse-borne relapsing fever, or 500 mg po every 6 hours for tick-borne relapsing fever.
- Jarisch-Herxheimer reaction may occur after antibiotic treatment, especially with penicillins.

ONGOING CARE
FOLLOW-UP RECOMMENDATIONS
Careful follow-up is necessary for patients with relapsing fever, due to the high probability of recurrence of the syndrome.

PROGNOSIS
The case-fatality rates for untreated relapsing fever are 4–40% for louse-borne relapsing fever and 2–5% for tick-borne relapsing fever.

COMPLICATIONS
- Liver damage, arrhythmias due to myocarditis, and cerebral hemorrhage are the main causes of death.
- Acute respiratory distress syndrome
- Meningitis and meningoencephalitis can result in hemiplegia or aphasia
- Cranial neuritis
- Iridocyclitis, panophthalmitis

REFERENCE
1. Hasin T, Davidovitch N, Cohen R, et al. Postexposure treatment with doxycycline for the prevention of tick-borne relapsing fever. *N Eng J Med* 2006;355(2):148–155.

ADDITIONAL READING
- Barbour Borgnolo G, Hailu B, Ciancarelli A, et al. Louse-borne relapsing fever. A clinical and an epidemiological study of 389 patients in Asella Hospital, Ethiopia. *Trop Geogr Med* 1993;45:66–69.
- Cadavid D, Barbour AG. Neuroborreliosis during relapsing fever: Review of the clinical manifestations, pathology, and treatment of infections in humans and experimental animals. *Clin Infect Dis* 1998;26(1):151–164.
- Dworkin MS, Schwan TG, Anderson DE Jr, et al. Tick-borne relapsing fever. *Infect Dis Clin North Am* 2008;22(3):449–468, viii.

CODES

ICD9
- 087.0 Relapsing fever, louse-borne
- 087.1 Relapsing fever, tick-borne
- 087.9 Relapsing fever, unspecified

CLINICAL PEARLS
- Relapsing fever occurs in two major forms: Louse-borne (or epidemic) caused by *B. recurrentis*, and tick-borne (or endemic) caused by *B. hermsii* and other species.
- Giemsa or Wright stain reveals the spirochetes in blood during periods of spirochetemia.
- Tetracycline or doxycycline is recommended for treatment. Meningitis or encephalitis should be treated with penicillin G or ceftriaxone.

RESPIRATORY SYNCYTIAL VIRUS INFECTION

Evridiki K. Vouloumanou
Petros I. Rafailidis
Matthew E. Falagas

 BASICS

DESCRIPTION
Respiratory syncytial virus (RSV) causes lower respiratory tract infections in children and adults (contagious), and is particularly severe in infants and children with congenital heart disease, in immunocompromised adults, and in the elderly. The main clinical manifestation is acute bronchiolitis in children.

EPIDEMIOLOGY
Incidence
- In 2005, the estimated new episodes of RSV-associated acute lower respiratory tract infections occurring in children younger than 5 years worldwide was 33.8 (95% CI 19.3–46.2) million (1).
- In 2005, 66,000–199,000 children younger than 5 years died from RSV-associated acute lower respiratory tract infection (1).
- The peak incidence of severe RSV disease occurs at age 2–8 months.
- Elderly adults are also commonly infected from RSV. Specifically, attack rates are approximately 5–10% per year (2).

Prevalence
By 24 months of age, most children will have acquired at least one RSV infection (3).

RISK FACTORS
- Day-care attendance/older siblings in day care
- Lower socioeconomic conditions
- Male sex,
- Age <6 months
- Exposure to passive smoking
- Birth during the first half of the RSV season
- Crowding
- Prematurity
- Immunosuppression due to chemotherapy or transplantation
- Chronic lung disease (including cystic fibrosis and bronchopulmonary dysplasia)
- Congenital heart disease (4,5).

GENERAL PREVENTION
- Vaccines are not yet available.
- Reduction of the virus spread to others by frequent hand washing and not sharing items with patients with a RSV infection.
- Glove and gown precautions may result in a substantial reduction of the nosocomial transmission of RSV (6).
- Passive immunization with intravenous gamma globulin (IVIG) and specific RSV-IVIG for patients at risk for severe RSV infection (7).

- Palivizumab is a specific monoclonal antibody for RSV that may be administered for prophylaxis to patients that are at risk for the development of severe RSV infection, such as premature infants (8).
- Motavizumab is an investigational enhanced-potency humanized monoclonal antibody for RSV. Data from in vitro and in vivo studies suggest that motavizumab has greater anti-RSV activity compared to palivizumab (9).

PATHOPHYSIOLOGY
The RSV virus spreads from the upper to the lower respiratory tract transferred from cell-to-cell through "bridges" located inside the cytoplasm that are called "syncytia."

COMMONLY ASSOCIATED CONDITIONS
- RSV prophylaxis in nonatopic children has been suggested to decrease the relative risk of recurrent wheezing by 80%. However, it does not seem to have any effect in infants with an atopic family history (10).
- Severe early bronchiolitis due to RSV is associated with increased prevalence of allergic asthma that persists into early adulthood (11).

 DIAGNOSIS

HISTORY
- Incubation period may vary from 2–8 days.
- RSV is transmitted by contact with infected secretions through hand-to-hand spread and/or fomites as well as through respiratory droplets.
- Initially, children and adults have symptoms suggestive of an upper respiratory–like infection that progresses rapidly to cough, coryza, and wheezing.
- Fever is typically low-grade. However, children may have high fever.
- Over time, children may develop a deepening cough, with spasms (bronchiolitis) and wheezing.
- Croup may occur in 10% of cases, but is usually mild.
- Otitis media may be present (40% of RSV infection cases).
- Elderly adults commonly develop bronchopneumonia as a complication of RSV.

PHYSICAL EXAM
- Infants with RSV lower respiratory tract infection: Rales (diffuse small airway disease).
- Tachypnea
- Cyanosis
- Associated otitis media
- Assessment of the hydration status (skin turgor, capillary refill, mucous membranes) is important particularly for infants with RSV infection.

DIAGNOSTIC TESTS & INTERPRETATION
Lab
Initial lab tests
- Arterial blood gas, oxygen saturation measurement, serum electrolytes, and CBC count.
- Rapid tests are available for screening of respiratory secretions.

Follow-Up & Special Considerations
- Indirect immunofluorescence assays
- Enzyme-linked immunosorbent assay
- Serologic diagnosis is available for community-screening purposes.
- Nasal washings can be sent for viral culture.

Imaging
Initial approach
Chest x-rays: Hyperinflated lung fields, focal atelectases, pulmonary infiltrates).

Follow-Up & Special Considerations
Expiratory CT: Evidence of small-airway disease of the lungs: Air trapping.

Diagnostic Procedures/Other
Lung tissue biopsy: Mononuclear cell and neutrophil infiltration of the peribronchiolar areas, areas of atelectasis, infiltrates.

DIFFERENTIAL DIAGNOSIS
- Asthma
- Acute bronchitis/chronic bronchitis
- Pneumonia
- Influenza
- Parainfluenza
- Croup
- Human metapneumovirus
- Neonatal sepsis

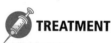 **TREATMENT**

MEDICATION
- Nebulized ribavirin is approved for treatment of severe RSV infection: 6 g of lyophilized ribavirin powder dissolved in 300 mL of distilled water and administered for nebulization by a small-particle aerosol generator over 12–20 hours per day for 3–7 days. However, the available evidence is insufficient to support a substantial beneficial effect (12). Furthermore, secondary toxicity to health care workers has been reported and the cost/benefit of the medication has also to be taken into account. Nevertheless, pediatricians may consider the administration of ribavirin in severe cases of RSV infection, especially so in immunocompromised children, congenital heart disease, and hemodynamic instability.
- Treatment with intravenous palivizumab alone or in combination with ribavirin has also been reported to be acceptably safe and was associated with decreased mortality in high-risk children with RSV infection (13).

ADDITIONAL TREATMENT
Additional Therapies
- A multidrug regimen of regimen of inhaled ribavirin, corticosteroids, and IVIG (with or without palivizumab) was reported to be both effective and safe for the treatment of adult heart and heart–lung transplants with RSV infections (14).
- RNA Interference Therapy (ALN-RSV01) appears to be a safe and potentially beneficial for long-term allograft function in lung transplant patients with RSV infection.

IN-PATIENT CONSIDERATIONS
Initial Stabilization
- Supportive therapy (oxygen administration, fluid replacement, bronchodilators).
- Mechanical ventilation or intubation.

 ONGOING CARE

FOLLOW-UP RECOMMENDATIONS
None required unless bronchospasm develops on a recurrent or permanent basis.

PROGNOSIS
- Recovery and hospital discharge occurs typically in 3–4 days in children hospitalized due to an RSV infection.
- Population-based studies suggested that RSV infections result in the intermediate care units (IMC) or intensive care units (ICU) admissions of approximately 1–2% of each annual birth cohort (15).
- RSV infection is associated with considerable mortality in infants, high-risk adults, and elderly individuals (1,2).

COMPLICATIONS
- Development of asthma is possibly connected to recurrent RSV infections in childhood.
- Bacterial pneumonia or otitis
- Neurologic complications (including encephalopathy, seizures) (16).
- A potential association between previous RSV infection and acute myocardial infarction has also been suggested (17).

REFERENCES

1. Nair H, Nokes DJ, Gessner BD, et al. Global burden of acute lower respiratory infections due to respiratory syncytial virus in young children: A systematic review and meta-analysis. *Lancet* 2010;375:1545–1555.
2. Falsey AR, Walsh EE. Respiratory syncytial virus infection in elderly adults. *Drugs Aging* 2005;22: 577–587.
3. Glezen WP, Taber LH, Frank AL, et al. Risk of primary infection and reinfection with respiratory syncytial virus. *Am J Dis Child* 1986;140: 543–546.
4. Figueras-Aloy J, Carbonell-Estrany X, Quero J. IRIS Study Group. Case-control study of the risk factors linked to respiratory syncytial virus infection requiring hospitalization in premature infants born at a gestational age of 33–35 weeks in Spain. *Pediatr Infect Dis J* 2004;23:815–820.
5. Simoes EA. Environmental and demographic risk factors for respiratory syncytial virus lower respiratory tract disease. *J Pediatr* 2003;143: S118–S126.
6. Leclair JM, Freeman J, Sullivan BF, et al. Prevention of nosocomial respiratory syncytial virus infections through compliance with glove and gown isolation precautions. *N Engl J Med* 1987;317:329–334.
7. Groothuis JR, Levin MJ, Rodriguez W, et al. Use of intravenous gamma globulin to passively immunize high-risk children against respiratory syncytial virus: Safety and pharmacokinetics. The RSVIG Study Group. *Antimicrob Agents Chemother* 1991;35:1469–1473.
8. Rogovik AL, Carleton B, Solimano A, et al. Palivizumab for the prevention of respiratory syncytial virus infection. *Can Fam Physician* 2010;56:769–772.
9. Mejías A, Chávez-Bueno S, Ríos AM, et al. Comparative effects of two neutralizing anti-respiratory syncytial virus (RSV) monoclonal antibodies in the RSV murine model: Time versus potency. *Antimicrob Agents Chemother* 2005; 4700–4707.
10. Simões EA, Carbonell-Estrany X, Rieger CH, et al; Palivizumab Long-Term Respiratory Outcomes Study Group. The effect of respiratory syncytial virus on subsequent recurrent wheezing in atopic and nonatopic children. *J Allergy Clin Immunol* 2010;126:256–262.
11. Sigurs N, Aljassim F, Kjellman B, et al. Asthma and allergy patterns over 18 years after severe RSV bronchiolitis in the first year of life. *Thorax* 2010;65:1045–1052.
12. Ventre K, Randolph AG. Ribavirin for respiratory syncytial virus infection of the lower respiratory tract in infants and young children. *Cochrane Database Syst Rev* 2007;(1):CD000181.
13. Chávez-Bueno S, Mejías A, Merryman RA, et al. Intravenous palivizumab and ribavirin combination for respiratory syncytial virus disease in high-risk pediatric patients. *Pediatr Infect Dis J* 2007;26:1089–1093.
14. Liu V, Dhillon GS, Weill D. A multi-drug regimen for respiratory syncytial virus and parainfluenza virus infections in adult lung and heart-lung transplant recipients. *Transpl Infect Dis* 2010;12: 38–44.
15. Berger TM, Aebi C, Duppenthaler A, et al. Swiss Pediatric Surveillance Unit. Prospective population-based study of RSV-related intermediate care and intensive care unit admissions in Switzerland over a 4-year period (2001–2005). *Infection* 2009;37:109–116.
16. Sweetman LL, Ng YT, Butler IJ, et al. Neurologic complications associated with respiratory syncytial virus. *Pediatr Neurol* 2005;32:307–310.
17. Guan XR, Jiang LX, Ma XH, et al. Respiratory syncytial virus infection and risk of acute myocardial infarction. *Am J Med Sci* 2010;340: 356–359.

ADDITIONAL READING

- Prodhan P, Sharoor-Karni S, Lin J, et al. Predictors of respiratory failure among previously healthy children with respiratory syncytial virus infection. *Am J Emerg Med* 2011;29:168–173.
- Medrano López C, García-Guereta L; CIVIC Study Group. Community-acquired respiratory infections in young children with congenital heart diseases in the palivizumab era: The Spanish 4-season civic epidemiologic study. *Pediatr Infect Dis J* 2010;29: 1077–1082.
- American Academy of Pediatrics Subcommittee on Diagnosis and Management of Bronchiolitis. Diagnosis and management of bronchiolitis. *Pediatrics* 2006;118:1774–1793.

 CODES

ICD9
- 079.6 Respiratory syncytial virus (rsv)
- 466.11 Acute bronchiolitis due to respiratory syncytial virus (rsv)
- 480.1 Pneumonia due to respiratory syncytial virus

CLINICAL PEARLS

- RSV is considered as the most important cause of acute lower respiratory tract infection in infants and young children.
- RSV infection also has a considerable burden in adults, particularly elderly individuals and transplant patients.
- Palivizumab may be administered for prophylaxis to patients at risk for the development of severe RSV infection.
- A potential association between early RSV infection and subsequent wheezing, asthma, and/or atopy has been suggested.

RHEUMATIC FEVER

Petros I. Rafailidis
Matthew E. Falagas

BASICS

DESCRIPTION
Rheumatic fever is a clinical syndrome that occurs following group A streptococcal pharyngitis. A constellation of signs and symptoms is associated with this illness, and they range from arthritis and atypical fleeting rashes to pancarditis with cardiac valve dysfunction (1).

EPIDEMIOLOGY
Incidence
- Rheumatic fever is a worldwide disease.
- It accounts for 40% of the heart disease in developing countries.
- Rates in the US have dropped secondary to antibiotic use.
- The estimated incidence within the US is 0.5 per 100,000.
- Rheumatic fever is a disease of the childhood, usually affecting children aged 6–15 years.
- One-third of cases occur after a subacute or asymptomatic case of group A streptococcal pharyngitis.
- The attack rate following untreated cases of streptococcal pharyngitis ranges from 0.4–3.0%.
- Epidemics of disease reflect the specific strain of *Streptococcus* present in the community.

Prevalence
In the US, the prevalence is ~2/10,000 (1) and it is more common in Hispanics.

RISK FACTORS
- Overcrowding
- History of rheumatic fever

Genetics
A variety of HLA-associations, B cell alloantigens (D 8/17 positive) or immune gene polymorphisms (TNF-a promoter) have been implicated in patients with susceptibility; however, the issue remains to be elucidated) (1).

GENERAL PREVENTION
- For streptococcal pharyngitis, penicillin treatment for 10 days prevents rheumatic fever. Penicillin can be given up to 9 days following the start of sore throat.
- Patients with a history of rheumatic fever have a high chance of developing recurrent disease and need secondary prophylaxis.
- Many possible regimes are available, including benzathine penicillin G, to be given intramuscularly every month. Alternatives also include sulfadiazine orally, penicillin VK orally, or erythromycin orally.
- Patients with valvular disease require antibiotic prophylaxis for dental procedures.

PATHOPHYSIOLOGY
Molecular mimicry between *Streptococcus* group A infections and host tissues elicits a generalized autoimmune response (2)

ETIOLOGY
- Group A streptococcal pharyngitis initiates rheumatic fever. The incubation time is 1–5 weeks, with an average of 19 days.
- Specific strains (including 1, 3, 5, 6, and 18) have been associated with this disease.
- Pathogenesis is related to antibodies that cross-react between streptococcal antigens and heart valves.

DIAGNOSIS

HISTORY
- Patients may report a variety of symptoms such as: Fever, skin manifestations and involuntary movements, fatigue, dyspnea, and ankle edema.
- The diagnosis of rheumatic fever is a clinical diagnosis, and there are many diseases with which it may be confused. This is especially true if the rheumatic fever is chronic or recurrent, in which case, manifestations may be less obvious.
- Clinical diagnosis is made with two major criteria, or one major criteria and two minor criteria plus laboratory confirmed evidence of antecedent streptococcal infection.
- The symptoms, if untreated, last an average of 3 months but may last up to 6 months in the case of carditis.

PHYSICAL EXAM
Major Criteria
- Polyarthritis in 75%
- Carditis in 50%
- Chorea in 15%
- Subcutaneous nodules in fewer than 10%
- Erythema marginatum in fewer than 10%

Polyarthritis
- Rheumatic fever often begins with fevers and polyarthritis.
- It involves the knees, ankles, elbows, and wrists. Most children have multiple joints involved. They may have arthralgias or frank arthritis.
- Symptoms resolve within 1 month.

Carditis
- Pancarditis may be silent.
- On occasions, patients present with congestive heart failure.
- Most acute valvular disease presents with mitral regurgitation and, to a lesser extent, aortic regurgitation.

Chorea
- Chorea is defined as irregular, purposeless (dancing-like) movement of the muscles.
- It may occur at all times of the day, and it includes the face and extremities.
- Chorea is often present, along with carditis and arthritis.

Subcutaneous Nodules
- Painless nodules appear over tendons, often near the joints.
- They may be as large as 2 cm.
- They occur often in conjunction with carditis.

Erythema Marginatum
- These irregular areas of erythema may be macular and are often present on the trunk and extremities.
- The rash is evanescent and may be hard to detect.

Minor Criteria
- Fever
- Arthralgias without frank arthritis
- Laboratory evidence that can constitute minor criteria includes a prolonged PR interval or elevated, acute-phase reactants such as an elevated erythrocyte sedimentation rate or C-reactive protein.

DIAGNOSTIC TESTS & INTERPRETATION
Lab
Initial lab tests
- Evidence of a recent streptococcal infection needs to be determined (however, this is not required for the case of Sydenham's chorea or indolent carditis).
- A positive throat culture or a serum ASO titer >200 Todd units/mL is necessary.
- Other serologic tests that should be elevated following a significant streptococcal infection include an antihyaluronidase antibody or anti-DNAse B.
- A rapid streptococcal antigen test may be positive.
- Should all serology be negative, the diagnosis needs to be questioned.

Follow-Up & Special Considerations
In acute rheumatic carditis, levels of troponin-I and of troponin T are usually normal (3,4).

Imaging
Initial approach
Echocardiography may be especially helpful to document clinical findings and detect potential pathology (5,6)

Follow-Up & Special Considerations
Echocardiography may be needed in case of deterioration.

Pathological Findings
Patients with rheumatic fever have inflammatory lesions in connective tissue and Aschoff nodules in the myocardium. This is a pancarditis involving all parts of the heart.

DIFFERENTIAL DIAGNOSIS
- Primary rheumatologic illness, such as juvenile rheumatoid arthritis and lupus.
- Infections such as Lyme disease, gonococcal arthritis, and endocarditis.
- Viral diseases such as rubella and coxsackievirus A or B.
- Other illnesses, such as drug reactions, sickle cell crisis, sarcoidosis, inflammatory bowel disease, and leukemia.
- Acute myocardial infarction (7).

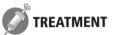

TREATMENT
MEDICATION
First Line
- Treatment with salicylates is necessary.
- Steroids are used if inflammation cannot be reduced with salicylates alone.
- Steroids are used when carditis leads to congestive heart failure.
- Aspirin is often given in high doses for 8 weeks. Start with 90 to 100 mg/kg/d and decrease after 2 weeks to 60–70 mg/kg/day. When used in conjunction with steroids (prednisone 40–60 mg/d), aspirin should be continued for 4 weeks after steroids are finished (usually steroids are given over a 1-month period).

Second Line
- Secondary prophylaxis is a mainstay in the management of rheumatic fever. Compliance with this is a crucial factor regarding prognosis of rheumatic fever.
- In rheumatic fever with carditis and residual valvular pathology, prophylaxis should be provided for 10 years or until the patient is 40 years old (select the longest duration option), while some patient will need lifelong prophylaxis (depending on the probability of being exposed to group A streptococci [teachers, children, and closed community residents] and the multitude of previous attacks.
- In case there is carditis but without remaining cardiac pathology, prophylaxis for 10 years or up to when the patient is 21 years old (select the longest duration option).
- In case there is rheumatic fever without carditis, give prophylaxis for 5 years or up to when the patient is 21 years old (whichever is longer).
- Sole manifestation of Sydenham's chorea is sufficient to warrant prophylaxis.

ADDITIONAL TREATMENT
Issues for Referral
Failure of medical treatment needs prompt referral to a cardiothoracic surgeon.

Additional Therapies
Extracorporeal support (8) may be a valuable intermediate management option before surgery (if needed).

SURGERY/OTHER PROCEDURES
- Rheumatic fever remains a significant cause of need for cardiac surgery.
- Cusp extension of the aortic valve for aortic insufficiency (9).
- Mitral valve commissurotomy is among the most common procedures performed. For patients surviving over 20 years, reoperation is needed (8).

IN-PATIENT CONSIDERATIONS
Admission Criteria
- Patients with signs of carditis, Sydenham's chorea, or severe symptomatology.
- Gastrointestinal bleeding due to therapy.

Discharge Criteria
- Symptom control
- No heart failure

ONGOING CARE
FOLLOW-UP RECOMMENDATIONS
In patients with carditis, follow up with the pediatrician and pediatric cardiologist.

Patient Monitoring
Echocardiography monitoring may be needed in cases of carditis.

PATIENT EDUCATION
Education regarding secondary prophylaxis

PROGNOSIS
- ~14.8 per 100,000 of hospitalized children annually for acute rheumatic fever with a median length of hospital stay of 3 days and an in-hospital mortality of 0.6% (10).
- Recurrences may occur.

COMPLICATIONS
- Valve dysfunction, leading to refractory heart failure.
- Patients may develop endocarditis.

REFERENCES
1. Bryant PA, Robins-Browne R, Carapetis JR, et al. Some of the people, some of the time: Susceptibility to acute rheumatic fever. *Circulation* 2009;119:742–753.
2. Lee JL, Naguwa SM, Cheema GS, et al. Acute rheumatic fever and its consequences: A persistent threat to developing nations in the 21st century. *Autoimmun Rev* 2009;9:117–123.
3. Williams RV, Minich LL, Shaddy RE, et al. Evidence for lack of myocardial injury in children with acute rheumatic carditis. *Cardiol Young* 2002;12:519–523.
4. Alehan D, Ayabakan C, Hallioglu O. Role of serum cardiac troponin T in the diagnosis of acute rheumatic fever and rheumatic carditis. *Heart* 2004;90:689–690.
5. Crain FE, Pham N, Wagoner SF, et al. Fulminant valvulitis from acute rheumatic fever: Successful use of extracorporeal support. *Pediatr Crit Care Med* 2011;12:e155–158.
6. Veasy LG. Time to take soundings in acute rheumatic fever. *Lancet* 2001;357:1994–1995.
7. Boruah P, Shetty S, Kumar SS. Acute streptococcal myocarditis presenting as acute ST-elevation myocardial infarction. *J Invasive Cardiol* 2010;22:E189–E191.
8. DiBardino DJ, ElBardissi AW, McClure RS, et al. Four decades of experience with mitral valve repair: Analysis of differential indications, technical evolution, and long-term outcome. *J Thorac Cardiovasc Surg* 2010;139:76–83.
9. Myers PO, Tissot C, Christenson JT, et al. Aortic valve repair by cusp extension for rheumatic aortic insufficiency in children: Long-term results and impact of extension material. *J Thorac Cardiovasc Surg* 2010;140:836–844.
10. Miyake CY, Gauvreau K, Tani LY, et al. Characteristics of children discharged from hospitals in the United States in 2000 with the diagnosis of acute rheumatic fever. *Pediatrics* 2007;120:503–508.

ADDITIONAL READING
- Carapetis JR, McDonald M, Wilson NJ. Acute rheumatic fever. *Lancet* 2005;366:155–168.

 ## CODES
ICD9
- 034.0 Streptococcal sore throat
- 390 Rheumatic fever without mention of heart involvement

CLINICAL PEARLS
- As the disease has become rare, physicians have to remain vigilant not to miss a diagnosis of this treatable condition.
- In chronic cases, the indolent nature of the carditis should not lure the physician into a false sense of security.

ROCKY MOUNTAIN SPOTTED FEVER

Mary L. Pisculli (E. Mylonakis, Editor)

 BASICS

DESCRIPTION
Rocky Mountain spotted fever (RMSF) is an acute and often fatal tick-borne infection caused by the intracellular bacterium *Rickettsia rickettsii*.

EPIDEMIOLOGY
Incidence
- RMSF is a reportable disease in the US; approximately 500–2,100 new cases of RMSF are reported annually. Although cases were reported from 46 states and the District of Columbia during the period from 2000–2007, 5 states (North Carolina, Oklahoma, Arkansas, Tennessee, and Missouri) accounted for 64% of all RMSF cases. Few cases are from the Rocky Mountain States.
- RMSF has been documented in Canada, Mexico, and in Central and South America.

RISK FACTORS
- RMSF onset follows a seasonal trend with the majority of cases occurring during the spring and summer months when tick activity is at its peak.
- The highest incidence is in children <10 years (peak age group is 5–9 years) and among adults aged 40–64 years.
- American Indians have the highest incidence of infection compared to other ethnic/racial groups. Incidence is also high among males and whites.
- Residence in wooded areas or areas with high grass and exposure to dogs increases the risk of *R. rickettsii* infection.

Genetics
Glucose-6-phosphate dehydrogenase deficiency in African–American men is associated with fulminant RMSF.

GENERAL PREVENTION
- Avoid tick habitats such as wooded areas, high grass fields, and stream banks.
- Frequently check for any attached ticks and wear protective clothing when venturing into tick-infested habitats. Consider the use of tick repellants such as DEET and permethrin.
- Remove attached ticks properly to reduce the likelihood of *R. rickettsii* transmission.
  - Grasp the tick carefully with fine forceps as close to the point of attachment as possible and pull straight outward to remove the tick.

PATHOPHYSIOLOGY
- Following inoculation by a tick bite, *R. rickettsii* enters endothelial cells and spreads contiguously to form a network of infected endothelial cells in the skin and internal organs.
  - Widespread vasculitis results in increased endothelial permeability and activation of the coagulation system causing edema, hypovolemia, and ischemia.

ETIOLOGY
- *R. rickettsii* is an obligate intracellular pleomorphic gram-negative coccobacillus that is transmitted from the salivary glands of feeding adult ticks. Transmission requires an attachment time of 4–6 hours, but may potentially require as long as 24 hours.
- The primary vectors are *Dermacentor variabilis*, the American dog tick, in the eastern two-thirds of the US and California, and *Dermacentor andersoni*, the Rocky Mountain wood tick, in the Western US.
- RMSF is also transmitted by *Rhipicephalus sanguineus*, the brown dog tick, in Mexico and Arizona, and by *Amblyomma cajennense*, the Cayenne tick, in Central and South America.

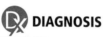 **DIAGNOSIS**

HISTORY
- The incubation period of RMSF is 2–14 days (mean, 7 days).
- The disease is initially characterized by sudden onset of fever and severe headache, usually accompanied by myalgias and malaise. Gastrointestinal complaints, including nausea, vomiting, and abdominal pain are frequently present. Neurologic manifestations may range from seizures to encephalitis.
- 30–40% of patients with RMSF do not report a history of recent tick bite.

PHYSICAL EXAM
- The classic triad of fever, rash, and history of exposure to ticks is found in only 3% during the first 3 days of illness.
- 60–70% of confirmed cases develop the triad within 2 weeks of the tick bite.

- A rash typically appears 2–5 days after the onset of fever and is initially characterized by small, blanching erythematous macules on the wrists and ankles before subsequent progression to the palms and soles. The rash then spreads to the arms, legs, and trunk and evolves into a petechial rash.
  - Onset of rash may be delayed and approximately 10% of patients do not develop a rash (Rocky Mountain "spotless" fever).
  - The rash may be difficult to detect in persons with dark skin.
- Ocular involvement includes conjunctivitis (30% of cases), retinal vein engorgement, flame hemorrhages, arterial occlusion, and papilledema.
- Neurologic manifestations (40% of cases) include lethargy, photophobia, meningismus, transient deafness, amnesia, and bizarre behavior.
- Hepatomegaly is noted in 12–25% of cases.
- Cough and pulmonary findings consistent with pneumonia have also been observed.

DIAGNOSTIC TESTS & INTERPRETATION
Lab
- A high index of suspicion is required as antibodies to *R. rickettsii* are not detectable until 7–10 days after disease onset.
- The indirect fluorescent antibody test is currently considered the gold standard serologic test for RMSF, although it cannot distinguish between infection with *R. rickettsii* and other spotted-fever rickettsiae.
  - A fourfold increase in paired samples or a convalescent titer >1:64 is considered diagnostic.
- Qualitative ELISA assays have become increasingly used in cases of suspected RMSF, although background seroprevalence for antibodies to *R. rickettsii* in the southeastern US can be as high as 20% among healthy adults.
- The most common laboratory abnormality associated with RMSF is thrombocytopenia. WBC is highly variable and has little utility in diagnosing or excluding RMSF.
- Other nonspecific laboratory abnormalities include hyponatremia, azotemia, increased serum transaminases, bilirubin, and creatinine kinase levels.

Imaging
- Chest x-ray may demonstrate focal infiltrates or interstitial edema.
- CT or MR imaging studies in cases of encephalopathy associated with RMSF may typically show generalized cerebral edema.

Diagnostic Procedures/Other
- Cerebrospinal fluid analysis is usually characterized by a lymphocytic pleocytosis.
- Electrocardiographic abnormalities range from atrial fibrillation to nonspecific ST wave changes.

Pathological Findings
The only specific test currently available to diagnose RMSF in its early stages is a direct immunofluorescence examination of skin biopsy samples for *R. rickettsii* antigens. The test is available from the Centers for Disease Control and Prevention (CDC) but is impractical and not widely used.

DIFFERENTIAL DIAGNOSIS
- Early in the illness, when medical attention usually is first sought, RMSF is difficult to distinguish from many tick-borne and non–tick-borne diseases including self-limiting viral infections, bacterial sepsis, respiratory tract infection, meningococcemia, disseminated gonococcal infection, secondary syphilis, typhoid fever, leptospirosis, ehrlichiosis, toxic shock syndrome, drug hypersensitivity, idiopathic thrombocytopenic purpura, and thrombotic thrombocytopenic purpura.
- Central nervous system infections, including bacterial and viral meningoencephalitis, should be considered in the presence of seizures, coma, and neurologic signs.

 TREATMENT

MEDICATION
First Line
- Tetracyclines are highly effective against rickettsial diseases and doxycycline is considered the drug of choice for nearly all patients.
  - Doxycycline should be administered at a dosage of 200 mg per day in 2 divided doses for adults and 2.2 mg/kg per dose given twice daily for children weighing <45 kg. The drug may be given orally or intravenously for 5–7 days and until 48 hours after the resolution of fever.

Second Line
- Chloramphenicol is the only other drug with proven efficacy for the treatment of RMSF and is the drug of choice in pregnant women.
- Chloramphenicol is administered at a dose of 50–75 mg/kg per day, divided into 4 doses, for 7 days or for at least 48 hours after the resolution of fever.

Pediatric Considerations
Both the American Academy of Pediatrics and CDC recommend doxycycline as the treatment of choice for children <9 years old for presumed or confirmed RMSF infection despite the small risk of permanent teeth staining with brief courses of tetracyclines.

Pregnancy Considerations
- Chloramphenicol is the recommended treatment for suspected RMSF in pregnant women.
  - Administration of chloramphenicol to pregnant women near term may result in grey baby syndrome.
  - Life-threatening situations may necessitate the use of doxycycline in pregnancy.

IN-PATIENT CONSIDERATIONS
Initial Stabilization
- The most seriously ill patients are managed in intensive care units, with careful supportive care.
- Intravenous antibiotic administration is often indicated for hospitalized patients, particularly those with vomiting, unstable vital signs, or neurologic symptoms.
- In the most severe cases, shock results in acute tubular necrosis–induced renal failure, which may require hemodialysis.

Admission Criteria
Approximately one-fourth of patients with suspected RMSF require hospitalization. Patients with neurologic symptoms, elevated creatinine, vomiting, or unstable vital signs should be admitted to the hospital if RMSF is suspected.

 ONGOING CARE

PROGNOSIS
- In the US, 5% of confirmed cases of RMSF have a fatal outcome and fatality rates of 20% have been reported for untreated cases. Age >60 years, delay in antibiotic treatment beyond the first 5 days of illness, lack of tetracycline treatment, treatment with chloramphenicol only, presence of neurologic symptoms, and an elevated serum creatinine are each associated with increased mortality.
- Delays in diagnosis are associated with increased rates of fatality for RMSF; the decision to treat should not be delayed awaiting laboratory confirmation.
- Although survivors of RMSF usually return to their previous state of health, patients who have been severely ill may sustain permanent sequelae, including neurologic deficits, and may need to have gangrenous extremities amputated.

COMPLICATIONS
Life-threatening complications of RMSF include meningitis/encephalitis, renal failure, adult respiratory distress syndrome, and coagulopathy.

ADDITIONAL READING
- Chapman AS, Bakken JS, Folk SM, et al. Diagnosis and management of tick-borne rickettsial diseases: Rocky Mountain spotted fever, ehrlichiosis, and anaplasmosis – United States: A practical guide for physicians and other health-care and public health professionals. *MMWR Recomm Rep* 2006; 55(RR-1):1–27.
- Dantas-Torres F. Rocky Mountain spotted fever. *Lancet Infec Dis* 2007;7(1):724–732.
- Minniear TD, Buckingham SC. Managing Rocky Mountain spotted fever. *Expert Rev Anti Infec Ther* 2009;7(9):1131–1137.
- Sexton DJ, Kaye KS. Rocky Mountain spotted fever. *Med Clin North Am* 2002;86(2):351–360.
- Anonymous. Case records of the Massachusetts General Hospital. Weekly clinicopathological exercises. Case 32–1997. A 43-year-old woman with rapidly changing pulmonary infiltrates and markedly increased intracranial pressure. *N Engl J Med* 1997;337:1149–1156.
- Conlon PJ, Procop GW, Fowler V, et al. Predictors of prognosis and risk of acute renal failure in patients with Rocky Mountain spotted fever. *Am J Med* 1996;101:621–626.
- Drage LA. Life-threatening rashes: Dermatologic signs of four infectious diseases. *Mayo Clin Proc* 1999;74:68–72.
- Spach DH, Liles WC, Campbell GL, et al. Tick-borne diseases in the United States. *N Engl J Med* 1993;329:936–947.
- Walker D, Raoult D, Brouqui P, et al. Rickettsia, mycoplasma, and chlamydia. In: Fauci AS, Braunwald E, Isselbacher KJ, et al., eds. *Harrison's principles of internal medicine*, 14th ed. New York: McGraw-Hill, 1998:1045–1052.

 CODES

ICD9
082.0 Spotted fevers

CLINICAL PEARLS
- Rash may not be apparent for several days after onset of symptoms and 10% of patients may never exhibit a rash.
- Early clinical (and epidemiologic) diagnosis is critical.
- Doxycycline is the drug of choice for treating suspected cases of RMSF, even in children.

ROUNDWORMS, INTESTINAL

Abiola C. Senok
Atef M. Shibl
Paschalis Vergidis
Matthew E. Falagas

 BASICS

DESCRIPTION
Roundworms are clinically important intestinal nematodes transmitted to humans by the ingestion of contaminated food or by skin penetration following contact with contaminated soil.

EPIDEMIOLOGY
Prevalence
- Trichuriasis
  - Worldwide infection with estimated 800 million cases
  - In the US, infections occurs mainly in the rural southeastern states
  - Humans are the principal host
  - Prevalent in poor communities with poor sanitary conditions
- Enterobiasis
  - Worldwide distribution but more prevalent in temperate regions
  - Most common helminthic infection in the US with estimated 40 million cases
  - Spans all socioeconomic classes and prevalent in group or overcrowded settings
  - Children are mostly affected and infection sspreads rapidly to other household members
- Ascariasis
  - Most common human helminthic infection affecting 1 billion people globally
  - Worldwide distribution
  - Prevalent in rural areas of Southeastern US
  - Infection mainly seen in young children
- Hookworm infection
  - Seen in tropical and subtropical regions
  - Second commonest human helminthic infection
  - Affects up to 25% of the world population
- Strongyloidiasis
  - Distribution in tropical and subtropical areas
  - More prevalent in rural areas, institutional settings, and lower socioeconomic groups.

RISK FACTORS
- Ingestion of food contaminated with ova
- Contact with contaminated soil

GENERAL PREVENTION
- Proper hand washing after defecation and before handling food
- Proper washing, peeling, or cooking of all fresh fruits and vegetables before consumption
- Proper disposal of sewage
- For hookworm infection and strongyloidiasis, proper foot wear particularly when there is contact with potentially contaminated soil

PATHOPHYSIOLOGY
- Trichuriasis
  - Contact with mature eggs occurs through contaminated soil
  - Ingested eggs hatch in the intestine and larvae migrate to the cecum
  - Adult worm resides in the cecum and ascending colon
  - Life span of adult worm is about 1 year
- Enterobiasis
  - Adult worm resides in the terminal ileum and cecum. Migrates to the perineal area to lay eggs during the night
  - Pruritus leads to scratching and auto-reinfection
  - Person-to-person transmission through handling of contaminated clothes or bed linen
  - Life span of adult worm is about 2 months
- Ascariasis
  - Largest human intestinal nematode. Adult worms measure up to 35 cm
  - Eggs passed in stool remain in the soil and become infectious in 3–12 weeks; eggs can survive in soil for years
  - Ingested eggs hatch to give the rhabditiform larvae. These penetrate the small bowel, migrate by the bloodstream into the lungs and break out into the alveoli. They are swallowed and develop into adults in the small intestine
  - Reside in the small intestine with a life span of 1–2 years

- Hookworm infection
  - Larvae in contaminated soil enter the patient by skin penetration. They migrate to the lung through the bloodstream where they penetrate the alveoli. The larvae are then swallowed and hook on to the small intestinal mucosa
  - Adult worms are 1 cm long and can live for decades
- Strongyloidiasis
  - Rhabditiform larvae are shed in stool and develop in the soil into infectious filariform larvae or adult free-living worms
  - Infection occurs by skin penetration following contact with contaminated soil
  - Autoinfection occurs when rhabditiform larvae transform into infective filariform larval form in the intestine
  - Filariform larvae penetrate the bowel wall, migrate to the lungs in the bloodstream, penetrate through the alveoli, and are swallowed
  - Adult worm lives in the upper small intestine

ETIOLOGY
- *Trichuris trichiura* or whipworm
- *Enterobius vermicularis* or pinworm
- *Ascaris lumbricoides*
- *Necator americanus* and *Ankylostoma duodenale* cause hookworm infections
- *Strongyloides stercoralis*

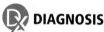 **DIAGNOSIS**

DIAGNOSTIC TESTS & INTERPRETATION
Lab
- Trichuriasis
  - Stool microscopy for characteristic ova (thick-shelled with a pair of polar plugs)
- Enterobiasis
  - Cellophane-tape slide (scotch-tape) test for identification of the characteristic elongated oval shaped eggs

- Ascariasis
  - Stool microscopy for eggs that are rounded and thick shelled
  - Eosinophilia during the pulmonary phase
- Hookworm infection
  - Stool microscopy for eggs (thin-shelled, colorless; 60–75 μm × 35–40 μm)
  - Eosinophilia during the migration phase
  - Blood tests for iron deficiency anemia
- Strongyloidiasis
  - Identification of rhabditiform larva in stool
  - Eosinophilia, which is usually present during the acute and chronic stages
  - Strongyloidiasis: Immunodiagnostic assay is indicated when the organism cannot be demonstrated in suspected infections

DIFFERENTIAL DIAGNOSIS
Rule out other intestinal helminthic infections.

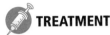 TREATMENT

MEDICATION
- Trichuriasis
  - Albendazole 400 mg PO daily for 3 days in light and moderate infections. Treat for 5–7 days for heavy infections (1).
  - Mebendazole 100 mg b.i.d PO for 3 days or 500 mg once.
- Enterobiasis
  - Albendazole 400 mg single dose PO, repeat in 2 weeks due to risk of reinfection and autoinfection.
  - Mebendazole 100 mg single dose PO repeat in 2 weeks
  - Alternative: Pyrantel pamoate 11mg/kg (max. 1 g) PO once, repeat in 2 weeks
- Ascariasis
  - Albendazole 400 mg single dose PO (2)
  - Mebendazole 100 mg b.i.d PO for 3 days
- Hookworm infection
  - Albendazole 400 mg single dose PO (2)
  - Mebendazole 100 mg b.i.d. PO for 3 days or 500 mg once
  - Alternative: Pyrantel pamoate 11 mg/kg (max. 1 g) PO for 3 days

- Strongyloidiasis
  - Ivermectin 200 μg/kg/d PO for 2 days, may repeat course in 14 days (3).
  - Albendazole 400 mg PO daily for 3 days, may repeat course in 14–21 days
  - Alternative: Thiabendazole 25 mg/kg b.i.d PO for 2 days
  - Hyperinfection cases should be treated with ivermectin for 7–14 days

 ONGOING CARE

FOLLOW-UP RECOMMENDATIONS
- Follow-up stool analysis to ensure worm has been eradicated and to detect any reinfection
- For enterobiasis, all family members should be treated. All bed linen should be washed.

PATIENT EDUCATION
Understand general preventive measures

PROGNOSIS
Prognosis is good with early diagnosis and adequate antihelminthic drugs

COMPLICATIONS
- Trichuriasis
  - Painful rectal prolapse in patients with heavy worm burden
- Enterobiasis
  - Perianal excoriations and bacterial superinfection
  - Ectopic disease with migration of adult worms to the female genital tract and abdominal cavity
- Ascariasis
  - Intestinal obstruction
  - Malnutrition
- Hookworm infection
  - Severe iron deficiency anemia
  - Malabsorption and failure to thrive
- Strongyloidiasis
  - Hyperinfection syndrome in immunocompromised patients
  - Sepsis and abdominal pain as a consequence of microperforation of intestine by migrating larvae

REFERENCES

1. Sirivichayakul C, Pojjaroen-Anant C, Wisetsing P, et al. The effectiveness of 3, 5 or 7 days of albendazole for the treatment of *Trichuris trichiura* infection. *Ann Trop Med Parasitol* 2003;97(8): 847–853.
2. Keiser J, Utzinger J. Efficacy of current drugs against soil-transmitted helminth infections: Systematic review and meta-analysis. *JAMA* 2008;299(16):1937–1948.
3. Marti H, Haji HJ, Savioli L, et al. A comparative trial of a single-dose ivermectin versus three days of albendazole for treatment of *Strongyloides stercoralis* and other soil-transmitted helminth infections in children. *Am J Trop Med Hyg* 1996; 55(5):477–481.

ADDITIONAL READING

- Greiner K, Bettencourt J, Semolic C, et al. Strongyloidiasis: A review and update by case example. *Clin Lab Sci* 2008;21:82–88.
- Horton J. Human gastrointestinal helminth infections: Are they now neglected diseases? *Trends Parasitol* 2003;19:527–531.

 CODES

ICD9
- 127.0 Ascariasis
- 127.3 Trichuriasis
- 127.4 Enterobiasis

CLINICAL PEARLS

- Hookworms are distributed globally. Prevalence is higher in poor communities.
- Complications may arise due to migratory larval forms or in heavy worm infestations.
- Prognosis is good with early diagnosis and adequate antihelminthic drugs

R

RUBELLA (GERMAN MEASLES)

Petros I. Rafailidis
Matthew E. Falagas

 BASICS

DESCRIPTION
Rubella, or German measles, is an infection due to an enveloped RNA virus of the togavirus family.

EPIDEMIOLOGY
Incidence
- Approximately 1/100,000 in the US. The disease is seen in groups of people who are unvaccinated or in people who immigrate from developing countries.
- The worldwide incidence of rubella has decreased by 82% during the last decade (1).

Prevalence
- Since 1969, when the vaccine for rubella became available, it has become a very rare disease (almost near elimination in the US)
- In areas where vaccination is not adhered to, the disease is often seen in young adults.

RISK FACTORS
The greatest risk factor is not having been vaccinated for this disease.

GENERAL PREVENTION
- Live attenuated vaccine was licensed in 1969.
- At present, vaccine is given twice in childhood as a measles–mumps–rubella vaccine (MMR): At age 1 year, and again when starting school, at age 4–6 years.
- Serologic screening should be done for women prior to marriage and at the first prenatal visit.
- If the prenatal serology reveals no history of previous infection or immunization, the patient should be checked again after delivery and revaccinated if it still negative.
- The vaccine is not given to seronegative pregnant women.
- The vaccine is safe for HIV-positive women, but it should not be given to women on chemotherapy or those having bone marrow transplants.
- Avoid pregnancy for 28 days after vaccination against rubella (2)[A].

- In case of inadvertent vaccination against rubella during pregnancy, the woman should be counseled regarding the theoretical risks of vaccination. However, the vaccination should not automatically lead to pregnancy termination (3).
- Patients with rubella should be isolated for up to 1 week after the rash appears.
- The use of immunoglobulin as prophylaxis against rubella in a seronegative pregnant woman is dubious and cannot be justified.

PATHOPHYSIOLOGY
Incubation is from 2–3 weeks.

ETIOLOGY
- Rubella is spread as an upper respiratory infection.
- It is a childhood disease, with a peak incidence between the ages of 5 and 14 years.
- The disease is mild in nature, but it can be devastating to the fetus in utero.
- The risk of developing congenital rubella is greatest in the first 16 weeks of gestation. The mother may be asymptomatic.
- Disease in the fetus or neonate can be transient, permanent, or delayed.
- Infants with congenital rubella shed virus for as long as 2 years after birth.

DIAGNOSIS

HISTORY
Patients note a mild, nonspecific upper respiratory infection syndrome with fevers and coryza.

PHYSICAL EXAM
- After this acute phase, patients may have red macules on the soft palate, followed by a morbilliform rash on the face, often starting in the posterior auricular region. This spreads down over the entire body over the next 2 days and coalesces. The rash may be pruritic. Lymphadenopathy in the postauricular and occipital regions is common early in the infection (4).

- Conjunctivitis
- Following the rash, the patient may develop arthralgias, which last 5–10 days or longer.
- Manifestations of congenital rubella syndrome (5), which may be progressive over the first 5 years of life, include the following:
  - Stillbirth
  - Growth retardation
  - Mental retardation
  - Deafness
  - Cataracts
  - Retinopathy
  - Patent ductus arteriosus
  - Pulmonary artery hypoplasia
  - Hepatosplenomegaly
  - Diabetes
  - Thyroid disorders

DIAGNOSTIC TESTS & INTERPRETATION
Lab
Initial lab tests
The white blood cell count may be low, with increased atypical lymphocytes.

Follow-Up & Special Considerations
- Serology is used most often for confirmation of the diagnosis (6).
- IgM antibodies can be detected a few days into the illness and for up to 1 month following the rash.
- False–positives may be noted for most serologic tests. Infections due to measles, CMV, EBV, parvovirus, and rheumatoid factor may give false–positive IgM for rubella.
- An IgG avidity is helpful to differentiate reinfection from primary infection (7).
- A positive serologic test has to be confirmed by PCR or Western Blot in case the diagnosis has clinical implications (termination of pregnancy) (8).

- PCR in oral fluid is positive during the disease and is especially helpful for the first 2–4 days after the initial manifestation of the rash. However, PCR may miss some cases (9). Oral fluid testing for IgM, IgG antibodies is also a helpful tool.
- Cultures of the throat, nasopharynx, or amniotic fluid can be performed in some laboratories (10).
- A PCR assay for detection of viral RNA in blood, amniotic fluid, or fetal blood or fetal cord blood is available.

DIFFERENTIAL DIAGNOSIS
- Enterovirus
- Parvovirus B19
- HIV
- Measles
- Scarlet fever
- Drug reactions

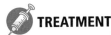 TREATMENT

MEDICATION
There is no treatment for rubella or congenital rubella.

 ONGOING CARE

FOLLOW-UP RECOMMENDATIONS
- Children with the congenital rubella syndrome require close follow-up by pediatric specialists.
- In addition, when hospitalized, patients need to be isolated until the virus is no longer being shed.

PATIENT EDUCATION
A new quadruple vaccine (MMRV) which in addition to the protection provided by the MMR vaccine is also active against varicella is available.

This is preferred as first dose for children >4 years and as the second dose for any age between 15 months-12 years. It can also be administered as a first dose at the age of 12–47 months; however, a twofold relative risk for febrile convulsions has been reported at this younger age and the CDC recommends separate vaccinations for the first dose in this age group (i.e., MMR followed by Varicella vaccination instead of MMRV).

PROGNOSIS
Prognosis is excellent for the vast majority of patients with rubella, except for the congenital form.

COMPLICATIONS
- Congenital rubella is a serious multisystem disease, and the option of therapeutic abortion should be considered when a pregnant woman develops it; a firm and rapid diagnosis is needed (11). Deafness is the most common complication.
- Acute disseminated encephalomyelitis is a very rare complication (12).
- Thrombocytopenia

REFERENCES

1. Centers for Disease Control and Prevention (CDC). Progress toward control of rubella and prevention of congenital rubella syndrome—worldwide, 2009. *MMWR Morb Mortal Wkly Rep* 2010; 59:1307–1310.
2. CDC. Notice to readers: Revised ACIP recommendation for avoiding pregnancy after receiving a rubella-containing vaccine. *MMWR Morb Mortal Wkly Rep* 2001;50:1117.
3. CDC. General recommendations on immunization: Recommendations of the Advisory Committee on Immunization Practices (ACIP). *MMWR Morb Mortal Wkly Rep* 2006;55:32–33.
4. Chantler JK, Ford DK, Tingle AJ. Persistent rubella infection and rubella-associated arthritis. *Lancet* 1982;1:1323–1325.
5. Cooper LZ. The history and medical consequences of rubella. *Rev Infect Dis* 1985;7(Suppl 1):S2–S10.
6. Canepa P, Valle L, Cristina E, et al. Role of congenital rubella reference laboratory: 21-months-surveillance in Liguria, Italy. *J Prev Med Hyg* 2009;50:221–226.
7. Bellin E, Safyer S, Braslow C. False positive IgM-rubella enzyme-linked immunoassay in three first trimester pregnant patients. *Pediatr Infect Dis J* 1990;9:671–672.
8. Grüninger T, Wunderli W, Böhlen-Bodmer AE, et al. False rubella diagnosis in pregnancy by IgM enzyme immunoassay. *Gynakol Geburtshilfliche Rundsch* 1992;32:208–210.
9. Hofmann J, Liebert UG. Significance of avidity and immunoblot analysis for rubella IgM-positive serum samples in pregnant women. *J Virol Methods* 2005;130:66–71.
10. Manikkavasagan G, Bukasa A, Brown KE, et al. Oral fluid testing during 10 years of rubella elimination, England and Wales. *Emerg Infect Dis* 2010;16:1532–1538.
11. Levin MJ, Oxman MN, Moore MG, et al. Diagnosis of congenital rubella in utero. *N Engl J Med* 1974;290:1187.
12. Noorbakhsh F, Johnson RT, Emery D, et al. Acute disseminated encephalomyelitis: Clinical and pathogenesis features. *Neurol Clin* 2008;26: 759–780, ix.

ADDITIONAL READING

- Forrest JM, Turnbull FM, Sholler GF, et al. Gregg's congenital rubella patients 60 years later. *Med J Aust* 2002;177:664–667.
- Ainsworth E, Debenham P, Carrol ED, et al. Referrals for MMR immunisation in hospital. *Arch Dis Child* 2010;95:639–641.

 CODES

ICD9
056.9 Rubella without mention of complication

CLINICAL PEARLS

- The role of vaccination against rubella is paramount and has resulted to near elimination of the disease.
- A vaccinated person may still be afflicted by rubella rarely.
- The vaccine has to be given subcutaneously. Inadvertent intramuscular injection counts as a dose administration and does not have to be repeated.
- Only the diluent for the vaccine is appropriate, so do not use distilled water instead.
- After the 16th week of pregnancy, the risk for rubella infection of the fetus is negligible, if any.
- A child allergic to eggs can still receive the vaccine with specialist advice, but not necessarily in the hospital environment.
- Administration of other live vaccines can be given at the same day with that of MMR. However, if this is not the case then a 4 week period must apart the 2 vaccinations. The same holds true for the tuberculin skin testing.

SCABIES

Abdul Ghafur
Matthew E. Falagas

 BASICS

DESCRIPTION
Scabies is an infestation by the mite *Sarcoptes scabiei var hominis*.

EPIDEMIOLOGY
- Worldwide annual prevalence has been estimated at 300 million cases, although no consensus exists about this number (1).
- There are approximately 1 million cases of scabies in the US annually.
- 1–10% of the global population is estimated to be infected with scabies.
- Both genders, all ages, and all socioeconomic and ethnic groups are affected.
- More common in the developing world.

RISK FACTORS
Crusted (Norwegian) scabies more common in men who have sex with men, HTLV-1 infection, corticosteroid therapy, malnutrition, and Down syndrome.

Genetics
No genetic predisposition.

GENERAL PREVENTION
- Treatment of infested patients and contacts
- Hot wash, dry sterilization, or disposal of the clothing and bedding.
- Better hygiene and healthcare provisions for the less privileged.
- Observe safe-sex precautions.
- Avoid contact with an infected person.

PATHOPHYSIOLOGY
- Female mites burrow into the skin, lay eggs, larvae develop, and mature to adult mites.
- Incubation period is 3–6 weeks in initial infestations, but can be as short as a few days in re-infestations.

ETIOLOGY
Scabies mite spread by close direct contact and also through fomites.

COMMONLY ASSOCIATED CONDITIONS
More common in immunocompromised, institutionalized elderly, homeless and mentally retarded.

 DIAGNOSIS

HISTORY
Intense, generalized itching, worse at night.

PHYSICAL EXAM
- Scratch marks, erythematous papules, and linear burrows are found in interdigital areas (finger and toe webs) flexor aspects of wrists, elbows, axillae, periumbilical skin, pelvic girdle, buttocks, genitalia, breasts, ankle, and feet.
- Head, neck, and face are usually spared in adults. However, the hairline, forehead, and neck may be afflicted at the extremes of age (infants and the elderly).
- Norwegian scabies appears as psoriasiform papular lesions of the scalp, face, neck, hands, feet, and nails.
- Nodular scabies lesions are seen in the groin and axillae as violaceous pruritic nodules.

DIAGNOSTIC TESTS & INTERPRETATION
Lab
- Diagnosis by history and clinical examination is the norm.
- Skin scraping of the burrow may be examined under a microscope to look for the mites, mite eggs, or feces. Use a needle or blade to scrape skin from linear burrows on interdigital areas, wrists, ankles, or penis. Suspend the specimen in immersion oil. Cover with a glass coverslip. Examine under a high, dry microscope lens.
- A handheld dermoscope (10 times magnification) aids greatly in identification (2).
- Videodermoscopy may enhance diagnostic ability further (3).
- Skin biopsy in atypical cases.

DIFFERENTIAL DIAGNOSIS
- Dermatitis herpetiformis
- Drug reactions
- Eczema
- Pediculosis corporis
- Lichen planus
- Pityriasis rosea.

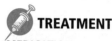 **TREATMENT**

MEDICATION
First Line
- Patient and close contacts (>2 months and nonpregnant) should be simultaneously treated, even if asymptomatic.
- 5% permethrin cream (30 g), apply from neck down, and wash off after 12 hours. Second application may be needed if living mites are observed at 2 weeks time after the first application. Not to be used for children <2 months of age (4).
- 10% crotamiton: Apply from neck down. Repeat in 48 hours. A cleansing bath is allowed 48 hours after this second application. May be repeated in 7–10 days.

- 10–25% benzoyl benzoate lotion (5).
- Precipitated sulfur (7%) in petroleum jelly is a safe therapy for very young infants, and pregnant and lactating women. It is applied on 3 consecutive days. It is left on for 24 hours after application and then washed off before the next application (4).

Second Line
- 1% lindane: Use only if other measures have failed (including no tolerance of treatment). Use only in adults >50 kg: 30 mL will suffice for the application of a thin layer of the medication from the neck downward, while 60 mL may be needed for larger body size adults. Due to neurotoxicity concerns, do not use in adults weighing <50 kg. Use is not recommended in the elderly, adolescents, and children (4).
- Oral ivermectin 200 μg/kg with optional second dose after 2 weeks (6). Not FDA approved in the US. Not recommended for children under 6 yrs of age.

ADDITIONAL TREATMENT
General Measures
Antihistamines for relief from itching.

Issues for Referral
- Dermatology opinion for atypical cases.
- Assessment of immune function in patients with Norwegian scabies.

Additional Therapies
- Wash clothing and bed linen in hot water.
- All carpets and upholstered furniture should be vacuumed and vacuum bags immediately discarded.

ONGOING CARE

FOLLOW-UP RECOMMENDATIONS
Patients may experience pruritus up to 2 weeks after successful treatment. If itching persists beyond this period, reassess the patient. Retreatment of the patient and contacts may be required.

DIET
Correction of malnutrition.

PATIENT EDUCATION
Patient and all close contacts should be treated simultaneously.

PROGNOSIS
95% cure rate with topical permethrin treatment.

COMPLICATIONS
- Secondary bacterial infection due to *Streptococcus pyogenes* or *Staphylococcus aureus*.
- Flaring of preexisting eczema.

REFERENCES

1. Chosidow O. Clinical practices. Scabies. *N Engl J Med* 2006;354:1718–1727.
2. Dupuy A, Dehen L, Bourrat E, et al. Accuracy of standard dermoscopy for diagnosing scabies. *J Am Acad Dermatol* 2007;56:53–62.
3. Micali G, Lacarrubba F, Tedeschi A. Videodermatoscopy enhances the ability to monitor efficacy of scabies treatment and allows optimal timing of drug application. *J Eur Acad Dermatol Venereol* 2004;18:153–154.
4. Currie BJ, McCarthy JS. Permethrin and ivermectin for scabies. *N Engl J Med* 2010;362:717–725.
5. Strong M, Johnstone PW. Interventions for treating scabies. *Cochrane Database Syst Rev* 2007;(3): CD000320.
6. Ly F, Caumes E, Ndaw CA, et al. Ivermectin versus benzyl benzoate applied once or twice to treat human scabies in Dakar, Senegal: A randomized controlled trial. *Bull World Health Organ* 2009;87:424–430.

ADDITIONAL READING

- Mytton OT, McGready R, Lee SJ, et al. Safety of benzyl benzoate lotion and permethrin in pregnancy: A retrospective matched cohort study. *BJOG* 2007;114:582–587.

 CODES

ICD9
133.0 Scabies

CLINICAL PEARLS

- Apply the medication before night sleep. Dress and linen should be washed in hot water or dry-cleaned.
- Treat the patient and the close contacts.
- Epidemics may occur in hospitals and nursing care homes.

SCARLET FEVER

Petros I. Rafailidis
Matthew E. Falagas

 BASICS

DESCRIPTION
Rash produced by erythrogenic toxin of group A *Streptococcus* typically during a case of pharyngitis.

EPIDEMIOLOGY
Incidence
- Scarlet fever often occurs in children aged 2–10 years. It is rare in adults.
- The epidemiology is similar to that of streptococcal pharyngitis.
- Only 1 in 10 patients with streptococcal pharyngitis will develop scarlet fever.

Prevalence
- The prevalence of scarlet fever has decreased significantly (1).
- However, a lifetime scarlet fever prevalence of 23.5% has been reported in Germany (2).
- Late fall through early spring in temperate-cool climate (parallels pharyngitis).

RISK FACTORS
- Wounds
- Burns
- Carrier of streptococcus (anus, pharynx), that is, surgeon, cook, and school pupils (3).
- Varicella
- Family member or close contact (roommate, military recruit).

GENERAL PREVENTION
Early treatment of streptococcal pharyngitis may abort scarlet fever and decrease the occurrence of epidemics.

PATHOPHYSIOLOGY
Enhancement by the pyrogenic exotoxin of hypersensitivity to streptococcal products (4).

ETIOLOGY
- Pyrogenic exotoxin or erythrogenic toxin A, B, C is at times produced by group A *Streptococcus*. The initial infection is often pharyngitis; however, skin infections, pelvic infections, and puerperal infections may produce the syndrome.
- Emergent strains of streptococci have been associated with recent outbreaks (5).

 DIAGNOSIS

HISTORY
- Incubation of streptococcal pharyngitis is 1–7 days.
- Fever
- Sore throat
- Diffuse muscle, joint pains
- Nausea, vomiting, abdominal pain
- History of burn or wound or recent surgical operation.

PHYSICAL EXAM
- Fever, chills
- Patients have pharyngitis or tonsillitis, with exudate and petechiae over the soft palate.
- Cervical lymphadenopathy
- Rash occurs on the second day of illness. Rash begins on the neck and upper chest and spreads over the body. Palms and soles are spared.
- When the rash is present on the face, it characteristically spares the area around the lips (perioral pallor).
- Rash is erythematous and blanches with pressure.
- Petechiae may be present.
- Pastia's lines are linear areas of deeper erythema (confluent areas of petechia) around skin folds. A positive Rumpel–Leede test may be present.
- Occasionally, a sandpaper texture is noted over the rash.
- Initially a white strawberry is noted: White coating through which the papillae emerge. This lasts for 4–5 days and then as the white coating is shed, a red "strawberry" (or raspberry) tongue is noted.
- Rash usually lasts 6–9 days.
- Desquamation occurs when the rash fades, and can last for weeks.
- Desquamation starts on the face and progresses down the trunk. Desquamation occurs on the hands and feet last. Usually lasts ~ 3 weeks.
- Of interest is the occasional presence of abdominal pain and vomiting.
- Signs of skin infection may be present instead of pharyngitis: Pyoderma.
- Careful examination of the skin is required carefully for infected wounds or burns.

DIAGNOSTIC TESTS & INTERPRETATION
Diagnostic Procedures/Other
- Clinical diagnosis in a patient with culture-positive Streptococcus pharyngitis.
- Leukocytosis can be present during the acute stages of illness.
- Eosinophilia of 5–10% is present during the desquamative phase.
- Streptococcal rapid antigen test.

Follow-Up & Special Considerations
- Serology against a variety of streptococcal antigens (including streptolysin O, hyaluronidase, DNAse) may help to make the diagnosis.
- One must be aware that antibodies to streptococcal antigens may remain elevated for a very long duration (up to years) and thus acute and convalescent antibodies titer should become fourfold.
- Pharyngeal culture.

DIFFERENTIAL DIAGNOSIS
- Viral rash
- Drug rash
- Toxic shock syndrome (hemodynamic instability and multisystem involvement)
- Kawasaki syndrome
- Sunburn
- Staphylococcal scarlet fever (6)
- Yersinia enterocolitica infection

TREATMENT

MEDICATION

- For pharyngitis, penicillin for 10 days or erythromycin for 10 days is sufficient.
- Clindamycin or amoxicillin-clavulanate are valuable agents in case there is no improvement with penicillin.

IN-PATIENT CONSIDERATIONS

Initial Stabilization
Treat an asymptomatic carrier if there is an outbreak in closed community (school, military, or hospital).

Admission Criteria
- If complications of scarlet fever arise.
- Associated with surgery.
- Associated with puerperal or pelvic infection.
- If streptococcal toxic shock has not been excluded.

Nursing
- If hospitalization is needed patient is not contagious after 24 hours of antibiotic treatment.
- Transmission is through respiratory droplets.

ONGOING CARE

FOLLOW-UP RECOMMENDATIONS
Only if deterioration occurs despite treatment: Need to exclude streptococcal toxic shock.

PROGNOSIS
- Is excellent, if treated appropriately. Scarlet fever after trauma.
- Severe illness leading to death is very rare if antibiotics are given early in the disease.
- Recurrences of scarlet fever may occur (7).

COMPLICATIONS

- Acute rheumatic fever can occur after any streptococcal pharyngitis (~3 weeks later).
- Acute glomerulonephritis (~10 days to 2 weeks later after pharyngitis or skin infection, associated with streptococcal glyceraldehyde-3-phosphate-dehydrogenase, streptococcal pyrogenic exotoxin B, and its zymogen precursor) (8)
- Peripharyngeal abscess
- Retropharyngeal abscess
- Otitis media
- Mastoiditis
- Meningitis
- Pneumonia
- Bacteremia
- Osteomyelitis
- Periprosthetic breast abscess (9)
- Hepatitis (10)
- Gallbladder hydrops

REFERENCES

1. Duncan CJ, Duncan SR, Scott S. The dynamics of scarlet fever epidemics in England and Wales in the 19th century. *Epidemiol Infect* 1996;117:493–499.
2. Kamtsiuris P, Atzpodien K, Ellert U, et al. Prevalence of somatic diseases in German children and adolescents. Results of the German Health Interview and Examination Survey for Children and Adolescents (KiGGS). *Bundesgesundheitsblatt Gesundheitsforschung Gesundheitsschutz* 2007;50:686–700.
3. Yang SG, Dong HJ, Li FR, et al. Report and analysis of a scarlet fever outbreak among adults through food-borne transmission in China. *J Infect* 2007;55:419–424.
4. Wannamaker LW. Streptococcal toxins. *Rev Infect Dis* 1983;5(Suppl 4):S723–S732.
5. Su YF, Wang SM, Lin YL, et al. Changing epidemiology of Streptococcus pyogenes emm types and associated invasive and noninvasive infections in Southern Taiwan. *J Clin Microbiol* 2009;47:2658–2661.
6. Lo WT, Tang CS, Chen SJ, et al. Panton-Valentine leukocidin is associated with exacerbated skin manifestations and inflammatory response in children with community-associated staphylococcal scarlet fever. *Clin Infect Dis* 2009;49:e69–e75.
7. Chiesa C, Pacifico L, Nanni F, et al. Recurrent attacks of scarlet fever. *Arch Pediatr Adolesc Med* 1994;148:656–660.
8. Rodríguez-Iturbe B, Batsford S. Pathogenesis of poststreptococcal glomerulonephritis a century after Clemens von Pirquet. *Kidney Int* 2007;71:1094–1104.
9. Persichetti P, Langella M, Marangi GF, et al. Periprosthetic breast abscess caused by Streptococcus pyogenes after scarlet fever. *Ann Plast Surg* 2008;60:21–23.
10. Elishkewitz K, Shapiro R, Amir J, et al. Hepatitis in scarlet fever. *Isr Med Assoc J* 2004;6:569–570.

ADDITIONAL READING

- Hahn RG, Knox LM, Forman TA. Evaluation of poststreptococcal illness. *Am Fam Physician* 2005;71:1949–1954.
- Stevens DL, Tanner MH, Winship J, et al. Severe group A streptococcal infections associated with a toxic shock-like syndrome and scarlet fever toxin A. *N Engl J Med* 1989;321:1–7.
- Warrack JS. The differential diagnosis of scarlet fever, measles and rubella. *Br Med J* 1918;2:486–488.

 CODES

ICD9
- 034.0 Streptococcal sore throat
- 034.1 Scarlet fever

CLINICAL PEARLS

- Pay great attention in differentiating from toxic shock syndrome, which necessitates immediate hospital admission.
- It is important to include scarlet fever in the differential diagnosis of children with fever and rash.
- It is important to educate the patient that completion of treatment is absolutely necessary even if symptoms and signs are cured before the 10 day penicillin regimen.

S

SCHISTOSOMIASIS

Paschalis Vergidis
Matthew E. Falagas

 BASICS

DESCRIPTION
Schistosomiasis (or bilharziasis) is one of the most widespread parasitic infections. Humans are the principal hosts for a number of blood flukes of the class Trematoda.

EPIDEMIOLOGY
Prevalence
- Human schistosomiasis affects about 200 million people worldwide.
- *Schistosoma mansoni*
  – Found throughout Africa: Risk of infection in freshwater in southern and sub-Saharan Africa. Transmission also occurs in the Nile River valley in Sudan and Egypt.
  – South America: Including Brazil, Suriname, and Venezuela.
  – Caribbean (risk is low): Antigua, Dominican Republic, Guadeloupe, Martinique, Montserrat, and Saint Lucia.
- *Schistosoma haematobium*
  – Found throughout Africa: Risk of infection in freshwater in southern and sub-Saharan Africa. Transmission also occurs in the Nile River valley in Egypt and the Maghreb region of North Africa.
  – Found in areas of the Middle East.
- *Schistosoma japonicum* found in Indonesia and parts of China and Southeast Asia.
- *Schistosoma mekongi* found in Cambodia and Laos.
- *Schistosoma intercalatum* found in parts of Central and West Africa.

RISK FACTORS
Skin contact with freshwater containing cercarial larvae.

GENERAL PREVENTION
- Improve sanitation so that eggs do not pass into areas where snails reside.
- Reduce snail populations with molluscicides.
- Prohibit swimming in contaminated waters.

PATHOPHYSIOLOGY
- Infection in humans (definitive host) occurs when cercariae penetrate through the skin. They migrate to the venous circulation and liver and develop into adult worms.
- Worms are about 1–2 cm in length and are of separate sex. It is estimated that the worm can survive for as long as 30 years.
- *S. mansoni*, *S. japonicum*, and *S. mekongi* worms live in the terminal venules of the portal and mesenteric blood vessels.
- *S. haematobium* lives within the vesical plexus around the bladder.
- Half of the eggs pass through the bladder wall or the intestinal wall, out into the environment.
- The remainder of the eggs stays locally or passes along the blood vessels.
- Once eggs are passed into fresh water, they develop into motile miracidia that live within snails (intermediate host).
- After 4–6 weeks, the miracidia evolve into cercariae, by which they can pass into the water and infect humans.

ETIOLOGY
- *S. mansoni*, *S. japonicum*, *S. mekongi*, *S. haematobium*, and *S. intercalatum* make up the group that infects humans.
- *S. mansoni* and *S. japonicum* cause: Katayama fever, hepatic perisinusoidal egg granulomas, periportal fibrosis, portal hypertension, and occasional embolic egg granulomas in brain or spinal cord.
- *S. haematobium* causes: Hematuria, scarring, bladder calcification, squamous cell bladder carcinoma, and occasional embolic egg granulomas in brain or spinal cord.

 DIAGNOSIS

HISTORY
Acute Schistosomiasis
- Schistosome dermatitis ("swimmer's itch").
- In those exposed for the first time, the rash disappears quickly. In those previously exposed, the rash may persist.
- 2–12 weeks after infection, patients develop fevers associated with chills, headaches, myalgias, abdominal pain, and cough (Katayama fever). Occasionally, hematochezia.
- Acute disease is particularly associated with *S. mansoni*, and *S. japonicum* and occurs during oviposition due to the antigenic stimulation produced by the laying of the eggs. It resembles serum sickness.
- Neurologic disease may occur due to eosinophil toxicity with vasculitis and small vessel thrombosis.
- Symptoms regress after 2–10 weeks.

Chronic Schistosomiasis
- Chronic disease is more common in endemic areas. Disease may last many years.
- Intestinal involvement: Patients may note abdominal pain and diarrhea.
- Hepatic involvement: Over years, eggs that pass through the liver lead to formation of granulomas and portal hypertension. Over many years, patients may develop decompensated liver disease, abdominal distention due to ascites, or hematemesis due to variceal bleeding.
- Pulmonary involvement: Eggs that bypass the liver in patients with portal hypertension can lodge in the lungs and produce dyspnea due to pulmonary hypertension.
- Urinary involvement: Patients with *S. haematobium* pass eggs into the genitourinary system. Reaction to the eggs can lead to urinary obstruction, bladder dysfunction, and hematuria. Renal failure may occur as a late event.
- Genital involvement: In males, epididymis, testicles, spermatic chord, or prostate can be involved. In females, ulcerative lesions of the vulva, vagina, and cervix may occur.
- Neurologic involvement: Eggs of *S. japonicum* can pass into vessels of the brain, causing seizures, or into the spinal cord, causing transverse myelitis.

PHYSICAL EXAM
Acute Schistosomiasis
- Urticaria followed by a maculopapular skin rash, lasting 24–48 hours, occurs in the location of the skin penetration by the cercariae ("swimmer's itch").
- Hepatosplenomegaly
- Diffuse lymphadenopathy

Chronic Schistosomiasis
- Abdominal tenderness
- Hepatomegaly from granulomas around embolized eggs
- Ascites
- Heme-positive stool
- Paralysis (with spinal cord involvement)

DIAGNOSTIC TESTS & INTERPRETATION
Lab
Initial lab tests
- Liver function tests are frequently normal.
- Eosinophilia is observed in most cases.
- Anemia due to chronic blood loss is mild.
- Eggs can be isolated from the urine or stool of infected patients.
  – Microscopy is useful for species detection.
  – Maximal egg excretion occurs between 10 am–2 pm.
  – Simple smear can detect heavy infections. Concentration or repeated examinations are usually needed.
    ○ *S. mansoni* eggs have a prominent lateral spine.
    ○ *S. haematobium* eggs have a prominent terminal spine.
    ○ *S. japonicum* eggs have a small inconspicuous spine.
    ○ *S. mekongi* eggs resemble those of *S. japonicum* but are smaller.
    ○ *S. intercalatum* has a terminal spine but is larger than *S. haematobium*.
- Serologic antibody tests are available. These cannot distinguish recent from past infections. Tests are not standardized.
  – Falcon assay screening test–enzyme-linked immunosorbent assay (FAST-ELISA) is 99% specific for all species and has a sensitivity of 99% for *S. mansoni* infection, 95% for *S. haematobium*, but less than 50% for *S. japonicum*.
  – If concern for *S. haematobium* and *S. japonicum* infections, use immunoblots with species-specific antigens.
  – In acute disease, serologic tests may become positive before egg excretion.
  – Reagent strip to detect schistosome antigens in urine has sensitivity >85%.
- PCR to detect schistosome DNA in stool or urine. In one study, sensitivity was 94.4%, specificity 99.9%.

Follow-Up & Special Considerations
- In chronic disease, test for coinfection with hepatitis B or C.
- In HIV infected patients, treatment of schistosomiasis leads to a decrease in HIV viral load and an increase in CD4 cell counts.

Imaging
- Abdominal ultrasound may reveal periportal fibrosis and hepatosplenomegaly in late *S. japonicum* and *S. mansoni* infections.
- Plain radiography may show calcification of the bladder wall in *S. haematobium* infections ("fetal head" calcification).
- Renal ultrasound may reveal hydroureter and hydronephrosis.
- Intravenous pyelogram may show ureteric strictures.
- CT or MRI of brain/spine in suspected neurologic involvement.

Diagnostic Procedures/Other
Endoscopy for esophageal varices.

Pathological Findings
In chronic disease: Periportal or Symmers "pipestem" hepatic fibrosis occurs after years of infection.

DIFFERENTIAL DIAGNOSIS
- Visceral larva migrans
- Paragonimiasis
- Clonorchiasis
- Visceral leishmaniasis

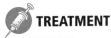
TREATMENT

MEDICATION
All infected patients should be treated since worms can survive for years.

First Line
- Praziquantel 20 mg/kg twice per day in 4-hour intervals for 1 day for *S. mansoni* and *S. haematobium*.
- Praziquantel 20 mg/kg 3 times per day in 4-hour intervals for 1 day for *S. mekongi* and *S. japonicum*.
- Praziquantel cures more than 80% of infections (1). Concerns about drug resistance have been raised (2).

Pregnancy Considerations
Praziquantel should be administered in endemic areas (3). Would defer treatment until after the first trimester.

Second Line
- Metrifonate 10 mg/kg orally every 14 days for 3 doses. No longer routinely used.
- Oxamniquine 15 mg/kg orally twice daily for 2 days. No longer routinely used.

ADDITIONAL TREATMENT
Additional Therapies
- Adjunctive use of glucocorticoids is considered in Katayama fever and neurologic disease.
- Propranolol and/or sclerotherapy for esophageal varices.

ONGOING CARE

FOLLOW-UP RECOMMENDATIONS
- Following treatment, patients should be observed for ongoing liver disease and genitourinary dysfunction.
- Single treatment is usually curative. Repeat treatment may occasionally be required after 2–4 weeks.
- Re-treatment is also indicated if reexposure and re-infection.

Patient Monitoring
- After therapy, monitor eosinophil count and examine stool or urine for eggs.
- Serologic test remains positive for prolonged periods post treatment.

PATIENT EDUCATION
Educate travelers or those living in endemic areas to reduce exposure risk.

PROGNOSIS
- Most patients improve with treatment.
- Heavy infection during acute schistosomiasis may be fatal.
- Patients with chronic schistosomiasis who are coinfected with hepatitis B or C have worse prognosis.
- Death may occur due to liver failure or due to variceal bleeding.

COMPLICATIONS
- Potential coinfections:
  – Recurrent bacteremia
  – Typhoid or non-typhoidal salmonellosis. Illness is indolent with persistent fever.
  – Hepatitis B, C
  – Malaria
  – Possible increased risk for acquisition of HIV infection
- Colonic polyposis may be caused by infection with *S. mansoni*.
- Gastrointestinal bleeding.
- Periportal hepatic fibrosis may occur due to formation of granulomas within the portal veins.
- Obstructive uropathy.
- Pulmonary hypertension.
- Cor pulmonale.
- Chronic infection with *S. haematobium* leads to squamous cell carcinoma of the bladder.
- Eggs can travel through Batson's plexus into the central nervous system and lead to myelitis.

REFERENCES
1. Berhe N, Gundersen SG, Abebe F, et al. Praziquantel side effects and efficacy related to *Schistosoma mansoni* egg loads and morbidity in primary school children in north-east Ethiopia. *Acta Trop* 1999;72(1):53–63.
2. Stelma FF, Talla I, Sow S, et al. Efficacy and side effects of praziquantel in an epidemic focus of Schistosoma mansoni. *Am J Trop Med Hyg* 1995;53(2):167–170.
3. Adam I, Elwasila E, Homeida M. Praziquantel for the treatment of schistosomiasis mansoni during pregnancy. *Ann Trop Med Parasitol* 2005;99(1):37–40.

ADDITIONAL READING
- Ross AG, Vickers D, Olds GR, et al. Katayama syndrome. *Lancet Infect Dis* 2007;7(3):218–224.
- Ross AG, Bartley PB, Sleigh AC, et al. Schistosomiasis. *N Engl J Med* 2002;346(16):1212–1220.

CODES

ICD9
120.9 Schistosomiasis, unspecified

CLINICAL PEARLS
- *S. mansoni* and *S. japonicum* may cause Katayama fever and portal hypertension.
- *S. haematobium* causes hematuria, bladder calcification, and squamous cell carcinoma.
- Demonstration of eggs in urine/stool is required for diagnosis and species identification. Serology does not distinguish between recent and past infection.

S

SEPTIC ARTHRITIS

Petros I. Rafailidis
Matthew E. Falagas

 BASICS

DESCRIPTION
Joint inflammation caused by various infectious agents: Viruses, bacteria, mycobacteria, and fungi.

EPIDEMIOLOGY
Incidence
- 4–10 per 100,000 patient-years (1). May be multifold (7–10 times higher) if preexisting rheumatoid arthritis (RA) or prosthetic joint.
- More common in children.

RISK FACTORS
- Prior arthritic condition
- Trauma or animal bites
- Diabetes
- Cancer
- Immunosuppression
- Intra-articular injections ($\sim$1 in 10,000)
- Joint surgery
- Intravenous drug use

GENERAL PREVENTION
Vaccination against *Streptococcus pneumoniae* and *Haemophilus influenzae*

PATHOPHYSIOLOGY
Invasion through trauma or extension of adjacent infection or bacteremia. Depends on the pathogen; *Staphylococcus aureus* secretes toxins and enzymes and also leads through interaction with B cells, T cells, and macrophages to secretion of interleukins and TNFa (1).

ETIOLOGY
Bacterial
- Hematogenous spread of bacteria, especially in cases of endocarditis.
- *S. aureus* leads to both monoarticular and polyarticular disease (2).
- Group A *Streptococcus* often leads to monoarticular disease.
- Group B *Streptococcus* is seen in diabetics and in elderly patients.
- *S. pneumoniae* remains an important pathogen (3).
- Gram-negative organisms are seen in elderly patients who may have had an episode of bacteremia and in immunosuppressed patients.
- *Neisseria gonorrhoeae* is the most common cause of septic arthritis in young adults.
  - Patients often present with a monoarticular process.
  - Arthralgias without frank arthritis are seen in the disseminated gonococcal syndrome.
- Lyme arthritis must be considered in patients who have had a history of tick bites and who live in endemic areas.
- Chronic monoarticular arthritis can be seen with tuberculosis, atypical mycobacterial infections, and chronic fungal infections such as *Coccidioides immitis* and *Sporothrix schenckii*.

Viral Arthritis
- Hepatitis B virus
- Rubella
- Mumps
- Varicella
- Rubeola
- Adenovirus
- Parvovirus B19

COMMONLY ASSOCIATED CONDITIONS
Rule out coexisting osteomyelitis.

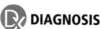 **DIAGNOSIS**

HISTORY
- Pain with limitation of joint motion
- Fever
- Swelling and red joint
- In the pediatric patient:
  - Unwillingness to move the limb (pseudoparalysis)
  - Inability to bear weight

PHYSICAL EXAM
- Fevers (not present in $\sim$20%)
- Swelling with effusions and erythema and warmth
- Knee joint affected most, followed by hip and shoulder joints.
- Infection of joints in the wrist associated with tenosynovitis suggests gonorrhea.
- Solitary joint infection in the hand may be the result of cat or other animal bites.
- Infection of the sternoclavicular of sacroiliac joints is seen in intravenous drug users.
  - Pseudomonas is often isolated.
- Viral etiology often affects multiple joints.

DIAGNOSTIC TESTS & INTERPRETATION
Lab
Initial lab tests
- Elevated erythrocyte sedimentation rate (3,4).
- Elevated C-reactive protein and procalcitonin.
- White blood cells may be increased with a polymorphonuclear predominance, or may be normal.
- Glucose in synovial fluid may be $<\frac{1}{2}$ of serum
- Anemia, if infection is chronic.
- Turbid synovial fluid with leukocyte count in synovial fluid is $>50,000$ cells/mm^3 in the majority of patients, with $>75\%$ of the cells polymorphonuclear in origin. However, one must not refute the possibility of septic arthritis if leukocytes are below the 50000 cutoff (5).
- Synovial fluid with Gram stains revealing organisms in one-third of patients.
- Synovial fluid cultures are positive in up to 90% of patients.
- PCR testing of the synovial fluid for specific organisms may be needed (i.e., *Kingella kingae*).

- Blood cultures are positive for the organism causing the septic arthritis in one-third of patients.
- Positive triple-phase bone scan
- Note: The scan can reveal a probable osteomyelitis, but it cannot resolve whether the process is infectious (neoplastic or traumatic) or whether the process has entered the joint.

Follow-Up & Special Considerations
- ESR and serum CRP levels.
- Repeat examination of the synovial fluid may be required not only for therapeutic but also for diagnostic reasons.

Imaging
Initial approach
- x-rays show
  - Periarticular soft-tissue swelling
  - Fat-pad edema
  - Joint-space widening or narrowing
  - Bone destruction is rarely noted, except when the infection is chronic.
- Computed tomography is helpful in revealing joint effusions.
- Magnetic resonance imaging of the afflicted joint is the best available method for the diagnosis of septic arthritis as it will give additional information regarding any involvement of the adjacent bone (i.e., presence of osteomyelitis). Make sure that if prosthetic material in the joint is present, it is compatible for the patient to undergo the test.

Follow-Up & Special Considerations
A repeat MRI may be necessary if response is not adequate.

Diagnostic Procedures/Other
Synovial tissue biopsy: Send for culture and histology (including stains for infectious culprits).

Pathological Findings
Polymorphonuclear leukocyte infiltrate of the synovial tissue and congested vessels. Gram stain may show bacteria induction of Toll-like receptors 2 and 4 and of human defensin 2 (6).

DIFFERENTIAL DIAGNOSIS
- Collagen vascular diseases (predominantly RA and juvenile RA).
- Trauma
- Crystal induced (pseudogout or gout).
- Toxic synovitis (7).
- Rheumatic fever
- Seronegative spondyloarthropathies

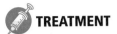

TREATMENT

MEDICATION

First Line

- Joint aspiration for recurrent effusions for the first 5–7 days, if necessary. This is a mainstay of therapy. Involve an orthopedic surgeon early if infected prosthesis and for difficulty to access the joint (hip or shoulder).
- For acute monoarticular arthritis or for septic arthritis in a patient with RA:
  - If Gram stain suggests *S. aureus*: Nafcillin or a second-generation cephalosporin have been suggested in the past empirically until cultures are available. In this era of increased rates of methicillin-resistant *S. aureus* (MRSA), physicians may need to resort to other antibiotics, until susceptibility testing results are available. If these show susceptibility to nafcillin (1–2 g every 4 hours) or cefazolin (1–1, 5 g) every 6 hours, then one can deescalate.
  - For community-acquired MRSA, treatment may include trimethoprim-sulfamethoxazole or clindamycin or ciprofloxacin or levofloxacin or minocycline or tetracycline.
  - Regarding hospital associated MRSA infection: Vancomycin 1 g every 12 hours. Pay attention to guidelines regarding vancomycin use. Teicoplanin for IV use (10 mg/kg daily) is available in Europe as an alternative to vancomycin.
  - If response to vancomycin is not adequate then one should consider other options such as linezolid or daptomycin, although more data on their role are needed.
  - If *Streptococcus* spp. (including *S. pneumoniae*), Penicillin in adults $24*10^6$ units daily (in divided doses every 4–6 hours); resistance to penicillin may necessitate use of ceftriaxone 2 g IV OD (in rare cases vancomycin may be needed) (1).
  - If Gram stain show gram-negative bacteria: A third-generation cephalosporin such as ceftriaxone 2 g IV OD or cefotaxime. Be aware of local data regarding ESBL producers as carbapenems may be needed.
  - If Gram stain does not show any organisms: Vancomycin plus Ceftriaxone or Cefotaxime or Ceftazidime.
- Duration of treatment is 2 weeks of intravenous antibiotics followed by an oral regimen for another 2–4 weeks (1)[A] (exception is gonococcal septic arthritis). Shorter duration regimens for children have been used (8).
- For gonococcal arthritis
  - Ceftriaxone 1–2 g IV once daily for 10 days.
- For *animal-bite* infections
  - Ampicillin/sulbactam 3 g every 6 hours IV.
- For *Lyme* arthritis
  - Doxycycline 100 mg BD for 1 month or ceftriaxone for 14 days.

ADDITIONAL TREATMENT

Issues for Referral

Orthopedic surgical drainage of the joint is needed if no improvement in the first 2 days or if removal of an infected prosthesis is needed.

Additional Therapies

Corticosteroids have been used as an adjunctive agent in children (0.2 mg/kg every 12 hours for 6 days) (1).

SURGERY/OTHER PROCEDURES

Removal of an infected prosthetic joint may be necessary (and joint replacement at the same time or after an interval of antimicrobial treatment).

IN-PATIENT CONSIDERATIONS

Initial Stabilization

Required if generalized sepsis.

Admission Criteria

- Septic arthritis is an indication for admission.
- In selected patients, one may consider outpatient parenteral antibiotic treatment.

Discharge Criteria

Completion of 2 weeks of intravenous antibiotic treatment with patient improving.

ONGOING CARE

FOLLOW-UP RECOMMENDATIONS

- Patients should have follow-up with physical therapy.
- Any recurrence of effusions should be tapped and recurrent arthritis ruled out.

Patient Monitoring

Measurement of CBC, CRP, liver function tests, and serum creatinine at regular intervals during antibiotic treatment at home.

PROGNOSIS

In adults, chronic disability occurs in 50% of patients. Worse prognosis if bacteremia or immunosuppression.

COMPLICATIONS

- Long-term complications
  - Worsening of arthritis
  - Joint-space narrowing
  - Ankylosis
  - Articular dysfunction or destruction
- Sepsis (systemic)
- Impairment of growth in children

REFERENCES

1. Mathews CJ, Weston VC, Jones A, et al. Bacterial septic arthritis in adults. *Lancet* 2010;375: 846–855.
2. Young TP, Maas L, Thorp AW, et al. Etiology of septic arthritis in children: An update for the new millennium. *Am J Emerg Med* 2010 (Epub ahead of print).
3. Ross JJ, Saltzman CL, Carling P, et al. Pneumococcal septic arthritis: Review of 190 cases. *Clin Infect Dis* 2003;36:319–327.
4. Ernst AA, Weiss SJ, Tracy LA, et al. Usefulness of CRP and ESR in predicting septic joints. *South Med J* 2010;103:522–526.
5. McGillicuddy DC, Shah KH, Friedberg RP, et al. How sensitive is the synovial fluid white blood cell count in diagnosing septic arthritis? *Am J Emerg Med* 2007;25:749–752.
6. Varoga D, Klostermeier E, Paulsen F, et al. The antimicrobial peptide HBD-2 and the Toll-like receptors-2 and -4 are induced in synovial membranes in case of septic arthritis. *Virchows Arch* 2009;454:685–694.
7. Sultan J, Hughes PJ. Septic arthritis or transient synovitis of the hip in children: The value of clinical prediction algorithms. *J Bone Joint Surg Br* 2010;92:1289–1293.
8. Peltola H, Pääkkönen M, Kallio P, et al. Short- versus long-term antimicrobial treatment for acute hematogenous osteomyelitis of childhood: Prospective, randomized trial on 131 culture-positive cases. *Pediatr Infect Dis J* 2010;29:1123–1128.

ADDITIONAL READING

- Rybak MJ, Lomaestro BM, Rotschafer JC, et al. Vancomycin therapeutic guidelines: A summary of consensus recommendations from the infectious diseases Society of America, the American Society of Health-System Pharmacists, and the Society of Infectious Diseases Pharmacists. *Clin Infect Dis* 2009;49:325–327.

CODES

ICD9

- 711.00 Pyogenic arthritis, site unspecified
- 711.05 Pyogenic arthritis involving pelvic region and thigh
- 711.06 Pyogenic arthritis involving lower leg

CLINICAL PEARLS

- Septic arthritis is a medical emergency.
- Don't rely absolutely on laboratory values, that is,
  - Gram-stain may be negative, leukocyte number may be below the 50,000/mm³ cutoff. Even the synovial fluid culture may not detect microorganisms.
- Septic arthritis may coexist with trauma, crystal induced or preexisting rheumatic disease.

SHIGELLOSIS

Jason B. Harris (E. Mylonakis, Editor)

 BASICS

DESCRIPTION
Shigellosis is caused by the bacterium *Shigella*, and is characterized by diarrhea, fever, nausea, cramps, and tenesmus.

EPIDEMIOLOGY
Incidence
- In the US, the incidence of shigellosis is approximately 7 cases per 100,000 population.
- Globally, shigellosis is more common. Shigella spp. infects over 150 million people and causes 100,000 deaths each year worldwide.
- Epidemic shigellosis occurs most frequently in overcrowded population with inadequate sanitation.
- Direct spread is by the fecal–oral route; indirect spread is by contaminated food and inanimate objects. Water-borne disease is unusual. Flies may serve as mechanical vectors.
- As few as 10 organisms may cause infection.
- Shigellosis is communicable during acute infection and while the infectious agent is present in feces (usually no longer than 4 weeks).

RISK FACTORS
- The majority of cases of shigellosis occur in children.
- Secondary attack rates in household contacts may be as high as 40%.
- Those at greater risk include children in daycare centers, foreign travelers to certain countries, and persons living in institutions.
- In developed countries, outbreaks commonly occur in prisons, institutions for children, childcare centers, psychiatric hospitals, crowded camps, and among men who have sex with men (MSM).

GENERAL PREVENTION
- Cases of shigellosis should be reported to local public health authorities.
- General recommendations include the use of safe drinking water, eating properly cooked foods and, hand washing.
- Infected food-handlers and childcare workers, children attending daycare, and patient care providers should be treated with appropriate antibiotics and should be restricted from their work activities until 2 stool samples have been tested and are negative for *Shigella*.
- Symptomatic contacts of shigellosis patients should be excluded from food handling and the care of children or patients until investigated.
- Stool cultures from contacts need only be confined to food-handlers and those in situations in which the spread of infection is particularly likely (day care centers, hospitals, and institutions).

PATHOPHYSIOLOGY
- The incubation period usually ranges from 1–3 days but may last up to 7 days.
- Shigellosis is an infection of the distal ileum and colon.
- Shigella invades and destroys colonic epithelial cells, resulting in tissue destruction and a local and systemic inflammatory response.

ETIOLOGY
- *Shigella* species are small, gram–negative rods that are members of the family *Enterobacteriaceae*. They are nonmotile and non-encapsulated.
- Four distinct *Shigella* species cause infection, with clinical presentations varying by species and serotype.
- *S. dysenteriae* type 1 is associated with epidemic dysentery, and has the highest risk of mortality. In addition, *S. dysenteriae* produces Shiga toxin that is associated with the risk of hemolytic uremic syndrome (HUS).
- *S. flexneri* is the most common species in developing countries and is associated with severe disease.
- *S. sonnei* is the most common species in developed countries and causes milder disease.
- *S. boydii* is a less common cause of shigellosis.

COMMONLY ASSOCIATED CONDITIONS
- Shigellosis is associated with several potentially life-threatening metabolic, neurologic, and abdominal complications.
- Dehydration and hypoglycemia are more common complications in young children.
- Rectal prolapse and fecal incontinence may result from severe tenesmus.
- Intestinal obstruction, which occurs in about 3% of patients, is a poor prognostic sign, not infrequently associated with death or the development of HUS.
- HUS is a well-described complication of *S. dysenteriae* type I infection in childhood.
- Seizures are common in young children with severe shigellosis and may be associated with fever (febrile convulsions), metabolic abnormalities, or encephalopathy.

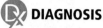 **DIAGNOSIS**

HISTORY
- The hallmark of severe shigellosis is dysentery, which is the frequent, painful passage of small volume stools that consist of mucus, blood, inflammatory cells, and fecal matter.
- The passage of stools is accompanied by tenesmus and cramping.
- Watery diarrhea, rather than dysentery, may often be the initial intestinal symptom.
- Other common symptoms include
  - Fever
  - Stomach cramps and/or
  - Nausea and/or vomiting
- Severe cases may cause dehydration (loss of fluids) or convulsions (in young children).

PHYSICAL EXAM
- Findings on physical examination are nonspecific and include a variable degree of systemic toxemia, fever, abdominal tenderness, especially over the lower abdominal quadrants, and hyperactive bowel sounds.
- Rectal examination or proctoscopy is generally painful. Sigmoidoscopy reveals a friable, hyperemic rectal mucosa, increased mucus secretion, and areas of ecchymosis. Ulcerations of the rectal mucosa are seen after several days of illness.

DIAGNOSTIC TESTS & INTERPRETATION
Lab
- The presence of fecal leukocytes is suggestive of a bacterial etiology of diarrhea.
- Patients presenting with bloody diarrhea should have a stool culture performed to determine whether they are infected with *Shigella* spp. Most people pass *Shigella* in their feces for 1–2 weeks (without treatment).
- Blood cultures are positive in up to 4% of patients with shigellosis.
- Patients presenting with watery diarrhea may not need a stool culture since supportive care and hydration is needed, and specific antimicrobial therapy is rarely required.
- The total white blood cell count may occasionally demonstrate leukopenia; up to 5% children may have a leukemoid reaction ($>50,000$ WBC/mm^3).
- Diarrhea usually causes isosmotic dehydration with metabolic acidosis and significant potassium loss. Thirst from dehydration can lead to a proportionately excessive water intake, causing hypotonicity.
- Hypoglycemia is a common complication of severe shigellosis and may be profound.
- Most people pass *Shigella* in their feces for 1–2 weeks (without treatment).

Imaging
Abdominal imaging (such as abdominal CT scan) should be reserved for evaluating potential complications in patients with signs of peritonitis. These include toxic colitis and intestinal perforation.

Pathological Findings
Biopsies from patients with shigellosis demonstrate inflammatory infiltrates, with sheets of neutrophils and plasma cells.

DIFFERENTIAL DIAGNOSIS
- In mild cases, presenting with acute watery diarrhea, the illness is indistinguishable from numerous other bacterial, viral, and protozoan infections that cause diarrhea.
- In patients who present with dysentery (stools containing visible blood and mucus), the differential diagnosis includes enteroinvasive and enterohemorrhagic *Escherichia coli*, *Salmonella*, *Yersinia*, *Campylobacter*, *Clostridium difficile* and amebiasis.

 ## TREATMENT
MEDICATION
First Line
- Antibiotics are always indicated in patients presenting with dysentery caused by *Shigella* spp.
- The initial choice of antibiotics depends on local susceptibility patterns.
- In patients who can tolerate oral antibiotics, first line therapies include ciprofloxacin or azithromycin.
- Ciprofloxacin can be given at a dose of 500 mg b.i.d for 3 consecutive days in adults.
- Azithromycin (500 mg of azithromycin on day 1, followed by 250 mg once daily for 4 days) is effective in the treatment of moderate to severe shigellosis caused by multidrug-resistant *Shigella* strains.
- A pediatric dosage schedule for azithromycin is 15 mg/kg (up to 500 mg) initially, followed by 10 mg/kg/d (up to 250 mg) on the subsequent 4 days.

Second Line
- Oral cephalosporins are not effective agents in the treatment of shigellosis.
- Trimethoprim-sulfamethoxazole, double-strength, b.i.d PO for 3 doses is another alternative for strains that are proven susceptible (most are resistant).
- In children, parenteral (IV) therapy is often needed secondary to severe disease. In such cases, ceftriaxone can be given at a dose of 50 mg/kg as a single daily dose for 5 days in children.

ADDITIONAL TREATMENT
General Measures
- In shigellosis, as in any diarrheal illness, proper fluid replacement is the mainstay of treatment.
- The use of intestinal antimotility drugs, including diphenoxylate (Lomotil), should be avoided in adult patients with severe disease, and never used in children.

- In children in developing countries, supplemental zinc reduces the severity and duration of the acute infection and recurrence. 20 mg of elemental zinc once daily for 10–14 days for children 7–59 months old, and 10 mg per day for infants 6 months or less, is recommended for children with shigellosis in developing countries.

SURGERY/OTHER PROCEDURES
Surgical management is limited to complications such as intestinal perforation and toxic megacolon.

IN-PATIENT CONSIDERATIONS
Initial Stabilization
Initial stabilization if needed includes immediate supportive management of severe dehydration, acute metabolic derangements, and seizures if present.

Admission Criteria
- The majority of cases of shigellosis are self-limited and do not require hospitalization.
- Indications for admission include toxic appearance or complications such as severe dehydration, hypoglycemia, HUS, intestinal obstruction, or encephalopathy.

IV Fluids
- Isotonic fluids (e.g. normal saline or Ringer's lactate) should be given to patients with severe dehydration.
- Non-isotonic and colloidal fluids (such as D5 1/4 NS) should **never** be given to dehydrated patients, because they may precipitate additional intracellular fluid losses in patients with severe dehydration.
- Dextrose should be given to patients with hypoglycemia (and added to replacement fluids of patients with dehydration and hypoglycemia).

Discharge Criteria
Patients demonstrating clinical improvement on an acceptable antibiotic regimen can be considered for discharge.

 ## ONGOING CARE

FOLLOW-UP RECOMMENDATIONS
Close follow-up of patients with dysentery is needed to ensure improvement. Symptoms should begin to improve 1–2 days after initiation of appropriate antimicrobial therapy and proper supportive care.

DIET
The diet of patients with uncomplicated shigellosis should not be restricted. Feeding with a high protein diet if possible can ameliorate the nutritional deterioration that follows shigellosis in children.

PATIENT EDUCATION
- Patients should be educated about the role of proper hand washing and food preparation in the prevention of shigellosis.
- Additional information geared toward patients is available through the Centers for Disease Control and Prevention website. http://www.cdc.gov/nczved/divisions/dfbmd/diseases/shigellosis/

PROGNOSIS
Shigellosis is usually a self-limited disease; in the absence of complications at presentation, prognosis is good.

COMPLICATIONS
- Dehydration
- Hypoglycemia
- Rectal prolapse
- Toxic megacolon
- Hemolytic uremic syndrome
- Encephalopathy
- Reactive arthritis

ADDITIONAL READING
- Pawlowski SW, Warren CA, Guerrant R. Diagnosis and treatment of acute or persistent diarrhea. *Gastroenterology* 2009;136(6):1874–1886.
- Prince Christopher RH, David KV, John SM, et al. Antibiotic therapy for Shigella dysentery. *Cochrane Database Syst Rev* 2010;(8):CD006784.

 ### See Also (Topic, Algorithm, Electronic Media Element)

- Acute diarrhea

 ## CODES

ICD9
- 004.0 *Shigella dysenteriae*
- 004.1 Shigella flexneri
- 004.9 Shigellosis, unspecified

CLINICAL PEARLS
- The diagnosis of shigellosis should be considered in patients presenting with acute bloody diarrhea.
- A stool culture for *Shigella*, *Salmonella*, *Yersinia*, *Campylobacter* and *E. coli* O157 should be performed as part of the evaluation of patients presenting with acute bloody diarrhea.
- Unlike other bacterial causes of acute bloody diarrhea, antibiotics are indicated in patients with culture proven shigellosis.
- Empiric antibiotics should be avoided in patients presenting with bloody diarrhea unless they are toxic appearing.

S

SINUSITIS

Drosos E. Karageorgopoulos
Petros I. Rafailidis
Matthew E. Falagas

 BASICS

DESCRIPTION
- Sinusitis (or rhinosinusitis) is a symptomatic inflammation of the paranasal sinuses (maxillary, ethmoid, frontal, and/or sphenoid)
- Classification of sinusitis with regard to duration of symptoms and signs (1):
  - Acute sinusitis (2): Less than 4 weeks.
  - Subacute sinusitis: More than 4 weeks but less than 3 months.
  - Chronic sinusitis: 3 months or longer.
  - Acute exacerbation of chronic sinusitis: Sudden worsening of symptoms or new symptoms, with return to baseline
  - Recurrent acute sinusitis: 4 or more episodes of acute sinusitis within 1 year, without persistent symptoms between the episodes
- Classification of chronic sinusitis:
  - Chronic sinusitis with nasal polyposis
  - Allergic fungal sinusitis
  - Chronic sinusitis without nasal polyposis
- Classification of fungal sinusitis:
  - Fungal colonization (fungus ball)
  - Allergic fungal sinusitis
  - Invasive fungal sinusitis (acute, in immunocompromised patients, or chronic, in immunocompetent patients)

EPIDEMIOLOGY
Incidence
5–13% (for children) and 0.5–2% (for adults) of acute viral upper respiratory tract infections are complicated by secondary bacterial sinusitis

Prevalence
- Sinusitis (any type) affects 1 in 7 adults in the US
- Chronic sinusitis: More common in young and middle-aged adults than in children

RISK FACTORS
- Allergic rhinitis
- Anatomic abnormalities (congenital choanal atresia, septal deviation), foreign bodies, nasal polyps, tumors
- Air pollutants, tobacco smoke, chemicals
- Impaired mucociliary clearance (e.g., cystic fibrosis)
- Granulomatous disease
- Immunodeficiency
- Nosocomial sinusitis: Prolonged presence of endotracheal or nasogastric tubes
- Specific for zygomycosis: Diabetic ketoacidosis, deferoxamine therapy, and iron overload

PATHOPHYSIOLOGY
- Viral infection of the nasal mucosa spreads to the paranasal sinuses (3). Mucosal edema, increased secretions and inflammatory fluid, and impaired mucociliary clearance lead to sinus obstruction. Secondary bacterial infection may ensue
- Chronic sinusitis with nasal polyposis:
  - Immune hyper-responsiveness (Th2 type) to colonizing *Staphylococcus aureus*
- Allergic fungal sinusitis: Chronic allergy to colonizing fungi

ETIOLOGY
- Acute sinusitis (community-acquired):
  - Viruses: Rhinovirus, influenza virus, and parainfluenza virus
  - Bacteria: *Streptococcus pneumoniae*, *Haemophilus influenzae* (nontypeable strains), and Moraxella catarrhalis (particularly in children). Less frequently, *S. aureus* or *Streptococcus* spp.
- Odontogenic infection: Aerobic bacteria and anaerobes of the oral flora
- Immunocompromised host: Fungi and *P. aeruginosa* are common pathogens
- Subacute and recurrent sinusitis: As for acute sinusitis plus *S. aureus* and anaerobes (Peptostreptococcus spp., Fusobacterium spp., pigmented Prevotella spp., and Porphyromonas spp.)
- Chronic sinusitis (including acute exacerbations): *S. pneumoniae*, *H. influenzae*, anaerobes, *S. aureus*, gram–negative bacilli
- Nosocomial sinusitis: Gram-negative bacilli, *S. aureus*, anaerobes, occasionally yeasts
- Invasive fungal sinusitis: Acute disease mainly due to Aspergillus spp. or Zygomycetes (Rhizopus spp., Mucor spp., and Rhizomucor spp.). In chronic disease, consider additionally Fusarium spp., *Pseudallescheria boydii*, dematiaceous fungi

COMMONLY ASSOCIATED CONDITIONS
Chronic sinusitis with nasal polyposis is associated with asthma and aspirin sensitivity

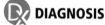 DIAGNOSIS

HISTORY
- Duration, severity, and clinical course
- Symptoms:
  - Nasal congestion and obstruction
  - Discolored (purulent) nasal or postnasal discharge
  - Pressure, fullness or pain over sinus areas, particularly when bending forward
  - Hyposmia or anosmia
  - Maxillary tooth pain, fever, headache, cough, foul smelling breath
- Symptom or signs cannot reliably differentiate between viral and bacterial acute sinusitis
- Risk factors or associated conditions
- Environmental exposures
- Prior treatments

PHYSICAL EXAM
- Tenderness over sinuses or pain when bending forward
- Tenderness by percussion of maxillary tooth
- Necrotic eschars in nasal passages or palate suggest invasive fungal sinusitis
- Anterior rhinoscopy
- Transillumination (limited diagnostic value)

DIAGNOSTIC TESTS & INTERPRETATION
Imaging
Initial approach
- Acute sinusitis:
  - Radiological imaging cannot reliably differentiate between viral and bacterial sinusitis
  - Plain sinus x-rays are not very accurate
  - Radiological signs of acute sinusitis include mucosal edema (at least 4 mm thickening), presence of air–fluid level, or sinus opacification
- Chronic sinusitis:
  - Sinus CT scan documents sinus involvement
  - CT findings include mucosal thickening, obstruction of the ostiomeatal complex, polyps, sinus opacification
- Invasive fungal sinusitis: CT scan can show bony erosion or invasion of surrounding structures

Follow-Up & Special Considerations
- Acute sinusitis:
  - Imaging if complications are suspected or to evaluate treatment failures
  - CT scan is the imaging modality of choice
  - MRI to evaluate complications of sinusitis (particularly intracranial ones)
- Chronic sinusitis: MRI can help delineate the nature of CT abnormalities

Diagnostic Procedures/Other
- Culture obtained by antral puncture is the gold standard
- Culture of middle meatal secretions by endoscopy is an alternative to antral puncture for adults
- Culture of nasal secretions is not reliable
- Acute sinusitis:
  - Culture recommended for complicated cases, unusually severe sinusitis, failure of empirical antimicrobials, serious immunodeficiency, nosocomial sinusitis, suspected antimicrobial drug resistance or unusual pathogen
- Nosocomial sinusitis: Cultures generally recommended for positive imaging signs and persistent, unexplained fever, despite general measures and empirical antimicrobial therapy
- Chronic sinusitis:
  - Anterior rhinoscopy or nasal endoscopy can document the presence of sinus inflammation or nasal polyps
  - Consider culture for serious persistent symptoms despite appropriate management
- Invasive fungal sinusitis: Urgent nasal endoscopy with biopsy and culture

DIFFERENTIAL DIAGNOSIS
- Common cold
- Allergic or nonallergic rhinitis
- Atrophic rhinitis (due to surgery, radiation)
- Tumors
- Granulomatous disease (e.g., Wegener's granulomatosis, Churg-Strauss syndrome, sarcoidosis, and rhinoscleroma)
- Intranasal cocaine abuse
- Cerebrospinal fluid leak
- Additionally in children: Nasal foreign bodies, adenoid hypertrophy, pertussis in catarrhal stage, and congenital syphilis

TREATMENT

MEDICATION
- Acute sinusitis:
  - Antibiotics have a modest therapeutic benefit over placebo in adults (4)
  - Antibiotics are reserved for persistent symptoms after 7–10 days, progressive or severe symptoms, worsening symptoms after initial improvement, or risk for complications (e.g., immunodeficiency)
  - Recommended duration is 7–14 days, depending on clinical response (5)
  - Respiratory fluoroquinolones (e.g., moxifloxacin, levofloxacin) are effective but can be reserved as second-line therapy (6)
  - Amoxicillin-clavulanate also effective, particularly for high dose (up to 90 mg/kg/d based on the amoxicillin component for children and 2 1 g/62.5 mg extended-release tablets b.i.d for adults)
  - Amoxicillin: Recommended as first-line therapy in patients without risk factors; not active against beta-lactamase producing *H. influenzae* or *M. catarrhalis*; high-dose amoxicillin active against penicillin-non-susceptible *S. pneumoniae*
  - Second or oral third generation cephalosporins (e.g., cefuroxime-axetil, cefdinir, and cefpodoxime)
  - Penicillin allergy (type I hypersensitivity): Respiratory fluoroquinolones, macrolides (e.g., clarithromycin, azithromycin) or trimethoprim-sulfamethoxazole
- Acute sinusitis associated with dental infection: Treatment should additionally cover oral anaerobes
- Chronic sinusitis:
  - Antibiotics are primarily used in the beginning of therapy or for acute exacerbations
  - Duration is 3 weeks or longer according to clinical response
  - Antimicrobials active against anaerobes (such as amoxicillin-clavulanate or moxifloxacin) are preferred
  - Clindamycin can be used, particularly if methicillin-resistant *S. aureus* is suspected
  - Other options: Combination of metronidazole with a cephalosporin, levofloxacin, a macrolide, or trimethoprim-sulfamethoxazole
  - Nasal glucocorticoids important (budesonide, fluticasone, mometasone, triamcinolone)
  - Consider systemic glucocorticoids if nasal glucocorticoids fail, for severe edema, or large polyps
- Nosocomial sinusitis: Empirical antimicrobial therapy as for ventilator-associated pneumonia
- Invasive fungal sinusitis:
  - Long-term antifungal therapy in addition to surgical resection
  - Empirical therapy: Lipid formulations of amphotericin B or amphotericin B deoxycholate
  - Voriconazole for aspergillosis
  - Posaconazole as oral step-down therapy for zygomycosis

ADDITIONAL TREATMENT
General Measures
- Acute sinusitis: Nasal irrigation with hypertonic saline
- Nosocomial sinusitis: Remove endotracheal or nasogastric tubes
- Chronic sinusitis: Saline nasal irrigation or nasal sprays

Issues for Referral
- Periorbital edema
- Diplopia or other visual changes
- Severe headache
- Neurological symptoms/signs
- Pathogen with antimicrobial resistance
- Need for obtaining culture
- Immunodeficiency
- Odontogenic infection

Additional Therapies
- Analgesics (acetaminophen) or nonsteroidal anti-inflammatory drugs
- Nasal decongestants (e.g., oxymetazoline)
- Nasal corticosteroids (e.g., mometasone)
- Nasal anticholinergics (ipratropium bromide)
- Systemic H1 antihistamines (for allergic underlying disease)
- Mucolytics

SURGERY/OTHER PROCEDURES
- Acute sinusitis: Surgical drainage may be required for extension to adjacent tissues or intracranial sites
- Chronic sinusitis: Surgery can be elected when medical management fails
- Allergic fungal sinusitis: Sinus surgery can demonstrate the presence of allergic mucin (microscopically contains degranulating eosinophils)
- Fungal colonization: Surgical removal of the fungus ball and correction of sinus obstruction
- Invasive fungal sinusitis: Urgent surgical debridement of affected tissues is required

IN-PATIENT CONSIDERATIONS
Admission Criteria
- Severe infection
- Patients unable to take oral drugs
- Suspected complications
- Immunocompromised host

 ONGOING CARE

FOLLOW-UP RECOMMENDATIONS
- Chronic sinusitis:
  - Smoking cessation
  - Consider allergy evaluation for most patients
  - Consider underlying immune deficiency if recurrent sinopulmonary infections

PATIENT EDUCATION
Use of nasal decongestants for more than 3 days should be avoided due to the risk for rhinitis medicamentosa

PROGNOSIS
- Acute sinusitis:
  - Acute viral sinusitis typically resolves within 7–10 days
  - Patients on antibiotics improve within 2–3 days

COMPLICATIONS
- Preseptal or orbital cellulitis: Usually secondary to ethmoid sinusitis
- Subperiosteal abscess of frontal bone (Pott's puffy tumor) associated with frontal sinusitis (more common in children)
- Intracranial complications (brain abscess, meningitis, septic cavernous sinus thrombosis, epidural abscess, subdural empyema)

REFERENCES
1. Lanza DC, Kennedy DW. Adult rhinosinusitis defined. *Otolaryngol Head Neck Surg* 1997;117:S1–S7.
2. Piccirillo JF. Clinical practice. Acute bacterial sinusitis. *N Engl J Med* 2004;351:902–910.
3. Benninger MS, Ferguson BJ, Hadley JA, et al. Adult chronic rhinosinusitis: Definitions, diagnosis, epidemiology, and pathophysiology. *Otolaryngol Head Neck Surg* 2003;129:S1–S32.
4. Falagas ME, Giannopoulou KP, Vardakas KZ, et al. Comparison of antibiotics with placebo for treatment of acute sinusitis: A meta-analysis of randomised controlled trials. *Lancet Infect Dis* 2008;8:543–552.
5. Falagas ME, Karageorgopoulos DE, Grammatikos AP, et al. Effectiveness and safety of short vs. long duration of antibiotic therapy for acute bacterial sinusitis: A meta-analysis of randomized trials. *Br J Clin Pharmacol* 2009;67:161–171.
6. Karageorgopoulos DE, Giannopoulou KP, Grammatikos AP, et al. Fluoroquinolones compared with beta-lactam antibiotics for the treatment of acute bacterial sinusitis: A meta-analysis of randomized controlled trials. *CMAJ* 2008;178:845–854.

CODES

ICD9
- 461.0 Acute maxillary sinusitis
- 461.9 Acute sinusitis, unspecified
- 473.9 Unspecified sinusitis (chronic)

CLINICAL PEARLS
- Knowing when to refer the patient with sinusitis is of paramount significance
- A 7-day regimen could suffice in cases where antibiotic treatment is deemed necessary.
- Beware of missing a diagnosis of cocaine abuse or Wegener's granulomatosis.

SPINAL EPIDURAL ABSCESS

Erica S. Shenoy (E. Mylonakis, Editor)

 BASICS

DESCRIPTION
Spinal epidural abscess (SEA) is a collection of pus in the epidural space (between the dura and the vertebral bodies), often as a result of local extension from vertebral osteomyelitis.

EPIDEMIOLOGY
Incidence
- SEA accounts for 2.5–3 cases per 10,000 hospital admissions.
- The incidence has increased dramatically over the past 3 decades, which has been attributed to increase in intravenous drug use (IVDU) as well as invasive spinal procedures.

RISK FACTORS
- Intravenous drug use (IVDU)
- Diabetes mellitus
- Immunosuppression (i.e. HIV, malignancy, immunosuppressive medications)
- Renal insufficiency
- Alcohol abuse, spinal abnormalities (i.e., degenerative disc disease)
- Spinal trauma
- Prior intervention (epidural analgesia, spinal injections, lumbar puncture, needle biopsy, etc.)
- Bacteremia, indwelling IV catheters, and endocarditis

SEA is more common in men than in women.

GENERAL PREVENTION
There are no prevention strategies except mitigation of risk factors.

PATHOPHYSIOLOGY
Up to 30% of SEA are caused by extension of local infection into the epidural space. About 50% are the result of hematogenous spread. Between 15–22% of SEA are thought to be secondary to invasive procedures or instrumentation such as epidural anesthesia, biopsies, lumbar punctures, etc. Cord compression is the feared complication and results from direct impingement by the abscess on the cord.

ETIOLOGY
The majority of cases are caused by *Staphylococcus aureus*, accounting for approximately 60% of cases, a growing number of which are the result of methicillin-resistant *S. aureus* (MRSA). After *S. aureus*, streptococci (10%), enterobacteriaceae (10%), coagulase-negative staphylococci (3–5%), Bacteroides spp. and other anaerobes (2%), Pseudomonas spp. (2%), mycobacteria (<1% in the US), polymicrobial (5–10%), and unknown (6–10%). Less common organisms include Acinetobacter, Enterococci, Actinomyces spp., Nocardia spp., Brucella spp., Candida spp., Coccidioides spp., Aspergillus spp., Blastomyces spp. and Sporothrix spp.

 DIAGNOSIS

HISTORY
- Patients present with back or neck pain (70–90%).
- If untreated, pain can progress to radiculopathy, then motor weakness, loss of bowel and bladder continence, decreased sensation, and paralysis. Back pain may represent the only symptom, and the absence of fever or neurological deficits should not rule out SEA.
- The history may elicit risk factors including prior injury or intervention that may predispose the patient to development of SEA.
- The time course of onset of symptoms can be highly variable—from hours to days, or from weeks to months.

PHYSICAL EXAM
- Fever may be noted in approximately 32% of patients.
- Examination should focus on assessing for portals of entry, and a complete neurological examination including evaluation of weakness, sensory function, reflex abnormalities, and sphincter tone.

DIAGNOSTIC TESTS & INTERPRETATION
Lab
Initial lab tests
- Basic laboratory tests including complete blood count (CBC) with differential (which may demonstrate a leukocytosis with left shift), erythrocyte sedimentation rate (ESR) and C-reactive protein (CRP), and blood cultures prior to the administration of antibiotics should be obtained.
- Identification of the pathogen is accomplished through CT guided aspiration or in the process of surgical decompression and drainage. Multiple cultures should be sent for Gram stain and culture, anaerobic culture, fungal stain and culture, AFB stain and mycobacterial culture as well as pathology.

Follow-Up & Special Considerations
ESR and CRP can be followed longitudinally as markers of successful treatment of disease, progression, or recrudescence.

Imaging
Initial approach
Magnetic resonance imaging (MRI) with gadolinium is the gold standard in the diagnosis of SEA, though if not available, computed tomography (CT) may be of some utility.

Follow-Up & Special Considerations
MRI can also be used to follow resolution of the lesion during the treatment period and afterwards.

Diagnostic Procedures/Other
- CT guided aspiration may be useful in identifying an organism
- Surgical decompression and drainage are necessary in some cases of SEA and should be performed on an emergent basis in the case of any evidence of neurological compromise.

DIFFERENTIAL DIAGNOSIS
- Malignancy
- Guillain-Barré syndrome
- Diskitis
- Compression fracture

TREATMENT

MEDICATION
- Empiric treatment should include an anti-staphylococcal agent as well as an agent directed at gram–negative bacilli. Vancomycin is recommended pending isolation of the organism and determination of susceptibilities. A third generation cephalosporin such as Cefepime or Ceftazidime, or a carbapenem can be used for gram–negative coverage.
- Once an organism is identified and susceptibilities are known, antimicrobial therapy can be tailored. Duration is generally between 4–8 weeks.

ADDITIONAL TREATMENT
General Measures
SEA is managed using a combined medical and surgical approach.

Issues for Referral
Patients should be referred to centers with expertise in orthopedic/spinal surgery as well as infectious disease.

SURGERY/OTHER PROCEDURES
- Surgical decompression and drainage is necessary in patients with evidence of neurological compromise and should be undertaken immediately. Once paralysis occurs, the chance of reversing neurological damage at time points greater than 24 hours is decreased.
- Medical management alone can be considered in cases where there is no evidence of neurological involvement, an organism has been identified, and when patients can be followed closely, as well as in cases where the patient is a high surgical risk.
- One recent retrospective review of a 10 year experience in managing SEA found no statistically significant difference in patient outcomes in those patients management with CT guided aspiration plus antibiotics and those managed with surgical intervention and antibiotics.

 ONGOING CARE

FOLLOW-UP RECOMMENDATIONS
Patient Monitoring
- Patients not undergoing surgical decompression and drainage should be monitored closely for evidence of neurological compromise.
- Patients undergoing treatment should be monitored as well for recrudescence of infection.

PROGNOSIS
- Advances in diagnosis and treatment have reduced what was once a fatal infection to a treatable disease, though the mortality rate is still in the range of 2–20%.
- Only 45% of patients experience a full recovery.
- Recovery can take place up to a year from the initial injury.

COMPLICATIONS
- Persistent neurological deficits, including paralysis.
- Death

ADDITIONAL READING
- Wallace MR, Rana A, Yadavalli GK. Epidural Abscess. *EMedicine Infectious Diseases*, 2009. http://emedicine.medscape.com/article/232570-overview. Accessed August 2, 2011.
- Tunkel AR. Subdural empyema, epidural abscess, and supurative intracranial thrombophlebitis. In Mandell, Douglas and Bennett, eds. *Principles and Practice of Infectious Diseases*, 7th ed. 2009.
- Karikari IO, Powers CJ, Reynolds RM, et al. Management of a spontaneous epidural abscess: A single-center 10-year experience. *Neurosurgery* 2009;65:919–924.

- Baker AS, Ojemann RG, Swartz MN, et al. Spinal epidural abscess. *N Engl J Med* 1975;293:463–468.
- Darouiche RO, Hamill RJ, Greenberg SB, et al. Bacterial spinal epidural abscess. Review of 43 cases and literature survey. *Medicine* 1992;71:369–385.
- Hlavin ML, Kaminski HJ, Ross JS, et al. Spinal epidural abscess: A ten-year perspective. *Neurosurgery* 1990;27:177–184.

CODES

ICD9
324.1 Intraspinal abscess

CLINICAL PEARLS
- Spinal epidural abscess should be suspected in patients with back pain, even in the absence of fever or neurological symptoms, especially if any risk factors are present.
- Every effort should be made to identify an organism.
- Management involves both medical and surgical approaches.

SPOROTRICHOSIS

Michael K. Mansour (E. Mylonakis, Editor)

 BASICS

DESCRIPTION

- Sporotrichosis is an endemic dimorphic fungal infection caused by *Sporothrix schenckii*, and it occurs in four forms: lymphocutaneous, fixed cutaneous, cutaneous disseminated, and systemic.
- Lymphocutaneous sporotrichosis is the most common manifestation due to the nature of exposure (traumatic inoculation).

EPIDEMIOLOGY

Incidence

- Most case reports come from the tropical and subtropical regions of the Americas.
- Exposure to plants such as rosebushes, barberry, sphagnum moss, contaminated mine timbers, hay, and other sharp vegetation may result in inoculation.
- Zoonotic exposure has been described following contact with horses, fish, birds, reptiles, armadillos, cats, dogs, and rats and is a possible source of sporotrichosis. Cats are the leading cause.
- An outbreak was associated with stored hay or hay bales harvested in the US Plains states. Outbreaks are possible, given adequate intensity of exposure, and may be difficult to recognize because of the delayed presentation of clinical illness.

RISK FACTORS

- Outbreaks have been associated with hay (Plains states), sphagnum moss (Wisconsin), and infected timber (gold mine, South Africa). Outbreaks are possible, given adequate intensity of exposure, and may be difficult to recognize because of the delayed presentation of clinical illness.

- Lymphocutaneous sporotrichosis is more common among the following:
  - Farmers
  - Florists
  - Gardeners
  - Horticulturists
  - Veterinarians (usually because of possible spread from cats)
- The extracutaneous and disseminated forms of the disease are uncommon and occur in immunocompromised individuals. Conditions which may predispose to disseminated infection include:
  - Alcoholism
  - Diabetes mellitus
  - Immunosuppression (due to steroid use, advanced HIV, chemotherapy, etc.)
  - COPD

GENERAL PREVENTION

Skin protection and care following skin trauma outdoors is often sufficient to avoid sporotrichosis.

ETIOLOGY

S. schenckii is a dimorphic fungus that, at room temperature, exists as branching hyphae, and in tissue, the organism exists as a yeast that is 4–6 μm in diameter, sometimes with a single bud or, infrequently, with multiple buds.

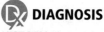 **DIAGNOSIS**

HISTORY

- Insidious onset skin lesion.
- Likely to present with significant outdoor activity and exposures.
- Broad presentations from individuals with an immunocompromised state.

PHYSICAL EXAM

- A papular lesion develops after the incubation period that is usually 1–12 weeks. The lesion may change from red to violaceous and ulceration follows, with discharge of a sero-sanguineous exudate. The lesion can persist for decades without spread.
- Secondary lesions develop along lymphatic channels.
- The papule can progress to form a pustule and then a nodule. The nodule is not tender (pain indicates a secondary bacterial infection).
- Papules and nodules that are irregularly distributed over the body indicate cutaneous disseminated form.
- Some patients present with joint involvement. The joint is swollen and painful on motion and, after weeks or months, a sinus tract may develop.
- Pulmonary infection results from inhalation or aspiration of the fungus.

DIAGNOSTIC TESTS & INTERPRETATION

Lab

- Diagnostics are limited to culture of cutaneous or disseminated sites.
- There is no accepted serologic testing available.

Diagnostic Procedures/Other
- Multiple biopsies may need to be obtained for diagnosis due to low organism burden.
- Attempts at culturing should include Sabouraud agar.
- Organisms can be stained with periodic acid–Schiff and Gomori-methenamine silver (difficult to see on hematoxylin and eosin).
- Appear to be 3–5 microns, cigar-shaped organisms with multiple buds.

Pathological Findings
Histopathologic findings of sporotrichosis include the identification of round to oval spores measuring 4–6 μm in diameter on periodic acid–Schiff stain; the spores stain stronger in the periphery of the lesion.

DIFFERENTIAL DIAGNOSIS
- Cutaneous sporotrichosis can mimic infection due to nocardia, non-tuberculous mycobacteria (i.e. *M. marinum*), leishmaniasis, tularemia, and lymphocutaneous disease due to *Staphylococcus aureus* or *Streptococcus pyogenes*, and other pathogens.
- The differential diagnosis of pulmonary sporotrichosis includes mycobacterial infections due to both *Mycobacterium tuberculosis* and other mycobacteria, histoplasmosis, coccidioidomycosis, and sarcoid.

 TREATMENT

MEDICATION
Azoles
- Mainstay of treatment has been potassium iodide for many years, but itraconazole is now accepted first line therapy.
- Therapeutic serum itraconazole levels need to be confirmed since the drug has variable absorption.
- Itraconazole is more effective then fluconazole or ketoconazole.
- Voriconazole is not effective.
- Little data on the use of posaconazole.
- Terbinafine can be used at high doses.
- May need to extend up to 8 weeks of treatment beyond resolution of cutaneous lesions to minimize risk of relapse.

Potassium Iodide
- Formulated in a saturated solution and can be dropped into liquids for ingestions.
- Start with small dose and increase over successive days.
- Affordable and provides good alternative to patients unable to secure more expensive therapies such as azoles.
- Common side-effects include nausea, rashes, parotid gland enlargement, and excessive lacrimation.

ADDITIONAL TREATMENT
General Measures
- Disseminated sporotrichosis is usually treated with intravenous amphotericin.
- Osteoarticular infections may require prolonged courses with higher dose antifungal agents even up to 1 year.

Issues for Referral
Orthopedic referral may be required for complicated infections of joints.

COMPLEMENTARY & ALTERNATIVE THERAPIES
Cutaneous sporotrichosis can be treated with local heat.

 ONGOING CARE

PATIENT EDUCATION
- Counsel patients regarding exposure risk.
- Specific counseling about handling of animals, specifically cats, which may be a main source of human exposure.

PROGNOSIS
Cutaneous sporotrichosis generally has an excellent prognosis, whereas a high mortality is associated with pulmonary manifestations.

COMPLICATIONS
Osteoarticular or meningitis due to sporotrichosis may require prolonged treatment.

ADDITIONAL READING
- Sporothrix schenckii. In: Mandell GL, Bennett JE, Dolin R, eds. *Principles and practice of infectious diseases*. New York: Churchill Livingstone, 2004.
- Schubach A. Epidemic cat-transmitted sporotrichosis. *N Engl J Med* 2005;353(11): 1185–1886.

 CODES

ICD9
117.1 Sporotrichosis

CLINICAL PEARLS
- *S. schenckii* is a dimorphic fungus that usually causes cutaneous infections.
- Immunocompromised patients can experience disseminated infections including cavitating pulmonary lesions, or even meningitis.
- Mainstay of treatment is oral potassium iodide or itraconazole with excellent prognosis.

S

STOMATITIS

Paschalis Vergidis
Matthew E. Falagas

 BASICS

DESCRIPTION
- Generalized or local inflammation of the oral mucosa of infectious or noninfectious etiology
- May be a manifestation of systemic disease

EPIDEMIOLOGY
Prevalence
- Recurrent aphthous stomatitis, herpetic stomatitis, and hand-foot-and-mouth disease are common.
- Other infections are uncommon, except for oral candidiasis in immunocompromised hosts or patients who receive broad-spectrum antibiotics.
- Herpangina, hand-foot-and-mouth disease, and primary herpetic stomatitis are more common in children.
- Acute necrotizing ulcerative gingivitis/stomatitis (or trench mouth or Vincent's stomatitis) usually affects teenagers and young adults.
- Noma (or gangrenous stomatitis or cancrum oris) is characterized by destruction of soft tissue and bone. Noma is more common in children with malnutrition in Sub-Saharan Africa.

RISK FACTORS
- Smoking
- Antibiotics, immunosuppressive agents
- HIV infection and neoplastic causes of immunosuppression
- Alcohol

GENERAL PREVENTION
- Avoidance of smoking
- Careful oral hygiene of dentures; removal of complete dentures during sleep

ETIOLOGY
- Several infectious causes
  - *Candida* infection (thrush) of the oral mucosa (tongue, buccal mucosa, palate, gums) is frequently seen in diabetics, patients who receive systemic or inhaled corticosteroids, antibiotics, chemotherapy, or patients with impaired cellular immunity (e.g., HIV).

- The cause of recurrent aphthous stomatitis is unknown.
  - Viruses, such as herpes simplex virus 1 and 2 and coxsackievirus (herpangina and hand-foot-and-mouth disease) are common causes of stomatitis.
  - Acute necrotizing ulcerative gingivitis/stomatitis (Vincent's angina or trench mouth) caused by *Prevotella intermedia*, *Fusobacterium* spp. and oral spirochetes.
  - Noma (gangrenous stomatitis) is considered to be caused by fusospirochetal organisms, such as *Borrelia vincentii* and *Fusobacterium nucleatum*. *Prevotella melaninogenica* may also be present.
- Noninfectious causes
  - Allergy (drugs, contact, food)
  - Vitamin deficiency: Riboflavin (vitamin B2) deficiency causes angular stomatitis; niacin deficiency causes pellagra.
  - Smoking (nicotinic stomatitis)
  - Traumatic (e.g., dentures)
  - Systemic diseases (Behçet's disease, uremia, collagen diseases, vascular disease, and anemia)

 DIAGNOSIS

HISTORY
- Clinical manifestations vary, depending on the cause of stomatitis.
- Some patients may complain of general symptoms, such as fever and malaise.
- Oral/gingival pain or tenderness may be present. Oral lesions depend on the etiology of stomatitis.

PHYSICAL EXAM
- Oral candidiasis (thrush) may appear as removable, creamy-white, curd-like patches (pseudomembranous type) or red, friable plaques (erythematous type).
- Round, clearly defined, small painful intraoral ulcers are seen in aphthous stomatitis. These heal without scarring.

- Primary herpetic stomatitis occurs primarily in children and is characterized by fever, malaise, and fatigue, followed by vesicular oral lesions. Mucocutaneous herpes simplex virus infection (usually type 1) may appear as vesicles, which form moist ulcers a few days later. Lesions are bordered by an inflammatory, erythematous base.
- Recurrent herpetic stomatitis may be precipitated by sunlight, emotional stress, or systemic illness.
- Herpangina presents with fever followed by sore throat and dysphagia. Vesicles and ulcers with erythematous rings (typically 5) are seen. These are located on the soft palate and uvula, tonsils, or posterior pharyngeal wall. On the contrary, herpetic gingivostomatitis occurs in the anterior oral cavity.
- Hand-foot-and-mouth disease is usually a mild illness. Buccal and lip ulcers are seen. Cutaneous lesions commonly occur on hands, feet, but also buttocks and groin.
- Vincent's angina presents with gingival necrosis, mainly in the interdental papilla. Results in a marginated, punched-out, and eroded appearance. A superficial grayish pseudomembrane is formed. Halitosis is present.
- Noma is more focal and destructive than acute necrotizing gingivitis.

DIAGNOSTIC TESTS & INTERPRETATION
Lab
- Cultures and stains of abnormal exudate specimens may be of diagnostic help. However, diagnosis should be based on clinical manifestations.
- Budding yeasts with or without pseudohyphae are seen in thrush.
- For herpetic stomatitis: Tzanck smear shows multinucleated giant cells. Other diagnostic tests include direct immunofluorescence, PCR, and viral culture.

Diagnostic Procedures/Other

Biopsy and histologic examination should be performed on all suspicious or chronically recurrent oral lesions, or if lesions fail to heal, to rule out oral malignancies.

DIFFERENTIAL DIAGNOSIS

- Herpetic stomatitis
- Herpangina, hand-foot-and-mouth disease (Coxsackie virus)
- Recurrent aphthous stomatitis
- Necrotizing ulcerative gingivitis/stomatitis and noma
- Thrush (candidal stomatitis)

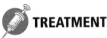 TREATMENT

MEDICATION

First Line

- Treatment is usually symptomatic.
- Topical treatment for mild oral candidiasis (1): Nystatin suspension (400,000–600,000 units 4 times daily), nystatin troche (200,000–400,000 units 4–5 times daily), or clotrimazole troche (10 mg troche dissolved 5 times daily) for 7–14 days (B-II). For moderate-to-severe disease: Fluconazole (100–200 mg daily) for 7–14 days (A-I). Local relief may be achieved by chlorhexidine mouth rinses.
- Antiseptic mouthwashes may be of help to reduce secondary bacterial infection of recurrent aphthous stomatitis. Local anesthetics may be used for pain relief.
- Oral acyclovir (200 mg 5 times a day) or valacyclovir may be necessary for treatment of herpetic stomatitis in immunosuppressed patients. (Intravenous acyclovir should be considered in severely immunosuppressed patients.)
- Oral lesions due to Coxsackie virus usually require no specific treatment.
- Necrotizing ulcerative gingivitis/stomatitis and noma require antibiotic therapy, using penicillin or metronidazole.

Second Line

- Topical or systemic steroids are used for extensive recurrent aphthous stomatitis. Thalidomide for severe recurrent disease, particularly in HIV-infected patients.
- Acyclovir-resistant herpes simplex virus isolates in HIV-positive patients should be treated with foscarnet (40–60 mg/kg IV t.i.d, adjusted for renal function).
- Acyclovir 200 mg 3 times daily or 400 mg twice daily, famciclovir 250 mg twice daily, or valacyclovir 500 mg daily (2) is used in cases of recurrent herpetic stomatitis (when there are more than 5 episodes per year).

ADDITIONAL TREATMENT

Additional Therapies

- Cessation of smoking
- Care of problematic denture
- Topical anesthetics/analgesics
- In noma, correct malnutrition. Loose teeth and sequestra need to be removed.

SURGERY/OTHER PROCEDURES

- Local debridement in necrotizing gingivitis
- Severe facial deformity and mutilation in noma require cosmetic surgery.

IN-PATIENT CONSIDERATIONS

Admission Criteria

- Usually outpatient management
- If stomatitis is severe and the patient cannot take oral, hospitalization may be needed.
- Hospitalization may be needed if stomatitis appears as a complication of severe immunosuppression.

 ONGOING CARE

FOLLOW-UP RECOMMENDATIONS

- Viral (herpetic or Coxsackie virus stomatitis) and episodes of recurrent aphthous stomatitis usually resolve in 7–14 days.
- Persistent, recurrent, or suspicious lesions require biopsy.

DIET

- If the oral lesions are severe and make chewing impossible, the administration of liquids (orally or intravenously) may be necessary.
- Spicy foods may need to be avoided.

COMPLICATIONS

- CNS or ocular involvement in herpetic infection
- Noma may be life-threatening if underlying conditions are severe.

REFERENCES

1. Pappas PG, Kauffman CA, Andes D, et al. Clinical practice guidelines for the management of candidiasis: 2009 update by the Infectious Diseases Society of America. *Clin Infect Dis* 2009;48(5): 503–535.
2. Baker D, Eisen D. Valacyclovir for prevention of recurrent herpes labialis: 2 double-blind, placebo-controlled studies. *Cutis* 2003;71(3): 239–242.

ADDITIONAL READING

- Berthold P. Noma: A forgotten disease. *Dent Clin North Am* 2003;47:559–574.
- McBride DR. Management of aphthous ulcers. *Am Fam Physician* 2000;62:149–154, 160.

 CODES

ICD9

- 054.2 Herpetic gingivostomatitis
- 528.00 Stomatitis and mucositis, unspecified
- 528.2 Oral aphthae

S

CLINICAL PEARLS

- Thrush is frequently seen in diabetics, patients who receive systemic or inhaled corticosteroids, antibiotics, chemotherapy, or patients with impaired cellular immunity (e.g., HIV).
- Herpangina caused by Coxsackie virus presents with vesicles and ulcers located on the soft palate and uvula, tonsils, or posterior pharyngeal wall. On the contrary, herpetic gingivostomatitis occurs in the anterior oral cavity.
- Noma is a public health concern in children with malnutrition in Sub-Saharan Africa.

STRONGYLOIDIASIS

Paschalis Vergidis
Matthew E. Falagas

 BASICS

DESCRIPTION
The intestinal nematode *Strongyloides stercoralis* is common worldwide. Infection starts after larval skin penetration. The parasite can complete its life cycle within the human host; hence the number of adult worms can increase substantially through autoinfection.

EPIDEMIOLOGY
Prevalence
- 3–100 million people may be infected worldwide.
- Less common than other intestinal nematodes.
- Usual locations for infection are tropical, poor, and underdeveloped countries.
- There is a high prevalence in parts of Brazil, Colombia, and Southeast Asia.
- Autoinfection of people in developed countries may occur for up to 40 years.

RISK FACTORS
- Persons residing in or visiting endemic areas
- People who walk barefoot or in other ways are in contact with contaminated soil where larvae may reside.
- Immunosuppression: Solid organ or hematopoietic stem cell transplantation, hematologic malignancies, corticosteroids, TNF-alpha blockers, and cytotoxic medications. Even short courses of steroids have led to hyperinfection syndrome. Relatively few cases of complicated disease in patients coinfected with HIV.
- HTLV-1 coinfection is a risk factor for disseminated strongyloidiasis.

GENERAL PREVENTION
- Adequate sanitation can prevent many cases of this disease.
- Avoid working barefoot in endemic areas.
- Pre-transplant serology testing in patients with relevant epidemiologic history. Treat asymptomatic infection prior to transplantation.

PATHOPHYSIOLOGY
- Adult female worms (2 mm in length) live within the human intestinal wall, at the level of the duodenum and jejunum.
- Eggs hatch in the intestine, and rhabditiform larvae pass in the stool or transform into filariform larvae within the intestine.
- These larvae may live for weeks in the soil.
- Filariform larvae may invade the skin and migrate.
- Filariform larvae within the bowel, reenter the host through the colonic mucosa or perianal skin, and complete their life cycle without leaving the host
- Larvae migrate into cutaneous blood vessels to gain access to the lungs.
- Complicated strongyloidiasis occurs with accelerated autoinfection in which the number of worms increases tremendously and the worms are detectable in extraintestinal regions, especially the lungs. The parasite can disseminate to the brain, kidneys, or liver.
- Person-to-person transmission can occur in day care centers, mental institutions, and among men who have sex with men.

ETIOLOGY
- *Strongyloides stercoralis* (globally distributed)
- *Strongyloides fuelleborni* (found sporadically in Africa, Papua New Guinea)

 DIAGNOSIS

HISTORY
- It takes 25–30 days for the worm to invade the skin, travel to the intestine by the lungs, and start to produce eggs.
- Cutaneous manifestations include a slightly raised, pruritic and irregular track under the skin, resembling cutaneous larva migrans.
- Gastrointestinal symptoms are mild and may include diarrhea, cramping, diffuse pain and weight loss. Symptoms may be more severe in children, with signs of malabsorption and vitamin B_{12} deficiency on rare occasions.

- Pulmonary disease is associated with a Loeffler-like syndrome. The patient has bronchospasm and cough.
- In hyperinfection, disruption of the mucosal patterns, ulcerations, and paralytic ileus may occur. The syndrome can produce overwhelming pneumonitis, leading to acute respiratory distress syndrome. The syndrome can cause polymicrobial sepsis or meningitis with enteric pathogens.

PHYSICAL EXAM
- In acute strongyloidiasis, pruritic erythematous papules appear at the site of larval skin penetration, usually the feet.
- In chronic disease, rapidly progressive serpiginous wheals begin perianally and extend to the buttocks (larva currens). These occur due to autoinfection.

DIAGNOSTIC TESTS & INTERPRETATION
Lab
- Moderate eosinophilia may be seen in the 10–25% range, but may be absent in overwhelming disease states.
- Identify adult worms or rhabditiform larvae in stool and duodenal aspirates. Shedding of the larvae may be light and require many specimens to make the diagnosis.
- Stool nutrient agar plate "culture" is more sensitive than direct smear. Stool sample is placed on agar plate and incubated for at least 2 days. As the larvae crawl over the agar, they carry bacteria with them, creating visible tracks.
- Real-time PCR to detect *Strongyloides* DNA in fecal samples (1).
- Serology (ELISA). Sensitivity reaches 95% in the immunocompetent host. Lower in immunocompromised patients.
- Identify larvae in a duodenal biopsy (usually recommended for rapid diagnosis in children with overwhelming disease).
- Suspect hyperinfection syndrome in gram-negative or polymicrobial sepsis or meningitis with enteric organisms (usually *E. coli*, *Klebsiella*) and no obvious source.

Imaging
- Upper gastrointestinal series are usually nonspecific but may show mucosal edema of the small intestine.
- Chest x-ray findings range from lobar pneumonia, interstitial infiltrates, or, in cases of massive infection, acute respiratory distress syndrome.

Diagnostic Procedures/Other
Duodenal aspirate, biopsy, or the string test may be needed to find the larvae.

DIFFERENTIAL DIAGNOSIS
- Ascaris, ancylostomiasis, and cutaneous larva migrans
- Disseminated disease may resemble atypical pneumonia or tropical pulmonary eosinophilia.

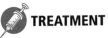 TREATMENT

MEDICATION
First Line
Ivermectin 200 μg/kg/d oral for 2 consecutive days (2) or two single doses 2 weeks apart.

Second Line
- Albendazole 400 mg oral for 3 days
- Thiabendazole 25 mg/kg oral b.i.d for 2 days

Hyperinfection Syndrome
- Ivermectin for 7–14 days.
- In patients with ileus and persistent active infection and no acceptable serum levels of ivermectin, one may consider as a compassionate treatment after obtaining informed consent from the patient (or other legally appointed person by the patient), use of a veterinary parenteral formulation of ivermectin or per rectal ivermectin (3–5).
- Patients also require supportive care and appropriate antibacterial treatment for sepsis.

ADDITIONAL TREATMENT
Additional Therapies
Decrease immunosuppression in transplant recipients and other immunocompromised patients.

 ONGOING CARE

FOLLOW-UP RECOMMENDATIONS
- Check stool samples 2 weeks after completion of antiparasitic treatment. If larvae identified, repeat therapy.
- In disseminated disease, obtain stool studies daily during treatment. Continue treatment until symptoms resolve and stool tests negative for at least 2 weeks.
- Follow serology to monitor response to treatment (6). Antibody titers decrease within 6–12 months.
- Monitor for resolution of eosinophilia.

PROGNOSIS
Hyperinfection syndrome is potentially fatal.

COMPLICATIONS
Hyperinfection syndrome may lead to respiratory failure or sepsis.

REFERENCES

1. Verweij JJ, Canales M, Polman K, et al. Molecular diagnosis of *Strongyloides stercoralis* in faecal samples using real-time PCR. *Trans R Soc Trop Med Hyg* 2009;103:342–346.
2. Igual-Adell R, Oltra-Alcaraz C, Soler-Company E, et al. Efficacy and safety of ivermectin and thiabendazole in the treatment of strongyloidiasis. *Expert Opin Pharmacother* 2004;5(12):2615–2619.
3. Turner SA, Maclean JD, Fleckenstein L, et al. Parenteral administration of ivermectin in a patient with disseminated strongyloidiasis. *Am J Trop Med Hyg* 2005;73:911–914.
4. Fusco DN, Downs JA, Satlin MJ, et al. Non-oral treatment with ivermectin for disseminated strongyloidiasis. *Am J Trop Med Hyg* 2010;83: 879–883.
5. Grein JD, Mathisen GE, Donovan S, et al. Serum ivermectin levels after enteral and subcutaneous administration for Strongyloides hyperinfection: A case report. *Scand J Infect Dis* 2010;42:234–236.
6. Page WA, Dempsey K, McCarthy JS. Utility of serological follow-up of chronic strongyloidiasis after anthelminthic chemotherapy. *Trans R Soc Trop Med Hyg* 2006;100(11):1056–1062.

ADDITIONAL READING
- Siddiqui AA, Berk SL. Diagnosis of *Strongyloides stercoralis* infection. *Clin Infect Dis* 2001;33(7): 1040–1047.

S

 CODES

ICD9
127.2 Strongyloidiasis

CLINICAL PEARLS
- Patients with strongyloidiasis may present with asymptomatic eosinophilia.
- *Strongyloides* can cause overwhelming infection in the immunocompromised host (hyperinfection syndrome). Consider if polymicrobial sepsis/ meningitis with enteric organisms and no obvious source.
- Treatment of choice is ivermectin.

SUPERFICIAL SKIN AND SOFT-TISSUE INFECTIONS

Michael N. Mavros
Paschalis Vergidis
Matthew E. Falagas

 BASICS

DESCRIPTION
- Superficial skin and soft-tissue infections occur just below the stratum corneum, in the hair follicles, or apocrine glands, and below the epidermis, penetrating the dermis to subcutaneous (SC) tissues.
- The disease can manifest as:
  - impetigo (epidermis)
  - folliculitis (dermis)
  - furunculosis (dermis)
  - simple abscess (dermis and SC tissue)
  - erysipelas (dermis and SC tissue)
  - cellulitis (deeper SC tissue)
- SSTIs can be classified as:
  - Uncomplicated: Superficial, respond to a single course of antibiotics or simple drainage (impetigo, folliculitis, simple abscess, erysipelas, superficial cellulitis).
  - Complicated (cSSTI): Involve deeper soft tissue, require surgical intervention (complicated abscess, complicated cellulitis, infected ulcers/wounds), or occur in a patient with a significant comorbidity that complicates response to treatment.

EPIDEMIOLOGY
Incidence
- Impetigo:
  - 10–20 cases per 1,000 persons-years (1).
  - May occur in outbreaks; most common in children and elderly, and in areas with poor sanitation.
- Erysipelas:
  - 0.1–2.0 cases per 1,000 patient-years (1).
  - Most common during 6th–7th decade of life, female predominance; 80% of cases in lower limbs.
- Cellulitis:
  - ~20 cases per 1,000 patient-years.
  - Most common during 6th decade of life; 40–70% of cases in lower limbs.

RISK FACTORS
- Immune deficiency predisposes to all SSTIs.
- Impetigo: Lower SES (poor sanitation), tropic climate (1,2).
- Folliculitis (& furunculosis): S. aureus carriage, poor hygiene (1,2).
- Erysipelas/cellulitis: Disruption of the cutaneous barrier, lymphedema, local venous stasis, or chronic edema, obesity, previous episode of cellulitis (only predisposes to cellulitis) (2).

GENERAL PREVENTION
- Improvement of sanitary conditions.
- Prompt treatment of comorbidities (i.e., venous stasis, obesity).
- Proper foot care for diabetics and patients with tinea pedis, lymphedema, or venous insufficiency.
- Standard infection control measures should be followed by health-care personnel to reduce transmission of methicillin-resistant S. aureus (MRSA).

PATHOPHYSIOLOGY
- Bacteria invade through a break in the skin (e.g., trauma, insect bite, or cutaneous disease).
- Infection then:
  - Gets localized (folliculitis, furunculosis, simple abscess)
  - Spreads at the site of inoculation (erysipelas, cellulitis), or at a distant site (cellulitis, usually in immunocompromised patients)
- In impetigo, the exfoliating toxins of S. aureus cause dermal necrosis.
- In erysipelas, the infection can rapidly spread through the course of the lymphatics.

ETIOLOGY
- Impetigo: S. aureus and/or GAS (Group A Streptococcus) (1,2).
- Folliculitis (& furunculosis): S. aureus (1,2)
- Simple abscess: S. aureus, polymicrobial (1,2)
- Erysipelas-cellulitis (1,2):
  - Usually GAS
  - Rarely other bacteria (e.g., S. aureus, P. multocida from animal bites, A. hydrophila from fresh water, Vibrio spp. from saltwater, other gram-negative bacteria).
- S. aureus is the most common pathogen overall, followed by GAS.
- Alarmingly increasing incidence of community-acquired MRSA (CA-MRSA) (2).

COMMONLY ASSOCIATED CONDITIONS
Colonization of the host (skin flora, nasopharyngeal flora) with S. aureus and/or GAS.

 DIAGNOSIS

HISTORY
Contact sports, crowded living conditions, and poor hygiene predispose to colonization with CA-MRSA.

PHYSICAL EXAM
- Impetigo:
  - Bullous (itchy superficial flaccid bullae)
  - Nonbullous (itchy thin-walled vesicles and pustules, on an erythematous base)
  - usually on face or extremities
  - common in hot, humid environment
- Folliculitis: Vesicles and lesions involving hair follicles.
- Furuncle (boil): Firm, discrete nodules, due to infection of hair follicles
- Carbuncle:
  - Extension and coalescence of furuncles causes an inflammatory, purulent mass
  - usually on the back of the neck, on the back, or the thigh.

- Erysipelas:
  - Raised, fiery-red, indurated painful plaque with a "peau d'orange" appearance
  - sharply demarcated, advancing margins
  - usually in the extremities, followed by the face (especially over the bridge of the nose or the cheeks)
  - Often systemic manifestations (malaise, fever, chills)
- Recurrent erysipelas:
  - Chronic edema from lymphatic or venous obstruction
  - Begins with painful red lesion, advancing rapidly up the limb
  - Systemic manifestations (malaise, fever, chills)
- Cellulitis:
  - Erythematous, hot, edematous, and tender lesions
  - Borders are poorly demarcated, not elevated
  - Systemic manifestations (malaise, fever, chills, toxicity)

DIAGNOSTIC TESTS & INTERPRETATION
Lab
Initial lab tests
- Diagnosis is primarily clinical.
- CBC (complete blood count), BMP (basic metabolic panel), and CRP (C-reactive protein) may be obtained if invasive disease is suspected.

Follow-Up & Special Considerations
Blood cultures and cultures of needle aspiration of the lesions are rarely recommended (e.g., in outbreaks of impetigo to identify MRSA, in patients with diabetes mellitus, malignancy, and unusual predisposing factors, such as immersion injury, animal bites, neutropenia, and immunodeficiency) (2).

Imaging
- Imaging is rarely useful in SSTIs.
- Ultrasonography may aid in guiding needle aspiration.
- CT or MRI may aid in ruling out a necrotizing infection and osteomyelitis.

Diagnostic Procedures/Other
Incision and drainage of abscesses provides a material for culture, which will guide antibiotic therapy, if necessary.

DIFFERENTIAL DIAGNOSIS
- Infectious:
  - Herpes simplex/zoster
  - Erysipeloid (E. rhusiopathiae)
  - Ecthyma gangrenosum (P. aeruginosa)
  - Necrotizing soft-tissue infections
- Noninfectious (3):
  - Contact dermatitis
  - Gout
  - Insect stings or bites
  - Drug reactions
  - Superficial thrombophlebitis
  - DVT (Deep venous thrombosis)
  - Eosinophilic cellulitis (Wells syndrome)
  - Acute lipodermatosclerosis
  - Lymphedema

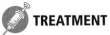

TREATMENT

MEDICATION

First Line
- Impetigo (1,2):
  – Mild: Topical mupirocin, fusidic acid, or retapamulin.
  – Moderate/severe: PO dicloxacillin or cephalexin
- Furunculosis (1,2):
  – Primary therapy is drainage.
  – When eradication of staphylococcal carriage is indicated (in recurrent impetigo and outbreaks), either topical mupirocin (in the anterior nares) or PO clindamycin may be used.
- Simple abscess (1,2):
  – Primary therapy is drainage.
  – If there are multiple abscesses or impaired host defences, doxycycline, minocycline, clindamycin, or TMP/SMX can be used.
- Erysipelas (1,2):
  – PO penicillin V or IV penicillin G (depending on severity)
  – If *S. aureus* is suspected, PO dicloxacillin or cephalexin should be preferred.
- Cellulitis (1,2):
  – PO dicloxacillin, cephalexin, clindamycin, or erythromycin
  – Severe: IV nafcillin, cefazolin (for penicillin-allergic patients, use clindamycin or vancomycin)
  – For uncomplicated erysipelas/cellulitis, a 5-day course appears as effective as a 10-day course.
- For CA-MRSA (2):
  – Doxycycline or minocycline (not in children ≤8 years old and in pregnant women)
  – Clindamycin (potential for emergence of resistance)
  – Linezolid, daptomycin, vancomycin are highly effective but should be reserved for hospitalized patients not responding to other antibiotics.
- Resistance to macrolides is increasing.

Second Line
- Impetigo (1,2):
  – Mild: Topical bacitracin and neomycin are considerably less effective than mupirocin.
  – Moderate/severe: PO clindamycin, amoxicillin/clavulanate.
- Erysipelas (1,2): PO amoxicillin or IV amoxicillin or cefazolin (depending on severity)
- For CA-MRSA (1,2):
  – TMP/SMX (Trimethoprim-sulfamethoxazole)
  – Levofloxacin, gatifloxacin, moxifloxacin

ADDITIONAL TREATMENT
General Measures
- Impetigo: Removal of infected crusts with soap and water.
- Furunculosis (1,2):
  – Small furuncles: Moist heat is sufficient
  – Large furuncles/carbuncles: Incision & drainage (PO antibiotics not necessary in the absence of systemic symptoms)
  – Control of outbreaks: Bathing with chlorhexidine, enhanced sanitation, and eradication of staphylococcal carriage.
  – Recurrent furunculosis: Eradication of carriage through either topical mupirocin (in the anterior nares), or PO clindamycin.

- Recurrent erysipelas/cellulitis (1,2):
  – Prophylactic IM penicillin G, or PO penicillin V, or erythromycin may be beneficial.
  – Providing patient with PO antibiotics to begin when symptoms of infection appear may be beneficial.
- Elevation of the affected limb to reduce edema and promote recovery.

Issues for Referral
Immediate referral to a surgeon if a necrotizing soft tissue infection is suspected.

Additional Therapies
Physiotherapy to improve muscle tone and venous return.

COMPLEMENTARY & ALTERNATIVE THERAPIES
For selected cases of uncomplicated erysipelas and cellulitis, systemic corticosteroids may be beneficial (2).

SURGERY/OTHER PROCEDURES
- Large furuncles/carbuncles:
  – Incision and drainage
- Abscess:
  – Incision and drainage alone is adequate for abscesses with a diameter of <5 cm.
  – If severe systemic symptoms occur, antibiotics should be administered.
- Immediate surgery is critical when the infection expands causing tissue necrosis, and cannot be controlled with antibiotics.

IN-PATIENT CONSIDERATIONS
Admission Criteria
Most patients with erysipelas/cellulitis don't need hospitalization (1).

Discharge Criteria
Patients with severe erysipelas/cellulitis admitted for IV therapy can be discharged and continued on oral antibiotics if they show marked improvement (outlining the borders of the erythema may aid in evaluating response to therapy).

ONGOING CARE

FOLLOW-UP RECOMMENDATIONS
- Patients with impetigo should follow up with their physician if the lesions do not improve with treatment.
- Patients with cellulitis should be followed up within 48–72 hours to confirm response to treatment.

PATIENT EDUCATION
For impetigo and folliculitis, patients can be educated to improve sanitary conditions, if applicable.

PROGNOSIS
- SSTIs may recur, but prognosis is excellent for promptly treated, uncomplicated cases.
- Very rarely, a SSTI may progress to a necrotizing soft-tissue infection, which is a life-threatening condition.

COMPLICATIONS
- Impetigo very rarely gives rise to post-streptococcal glomerulonephritis (not prevented by proper treatment).
- Erysipelas/cellulitis:
  – Abscess formation
  – Recurrence in ~20% of cases (recurrent episodes may cause lymphedema).
  – Lymphangitis or thrombophlebitis.
  – Rare: Bacteremia with seeding of distant sites, endocarditis
  – Infection may occasionally spread to deeper tissues causing a necrotizing soft-tissue infection.

REFERENCES
1. Bernard P. Management of common bacterial infections of the skin. *Curr Opin Infect Dis* 2008;21:122–128.
2. Stevens DL, Bisno AL, Chambers HF, et al. Practice guidelines for the diagnosis and management of skin and soft-tissue infections. *Clin Infect Dis* 2005;41:1373–1406.
3. Falagas ME, Vergidis PI. Narrative review: Diseases that masquerade as infectious cellulitis. *Ann Intern Med* 2005;142:47–55.

ADDITIONAL READING
- Stryjewski ME, Chambers HF. Skin and soft-tissue infections caused by community-acquired methicillin-resistant *Staphylococcus aureus*. *Clin Infect Dis* 2008;46(Suppl 5):S368–S377.

CODES

ICD9
- 684 Impetigo
- 686.9 Unspecified local infection of skin and subcutaneous tissue
- 704.8 Other specified diseases of hair and hair follicles

CLINICAL PEARLS
- SSTIs are very common and, when uncomplicated, carry an excellent prognosis.
- Increasing incidence of CA-MRSA may warrant modifications in the standard regimens.
- Physicians should be alert for signs of progression of the infection with tissue necrosis (NSTI), which requires surgical exploration.

S

SURGICAL SITE INFECTIONS

Jatin M. Vyas (E. Mylonakis, Editor)

 BASICS

DESCRIPTION

- Surgical site infection (formerly termed surgical wound infection) is characterized as having any of the following:
  - A purulent exudate draining from a surgical site.
  - A positive fluid culture obtained from a surgical site that was closed primarily.
  - The surgeon's diagnosis of infection.
  - A surgical site that requires reopening.
- Further classifications can be made based on the site of infection:
  - Superficial incisional infection when it occurs within 30 days after the operation, and it involves only skin or subcutaneous tissue and one of the following:
    - Purulent drainage from the superficial incision
    - Organisms isolated from an aseptically obtained sample from the superficial incision
    - Clinical diagnosis by a clinician
  - Deep superficial incisional when it occurs within 30 days after the operation (or up to 1 year if the implant is in place), it appears to be related to the operation, and it involves deep soft tissues and one of the following:
    - Purulent drainage from the deep tissues of the surgical site
    - Signs of abscess or other signs (e.g., radiologic) of infection involving the deep tissues
    - Clinical diagnosis by a clinician
  - Organ/space when it occurs within 30 days after the operation (or up to 1 year if implant is in place), it appears to be related to the operation, and it involves any parts of the anatomy except the incision and one of the following:
    - Purulent drainage from a drain that is placed into the organ/space
    - Organisms isolated from an aseptically obtained sample from the organ/space
    - Signs of abscess or other signs (e.g., radiologic) of infection involving the organ/space
    - Clinical diagnosis by a clinician

EPIDEMIOLOGY

Incidence

- Surgical site infections account for approximately 15% of all nosocomial infections and are the second most common nosocomial infections.
- Among surgical patients, surgical site infections are the most common nosocomial infections, accounting for approximately 40% of all such infections. Of these surgical site infections, two-thirds are confined to the incision, and one-third involves organs or spaces accessed during the operation.

- A 2002 analysis showed that each surgical site infection resulted in 12 additional postoperative hospital days, doubling the rehospitalization rate and increasing the cost by 300%.
- Many surgical site infections are detected after the patient is discharged from the hospital.
- From 1991 to 1995, the incidence of surgical site infections caused by fungi increased from 0.1 to 0.3 per 1,000 discharges.

RISK FACTORS

- In general, 3 main risk factors for surgical site infections are as follows:
  - The nature and number of organisms contaminating the surgical site
  - The general health status of the patient including the presence or absence of comorbidities
  - The skill and technique of the surgeon
- Patient characteristics associated with an increased risk of a surgical site infection include the following:
  - Cigarette smoking
  - Coincident remote site infections or colonization
  - Diabetes
  - Extremes of age
  - Duration of surgery (longer time translates into higher risk)
  - Long preoperative length of stay
  - Obesity
  - Poor nutritional status
  - Preoperative shaving of the field, especially if performed 24 hours or more, prior to the operation
  - Presence of a drain
  - Presence of an untreated remote infection
  - Systemic steroid use or other immunomodulatory agent
  - Preoperative nasal carriage or colonization at other sites with *S. aureus*

GENERAL PREVENTION

- Advances in infection control practices include improved operating room ventilation, sterilization methods, barriers, surgical technique, and availability of antimicrobial prophylaxis.
- Preventive antibiotics (usually administered once, within 2 hours prior to the operation)
  - Hysterectomy: Cefazolin 1–2 g IV or cefoxitin 1–2 g IV.
  - Upper gastrointestinal tract: Cefazolin 1–2 g IV or cefoxitin 1–2 g IV.
  - Lower gastrointestinal tract
    - Elective: The vast majority of surgeons use antibiotics and mechanical cleansing for preoperative preparation for elective colon resection. The most popular regimen in the US has been oral neomycin-erythromycin base, along with cefoxitin IV.
    - Emergency: Cefoxitin 1–2 g IV or cefoxitin 1–2 g IV, and metronidazole 500 mg IV or cefotetan 1–2 g IV.
  - Cardiovascular: Cefazolin 1 g t.i.d for up to 24–48 hours or vancomycin 1 g IV b.i.d for up to 48 hours (the use of vancomycin is also discussed below)

- A preoperative antiseptic shower or bath decreases skin microbial colony counts.
- The routine use of vancomycin in surgical antibiotic prophylaxis is not recommended. However, vancomycin may be the agent of choice in certain clinical circumstances, such as risk factors for postoperative methicillin-resistant *S. aureus* (MRSA) infection (such as recent hospitalization, renal disease, or diabetes).
- Preventing hypothermia can prevent surgical site infections.
- The Centers for Disease Control and Prevention recommendations for the prevention of surgical site infections include the following:
  - Whenever possible, identify and treat all infections remote to the surgical site before elective operation.
  - Adequately control serum blood glucose levels in all diabetic patients and avoid hyperglycemia perioperatively.
  - Encourage tobacco cessation.
  - Keep the preoperative hospital stay as short as possible while allowing for adequate preoperative preparation of the patient.
  - Administer a prophylactic antimicrobial agent only when indicated.
  - Use delayed primary skin closure or leave an incision open to heal by second intention if the surgeon considers the surgical site to be heavily contaminated.

ETIOLOGY

- For most surgical site infections, the source of pathogens is the endogenous flora.
- The dose of contaminating microorganisms required to produce infection may be much lower when foreign material is present at the site.
- Pathogens isolated from surgical site infections mainly include the following:
  - *Staphylococcus aureus*
  - Coagulase-negative staphylococci
  - *Streptococcus* spp.
  - Enterobacteriaceae (usually *Escherichia coli*)
  - *Enterococcus* spp.
  - *Bacteroides* spp. and other anaerobes are associated with surgery involving the gastrointestinal and female genital tracts.
- An increasing proportion of surgical site infections are caused by antimicrobial-resistant pathogens, such as MRSA or *Candida albicans*.
- Outbreaks or clusters of surgical site infections have also been caused by unusual pathogens, such as *Rhizopus oryzae*, *Clostridium perfringens*, Rhodococcus bronchialis, *Nocardia* spp., and *Legionella* spp. These rare outbreaks have been traced to contaminated adhesive dressings, elastic bandages, colonized surgical personnel, tap water, or contaminated disinfectant solutions.
- Unusual pathogens or cluster of infections should be reported to the local infection control office.

DIAGNOSIS

HISTORY
- Fever is often present, especially in deep incisional or organ/space surgical site infections and it can be the only presenting symptom.
- Excessive pain at the surgical site
- Drainage from the surgical site
- Chills or rigors
- Tenderness at the site of surgery

PHYSICAL EXAM
- A surgical wound should be examined for erythema extending more than 2 cm beyond the margin of the wound, localized tenderness and induration, fluctuance, drainage of purulent material, and dehiscence of sutures.
- Mechanical factors, as well as infection, can cause wound dehiscence.
- Sternal wounds following cardiac surgery are of special concern because the consequences of infection can be severe. The surface of the wound may not present an obvious cause for concern, but, in some patients, ongoing fevers and especially the development of rocking or instability of the sternum may be sufficient cause for surgical exploration of the wound.

DIAGNOSTIC TESTS & INTERPRETATION
Lab
- Persistent leukocytosis is a common laboratory finding.
- Drainage and microbiologic evaluation of the exudate (Gram stain and aerobic and anaerobic cultures) as well as blood cultures can help identify the pathogen(s).

Imaging
Initial approach
Imaging of the surgical area (usually with the use of computed tomography) is often helpful in evaluating the presence and the extent of collection(s).

Follow-Up & Special Considerations
Drainage and sampling of an abscess for Gram stain and culture is typically required.

TREATMENT

MEDICATION
First Line
- Superficial incisional surgical site infection: Amoxicillin/clavulanate (500 mg t.i.d) or dicloxacillin (100 mg PO b.i.d), with or without fluoroquinolone (e.g., levofloxacillin 500 mg PO once daily)
- Deep superficial or organ/space surgical site infections are typically driven by the microbiology of the infection. Empiric coverage may include any of the following: Ampicillin-sulbactam (3 g IV q.i.d), or piperacillin-tazobactam (3.375 g IV t.i.d; higher doses are needed for covering *Pseudomonas* spp.), or ticarcillin-clavulanate. For surgery involving the gastrointestinal or female genital tracts, consider also cefoxitin (1 g IV t.i.d) or imipenem (500 mg IV q6h).
- Surgical drainage is often necessary.
- Duration of treatment depends on the site and extent of infection, presence of drains, response to treatment, surgical management, and the causative microorganism.

SURGERY/OTHER PROCEDURES
Re-exploration of the surgical site may be required to drain an abscess or improve wound healing.

ONGOING CARE

FOLLOW-UP RECOMMENDATIONS
- If gastrointestinal leakage is identified at the time of the operation, then the continuation of the antibiotic agents from 1–3 days is usually recommended.
- Leaving the operative wound open, packed with saline-soaked gauze, decreases the incidence of postoperative wound infection in high-risk patients.

PATIENT EDUCATION
Please return to the surgeon or your PCP if you develop fevers or redness near the surgical wound site.

COMPLICATIONS
- Patients with a deep surgical site infection have a significantly increased mortality rate, with a risk ratio of 1.7.
- Mediastinitis or sternal osteomyelitis is a severe complication of cardiac surgery.
- Infection of wounds associated with the placement of prosthetic devices can lead to infection of the prosthesis, and generally requires surgical removal of the device.

ADDITIONAL READING
- Bratzler DW, Hunt DR. The surgical infection prevention and surgical care improvement projects: National initiatives to improve outcomes for patients having surgery. *Clin Infect Dis* 2006;43: 322.
- Antimicrobial prophylaxis for surgery. *Treat Guidel Med Lett* 2009;7:47–52.

CODES

ICD9
998.59 Other postoperative infection

S

SYPHILIS

Paschalis Vergidis
Matthew E. Falagas

 BASICS

DESCRIPTION
Syphilis is a sexually transmitted infection caused by *Treponema pallidum*. Disease progression is divided into overlapping stages of primary, secondary, latent, and tertiary.

EPIDEMIOLOGY
Incidence
- In the US, the number of cases of early syphilis increased in 2001 for the first time since 1990, and this trend has continued through 2007. From 2000 to 2007, the incidence rate increased from 2.1 to 3.7 cases per 100,000 population.
- Rates are higher among men who have sex with men and African–American men and women.
- There is a relatively high rate of HIV coinfection in persons with syphilis.

RISK FACTORS
- Unsafe sexual practices
- Multiple partners
- Anonymous sex
- Injection drug use
- Exchanging sex for money
- Syphilis and HIV infection enhance the acquisition and transmission of one another (1).

GENERAL PREVENTION
Safe sex practices (barrier methods for vaginal, anal, and oral sex)

PATHOPHYSIOLOGY
- Syphilis is transmitted through direct contact with an active lesion. Only mucocutaneous lesions are infectious; they are seen in primary and secondary stages. Disease can spread by kissing or touching infectious lesions.
- After penetrating the skin or mucous membranes, *T. pallidum* enters the lymphatics and bloodstream and disseminates.
- Syphilis is also transmitted transplacentally.
- The disease is rarely transmitted through blood product transfusion.

ETIOLOGY
Treponema pallidum spirochete

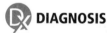 **DIAGNOSIS**

HISTORY
- Primary syphilis has an incubation period of 2–4 weeks. Characterized by primary chancre.
- Secondary syphilis: 3–6 weeks after disappearance of primary lesion. Characterized by protean manifestations and diffuse rash. Malaise, headaches, sore throat, fever, weight loss, and musculoskeletal pain may develop.
- After resolution of secondary signs, the patient enters a latent phase. Disease can still progress. Infection can be demonstrated only by serologic testing.

- Early latent: Initial infection has occurred within the previous 12 months. Patient potentially infectious. Relapse possible.
- Late latent: Initial infection has occurred more than 1 year previously. Transmission or relapse very unlikely.
- Late syphilis of unknown duration: If past serologic testing not available.
- Tertiary syphilis: 5–25 years of latent syphilis. The patient may have not developed symptomatic primary or secondary disease.
- Neurosyphilis can occur at any stage. Typically, meningitis, and meningovascular involvement occurs in early disease. General paralysis and tabes dorsalis occurs in late disease.

PHYSICAL EXAM
Primary Syphilis
- Papule, 5–15 mm diameter, sharply demarcated, elevated, smooth, firm, and nonpurulent. The lesion quickly erodes and becomes indurated. Regional lymphadenopathy may be present.
- Papule generally painless; appears at site of inoculation: External genitalia, anal area, lips, oral cavity, breasts, or fingers.

Secondary Syphilis
- 3–6 weeks after disappearance of primary lesion, but, occasionally, primary lesion still present
- Rash in approximately 90% of patients
- Rash begins as faint, rose-pink, macular, rounded lesions up to 1-cm diameter. Lesions begin in the trunk and proximal extremities.
- Gradually becomes red and papular, spreading to entire body, including palms and soles
- Nonpruritic macular, maculopapular, papular, or pustular lesions may be seen. Vesicular lesions are only present in congenital syphilis
- Generalized painless lymphadenopathy (70% of patients). Involvement of the epitrochlear lymph nodes is a unique finding.
- Mucosal lesions, mainly oral patches (20% of patients)
- Condylomata lata (broad, flat, exophytic lesions) in warm, moist areas; typically perianal. These are highly infectious.
- Focal alopecia, loss of eyebrows or beard
- Hepatitis
- Infiltration or induration of the gastrointestinal tract
- Arthritis, osteitis, periosteitis
- Immune complex glomerulonephritis

Tertiary Syphilis
- Cardiovascular involvement of ascending aorta, leading to aortic aneurysm and aortic valve regurgitation
- Gummas in skin, bone or internal organs. Skin gummas present as ulcers or heaped up granulomatous lesions of varying size.

Neurosyphilis
- Asymptomatic neurosyphilis: Cerebrospinal fluid (CSF) abnormalities in the absence of symptomatic neurologic disease
- Symptomatic aseptic meningitis
- Anterior uveitis, posterior uveitis, interstitial keratitis, iritis, optical neuritis, and retinal necrosis
- Sensorineural sudden or progressive hearing loss, tinnitus, vertigo, and dysequilibrium
- Other cranial abnormalities
- Brain or spinal cord infarction
- General paresis: Progressive dementia (usually 10–25 years after infection)
- Tabes dorsalis: Sensory ataxia, pupillary abnormalities, sudden, severe pains in extremities, back, or face (usually 20 years after infection)
- Argyll-Robertson pupil: Small, not reactive to light, contracts normally to accommodation.

DIAGNOSTIC TESTS & INTERPRETATION
Lab
Direct detection
- Dark-field examination. Detects *T. pallidum* upon characteristic morphology and motility. Can be used for primary and secondary lesions (except for oral lesions).
- Immunofluorescence
- Polymerase chain reaction (PCR)

Serology
- A presumptive diagnosis is made with use of a treponemal and a non-treponemal test. The use of only one type of serologic test is insufficient.
- The traditional algorithm employs a non-treponemal test (such as rapid plasma reagin [RPR]) to screen patients and a treponemal test to confirm reactive tests.
- In recent years, laboratories have switched to screening populations with treponemal tests (typically, enzyme immunoassay).
- Individuals with a positive treponemal screening test should have a standard non-treponemal test with titer performed. If the non-treponemal test is negative, then the laboratory should perform a different treponemal test to confirm the results of the initial test.
- Non-treponemal tests
  – Rapid Plasma Reagin (RPR)
  – Venereal Disease Research Laboratory (VDRL)
  – Toluidine Red Unheated Serum Test (TRUST)
    ○ Nonspecific for syphilis
    ○ Yield false–positives in older age, pregnancy, intravenous drug use, autoimmune diseases, and non-syphilis treponemal infection
    ○ Titer correlates with disease activity.
- Treponemal tests
  – *T. pallidum* immobilization assay (TPI)
  – Fluorescent treponemal antibody absorption (FTA-ABS)
  – *T. pallidum* hemaglutination assay (TPHA)
  – *T. pallidum* passive particle agglutination assay (TPPA)
  – Enzyme Immunoassay (EIA)

○ More specific than nontreponemal tests
○ Titers do not correlate with disease activity.
- Patients with latent syphilis with any of the following should have a CSF examination:
  – Neurologic or ophthalmic signs or symptoms
  – Evidence of active tertiary syphilis (e.g., aortitis, gumma)
  – Serologic nonresponse to treatment
- In HIV coinfected patients, CSF examination should be performed if any of the following (2):
  – Late latent syphilis or syphilis of unknown duration, regardless of CD4 count or RPR titer.
  – CD4 count ≤350 cells/mL and/or RPR titer ≥1:32, regardless of syphilis stage.
  – Serologic nonresponse to syphilis therapy.
- Syphilitic meningitis: Lymphocytic pleocytosis (typically <100 cells/μL), elevated protein concentration (usually <100 mg/dL), a reactive CSF–VDRL.
  – Note: CSF–VDRL may be nonreactive in late syphilis (i.e., tabes dorsalis)

DIFFERENTIAL DIAGNOSIS
- **Infectious**
  – Genital herpes
  – Chancroid
  – Acute HIV infection
  – Venereal warts
  – Scabies
  – Molluscum contagiosum
  – Folliculitis
  – Lymphogranuloma venereum (rare)
  – Granuloma inguinale/donovanosis (rare)
  – Mycobacteria (rare)
  – Fungi (rare)
  – Parasites (rare)
- **Noninfectious**
  – Malignancy
  – Benign lesions
  – Fixed drug eruption
  – Erythema multiforme
  – Dermatitis herpetiformis
  – Behçet's syndrome

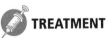 TREATMENT

MEDICATION
First Line
- Primary and secondary syphilis
  – Benzathine penicillin 2.4 million U IM one time
  – Retreatment (if failure): 2.4 million U IM weekly for 3 weeks
- Latent Syphilis
  – Early latent: Benzathine penicillin 2.4 million U IM one time. Retreatment: 2.4 million U IM weekly for 3 weeks
  – Late latent or unknown duration: Benzathine penicillin 2.4 million U IM weekly for 3 weeks
- Tertiary syphilis
  – Benzathine penicillin 2.4 million U IM weekly for 3 weeks
- Neurosyphilis
  – Aqueous penicillin G 18–24 million units per day, administered as 3–4 million units IV every 4 hours or continuous infusion, for 10–14 days.

Second Line
- Primary and secondary Syphilis
  – Doxycycline 100 mg orally twice daily for 14 days (3).
  – Tetracycline 500 mg 4 times daily for 14 days.
  – Azithromycin 2 g oral single dose (4).
  – Note: *T. pallidum* chromosomal mutations associated with azithromycin resistance and treatment failures have been documented in several geographical areas in the US (5).
- Latent Syphilis
  – Doxycycline 100 mg orally twice daily for 28 days
  – Tetracycline 500 mg orally 4 times daily for 28 days
- Neurosyphilis
  – Procaine penicillin 2.4 million units IM once daily plus probenecid 500 mg orally 4 times a day, both for 10–14 days.

Pregnancy Considerations
Parenteral penicillin G is the only therapy with documented efficacy during pregnancy. Pregnant women with syphilis in any stage who report penicillin allergy should be desensitized.

ALERT
- Jarisch–Herxheimer reaction is a possible acute febrile treatment reaction. Characterized by headache, myalgia, fever, and other symptoms.
- Usually occurs within 24 hours after treatment initiation. Can occur at any stage but most frequently in early syphilis.

 ONGOING CARE

FOLLOW-UP RECOMMENDATIONS
- Evaluate sex partners clinically and serologically.
- Treat partners as appropriate to stage of disease if seropositive.
- Persons who were exposed within 90 days preceding the diagnosis of primary, secondary, or early latent syphilis in a sex partner might be infected even if seronegative; therefore, such persons should be treated presumptively.
- Failure of non-treponemal test titers to decline fourfold within 6–12 months after therapy for primary or secondary syphilis may be indicative of treatment failure
- However, >15% of patients with early syphilis treated with the recommended therapy will not achieve the two dilution decline at 1 year
- Patients with late syphilis or neurosyphilis should have serum non-treponemal titers measured at 3 and 6 months followed thereafter at 6-month intervals for up to 2 years or until the serology reverts to nonreactive. Titers should fall fourfold within a year, and continue to fall thereafter.
- For neurosyphilis: Repeat CSF analysis recommended every 6 months until the cell count has normalized

REFERENCES
1. Buchacz K, Klausner JD, Kerndt PR, et al. HIV incidence among men diagnosed with early syphilis in Atlanta, San Francisco, and Los Angeles, 2004 to 2005. *J Acquir Immune Defic Syndr* (1999) 2008;47(2):234–240.
2. Ghanem KG, Moore RD, Rompalo AM, et al. Lumbar puncture in HIV-infected patients with syphilis and no neurologic symptoms. *Clin Infect Dis* 2009;48(6):816–821.
3. Ghanem KG, Erbelding EJ, Cheng WW, et al. Doxycycline compared with benzathine penicillin for the treatment of early syphilis. *Clin Infect Dis* 2006;42(6):e45–e49.
4. Hook EW 3rd, Behets F, Van Damme K, et al. A phase III equivalence trial of azithromycin versus benzathine penicillin for treatment of early syphilis. *J Infect Dis* 2010;201(11):1729–1735.
5. Mitchell SJ, Engelman J, Kent CK, et al. Azithromycin-resistant syphilis infection: San Francisco, California, 2000–2004. *Clin Infect Dis* 2006;42(3):337–345.

ADDITIONAL READING
- Workowski KA, Berman S. Sexually transmitted diseases treatment guidelines, 2010. *MMWR Recomm Rep* 2010;59(RR-12):1–110.

 CODES

ICD9
- 091.2 Other primary syphilis
- 091.9 Unspecified secondary syphilis
- 097.9 Syphilis, unspecified

CLINICAL PEARLS
- Syphilis and HIV infection enhance the acquisition and transmission of one another.
- The differential diagnosis of genital ulcers should include genital herpes, syphilis, and chancroid.

S

TETANUS
Jason B. Harris (E. Mylonakis, Editor)

 BASICS

DESCRIPTION
Tetanus is characterized by persistent tonic spasms caused by *Clostridium tetani* and is divided into 4 clinical types:
- Generalized
- Localized
- Cephalic
- Neonatal

EPIDEMIOLOGY
Incidence
- The overall incidence of tetanus in the US is estimated at 0.16 cases per million (an average of approximately 40 cases per year). The incidence is similarly low in other developed countries with high vaccination rates.
- The incidence is much higher in developing countries, with a global incidence estimated at over 1,000,000 cases annually.
- Although tetanus has been described in fully immunized persons, the incidence of disease in this population is extremely low.

RISK FACTORS
- The majority of cases of nonneonatal tetanus are associated with soft-tissue injury.
- In developed countries, the major risk factor is age, as increasing age is associated with declines in immunity. Persons over age 60 are at highest risk.
- Non-vaccinated children are at higher risk.
- Injection drug use is another risk factor for tetanus.

GENERAL PREVENTION
- The Advisory Committee on Immunization Practices recommends a routine 5-dose primary series of DTaP (diphtheria, tetanus, and acellular pertussis) vaccine during childhood, and adolescents and adults should receive a regular booster vaccine containing tetanus toxoid every 10 years.
- For potentially contaminated or major wounds (including bite wounds and puncture wounds, avulsions, and wounds contaminated with foreign material), tetanus immune globulin and tetanus toxoid should be administered to patients who have had 2 or fewer primary immunizations.
- Tetanus toxoid alone can be given to those who have completed a primary immunization series but who have not received a booster for more than 5 years.

- Almost 70% of a random sample of Americans 6 or more years of age have protective levels of tetanus antibodies. However, by the age of 60–69 years, the prevalence of protective antibodies is less than 50% and by the age of 70 about 30%. Tetanus toxoid is a very effective immunogen that stimulates a protective response in virtually all immunocompetent subjects to whom it is administered. Studies in former military personnel have shown that up to 88% have protective antibody levels 15 years after vaccination.
- The World Health Organization is now promoting vaccination of all women of childbearing age by screening a woman's tetanus toxoid vaccine status at every contact with the health services.
- Some patients with humoral immune deficiencies may not respond adequately to toxoid injection and should receive passive immunization for tetanus-prone injuries, regardless of the period since the last booster.

PATHOPHYSIOLOGY
- *C. tetani* produces tetanospasmin (tetanus toxin), a potent inhibitor of neurotransmitter release.
- *C. tetani* does not grow or produce toxin in healthy tissue, which is why disease typically occurs in the setting of injury or devitalized tissue (such as the umbilical cord stump in the case of neonatal tetanus).
- The ultimate effect of the toxin is the blockade of inhibitory impulses to motor neurons, resulting in spastic paralysis.

ETIOLOGY
The etiologic agent of tetanus is *C. tetani*, an anaerobic bacterium that is widely present in the environment.

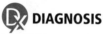 **DIAGNOSIS**

HISTORY
- Generalized tetanus is the most commonly recognized form and has an insidious onset, over several days.
- Generalized disease often begins with trismus (lockjaw), which causes a smile or grimace (risus sardonicus). Abdominal rigidity is present. The patient does not lose consciousness and experiences severe pain during each spasm. During the spasm, the upper airway can be obstructed, or the diaphragm may participate in the general muscular contraction.

- The initial manifestation may be of "local tetanus," in which the rigidity affects only 1 part or area of the body in which the *Clostridium*-containing wound is located. This mild picture may progress to generalized tetanus.
- Localized tetanus involves rigidity of the muscles associated with the site of spore inoculation.
- Cephalic tetanus involves spasm of the cranial motor nerves associated with head and neck injuries, often first manifested as dysphagia or trismus.
- Neonatal tetanus occurs in infants born to insufficiently immunized mothers, and the first symptoms are often inability to suck adequately before progressing to generalized spasms and rigidity. The disease usually develops within the first 2 weeks of life.

PHYSICAL EXAM
- The wound may seem insignificant at the time of the injury and may even appear well healed at the time of the neurologic disease.
- Early on, the patient may report a "sore throat" with dysphagia.
- With severe tetanus, there is opisthotonos, flexion of the arms, extension of the legs, periods of apnea due to spasm of the intercostal muscles and diaphragm, and rigidity of the abdominal wall.
- Later in the disease, autonomic dysfunction develops, with hypertension and tachycardia alternating with hypotension and bradycardia.

DIAGNOSTIC TESTS & INTERPRETATION
Tetanus has to be diagnosed clinically. A history of a soil-contaminated puncture wound should be sought, as there are no specific diagnostic laboratory tests.

Lab
Blood counts and blood chemical findings are unremarkable.

Imaging
Imaging studies of the head and spine reveal no abnormalities.

DIFFERENTIAL DIAGNOSIS
- Strychnine poisoning is the only condition that truly mimics tetanus.
- Dystonic reactions to neuroleptic drugs or other central dopamine antagonists may be confused with the neck stiffness of tetanus.
- A number of conditions (including dental and other local infections, hysteria, neoplasms, encephalitis, etc.) may produce trismus, and should be sought, but do not cause the other manifestations of tetanus.

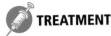 TREATMENT

MEDICATION
- Since the effect of the toxin is not reversible, supportive care and the control of muscle spasms are the mainstays of therapy and prevent life-threatening complications of tetanus.
- Benzodiazepines have emerged as the mainstay of symptomatic therapy for tetanus.
- To prevent spasms that last more than 5–10 seconds, diazepam is administered intravenously. The usual dosage is 10–40 mg every 1–8 h.
- Magnesium sulfate given by continuous infusion improves autonomic instability.
- Neuromuscular blocking agents (paralytic drugs) including vecuronium (by continuous infusion) or pancuronium (by intermittent injection) are necessary when sedation alone is insufficient.
- Sedative-hypnotics, narcotics, inhalational anesthetics, neuromuscular blocking agents, and centrally acting muscle relaxants, such as intrathecal baclofen, have been used.

ADDITIONAL TREATMENT
General Measures
Supportive therapy includes ventilatory support and pharmacologic agents that treat reflex muscle spasms, rigidity, and tetanic seizures.

Additional Therapies
- Passive immunization with human tetanus immunoglobulin shortens the course of tetanus and may lessen its severity. A single dose of 3000–6000 IU is recommended, although 500 U is recommended by some experts and may be as effective as larger doses.
- A study comparing oral metronidazole with intramuscular penicillin showed better survival, shorter hospitalization, and less progression of disease in the metronidazole group (0.5 g every 6 h or 1.0 g every 12 h i.v. for 7–10 days).
- A dose of tetanus–diphtheria vaccine should be administered (usually 1 upon discharge), with another dose of toxoid 4 weeks later.

SURGERY/OTHER PROCEDURES
All patients with soft-tissue injuries should undergo wound exploration and debridement to remove or reduce the number of toxin-producing organisms.

IN-PATIENT CONSIDERATIONS
Initial Stabilization
In cases of generalized tetanus, autonomic instability and generalized spasms are life threatening and require ICU level intensive care and monitoring.

 ONGOING CARE

FOLLOW-UP RECOMMENDATIONS
Patients with generalized tetanus require several weeks to recover and may require intensive supportive care.

DIET
Patients have high nutritional demands. Percutaneous endoscopic gastrostomy (PEG) facilitates prolonged enteral feeding regimens in patients.

PROGNOSIS
- The mortality rate in mild and moderate tetanus is presently about 6%, and, for severe generalized tetanus and neonatal tetanus, mortality rates may exceed 50%.
- Tetanus survivors often have serious psychological problems related to the disease and its treatment, which persist after recovery and may require psychotherapy.

COMPLICATIONS
Sympathetic overactivity has become the major cause of death in the intensive care unit. Sympathetic hyperactivity is usually managed with labetalol 0.25–1.0 mg/min, as needed for blood pressure control, or morphine 0.5–1.0 mg/kg/h by continuous infusion.

ADDITIONAL READING
- Fontanilla JM, Kirkland KB, Cotter JG, et al. Ability of healthcare workers to recall previous receipt of tetanus-containing vaccination. *Infect Control Hosp Epidemiol* 2010;31(6):647–649.
- Thwaites CL, Farrar JJ. Preventing and treating tetanus. *BMJ* 2003;326:117.
- Thwaites CL, Yen LM, Loan HT, et al. Magnesium sulphate for treatment of severe tetanus: A randomised controlled trial. *Lancet* 2006;368:1436.

 CODES

ICD9
037 Tetanus

CLINICAL PEARLS
- The diagnosis of tetanus is suspected on clinical grounds in patients with muscle spasms.
- The mainstay of therapy is aggressive supportive care including the control of spasms and autonomic instability.

THROMBOPHLEBITIS

Jatin M. Vyas (E. Mylonakis, Editor)

 BASICS

DESCRIPTION

- Suppurative, or septic, thrombophlebitis is inflammation of a vein due to microorganisms associated with thrombus formation and bacteremia.
- Suppurative thrombophlebitis is divided into the following categories:
  – Superficial
  – Central (including pelvic)
  – Intracranial, that is, defined by the simultaneous presence of venous thrombosis and suppuration in the intracranial compartment
  – Portal vein
- Suppurative thrombophlebitis occurs infrequently in bacteremia associated with central venous catheters such as PICC lines.

EPIDEMIOLOGY
Incidence
- Superficial suppurative thrombophlebitis accounts for up to 10% of nosocomial infections, and the estimated incidence is about 88 cases per 100,000 discharges. It is usually a result of a skin and soft-tissue infection or an indwelling intravenous catheter. Most common culprits are indwelling intravenous catheters that have been in place for 3 or more days.
- The incidence is higher when indwelling intravenous catheters are inserted in the lower extremities.
- Burn patients are at highest risk for developing suppurative thrombophlebitis, followed by patients with neoplastic diseases and those on steroid therapy.
- The overall incidence of septic pelvic thrombophlebitis is 1 in 2,000 to 1 in 3,000 deliveries. The incidence is about 1 in 9,000 after vaginal delivery, 1 in 800 after cesarean section or major gynecologic surgery, and 1 in 200 after septic abortion.
- Pelvic suppurative thrombophlebitis usually presents 1–2 weeks postpartum or postoperatively.

RISK FACTORS
For septic pelvic thrombophlebitis,
- Cesarean section
- Pregnancy
- Pelvic infection
- Induced abortion
- Pelvic surgery
- Uterine fibroids
- Underlying malignancy
- Hormonal stimulation

GENERAL PREVENTION
- The cannulation of the lower extremity should be avoided. Cannulae, intravenous fluid bottles, and connecting tubing should be replaced every 48–72 hours.
- Strategies to block microbial access to the transcutaneous tract, such as use of more potent cutaneous antiseptic agents, topical application of antimicrobial agents, use of central venous catheters coated with antibiotics (such as minocycline and rifampin), or attachment of a subcutaneous silver-impregnated cuff, have helped reduce the incidence of catheter-related infection.
- The recent Centers for Disease Control and Prevention guidelines for the prevention of catheter-related infections recommend the use of antimicrobial-impregnated venous catheters for patients with a high rate of infection after full adherence to other infection-control measures, such as maximal sterile barrier precautions.

ETIOLOGY
- The pathogenesis of suppurative thrombophlebitis is unclear, but probably a thrombus acts as a nidus for bacteria that gain access to the site from another focus. The route of spread of organisms to the inflamed vein may be through migration from the skin between the catheter wall and perivascular tissue, from contaminated intravenous fluid, or through hematogenous dissemination from an infected focus elsewhere. The relative contribution of these 3 routes, however, is unknown.
- In pelvic suppurative thrombophlebitis, the ovarian vein and the inferior vena cava are usually affected. Thrombus formation may result from stasis and/or be due to the hypercoagulable state of parturition. In a second stage, microorganisms (such as *Bacteroides* spp., *Streptococcus* spp, and *Enterobacteriaceae* such as *Escherichia coli*) from the vaginal or the perineal flora gain access to the thrombus.

- Septic thrombosis of the portal vein is usually associated with hepatic abscess, and an obvious extrahepatic source is often absent.
- Suppurative intracranial thrombophlebitis may begin in veins and/or venous sinuses and can occur in the following ways:
  – Following infection of the paranasal sinuses, middle ear, mastoid, facial skin, or oropharynx
  – In the presence of epidural abscess, subdural empyema, or bacterial meningitis
  – After metastatic spread of infection from a distant site
  – The usual predisposing conditions for the development of cavernous sinus thrombosis are paranasal sinusitis or infections of the face or mouth.
- The organisms most often isolated from superficial suppurative thrombophlebitis are the following:
  – Staphylococcus aureus
  – Coagulase-negative staphylococci
  – Enterobacteriaceae
  – Pseudomonas aeruginosa
  – Enterococcus spp.
  – Candida spp.
- The recovery of anaerobic bacteria is rarely reported.
- In suppurative intracranial thrombophlebitis, the most common bacterial pathogens depend on the initial source of infection; with sinusitis, they are staphylococci, aerobic and/or microaerophilic streptococci, gram-negative bacilli, and/or anaerobes, whereas *S. aureus* predominates when a facial infection is the source.
- *S. aureus* is the most important associated pathogen in patients with cavernous sinus thrombosis and is isolated in more than two-thirds of cases. Less common isolates include streptococci, pneumococci, gram-negative bacilli, and *Bacteroides* spp. In the appropriate clinical setting, fungal pathogens, such as *Aspergillus*, *Mucor*, and *Rhizopus* spp., should be considered. (See "Sinusitis," for details.)

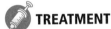 **DIAGNOSIS**

HISTORY
- Fever is present in 70% of the cases of suppurative thrombophlebitis, but rigors are rare.
- Patients with suppurative thrombophlebitis of the thoracic central veins usually present with systemic symptoms of bacteremia and sepsis and with minor or no local findings.
- Pelvic suppurative thrombophlebitis usually presents with high fever, chills, anorexia, nausea, and vomiting.
- The clinical presentation of suppurative intracranial thrombophlebitis is variable and can include focal or generalized seizures or symptoms of increased intracranial pressure.
- The most common complaints in patients with cavernous sinus thrombosis include fever, periorbital swelling, and headache. Other symptoms include change in mental status, diplopia, tearing, photophobia, drowsiness.

PHYSICAL EXAM
- Local findings are usually present in superficial suppurative thrombophlebitis and include erythema, lymphangitis, tenderness, and warmth. However, these signs can be difficult to identify, especially in burn patients.
- Patients with pelvic suppurative thrombophlebitis can demonstrate flank or lower abdominal tenderness.
- The clinical presentation of suppurative intracranial thrombophlebitis is variable, and various focal neurologic findings can be seen.
- For patients with cavernous sinus thrombosis, papilledema, ptosis, proptosis, chemosis, periorbital edema, and weakness of the extraocular muscles can be seen. Lateral gaze palsy may be an early neurologic finding.

DIAGNOSTIC TESTS & INTERPRETATION
Lab
Initial lab tests
- Superficial suppurative thrombophlebitis can induce bacteremia in 80–90% of the cases, and thus blood cultures should be obtained in all patients suspected of this disease
- CBC with differential
- ESR
- CRP

Follow-Up & Special Considerations
Surveillance blood cultures should be obtained after cessation of antimicrobial therapy to ensure that there has been no relapse of infection.

Imaging
- The utility of computed tomography and magnetic resonance imaging in the diagnosis of septic phlebitis has been shown in a number of reports. Especially, computed tomography with intravenous contrast has been found useful in the diagnosis of suppurative thrombophlebitis of the great veins (including pelvic suppurative thrombophlebitis) and the portal vein.
- Magnetic resonance imaging is the diagnostic procedure of choice for the evaluation of patients with suspected suppurative intracranial thrombophlebitis, and yield improves with magnetic resonance angiography.
- The diagnosis of deep central vein suppurative thrombophlebitis in the thorax can also be supported by venography.

 TREATMENT

MEDICATION
First Line
- Superficial suppurative thrombophlebitis can be fatal if left untreated, and prompt diagnosis and treatment is indicated. Most patients respond to antimicrobial treatment. Excision of the infected vein should be considered only when persistent bacteremia and sepsis is present, despite antibiotics.
- When infection of a venous catheter is suspected, it should be removed and cultured.
- Empiric antibiotic therapy.
- Superficial suppurative thrombophlebitis: Vancomycin. A third-generation cephalosporin with activity against *Pseudomonas* (such as ceftazidime) or an aminoglycoside should be added in immunocompromised or burn patients.
- Septic pelvic vein thrombophlebitis: Metronidazole (500 mg i.v. q.i.d.) with a third-generation cephalosporin; or monotherapy with imipenem (500 mg i.v. q.i.d.) or cefoxitin. Intravenous heparin has been recommended though it is not universally used.

- Suppurative intracranial thrombophlebitis: Nafcillin or oxacillin (2 g every 4 h i.v.) and a third-generation cephalosporin with activity against *Pseudomonas* (such as ceftazidime 2 g every 8 h i.v.). Vancomycin can replace nafcillin for the management of methicillin-resistant staphylococci.
- Concomitant use of heparin is controversial in suppurative intracranial thrombophlebitis, and the use of anticoagulation should be decided on a case-by-case basis.

 ONGOING CARE

FOLLOW-UP RECOMMENDATIONS
All patients and especially those at higher risk, such as burn patients who develop bacteremia or other systemic infection, should undergo careful examination of all previously cannulated veins.

COMPLICATIONS
Acute bacterial endocarditis, sepsis, pneumonia, or metastatic abscess can result from suppurative thrombophlebitis.

ADDITIONAL READING
- Garcia J, Aboujaoude R, Apuzzio J, et al. Septic pelvic thrombophlebitis: Diagnosis and management. *Infect Dis Obstet Gynecol* 2006; 2006:15614.
- Mermel LA, Allon M, Bouza E, et al. Clinical practice guidelines for the diagnosis and management of intravascular catheter-related infection: 2009 update by the Infectious Diseases Society of America. *Clin Infect Dis* 2009;49:1.
- Southwick FS, Richardson EP Jr, Swartz MN. Septic thrombosis of the dural venous sinuses. *Med (Baltimore)* 1986;65:82.

CODES

ICD9
- 451.9 Phlebitis and thrombophlebitis of unspecified site
- 790.7 Bacteremia

T

THYROIDITIS, INFECTIOUS
Rachel P. Simmons (E. Mylonakis, Editor)

 BASICS

DESCRIPTION
- Acute suppurative thyroiditis (also termed infectious, pyogenic, or bacterial) is painful thyroid inflammation with suppuration and abscess formation caused by an infection.
- Painful subacute thyroiditis (also termed subacute granulomatous, granulomatous, pseudogranulomatous, giant-cell, or de Quervain's) is a condition characterized by self-limited painful enlargement of the thyroid gland.

EPIDEMIOLOGY
Incidence
- Acute suppurative thyroiditis is rare and accounts for less than 1% of all thyroid disease.
- It affects both children and adults and occurs in both sexes equally.
- Painful subacute thyroiditis is the most common cause of thyroid pain.
- Painful subacute thyroiditis affects adults, typically in the second-to-sixth decades of life, and occurs 5 times more commonly in women than in men.
- Painful subacute thyroiditis occurs more frequently in the summer (2).

RISK FACTORS
- Infections of the thyroid are rare because of its protective capsule, lymphatic drainage, high iodine concentration, and abundant blood supply.
- Patients with AIDS, transplant recipients, or those receiving chemotherapy, steroid treatment, or other immunosuppressants are at increased risk of pyogenic thyroiditis.
- Congenital anomalies of the head and neck such as pyriform sinus fistula and pre-existing thyroid conditions such as thyroid cancer or goiter have been associated with increased risk of acute suppurative thyroiditis.

Genetics
Subacute painful thyroiditis has been associated with the haplotype, HLA-Bw35.

PATHOPHYSIOLOGY
- Pyogenic thyroiditis usually arises from adjacent structures, such as the oropharynx or lymph nodes, or from congenital abnormalities, such as a persistent thyroglossal duct or piriform sinus fistulae or branchial cleft abnormalities.
- Infection can also occur by means of hematogenous spread associated with pyelonephritis, prostatitis, esophageal perforation, otitis, endocarditis, postpartum infection or dental infection, or after direct trauma.
- Intravenous drug use is also cause of hematogenous spread.
- Direct traumas from foreign bodies (fine-needle aspiration, chicken-bone penetration or fish-bone penetration, tooth pick ingestion) have been identified as potential causes.
- Subacute thyroiditis often follows a viral upper respiratory tract infection though direct evidence of a viral etiology has not been demonstrated.

ETIOLOGY
- The most common pathogens associated with pyogenic thyroiditis are the following:
  - *Streptococcus* spp.
  - *Staphylococcus aureus* (including methicillin-resistant *Staphylococcus aureus*—MRSA)
- Less common organisms that lead to pyogenic thyroiditis include the following:
  - *Acinetobacter* spp.
  - *Actinomyces* spp.
  - *Aspergillus* spp.
  - *Bacteroides* spp.
  - *Candida* spp.
  - *Coccidioides immitis*
  - *Echinococcus* spp.
  - *Eikenella corrodens*
  - *Escherichia coli*
  - *Fusobacterium* spp.
  - *Haemophilus influenzae*
  - *Histoplasma* spp.
  - *Klebsiella* spp.
  - *Mycobacterium tuberculosis*
  - *Mycobacterium avium intracellulare*
  - *Nocardia* spp.
  - *Pasteurella multocida*
  - *Peptostreptococcus* spp.
  - *Pneumocystis* spp.
  - *Pseudallescheria boydii*
  - *Pseudomonas aeruginosa*
  - *Streptococcus viridans*
  - *Salmonella* spp.
- Approximately one-third of all cases are polymicrobial.
- Patients with AIDS may present with thyroiditis due to unusual organisms, such as *Pneumocystis jiroveci* (formerly *Pneumocystis carinii*).
- Immunocompromised patients are more prone to present with an infectious thyroiditis from uncommon pathogens including *Acinetobacter*, *Mycobacterium*, *Coccidioides*, *Salmonella*, *Pseudomonas*, *Nocardia*, *Pneumocystis*, *Haemophilus*, and *Candida*, and filamentous fungi.

℞ DIAGNOSIS

HISTORY
- Pyogenic thyroiditis is characterized by acute anterior neck pain and swelling and fever.
- In patients with AIDS or suppressed immune systems or in infections due to mycobacteria or fungi, the presentation of suppurative thyroiditis can be more insidious.
- A history of any immunosuppressing medications or conditions should be elicited.
- Subacute thyroiditis presents with the slow onset of thyroid pain and tenderness, along with nonspecific symptoms such as myalgia, fatigue, and low-grade fever.
- Up to half of patients with subacute painful thyroiditis will have symptoms of thyrotoxicosis.

PHYSICAL EXAM
- Clinical signs of pyogenic thyroiditis include fever, thyroid tenderness, symmetrical or asymmetrical neck swelling, anterior neck erythema and warmth, dysphonia, and pharyngitis.
- A thorough examination to identify other sites of infection should be undertaken.
- Physical findings in subacute thyroiditis include diffuse tenderness and enlargement of the thyroid.

DIAGNOSTIC TESTS & INTERPRETATION
Lab
Initial lab tests
- In pyogenic thyroiditis, initial laboratory evaluation includes complete blood count with differential, electrolytes, blood urea nitrogen, creatinine, liver function tests, and thyroid function studies.
- Leukocytosis is often present. Thyroid function tests are frequently normal though thyrotoxicosis can be present due to destruction of thyroid follicles and subsequent release of thyroxine and triiodothyronine.
- HIV screening.
- Blood cultures and urine cultures (if symptoms or history to suggest urinary tract infection) should be performed to identify the causative pathogen.
- Usual laboratory findings in subacute thyroiditis include a high erythrocyte sedimentation rate and c-reactive protein.
- Early in the course of subacute painful thyroiditis, patients may be mildly thyrotoxic. Later, as glandular hormone is depleted, patients pass through a hypothyroid phase.
- In subacute painful thyroiditis, thyroid function can take up to 1 year to normalize.
- Approximately 5% of patients will have persistent hypothyroidism requiring replacement.

Imaging
Initial approach
- CT scan of the neck with intravenously administered contrast is the test of choice for the diagnosis of acute suppurative thyroiditis. CT imaging also helps define the surrounding anatomy and can identify congenital anomalies.
- Consider including a CT of the chest to evaluate for the extension of the infection into the mediastinum.
- Thyroid ultrasonography can also identify a thyroid abscess though with less sensitivity as a CT scan, and it provides a less comprehensive evaluation of the surrounding structures.
- Direct visualization with fiberoptic laryngoscopy can identify a pyriform sinus fistula.
- 24-hour radioactive iodine uptake (RAIU) is usually normal in pyogenic thyroiditis.
- In subacute painful thyroiditis, 24-h RAIU is reduced (less than 5%).
- If the patient deteriorates clinically, consider repeat CT scan of the neck to evaluate for extension of the abscess or complications.
- Follow-up ultrasound or CT scan of the neck may be helpful to ensure resolution of the infection prior to stopping antibiotics in acute suppurative thyroiditis.

Diagnostic Procedures/Other
Fine-needle aspiration of an abscess can make the diagnosis. Gram's stain and culture of the aspirated material should be performed to identify the causative pathogen.

Pathological Findings
- The pathologic findings in acute suppurative thyroiditis are abscess formation and bacteria, fungi, or mycobacteria on appropriate tissue stains.
- In painful thyroiditis, histopathologic evaluation shows multinucleated giant cells, granuloma formation, and mononuclear cell infiltrate.

DIFFERENTIAL DIAGNOSIS
- The differential diagnosis of acute pyogenic thyroiditis includes deep neck space infections, neck trauma, parathyroid hemorrhage, thyroglossal duct cyst infection, aggressive thyroid cancer, thyroid cyst rupture or hemorrhage (1).
- Imaging of the neck and fine-needle aspiration of an abscess or cystic structure can differentiate between these conditions.
- The differential diagnosis of painful subacute thyroiditis include other forms of thyroiditis, such as Hashimoto's thyroiditis, painless postpartum thyroiditis, painless sporadic thyroiditis and Reidel's thyroiditis, thyroid cancer, Graves' disease, and drug-induced thyroiditis.
- History, examination, thyroid peroxidase antibody testing, serum inflammatory markers, thyroid function testing, 24-h RAIU, and fine-needle aspiration differentiate subacute thyroiditis from these other causes of thyroiditis.

 ## TREATMENT

MEDICATION
- Empirical treatment with broad-spectrum intravenous antibiotics should be initiated promptly when acute suppurative thyroiditis is suspected.
- Patient history (such as colonization with MRSA), severity of infection, local antibiotic resistance patterns, antibiotic allergies, and possible site of primary infection guide antibiotic choice.
- A potential empiric antibiotic regimen for immunocompetent patients who can tolerate penicillin is a penicillinase-resistant penicillin in combination with a β-lactamase inhibitor (piperacillin/tazobactam or ampicillin/sulbactam) plus vancomycin if MRSA is a concern (1).
- In a patient with AIDS or an impaired immune system, consider opportunistic infections and unusual pathogens and treat accordingly.
- Contaminant with antibiotics, obtain early surgical evaluation.
- When culture and sensitivity reports are available, tailor antibiotics accordingly.
- Duration of antibiotics is dependent on the clinical course, the organism, bioavailability of the antibiotic, and underlying cause. The course is typically no shorter than 2 weeks and can be as long as 8 weeks.

- For painful subacute thyroiditis, the goal of therapy is to ameliorate the symptoms.
- Nonsteroidal antiinflammatory drugs or salicylates can be used to treat mild or moderate forms of the disorder.
- In more severe cases, glucocorticoids can be prescribed to rapidly treat symptoms.
- Prednisone may be initiated at dosages of 40–60 mg daily, with a gradual reduction in dosage thereafter over several weeks.

ADDITIONAL TREATMENT
General Measures
- Timely drainage either surgically or by ultrasound-guided fine-needle aspiration is paramount in acute suppurative thyroiditis.
- Systemic inflammatory response syndrome or septic shock associated with acute suppurative thyroiditis is managed with ICU monitoring, fluid resuscitation, antibiotics, prompt drainage, and vasoactive medications as needed.
- Monitor the airway in acute suppurative thyroiditis.

Issues for Referral
Acute suppurative thyroiditis is a rare, potentially life-threatening illness, and early input from ENT, infectious diseases, and endocrine experts is recommended.

Additional Therapies
- If symptomatic thyrotoxicosis develops during painful subacute thyroiditis, a beta blocker can be initiated.
- A minority of patients with symptomatic hypothyroidism in the hypothyroid phase of the painful subacute thyroiditis will require thyroid hormone replacement.

SURGERY/OTHER PROCEDURES
- Prompt surgical drainage and debridement of necrotic tissues is recommended in acutely ill patients with acute suppurative thyroiditis. Partial or total thyroidectomy may be required.
- If a fistula is identified, the surgical resection or obliteration of the fistula is recommended.

IN-PATIENT CONSIDERATIONS
Initial Stabilization
Assess and stabilize airway and cardiac system in acute suppurative thyroiditis.

Admission Criteria
- Patients with acute suppurative thyroiditis should be admitted to the hospital for monitoring, initiation of intravenous antibiotics, and expedited workup.
- Patients with painful subacute thyroiditis can be managed as outpatients.

Admission Criteria
Patients may be discharged when fevers have abated for more than 24 h, vital signs are normal, the abscess has been adequately drained, and an antibiotic and follow-up plans are in place.

 ## ONGOING CARE
FOLLOW-UP RECOMMENDATIONS
- In painful subacute thyroiditis, a hypothyroid phase often follows subacute thyroiditis
- During the period of transient hypothyroidism, thyroid hormone replacement is provided if symptomatic. It can usually be discontinued subsequently as 5% of patients remain persistently hypothyroid.
- Recurrences occur in approximately 2% of patients with subacute thyroiditis.

Patient Monitoring
- If a patient requires intravenous antibiotics for the duration of therapy, send weekly monitoring labs per guidelines or package insert.
- In subacute painful thyroiditis, thyroid function monitoring is important for 1 year following diagnosis.

PATIENT EDUCATION
Patients with subacute painless thyroiditis should be aware of the symptoms of hyper- and hypothyroidism.

PROGNOSIS
Outcome in pyogenic thyroiditis is usually favorable, with complete recovery expected in most cases. Fatal cases have been associated with delays in diagnosis.

COMPLICATIONS
- Complications of pyogenic thyroiditis include destruction of the thyroid and parathyroid glands, internal jugular vein thrombophlebitis, vocal cord paralysis, hypothyroidism (usually transient), tracheal involvement, hematologic spread to other organs including mediastinitis, and sepsis.
- Risk of complications increases with delay in diagnosis.

REFERENCES
1. Paes JE, Burman KD, Cohen J, et al. Acute bacterial suppurative thyroiditis: A clinical review and expert opinion. *Thyroid* 2010;20:247–255.
2. Pearce, et al. Thiroiditis. *N Engl J Med* 2003; 348(26):46–55.

 ## CODES

ICD9
245.0 Acute thyroiditis

CLINICAL PEARLS
Acute suppurative thyroiditis is potentially life threatening and is managed with a combination of antibiotics and early drainage.

TOXIC SHOCK SYNDROME

Jason B. Harris (E. Mylonakis, Editor)

BASICS

DESCRIPTION
- Toxic shock syndrome (TSS) is a severe, life-threatening illness caused by toxin produced by to *Staphylococcus aureus* (staphylococcal TSS) or *Streptococcus pyogenes* (streptococcal TSS).
- TSS is characterized by acute onset of fever, erythrodermal rash, and hypotension, with multiorgan involvement usually manifested by diarrhea, vomiting, and myalgia, followed by desquamation during the early convalescent period.

EPIDEMIOLOGY
Incidence
- The incidence of staphylococcal TSS in the US is estimated to be 1–3 cases per 100,000.
- The incidence of streptococcal TSS in the North America is estimated to be 3.5 cases per 100,000.

RISK FACTORS
- 50% of cases of staphylococcal TSS occur in menstruating women using tampons. Tampon use is the major risk factor staphylococcal TSS.
- Although tampon use is the most common setting for TSS, the disease can also complicate the use of barrier contraceptives, the puerperium, septic abortion, and nonobstetric gynecologic surgery.
- The remaining 50% of cases of staphylococcal TSS occurrence are distributed among individuals of both sexes and all ages. Nonmenstrual TSS can complicate skin lesions of many types (such as chemical or thermal burns, insect bites, etc.), surgical wound infections, nasal packing, bacteremia, musculoskeletal infections, and respiratory infections.
- Menstrual and nonmenstrual cases are clinically indistinguishable.
- Streptococcal TSS occurs most commonly in the setting of invasive soft-tissue infections (80% of cases), such as necrotizing fasciitis, myonecrosis, and cellulitis.
- Risk factors for invasive streptococcal infection include minor trauma, including wounds and soft-tissue injury, surgical procedures, varicella, nonsteroidal anti-inflammatory drug (NSAID) use, and close contact with another patient with invasive streptococcal infection.

PATHOPHYSIOLOGY
- TSS is a bacterial toxin-mediated disease.
- Tampons are nidus for *S. aureus* colonization in menstrual-associated TSS.
- Certain streptococcal and staphylococcal toxins (see etiology below) stimulate a large portion of lymphocytes to synthesis of cytokines such as tumor necrosis factor-alpha, interleukin-1beta, and interleukin-6. These cytokines mediate fever, shock, and tissue injury.
- These toxins are known as superantigens because they can directly activate large portions of T-lymphocytes to secrete cytokines by binding directly to the T-cell receptor.

ETIOLOGY
- The vast majority of cases (>90%) of staphylococcal TSS is mediated by *S. aureus* which produces toxic shock syndrome toxin-1 (TSST-1). A small number of cases are associated with other staphylococcal exotoxins.
- For illness to develop, an individual must be colonized or infected with a toxigenic strain of *S. aureus* and must lack a protective level of antibody to the toxin made by that strain.
- Streptococcal TSS is caused by infection with group A *Streptococcus (S. pyogenes)* and the production of streptococcal pyrogenic exotoxins A, B, and C.

COMMONLY ASSOCIATED CONDITIONS
Streptococcal TSS is typically associated with bacteremia and/or a pyogenic focus of invasive infection including necrotizing fasciitis, cellulitis, or soft-tissue abscess.

DIAGNOSIS

HISTORY
TSS is an acute illness, the onset of symptoms is typically acute and rapidly progressive over a period of 48–72 h.

CDC case definition of staphylococcal toxic shock syndrome
- Fever: Temperature of 38.9°C (102°F) or higher
- Rash: Diffuse macular erythroderma ("sunburn" rash)
- Hypotension: Systolic blood pressure of less than 90 mm Hg, or orthostatic hypotension

- Involvement of at least 3 of the following organ systems:
  - Gastrointestinal: Vomiting or diarrhea at onset of illness
  - Muscular: Severe myalgias or serum creatine phosphokinase level at least twice the upper limit of normal
  - Mucous membranes: Vaginal, oropharyngeal, or conjunctival hyperemia
  - Renal: Blood urea nitrogen or creatinine level at least twice the upper limit of normal or pyuria
  - Hepatic: Total serum bilirubin or aminotransferase level at least twice the upper limit of normal
  - Hematologic: Thrombocytopenia
  - Central nervous: Disorientation or alteration in consciousness but no focal neurological signs at a time when fever and hypotension are absent
  - Desquamation: 1–2 weeks after the onset of illness (typically palms and soles)
  - Evidence against an alternative diagnosis: Negative results of cultures of blood, throat, or CSF (if performed); no rise in titers of antibody to the agents of Rocky Mountain spotted fever, leptospirosis, and rubeola (if obtained)
- Often in staphylococcal TSS, there is no immediately obvious focus

Case definition of streptococcal toxic shock syndrome
- I. Isolation of group A streptococcus (*S. pyogenes*) from a normally sterile site (e.g., blood, cerebrospinal fluid, peritoneal fluid, or tissue biopsy specimen) or from a non-sterile site (e.g., throat, sputum, vagina, open surgical wound, or superficial skin lesion)
and
- II. Hypotension: Systolic pressure 90 mm Hg or less in adults or lower than the fifth percentile for age in children and multiorgan involvement including 2 or more of the following signs:
  - Renal impairment: Creatinine concentration 177 μmol/L (2 mg/dL) or greater for adults or 2 times or more the upper limit of normal for age
  - Coagulopathy: Platelet count 100,000/mm³ or less or disseminated intravascular coagulation
  - Hepatic involvement: Elevated alanine transaminase, aspartate transaminase, or total bilirubin concentrations 2 times or more the upper limit of normal for age
  - Adult respiratory distress syndrome
  - A generalized erythematous macular rash that may desquamate
  - Soft-tissue necrosis, including necrotizing fasciitis or myositis or gangrene

PHYSICAL EXAM
- Physical exam findings are often limited in cases of TSS.
- The predominant physical exam finding in staphylococcal TSS is the diffuse erythroderma rash.
- Desquamation is a late finding (1–2 weeks after illness).
- In any case of possible TSS, a gynecologic exam should be performed and tampons should be removed.
- In contrast in streptoccocal TSS, there is often an obvious soft-tissue focus of infection.

DIAGNOSTIC TESTS & INTERPRETATION
Lab
- Usual laboratory abnormalities of TSS are listed in the diagnostic criteria above and include azotemia, hypoalbuminemia, hypocalcemia, hypophosphatemia, creatine phosphokinase elevation, leukocytosis or leukopenia with a left shift, thrombocytopenia, and pyuria.
- A blood culture should be performed in patients presenting with acute fever, rash, hypotension, and multiorgan failure to evaluate other potential bacterial causes of illness including meningococcemia and Gram-negative sepsis.
- In contrast to staphylococcal TSS, more than 60% of patients with streptococcal TSS have bacteremia.

DIFFERENTIAL DIAGNOSIS
- Meningococcemia
- Gram-negative bacteremia
- Rocky Mountain spotted fever
- Leptospirosis
- Measles
- Kawasaki's disease
- Heat stroke

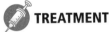 TREATMENT

MEDICATION
First Line
- Empiric treatment for staphylococcal TSS includes vancomycin (15 mg/kg/q12 in adults) and clindamycin (600 mg i.v. q8 in adults) to reduce toxin production.
- If an isolate is available for sensitivity testing and is shown to be methicillin susceptible, then semisynthetic penicillins (nafcillin or oxacillin 2 g i.v. every 6 h) plus clindamycin is recommended.
- Empiric treatment for streptococcal TSS consists of penicillin G (24 million units/d intravenously) and clindamycin (900 mg i.v. every 8 h).
- Duration of therapy varies, but, in uncomplicated cases, a 14-day course of therapy is reasonable.

Second Line
- For staphylococcal TSS, alternative agents include linezolid.
- For streptococcal TSS, ceftriaxone (2 g i.v. once daily) is a less-well-studied alternative to penicillin G.

ADDITIONAL TREATMENT
General Measures
- Supportive care is the most critical aspect of care for patients with TSS.
- Appropriate treatment of shock may require extensive fluid requirements (up to 20 L/day). Vasopressors are also often required.

Additional Therapies
- Patients with streptococcal TSS appear to benefit from IVIG (intravenous immunoglobulin) which may neutralize or dampen the effect of toxin. The dose of IVIG recommended for streptococcal TSS is 1 gram/kg on day 1 followed by 0.5 g/kg days 2 and 3.
- Patients with severe staphylococcal TSS may also benefit from IVIG, however, evidence for its efficacy is anecdotal.
- There is not currently sufficient evidence to support the routine use of steroids in TSS.

SURGERY/OTHER PROCEDURES
- Treatment of both staphylococcal and streptococcal TSS should always prompt the immediate identification and removal of the source of the infection (surgical debridement or drainage, or removal of nasal packing or tampon), initiation of effective antibiotic therapy, and appropriate supportive care.
- In the majority of cases of streptococcal TSS, a surgical drainage or debridement procedure is needed.

IN-PATIENT CONSIDERATIONS
Initial Stabilization
Patients with TSS should be admitted to an ICU

Admission Criteria
Patients with TSS should be admitted to an ICU for hemodynamic and respiratory support and monitoring

IV Fluids
Extensive isotonic fluids are usually required for patients with TSS.

Discharge Criteria
Patients should be afebrile and hemodynamically stable without additional supportive care requirements.

 ONGOING CARE

FOLLOW-UP RECOMMENDATIONS
- In patients with staphylococcal TSS and nasal carriage of S. aureus, it is reasonable to attempt to eradicate carriage using a regimen including intranasal mupirocin.
- Chemoprophylaxis of household contacts of patients with Streptococcal TSS who are >65 years of age, have diabetes or HIV infection or other immunodeficiency should be considered. Chemoprophylaxis is not recommended in schools or child care facilities.

PATIENT EDUCATION
- Staphylococcal TSS recurs in as many as 40% of cases.
- Among women with staphylococcal TSS, tampons and barrier contraceptives should be avoided in women in whom seroconversion does not occur after an acute illness.

PROGNOSIS
- Mortality in cases of staphylococcal TSS is less than 5%. Most deaths occur within the first few days of hospitalization.
- Mortality rates are higher in cases of streptococcal TSS, possibly reflecting its association with an invasive pyogenic focus of infection.

COMPLICATIONS
- Numerous complications can result from shock and end organ involvement including:
  – ARDS
  – Acute renal failure
  – DIC
  – Waterhouse–Friderichsen syndrome

ADDITIONAL READING
- Darenberg J, Ihendyane N, Sjolin J, et al. Intravenous immunoglobulin G therapy in streptococcal toxic shock syndrome: A European randomized, double-blind, placebo-controlled trial. *Clin Infect Dis* 2003;37:333.
- Lappin E, Ferguson AJ. Gram-positive toxic shock syndromes. *Lancet Infect Dis* 2009;9(5):281–290
- Larkin EA, Carman RJ, Krakauer T, et al. *Staphylococcus aureus*: The toxic presence of a pathogen extraordinaire. *Curr Med Chem* 2009;16(30):4003–4019.

 CODES

ICD9
- 040.82 Toxic shock syndrome
- 041.10 Staphylococcus infection in conditions classified elsewhere and of unspecified site, staphylococcus, unspecified

CLINICAL PEARLS
- TSS should be considered in patients with acute and profound hypotension, fever, and evidence of multiorgan involvement.
- It is always critical to exclude other life-threatening causes of fever and shock (such as meningococcemia).
- All patients with TSS should be thoroughly evaluated for a potential nidus of staphylococcal or streptococcal infection. This is usually obvious in the case of streptococcal TSS.

TOXOPLASMOSIS

Luisa M. Stamm (E. Mylonakis, Editor)

 BASICS

DESCRIPTION
- Toxoplasmosis is an infection caused by the intracellular protozoan *Toxoplasma gondii*.
- Infection is usually asymptomatic in immunocompetent patients.
- Severe infections usually occur in an immunocompromised patient or by the transplacental passage of parasites from an infected woman to fetus (congenital toxoplasmosis).
- When symptoms occur, they range from a mild, self-limited disease to a fulminant disseminated disease that affects the following:
  - Central nervous system (CNS)
  - Eyes
  - Lymph nodes
  - Skeletal or cardiac muscle
  - Lungs
  - Liver

EPIDEMIOLOGY
Incidence
- Toxoplasmosis in immunocompetent patients
  - The incidence increases with age and is similar between sexes.
- Toxoplasmosis in HIV-infected patients
  - The greatest incidence is seen among patients with a low CD4 T-cell count (<100 cells/mm^3)
  - In areas with high seroprevalence for toxoplasmosis, 25–50% of all AIDS patients, who are not receiving antiretroviral therapy or prophylaxis, will develop CNS toxoplasmosis.
- Congenital toxoplasmosis
  - Only 1 of 5 pregnant women infected with *T. gondii* develops clinical signs.
  - Women who are seropositive before pregnancy usually are protected.
  - If the acute infection in an infected woman goes untreated, congenital infection occurs in approximately 15% of fetuses during the first trimester, 30% of fetuses during the second trimester, and 60% of fetuses during the third trimester.
  - The earlier in the pregnancy the transmission, the more severe the outcome is.

Prevalence
The seroprevalence depends on geographic location and the age of the population. In the US, it varies between 3% to >50%, while in tropical countries and in areas of Western Europe, it is up to 90%.

RISK FACTORS
- Because cats are the definitive host of *T. gondii*, owning a cat is a risk factor for disease.
- Additional risk factors include eating undercooked meat or contaminated vegetables in areas of high prevalence.
- Seronegative patients receiving solid organs from seropositive donors are at risk for acquiring disease.
- Reactivation occurs in immunocompromised patients.

Genetics
- Basic research with mice suggest that genetic factors in the host contribute to disease caused by *T. gondii*.
- In particular, certain HLA class II genes correlate with particular outcomes of CNS toxoplasmosis in AIDS patients.

GENERAL PREVENTION
- HIV-infected patients
  - All HIV-infected persons should be tested for IgG antibody to *T. gondii* soon after the diagnosis of HIV infection.
  - Toxoplasma-seropositive patients with CD4 T-cell counts <100 cells/mm^3 should receive prophylaxis for toxoplasmosis.
  - The doses of trimethoprim–sulfamethoxazole (TMP/SMX) recommended for *Pneumocystis carinii* pneumonia appear also to be effective prophylaxis for *T. gondii*.
  - A combination of dapsone and pyrimethamine with folinic acid or atovaquone is an alternative.
  - Primary prophylaxis should continue until CD4 T-cell count is greater than 200 cells/mm^3 for 3 months.
- Other immunocompromised patients
  - Post transplantation of bone marrow and solid organs, high-risk patients should receive TMP/SMX.
- Pregnant patients
  - Seronegative pregnant women and other individuals at risk should be advised not to eat raw or undercooked meat, unpasteurized dairy products and should wash fruits and vegetables well.
  - They should wash their hands after contact with raw meat and contact with soil.
  - They should wear gloves while changing a cat's litter box, or, preferably, it should be changed by a non-pregnant, HIV-negative person.

PATHOPHYSIOLOGY
- There are 2 stages in the life cycle of *T. gondii*:
  - The sexual phase results in the formation of oocysts in the cat's intestine. Oocysts are excreted in the feces, sporulation occurs, and may remain infectious for many months.
  - Sporulated oocysts are ingested by an intermediate host (e.g., a human). Bradyzoites or sporozoites are released and transform to rapidly dividing tachyzoites, which can infect any organ.

ETIOLOGY
- Cats are the definitive hosts for *T. gondii*.
- Humans and other animals, such as sheep and pigs, become infected when they ingest oocysts shed in the feces of cats.
- Additionally, humans become infected by eating raw or undercooked meat containing tissue cysts.

COMMONLY ASSOCIATED CONDITIONS
Serious disease is associated with immunocompromised states such as AIDS with CD4 T-cell count <100 cells/mm^3, hematologic malignancy, solid organ transplant and those receiving immunosuppressive therapy with high-dose corticosteroids and TNF-α (tumor necrosis factor) inhibitors.

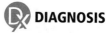 **DIAGNOSIS**

HISTORY
- **Immunocompetent Patients**
  - Immunocompetent patients who newly acquire infection are asymptomatic in 80–90% of cases. Among symptomatic patients, lymphadenopathy is the most common presentation. The clinical course is self-limited.
  - Less common presenting symptoms are:
    - Fever
    - Myalgias
    - Arthralgias
    - Malaise
    - Sore throat
    - Maculopapular rash
    - Night sweats
    - Abdominal pain
    - Confusion
    - Symptoms of myocarditis, pericarditis, or polymyositis
  - Toxoplasma causes near about 30–35% of cases of chorioretinitis in the US. Interestingly, most cases are from congenital infection. Patients usually develop symptoms during the second and third decades of life. Patients may present with the following:
    - Blurred vision
    - Scotoma
    - Ocular pain
    - Photophobia
    - Epiphora
- **Immunocompromised Patients**
  - A newly acquired or reactivated infection in immunocompromised patients usually involves the CNS, and less often, the lung (pneumonitis), the eye (chorioretinitis), or the heart. Cases of gastrointestinal, liver, skin, or multiorgan involvement also have been reported.
  - Symptoms of CNS infection are usually subacute and include the following:
    - Headache
    - Seizures
    - Weakness or numbness
    - Visual field complaints
    - Confusion
    - Imbalance
    - Difficulty with speech
    - Stiff neck
    - Fever
  - Extracerebral toxoplasmosis which is less common among patients with HIV infection involves the lungs and/or the eyes in more than 75% of the cases, and it may develop among patients seronegative for *T. gondii*.
  - Toxoplasmic pneumonitis usually presents with fever, dyspnea, and nonproductive cough.
  - Ocular toxoplasmosis presents with the same symptoms as in immunocompetent patients, but it can progress more rapidly.

- **Congenital toxoplasmosis**
  - Presentation is variable. There may be no sequelae, or sequelae may develop at various times after birth.
  - Premature infants may present with CNS or ocular disease.
  - Full-term infants usually develop milder disease, with hepatosplenomegaly and lymphadenopathy.

PHYSICAL EXAM
- CNS infection is associated with cranial nerve defects, visual field defects, mental status changes, cerebellar signs, meningismus, and sensory or motor disturbances.
- In immunocompetent patients, cervical lymph nodes are most commonly involved, but any or all lymph node groups may be enlarged. Nodes are usually discrete, non-tender, less than 3 cm in diameter, and non-suppurative.
- In patients with chorioretinitis, ophthalmologic examination reveals yellow–white, cotton-like patches with indistinct margins of hyperemia. Lesions are usually multiple and develop distinct borders and black spots within the retina.
- Patients may have hepatomegaly.

DIAGNOSTIC TESTS & INTERPRETATION
Diagnosis is usually based on a compatible clinical picture, neuroimaging findings, and serology. Definitive diagnosis is based on pathology.

Lab
- *T. gondii*-specific IgG and IgM levels are part of the initial work up for toxoplasmosis and aid in determining whether infection is acute or a reactivation. However, approximately 20% of patients have no detectable antibodies, and the titer does not always rise during infection. Negative serology does not rule out infection, but a rising titer may be of diagnostic significance.
- Parasitemia may be detected in tissue culture in a proportion of patients with acute infection.
- Evaluation of other body fluids including bronchoalveolar lavage, cerebrospinal fluid (CSF), or amniotic fluid by direct examination (by Giemsa or immunofluorescence) can demonstrate tachyzoites.
- Polymerase chain reaction (PCR) of body fluids is possible but not often used because test performance varies greatly.
- CSF analysis usually reveals elevated protein and mild pleocytosis.

Imaging
- On neuroimaging, the abscesses of cerebral toxoplasmosis are typically multiple, located in the cortex or deep nuclei (thalamus and basal ganglia), surrounded by edema, and enhance in a ring-like pattern with contrast.
- Magnetic resonance imaging (MRI) has greater sensitivity than computed tomography (CT) for detection of smaller lesions in this population.
- After fetal infection, neuro-imaging reveals CNS calcifications and ventricular dilation.

Diagnostic Procedures/Other
- Definitive diagnosis of CNS toxoplasmosis requires brain biopsy or identification of the microorganism in CSF by Wright–Giemsa stain.
- Currently, brain biopsy is indicated for patients with focal enhancing cerebral lesions seen on CT and MRI who do not respond to a trial of empiric anti-toxoplasmosis therapy, for patients who are showing rapid clinical deterioration with neuroimaging, or for patients whose serology is not suggestive of toxoplasmosis.
- Chest X rays are abnormal in more than half of the patients with pulmonary toxoplasmosis.

DIFFERENTIAL DIAGNOSIS
- For immunocompetent patients with lymphadenopathy, the differential includes Epstein-Barr virus (EBV), cytomegalovirus (CMV), and acute HIV infection.
- For HIV-positive patients with CNS lesions, the differential includes lymphoma, cryptococcal and mycobacterial disease, bacterial abscess, and progressive multifocal leukoencephalopathy.

 TREATMENT

MEDICATION
First Line
- Drugs, dosages, and treatment duration for extracerebral toxoplasmosis, such as ocular, pulmonary, or disseminated, are the same as for CNS involvement.
- The combination of pyrimethamine plus sulfadiazine is the regimen of choice for acute therapy.
- For acute therapy, the usual dose are:
  - Sulfadiazine 1–1.5 g p.o. q.i.d.
  - Pyrimethamine loading dose 200 mg p.o. × 1, followed by 75 mg p.o. per day.
- Folinic acid should always be co-administered with pyrimethamine to prevent the folinic acid deficiency and ameliorate the hematologic toxicity of pyrimethamine.
- Duration of treatment should be individualized, but it usually is for 6–8 weeks.

Second Line
- Pyrimethamine (accompanied by folinic acid) combined with clindamycin, clarithromycin, azithromycin, or atovaquone are acceptable alternatives.
- TMP–SMX alone may also be used.

ADDITIONAL TREATMENT
General Measures
For patients for whom there is a strong suspicion of cerebral toxoplasmosis, a trial of empiric therapy prior to definitive diagnosis is reasonable.

Additional Therapies
- For acute infection in pregnant women, spiramycin or a combination of sulfadiazine and pyrimethamine with leucovorin is used.
- For congenital toxoplasmosis, toxoplasmic meningitis with evidence of high intracranial pressures and chorioretinitis, steroids can be added until CSF protein normalizes, and impending herniation and/or vision-threatening inflammation resolves.

 ONGOING CARE

FOLLOW-UP RECOMMENDATIONS
After induction treatment, HIV-infected patients should receive suppression therapy with pyrimethamine (25–50 mg p.o. per day) and sulfadiazine (500–1000 g p.o. per day) until CD4 T-cell count is greater than 200 cells/mm^3 for 6 months.

Patient Monitoring
- Careful ophthalmologic examination is essential for newborns with suspected congenital infection.
- Patients with CNS disease should be carefully monitored for improvement with serial exams and imaging.
- Additionally, patients should be monitored for adverse effects of the medications (pyrimethamine causes rash and bone marrow suppression; sulfadiazine causes rash, GI disturbances, leukopenia, hepatitis and renal failure).

PATIENT EDUCATION
Pregnant patients and seronegative HIV-positive patients should be educated by their doctors regarding prevention of primary disease.

PROGNOSIS
80–90% of patients with AIDS will have a radiographic and/or clinical response within 7–10 days. If patients do not improve, brain biopsy should be pursued. Relapses of ocular toxoplasmosis occur in up to one-third of patients.

COMPLICATIONS
Ocular toxoplasmosis can lead to loss of central vision, nystagmus, or strabismus.

 CODES

ICD9
130.9 Toxoplasmosis, unspecified

CLINICAL PEARLS

- CNS infection toxoplasmic is the most common presentation of toxoplasma in patients with AIDS, usually in patients with CD4 T-cell count less than 100 and with multiple ring-enhancing lesions on brain MRI.

T

TRACHOMA
Luisa Stamm (E. Mylonakis, Editor)

 BASICS

DESCRIPTION
- Trachoma is a chronic follicular conjunctivitis due to infection by *Chlamydia trachomatis*.
- In non-endemic areas, organisms can be transmitted from the genital tract to the eye, causing inclusion conjunctivitis syndrome.
- Active infection with *C. trachomatis* is seen in young children whereas the resulting scarring and blindness are seen in adults.

EPIDEMIOLOGY
- Trachoma is hyper-endemic in the poor, remote, rural regions of Africa, Asia, Central and South America, Australia, and the Middle East.
- Trachoma is directly transmitted from the eye, nose, and throat of infected people via hands (particularly among young children and the women who look after them), flies, and towels.
- In younger children, boys and girls are equally affected. As adults, women are 2–6 times more likely to be infected because of repeat exposure to infected children.

Prevalence
- 84 million people are affected by trachoma, 8 million of whom are visually impaired.
- 1.3 million people are blind as a result of trachoma which is the leading infectious cause of blindness worldwide.

RISK FACTORS
- The largest risk factor for trachoma infection is living in a hyper-endemic area which has overcrowding, proximity to cattle, poor hygiene, high density of flies, seasonal epidemics of bacterial or viral conjunctivitis, and dry, dusty environments with an inadequate supply of water.
- Eye infection with genital *C. trachomatis* strains occur among sexually active young adults.

GENERAL PREVENTION
- Community-based strategies for improving hygiene in children can reduce the prevalence of trachoma, and school teachers and health workers should propagate this message.
- Health education is directed at communities with a high prevalence of inflammatory disease and focuses on the need for daily face washing, the use of latrines, and the proper disposal of refuse.

PATHOPHYSIOLOGY
- *C. trachomatis* has a predilection for cells of the conjunctiva.
- After years of repeat infection, the conjunctiva scar and cause eyelid deformities, particularly entropion where lids turn inwards and trichiasis where lashes turn inwards, which then cause corneal exposure and ulceration and ultimately blindness.

ETIOLOGY
Serovars A, B, Ba, and C are associated with trachoma, and serovars D through K cause the inclusion conjunctivitis syndrome.

 DIAGNOSIS

HISTORY
- Both endemic trachoma and inclusion conjunctivitis syndrome present initially as a mild conjunctivitis; many are asymptomatic and few have mucopurulent discharge.
- Neonatal chlamydial conjunctivitis has an acute onset and often produces a profuse mucopurulent discharge.
- Patients with trachoma can develop dryness of the eyes, due to destruction of the lacrimal ducts, and lacrimal gland.
- Most important aspects of history in adults are living in endemic area, changes in eyelids, and visual complaints.

PHYSICAL EXAM
- In an endemic area, diagnosis is based upon clinical manifestations seen with a 2.5× magnifying glass and good light. The everted upper lid and cornea should be examined carefully.
- In children, follicles that are white foci of inflammatory material are seen on the upper tarsal conjunctiva. Scar tissue forms leading to entropion and trichiasis. Arlt's line is a horizontal line of conjunctival scarring along the superior palpebral conjunctiva.
- Eventually, the corneal epithelium is abraded and may ulcerate, with subsequent corneal scarring, corneal pannus (inflammation with leukocytic infiltration and superficial vascularization), corneal haze, and blindness. Hebert's pits are ulcers in the cornea filled with clear epithelial tissue.
- Inclusion conjunctivitis syndrome is frequently associated with corneal inflammation in the form of discrete opacities (infiltrates), punctate epithelial erosions, and minor degrees of superficial corneal vascularization.

DIAGNOSTIC TESTS & INTERPRETATION
Lab
- Demonstration of chlamydiae by Giemsa- or immunofluorescent-stained smears, by isolation in cell cultures, or by DNA-based tests constitutes definitive evidence of infection.
- DNA amplification techniques to detect chlamydial infections may be used.

Pathological Findings
See "Physical Exam"

DIFFERENTIAL DIAGNOSIS
- The differential diagnosis of trachoma includes multiple infections due to viruses, bacteria, parasites, and fungi (see Section II chapter, "Conjunctivitis" for details).
- Specifically, in addition to *C. trachomatis* and *Neisseria gonorrhoeae*, the other important infectious causes of conjunctivitis in newborns include *Haemophilus influenzae*, *Streptococcus pneumoniae*, and herpes simplex virus.

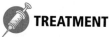 **TREATMENT**

MEDICATION
First Line
- Single-dose azithromycin therapy (20 mg/kg orally) is the treatment of choice (efficacy almost 80% at 6-month follow-up).
- Because concomitant pharyngeal infection is often present, neonatal chlamydial conjunctivitis should be treated with oral antimicrobials in order to prevent chlamydial pneumonia.

Second Line
- Topical tetracycline eye ointment 1% b.i.d. for at least 6 weeks, or on 5 consecutive days a month for 6 months, can be administered.
- Oral doxycycline 100 mg p.o. b.i.d. for 21 days and tetracycline 250 mg p.o. q.i.d. for 14 days are alternatives (to be avoided in young children).

ADDITIONAL TREATMENT

General Measures

- In communities where more than 10% of children of age 1–9 years have active trachoma, mass community-based chemotherapy followed by annual treatment for 3 years is recommended by the World Health Organization (WHO). After which time, prevalence should be re-assessed.
- In communities where prevalence is 50% among children, biannual treatment is necessary.
- The WHO has formed the Global Elimination of Trachoma by the Year 2020 campaign in 1998. This campaign is based on the SAFE strategy:
  - Surgery for in-turned eyelids with simplified procedures, often performed by non-specialist personnel
  - Antibiotic treatment (either oral azithromycin or topical tetracycline) for entire communities to reduce the prevalence of *C. trachomatis* and to lower transmission rates
  - Face washing and improved hygiene in young children
  - Environmental improvements: Providing safe water and better disposal of animal and human feces to reduce the population of eye-seeking flies that transmit infections

SURGERY/OTHER PROCEDURES

- Bimalar tarsal rotation is the surgery for trichiasis, which can improve vision, but it is unclear whether it can prevent blindness.
- Surgery is recommended by the WHO in endemic areas but is often not implemented because of a lack of patient awareness, availability, funds, and transportation.

 ## ONGOING CARE

FOLLOW-UP RECOMMENDATIONS

- Acute relapse of old trachoma occasionally follows treatment with cortisone eye ointment or develops in very old persons who were exposed in their youth.
- A considerable percentage of the patients with inclusion conjunctivitis have a concomitant genital chlamydial infection, and a majority of them have no genital symptoms. It is recommended that both patients and their sexual partners be referred for routine examination and systemic treatment when indicated.

Patient Monitoring

In endemic areas receiving mass antibiotic treatment, children should be reassessed by physical exam after 3 years of treatment. If prevalence becomes less than 5%, treatment can then be given to affected individuals and their household contacts only.

PATIENT EDUCATION

- Patient education at the community level focuses on promoting face washing, fly control, modifying water use, latrine use, and proximity of living to animals.
- Additionally, patients are taught regarding the benefits of surgery for trichiasis.

PROGNOSIS

Prognosis is good if patients are treated early in infection. The risk of blindness is higher with repeat infections and chronic inflammation.

COMPLICATIONS

- Entropion and trichiasis lead to corneal ulceration, scarring, and vascularization and may result in visual loss.
- If untreated, inclusion conjunctivitis may persist for weeks to years.
- Inclusion conjunctivitis can lead to conjunctival scarring especially among patients who received prolonged therapy with topical glucocorticoids.
- Recurrent eye infections develop most often in patients whose sexual consorts are not treated with antimicrobials.

REFERENCES

1. Kuper H, Solomon AW, Buchan J, et al. A critical review of the SAFE strategy for the prevention of blinding trachoma. *Lancet Infect Dis* 2003;3:372.
2. Solomon AW, Holland MJ, Alexander ER, et al. Mass treatment with a single-dose azithromycin for trachoma. *N Engl J Med* 2004;351:1962.

 ## See Also

WHO website: http://www.who.int/topics/trachoma/en/

 ## CODES

ICD9

- 076.9 Trachoma, unspecified
- 079.88 Other specified chlamydial infection

CLINICAL PEARLS

- Trachoma is the leading infectious cause of blindness in the world.
- Treatment and eradication in endemic areas requires community-based interventions.

TRAVELER'S DIARRHEA

Paschalis Vergidis
Matthew E. Falagas

 BASICS

DESCRIPTION

Traveler's diarrhea is the most common illness affecting travelers. Primary source is fecally contaminated food or water. The risk is associated with hygiene practices, handling, and preparation of food.

EPIDEMIOLOGY

Incidence

- Between 20 and 50% of international travelers develop diarrhea.
- Attack rates are similar in men and women.
- Risk depends on destination.
  - High risk areas: Greater than 50% occurrence
    ○ Latin America (21%–80%)
    ○ Asia and the Middle East (21%–80%)
    ○ Africa (36%–62%)
  - Intermediate risk areas: 10–20%
    ○ Southern Europe
    ○ Israel
    ○ Select Caribbean islands
  - Low risk areas: Less than 8%
    ○ Canada
    ○ US
    ○ Northern Europe
    ○ Australia
    ○ New Zealand
    ○ Japan
    ○ Majority of the Caribbean islands

RISK FACTORS

- Travel to higher risk countries
- Immunocompromised travelers
- Patients with inflammatory bowel disease
- Persons with reduced gastric acidity (such as those taking proton-pump inhibitors)
- Students, itinerant tourists
- Failure to adhere to dietary precautions
- Pregnant women may be at higher risk of traveler's diarrhea because of lowered gastric acidity and increased gastrointestinal transit time

GENERAL PREVENTION

- Avoid the following:
  - Tap water, even for brushing teeth
  - Ice, unless made from purified water
  - Unpasteurized dairy products
  - Raw or undercooked meat or fish
  - Uncooked fruits and vegetables unless they can be peeled
  - Lettuce or other leafy raw vegetable (such as spinach)
  - Food from street vendors
- Boiling is the best way to purify water.
- Iodination or chlorination is acceptable but does not kill *Cryptosporidium* or *Cyclospora*.
- Bottled water is safe if cap and seal are intact.

- Indications for the use of chemoprophylaxis (1):
  - Important trip (the purpose of which might be ruined by a short-term illness)
  - Underlying illness that might be worsened by diarrhea
  - Underlying condition which may make the individual more susceptible to diarrhea
  - Previous bouts of traveler's diarrhea which suggest increased susceptibility to illness
- Antibiotic prophylaxis: Effective but not generally recommended due to risk of emergence of resistance and side effects.
  - Rifaximin (A) (200 mg once or twice a day with major meals for the duration of the trip)
  - Ciprofloxacin (A) (500 mg/d for the duration of the trip). Increasing resistance to fluoroquinolones may limit use
- Nonantibiotic prophylaxis:
  - Role of probiotics not established [*Lactobacillus* GG (BI) and *Saccharomyces boulardii* (CI)]
  - The best studied drug is bismuth subsalicylate (AI) (two 262-mg tablets or 60 mL four times daily for up to 3 weeks)
  - Note: Bismuth subsalicylate not recommended for persons taking anticoagulants or other salicylates. Avoid in persons taking doxycycline for malaria prophylaxis, as it interferes with absorption
- Administration of cholera vaccine is not routinely recommended.
- The oral cholera vaccine (Dukoral) has limited efficacy against enterotoxigenic *Escherichia coli* (2), as the *Vibrio cholerae* whole cell/recombinant cholera toxin B subunit is antigenically similar to the heat labile enterotoxin.

ETIOLOGY

- Bacterial (80–90%)
  - *E. coli* (mainly enterotoxigenic, but enteroaggregative are increasingly recognized)
  - Campylobacter
  - Salmonella (nontyphoid)
  - *Shigella*
  - *Aeromonas* spp.
  - *Plesiomonas shigelloides*
  - Vibrio (non-cholerae)
- Viral (5–8%)
  - Rotavirus
  - Norovirus
- Parasitic (about 10% in longer-term travelers)
  - *Giardia lamblia*
  - *Entamoeba histolytica*
  - *Cryptosporidium parvum*
  - *Cyclospora cayetanensis*
  - *Isospora belli*
  - *Balantidium coli*
- Toxigenic *E. coli*: Contaminated food and beverages
- Rotavirus: Endemic in tropics

- Noroviruses: Camps, cruise ships
- Giardia: Protozoa in contaminated water and food prevalent in developing countries, wilderness
- *E. histolytica*: Amoeba in contaminated water or vegetables prevalent in developing countries
- *Cryptosporidium*: Protozoa parasite in contaminated water prevalent in developing countries and young animals, farm animals
- *Cyclospora*: Protozoa in food and water worldwide
- *Isospora belli*: Subtropical climates and developing countries

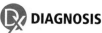 **DIAGNOSIS**

HISTORY

- Bacterial and viral pathogens have an incubation period of 6–48 h.
- Protozoa have an incubation period of 1–2 weeks. Infection with *Cyclospora cayetanensis* can present early in areas of high risk.
- There are 3 forms of the disease:
  - *Classic*. Passage of 3 or more unformed stools in a 24-h period plus at least 1 of the following symptoms: Nausea, vomiting, abdominal pain or cramps, fever, blood in stools
  - *Moderate*. Passage of 1 or 2 unformed stools in 24 h plus at least 1 of the above symptoms or more than 2 unformed stools in 24 h without other symptoms
  - *Mild*. Passage of 1 or 2 unformed stools in 24 h without other symptoms
- *Bacterial diarrhea*. Sudden onset of symptoms ranging from mild cramps and urgent loose stools, to severe abdominal pain, fever, vomiting, and bloody diarrhea.
- Tenesmus is uncommon.
- *Viral diarrhea*. Similar symptoms to bacterial diarrhea. Vomiting prominent with norovirus infection.
- *Protozoal diarrhea*. More gradual onset of low-grade symptoms, with 2–5 loose stools per day.
- Untreated bacterial diarrhea lasts 3–5 days. Viral diarrhea lasts 2–3 days. Protozoal diarrhea can persist for weeks to months without treatment.

PHYSICAL EXAM

- Watery, loose stools
- Bloody stools (2–10%)
- Abdominal tenderness

DIAGNOSTIC TESTS & INTERPRETATION
Lab
Initial lab tests
- Diagnosis is generally based on travel history and clinical symptoms. Treatment is empiric.
- Obtain a stool specimen for culture in patients with fever and colitis.
- Check for parasites if symptoms have persisted for more than 10–14 days.

DIFFERENTIAL DIAGNOSIS
- Food poisoning (ingestion of preformed toxins)
- Shellfish poisoning
- Scombroid poisoning
- Ciguatera poisoning

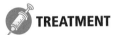 TREATMENT

Traveler's diarrhea is a self-limiting illness. Treatment is designed to reduce symptoms and shorten illness limiting the duration of inconvenience.

MEDICATION
First Line
- Ciprofloxacin 500 mg twice per day p.o. for 3 days (AI) (3)
- Amebiasis: Metronidazole 500–750 mg p.o. 3 times daily for 10 days, followed by an agent to eliminate luminal cysts: Iodoquinol 650 mg p.o. 3 times daily for 20 days or paromomycin 500 mg p.o. 3 times daily for 7 days
- Giardiasis: Metronidazole 250 mg p.o. 3 times daily for 5 days

Second Line
- Azithromycin 1 g p.o. (single dose) (AI) (4). To be considered in travelers to Southeast Asia where quinolone resistance to *Salmonella, Campylobacter* is emerging.
  - Note: Azithromycin is safe to use in pregnant women and children
- Newer fluoroquinolones (e.g., levofloxacin 500 mg p.o. daily for 3 days).
- Rifaximin 200 mg p.o. twice daily for 3 days is an alternative for afebrile non-dysenteric traveler's diarrhea (AI) (5).
- Trimethoprim–sulfamethoxazole, ampicillin, doxycycline not recommended due to widespread resistance.

Pregnancy Considerations
- Quinolones generally are not advised during pregnancy, but azithromycin is safe.
- Although rifaximin is not absorbed, the safety of this medication in pregnant women has not been established.
- Loperamide may be used, but bismuth subsalicylate should be avoided.

ADDITIONAL TREATMENT
General Measures
Replacement of fluids and electrolytes is the cornerstone of treatment in traveler's diarrhea.

Pediatric Considerations
Infants and younger children are at higher risk for developing dehydration which is best prevented by the use of oral rehydration solution.

Additional Therapies
- Loperamide 2 mg, up to 2 tablets 4 times daily (AI).
  - Avoid if presence of hematochezia, fever >38°C in young children.
  - Loperamide can be combined with a quinolone for moderate-to-severe cases (6).
- Bismuth subsalicylate (AI): Two 262-mg tablets or 60 mL up to 4 times per day.
- Opiates and diphenoxylate are effective but may have neurological adverse effects and are poorly tolerated by elderly persons.

 ONGOING CARE

DIET
Refeeding with slight restrictions (avoid coffee, alcohol, carbonated beverages, dairy products)

PATIENT EDUCATION
- Pre-travel counseling:
  - Provide instructions regarding food and beverage selection
  - Use of non-antimicrobial agents or antibiotics for prophylaxis
  - Advise to use hand-sanitizing solutions or gels (containing at least 60% alcohol) to clean hands before eating

PROGNOSIS
- Not fatal; usually a self-limited illness.
- In severe episodes, dehydration may pose a greater health risk, especially in children and older adults.

COMPLICATIONS
- Reactive arthritis.
- Guillain–Barré syndrome after *Campylobacter* infection.
- Post-infectious irritable bowel syndrome.

REFERENCES
1. DuPont HL, Ericsson CD, Farthing MJ, et al. Expert review of the evidence base for prevention of travelers' diarrhea. *J Travel Med* 2009;16:149–160.
2. Wiedermann G, Kollaritsch H, Kundi M, et al. Double-blind, randomized, placebo controlled pilot study evaluating efficacy and reactogenicity of an oral ETEC B-subunit-inactivated whole cell vaccine against travelers' diarrhea (preliminary report). *J Travel Med* 2000;7:27–29.
3. Petruccelli BP, Murphy GS, Sanchez JL, et al. Treatment of traveler's diarrhea with ciprofloxacin and loperamide. *J Infect Dis* 1992;165:557–560.
4. Adachi JA, Ericsson CD, Jiang ZD, et al. Azithromycin found to be comparable to levofloxacin for the treatment of US travelers with acute diarrhea acquired in Mexico. *Clin Infect Dis* 2003;37(9):1165–1171.
5. Taylor DN, Bourgeois AL, Ericsson CD, et al. A randomized, double-blind, multicenter study of rifaximin compared with placebo and with ciprofloxacin in the treatment of travelers' diarrhea. *Am J Trop Med Hyg* 2006;74(6):1060–1066.
6. Ericsson CD, DuPont HL, Mathewson JJ. Optimal dosing of ofloxacin with loperamide in the treatment of non-dysenteric travelers' diarrhea. *J Travel Med* 2001;8(4):207–209.

ADDITIONAL READING
- Hill DR, Ericsson CD, Pearson RD, et al. The practice of travel medicine: Guidelines by the Infectious Diseases Society of America. *Clin Infect Dis* 2006;43(12):1499–1539.

 CODES

ICD9
- 009.2 Infectious diarrhea
- 009.3 Diarrhea of presumed infectious origin

CLINICAL PEARLS
- Disease most commonly occurs in resource-poor countries but may occur in developed countries.
- Empiric self-treatment is usually required in resource-poor settings.
- Consider traveler's diarrhea in a person who develops symptoms up to 2 weeks after return.

TRICHINOSIS

Paschalis Vergidis
Matthew E. Falagas

 BASICS

DESCRIPTION
Trichinella spiralis is a nematode that infects domestic and wild pigs, polar bears, walruses, and foxes. Infection in humans is due to larval migration into striated muscle, brain, and heart.

EPIDEMIOLOGY
Incidence
- 5–15 symptomatic cases occur in the US each year (1).
- The decline in reported cases is a result of improved observance of standards and regulations in the pork industry.
- Cases still occur among consumers of wild game meat and noncommercial pork.

Prevalence
Disease is found worldwide. Prevalence is highest in Mexico, Argentina, Bolivia, China, Thailand, the former Soviet Union, and parts of Central Europe.

RISK FACTORS
Eating undercooked pork; outbreaks have been noted due to eating undercooked sausages

GENERAL PREVENTION
- Pork should be cooked properly at all times. This means that the temperature during cooking should be above 550°C until there is no trace of blood.
- Cysts in pork will not survive freezing at −15°C for 20 days.

PATHOPHYSIOLOGY
- *T. spiralis* lives in the small intestine of carnivores such as swine.
- Infection in humans is the result of eating undercooked meat, usually pork or bear meat, containing encysted larvae.
- Upon ingestion, the larvae develop into adult worms.
- Larvae produced by the adult worms penetrate the intestines within 2–3 weeks and travel via lymphatics and the blood into striated muscles, where they encyst. New larvae also disseminate to heart and brain.
- Adult worms are excreted in stool.

ETIOLOGY
- Nematodes of the genus *Trichinella*, most commonly *T. spiralis*, a small worm (males, 1.6 mm; females, 3.0 mm).
- Other species: *T. nativa, T. britovi, T. nelsona, T. murrelli, T. pseudospiralis*.

 DIAGNOSIS

HISTORY
- Most infections are asymptomatic.
- Diarrhea of varying severity occurs after the adult worm enters the intestine.
- On occasion, the patient has nausea and vomiting.
- At the time of larval invasion, the patient may have high fevers, severe myalgias, headache, and periorbital edema.
- Pain in the extraocular muscles is noted frequently.
- A dry cough may be present.
- Symptoms often last for weeks (up to 2–3 months).

PHYSICAL EXAM
- Periorbital (including palpebral) edema is a hallmark feature. May be associated with chemosis and proptosis.
- Facial edema.
- Urticarial and maculopapular rash.
- Muscle weakness and tenderness. Peripheral muscles may also appear swollen.
- Subconjunctival, subretinal, or subungual hemorrhages.
- Migration of the larvae through the heart may lead to congestive heart failure and sudden death.
- Larval passage through the central nervous system leads to meningitis and encephalitis.

DIAGNOSTIC TESTS & INTERPRETATION
Lab
- Eosinophilia is present in the muscle stage of infection.
- Immunoglobulin E levels may be increased.
- Muscle enzymes, such as creatine phosphokinase, aldolase, and lactate dehydrogenase, are elevated in severe illness. Myoglobinuria may be present.

- Among serologic tests, Enzyme-linked immunosorbent assay (ELISA) is the most sensitive. Serology can take 3 weeks to become positive after ingestion of the larvae.
- Serology may remain positive for 1 year or more after resolution of infection. Infection with other helminthes may cause false positive results.
- Indirect immunofluorescence has been used less frequently.
- To avoid cross-reactions when using ELISA, Western Blot techniques have been used, such as immunoelectrotransfer blot assay using excretory secretory products of *T. spiralis* to detect reactivity with patient's serum (2).
- PCR amplification of larvae products.

Imaging
- Muscle calcifications on plain radiographs indicate old infection.
- Orbital CT scan in patients with chemosis/proptosis to rule out other etiologies.
- MRI of the brain: Small cortical infarcts.

Diagnostic Procedures/Other
- On occasion, a muscle biopsy reveals larval organisms (free or encapsulated).
- Yield is highest in symptomatic muscles near a tendinous insertion.
- ECG: Repolarization changes or bundle branch block.
- Echocardiogram: To detect effusion.
- Serum troponin: May be increased.
- Serum albumin: May be decreased.

Pathological Findings
Disappearance of sarcomere myofibrils in a new phenotype host cell (nurse cell), encapsulation of larvae, and the formation of a capillary network surrounding the infected cell are the primary findings in striated muscle biopsy (3). Few months later, calcification of the collagen capsule and then of the "nurse cell" and the larvae occurs. Despite this host response, some larvae survive for years.

DIFFERENTIAL DIAGNOSIS
Infectious
- Viral infections (such as influenza, measles) and bacterial infections (such as scarlet fever, typhoid fever, and typhus) may appear clinically similar
- Schistosomiasis
- Strongyloidiasis
- Toxocariasis
- Visceral larva migrans
- Neurocysticercosis

Noninfectious
- Angioneurotic edema can be confused with the periorbital edema
- Myopathies
- Dermatomyositis
- Hypereosinophilic syndrome

 TREATMENT

MEDICATION
- Upon diagnosis, institute treatment as soon as possible (4).
- Anti-parasitic medications are active against the adult worm, not the larvae (5,6).

First Line
- Albendazole 400 mg p.o. b.i.d. for 8–14 days.
- Mebendazole (6) 200–400 mg t.i.d. by mouth for 3 days, then 400–500 mg t.i.d. by mouth for 10 days.

Second Line
- Thiabendazole (7): Treatment duration is 2–5 days for all dose regimens; the dose regimen varies according to weight: >68 kg: 1.5 g b.i.d.; 57–67 kg: 1.25 g b.i.d.; 46–56 kg: 1 g b.i.d.; 35–45 kg: 0.75 g b.i.d.; 23–34: 0.5 g b.i.d.; 13.6–22 kg: 0.25 g b.i.d.
- For the treatment of the intestinal stage of trichinellosis: Pyrantel 10 mg/kg per day for 4 consecutive days.

Pediatric Considerations
Albendazole and mebendazole are not approved for use in children under the age of 2 years.

Pregnancy Considerations
- Severe trichinellosis during pregnancy should be treated with corticosteroids.
- Albendazole and mebendazole not approved for use in pregnancy.

ADDITIONAL TREATMENT
General Measures
- In patients with symptoms of myositis, bed rest with supportive care is necessary.
- Treatment with analgesics/antipyretics is also recommended.

Additional Therapies
- Prednisone 60 mg p.o. every day for 14 days can be used in patients with very severe disease, especially those with heart failure or encephalitis.
- Anticoagulants have been used in cases of cardiovascular thrombosis.

 ONGOING CARE

PROGNOSIS
- Infection often subsides with encystment of larvae, although encysted larvae remain viable.
- Death may occur in severe myocarditis.

COMPLICATIONS
- Pulmonary involvement
  - Direct involvement with passage of larvae through the lungs
  - Myositis involving pulmonary muscle
  - Secondary pneumonia
- Congestive heart failure
- Thrombus of the cardiovascular system (8)
- Meningitis, encephalitis
- Nephritis

REFERENCES
1. Kennedy ED, Hall RL, Montgomery SP, et al. Trichinellosis surveillance – United States, 2002–2007. *MMWR Surveill Summ* 2009;58:1–7.
2. Yera H, Andiva S, Perret C, et al. Development and evaluation of a Western blot kit for diagnosis of human trichinellosis. *Clin Diagn Lab Immunol* 2003;10:793–796.
3. Dupouy-Camet J, Paugam A, De Pinieux G, et al. *Trichinella murrelli*: Pathological features in human muscles at different delays after infection. *Parasite* 2001;8:S176–S179.
4. Gottstein B, Pozio E, Nöckler K. Epidemiology, diagnosis, treatment, and control of trichinellosis. *Clin Microbiol Rev* 2009;22:127–145.
5. Pozio E, Sacchini D, Sacchi L, et al. Failure of mebendazole in the treatment of humans with *Trichinella spiralis* infection at the stage of encapsulating larvae. *Clin Infect Dis* 2001;32:638–642.
6. Watt G, Saisorn S, Jongsakul K, et al. Blinded, placebo-controlled trial of antiparasitic drugs for trichinosis myositis. *J Infect Dis* 2000;182:371–374.
7. Cabié A, Bouchaud O, Houzé S, et al. Albendazole versus thiabendazole as therapy for trichinosis: A retrospective study. *Clin Infect Dis* 1996;22:1033–1035.
8. Tint D, Cocuz ME, Ortan OF, et al. Cardiac involvement in trichinellosis: A case of left ventricular thrombosis. *Am J Trop Med Hyg* 2009;81:313–316.

ADDITIONAL READING
- Dupouy-Camet J, Kociecka W, Bruschi F, et al. Opinion on the diagnosis and treatment of human trichinellosis. *Expert Opin Pharmacother* 2002;3:1117–1130.
- Murrell KD, Pozio E. Trichinellosis: The zoonosis that won't go quietly. *Int J Parasitol* 2000;30:1339–1349.

 CODES

ICD9
124 Trichinosis

CLINICAL PEARLS
- For patients who present with myositis and eosinophilia, the diagnosis of trichinosis should be considered.
- Periorbital edema (including palpebral edema) often associated with chemosis is a characteristic physical finding in trichinosis.
- Severe complications include congestive heart failure and encephalitis.

T

TRYPANOSOMIASIS: AMERICAN (CHAGAS DISEASE) AND AFRICAN (SLEEPING SICKNESS)

Paschalis Vergidis
Matthew E. Falagas

 BASICS

DESCRIPTION
Trypanosomiasis is a zoonotic protozoal disease transmitted to humans by blood-sucking insect vectors. It produces various acute and chronic diseases in humans.

EPIDEMIOLOGY
Incidence
- The estimated global annual infection rate with *Trypanosoma cruzi* is 300,000.
- In 1999, 45,000 cases of African trypanosomiasis were reported to WHO.

Prevalence
- An estimated 16–18 million people are infected with *Trypanosoma cruzi*.
- *T. cruzi* is present in South and Central America, Mexico, and the southern US. The majority of cases are reported from Brazil. Autochthonous disease is extremely rare in the US.
- It is estimated that at least 300,000 to 500,000 people have African trypanosomiasis. The disease is endemic in Sub-Saharan Africa. Approximately 80% of cases occur in Congo.

RISK FACTORS
- Chagas disease is prevalent in poor rural areas where the reduviid bug takes to houses made of clay or mud brick.
- Chagas disease may reactivate in immunosuppressed patients, such as those with organ transplantation or HIV.

GENERAL PREVENTION
- Adequate housing and avoidance of infestations of the insect vectors, especially in bedrooms, are needed in Latin America, primarily in the poor rural areas.
- Insect repellents for travelers. No vaccine is available.
- Blood for transfusion should be screened for *T. cruzi* in high-risk areas. Blood donors are currently screened in the US.

PATHOPHYSIOLOGY
- *T. cruzi* is transmitted by blood-sucking insects (kissing bugs), in the insects' feces. From there, the infectious trypomastigotes enter the human body through breaks in the skin and are transformed into amastigotes.
- *T. cruzi* also can be transmitted by blood transfusions or organ transplantation.
- *T. cruzi* has been transmitted in utero, and is associated with fetal demise and fetal abnormalities.
- Oral transmission has been reported after ingestion of contaminated food.
- Human African trypanosomiasis is caused by trypanosomes transmitted by the tsetse fly.

ETIOLOGY
- *T. cruzi* causes Chagas disease in 10–30% of those infected.
- *Trypanosoma brucei gambiense* causes West African disease.
- *T. brucei rhodesiense* causes East African disease.

DIAGNOSIS

HISTORY
- Acute symptoms of Chagas disease occur 1 week after contact with the parasite. Usually a mild illness occurring in young children.
- Chronic Chagas disease takes years to decades to cause significant illness.
- Symptoms suggestive of heart disease:
  – Palpitations
  – Syncope, presyncope
  – Symptoms of congestive heart failure
  – Thromboembolic phenomena
  – Atypical chest pain
- Symptoms of West African trypanosomiasis occur 1 to 2 weeks following the insect bite.
- Symptoms of East African trypanosomiasis occur a few days following the insect bite.

PHYSICAL EXAM
ACUTE CHAGAS DISEASE
- A small, indurated papule with erythema and local lymphadenopathy occurs at the site of invasion by the organism (chagoma).
- When contact is made from the organism to the conjunctiva, periocular or palpebral edema occurs (Romaña sign). This is a classic sign of acute Chagas disease.
- Fevers, constitutional symptoms, lymphadenopathy, and splenomegaly can occur and usually resolve within weeks.
- Central nervous system symptoms and myocarditis are rare complications at this stage.

CHRONIC CHAGAS DISEASE
- Develops years after the initial infection. Most commonly it involves the heart.
- Cardiomyopathy develops and is associated with heart failure and/or arrhythmias, which are often fatal.
- Patients develop megaesophagus and dysphagia.
- Aspiration is common.
- Colonic dysfunction with megacolon occurs.

WEST AFRICAN TRYPANOSOMIASIS
Stage I (hemolymphatic)
- A painful, indurated chancre develops within 1 to 2 weeks following the tsetse fly bite. The chancre may ulcerate.
- Several weeks to several months after the initial infection, patients develop fevers associated with nontender lymphadenopathy.
- Marked constitutional signs occur at this stage, along with pruritus, arthralgias, transient edema of the face and extremities, and round erythematous rashes with internal clearing.

Stage II (meningoencephalitic)
- Several months to years after the initial infections, patients can develop CNS signs of lethargy, somnolence, and personality changes. Severe headache, ataxia, fasciculations, and choreiform movements occur at this stage.
- Neurologic signs progress slowly to stupor, coma, and death.

EAST AFRICAN TRYPANOSOMIASIS
- Acute disease with early CNS involvement and duration of less than 9 months.
- Patients develop fevers, malaise, headache and rash within weeks, as opposed to months, after the tsetse fly bite.

DIAGNOSTIC TESTS & INTERPRETATION
Lab
Initial lab tests
ACUTE CHAGAS DISEASE
- Finding circulating parasites in the blood confirms the diagnosis.
- Wet preparations and Giemsa stains of anticoagulated blood or buffy coat (thin and thick smears) should be obtained.
- The organisms are motile. Detection occurs 50% of the time.
- IgM serology not useful for diagnosing acute disease.
- PCR assays have been developed. These have variable sensitivity and are not commercially available.

CHRONIC CHAGAS DISEASE
- Serology is used to detect IgG antibodies to the organism (ELISA, indirect hemagglutination, indirect immunofluorescence).
- Many false-positive tests occur. Hence, samples should be tested by 2 different assays.

AFRICAN TRYPANOSOMIASIS
- Fluid from chancres or aspirated fluid from lymph nodes should be prepared with Giemsa stains to search for organisms.
- Wet preparations and Giemsa stains of blood may reveal the organism.
- Card agglutination tests for trypanosomes (CATT) can be used for screening purposes. The test takes less than 10 min, can be conducted in the field, and is highly sensitive.
- Lumbar puncture should be performed in all suspected or proven cases. Cerebrospinal fluid analysis shows pleocytosis and elevated protein.

Imaging
- Barium swallow/enema for patients with symptoms suggestive of esophageal/colonic involvement.
- 2-D echocardiography if concern for cardiac disease

Diagnostic Procedures/Other
- Resting electrocardiogram (ECG) with 30-sec lead II rhythm strip.
- If symptoms or abnormal resting ECG findings, proceed to ambulatory 24-hour ECG monitoring, exercise testing, and echocardiography.
- Esophageal manometry
- Upper endoscopy not indicated for diagnosis of megaesophagus. Only if concern for esophageal carcinoma.

Pathological Findings

- In chronic Chagas heart disease, there is marked bilateral ventricular enlargement (more on the right side than the left). There is also thinning of the ventricular walls, apical aneurysms, and mural thrombi.
- Microscopically there is widespread lymphocytic infiltration, diffuse interstitial fibrosis, and atrophy of myocardial cells.
- In megaesophagus/megacolon there is dilation and muscular hypertrophy with marked reduction of neurons in the myenteric plexus.

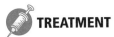

TREATMENT

MEDICATION

- Indications for antitrypanosomal treatment:
  - Acute Chagas disease (AII) (1)
  - Early congenital infection (AII)
  - Reactivation after immunosuppression (AII)
  - Children with chronic Chagas disease (aged ≤12 years AI, 13–18 years AIII) (2)
  - For adults 19–50 years without advanced cardiomyopathy treatment should be offered (BII)
  - Impending immunosuppression (e.g., before organ transplantation) (BII)
- Younger patients have higher probability of parasitologic cure.
- For adults, data suggest that treatment may prevent progression to cardiomyopathy (3).
- Antitrypanosomal treatment not indicated in patients with cardiomyopathy or megaesophagus.

CHAGAS DISEASE

- Benznidazole 5–7 mg/kg/d orally in 2 divided doses for 60 days. Better tolerated than nifurtimox.
- Nifurtimox 8–10 mg/kg/d orally in 4 divided doses over a 90- to 120-day period.
- Both drugs can be obtained from the Centers for Disease Control.

WEST AFRICAN TRYPANOSOMIASIS

- Stage I
  - Pentamidine isoethionate 4 mg/kg/d i.m. or i.v. each day for 10 days. I.m. injections painful. I.v. route preferred
- Stage II
  - Eflornithine 400 mg/kg/d i.v. in four divided doses for 14 days. Less toxic than melarsoprol.

EAST AFRICAN TRYPANOSOMIASIS

- Stage I
  - Suramin 100 mg i.v. test dose, followed by 1 g i.v. days 1, 3, 7, 14, and 21. Immediate hypersensitivity reaction can occur after injection. Test dose given due to risk of anaphylaxis.
- Stage II
  - Melarsoprol 2.0 to 3.6 mg/kg/d i.v. in days 1, 2, 3, followed by 3.6 mg/kg/d in days 11, 12, 13, and days 21, 22, 23. Studies have also shown the effectiveness of a 10-day melarsoprol treatment which decreases treatment duration and drug amount.

ONGOING CARE

FOLLOW-UP RECOMMENDATIONS

- Infected patients who did not receive treatment should be followed closely for signs of cardiac dysfunction, arrhythmias, and signs of achalasia and megacolon.
- Adults should have yearly comprehensive evaluations that include history, physical exam, and ECG.

Patient Monitoring

Offer diagnostic screening to:

- Children of seropositive women
- Family members of patients
- Individuals with a history of potential exposure to the parasite in endemic settings

PATIENT EDUCATION

Persons infected with *T. cruzi* should be counseled not to donate blood.

PROGNOSIS

- 20–30% of infected persons will progress to heart failure.
- Congestive heart failure and left ventricular ejection fraction <30% have a <30% survival at 2–4 years.
- The presence of an apical aneurysm is associated with a high risk of stroke.
- Cause of death: Sudden death due to ventricular arrhythmias or complete heart block, intractable congestive heart failure, or embolic phenomena.
- Outcome of heart transplantation better in patients with Chagas disease compared to ischemic or idiopathic dilated cardiomyopathy (4).

COMPLICATIONS

- Chronic Chagas disease causes cardiomyopathy and megaesophagus and megacolon.

REFERENCES

1. de Andrade AL, Zicker F, de Oliveira RM, et al. Randomised trial of efficacy of benznidazole in treatment of early *Trypanosoma cruzi* infection. *Lancet* 1996;348(9039):1407–1413.
2. Sosa Estani S, Segura EL, Ruiz AM, et al. Efficacy of chemotherapy with benznidazole in children in the indeterminate phase of Chagas' disease. *Am J Trop Med Hyg* 1998;59(4):526–529.
3. Viotti R, Vigliano C, Lococo B, et al. Long-term cardiac outcomes of treating chronic Chagas disease with benznidazole versus no treatment: A nonrandomized trial. *Ann Intern Med* 2006; 144(10):724–734.
4. Bocchi EA, Fiorelli A. The paradox of survival results after heart transplantation for cardiomyopathy caused by *Trypanosoma cruzi*. First Guidelines Group for Heart Transplantation of the Brazilian Society of Cardiology. *Ann Thorac Surg* 2001; 71(6):1833–1888.

ADDITIONAL READING

- Bern C, Montgomery SP, Herwaldt BL, et al. Evaluation and treatment of Chagas disease in the United States: A systematic review. *JAMA* 2007; 298(18):2171–2181.
- Rodriques Coura J, de Castro SL. A critical review on Chagas disease chemotherapy. *Mem Inst Oswaldo Cruz* 2002;97(1):3–24.
- Brun R, Balmer O. New developments in human African trypanosomiasis. Current opinion in infectious diseases. 2006 Oct;19(5):415–20.

CODES

ICD9

- 086.0 Chagas' disease with heart involvement
- 086.1 Chagas' disease with other organ involvement
- 086.2 Chagas' disease without organ involvement
- 086.5 African trypanosomiasis, unspecified

TUBERCULOSIS

Emily P. Hyle (E. Mylonakis, Editor)

 BASICS

DESCRIPTION
Any infection caused by *Mycobacterium tuberculosis*

Geriatric Considerations
Older patients are at increased risk for atypical presentations of reactivation disease.

Pediatric Considerations
- TB is among the top 10 causes of death in children worldwide.
- Children progress more rapidly from initial infection to active disease with TB.
- Definitive diagnosis with early morning gastric lavage, induced sputum, or nasopharyngeal aspirate; however, clinical suspicion must remain high as diagnostics are often limited.
- Treatment is similar as with adults, although drug dosing may be affected as underdosing may occur given increased metabolism of children in comparison to adults.

Pregnancy Considerations
- Pregnancy does not affect the progression of TB; as a result, only those women at high risk for active TB should undergo diagnostics.
- If latent TB treatment (LTBI) treatment is pursued because of concern for increased risk of progression to active TB, isoniazid (INH) should be used with careful monitoring given increased risks of INH-hepatitis in this population.
- When an expectant mother is diagnosed with active TB, rifampin, isoniazid, and ethambutol can be used for combination therapy in pregnancy and lactation with close follow-up. Pyrazinamide is not used.
- Congenital TB is rare and occurs through hematogenous spread to the fetus. Neonatal TB is more common given close proximity of mother with child when breast feeding. Mortality of both congenital and neonatal TB is near 50%.

EPIDEMIOLOGY
Incidence
- 12,000 cases annually in US (4.2/100,000) (3).
- 8.9–9.9 million cases worldwide (2008).
- 1.3 million deaths (HIV-negative) and 0.52 million deaths (HIV-infected) worldwide annually.

Prevalence
- Fewer than 5% of cases is usually active after 1 year from exposure.
- Only 15% of people exposed develop active disease.
- Among immunocompromised and HIV-infected, risk of active infection is 10% per year.
- 9.6–13.3 million cases worldwide (estimated 2008 global prevalence).

RISK FACTORS
- Living in over-crowded environments.
- Homelessness.
- History of intravenous drug use (IDU) or EtOH.
- Diabetes (2–4 fold).
- Chronic renal disease (10–25 fold).
- Use of TNF-inhibitors (2–25 fold).
- Silicosis (30 fold).
- HIV (>100 fold).
- Poverty.
- Born outside US

Genetics
Polymorphisms are being studied to assess baseline increased risk for infection among exposed cases.

GENERAL PREVENTION
- Hospital/institutional: Negative pressure isolation for TB suspects with N95 masks for those who enter the room.
- Home: Surgical mask on patient while infectious; avoidance of immunocompromised or children <5 years old.
- Contact tracing and reporting to the local Department of Public Health are essential after a new diagnosis.

PATHOPHYSIOLOGY
- Spread by respiratory route.
- Killed by UV light.
- After tuberculi is inhaled into lungs, it can be cleared by the host's immune system, cause primary disease, or be controlled into asymptomatic latent disease that sometimes reactivates later on.

ETIOLOGY
- *M. tuberculosis* is a small aerobic bacillus that is slow-growing in the laboratory. Upon staining, the organism is acid-fast (AFB), appearing red on a Ziehl–Neelsen stain.
- Humans are the only reservoir for MTb.

 DIAGNOSIS

HISTORY
- Primary pulmonary TB: Cough and fevers but can be asymptomatic (2).
- Postprimary TB: Cough, fevers, night sweats with weight loss. Can include pleuritic chest pain and hemoptysis.
- Extrapulmonary TB: Includes adenitis, laryngitis (e.g., dysphagia and hoarseness), otitis media (e.g., otorrhea, perforation), meningitis (e.g., headaches, fevers, cranial nerve findings, meningismus often subacute), skeletal (Potts), GI (e.g., diarrhea, obstruction, pain), GU (often asymptomatic).
- Disseminated/miliary: Can be a subacute presentation or fulminant septic shock.

PHYSICAL EXAM
- Adenitis: Painless, erythematous, firm lymph nodes without fluctuance or drainage – often cervical (scrofula).
- Pulmonary: Dullness, fremitus, crackles.
- CNS: Cranial nerve deficits, meningismus.
- GI: Obstruction (especially at terminal ileum), ascites.

DIAGNOSTIC TESTS & INTERPRETATION
Lab
Initial lab tests
- Often normal in pulmonary TB.
- Anemia is often evident in disseminated disease, with either leukopenia or leukocytosis evident. Pancytopenia also occurs.
- Elevated alkaline phosphatase is often evident with granulomatous hepatitis caused by TB.

Follow-Up & Special Considerations
Careful follow-up of basic laboratories is essential when therapy is initiated, as many drugs cause toxicities to kidney or liver function or cell counts.

Imaging
Initial approach
- Chest XRay (CXR): Lower lobe involvement for primary disease with hilar lymphadenopathy; pleural effusion can result. In reactivation disease, apical disease is most frequent but can also include cavitation, solitary nodules, pleural effusion.
- Chest CT: Tree-in-bud pattern, cavities, nodules.

Follow-Up & Special Considerations
To follow response to treatment.

Diagnostic Procedures/Other
Latent disease
- Tuberculin skin tests (TSTs): In immunocompetent patients, induration greater than 15 mm in diameter suggests a very high likelihood of having TB. In patients with known TB risk, induration greater than 10 mm is positive. In immunocompromised patients, induration of greater than 5 mm is positive.
- False-positive TST can occur with cross-reaction to the Bacille Calmette–Guerin (BCG) used in immunization, but this is less common more than 10 years after immunization. Anyone at risk for infection with a TST greater than 10 mm should be considered infected regardless of BCG history.
- Interferon gamma-release assays (IGRAs) are increasingly used for diagnosis of latent or active infection. IGRAs are preferred for those patients with low likelihood of returning for TST-reading or history of BCG. TST remains referred for children <5 years old.

Active disease
- AFB smear and mycobacterial culture.
- For pTB: Sputum remains gold standard. Typically, >10,000 organisms/mL is necessary.
- Early AM-induced sputum is highest yield with 3 specimens recommended. Cumulative yield on smear is 64, 81, 91% and that on culture is 70, 90, and 91%.
- Bronchoscopy with post-bronchoscopy sputum has >90% yield.
- For extrapulmonary disease, smear/culture is less sensitive; histopathology from biopsy plays a key role.
- In HIV patients with low CD4 counts, blood cultures are positive in 75% of cases.
- TST can be negative in as many as 50% of patients with overwhelming disease (false-negative due to anergy).

Pathological Findings
Caseating granuloma.

DIFFERENTIAL DIAGNOSIS
- Sarcoidosis
- Atypical mycobacteria
- Lung abscess due to necrotizing pneumonias
- Endemic fungi (e.g. histoplasmosis)
- Lymphoma

TREATMENT

MEDICATION

Latent Disease Treatment
- Positive tuberculin test without evidence of disease (2).
  – Isoniazid 300 mg/d orally for 6 months
  – Pyridoxine supplements 50 mg/d orally are often given.
  – Alternatives to daily INH therapy
    ◦ INH 900 mg orally, 2 times per week for 12 months
    ◦ Rifampin 600 mg orally per day, plus ethambutol 15 mg/kg orally per day for 9–12 months
    ◦ Rifampin 600 mg orally per day, plus pyrazinamide 20 mg/kg/d for 6–12 months
    ◦ Shorter courses of rifampin and pyrazinamide for 2 months have proved effective in HIV-infected patients.
- Positive tuberculin test with abnormal chest x-ray or in an HIV-positive patient.
  – Isoniazid 300 mg/d orally for 12 months
  – Pyridoxine supplements 50 mg a day orally are often given.

Active Disease Treatment
First Line
- Pulmonary TB.
  – Total duration of drug therapy is 6 months.
  – 4 drugs for the first 2 months of treatment including isoniazid (INH) 300 mg p.o. daily, rifampin (RIF) 600 mg p.o. daily, pyrazinamide (PYR) 15–30 mg/kg p.o. daily, ethambutol (EMB) 15–25 mg/kg p.o. daily.
  – Then, INH and RIF for 4 additional months (total treatment of 6 months).
  – Extend to 9 months if cavitary disease is present or remains culture positive at 2 months.
  – Alternative: Streptomycin 15 mg/kg i.v. or i.m. may be used along with 3 or 4 other drugs in the treatment of TB.
  – Extrapulmonary TB: Same as for pulmonary TB, but the duration of therapy should be at least 12 months (INH plus rifampin for the last 10 months).
- Immunocompromised patients/HIV-infected patients with pulmonary disease or extrapulmonary disease.
  – Same as for HIV-negative patients. Some suggest treating extrapulmonary disease for at least 18 months.
  – Treatment for MDR-TB should be extended to 18–24 months.

Second Line
- Respiratory quinolones: Moxifloxacin, levofloxacin (1)
- Injectables: Amikacin, kanamycin
- Ethionamide
- Para-aminosalicylic acid (PAS)
- Cycloserine
- Linezolid

Drug Resistance
- Drug-resistant TB: Resistant to a first-line agent (e.g.; INH, RIF, PYZ, or EMB).
- Multi-drug resistant TB (MDR-TB): Resistant to both INH and RIF.
- Extremely drug resistant TB (XDR-TB): Resistant to both INH and RIF, as well as quinolones and injectable (aminoglycosides and/or capreomycin).

ADDITIONAL TREATMENT
Issues for Referral
- Concern for drug-resistant TB.
- Co-infection with HIV or viral hepatitis.

Additional Therapies
Steroids: Mortality benefit in TB meningitis but no effect on disability.

SURGERY/OTHER PROCEDURES
For pulmonary cavity disease especially with MDR-TB; resection should occur only after 1–3 months of active combination therapy.

IN-PATIENT CONSIDERATIONS
Admission Criteria
- For respiratory isolation or expedited workup.
- For those patients with severe disseminated or CNS disease.

Discharge Criteria
- 3 sequential smear-negative sputa.
- After 2 weeks of treatment, patients with smear-positive pulmonary TB are typically no longer infectious and can be discharged to continue therapy.

ONGOING CARE

FOLLOW-UP RECOMMENDATIONS
Close follow-up after completion of treatment is necessary given potential risk of relapse.

Patient Monitoring
- Complications of therapy include the following:
  – INH hepatitis: Risks approach 1% for patients above the age of 35 years.
  – Ethambutol ophthalmic toxicity: Optic neuritis; green–red discrimination should be tested on a monthly basis during therapy.
  – Streptomycin-induced ototoxicity: Ototoxicity and vestibular dysfunction can occur and be permanent.
  – Rifamycins interact with many drugs that require cytochrome P-450 metabolism.

DIET
- Malnutrition is a risk factor for the development of active disease.
- Vitamin D deficiency puts patients at risk for progression of TB.
- Iron overload may contribute to poor outcomes and acceleration of disease.

PATIENT EDUCATION
- Emphasis on medication adherence and follow-up.
- Review of drug toxicities and drug–drug interactions.

PROGNOSIS
With completion of sufficient therapy, outcomes are excellent.

COMPLICATIONS
Pulmonary TB: Hemoptysis, pneumothorax, bronchiectasis, pulmonary cavities with superinfection.

REFERENCES

1. Johnston JC, Shahadi NC, Sadatsafavi M, et al. Treatment outcomes of multidrug-resistant tuberculosis: A systematic review and meta-analysis. *PLoS One* 2009;4(9):e6914.
2. Mandell GL, Bennett JE, Dolin R. *Principles and practice of infectious diseases.* 7th ed. Philadelphia, PA: Churchill Livingstone/Elsevier, 2010.
3. http://www.who.int/tb/publications/factsheets/en/index.html

ADDITIONAL READING

- Jassal MS, Bishai WR. Epidemiology and challenges to the elimination of global tuberculosis. *CID* 2010;50(S3):S156–S154.
- Swaminathan S, Rekha B. Pediatric tuberculosis: Global overview and challenges. *CID* 2010;50(S3):S184–S194.

 See Also

- http://www.cdc.gov/mmwr/preview/mmwrhtml/rr5211a1.htm

CODES

ICD9
- 011.90 Unspecified pulmonary tuberculosis, confirmation unspecified
- 018.90 Unspecified miliary tuberculosis, unspecified examination
- 771.2 Other congenital infections specific to the perinatal period

CLINICAL PEARLS
- Infection control measures for active pulmonary or laryngeal tuberculosis are necessary.
- Resistant tuberculosis should be considered when in those previously treated or from a region with high rates of drug-resistance.

TULAREMIA

Paschalis Vergidis
Matthew E. Falagas

 BASICS

DESCRIPTION
Tularemia is a zoonotic infection caused by *Francisella tularensis*. The organism is responsible for a number of syndromes in humans that range from a plague-like ulceroglandular illness to pneumonia.

EPIDEMIOLOGY
Incidence
Tularemia is a rare disease, with fewer than 300 cases reported in the US annually.

Prevalence
- The disease occurs mainly in the Northern Hemisphere; it is not found in the UK. The disease has not been reported in Africa, South America, or Australia.
- Most cases in the US occur in the south central states Arkansas, Oklahoma, and Missouri.
- Tick-borne cases occur in the summer.
- Disease in the winter months is usually associated with skin contact with infectious organisms (hunting-associated cases).
- Infection is found to occur in over 100 species of small and large mammals, 25 species of birds, and 50 species of insects.
- Fish and amphibians may be infected.
- In the US, the rabbit is the most important reservoir of infection.
- Insects such as ticks, flies, and mosquitoes serve as vectors for disease in humans.
- Commonly found wood ticks, dog ticks, and lone star ticks are responsible for the majority of transmission in the US.

RISK FACTORS
High-risk professionals include hunters, farm workers, veterinarians, and laboratory workers.

GENERAL PREVENTION
- A live attenuated vaccine is available for people at high risk of infection. It does not provide complete protection but reduces the severity of disease.
- Protection from ticks is important.
- People who skin animals (hunters, trappers) should wear gloves.

PATHOPHYSIOLOGY
- Infection in humans can occur by one of the following routes:
  - Bite from an arthropod vector (tick or mosquito).
  - Skin contact with an infected carcass
  - Inhalation of the organism, particularly by laboratory workers. (May be used as an agent of bioterrorism)
  - Ingestion of meat contaminated with the bacterium
  - Bite from an animal (including pets) that harbors the organism in the oropharynx
- The organism spreads from the site of entry to regional lymph nodes. *Francisella* replicates within host macrophages and disseminates via a lymphohematogenous route. Bacteremia is common in the early phase.

ETIOLOGY
- *F. tularensis* is an aerobic gram-negative rod.
- The organism is virulent, and small numbers of organisms on the skin can invade and lead to systemic illness.
- The organism
  - Requires cysteine for growth
  - Produces a β-lactamase
  - Is resistant to freezing and may persist for weeks in dead animals
  - Is inactivated by heat

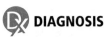 **DIAGNOSIS**

HISTORY
- The incubation period varies and averages 3–5 days.
- In most cases, cutaneous infection disseminates to regional lymph nodes prior to bacteremia.
- Bacteremia is associated with fever, chills, myalgias, headache, sore throat, and cough that continue for 1–4 days.
- Remission occurs for 1–3 days, followed by recurrent symptoms that can continue for several weeks.

PHYSICAL EXAM
- Fever may be associated with a pulse-temperature deficit.
- Some patients have a rash that begins as blotchy, macular, or maculopapular and progresses to pustular lesions.
  - Ulceroglandular
    - Accounts for 60–80% of cases.
    - Ulcers appear at the skin site of inoculation and start as a red, painful papule, progressing to necrotic ulcers, which leave a scar.
    - Regional lymph nodes become markedly enlarged and tender during this stage. They may stay enlarged for months.
    - Half of patients with the ulceroglandular form have evidence of pneumonia, effusions, or hilar adenopathy on chest x-ray.
  - Glandular
    - There is no identifiable skin lesion
  - Typhoidal
    - Typhoidal disease is rare and may lead to fever of unknown origin.
    - Presumably, the organism is ingested, but tick exposure may initiate the disease.
    - Ulcers and lymphadenopathy are usually absent.
    - Diarrhea is usually prominent.
    - Most patients with the typhoidal form have abnormalities on chest x-ray and pneumonitis.
  - Pneumonic
    - Associated with inhalation of the organism or hematogenous spread.
    - Patients present with a dry cough, pleuritic chest pain, fevers, and myalgias.
  - Oculoglandular
    - Inoculation in the eye may lead to an oculoglandular form of the illness.
    - Painful conjunctivitis with yellow conjunctival ulcers and preauricular or cervical lymphadenopathy occurs.
  - Oropharyngeal
    - Ingestion of the bacteria may lead to this rare form of disease.
    - The throat may contain a membrane that resembles diphtheria.
    - Cervical lymphadenopathy is extensive.

ALERT
F. tularensis is an agent of bioterrorism. Notify public health authorities in cases with unusual epidemiologic history.

DIAGNOSTIC TESTS & INTERPRETATION
Lab
- Modest elevation of the leukocyte count may occur
- Mild elevations of transaminases can be noted
- Sterile pyuria
- Rhabdomyolysis is a poor prognostic sign
- Diagnosis is often made serologically
  - Tularemia tube agglutination testing is the most commonly used test.
  - A single titer of 1:160 or higher is supportive of the diagnosis.
  - A fourfold increase in convalescent serum is also supportive.
  - Serologic tests may cross-react with *Salmonella*, *Brucella*, *Yersinia*, and *Legionella* species.
- Cultures require a media that contains cysteine
- Sputum gram stain usually does not demonstrate the organism
- Culture poses a risk for laboratory workers. Always notify laboratory personnel if tularemia is suspected so that they may take appropriate precautions

Imaging
- Chest x-rays often show patchy ill-defined infiltrates with pleural effusions.
- There is often associated hilar adenopathy.
- Nodular infiltrates 2–8 cm in size may be observed.

Diagnostic Procedures/Other
Lymph node biopsy is generally not required for diagnosis.

Pathological Findings
- Early tularemia: Areas of focal necrosis surrounded by neutrophils and macrophages.
- Late disease: Necrotic areas with caseating granulomata.

DIFFERENTIAL DIAGNOSIS
- Plague
- Typhoid fever
- Atypical pneumonia
- Q fever
- Psittacosis

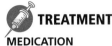

TREATMENT
MEDICATION
First Line
- Drug of choice: Streptomycin 7.5–10.0 mg/kg every 12 h; intravenous or intramuscular delivery for 7–14 days (1)
- Gentamicin 3–5 mg/kg/d, divided every 8 h i.v. for 7–14 days
- Chloramphenicol plus streptomycin used with central nervous system involvement (CNS penetration of aminoglycosides is erratic)

Second Line
The following alternatives are to be used with caution:
- Tetracycline 1 g every day for 15 days has been associated with recurrences.
- Erythromycin is possibly effective, but resistance has been noted.
- Quinolones are possibly effective; however, clinical experience is lacking.
- Third-generation cephalosporins are not effective.

ADDITIONAL TREATMENT
Additional Therapies
Debridement of superinfected necrotic lesions or surgical drainage of lymph nodes.

IN-PATIENT CONSIDERATIONS
Admission Criteria
- Septic shock
- Pneumonia
- Lung abscess
- Adult respiratory distress syndrome
- Meningitis

ONGOING CARE
PROGNOSIS
- Mortality as high as 33% without treatment.
- With appropriate treatment mortality is <4%.

COMPLICATIONS
- Disseminated disease may lead to renal or hepatic failure, meningitis, disseminated intravascular coagulation, shock, and death.
- Suppuration of lymph nodes may occur and be prolonged.
- Lung abscess or adult respiratory distress syndrome may complicate pulmonary tularemia.
- Other complications: Pericarditis, peritonitis, osteomyelitis, endocarditis.

REFERENCE
1. Urich SK, Petersen JM. *In vitro* susceptibility of isolates of *Francisella tularensis* types A and B from North America. *Antimicrob Agents Chemother* 2008;52:2276–2278.

ADDITIONAL READING
- Conlan JW. Vaccines against *Francisella tularensis*—Past, present and future. *Expert Rev Vaccines* 2004;3:307–314.
- Dennis DT, Inglesby TV, Henderson DA, et al. Tularemia as a biological weapon: Medical and public health management. *JAMA* 2001;285: 2763–2773.
- Eliasson H, Broman T, Forsman M, et al. Tularemia: Current epidemiology and disease management. *Infect Dis Clin North Am* 2006;20:289–311, ix.

CODES

ICD9
- 021.1 Enteric tularemia
- 021.2 Pulmonary tularemia
- 021.9 Unspecified tularemia

CLINICAL PEARLS
- Tularemia is a zoonotic infection that can occur after bite from an arthropod or animal, after inhalation, injection, or contact with a contaminated carcass.
- Treatment of choice is streptomycin. Gentamicin may also be used.
- If suspecting tularemia, always notify the microbiology laboratory for appropriate media and protection of personnel.

T

TYPHOID FEVER

Sarah Taimur
Paschalis Vergidis
Matthew E. Falagas

 BASICS

DESCRIPTION
Typhoid fever is a systemic illness caused by *Salmonella enterica* serotype *typhi*.

EPIDEMIOLOGY
Incidence
- There was an estimated 21 million new cases of typhoid fever with 200,000 deaths during 2000 worldwide (1).
- Regions with high incidence: South-central Asia and south-east Asia (>100/100,000 cases/year).
- Regions with medium incidence: Rest of Asia, Africa, Latin America and the Caribbean, and Oceania, except for Australia and New Zealand (10–100/100,000 cases/year).
- Regions with low incidence of typhoid fever: Europe, North America, and the rest of the developed world (<10/100,000 cases/year).
- In the US, approximately 300 cases are reported each year (2).

RISK FACTORS
- Recent typhoid fever in household (3)
- Lack of a toilet and soap in the household
- Younger age
- Female sex
- Use of ice cubes (endemic areas)
- Travel to an endemic area within 30 days before onset of illness
- Food from a street vendor (endemic areas)
- Achlorhydria, gastrectomy, use of histamine blockers and proton pump inhibitors (lowers infective dose)

GENERAL PREVENTION
- Hand washing
- Improved food and water hygiene
- Provision of adequate toilet facilities
- Monitor food handlers for chronic carrier stage
- Vaccination recommended for traveling to areas of moderate-to-high endemicity.
  - Live attenuated vaccine (Ty21a): 4 capsules taken 2 days apart, 1 week prior to potential exposure. Booster needed every 5 years.
  - Parenteral Vi capsular polysaccharide vaccine (Vi CPS): 1 dose taken i.m. 2 weeks prior to potential exposure. Booster needed every 2 years.

PATHOPHYSIOLOGY
- The mode of transmission is fecal–oral through the ingestion of contaminated food or water.
- Person-to-person transmission is uncommon. The organism can be transmitted sexually.
- The incubation period is usually 7–14 days.
- The bacteria have to survive exposure to gastric acid to reach the small intestine, where they adhere and then invade the intestinal mucosa at the Peyer's patches.
- Transportation follows to the intestinal lymphoid tissue and then to the reticuloendothelial cells of the liver and spleen.
- Bacteremia may follow with dissemination of the organism to intestinal and extraintestinal sites including liver, spleen, gallbladder, bone marrow, terminal ileum.

ETIOLOGY
S. enterica serotype *typhi* is a Gram-negative rod within the family of Enterobacteriaceae.

COMMONLY ASSOCIATED CONDITIONS
- Malnourishment
- Recent malaria infection
- Sickle cell disease
- HIV infection (association more robust for non-typhoidal salmonellosis)

 DIAGNOSIS

HISTORY
- Stages of disease
  - Week 1: The onset of bacteremia is marked by fever
  - Week 2: Abdominal symptoms and organomegaly with or without rash (rose spots)
  - Week 3: The patient is more toxic and may develop intestinal perforation/bleeding or extraintestinal complications
- Fever (93–100% of cases)
- Diarrhea (more common in children)
- Constipation (more common in adults)
- Abdominal pain (even distribution across age groups)
- Cough
- Headache
- Chest pain and/or palpitations
- Bone and joint pains or swelling
- Neck pain or stiffness
- Intermittent confusion
- Seizures (more common in children of 5 years of age or younger)

PHYSICAL EXAM
- Initially the fever is low grade, but by the second week it is often 39°C–40°C.
- Abdominal tenderness to severe distention
- Hepatomegaly and splenomegaly
- Relative bradycardia
- Rose spots: Faint, blanching erythematous maculopapular lesions (2–4 mm in diameter);. usually occur on the abdomen and chest and more rarely on the back, arms, and legs.
- Cervical lymphadenopathy
- Rales/rhonchi (Pneumonia more common in children of 5 years of age or younger)
- Meningismus
- New murmur
- Apathetic face
- Encephalopathy/psychosis
- Bone tenderness
- Joint swelling and tenderness

DIAGNOSTIC TESTS & INTERPRETATION
Lab
- Leukopenia (more common in older children/adults)
- Leukocytosis (most common in infants)
- Anemia (more common in infants/young children)
- Thrombocytopenia
- Elevated bilirubin and liver enzymes
- Positive fecal leukocytes
- Cultures
  - Blood (positive in 40–80%)
  - Bone marrow (positive in 90–100%)
  - Stool (positive in 30–40% of acute typhoid fever)
  - Biopsy specimens of rose spots (reported positive up to 62%)
  - Bile (positive in 57–70%)
- Widal test (serum antibodies to O and H antigens)
  - Highly variable yield
  - Can be falsely negative
  - Can cross-react with other Enterobacteriaceae
  - Primarily used in the developing world
- Other serological tests (not widely adopted)
  - IgG or IgM antibodies against outer membrane protein antigen of *S. typhi*
  - Anti-LPS hemagglutination tests
  - Reverse passive hemagglutination test (RPHA)
- PCR testing
  - Not routinely available
  - Can be done on blood, urine, or stool
  - Higher sensitivity than blood cultures (4)

Imaging
- Chest x-ray: Pulmonary infiltrates
- Abdominal imaging: Colitis with or without intestinal perforation

Diagnostic Procedures/Other
- Duodenal capsule string cultures (positive in approximately 60% of cases)
- Bone marrow aspiration: The most sensitive method of isolating the pathogen

Pathological Findings
Infiltration of tissues by macrophages (typhoid cells) containing bacteria, erythrocytes, and degenerated lymphocytes.

DIFFERENTIAL DIAGNOSIS
- Non-typhoidal *Salmonella* species
- *Salmonella paratyphi*
- *Yersinia enterocolitica*
- *Campylobacter fetus*
- Intraabdominal abscess
- Intestinal tuberculosis
- Malaria
- Viral hepatitis
- Bacterial pneumonia
- Bacterial endocarditis

TREATMENT

MEDICATION

First Line
- Resistance to fluoroquinolones is highest in the Indian subcontinent and increasing in South and East Asia. Injectable third-generation cephalosporins are often the empiric drug of choice when the possibility of fluoroquinolone resistance is high.

Uncomplicated typhoid fever
- Ciprofloxacin 500 mg p.o. every 12 h for 5–7 days
- Ofloxacin 400 mg p.o. every 12 h for 5–7 days
- Ceftriaxone 2 g i.v. daily for 10–14 days
- Cefixime 200 mg p.o. every 12 h for 7–14 days
- Azithromycin 1 g p.o. daily for 7 days

Severe typhoid fever
- Ciprofloxacin 400 mg i.v. every 12 h for 10–14 days
- Ceftriaxone 2 g i.v. every 12 h for 10–14 days
- Cefotaxime 2 g i.v. every 8 h for 10–14 days

Second Line
Uncomplicated typhoid fever
- Amoxicillin 1 g p.o. t.i.d for 14 days
- Azithromycin 1 g p.o. daily for 7 days
- Trimethoprim–sulfamethoxazole (TMP-SMX) 160/800 mg p.o. twice daily for 7 days
- Chloramphenicol 500 mg p.o. q.i.d. for 14–21 days

Severe typhoid fever
- Ampicillin 2 g i.v. every 6 hours for 14 days
- Chloramphenicol 1.5 g i.v. every 6 h for 14–21 days

Pregnancy Considerations
Data on treatment of typhoid fever in pregnancy are limited. Use of beta-lactams or macrolides is preferred.

ALERT
- Nalidixic acid-resistant *S. typhi* strains (NARST) have reduced susceptibility to fluoroquinolones (5). Incidence is highest in India, Pakistan, and Bangladesh.
- Multidrug-resistant strains of *S. typhi* (MDRST) with resistance to ampicillin, chloramphenicol, and TMP/SMX are seen worldwide (including the US)
  – 1999–2006: *S. typhi* strains in the US (6):
    ○ 12–15% MDRST
    ○ 35–40% NARST

ADDITIONAL TREATMENT
General Measures
- Intravenous hydration
- Other supportive care

SURGERY/OTHER PROCEDURES
Surgical correction indicated in intestinal perforation or other severe intraabdominal complications (such as uncontrollable bleeding)

IN-PATIENT CONSIDERATIONS
Admission Criteria
- Complicated typhoid fever
- Severe systemic illness
- Severe dehydration
- Pediatric or geriatric age group

 ONGOING CARE

FOLLOW-UP RECOMMENDATIONS
Clinical follow-up for detection of relapse and chronic carrier states

PATIENT EDUCATION
- Frequent hand washing with soap
- Consuming bottled or boiled water
- Avoid sharing food or water with other household members if recent infection
- Avoid food or drinks from street vendors
- Vaccination prior to travel to endemic area

PROGNOSIS
- Average case fatality rate is less than 1%
- Higher mortality among children younger than 1 year and the elderly

COMPLICATIONS
- Gastrointestinal bleeding (occurs in up to 10%)
- Gastrointestinal perforation (occurs in 1–3%). More common in adults –usually in the third week of illness.
- Hepatic, splenic abscess
- Pancreatitis
- Central nervous system disease (cerebral abscess, meningoencephalitis)
- Encephalopathy, delirium, psychotic state
- Cardiovascular disease (endocarditis, myocarditis, pericarditis, arteritis)
- Pulmonary disease (pneumonia, empyema)
- Genitourinary infections
- Musculoskeletal abscess (psoas abscess)
- Hemophagocytic syndrome
- Typhoid fever during pregnancy may lead to miscarriage
- Relapse typically occurs 2–3 weeks after resolution of fever (in 1–6% of cases)
- Chronic carrier state (more common in women, elderly, patients with cholelithiasis). Most carriers are asymptomatic.

REFERENCES
1. Crump JA, Luby SP, Mintz ED. The global burden of typhoid fever. *Bull World Health Organ* 2004;82(5): 346–353.
2. McNabb SJ, Jajosky RA, Hall-Baker PA, et al. Summary of notifiable diseases–United States, 2006. *Morb Mortal Wkly Rep* 2008;55(53):1–92.
3. Vollaard AM, Ali S, van Asten HA, et al. Risk factors for typhoid and paratyphoid fever in Jakarta, Indonesia. *JAMA*. 2004;291(21):2607–2615.
4. Hatta M, Smits HL. Detection of *Salmonella typhi* by nested polymerase chain reaction in blood, urine, and stool samples. *Am J Trop Med Hyg* 2007; 76(1):139–143.
5. Crump JA, Barrett TJ, Nelson JT, et al. Reevaluating fluoroquinolone breakpoints for *Salmonella enterica* serotype *Typhi* and for non-*Typhi* salmonellae. *Clin Infect Dis* 2003;37(1):75–81.
6. Lynch MF, Blanton EM, Bulens S, et al. Typhoid fever in the United States, 1999–2006. *JAMA* 2009;302(8):859–865.

ADDITIONAL READING
- Parry CM, Hien TT, Dougan G, et al. Typhoid fever. *N Engl J Med* 2002;347(22):1770–1782.
- Bhutta ZA. Current concepts in the diagnosis and treatment of typhoid fever. *BMJ* 2006;333(7558): 78–82.

CODES

ICD9
- 002.0 Typhoid fever
- 484.8 Pneumonia in other infectious diseases, classified elsewhere

CLINICAL PEARLS
- For individuals not residing in endemic areas, a travel history is crucial in the diagnosis of typhoid fever.
- The classic Widal test lacks sensitivity and specificity and may lead to overdiagnosis in endemic areas.
- Rising incidence of resistance to nalidixic acid and subsequent reduced susceptibility to fluoroquinolones among *S. typhi* isolates must be considered when treating patients.

T

TYPHUS

Petros I. Rafailidis
Matthew E. Falagas

BASICS

DESCRIPTION
Typhus comprises a group of diseases caused by rickettsias, characterized by fever and rash. These include murine (endemic) (1), epidemic (louse-borne, classic) (2), and scrub typhus (3), as well as Brill-Zinsser disease.

EPIDEMIOLOGY
Incidence
- The typhus group of rickettsioses (especially epidemic typhus) has been a major global health problem since the beginning of the 20th century, particularly in Eastern Europe during the 2 world wars. Spread of epidemics, depending on the spread of the arthropod vectors and the animal reservoirs, is favored by bad sanitary conditions and crowding.
- Epidemic typhus still occurs in the highlands of South America, Africa, and Asia; murine typhus has an endemic worldwide distribution, and scrub typhus occurs in the South Pacific, Asia, and Australia.
- Brill-Zinsser disease constitutes the recurrence of epidemic typhus, years after the primary attack. It mainly occurs among immigrant populations, particularly those originating from Eastern Europe. Brill-Zinsser disease patients may serve as a pool for recurrent epidemic typhus epidemics.
- All these diseases are transmitted to humans via arthropod bites (by contaminated insect feces, as the latter defecate during feeding, with the exception of mites, which directly inoculate R. tsutsugamushi during feeding); mites and fleas pass the rickettsias to their progeny, but infected lice die of intestinal obstruction within 1–3 weeks.

Prevalence
- Effective improvement in sanitary conditions and animal and insect control programs have led to almost complete elimination of epidemic typhus in the US during past decades.
- Murine typhus is still prevalent in the southeastern and Gulf Coast states (4).

RISK FACTORS
- Bad sanitary conditions
- Crowding
- Famine
- Wars (5)
- Refugee populations
- Prison inmates

GENERAL PREVENTION
- Control of animal reservoirs in high-prevalence areas
- Elimination of insect vectors
- Primary chemoprophylaxis has proved to be effective in preventing scrub typhus attacks and mounting an active immune response (single-dose chloramphenicol or tetracycline every 5 days, for an overall duration of 35 days)
- Vaccines against with variable effectiveness against epidemic typhus and scrub typhus are available (2,6).

PATHOPHYSIOLOGY
- The abrupt clinical presentation of louse-borne typhus starts about a week after the challenge, and, if untreated, the illness lasts for 2 weeks; the patient may recover fully after approximately 2 months.
- The incubation period ranges from 1–2 weeks for murine typhus and from 6–18 days for scrub typhus. Brill-Zinsser disease may appear years after the primary epidemic typhus attack.
- Organisms multiply at the site of entry before entering the bloodstream. Despite that, the initial local lesion can be seen only in scrub typhus.
- Rickettsemia develops late in the incubation period and precedes the onset of pyrexia.
- Vascular endothelial cell destruction and consequent damage in several organ systems (notably skin, cardiovascular, respiratory, central nervous, and liver) is the primary pathology found.

ETIOLOGY
- Rickettsias are small, pleomorphic, fastidious, obligate intracellular bacterial organisms.
- *Rickettsia typhi*, *Rickettsia prowazekii*, and *Orientia* (former Rickettsia) *tsutsugamushi* are the causative agents of murine, epidemic, and scrub typhus, respectively. Brill-Zinsser disease represents recurrence of epidemic typhus, years after the initial attack.
- All have a natural cycle involving an arthropod vector (fleas for *R. typhi*, lice, for *R. prowazekii*, mites for *O. tsutsugamushi*) and a vertebrate host (small rodents for *R. typhi*, humans and flying squirrels for *R. prowazekii*, wild rodents for *R. tsutsugamushi*).

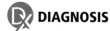 DIAGNOSIS

HISTORY
- The following are common in all forms of typhus:
  - Abrupt onset
  - Fever (102°F–104°F), chills and myalgias
  - Severe frontal headache
  - Altered mentation (i.e., delirium) and neurologic signs
  - Severe nausea and vomiting
  - Anorexia
  - Nonproductive cough and, occasionally, moderate hemoptysis
  - Tinnitus, transient deafness
  - The patient may recall lice, fleas, or mite exposure.

PHYSICAL EXAM
- Epidemic typhus
  - A macular rash that fades on pressure presents on about the fifth day of illness, starting from the axillary folds and the upper trunk and spreading centrifugally, becoming petechial and confluent, sparing the face, palms, and soles. There is no visible eschar.
- Murine typhus
  - Rash develops in only about 50% of patients between the third and fifth day of illness, and may involve both the trunk and extremities. It is usually macular or maculopapular; petechiae are rare (<10%). There is no visible eschar.
  - Splenomegaly may occur in about 25% of the patients.
- Brill-Zinsser disease is generally milder than epidemic typhus, resembling murine typhus in presentation.
- Scrub typhus
  - An erythematous, indurated lesion, surrounded by vesicles that subsequently ulcerate and form a black eschar, may be present at the inoculation site (<50% of cases); regional lymphadenopathy also may occur.
  - Ocular pain and conjunctival injection
  - A maculopapular rash appears about the fifth day of illness, involving the trunk and extremities.
  - Splenomegaly and generalized lymphadenopathy
  - In critically ill patients, signs of cardiovascular collapse (edema, hypovolemia) and severe neurologic signs may be prominent (3).

DIAGNOSTIC TESTS & INTERPRETATION
Lab
Initial lab tests
- Normochromic anemia and mild thrombocytopenia may be present.
- The WBC count is usually normal or slightly decreased.
- Clotting disorders may be present.
- Hypoproteinemia, hyponatremia, hypochloremia, and azotemia are the hallmarks of fulminant disease.

Follow-Up & Special Considerations
- Positive after the second week of illness
- The Weil-Felix reaction and complement fixation tests can be used for routine diagnosis; but they are not very sensitive and specific.
- The Weil-Felix reaction, employing OX-19 and OX-2 Proteus strains, is positive in epidemic, murine, and scrub typhus. A positive test is defined by either determination of a titer of 1 in 320 or greater or a fourfold rise in titer. The OX-19 reaction is negative or low-titer-positive in Brill-Zinsser disease.
- Further confirmation and specific identification can be made by indirect fluorescent antibody (IFA) and the latex agglutination test (LA), and by direct immunofluorescent tests.
- Western Blot in combination with cross-adsorption tests is needed to discern *R. prowazekii* from *R. typhi* (2)
- Tissue immunofluorescence can detect rickettsias several days after the initiation of specific antibiotic therapy.
- Early and effective antibiotic therapy may delay the maximum antibody response.
- PCR tests (real time PCR) to diagnose acute *R. prowazekii*, *R. typhi*, and *R. tsutsugamushi* infection have been developed (2).

Imaging
Depends on potentially afflicted organ, that is, chest x-ray, abdominal ultrasonography, and echocardiography.

Pathological Findings
Occlusive thrombosis with extravasation of leucocytes (1).

DIFFERENTIAL DIAGNOSIS
- Other rickettsial infections (i.e., Rocky Mountain spotted fever)
- Meningococcemia/bacterial meningitis
- Typhoid
- Secondary syphilis
- Leptospirosis
- Lyme disease
- Infectious mononucleosis
- Rubella
- Measles
- Flavivirus infections

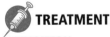

TREATMENT
MEDICATION
First Line
- Specific antibiotic chemotherapy for 5–7 days
  - Tetracycline 25–50 mg/kg/d in 4 equally divided oral or intravenous doses or doxycycline 100 mg orally or intravenously every 12 hours (for adults excluding pregnant)
  - Chloramphenicol 50–75 mg/kg/d in 4 equally divided oral or intravenous doses
- Treatment should be continued for 2–4 days after the resolution of fever in epidemic and murine typhus and in Brill-Zinsser disease. In scrub typhus, treatment should be continued for 3–7 days, and for 2 weeks in case treatment starts during the first 4–5 days of illness, to prevent relapse.

Second Line
- Epidemic typhus
  - Single-dose doxycycline (100 mg PO)
- Murine typhus
  - Ciprofloxacin, pefloxacin, and ofloxacin also may be used.
- Scrub typhus
  - Single-dose doxycycline (200 mg PO)
  - Ciprofloxacin also may be used.

ADDITIONAL TREATMENT
General Measures
Delouse the patient by bathing and boiling clothes and linens.

IN-PATIENT CONSIDERATIONS
Initial Stabilization
- Supportive treatment may be necessary in moderate and severe cases of epidemic and scrub typhus.
- Nutritional and blood transfusion support, careful management of electrolyte abnormalities, and dialysis if renal failure occurs.

Admission Criteria
Inability to take antibiotics orally or any major organ affliction (see complications).

Nursing
Careful nursing care to prevent aspiration pneumonia and xerostomia.

Discharge Criteria
Afebrile for 4 days with no major organ dysfunction.

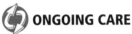

ONGOING CARE
FOLLOW-UP RECOMMENDATIONS
- Epidemic typhus is the most severe of the typhus group rickettsioses. If untreated, fever subsides after about 2 weeks, but the convalescence period may last up to 2–3 months. The mortality rate in untreated disease may be high (up to 60%), with a peak incidence in elderly patients.
- Brill-Zinsser disease resembles epidemic typhus but is generally more benign.
- Murine typhus is a more benign illness, and the mortality rate, even before the introduction of specific antibiotic therapy, may be as low as 1%.
- The mortality rate in untreated scrub typhus ranges from 1–60% in different series.
- Antibiotic therapy dramatically alters the prognosis of this disease. After initiation of therapy, patients become afebrile within 2–3 days.

PROGNOSIS
Relapses occur if treatment is delayed. A second course of treatment is usually effective.

COMPLICATIONS
- Cardiovascular collapse
- Renal impairment (prerenal azotemia), resulting occasionally in overt renal failure
- Hepatic insufficiency
- Pneumonitis, pulmonary edema, respiratory failure
- Endocarditis
- Upper gastrointestinal bleeding
- Superinfections (aspiration pneumonia, parotitis, gingivitis)
- Seizures and coma

REFERENCES
1. Green JS, Singh J, Cheung M, et al. A cluster of pediatric endemic typhus cases in Orange County, California. *Pediatr Infect Dis J* 2011;30:163–165.
2. Bechah Y, Capo C, Mege JL, et al. Epidemic typhus. *Lancet Infect Dis* 2008;8:417–426.
3. Kim DM, Kim SW, Choi SH, et al. Clinical and laboratory findings associated with severe scrub typhus. *BMC Infect Dis* 2010;10:108.
4. Dumler JS, Taylor JP, Walker DH. Clinical and laboratory features of murine typhus in south Texas, 1980 through 1987. *JAMA* 1991;266:1365–1370.
5. Raoult D, Dutour O, Houhamdi L, et al. Evidence for louse-transmitted diseases in soldiers of Napoleon's Grand Army in Vilnius. *J Infect Dis* 2006;193:112–120.
6. Chattopadhyay S, Richards AL. Scrub typhus vaccines: Past history and recent developments. *Hum Vaccin* 2007;3:73–80.

ADDITIONAL READING
- Civen R, Ngo V. Murine typhus: An unrecognized suburban vectorborne disease. *Clin Infect Dis* 2008;46:913–918.
- Lee HI, Shim SK, Song BG, et al. Detection of Orientia tsutsugamushi, the causative agent of scrub typhus, in a novel mite species, eushoengastia koreaensis, in Korea. *Vector Borne Zoonotic Dis* 2011;11:209–214.
- Kelly DJ, Richards AL, Temenak J, et al. The past and present threat of rickettsial diseases to military medicine and international public health. *Clin Infect Dis* 2002;34:S145–S169.

 CODES

ICD9
- 080 Louse-borne (epidemic) typhus
- 081.0 Murine (endemic) typhus
- 081.9 Typhus, unspecified

CLINICAL PEARLS
- Treat empirically and early before laboratory confirmation.
- Consider epidemic typhus and scrub typhus as diagnostic possibilities in the returning traveler with fever and in the patient with fever of unknown origin.

T

VIRAL HEPATITIS

Alejandro Restrepo
Eleftherios Mylonakis

 BASICS

DESCRIPTION
- Viral hepatitis is an acute and/or chronic inflammation and injury of the liver.
- Fulminant hepatitis is massive hepatic necrosis—usually associated with hepatitis B or C.

EPIDEMIOLOGY
Hepatitis A Virus (HAV)
- Infections per year: 125,000–200,000
- Worldwide infection
- Transmission: Most common is via fecal–oral route. Large outbreaks as well as sporadic cases have been traced to contaminated food and water. Sexual and parenteral transmission may occur
- Age: Rare in infants; increases with age, no sex predilection

Hepatitis B Virus (HBV)
- 350 million persons are infected with HBV worldwide
- Transmission: The major routes are by percutaneous exposure, blood transfusion, sexual contact, vertical and perinatal transmission
- In children, 90% develop chronic infection
- In adults, 5–10% develop chronic infection

Hepatitis C Virus (HCV)
- 180 million people are infected with HCV worldwide infection
- Transmission: The major routes are parenteral exposure, sexual contact, blood transfusion, and perinatal transmission
- There is risk of HCV infection in transplanted organ with HCV
- Chronic infection occurs in 80% of the cases

Hepatitis D Virus (HDV)
- Worldwide infection, with endemic areas in Middle East, Mediterranean countries, and South America
- In nonendemic areas, it can be transmitted by blood products and parenteral exposure
- It can present as coinfection (infect simultaneously with HBV), superinfection (superinfect a patient that already has HBV infection). HDV requires the infection with HBV for infection and replication

Hepatitis E Virus (HEV)
- Epidemiologic features resembling those of HAV. Infection occurs primarily in developing countries
- Transmission: Via fecal–oral

Hepatitis G Virus (HGV)
- Transmitted: Most common is via blood transfusion but vertical transmission and sexual has been documented
- No evidence that causes chronic disease

RISK FACTORS
HAV
- High-risk groups are: Those having employment in health care, intimate exposure, people traveling to underdeveloped endemic countries, men having sex with men, and people at day care centers

HBV
- History of multiple blood products, immigrants from endemic areas, hemodialysis, men who have sex with men, injection drug use, occupation exposure, transplant donors, cocaine use, health care workers, and travelers to endemic areas

HCV
- Injection drug users, multiple sexual partners, occupation exposure (needle stick or contact with blood products), hemodialysis, h/o multiple blood transfusions, transplant donors, patients with HIV. Other factors: Tattooing, piercing, inhaled cocaine

HDV
- Risk factors are similar to HBV (1)

HEV
- Risk factors are similar to HAV

GENERAL PREVENTION
HAV
- Good sanitation, hygiene, hand washing
- HAV vaccine 1 mL i.m. for adults; 2nd dose 6–12 months later. Should be considered in travelers, patient at high occupational risk (day care staff/children, custodial facility employees, sewage workers, military, food handlers), men who have sex with men, drug users, patients with chronic liver disease
- Immune globulin (passive immunization): 0.02 mL/kg i.m. (given 1–2 weeks after exposure prevents illness in 80–90%), give to unvaccinated people who are at risk of having hepatitis A

HBV
- Vaccines for HBV are effective and widely used (see section "Drugs and Vaccines"). Given to everyone, mainly in hemodialysis patients, health care workers, i.v. drug users, homosexuals, travelers to endemic areas, natives of Alaska, Asia and Pacific Islands, patients with multiple blood transfusions, transplant recipients, and all infants. 3 doses are usual (0, 1, and 6 months). The presence of HBsAb is indicative of vaccine immunity
- For unvaccinated persons sustaining an exposure to HBV, post-exposure prophylaxis with a combination of hepatitis B immunoglobulin (HBIG) and HBV vaccine is recommended
- Avoid sharing needles, razors, tooth brushes
- Avoid sexual contact

HCV
- There is no vaccine available for HCV
- Avoid sharing needles, razors, tooth brushes
- Avoid sexual contact
- Proper hygiene

HDV
- There is no vaccine or specific immunoglobulin available for HDV
- HDV can be prevented with HBV vaccination

HEV
- An HEV vaccine is undergoing clinical testing
- Good sanitation

PATHOPHYSIOLOGY
Acute viral hepatitis consists of multilobular infiltration with mononuclear cells, hepatic cell necrosis, hyperplasia of Kupffer cells, and cholestasis. It causes cell damage with hepatic cell degeneration and necrosis, cell dropout, and degeneration of hepatocytes

ETIOLOGY
HAV
- RNA virus from the picornavirus family

HBV
- DNA virus from the hepadnavirus family
- 8 genotypes have been identified from A to H

HCV
- RNA virus from the Flaviviridae family
- Genotype 1 accounts for 75% of the case in the US, and genotypes 2 and 3 account for 20–25%

HDV
- RNA virus that coinfects with HBV (or other hepadnavirus) and is an envelope of HBsAg
- HDV can either infect a person simultaneously with HBV or superinfect a person already infected with HBV

HEV
- RNA virus from the Caliciviridae family

HGV
- RNA virus from the Flaviviridae family

Other
- Other viruses can cause hepatitis, such as EBV, CMV, HSV, HIV, adenovirus, measles, and enterovirus

COMMONLY ASSOCIATED CONDITIONS
HAV
- Arthritis, urticaria, nephritis, anemia

HBV
Polyarteritis nodosa, arthritis, cryoglobulinemia, acrodermatitis, glomerulonephritis, aplastic anemia, and serum-like syndrome

HCV
- Mixed cryoglobulinemia, glomerulonephritis, porphyria cutanea tarda, skin lesions such as dermatitis, lichen planus, cutaneous necrotizing vasculitis, anemia, lymphoma, diabetes mellitus, and hepatocellular carcinoma

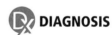 **DIAGNOSIS**

HISTORY
Incubation period:
- HAV: 15–45 days
- HBV: 1–6 months
- HCV: 15–160 days
- HDV: 1–6 months
- HEV: 15–60 days
- The prodromal symptoms of acute viral hepatitis are systemic and include: Alterations in olfaction and taste, anorexia, arthralgias, coryza, cough, fatigue, fever, headache, malaise, myalgias, nausea, and vomiting
- These constitutional symptoms may precede the onset of jaundice by 1–2 weeks

PHYSICAL EXAM
- A big number of patients with viral hepatitis never become icteric
- In acute viral hepatitis, splenomegaly and cervical adenopathy are present in 10–20% of patients and liver can have hepatomegaly with tenderness and discomfort in right upper quadrant area
- The duration of the posticteric phase is variable, ranging from 2 to 12 weeks

DIAGNOSTIC TESTS & INTERPRETATION
Lab
- Neutropenia and lymphopenia in acute viral hepatitis are transient and are followed by a relative lymphocytosis
- Atypical lymphocytes are common during the acute phase
- Serum aminotransferases increase during the prodromal phase of acute viral hepatitis. Peak levels vary, are usually reached at the time the patient is clinically icteric, and diminish progressively
- When jaundice appears, the serum bilirubin typically rises to levels ranging from 85 to 340 mol/L (5–20 mg/dL)
- Prolonged prothrombin time (PT) indicates a worse prognosis
- Hypoglycemia is noted occasionally in patients with severe viral hepatitis
- Serum alkaline phosphatase may be normal or only mildly elevated
- A diffuse but mild elevation of the gamma globulin fraction is common during acute viral hepatitis

HAV
- Acute: Detection of IgM anti- HAV antibodies
- Chronic: Detection of IgG HAV antibodies

HBV
- After infection with HBV, HBsAg becomes detectable first. This is followed by the antibody to core antigen (anti-HBc); usually persists for life
- About 3–5 months after exposure, HBsAg becomes undetectable, and there is a period of several weeks before the antibody (anti-HBsAg) becomes detectable. During this "window period," testing for IgM anti-HBc can establish the diagnosis
- Presence of HBeAg during chronic hepatitis B is associated with ongoing viral replication, infectivity, and inflammatory liver injury
- The presence of HBV DNA detected by PCR is a marker of viral replication

HCV
- For HCV infection, check antibodies against HCV (2). It does not confer immunity
- Anti-HCV antibodies can be negative in the 1st to 2 months after infection
- HCV RNA is detected by PCR and becomes positive in acute cases, mainly 1–2 weeks after infection
- In ongoing HCV, the recombinant immunoblot assay (RIBA) is an additional test used
- Detection of HCV genotypes is useful and influences treatment and prognosis. Genotype 2 and 3 have favorable prognosis compare to 1 (3)

HDV
- Check for HDV antibodies
- Detection of HDV RNA or HDV antigen in serum or liver

HEV
For HEV infection, check for detection of IgM-anti HEV and/or IgG anti-HEV antibodies (not done routinely, available at the CDC)

Imaging
Initial approach
Ultrasound of the liver may rule out obstruction and check liver ultrasound with dopplers

Follow-Up & Special Considerations
- Serial measurement of liver function tests. Prothrombin time (PT/INR) and albumin in fulminant disease and chronic hepatitis is needed.
- Appropriate serum viral markers are useful for evaluation of recovery or progression.
- Monitor for metabolic complications.
- In HAV usually resolves in 4 weeks and can have some cholestasis for weeks.

Diagnostic Procedures/Other
- Liver biopsy is rarely necessary or indicated in acute viral hepatitis, except when there is clinical evidence suggesting a diagnosis of chronic hepatitis and/or want to exclude other diseases
- Liver biopsy is important to see the degree of inflammation and fibrosis in patients with chronic hepatitis

DIFFERENTIAL DIAGNOSIS
For details, see the Section I chapter, "Jaundice and Fever."

 TREATMENT

MEDICATION
HAV
- Supportive care. Antiviral not indicated.

HBV
- For HBV infection: Interferon alfa (also pegylated interferon alfa 2A and 2 B), adefovir, lamivudine, entecavir, and telbivudine. HIV medications such as tenofovir and emtricitabine are also effective for HBV
- The goal of therapy is the clearance of HBV DNA levels, loss of HBeAg and HBsAg levels, and normalization of liver function tests
- Please review guidelines for patient who need treatment for HBV
- There is an increased rate of antiviral resistance to HBV. The most common medication associated with resistance is lamivudine (2)

HCV
- The combination of interferon-alfa (standard or pegylated interferon [PEG-IFN]) and ribavirin is the most common treatment used for the treatment of HCV. Other options are PEG-IFN monotherapy and interferon gamma. Duration of therapy is between 24 weeks and 1 year, but depends on the genotype, drug combination, and sustained viral response (SVR)
- Telaprevir and Boceprovir are protease inhibitors that are newly approved for the treatment of chronic Hepatitis C
- The goal is sustained virologic response, defined as clearance of the HCV RNA from 12 to 48 weeks
- Liver transplantation can be offered. Patients with chronic hepatitis C have done as well as any other subset of patients after transplantation, despite the fact that recurrent infection in the donor organ is the rule. In patients with chronic HBV, prophylactic use of hepatitis B immunoglobulin (HBIG) and medications such as lamivudine, adefovir, entecavir prior and after transplantation has been exercised to control the disease. Patients should be vaccinated with HAV and HBV prior to transplantation (3)

HDV
The treatment of choice is Interferon gamma

HEV
Supportive care. Antiviral not indicated

SURGERY/OTHER PROCEDURES
Liver transplantation is considered in patients with fulminant hepatitis, end stage liver disease and hepatocellular carcinoma

 ONGOING CARE

COMPLICATIONS
In acute fulminant hepatitis, the fatality is greater than 80% and patients with fulminant hepatitis are candidates for liver transplantation

HAV
- Case fatality rate in HAV is low (approximately 0.1%) but is higher among the elderly and patients with underlying debilitating disorders
- Few patients experience relapsing hepatitis weeks to months after apparent recovery from the acute episode

HBV
- In adults, 5–10% develop chronic hepatitis, 25% of the patients develop cirrhosis, and 1–4% progress to hepatocellular carcinoma
- Less than 1% HBV develop fulminant hepatitis
- The case fatality rate in HBV and HDV coinfection is approximately 5% and in HDV super-infection can be up to 20%

HCV
70–80% of patients develop chronic hepatitis, although only 20% develop cirrhosis. 1.5–3% develop hepatocellular carcinoma

HDV
If coinfection, disease is selflimited. In superinfection, can present with severe acute hepatitis and/or progression of chronic HDV infection

HEV
- Has a high mortality (around 20–30%) in pregnant women in the 2nd and 3rd trimester
- In outbreaks of water-borne HEV, in India and Asia, the case fatality rate is 1–2% and up to 20% in pregnant women

ADDITIONAL READING
- Ghany MG, Strader DB, Thomas DL, et al. Diagnoses, management, and treatment of hepatitis C, AASLD Practice Guidelines. *Hepatology* 2009;49 (4):1335–1475.
- Lok ASF, McMahon BJ. Chronic hepatitis B: Update 2009, AASLD Practice Guidelines. *Hepatology* 2009;50 (3):1–36.
- Wasley A, Grytdal S, Gallagher K. Centers for Disease Control and Prevention (CDC). Surveillance for acute viral hepatitis—United States, 2005. *MMWR Surveill Summ* 2007;56(3):1–24.

 CODES

ICD9
- 070.30 Viral hepatitis b without mention of hepatic coma, acute or unspecified, without mention of hepatitis delta
- 070.9 Unspecified viral hepatitis without mention of hepatic coma
- 573.3 Hepatitis, unspecified

WARTS

Paschalis Vergidis
Matthew E. Falagas

 BASICS

DESCRIPTION
Warts (verrucae) are benign viral tumors of the skin and mucous membranes and include cutaneous and genital warts. The virus is transmitted by direct contact, sexual contact, and autoinoculation.

EPIDEMIOLOGY
Incidence
- 7–10% of the population has warts
- Less common in blacks than in whites
- Cutaneous warts
  - Spread by direct contact with infected person or touch of contaminated material
  - Occur primarily in children and young adults
  - Especially common in handlers of meat, poultry, and fish
  - Fomites may be involved in the transmission of human papillomavirus (HPV) types that are associated with cutaneous warts
- Anogenital warts
  - Most common viral sexually transmitted disease (STD)

RISK FACTORS
- Meat, poultry, fish-handlers: Infection rates up to 50%
- Atopic dermatitis
- Unprotected sex with partner with anogenital HPV
- Men who have sex with men
- Defects in cell-mediated immunity predispose to extensive disease

GENERAL PREVENTION
- Avoid touching warts to prevent self-inoculation.
- Use footwear in public showers/pools.
- Avoid direct contact with persons with cutaneous warts.
- Adopt safe-sex practices to prevent anogenital warts.
- The quadrivalent vaccine (Gardasil) offers protection from genotypes 6, 11, 16, and 18 (1–2). Administered in 3 doses at 0, 2, and 6 months.
- The bivalent vaccine (Cervarix) offers protection from genotypes 16 and 18. Administered in 3 doses at 0, 1, and 6 months.
- HPV vaccination recommended for females aged 11–12 years. Also recommended for females aged 13–26 years who have not been previously vaccinated.
- The quadrivalent vaccine may be given to males aged 9–26 years to reduce the likelihood of acquiring genital warts.
- The vaccines do not affect disease present prior to immunization.
- Cervical cancer screening should be pursued as recommended, even in vaccinated women.
- Women with cervical dysplasia should be vaccinated to be protected from genotypes that they may have not acquired.

Pregnancy Considerations
HPV vaccine does not contain live virus. However, use in pregnancy is not recommended due to limited data.

ETIOLOGY
- HPV: Epitheliotropic DNA virus with 150 subtypes
- HPV 16 and HPV 18 cause 70% of cervical cancers
- HPV 6 and HPV 11 cause 90% of genital warts

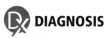 **DIAGNOSIS**

HISTORY
Incubation period: 1–20 months after exposure

PHYSICAL EXAM
Cutaneous
- Common warts: Hyperkeratotic papules with rough surface commonly seen on hands, fingers, elbows, but may be seen anywhere on the body
- Plantar warts: Painful, thrombosed capillaries beneath surface, bleed easily
- Juvenile/flat warts: Multiple papules with smooth surface and irregular contour

Anogenital
- Condylomata acuminata: Exophytic lesions varying in size and morphology
- Cervical, vaginal, vulvar: Exophytic lesions varying in size and morphology
- Cervical intraepithelial neoplasia: Nonadvanced lesion, often not visible to naked eye

Respiratory Papillomatosis
- Usually seen in children and related to ororespiratory exposure during vaginal birth. Can recur
- Signs of upper respiratory tract obstruction (hoarseness, stridor, respiratory distress). Site of obstruction is the larynx

DIAGNOSTIC TESTS & INTERPRETATION
Lab
- Diagnosis is based on typical appearance upon visual examination.
- Pap smear annually to detect cervical cancer associated with anogenital warts.
- To identify specific HPV type, a Southern blot, *in situ* hybridization, or polymerase chain reaction is used. Molecular diagnostic methods are not routinely used in the clinical laboratory.

Diagnostic Procedures/Other
- Biopsy recommended in those with atypical lesions, large lesions, in immunosuppressed patients and those who do not respond to therapy.
- Dilute solution of acetic acid (3–5%) to delineate disease before cervical biopsy. Lesions develop an acetowhite appearance.

Pathological Findings
Papillomatosis, acanthosis, parakeratosis, hyperkeratosis. Koilocytosis (cytoplasmic vacuolation of squamous cells) is less often seen in sites other than the cervix.

DIFFERENTIAL DIAGNOSIS
Infectious
- Fungal infection
- Molluscum contagiosum
- Secondary syphilis (anogenital only)

Noninfectious
- Squamous cell malignancies
- Skin cancer
- Actinic keratosis
- Callus (plantar only)

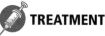 **TREATMENT**

- HPV is not clearly eradicated by any treatment.
- Warts often regress spontaneously.
  - Cutaneous warts in children, between 1 and 5 years (50% and 90%, respectively)
  - Anogenital warts, within 4 months (20%)
- The rate of recurrence of the anogenital type after treatment is high (<25% at 3 months).
- Most currently available therapies are not specific antiviral regimens, but rather are physically destructive or chemically cytotoxic to the superficial wart; some cause scarring.

MEDICATION
Cutaneous
- In light-skinned adults treat common, plantar, and palmar warts with liquid nitrogen. Treat dark-skinned adults with salicylic acid. (Liquid nitrogen can cause hypopigmentation.)
  - Salicylic acid plaster 40%
    - Self-treatment after demonstration by health care provider
    - Pare lesions before applying plaster; remove after 1–3 days; scrape off macerated skin for 2–3 weeks
- Flat warts
  - Topical 5-fluorouracil or retinoic acid
- Facial lesions (scarring is a concern)
  - Imiquimod
  - Intralesional immunotherapy with skin test antigens

Pediatric Considerations
In younger children treat common, plantar, and palmar warts with salicylic acid (liquid nitrogen is painful).

Anogenital
- External genital
  - Podophyllotoxin 0.5% (Podofilox) applied by patient twice per day for 3 days, followed by 4 days of no therapy (3). Repeat up to 4 weeks as needed. Treatment is effective in 45–88%. The health care provider should give the initial application or instruct the patient on how to do the initial application.
  - Imiquimod 5% cream applied by patient to warts 3 times a week at bedtime (4). Wash the area the next morning. Treat until lesions clear or for a total of 16 weeks.
  - Podophyllin 10–25% in a compound tincture of benzoin is effective: 32–79%, with recurrences of 27–65%. Must wash off thoroughly 1–4 hours after application. Administered by provider.
  - Trichloroacetic acid (TCA) or bichloroacetic acid (BCA) 80–90%. Administered by provider weekly for 4 weeks. A small amount should be applied only to warts and allowed to dry, at which time a white "frosting" develops. If an excess amount of acid is applied, the treated area should be powdered with talc, sodium bicarbonate, or liquid soap preparations to remove unreacted acid. Pain common in treatment.
  - Intralesional interferon-alpha used for refractory warts; effective 44–61%, with recurrence up to 67%.
- Perianal
  - Treat as for external genital (discussed previously), except that podophyllotoxin is contraindicated.
- Anal
  - Patients with warts on rectal mucosa should be referred to an expert.
  - TCA or BCA 80–90%.
- Urethral meatus
  - Podophyllin 10–25%. Wash off thoroughly 1–2 hours after application. Contraindicated in pregnancy.
- Cervical
  - Consult with an expert. High-grade squamous intraepithelial lesion should be excluded.
- Vaginal
  - TCA or BCA 80–90%.
  - Podophyllin 10–25%.

ADDITIONAL TREATMENT
Additional Therapies
Sex partners may benefit from evaluation for other STDs and education about HPV and STDs.

SURGERY/OTHER PROCEDURES
Cutaneous
- Cryotherapy with liquid nitrogen
  - Pain during and after procedure
  - Apply with a cotton swab, and retreat in 2–3 weeks, if necessary
  - Contraindicated in patients with Raynaud's phenomenon
- Filiform warts
  - Shave excision

Anogenital
- External genital
  - Cryotherapy with liquid nitrogen or cryoprobe is effective: 63–88%, with recurrence in 21–39%. Repeat applications every 1–2 weeks. Safe during pregnancy
  - Electrodesiccation or electrocautery. Contraindicated in patients with pacemakers. Local anesthesia required; pain common in treatment. Scarring is a concern
  - Carbon dioxide laser or surgery used for extensive warts
  - Surgery for extensive or refractory lesions
- Anal
  - Patients with warts on rectal mucosa should be referred to an expert
  - Cryotherapy with liquid nitrogen or TCA 80–90%
  - Cryoprobe is contraindicated
  - Surgery
- Urethral meatus
  - Cryotherapy with liquid nitrogen
- Vaginal
  - Cryotherapy with liquid nitrogen, not cryoprobe

Oral
- Treatment is not necessary unless warts are painful or cause a cosmetic problem
- Cryotherapy with liquid nitrogen, not cryoprobe
- Electrodesiccation or electrocautery
- Surgery

Respiratory Papillomatosis
- Endoscopic cryotherapy
- Laser therapy
- Intralesional cidofovir
- Avoid tracheostomy as papillomas can extend to tracheostomy site

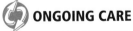 ## ONGOING CARE

FOLLOW-UP RECOMMENDATIONS
The initial Pap smear for women with genital warts should be followed at 6 months, then annually if the smear is negative.

COMPLICATIONS
- Cervical cancer is associated with anogenital warts.
- Recurrences result from reactivation of subclinical HPV rather than from reinfection.

Pregnancy Considerations
Anogenital warts tend to enlarge and become friable; cesarean section may be required if the size of genital warts obstructs the birth canal.

REFERENCES
1. The Future II Study Group. Quadrivalent vaccine against human papillomavirus to prevent high-grade cervical lesions. *N Engl J Med* 2007;356:1915–1927.
2. Garland SM, Hernandez-Avila M, Wheeler CM, et al. Quadrivalent vaccine against human papillomavirus to prevent anogenital diseases. *N Engl J Med* 2007;356:1928–1943.
3. Lacey CJ, Goodall RL, Tennvall GR, et al. Randomised controlled trial and economic evaluation of podophyllotoxin solution, podophyllotoxin cream, and podophyllin in the treatment of genital warts. *Sex Transm Infect* 2003;79:270–275.
4. Fife KH, Ferenczy A, Douglas JM Jr, et al. Treatment of external genital warts in men using 5% imiquimod cream applied three times a week, once daily, twice daily, or three times a day. *Sex Transm Dis* 2001;28(4):226–231.

ADDITIONAL READING
- Centers for Disease Control and Prevention. FDA licensure of quadrivalent human papillomavirus vaccine (HPV4, Gardasil) for use in males and guidance from the Advisory Committee on Immunization Practices (ACIP). *MMWR* 2010;59:630–632.
- Centers for Disease Control and Prevention. FDA licensure of bivalent human papillomavirus vaccine (HPV2, Cervarix) for use in females and updated HPV vaccination recommendations from the Advisory Committee on Immunization Practices (ACIP). *MMWR* 2010;59:626–629.
- Workowski KA, Berman SM. Sexually transmitted diseases treatment guidelines, 2010. *MMWR Recomm Rep* 2010;59(RR-12):110.

 ## CODES

ICD9
- 078.10 Viral warts, unspecified
- 078.11 Condyloma acuminatum
- 078.12 Plantar wart

CLINICAL PEARLS
- The quadrivalent HPV vaccine offers protection from genotypes 6, 11, and the carcinogenic types 16 and 18.
- Available therapies for warts are physically destructive or chemically cytotoxic agents.
- Cryotherapy with liquid nitrogen is most commonly used for cutaneous and anogenital warts.

W

WHIPPLE'S DISEASE

Paschalis Vergidis
Matthew E. Falagas

 BASICS

DESCRIPTION
Rare systemic disease caused by *Tropheryma whipplei*, manifesting with weight loss, diarrhea, lymphadenopathy, and neurologic symptoms.

EPIDEMIOLOGY
Incidence
The annual incidence since 1980 has been approximately 30 cases per year.

Prevalence
- Prevalence unknown. About 1000 cases have been reported to date, mainly from Western Europe and North America.
- Disease typically occurs in middle-aged white men.

RISK FACTORS
- Rapid progression in patients taking corticosteroids or other immunosuppressive medications.
  - Note: HIV-infected patients do not develop the disease.

Genetics
Disease associated with HLA B-27 haplotype

PATHOPHYSIOLOGY
- Invasion with *Tropheryma* has been demonstrated at several sites (intestinal epithelium, brain, liver, heart, lung, kidney). There is lack of inflammatory response.
- Malabsorption results from disruption of normal villous function.
- Isolated infection of cardiac valves may occur without other symptoms of Whipple's disease.

ETIOLOGY
T. whipplei, a gram-positive, non-acid-fast, periodic acid-Schiff positive bacillus, which is related to Actinomycetes

 DIAGNOSIS

HISTORY
- Prodromal stage: Protean symptoms and chronic nonspecific findings, mainly arthralgia and arthritis
- Steady-state stage: Weight loss, diarrhea or both, and other manifestations, since many organs can be involved
- Time between prodromal and steady-state stage is 6 years
- Fever
- Weight loss
- Diarrhea
- Abdominal pain
- Intermittent migratory, nondestructive arthritis
- Myalgias
- Psychiatric symptoms such as depression
- Hypothalamic involvement (polydipsia, hyperphagia, decreased libido, amenorrhea)

PHYSICAL EXAM
- Cachexia, muscle wasting
- Hypotension
- Steatorrhea
- Occult gastrointestinal bleeding. Frank hematochezia is rare
- Abdominal distention, ascites
- Hepatomegaly
- Splenomegaly
- Glossitis, angular cheilitis
- Skin hyperpigmentation
- Peripheral and abdominal lymphadenopathy
- Dyspnea
- Cardiac murmurs
- Cognitive changes, including dementia
- Cerebellar ataxia
- Seizures (partial or generalized)
- Nystagmus
- Myoclonus
- Supranuclear ophthalmoplegia
- Uveitis, retinitis
- Signs of adrenal insufficiency

DIAGNOSTIC TESTS & INTERPRETATION
Lab
- Anemia
- Leukocytosis, lymphopenia
- Thrombocytosis
- Prothrombin time may be prolonged due to Vitamin K malabsorption
- Elevated inflammatory markers
- Cerebrospinal fluid (CSF) pleocytosis and elevated protein
- Eosinophilia may be present
- Diagnosis is established with biopsy
- Immunohistochemical staining can be done
- Polymerase chain reaction (PCR) can be used to detect the organism in tissue samples (small bowel, cardiac valve tissue, lymph nodes, synovial tissue) and body fluids (blood, CSF)
  - Quantitative PCR of saliva and stool may be used for noninvasive screening (1)
  - Always test PCR in CSF if central nervous system (CNS) disease is suspected
  - PCR is performed in specialized laboratories
- The organism can be cultivated (2). Cultures are performed in specialized laboratories and are challenging because of the slow replication time
- Serology is not helpful due to lack of antibody response

Imaging
- Plain chest radiography may reveal pleural effusions
- Nonspecific findings in upper gastrointestinal series (small bowel dilation with or without prominent mucosal folds of the duodenum and jejunum) or abdominal CT scan
- Nonspecific T1, T2, FLAIR abnormalities in brain MRI

Diagnostic Procedures/Other
- Small bowel endoscopic biopsy. Multiple specimens should be obtained and stained with periodic acid-Schiff.
- Stereotactic brain biopsy is the last mean of diagnosis for CNS disease.

Pathological Findings
Specimens of small bowel biopsy demonstrate magenta-stained inclusions within macrophages of the lamina propria.

DIFFERENTIAL DIAGNOSIS
- Celiac disease
- Inflammatory bowel disease
- Sarcoidosis
- Small bowel lymphoma
- Nontuberculous mycobacterial infection
- Autoimmune diseases
- Reactive arthritis
- Familial Mediterranean fever
- Infective endocarditis
- Hyperthyroidism
- AIDS
- HIV enteropathy
- Alzheimer's disease
- Neurosarcoidosis
- Neurosyphilis

 TREATMENT

MEDICATION
First Line
- Initial treatment for 2–4 weeks (favor 4-week treatment for patients with endocarditis, neurologic disease, or relapse).
  – Ceftriaxone (2 g i.v. daily), or
  – Penicillin G (1.2 million U i.v. daily) plus streptomycin (1 g daily)
- Initial treatment should be followed by trimethoprim/sulfamethoxazole 160/800 mg p.o. twice daily for 1–2 years.

Second Line
- Tetracycline has high rate of disease relapse.
- For sulfa allergic patients: Doxycycline 100 mg p.o. twice daily plus hydroxychloroquine 200 mg p.o. 3 times daily.

ADDITIONAL TREATMENT
Additional Therapies
- Corticosteroids recommended for:
  – Patients with severe CNS disease
  – Patients with high fever despite antibiotic treatment

SURGERY/OTHER PROCEDURES
Surgical resection of infected valve is usually required.

 ONGOING CARE

FOLLOW-UP RECOMMENDATIONS
- Monitor weight.
- PCR can be used to document response to treatment. Histopathologic evaluation of post-treatment specimens does not predict clinical cure (3).
- Relapses occur in 30–40% of patients and represent incomplete eradication of the organism.
- Relapses should be treated with ceftriaxone (2 g i.v. twice daily) for 4 weeks followed by oral regimen for 1–2 years.

Patient Monitoring
- Jarisch–Herxheimer reaction has been described after treatment with intravenous antibiotics, especially penicillin.
- An immune reconstitution syndrome, manifested with high fever, has been described after initiating treatment. More common in patients with neurologic disease.

DIET
- No dietary changes are usually required.
- If malabsorption, provide supplemental fat-soluble vitamins.

PROGNOSIS
- If left untreated, disease is ultimately fatal, especially when there is neurologic involvement.
- Relapse occurs in 2–33% of cases after an average of 5 years, mainly with neurologic involvement.

COMPLICATIONS
- Pericarditis
- Myocarditis
- Culture-negative endocarditis (4)

REFERENCES

1. Fenollar F, Laouira S, Lepidi H, et al. Value of *Tropheryma whipplei* quantitative polymerase chain reaction assay for the diagnosis of Whipple disease: Usefulness of saliva and stool specimens for first-line screening. *Clin Infect Dis* 2008;47(5): 659–667.
2. Raoult D, Birg ML, La Scola B, et al. Cultivation of the bacillus of Whipple's disease. *N Engl J Med* 2000;342:620–625.
3. Ramzan NN, Loftus E Jr, Burgart LJ, et al. Diagnosis and monitoring of Whipple disease by polymerase chain reaction. *Ann Intern Med* 1997;126: 520–527.
4. Fenollar F, Lepidi H, Raoult D. Whipple's endocarditis: Review of the literature and comparisons with Q fever, *Bartonella* infection, and blood culture-positive endocarditis. *Clin Infect Dis* 2001;33:1309–1316.

ADDITIONAL READING

- Fenollar F, Puechal X, Raoult D. Whipple's disease. *N Engl J Med* 2007;356(1):55–66.
- Gerard A, Sarrot-Reynauld F, Liozon E, et al. Neurologic presentation of Whipple disease: Report of 12 cases and review of the literature. *Medicine* 2002;81(6):443–457.
- Schneider T, Moos V, Loddenkemper C, et al. Whipple's disease: New aspects of pathogenesis and treatment. *Lancet Infect Dis* 2008;8:179–190.

CODES

ICD9
040.2 Whipple's disease

CLINICAL PEARLS
- Manifestations of Whipple's disease include weight loss, diarrhea, lymphadenopathy, and neurologic symptoms.
- Isolated infection of cardiac valves may occur without other symptoms.
- Diagnosis is established with tissue biopsy. PCR can be used to detect the organism in tissue samples and body fluids.

W

YELLOW FEVER

Paschalis Vergidis
Matthew E. Falagas

 BASICS

DESCRIPTION
Yellow fever virus is a mosquito-borne infection. Manifestations range from self-limited illness to severe systemic disease associated with hemorrhage, liver dysfunction with profound jaundice, and fevers.

EPIDEMIOLOGY
Incidence
- Yellow fever virus is present in sub-Saharan Africa and tropical South America, between 15 degrees North and South latitudes (1).
- Disease may be sporadic or part of an outbreak.
- Underreporting of disease occurs
  - Africa: 5,000 cases per year reported in epidemic years. True incidence estimated to more than 200,000 per year.
  - South America: 100 cases per year in the past 25 years.
- Incidence is lower in South America compared to Africa because the mosquitoes that transmit the virus do not often come in contact with humans, and vaccination coverage in the indigenous population is high.
- For travelers, risk of illness is probably 10 times higher in urban West Africa than in South America.
  - West Africa: Virus transmission highest between July and October.
  - Brazil: Virus transmission highest between January and March.

RISK FACTORS
- Travel in endemic areas, especially during the rainy season
- Mosquito bites occurring while in endemic regions
- No prior immunization

GENERAL PREVENTION
- Eradication of the *Aedes aegypti* mosquito in tropical areas
- Avoidance of mosquito bites in endemic areas, especially during the rainy seasons (insect repellents, proper clothing).
- Vaccination with a live attenuated virus is effective.
- Immunization takes 7–10 days to be effective and is effective for 10 years.
- An international certificate of vaccination is required for entry to many endemic countries or from travelers arriving from certain endemic countries.

VACCINE ADVERSE REACTIONS
- Mild adverse events (headache, myalgia, low-grade fever) to yellow fever vaccine (YFV) are common
- YFV-associated neurological disease
  - 0.5 cases per 100,000 doses distributed
  - Encephalitis occurs primarily in infants younger than 6 months. May occur at any age.
  - Onset 4–27 days post vaccination
  - Rarely fatal
- YFV-associated viscerotropic disease
  - 0.3–0.5 cases per 100,000 doses distributed
  - Frequency higher in persons older than 60 years and those with history of thymus disease (thymoma, thymectomy, myasthenia gravis)
  - Onset in 2–5 days post vaccination
  - Severe illness (similar to wild-type disease) characterized by fever, hypotension, respiratory failure, lymphopenia, thrombocytopenia, elevated liver enzymes
  - Case fatality rate: 53%
- HIV-positive patients may be immunized if the CD4 count is greater than 200/mm^3 (2).
- Safety not established in pregnancy

PATHOPHYSIOLOGY
- Transmission to humans occurs via *A. aegypti* mosquitoes.
- Humans, along with nonhuman primates, comprise a reservoir of infection.
- The virus replicates initially in local lymph nodes. This is followed by rapid hematogenous dissemination and involvement of liver, kidneys, adrenals, and other organs.
- Hemorrhages occur due to thrombocytopenia, platelet dysfunction, and reduced synthesis of clotting factors.

ETIOLOGY
- Yellow fever virus is an RNA virus in the family Flaviviridae.
- The virus is enveloped and spherical.

DIAGNOSIS

HISTORY
- Incubation: 3–6 days
- The spectrum of disease ranges from asymptomatic to severe illness with death.
- The disease has three stages:
  - Infection
  - Remission
  - Intoxication
- The infection stage is noted by the onset of fever, chills, myalgias, back pain, severe headache, and prostration.

- Remission of symptoms occurs after 3–4 days of fever and lasts for hours to days.
- The intoxication stage is associated with recurrent fevers, mucosal hemorrhage, liver failure with jaundice, renal failure, and myocarditis. Hematemesis or hematochezia may occur. Disseminated intravascular coagulation (DIC) may occur.

PHYSICAL EXAM
- Relative bradycardia despite high fevers
- Conjunctival injection
- Jaundice
- Abdominal tenderness
- Hepatomegaly
- Petechiae, purpura. Mucosal, gastrointestinal bleeding
- The disease may evolve to septic shock and acute respiratory disease syndrome (ARDS)
- Confusion, seizures, coma are late neurological manifestations

DIAGNOSTIC TESTS & INTERPRETATION
Lab
- Nonspecific leukopenia and thrombocytopenia are often seen.
- Severe elevations of transaminases and bilirubin are seen in severe cases.
- Evidence of DIC
- Metabolic acidosis
- Azotemia, albuminuria
- Diagnosis is made by serology (IgM by ELISA). Hemagglutination inhibition and complement fixation tests are used infrequently
- Serology may be misleading due to cross-reactive antibodies with other flavivirus.
- Virus can be grown in cell culture.
- A polymerase chain reaction may be performed on blood samples of patients felt to be viremic. Not widely available
- Immunohistochemical staining of affected tissues (liver, kidney, myocardium) will provide the diagnosis.

Diagnostic Procedures/Other
- Liver biopsy contraindicated due to the risk of fatal hemorrhage.
- ECG: Sinus bradycardia without conduction defects, ST-T abnormalities

Pathological Findings
Liver: Apoptosis, steatosis, hepatic midzonal necrosis (3)

DIFFERENTIAL DIAGNOSIS
- Hemorrhagic fevers caused by a wide array of viruses, such as Ebola, Marburg, Lassa fever, Rift Valley fever, South American viral hemorrhagic fevers, and Congo-Crimean hemorrhagic fever.
- Viral encephalitides, such as Japanese encephalitis
- Acute hepatitis
- Dengue
- Malaria
- Typhoid fever
- Leptospirosis

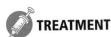

TREATMENT
MEDICATION
No specific antiviral therapy available

ADDITIONAL TREATMENT
General Measures
- Supportive measures in the intensive care unit are needed for the sickest patients.
- Treat metabolic abnormalities

Additional Therapies
- Non-hepatotoxic antipyretics
- Histamine-receptor antagonists, proton pump inhibitors, and sucralfate to prevent or ameliorate gastric bleeding
- Fresh frozen plasma, vitamin K for clotting abnormalities
- Hemodialysis for renal failure
- Endotracheal intubation, mechanical ventilation for ARDS.

IN-PATIENT CONSIDERATIONS
Initial Stabilization
- Treat hypovolemia, oliguria, hypoxemia, acid–base disturbances, electrolyte abnormalities.
- Vasopressor support as indicated

Admission Criteria
Hospitalize all patients with suspected yellow fever in non-endemic areas.

ONGOING CARE
FOLLOW-UP RECOMMENDATIONS
Patients surviving the illness have high antibody levels and are thus immune to recurrence of disease.

PATIENT EDUCATION
Inform patients about risk of severe adverse reactions due to yellow fever vaccine.

PROGNOSIS
Mortality rate in the intoxication stage is 20–50%.

COMPLICATIONS
- Bacterial infections in acutely ill patients account for much of the mortality associated with the infection.
- Myocarditis may lead to arrhythmias and late death.

REFERENCES
1. Barrett AD, Monath TP. Epidemiology and ecology of yellow fever virus. *Adv Virus Res* 2003;61: 291–315.
2. Tattevin P, Depatureaux AG, Chapplain JM, et al. Yellow fever vaccine is safe and effective in HIV-infected patients. *AIDS* (London, England) 2004;18:825–827.
3. Quaresma JA, Barros VL, Fernandes ER, et al. Reconsideration of histopathology and ultrastructural aspects of the human liver in yellow fever. *Acta Trop* 2005;94:116–127.

ADDITIONAL READING
- Barnett ED. Yellow fever: Epidemiology and prevention. *Clin Infect Dis* 2007;44:850–856.
- Barrett AD, Monath TP, Barban V, et al. 17D yellow fever vaccines: New insights. A report of a workshop held during the World Congress on medicine and health in the tropics, Marseille, France, Monday 12 September 2005. *Vaccine* 2007;25:2758–2765.
- Staples JE, Gershman M, Fischer M. Yellow fever vaccine: Recommendations of the Advisory Committee on Immunization Practices (ACIP). *MMWR Recomm Rep* 2010;59(RR-7):1–27.

 CODES

ICD9
060.9 Yellow fever, unspecified

CLINICAL PEARLS
- Manifestations of yellow fever range from asymptomatic to severe systemic disease which may be fatal.
- There is no specific antiviral treatment.
- Yellow fever vaccine is effective with an acceptable safety profile. YFV-associated neurological and viscerotropic disease are extremely rare.

Y

YERSINIA ENTEROCOLITICA INFECTIONS

Jatin M. Vyas (E. Mylonakis, Editor)

 BASICS

DESCRIPTION

The genus Yersinia includes the pathogens *Yersinia pestis* (the cause of plague), *Yersinia enterocolitica*, and *Yersinia pseudotuberculosis*. These gram-negative coccobacilli are facultative anaerobes. (The topic of plague is discussed in a separate chapter.)

EPIDEMIOLOGY

Incidence

- *Y. enterocolitica* is more common in Northern Europe. Infections have been documented in other parts of the world, including South America, Africa, and Asia.
- Between 1967 and 1996, more than 18,700 strains of Yersinia species, excluding *Y. pestis*, were recovered in Belgium from a variety of gastrointestinal and extraintestinal sites in patients. Acute enterocolitis was the most common clinical form of *Y. enterocolitica* infection, affecting primarily children younger than 5 years of age. Starting in 1967, there was a steady increase in isolations every year, with 305 cases in 1975 and up to 1,469 in 1986. From 1987 on, there was a clear decrease in the number of reported cases, although the number of participating laboratories and culture techniques remained constant. This significant decrease in the occurrence of *Y. enterocolitica* infections may be explained by changes in the slaughtering procedures and eating habits of the population.
- *Y. enterocolitica* is transmitted through food, animal contact, and contaminated blood products.
- Yersinia is the third most commonly isolated food-borne agent (after *Campylobacter* and *Salmonella*) in Belgium and the Netherlands.

RISK FACTORS

- A prospective case control study in Auckland, New Zealand, concluded that the risk of illness due to *Y. enterocolitica* is increased by contact with untreated water and consumption of pork.
- Patients with iron excess (such as those with beta-thalassemia) and those receiving desferrioxamine are at a higher risk for serious infection due to *Y. enterocolitica*.
- *Y. enterocolitica* septicemia is more common among patients with diabetes mellitus, severe anemia, hemochromatosis, cirrhosis, and malignancy, and very young or very old patients.
- The increased number of reported transfusion complications during recent years, caused by *Y. enterocolitica*–infected blood components, is probably related to the use of additive solutions for red-cell storage, which brings about a decrease in complement activity and prolonged storage.

GENERAL PREVENTION

Public health measures to control *Yersinia* infection should focus on the animal reservoirs in any particular location.

PATHOPHYSIOLOGY

The organism invades the intestinal epithelium using virulence factors after oral ingestion. It localizes to the Peyer's patches and then transported to regional lymph nodes within the mesentery.

ETIOLOGY

- *Y. enterocolitica* are gram-negative, non–lactose-fermenting, urease-positive bacilli.
- The natural reservoirs of *Y. enterocolitica* are animals, including rodents, rabbits, pigs, sheep, cattle, horses, dogs, and cats.

DIAGNOSIS

HISTORY

- *Y. enterocolitica* produces a spectrum of disease, including acute enterocolitis, terminal ileitis, and mesenteric adenitis.
- *Y. enterocolitica* infection in mesenteric lymph nodes can also cause necrotizing lymphadenitis.
- *Y. enterocolitica* can each produce an enteric fever–like illness, characterized by fever, headache, and abdominal pain.
- Symptoms typically start 4 days after ingestion with a range from 1–11.

PHYSICAL EXAM

There are no specific physical examination findings.

DIAGNOSTIC TESTS & INTERPRETATION
Lab
- Stool, mesenteric lymph node, or blood cultures may yield Yersinia, depending on the clinical syndrome.
- Fecal excretion of Yersinia may continue for weeks after symptoms have subsided. Leukocytes and, less commonly, blood or mucus may be present in the stool. Most patients with this syndrome are <5 years of age.
- Serologic tests are useful in diagnosing Yersinia infections though these are not widely available in the US. *Y. enterocolitica* and *Y. pseudotuberculosis* cross-react with each other and with other organisms. Agglutinating antibodies appear soon after onset of illness but generally disappear within 2–6 months.

 TREATMENT

MEDICATION
- The value of antimicrobial therapy in cases of enterocolitis and mesenteric adenitis due to *Y. enterocolitica* is unclear, because these infections are usually self-limited.
- Doxycycline or trimethoprim-sulfamethoxazole can be used for complicated gastrointestinal infections or focal extraintestinal infections.
- Patients with *Y. enterocolitica*–induced septicemia should receive antibiotic therapy. The drug of choice has not yet been identified, but ceftriaxone plus gentamicin or ciprofloxacin is suggested.

 ONGOING CARE

COMPLICATIONS
- Patients with *Y. enterocolitica*–induced septicemia, which has a mortality of 50% despite treatment, should receive antibiotic therapy. Arthritis or ankylosing spondylitis rarely occurs. This complication is much more likely to develop in individuals with the HLA-B27 antigen.
- A reactive polyarthritis is seen in 10–30% of adults with *Y. enterocolitica* infection.

ADDITIONAL READING

- Black RE, Slome S. Yersinia enterocolitica. *Infect Dis Clin North Am* 1988;2:625.
- Cover TL, Aber RC. Yersinia enterocolitica. *N Engl J Med* 1989;321:16.
- Tacket CO, Narain JP, Sattin R, et al. A multistate outbreak of infections caused by Yersinia enterocolitica transmitted by pasteurized milk. *JAMA* 1984;251:483.

 CODES

ICD9
008.44 Intestinal infection due to yersinia enterocolitica

Y

Section III

Microorganisms

Matthew E. Falagas
Eleftherios Mylonakis

Isaac Bogoch
Petros I. Rafailidis
Paschalis I. Vergidis

ABSIDIA CORYMBIFERA

GENUS Absidia

SPECIES

- *A. corymbifera* is the only human pathogenic species of *Absidia*.
- *A. corymbifera* was previously named *A. ramosa*.

MICROBIOLOGIC CHARACTERISTICS

- Filamentous fungus (mold)
- Similar to *Rhizopus* species
- Hyaline nonseptate hyphae
- Hyphae are wide (6–15 μm in diameter).
- Rapid growth in cultures (within 4 days); light gray to grayish-brown
- Grows at 25–45°C
- Belongs to the order Mucorales

EPIDEMIOLOGY

- Inhalation of sporangiospores is the most probable cause of infection.
- Ubiquitous
- May be a contaminant in cultures
- May cause severe infections, especially in immunocompromised patients
- Immunocompromised patients are at higher risk to develop infections.

INFECTIONS

- An infrequent cause of mucormycosis
- Mucormycosis may affect a wide range of anatomic sites.
- The most common forms of the infection are rhinocerebral, pulmonary, cutaneous, and disseminated.
- Meningitis (after head injury); rare
- Cutaneous infections
- Infections in patients with AIDS or other causes of immunosuppression

DIAGNOSIS

- Culture

TREATMENT

- Amphotericin B deoxycholate 1.0–1.5 mg/kg/d
- Appropriate total dose not known (2–4 g recommended or until correction of neutropenia in neutropenic patients)

ALTERNATIVE TREATMENT

- A lipid formulation of amphotericin B 3–5 mg/kg/d
- Posaconazole 800 mg/d

PREVENTION

- Avoidance of severe immunosuppression, if possible (e.g., appropriate management of HIV infection)

ACANTHAMOEBA SPECIES

GENUS Acanthamoeba

SPECIES

- *A. astronyxis*
- *A. castellanii*
- *A. culbertsoni*
- *A. divionensis*
- *A. glebae*
- *A. griffini*
- *A. healyi*
- *A. hatchetti*
- *A. palestinensis*
- *A. polyphaga*
- *A. rhysodes*

MICROBIOLOGIC CHARACTERISTICS

- Protozoon
- Free-living life cycle
- Ubiquity in the environment

EPIDEMIOLOGY

- Worldwide distribution
- Found in soil, fresh and brackish water, dust, hot tubs, and sewage
- Acquisition probably occurs by inhalation or direct contact with contaminated soil or water.
- Contaminated saline solutions or tap water rinses for care of contact lenses may transmit the pathogen.

INFECTIONS

- Granulomatous encephalitis in immunosuppressed patients
- Infections occur primarily in debilitated and immunocompromised persons; however, some patients have no demonstrable underlying disease or defect.
- Encephalitis (granulomatous) has an insidious onset and is usually chronic, lasting for more than a week and sometimes even months.
- Dendritic keratitis (mimicking herpes keratitis); trauma-related or keratitis related to infection transmitted with contact lenses contaminated by cleaning solutions
- Chronic ulcerative skin lesions, abscesses, or erythematous nodules

DIAGNOSIS

- Culture in special media
- Cysts can be visualized in sections of brain or corneal tissue or fresh CSF (rarely).
- Silver-methenamine, periodic acid-Schiff stains
- Serologic studies not useful
- May be identified on corneal scrapings or biopsy specimens by histopathologic examination, culture, or PCR

TREATMENT

- Pentamidine, azoles, sulfonamides, 5-fluorocytosine, and to a lesser extent amphotericin B are active against *Acanthamoeba* species *in vitro*.
- Combination of *in vitro* active drugs may be used. However, the appropriate treatment for encephalitis is unknown.
- Keratitis may be treated with a combination of topical agents. Primary regimen: Propamidine 0.1% and neomycin/gramicidin/polymyxin. Alternative: Biguanide 0.02% or chlorhexidine 0.02%.

PREVENTION

- Standard precautions for hospitalized patients are recommended.
- Avoid swimming in hot springs and other bodies of warm, polluted, fresh water.
- *Acanthamoeba* species are resistant at the usual concentrations of chlorine found in drinking water and swimming pools.
- Only sterile solutions should be used to clean contact lenses.

ACINETOBACTER SPECIES

GENUS Acinetobacter

SPECIES

- *A. baumannii*
- *A. calcoaceticus*
- *A. haemolyticus*
- *A. johnsonii*
- *A. junii*
- *A. lwoffii*
- *A. radioresistens*
- *Acinetobacter* spp. unnamed
- Others

MICROBIOLOGIC CHARACTERISTICS

- Aerobic, Gram-negative bacillus (rod-shaped during rapid growth, coccobacillary in the stationary phase), encapsulated, nonmotile
- It is a constituent of the normal skin and mucosa flora.

EPIDEMIOLOGY

- Worldwide distribution
- Common cause of nosocomial infection, especially in ICUs

INFECTIONS

- Pneumonia (alcoholics, nosocomial/ventilator-associated)
- Bacteremia
- Tracheobronchitis (children, tracheal intubation)
- Cellulitis (catheter-associated)
- Burn and wound infections (e.g., war wounds)
- Urinary tract infection (UTI) (after urinary catheterization or related to other causes of complicated UTI)
- Meningitis (especially after neurosurgical operations)

DIAGNOSIS

- Culture

TREATMENT

- Carbapenem (imipenem, meropenem). Cases of carbapenem resistance have been reported.
- Sulbactam has antibacterial activity against *Acinetobacter*. Tazobactam and clavulanic acid are less active than sulbactam.
- Third/fourth-generation cephalosporins, aminoglycosides, fluoroquinolones, doxycycline or tigecycline, and polymyxins are frequently active against *Acinetobacter*.
- In systemic or severe infections, amikacin or another active aminoglycoside may be added to the initially chosen drug.
- Local infection associated with a catheter (vascular, urinary, others) may be controlled by removing the catheter. However, antibiotics should also be given.
- *A. baumannii* is more resistant than other *Acinetobacter* species.

PREVENTION

- Adherence to infection control guidelines in hospitals, especially in ICUs

ACREMONIUM SPECIES

GENUS Acremonium

SPECIES

- Formerly called *Cephalosporium*
- About 100 species:
  - *A. alabamense*
  - *A. falciforme*
  - *A. kiliense* (the most common, medically important species)
  - *A. recifei*
  - *A. roseogriseum*
  - *A. strictum*

MICROBIOLOGIC CHARACTERISTICS

- Filamentous fungi (mold)
- Septate hyphae
- Similar to *Fusarium*, but growth is slower
- Some species can tolerate cycloheximide.
- Colonies are often white, velvety, cottony, or fasciculate and flat or slightly raised in the center.

EPIDEMIOLOGY

- *Acremonium* is associated with soil, insects, sewage, rhizospheres of plants, and other environmental substrates.

INFECTIONS

- Mycetoma (chronic skin and subcutaneous tissue infection)
- Onychomycosis
- Mycotic keratitis
- Colonization of soft contact lenses
- Rarely invasive infection
  - Invasive pulmonary disease
  - Meningitis
  - Cerebritis
  - Brain abscess
  - Prosthetic valve endocarditis
  - Midline granuloma
  - Osteomyelitis and posttraumatic arthritis
  - Postsurgery endophthalmitis
  - Peritonitis associated with peritoneal dialysis
  - Disseminated infection in neutropenic patients

DIAGNOSIS

- Culture

TREATMENT

- Amphotericin B is the mainstay of treatment. Novel azoles may be effective, but experience is limited.
- Surgical drainage or resection is helpful (when possible).

ACTINOBACILLUS SPECIES

GENUS Actinobacillus

SPECIES

- *A. actinomycetemcomitans*, formerly the major pathogen of the genus *Actinobacillus*, is now classified in the genus *Aggregatibacter*.
- *A. equuli*
- *A. hominis*
- *A. suis*
- *A. ureae*

MICROBIOLOGIC CHARACTERISTICS

- Aerobic, Gram-negative bacillus, nonmotile, coccoid to coccobacillary

EPIDEMIOLOGY

- Actinobacilli were first associated with cattle, but they have been recovered from other animals and humans.
- Several human infections occur after animal bites (e.g., horse bite).

INFECTIONS

- *A. actinomycetemcomitans*
- Endocarditis (part of the HACEK group, which includes *Haemophilus* species, *A. actinomycetemcomitans*, *Cardiobacterium* species, *Eikenella* species, and *Kingella* species)
- Wound infection
- Periodontitis: In this infection the organism is commonly recovered in conjuction with *Actinomyces israelii*.
- Animal bites
- Endophthalmitis
- *A. hominis*: Bacteremia (especially in patients with chronic lung disease and hepatic failure)
- *A. ureae*: Bacteremia, meningitis
- *A. suis* and *A. equuli*: Animal bite-related wound infections

DIAGNOSIS

- Culture
- On 1-day-old plates, colonies are translucent and 1–2 mm in diameter.
- *A. actinomycetemcomitans*: Relatively fastidious, obligate capnophile. Colonies on 1-day-old plates may be less than 0.5 mm in diameter but enlarge to 2–3 mm, sometimes with rough surfaces and pitting after several days of incubation.

TREATMENT

- HACEK endocarditis: Ceftriaxone

ALTERNATIVE TREATMENT

- Ampicillin or penicillin G plus a minoglycoside
- Ciprofloxacin
- Trimethoprim–sulfamethoxazole
- Azithromycin shows good activity *in vitro*.

ACTINOMADURA SPECIES

GENUS Actinomadura

SPECIES

- *A. madurae*
- *A. pelletieri*
- *A. latina*
- Others

MICROBIOLOGIC CHARACTERISTICS

- Filamentous bacterium
- Branched
- Gram-positive
- Aerobic

EPIDEMIOLOGY

- Mainly affecting humans in tropical and subtropical regions of the world
- Rare cause of infections in the US

INFECTIONS

- Actinomycetomas
- Chronic infection of skin, soft tissue, muscles, and bones
- Occasionally a cause of pulmonary or disseminated disease

DIAGNOSIS

- Culture

TREATMENT

- Infections due to *Actinomadura* are frequently refractory to antimicrobial therapy.
- Pulmonary or disseminated infection is managed with aggressive antimicrobial treatment. Streptomycin, with trimethoprim–sulfamethoxazole (TMP–SMX) or dapsone, has been associated with moderate success.
- Surgical resection is used in several cases to manage actinomycetomas.

ALTERNATIVE TREATMENT

- Combination of penicillin, gentamicin, and TMP–SMX followed by TMP–SMX and amoxicillin
- Amoxicillin-clavulanate
- Fusidic acid
- Clindamycin
- Carbapenems

ACTINOMYCES SPECIES

See Section II, "Actinomycosis"

AEROMONAS SPECIES

GENUS Aeromonas

SPECIES

- *A. caviae*
- *A. hydrophila*
- *A. schubertii*
- *A. veronii*
- Others

MICROBIOLOGIC CHARACTERISTICS

- Aerobic, Gram-negative, nonsporulating facultative anaerobic bacillus

EPIDEMIOLOGY

- Ubiquitous in fresh and brackish water and soil
- Aeromonads have been isolated in chlorinated tap water
- May be isolated from stools of asymptomatic carriers

INFECTIONS

- Gastroenteritis (usually mild but sometimes severe)
- Intraabdominal abscess
- Acute enteritis is common in patients with AIDS.
- Wound infection after exposure to contaminated water or bleeding with leeches (cellulitis, osteomyelitis, myonecrosis)
- Sepsis and necrotizing myositis or ecthyma gangrenosum in patients who are immunosuppressed
- Aspiration pneumonia (after drowning)
- Bacteremia and spontaneous peritonitis in patients with cirrhosis

DIAGNOSIS

- Culture

TREATMENT

- Third-generation cephalosporin, with or without an aminoglycoside
- Fluoroquinolones
- In patients with enteritis, appropriate volume and salt repletion is important.

ALTERNATIVE TREATMENT

- Imipenem, meropenem, ertapenem
- Aztreonam
- Trimethoprim–sulfamethoxazole
- Aminoglycoside
- Tetracycline, tigecycline

Microorganisms

AFIPIA SPECIES

GENUS Afipia

SPECIES
- *A. broomeae*
- *A. clevelandensis*
- *A. felis*

MICROBIOLOGIC CHARACTERISTICS
- Pleomorphic, aerobic, Gram-negative bacillus
- Better seen with silver strains

INFECTIONS
- Its role in human disease is unclear.
- It was thought to be the cause of cat-scratch disease for some time, but more recent data have proved that other agents (mainly *Bartonella* species) cause most cases of this infection.
- *A. felis* may cause a minority of cases of cat-scratch disease.

DIAGNOSIS
- Histology of affected lymph nodes

TREATMENT
- A macrolide antibiotic may be beneficial (no clear data).

ALCALIGENES SPECIES

GENUS Alcaligenes

SPECIES
- *A. denitrificans*
- *A. faecalis*
- *A. piechaudii*
- *A. xylosoxidans* (previously classified as *Achromobacter*, but recent 16S rRNA sequence analysis supports that the organism belongs to the genus *Achromobacter*)

MICROBIOLOGIC CHARACTERISTICS
- Aerobic, Gram-negative bacillus

EPIDEMIOLOGY
- Worldwide, rare infection

INFECTIONS
- Sepsis
- Localized infections
- It has been reported to be a rare cause of bacteremia secondary to contaminated intravenous fluids.

DIAGNOSIS
- Culture

TREATMENT
- Carbapenem (imipenem, meropenem)
- Ureidopenicillins

ALTERNATIVE TREATMENT
- Antimicrobial treatment may need to be modified based on results of *in vitro* susceptibility testing.
- Ceftazidime
- Trimethoprim–sulfamethoxazole
- Fluoroquinolones
- Colistin

ALPHAVIRUS

GROUP Alphavirus

SUBGROUPS
- Eastern equine encephalitis virus
- Western equine encephalitis virus
- Venezuelan equine encephalitis virus
- Ross River
- Chikungunya
- Mayaro
- O'nyong-nyong
- Sindbis
- Barmah Forest virus
- Others

MICROBIOLOGIC CHARACTERISTICS
- These viruses belong to the arboviruses group A.
- Single-stranded, positive RNA virus
- Icosahedral symmetry
- Enveloped

EPIDEMIOLOGY
- Alphaviruses cause vector-borne infections.
- Infections are usually transmitted to humans via mosquito bites.
- Rare infections
- Specific subgroups of alphaviruses are associated with infection in different parts of the world.
- Ross River virus is found in Australia and Tasmania, Papua-New Guinea, Indonesia, and the South Pacific Islands.
- Sindbis virus is found throughout Africa, Europe, and Australia.
- Barmah Forest virus is found in Australia.
- Chikungunya virus is found in sub-Saharan Africa, Southeast Asia, and the Philippines.
- O'nyong virus is found in sub-Saharan Africa.
- Mayaro virus is found in the forests of South America.

INFECTIONS
- Eastern equine, Western equine, and Venezuelan alphaviruses cause encephalitis.
- Other subgroups of alphaviruses, such as Chikungunya, usually cause epidemic outbreaks, with fever, macular or maculopapular rash, and polyarthralgia/polyarthritis.

DIAGNOSIS
- Cell culture
- Serology
- PCR

TREATMENT
- Symptomatic
- There is no specific treatment.
- Ribavirin has some activity *in vitro* against alphaviruses, but there is no controlled, published experience from clinical use.

PREVENTION
- Control of mosquitoes and other arthropods

ALTERNARIA SPECIES

GENUS Alternaria

SPECIES
- *A. alternata*
- *A. longipes*
- *A. tenuissima*
- Others

MICROBIOLOGIC CHARACTERISTICS
- Dematiaceous, filamentous fungi (mold)
- In histologic specimens, *Alternaria* may be found in several forms: Yeasts, pseudohyphae, or pigmented septate hyphae *in vivo*.
- Hyphae at 30°C in culture

EPIDEMIOLOGY
- Worldwide infection

INFECTIONS
- Phaeohyphomycosis involving skin and subcutaneous tissue
- Sinusitis and osteomyelitis in immunosuppressed patients
- Peritonitis in patients undergoing peritoneal dialysis
- Corneal infections (keratitis)
- Otitis media in agricultural field workers

DIAGNOSIS
- Identification of *Alternaria* from clinical specimens
- Isolation from culture

TREATMENT
- Amphotericin B i.v.
- Itraconazole
- Voriconazole

ALTERNATIVE TREATMENT
- Surgical management may be beneficial in cases of skin, subcutaneous tissue, or bone involvement.

ANAEROBIOSPIRILLUM

GENUS Anaerobiospirillum

SPECIES
- *A. succiniciproducens*
- *A. thomasii*

MICROBIOLOGIC CHARACTERISTICS
- Anaerobic, Gram-negative spiral-shaped bacillus

EPIDEMIOLOGY
- Rare cause of infections

INFECTIONS
- Bacteremia
- Gastroenteritis, especially in immunosuppressed persons

DIAGNOSIS
- Anaerobic culture

TREATMENT
- There are no good data for the optimal treatment.
- Chloramphenicol
- Metronidazole

ALTERNATIVE TREATMENT
- Doxycycline

ANCYLOSTOMA

GENUS Ancylostoma

SPECIES
- *A. braziliense* (hookworm of dogs and cats)
- *A. ceylanicum*
- *A. duodenale*

MICROBIOLOGIC CHARACTERISTICS
- Nematode helminth (round worm)

EPIDEMIOLOGY
- *A. braziliense*: Tropical and subtropical regions
- *A. ceylanicum*: More rare than the other 2 species (occurs in Southeast Asia)
- *A. duodenale*: Mediterranean coast of Europe and Africa, South America, India (especially in the northern part of the country), China, Southeast Asia, South Pacific

INFECTIONS
- Cutaneous larva migrans: A syndrome manifested by dermatitis, causing significant pruritus, may be the result of *A. braziliense* infection.
- *A. duodenale*: Hookworm (anemia, dyspepsia, diarrhea)

DIAGNOSIS
- Stool examination after concentration

TREATMENT
- *A. braziliense*: Albendazole 400 mg q12h for 3 days
- *A. duodenale*: Mebendazole 100 mg p.o. q12h for 3 days

ALTERNATIVE TREATMENT
- *A. braziliense*: Ivermectin 200 μ/kg/d p.o. for 1–2 days
- *A. duodenale*: Pyrantel pamoate 11 mg/d p.o. for 3 days. In severe parasitosis with anemia, repeat the same dose 8–14 days later.

ANGIOSTRONGYLUS SPECIES

GENUS Angiostrongylus

SPECIES
- *A. cantonensis*
- *A. costaricensis*

MICROBIOLOGIC CHARACTERISTICS
- Nematode helminth (round worm)

EPIDEMIOLOGY
- Southeast Asia and South Pacific for *A. cantonensis*
- Central and South America for *A. costaricensis*

INFECTIONS
- Angiostrongylosis, which is manifested by eosinophilic meningoencephalitis, keratitis, iritis, and blepharospasm, may be the result of *A. cantonensis* infection.
- *A. costaricensis* may lead to intestinal infection of varying severity, which ranges from an asymptomatic infection to persistent abdominal discomfort due to abdominal masses.

DIAGNOSIS
- CSF examination
- Serology

TREATMENT
- *A. cantonensis*: Corticosteroid treatment for 14 days.
- *A. costaricensis*: Surgical management may be necessary to remove abdominal masses.

ALTERNATIVE TREATMENT
- *A. cantonensis*: Unclear whether combination treatment with mebendazole or albendazole is beneficial.
- *A. costaricensis*: Thiabendazole 25 mg/kg p.o. q8h for 3 days. Repeat 3 times within 3 weeks.

ANISAKIS SPECIES

GENUS Anisakis

SPECIES
- Several species

MICROBIOLOGIC CHARACTERISTICS
- Nematode helminth (round worm)

INCUBATION PERIOD
- The patient may develop gastric symptoms a few hours after ingestion of infective larvae.
- It takes a few days to weeks after infection for small- and large-bowel symptoms to develop.

EPIDEMIOLOGY
- The infection occurs in people who eat raw, inadequately cooked, or inadequately treated (smoked, marinated, salted) saltwater fish, squid, or octopus.
- Common in Japan, Scandinavian countries, the Netherlands, and the Pacific coast of Latin America
- Increasing incidence in the US and Europe

INFECTIONS
- Gastric anisakiasis: Abdominal pain, nausea, and vomiting
- Intestinal disease: Lower abdominal pain and signs of obstruction

DIAGNOSIS
- Recognition of the parasite (a 2-cm-long larvae invading the oropharynx or the stomach)

TREATMENT
- Endoscopic removal of the parasite

ALTERNATIVE TREATMENT
- Surgical excision of lesions
- Possible treatment benefit of albendazole

APOPHYSOMYCES ELEGANS

GENUS Apophysomyces

SPECIES
- A. elegans

MICROBIOLOGIC CHARACTERISTICS
- Filamentous fungi (mold) with hyaline, nonseptate hyphae

EPIDEMIOLOGY
- Worldwide, rare infection

INFECTIONS
- Rare cause of mucormycosis. Can occur in the immunocompetent host
- Wound infection with secondary spread
- Invasive soft tissue infection of burns or wounds contaminated by soil
- Necrotizing fasciitis
- Osteomyelitis

DIAGNOSIS
- Culture
- Identification of the fungus in tissue biopsies

TREATMENT
- Amphotericin B

ALTERNATIVE TREATMENT
- There are no clear data for the effectiveness of itraconazole or other azoles.

ARCANOBACTERIUM SPECIES

GENUS Arcanobacterium

SPECIES
- A. haemolyticum
- A. pyogenes
- A. bernardiae

MICROBIOLOGIC CHARACTERISTICS
- Aerobic, Gram-positive bacillus

INCUBATION PERIOD
- Unknown

EPIDEMIOLOGY
- Worldwide, rare infection

INFECTIONS
- Pharyngitis (with erythematous morbilliform or scarlatiniform rash in about 50% of cases)
- A. haemolyticum may also cause endocarditis.

DIAGNOSIS
- Culture

TREATMENT
- Macrolides (erythromycin, azithromycin)

ALTERNATIVE TREATMENT
- Clindamycin
- Tetracycline

ARENAVIRAL HEMORRHAGIC FEVERS IN SOUTH AMERICA

GROUP Arenavirus

STRAINS
- Junin virus (Argentinian hemorrhagic fever)
- Machupo virus (Bolivian hemorrhagic fever)
- Guanarito virus (Venezuelan hemorrhagic fever)
- Sabia virus (Brazilian hemorrhagic fever)

MICROBIOLOGIC CHARACTERISTICS
- These viruses belong to the Tacaribe complex of Arenaviruses.
- They are Arenaviruses.
- They are related to the viruses of Lassa fever and lymphocytic choriomeningitis.

INCUBATION PERIOD
- 7–16 days

EPIDEMIOLOGY
- Occasional outbreaks have been reported from South American countries.
- Transmission to humans usually occurs via the inhalation of small-particle aerosols derived from contaminated excreta and saliva of rodents.
- They may be directly transmitted from person to person (rarely).

INFECTIONS
- These viruses cause acute illness, manifested by fever, headache, retro-orbital pain, sweating, conjunctival infection, myalgias, malaise, and prostration.
- In severe cases, hemorrhagic manifestations, CNS dysfunction, bradycardia, and hypotension may appear.
- Case fatality rates range from 10% to 30%.

DIAGNOSIS
- Isolation of the virus (virologic culture)
- Detection of viral antigens in blood or affected organs
- Serology tests which identify serum antibody against the causative virus

TREATMENT
- There are only few reported data on the treatment of these syndromes.
- Ribavirin is useful in all 4 hemorrhagic fevers caused by Arenaviruses.

ALTERNATIVE TREATMENT
- Specific immune plasma was shown to be effective in the treatment of Junin virus (Argentinian hemorrhagic fever) if given within 8 days of onset of disease.

PREVENTION
- Strict isolation of affected persons during the acute febrile period
- Rodent control

ASCARIS LUMBRICOIDES

GENUS Ascaris

SPECIES
- A. lumbricoides

MICROBIOLOGIC CHARACTERISTICS
- Nematode helminth (round worm, about 15–35 cm in length)

INCUBATION PERIOD
- The incubation period is prolonged. The life cycle of A. lumbricoides is 4–8 weeks.
- Feces contain eggs about 2 months after ingestion of embryonated eggs.

EPIDEMIOLOGY
- Very common infection worldwide, mainly in developing countries (and especially in tropical areas)
- Estimated prevalence of infected people about 1 billion worldwide

INFECTIONS
- Ascariasis (abdominal pain, pulmonary infiltrates, biliary tract obstruction, and eosinophilia). May present with intestinal obstruction
- Heavy infection may lead to severe nutritional problems.
- Transmission is usually by hand to mouth.

DIAGNOSIS
- Stool examination after concentration

TREATMENT
- Mebendazole 100 mg p.o. q12h for 3 days, or 500 mg p.o. (single dose)
- Albendazole 400 mg p.o. (single dose)

ALTERNATIVE TREATMENT
- Pyrantel pamoate 11 mg/kg (maximum dose 1 g) in a single dose
- Ivermectin 150–200 μg/kg (single dose)
- Nitazoxanide 500 mg p.o. q12h for 3 days

ASPERGILLUS SPECIES

See Section II, "Aspergillosis"

AUREOBASIDIUM SPECIES

GENUS Aureobasidium

SPECIES
- *A. pullulans*
- *A. mansoni*

MICROBIOLOGIC CHARACTERISTICS
- Dematiaceous, filamentous fungus (mold)
- Yeasts, pseudohyphae, or pigmented septate hyphae *in vivo*
- Hyphae in cultures at 30°C

EPIDEMIOLOGY
- Worldwide, rare infection

INFECTIONS
- Phaeohyphomycosis in immunosuppressed individuals
- Peritonitis in patients under peritoneal dialysis

DIAGNOSIS
- Culture
- Identification of the fungus in tissue biopsies

TREATMENT
- There are no good data for treatment.
- Amphotericin B is probably effective.
- Removal of the peritoneal dialysis catheter helps in the management of this fungal infection (in patients with peritonitis related to peritoneal dialysis).

ALTERNATIVE TREATMENT
- No data for clinical efficacy of azoles

BABESIA SPECIES

See Section II, "Babesiosis"

BACILLUS SPECIES

GENUS Bacillus

SPECIES
- *B. alvei*
- *B. anthracis* (the cause of anthrax, discussed in Section II)
- *B. cereus*
- *B. circulans*
- *B. laterosporus*
- *B. pseudoanthracis*
- *B. pumilus*
- *B. sphaericus*
- *B. subtilis*
- Others

MICROBIOLOGIC CHARACTERISTICS
- Aerobic, Gram-positive bacillus

INCUBATION PERIOD
- For the food poisoning syndrome, causing mainly vomiting, the incubation period is 1–6 hours; for the diarrhea syndrome, it is 6–24 hours.

EPIDEMIOLOGY
- Rice is the usual food related to *Bacillus* spp. food poisoning (emetic form).
- Meat or a vegetable is usually associated with the diarrhea syndrome caused by *Bacillus* species.

INFECTIONS
- Food poisoning and enterotoxic gastroenteritis (*B. cereus*)
- Bacteremia (in intravenous drug users or associated with intravenous lines)
- Meningitis, brain abscess
- Endocarditis
- Pneumonia
- Soft-tissue infections
- Conjunctivitis, keratitis ulcers, panophthalmitis

DIAGNOSIS
- Culture

TREATMENT
- There is no need for a specific antimicrobial treatment in patients with gastroenteritis due to *Bacillus* species.
- Vancomycin, with or without an aminoglycoside

ALTERNATIVE TREATMENT
- Imipenem
- Ciprofloxacin
- Tetracycline
- Clindamycin
- Macrolide
- *B. cereus* is resistant to most beta-lactam antibiotics.

PREVENTION
- Proper food handling reduces the risk of food poisoning due to *Bacillus* species.

BACTEROIDES SPECIES

GENUS Bacteroides

SPECIES
- *B. caccae*
- *B. capillosus*
- *B. distasonis*
- *B. eggerthii*
- *B. forsythus*
- *B. fragilis*
- *B. merdae*
- *B. ovatus*
- *B. putredinis*
- *B. stercoris*
- *B. tectum*
- *B. thetaiotaomicron*
- *B. uniformis*
- *B. ureolyticus*
- *B. vulgatus*
- Others

MICROBIOLOGIC CHARACTERISTICS
- Anaerobic, Gram-negative bacillus
- *Bacteroides* species are classified in the *B. fragilis* group and others.

EPIDEMIOLOGY
- Usual cause of infection where there is mixed etiology with aerobic and anaerobic organisms
- Many of the *Bacteroides* spp. are part of the normal gastrointestinal flora (i.e., *B. fragilis*).

INFECTIONS
- Intraabdominal and pelvic infections
- Pleuropulmonary
- Cervicofacial infection
- Brain abscess
- Sepsis
- Skin and soft-tissue infections (including surgical wounds)

DIAGNOSIS
- Anaerobic culture

TREATMENT
- Metronidazole

ALTERNATIVE TREATMENT
- Carbapenem (imipenem, meropenem, ertapenem, doripenem)
- Piperacillin–tazobactam
- Ticarcillin–clavulanate
- Ampicillin–sulbactam
- Cephamycin (cefoxitin, cefotetan)
- Tigecycline
- There is an increasing incidence of resistance in *Bacteroides* species.
- 20% of the *B. fragilis* group (particularly *B. distasonis* and *B. thetaiotaomicron*) and nearly 30% of *B. gracilis* are resistant to the cephamycins.
- Resistance to clindamycin is higher than 35%.
- 10% of *B. gracilis* are resistant to metronidazole.

BALANTIDIUM COLI

GENUS Balantidium

SPECIES
- *B. coli*

MICROBIOLOGIC CHARACTERISTICS
- Protozoon

INCUBATION PERIOD
- Unknown, but may be only several days

EPIDEMIOLOGY
- Worldwide distribiution
- Most frequent in Latin America, Southeast Asia, parts of the Middle East

INFECTIONS
- Most infections are asymptomatic
- Balantidiasis (colitis, dysentery)

DIAGNOSIS
- Stool examination (fresh and after concentration)

TREATMENT
- Tetracycline 500 mg q6h for 10 days

ALTERNATIVE TREATMENT
- Metronidazole 750 mg q8h for 5 days
- Iodoquinol 650 mg q8h for 20 days

BARTONELLA BACILLIFORMIS

See Section II, "Bartonellosis"

BARTONELLA HENSELAE

GENUS Bartonella

SPECIES
- B. henselae (formerly Rochalimanea henselae)

MICROBIOLOGIC CHARACTERISTICS
- Gram-negative coccobacillus of intracellular growth

INCUBATION PERIOD
- Usually 2–14 days from inoculation of the pathogen to primary skin lesion and 5–60 days from inoculation to lymphadenopathy

EPIDEMIOLOGY
- Worldwide infection

INFECTIONS
- Cat-scratch disease (local process with regional adenopathy, oculoglandular syndrome)
- Bacillary angiomatosis (skin lesions due to vascular proliferation), peliosis hepatica or splenic involvement, CNS lesions, lymph node involvement (especially in AIDS patients)
- Endocarditis
- Bacteremia

DIAGNOSIS
- Blood cultures using lysis-centrifugation methods
- Optimal growth in blood-enriched media
- Prolonged incubation (minimum, 2 weeks)
- Histopathology of cutaneous lesions is characteristic.
- Serology
- PCR

TREATMENT
- Cat-scratch disease usually has a benign course, with spontaneous improvement in a few weeks.
- Extensive lymphadenitis: Azithromycin 500 mg on day 1, then 250 mg/d p.o. on days 2–5
- Neuroretinitis: Doxycycline 100 mg q12h, rifampin 300 mg q12h for 4–6 weeks
- Endocarditis: Doxycycline 100 mg p.o. q12h for at least 6 weeks plus gentamicin 3 mg/kg/d i.v. for the first 2 weeks
- Bacillary angiomatosis/peliosis hepatis: Doxycycline 100 mg p.o. q12h for 3–4 months

ALTERNATIVE TREATMENT
- Erythromycin
- Clarithromycin

PREVENTION
- Avoid cat scratches

BARTONELLA QUINTANA

GENUS Bartonella

SPECIES
- B. quintana (formerly Rochalimanea quintana)

MICROBIOLOGIC CHARACTERISTICS
- Small coccobacillus of intracellular growth

INCUBATION PERIOD
- Usually 7–30 days

EPIDEMIOLOGY
- There are several endemic foci of the infection in many countries, including Poland, the former Soviet Union, and several African and South American countries.

INFECTIONS
- Trench fever
- Bacillary angiomatosis in immunosuppressed patients
- Bacteremia
- Endocarditis

DIAGNOSIS
- Blood cultures using lysis-centrifugation systems
- Cell cultures
- PCR

TREATMENT
- Bacteremia (without endocarditis): Doxycycline 100 mg p.o. q12h for 4 weeks plus gentamicin 3 mg/kg/d i.v. for the first 2 weeks
- Endocarditis: Doxycycline 100 mg p.o. q12h for at least 6 weeks plus gentamicin 3 mg/kg/d i.v. for the first 2 weeks
- Bacillary angiomatosis/peliosis hepatis: Doxycycline 100 mg p.o. q12h for 3–4 months

ALTERNATIVE TREATMENT
- Erythromycin, azithromycin

PREVENTION
- Destroy the vector (louse) to prevent transmission to humans

BASIDIOBOLUS RANARUM

GENUS Basidiobolus

SPECIES
- B. ranarum

MICROBIOLOGIC CHARACTERISTICS
- Filamentous fungus (mold)

EPIDEMIOLOGY
- Worldwide, rare infection
- More common in India, Indonesia, and Africa

INFECTIONS
- Nonulcerating nodular skin lesions in the subcutaneous tissue of chest, back, buttocks, and extremities

DIAGNOSIS
- Culture
- Identification of the fungus in tissue (biopsy)

TREATMENT
- Potassium iodide-saturated solution, 30 mg/kg/d for 6–12 months
- Spontaneous resolution has been observed occasionally.
- Surgical management may be helpful in difficult-to-treat cases with the use of antifungal agents.

ALTERNATIVE TREATMENT
- Trimethoprim–sulfamethoxazole
- Ketoconazole
- Amphotericin B i.v.

BAYLISASCARIS PROCYONIS

GENUS Baylisascaris

SPECIES
- B. procyonis

MICROBIOLOGIC CHARACTERISTICS
- Nematode parasite (round worm)

EPIDEMIOLOGY
- Rare infection in the US
- Humans are infected accidentally when they ingest infective eggs found in soil.
- Intestinal round worm of raccoon

INFECTIONS
- Visceral larva migrans
- Meningoencephalitic complications

DIAGNOSIS
- Histologic examination of surgically removed tissues

TREATMENT
- Directed laser therapy (ocular infection)
- Corticosteroids

ALTERNATIVE TREATMENT
- Diethylcarbamazine or ivermectin may be tried.

BILOPHILA WADSWORTHIA

GENUS Bilophila

SPECIES
- B. wadsworthia

MICROBIOLOGIC CHARACTERISTICS
- Anaerobic, Gram-negative bacillus

EPIDEMIOLOGY
- Isolated, usually, from mixed infections

INFECTIONS
- Peritonitis secondary to appendicitis
- Bacteremia
- Liver abscess

DIAGNOSIS
- Anaerobic culture

TREATMENT
- Metronidazole
- Clindamycin

ALTERNATIVE TREATMENT
- Carbapenem (imipenem, meropenem), piperacillin–tazobactam, or ticarcillin–clavulanate or cefoxitin

BIPOLARIS SPECIES

GENUS Bipolaris

SPECIES
- B. australiensis
- B. hawaiiensis
- B. spicifera

MICROBIOLOGIC CHARACTERISTICS
- Dematiaceous, filamentous fungus (mold)
- Rapidly growing, cottony, gray to black colonies
- Yeast, pseudohyphae, or septate and pigmented hyphae *in vivo*
- Hyphae grow at 30°C in culture.

EPIDEMIOLOGY
- Usually found in soil and plants
- Inoculation through a penetrating injury or by inhalation of conidia from the environment

INFECTIONS
- Occasionally, it causes infections in humans and animals.
- Mycotic infection in healthy and compromised hosts
- Infections of the eye (corneal)
- Subcutaneous infections
- Paranasal sinusitis in patients with allergic rhinitis and nasal polyposis
- Pulmonary infections
- Meningoencephalitis
- Disseminated manifestations in immunosuppressed patients

DIAGNOSIS
- Identification of the fungus in clinical specimens
- Culture

TREATMENT
- Infection of the cornea: Topical natamycin
- Subcutaneous infection: Amphotericin B i.v., flucytosine, ketoconazole, or itraconazole as complement for surgery
- Systemic infection: Amphotericin B i.v.

ALTERNATIVE TREATMENT
- Subcutaneous or systemic infection: Itraconazole, voriconazole (limited experience)
- Surgical excision of local lesions is important.

BLASTOCYSTIS HOMINIS

GENUS Blastocystis

SPECIES
- B. hominis

MICROBIOLOGIC CHARACTERISTICS
- Protozoon

EPIDEMIOLOGY
- Worldwide
- It is commonly found in stool specimens; however, its pathogenicity is unclear. It seems not to cause any disease in most cases of isolation.

INFECTIONS
- Self-limited, acute diarrhea

DIAGNOSIS
- Identification in stool specimen

TREATMENT
- Antibiotic treatment is indicated only if another enteropathogen is not isolated and a high number of *Blastocystis* is found in stools.
- Nitazoxanide 500 mg q12h for 3 days

ALTERNATIVE TREATMENT
- Metronidazole 1.5 g/d for 10 days
- Trimethoprim–sulfamethoxazole, 1 double-strength tablet q12h for 7 days
- Iodoquinol 650 mg q8h for 20 days

BLASTOMYCES DERMATITIDIS

See Section II, "Blastomycosis"

BLASTOSCHIZOMYCES CAPITATUS

GENUS Blastoschizomyces

SPECIES
- B. capitatus

MICROBIOLOGIC CHARACTERISTICS
- Yeast that can develop arthroconidia, hyphae, blastoconidia, and pseudohyphae

EPIDEMIOLOGY
- Rare infection
- Probably worldwide

INFECTIONS
- Disseminated forms with fungemia, skin lesions, and visceral abscesses in neutropenic patients
- Fungemia in intravenous drug users
- Surgical wound infections
- Prosthetic valve endocarditis

DIAGNOSIS
- Culture
- Identification of fungus in tissue biopsies

TREATMENT
- Amphotericin B i.v.
- Flucytosine has been used in combination with amphotericin B.

ALTERNATIVE TREATMENT
- Fluconazole 800 mg/d

BORDETELLA BRONCHISEPTICA

GENUS Bordetella

SPECIES
• B. bronchiseptica

MICROBIOLOGIC CHARACTERISTICS
• Aerobic, Gram-negative bacillus

EPIDEMIOLOGY
• Worldwide

INFECTIONS
• Pneumonia
• Tracheobronchitis
• Bacteremia

DIAGNOSIS
• Culture

TREATMENT
• In contrast to B. pertussis, B. bronchiseptica is usually resistant to macrolide antibiotics.
• Antipseudomonal beta-lactam agents are usually effective.

ALTERNATIVE TREATMENT
• Aminoglycoside, imipenem, doxycycline

BORDETELLA SPECIES

GENUS Bordetella

SPECIES
• B. parapertussis
• B. pertussis

MICROBIOLOGIC CHARACTERISTICS
• Aerobic, Gram-negative bacillus

EPIDEMIOLOGY
• Worldwide
• It may affect previously immunized patients, particularly adults.

INFECTIONS
• Whooping cough

DIAGNOSIS
• Culture in special medium (Bordet–Gengou)
• PCR
• Serology may be helpful.
• Antigen detection in nasopharyngeal exudate

TREATMENT
• Cough medicines, including codeine, are usually ineffective.
• Erythromycin 2 g/d in 4 divided doses for 14 days
• Azithromycin 500 mg on day 1, 250 mg on days 2–5
• Clarithromycin 500 mg q12h for 7 days

ALTERNATIVE TREATMENT
• Trimethoprim–sulfamethoxazole, 1 double-strength tablet q12h for 7 days

PREVENTION
• Respiratory isolation is required.

BORRELIA BURGDORFERI

See Section II, "Lyme Disease"

BORRELIA SPECIES

GENUS Borrelia

SPECIES
• B. hispanica
• B. mazzottii
• B. recurrentis
• B. venezuelensis
• Others

MICROBIOLOGIC CHARACTERISTICS
• Aerobic, Gram-negative bacillus

INCUBATION PERIOD
• The incubation period is 4–18 days, with a mean of 7 days.

EPIDEMIOLOGY
• Worldwide infection

INFECTIONS
• Relapsing fever (discussed in Section II)

DIAGNOSIS
• Identification with Giemsa or Wright stains or dark-field examination of peripheral blood smears (not available in most laboratories)
• PCR
• Serology (limited sensitivity and specificity)

TREATMENT
• Louse-borne infection: Tetracycline 500 mg (single dose), doxycycline 100 mg (single dose)
• Tick-borne infection: Tetracycline 500 mg q6h, doxycycline 100 mg q12h for 7 days

ALTERNATIVE TREATMENT
• Erythromycin
• Penicillin G or ceftriaxone (for meningitis, encephalitis)

BRUCELLA SPECIES

See Section II, "Brucellosis"

BRUGIA SPECIES

GENUS Brugia

SPECIES
• B. malayi
• B. timori

MICROBIOLOGIC CHARACTERISTICS
• Nematode helminth

EPIDEMIOLOGY
• B. malayi: India, China, Malaysia, Vietnam, Cambodia, Thailand (and other countries of Indochina), Korea, Papua New Guinea, various Pacific Islands
• B. timori: Indonesia

INFECTIONS
• Lymphatic filariasis
• Elephantiasis (lymphangitis, lymphedema, abscesses)

DIAGNOSIS
• Blood smear examination for detection of microfilariae (fresh, concentrated, or filtrated specimen)
• Thick smear staining with Giemsa or H&E stain for species identification
• Serology (antifilarial antibodies)

TREATMENT
• Diethylcarbamazine 2 mg/kg q8h for 12 days (for patients with microfilaremia: 50 mg on day 1, 50 mg q12h on day 2, 50 mg q8h on day 3, 100 mg q12h on day 4, and 100 mg q8h on day 5, for completion of a 12-day treatment period)
• Allergic reactions may occur during treatment, especially during the first few days of treatment.

ALTERNATIVE TREATMENT
• Diethylcarbamazine 6 mg/kg (single dose)
• Ivermectin 150 μg/kg (single dose)

BURKHOLDERIA MALLEI

GENUS Burkholderia

SPECIES
• B. mallei

MICROBIOLOGIC CHARACTERISTICS
• Aerobic, Gram-negative bacillus

INCUBATION PERIOD
• 1–5 days

EPIDEMIOLOGY
• B. mallei causes infection in equine animals. However, it is sometimes transmitted to humans.
• Rare human infection, mainly in Asia, Africa, and Central and South America
• Affected persons usually have a history of contact with horses, donkeys, or mules.

INFECTIONS
• Glanders (cutaneous infection with adenitis, pneumonia, or sepsis)

DIAGNOSIS
• Microscopic examination of exudates rarely reveals the pathogen.
• B. mallei cannot be distinguished by microscopic examination from B. pseudomallei.
• Culture or inoculation into animals
• Serology

TREATMENT
• There are limited data on the efficacy of antibiotics for glanders.
• Combination of imipenem and doxycycline may be beneficial.
• Surgical management is helpful in cases with suppurative lymphadenitis.

ALTERNATIVE TREATMENT
• Ceftazidime, gentamicin, imipenem, doxycycline, and ciprofloxacin all have reliable in vitro activity.

PREVENTION
• Unlike melioidosis, isolation of the affected person is indicated.
• Control of disease in horses

BURKHOLDERIA PSEUDOMALLEI

GENUS Burkholderia

SPECIES
• B. pseudomallei

MICROBIOLOGIC CHARACTERISTICS
• Aerobic, Gram-negative bacillus

INCUBATION PERIOD
• The first symptoms may appear quickly after infection (2–3 days).
• Most patients develop symptoms months to years after infection.

EPIDEMIOLOGY
• B. pseudomallei is a natural saprophyte isolated from soil, ponds, and market produce.
• It is unclear how humans contract the pathogen. Some experts believe that the most common mechanism is by soil contamination of skin abrasions.
• It is a rare cause of human infection, except in Thailand. A study from northeast Thailand reported that 40% of deaths from community-acquired septicemia were attributable to melioidosis (B. pseudomallei).

INFECTIONS
• Melioidosis (skin infection, with adenitis, pneumonia, or sepsis)
• Some patients may develop a secondary abscess in several organs.

DIAGNOSIS
• Culture or inoculation into animals
• Serology
• Locally developed antigen and DNA detection techniques used in endemic regions

TREATMENT
• Initial intensive therapy (mimimum of 10–14 days): Ceftazidime 2 g q6h or meropenem 1 g q8h or imipenem 1 g q6h. Any of the 3 may be combined with trimethoprim–sulfamethoxazole (TMP–SMX), 2 double-strength tablets (1600/320 mg) q12h.
• Addition of TMP–SMX is recommended in neurologic, cutaneous, bone, and prostatic disease.
• Eradication therapy (minimum of 3 months): TMP–SMX, 2 double-strength tablets q12h. May be combined with doxycycline 100 mg q12h.
• Surgical drainage of large abscesses

ALTERNATIVE TREATMENT
• Amoxicillin–clavulanate
• Ciprofloxacin, ofloxacin
• A significant proportion (10–80%) of B. pseudomallei species isolated from patients in Thailand are resistant to TMP–SMX.
• Patients with low-titer antibodies against the pathogen, but without any evidence of infection, do not require treatment.

BURKHOLDERIA SPECIES

GENUS Burkholderia

SPECIES
• B. cepacia complex: B. cenocepacia, B. multivorans, B. dolosa, B. cepacia and others
• B. gladioli
• B. pickettii

MICROBIOLOGIC CHARACTERISTICS
• Aerobic, Gram-negative bacillus

EPIDEMIOLOGY
• Recent studies in patients with cystic fibrosis have shown that B. cepacia is transmissible between humans.

INFECTIONS
• Bronchitis in patients with cystic fibrosis (B. cepacia, B. gladioli)
• Wound infection
• Sepsis in immunosuppressed patients or in association with central venous lines
• Outbreaks of bloodstream infections associated with contaminated intravenous products (B. pickettii)

DIAGNOSIS
• Culture

TREATMENT
• Several antipseudomonal agents are also active against B. cepacia complex. However, strains isolated from patients with cystic fibrosis have frequently higher minimal inhibitory concentration with these agents. Combination antimicrobial treatment is recommended.
• Ceftazidime, cefepime
• Meropenem, imipenem
• Piperacillin–tazobactam
• Ciprofloxacin
• Aminoglycosides

ALTERNATIVE TREATMENT
• Trimethoprim–sulfamethoxazole
• Nebulization of antimicrobial agents, such as meropenem or tobramycin

PREVENTION
• Patients with cystic fibrosis who are not colonized with B. cepacia complex should avoid contact with patients who are infected or colonized with the pathogen.

CALICIVIRUSES AND CALICI-LIKE VIRUSES

GROUP Calicivirus

GENOGROUPS
• There are 2 genera of caliciviruses causing disease in humans: Norovirus and Sapovirus

MICROBIOLOGIC CHARACTERISTICS
• Small, nonenveloped, single-stranded, positive RNA virus
• Icosahedral symmetry

INCUBATION PERIOD
• 12 hours–4 days

EPIDEMIOLOGY
• Common cause of human disease (norovirus)
• Transmitted from person to person (fecal–oral route), via contaminated food/water, fomites, and airborne droplets

INFECTIONS
• Calicivirus causes gastroenteritis in children and adults.

DIAGNOSIS
• Direct visualization in stools, using electron microscopy
• Enzyme immunoassay for detection of viral antigen in stool or antibody in serum
• Reverse transcriptase polymerase chain reaction (RT-PCR) for detection of viral RNA in stool
• Specific diagnosis usually not required in the management of acute gastroenteritis

TREATMENT
• Symptomatic

ALTERNATIVE TREATMENT
• There is no effective specific treatment with antiviral agents.

PREVENTION
• Contact precautions for diapered and/or incontinent children for the duration of illness.

CAMPYLOBACTER SPECIES

See Section II, "Campylobacter Infections"

CANDIDA SPECIES

See Section II chapters on Candida infections

CAPILLARIA SPECIES

GENUS Capillaria

SPECIES
- C. aerophila
- C. hepatica
- C. philippinensis

MICROBIOLOGIC CHARACTERISTICS
- Nematode helminth

EPIDEMIOLOGY
- C. philippinensis: Philippines, Thailand; rare elsewhere
- C. hepatica: Sporadic cases reported in several countries worldwide
- C. aerophila: Rare cases reported from the former Soviet Union

INFECTIONS
- C. philippinensis: Intestinal capillariasis
- C. hepatica: Hepatic capillariasis
- C. aerophila: Pulmonary capillariasis

DIAGNOSIS
- Identification of ova or larvae in the stool in cases of intestinal capillariasis
- Histopathology of liver biopsy in cases of hepatic capillariasis

TREATMENT
- Intestinal capillariasis: Mebendazole 200 mg p.o. q12h for 20 days
- Hepatic capillariasis: Thiabendazole

ALTERNATIVE TREATMENT
- Intestinal capillariasis: Albendazole 200 mg q12h for 10 days
- Hepatic capillariasis: Albendazole
- Pulmonary capillariasis: Mebendazole, albendazole

PREVENTION
- Avoid eating uncooked fish in endemic areas (for C. philippinensis)

CAPNOCYTOPHAGA SPECIES

GENUS Capnocytophaga

SPECIES
- C. canimorsus
- C. cynodegmi
- C. gingivalis
- C. granulosa
- C. haemolytica
- C. leadbetteri
- C. ochracea
- C. sputigena

MICROBIOLOGIC CHARACTERISTICS
- Microaerophilic, Gram-negative bacillus

INCUBATION PERIOD
- 1–5 days after inoculation

EPIDEMIOLOGY
- Capnocytophaga species can cause clinical infection in persons who have been bitten, scratched, or licked by dogs or cats.
- Splenectomy, alcoholism, and chronic pulmonary disease are known risk factors.
- Some Capnocytophaga species are part of the normal human flora.
- Neutropenic patients may develop septicemia due to these organisms.

INFECTIONS
- Wound infection after dog bite
- Sepsis (severe, with shock and diffuse intravascular coagulation in splenectomized patients)
- Purulent meningitis
- Endocarditis
- Septic arthritis
- Capnocytophaga species of the normal human oral flora may cause periodontitis and oral mucositis.

DIAGNOSIS
- Culture
- Finding Gram-negative bacilli within neutrophils

TREATMENT
- Combination of penicillin/beta-lactamase inhibitor
- Third-generation cephalosporin

ALTERNATIVE TREATMENT
- Carbapenems
- For milder infections: Clindamycin, doxycycline, or a fluoroquinolone
- C. granulosa and C. haemolytica often resistant to beta-lactams.

PREVENTION
- Preventive therapy with amoxicillin–clavulanate may be warranted for splenectomized patients bitten by dogs.

CHLAMYDIA SPECIES

GENUS Chlamydia

SPECIES
- C. trachomatis

MICROBIOLOGIC CHARACTERISTICS
- Gram-negative bacteria
- Obligate intracellular bacteria

EPIDEMIOLOGY
- Common cause of infection worldwide
- 500 million people are affected by ocular trachoma and approximately 7–9 million are blind due to the disease.
- The most common cause of bacterial sexually transmitted infection

INFECTIONS
- Anogenital infections (urethritis, proctitis, cervicitis, pelvic inflammatory disease)
- Conjunctivitis
- Infant pneumonia
- Lymphogranuloma venereum (serovars L_1, L_2, L_3)
- Trachoma

DIAGNOSIS
- Nucleic acid amplification techniques (such as PCR). Can be performed on urethral/cervical specimens and urine
- Antigen detection by ELISA or immunofluorescent staining
- Serology: Patients with lymphogranuloma venereum have complement-fixing antibody titers greater than 1:16.
- Cell culture (limited in research and reference laboratories)
- Intracytoplasmic inclusions in Giemsa-stained cell scrapings from the conjunctiva
- Cytology from endocervical scrapings

TREATMENT
- Nongonococcal urethritis/proctitis/cervicitis: Azithromycin 1 g (single dose) or doxycycline 100 mg q12h for 7 days
- Lymphogranuloma venereum: Doxycycline 100 mg p.o. q12h for 3 weeks

ALTERNATIVE TREATMENT
- Nongonococcal urethritis: Erythromycin 500 mg q6h or ofloxacin 300 mg q12h or levofloxacin 500 mg/d for 7 days

CHLAMYDOPHILA SPECIES

GENUS Chlamydophila
- C. pneumoniae (TWAR): Etiologic agent in a proportion of cases of community-acquired pneumonia
- C. psittaci: Causes psittacosis (see Section II, "Psittacosis")

MICROBIOLOGIC CHARACTERISTICS
- Gram-negative bacteria
- Obligate intracellular bacteria

EPIDEMIOLOGY
- C. pneumoniae spreads person to person.
- C. psittaci is common in birds and domestic animals. Infection in pet owners, animal handlers

INFECTIONS
- There is some evidence of the role of C. pneumoniae in the pathogenesis of atherosclerosis.

DIAGNOSIS
- Serology: Complement fixation and microimmunofluorescence
- Patients with psittacosis have complement-fixing antibody titers greater than 1:16.
- Antigen detection
- Molecular biology techniques (PCR)
- Cell culture

TREATMENT
- Pneumonia: Doxycycline 100 mg q12h for 10–14 days

ALTERNATIVE TREATMENT
- Azithromycin, clarithromycin
- Tetracycline
- Levofloxacin

CHROMOBACTERIUM VIOLACEUM

GENUS Chromobacterium

SPECIES
- *C. violaceum*

MICROBIOLOGIC CHARACTERISTICS
- Aerobic, Gram-negative bacillus

EPIDEMIOLOGY
- Worldwide, rare infection

INFECTIONS
- Traumatic wound infections
- Sepsis (mostly in neutropenic patients and in patients with chronic granulomatous disease)
- Pneumonia (after drowning)

DIAGNOSIS
- Culture

TREATMENT
- Doxycycline or a fluoroquinolone
- For severe infection: Imipenem or a ureidopenicillin in combination with an aminoglycoside

ALTERNATIVE TREATMENT
- Trimethoprim–sulfamethoxazole
- Aminoglycoside

CHROMOBLASTOMYCOSIS AGENTS

GENUS/SPECIES
- Chromoblastomycosis (chromomycosis or dermatitis verrucosa) may be caused by several fungal species, including the following:
  - *Cladophialophora (Cladosporium) carrionii*
  - *Fonsecaea compacta*
  - *Fonsecaea pedrosoi* (most common)
  - *Phialophora verrucosa*
  - *Rhinocladiella aquaspera*

MICROBIOLOGIC CHARACTERISTICS
- Dematiaceous, filamentous fungus (mold)
- Pigmented septate hyphae *in vivo*

INCUBATION PERIOD
- The incubation period is unknown; however, it is probably months.

EPIDEMIOLOGY
- Rare cause of infection
- There is a worldwide distribution of cases, although most of the cases occur in developing countries.
- It usually affects rural, barefooted agricultural workers in tropical and subtropical regions.

INFECTIONS
- Chromoblastomomycosis is manifested by chronic warty nodules or tumor-like masses of the subcutaneous tissue of the lower extremities (and sometimes in other areas of the body).
- Rarely, the infection spreads to muscle, CNS, or the lungs.

DIAGNOSIS
- The etiologic agents of chromoblastomycosis are seen in affected tissue as sclerotic bodies.
- Identification of responsible fungus is based on morphology and culture characteristics.

TREATMENT
- Optimal management has not been defined.
- Small skin and subcutaneous tissue lesions may be treated with excision or cryosurgery.
- Itraconazole may benefit some patients. Long-term treatment is usually necessary (for at least 6 months). Can be combined with cryosurgery or other local methods.

ALTERNATIVE TREATMENT
- Terbinafine
- Intravenous 5-fluorocytosine combined with amphotericin B may be necessary in patients with large lesions.
- The newer broad-spectrum azoles may be useful.

PREVENTION
- Wearing shoes and clothes decreases the probability of small puncture wounds.

CHRYSOSPORIUM PARVUM

GENUS Chrysosporium

SPECIES
- *C. parvum*

MICROBIOLOGIC CHARACTERISTICS
- Filamentous fungus (mold)
- Septate hyaline hyphae *in vivo*

EPIDEMIOLOGY
- Worldwide, rare infection

INFECTIONS
- Osteomyelitis
- Pulmonary infection
- Prosthetic valve endocarditis
- Rhinitis–sinusitis with occasional extension to the CNS
- Dissemination of infection in immunocompromised patients

DIAGNOSIS
- Culture of the fungus
- Identification of the fungus in tissue biopsies

TREATMENT
- Amphotericin B i.v.

CITROBACTER SPECIES

GENUS Citrobacter

SPECIES
- *C. amalonaticus*
- *C. freundii*
- *C. koseri*

MICROBIOLOGIC CHARACTERISTICS
- Aerobic, Gram-negative bacillus

EPIDEMIOLOGY
- Increasing importance as a cause of nosocomial infections

INFECTIONS
- Urinary tract infections
- Pulmonary infections
- Catheter-associated bacteremia
- Surgical wound infections
- Neonatal meningitis

DIAGNOSIS
- Culture of the pathogen

TREATMENT
- Third-generation cephalosporin
- Antipseudomonal penicillins
- Carbapenem (imipenem, meropenem)
- Fluoroquinolone
- The addition of an aminoglycoside to carbapenem or fluoroquinolone may be warranted in severe cases of *Citrobacter* infection.

ALTERNATIVE TREATMENT
- Aztreonam, or an aminoglycoside

CLONORCHIS SINENSIS (OPISTHORCHIS SINENSIS)

GENUS Clonorchis

SPECIES
- *C. sinensis*

MICROBIOLOGIC CHARACTERISTICS
- A trematode helminth

EPIDEMIOLOGY
- People are infected by eating raw or undercooked freshwater fish.
- Endemic in China, especially in the southeast part of the country. The infection is also a problem in Indochina, Taiwan, Korea, and Japan.
- Imported cases occur in other countries.

INFECTIONS
- Clonorchiasis (obstructive jaundice and cholangitis)
- Symptoms sometimes appear late after infection (many years later).
- Clonorchiasis is considered to be a risk factor for cholangiocarcinoma.

DIAGNOSIS
- Examination of concentrated stools or bile obtained with a duodenal aspirate
- Serologic tests (not widely available outside of endemic areas)

TREATMENT
- Praziquantel 25 mg/kg p.o. q8h for 1 day
- Albendazole 10 mg/kg/d for 7 days

PREVENTION
- Cook or irradiate freshwater fish.

CLOSTRIDIUM BOTULINUM

See Section II, "Botulism"

CLOSTRIDIUM DIFFICILE

See Section II, "Antibiotic and *Clostridium difficile*-associated Diarrhea"

CLOSTRIDIUM SPECIES

GENUS Clostridium

SPECIES
- *C. bifermentans*
- *C. butyricum*
- *C. clostridioforme*
- *C. histolyticum*
- *C. novyi*
- *C. perfringens*
- *C. ramosum*
- *C. septicum*
- *C. sordellii*
- Other species are discussed elsewhere (*C. difficile, C. botulinum*, and *C. tetani*)

MICROBIOLOGIC CHARACTERISTICS
- Anaerobic, Gram-positive bacillus

INCUBATION PERIOD
- For cases of food poisoning due to *Clostridium* species, the incubation period is 6–24 hours, usually 8–12 hours.

EPIDEMIOLOGY
- Worldwide infections

INFECTIONS
- Food poisoning
- Bacteremia
- Localized infections (polymicrobial) involving the biliary tract, intraabdominal abscesses, and soft tissues
- Gas gangrene (see Section II, "Gas Gangrene")
- Necrotizing enteritis
- Typhlitis in neutropenic patients and patients with AIDS
- Postpartum endometritis, with hypotension and shock (*C. sordellii*)
- The isolation of *C. septicum* from blood cultures or the onset of spontaneous gas gangrene should prompt the search for a colonic neoplasia or other structural lesions.

DIAGNOSIS
- Anaerobic culture
- Prolonged incubation of culture may be needed.

TREATMENT
- No antibiotic treatment is needed for cases of food poisoning.
- Penicillin G alone or with clindamycin for severe clostridial infections such as gas gangrene

ALTERNATIVE TREATMENT
- Metronidazole, carbapenem (imipenem, meropenem) clindamycin, or a tetracycline (agents with action against anaerobic bacteria)

CLOSTRIDIUM TETANI

See Section II, "Tetanus"

COCCIDIOIDES IMMITIS

See Section II, "Coccidioidomycosis"

COLORADO TICK FEVER VIRUS

GROUP Coltivirus

STRAINS
- Colorado tick fever virus
- Other tick-borne arboviral fevers include infections caused by Kemerovo virus, Nairobi sheep disease (Ganjam), Lipovnik, Quaranfil, Bhanja, Thogoto, and Dugde viruses.

MICROBIOLOGIC CHARACTERISTICS
- Double-stranded RNA
- Nonenveloped

INCUBATION PERIOD
- About 5 days

EPIDEMIOLOGY
- Colorado tick fever is endemic in the mountainous regions (altitude above 5000 ft) of Canada and the western US.
- Mode of transmission is by the bite of an infected tick.
- Persons engaged in recreational activities or occupations that increase the probability of tick bite in the endemic areas are at risk of developing Colorado tick fever.

INFECTIONS
- Colorado tick fever is an acute febrile illness.
- Encephalitis, meningitis, particularly in children

DIAGNOSIS
- Serology tests
- Cell culture

TREATMENT
- Symptomatic
- There is no specific antiviral treatment.

PREVENTION
- Protective measures to avoid tick bites

COMAMONAS SPECIES

GENUS Comamonas

SPECIES
- *C. acidovorans*
- *C. terrigena*
- *C. testosteroni* (most common)

MICROBIOLOGIC CHARACTERISTICS
- Aerobic, Gram-negative bacillus
- Low pathogenicity

EPIDEMIOLOGY
- Common environmental bacteria that can occasionally cause human infection
- An infrequent contaminant of cultures

INFECTIONS
- Endocarditis, especially in intravenous drug abusers
- Bacteremia in immunosuppressed patients
- Rarely a cause of keratitis, leading to corneal ulcers (usually *C. acidovorans*)

DIAGNOSIS
- Culture
- The physician should consider the possibility of contamination in cases of patients with positive cultures for *Comamonas*.

TREATMENT
- Little is known about the efficacy of antibiotics of different classes against *Comamonas* species.
- Few available data support the use of antipseudomonal agents.

CONIDIOBOLUS SPECIES

GENUS Conidiobolus

SPECIES
* *C. coronatus*

MICROBIOLOGIC CHARACTERISTICS
* Filamentous fungus (mold)
* Hyphae have few septa.

EPIDEMIOLOGY
* Distributed in tropical areas, particularly Central America, equatorial Africa, and India.

INFECTIONS
* Most common manifestation is entomophthoromycosis conidiobolae, a chronic granulomatous disease. This presents with nodular lesions of the nose, mouth, and perinasal tissues, which are frequently large and disfiguring.
* Mediastinitis
* Pericarditis

DIAGNOSIS
* Identification of the fungus in biopsy
* Culture of the fungus

TREATMENT
* There are scarce published data for the management of this fungal infection.
* Saturated potassium iodide solution, with or without trimethoprim–sulfamethoxazole, may be used in cases of skin and subcutaneous tissue disease.
* Surgical management may be done in patients with large disfiguring lesions.
* Azoles (fluconazole or ketoconazole) have been reported to help and may be used in patients with severe manifestation of entomophthoromycosis conidiobolae.

CORONAVIRUS

GROUP Coronavirus

MICROBIOLOGIC CHARACTERISTICS
* Single-stranded, positive RNA virus
* Enveloped virus

INCUBATION PERIOD
* Usually 2–4 days

EPIDEMIOLOGY
* Worldwide infection

INFECTIONS
* Common cold and other upper respiratory tract infections, such as sinusitis
* Rare cause of pneumonia in children or adults
* A novel coronavirus was the cause of SARS
* Diarrhea

DIAGNOSIS
* Efforts for specific diagnosis of coronavirus are not warranted for patients with common cold in clinical practice.
* PCR
* Antigen detection
* Direct visualization with electron microscopy

TREATMENT
* Symptomatic

PREVENTION
* Avoid crowded places during winter months.

CORYNEBACTERIUM DIPHTHERIAE

See Section II, "Diphtheria"

CORYNEBACTERIUM JEIKEIUM

GENUS Corynebacterium

SPECIES
* *C. jeikeium*

MICROBIOLOGIC CHARACTERISTICS
* Aerobic, Gram-positive bacillus

EPIDEMIOLOGY
* Worldwide rare infection

INFECTIONS
* Infections due to *C. jeikeium* are mainly seen in immunosuppressed patients, especially those with neutropenia and advanced infection with HIV.
* Sepsis
* Endocarditis
* Central venous catheter-associated infections
* Pneumonia
* Meningitis

DIAGNOSIS
* Culture

TREATMENT
* Vancomycin

ALTERNATIVE TREATMENT
* Penicillin G in combination with an antipseudomonal aminoglycoside

CORYNEBACTERIUM MINUTISSIMUM

GENUS Corynebacterium

SPECIES
* *C. minutissimum*

MICROBIOLOGIC CHARACTERISTICS
* Aerobic, Gram-positive bacillus

EPIDEMIOLOGY
* Common cause of skin infection

INFECTIONS
* Erythrasma
* A rare cause of endocarditis and sepsis, especially in neutropenic patients
* Subcutaneous tissue infections

DIAGNOSIS
* Culture
* Coral-red fluorescence with Wood's lamp in cases of erythrasma

TREATMENT
* Erythromycin 250 mg q6h for 14 days
* Vancomycin for systemic infections due to *C. minutissimum*

ALTERNATIVE TREATMENT
* Local treatment with 2% aqueous clindamycin is also effective in patients with erythrasma.
* Tetracycline 250 mg p.o. q6h

CORYNEBACTERIUM PSEUDOTUBERCULOSIS

GENUS Corynebacterium

SPECIES
- C. pseudotuberculosis

MICROBIOLOGIC CHARACTERISTICS
- Aerobic, Gram-positive bacillus

EPIDEMIOLOGY
- Rare cause of human infection, usually in persons exposed to animals

INFECTIONS
- Suppurative granulomatous lymphadenitis

DIAGNOSIS
- Culture in blood agar with 10% CO_2

TREATMENT
- Macrolide antibiotics
- Excision of infected lymph nodes

ALTERNATIVE TREATMENT
- Tetracycline or penicillin G

CORYNEBACTERIUM SPECIES

GENUS Corynebacterium

SPECIES
- C. bovis
- C. pilosum
- C. pseudodiphtheriticum
- C. striatum
- C. xerosis
- Others

MICROBIOLOGIC CHARACTERISTICS
- Aerobic, Gram-positive bacillus

EPIDEMIOLOGY
- Rare cause of infections

INFECTIONS
- Native or prosthetic valve endocarditis
- Rare cause of septicemia (seen more commonly in neutropenics)
- Pneumonia, tracheitis, other respiratory tract infections
- Infection of prosthetic materials

DIAGNOSIS
- Culture

TREATMENT
- Vancomycin plus an aminoglycoside in cases of endocarditis)
- Removal of the prosthetic material is frequently necessary.

ALTERNATIVE TREATMENT
- Modification of the initially chosen empiric regimen may be needed, based on the progress of the infection and *in vitro* antimicrobial susceptibility testing.
- Penicillin G, tetracycline, a macrolide, rifampicin, first-generation cephalosporin, or teicoplanin

CORYNEBACTERIUM UREALYTICUM

GENUS Corynebacterium

SPECIES
- C. urealyticum

MICROBIOLOGIC CHARACTERISTICS
- Aerobic, Gram-positive bacillus

INFECTIONS
- Rare cause of urinary tract infection
- It may cause chronic cystitis with deposits of phosphate ammonium magnesium crystals.
- Bacteremia has been reported rarely.

DIAGNOSIS
- Culture

TREATMENT
- Vancomycin

ALTERNATIVE TREATMENT
- Doxycycline

COXIELLA BURNETII

See Section II, "Q Fever"

COXSACKIEVIRUS

GROUP Enterovirus

TYPES
- There are several serotypes of coxsackievirus A and coxsackievirus B.

MICROBIOLOGIC CHARACTERISTICS
- Single-stranded, positive RNA virus
- Icosahedral symmetry
- Naked

EPIDEMIOLOGY
- Worldwide, common cause of infections

INFECTIONS
- Common cause of several types of syndromes, which are manifested by enanthems and exanthems, including a herpetiform rash (mouth-hand-foot syndrome)
- Upper respiratory infection
- Herpangina
- Pleurodynia
- Myopericarditis
- Acute hemorrhagic conjunctivitis
- Disseminated infection in newborns
- Meningitis, encephalitis, and, rarely, paralytic syndromes
- Chronic meningoencephalitis in immunosuppressed persons, especially in patients with agammaglobulinemia

DIAGNOSIS
- Virologic culture
- Serology tests
- PCR

TREATMENT
- Symptomatic

ALTERNATIVE TREATMENT
- There is no specific antiviral treatment.

PREVENTION
- Enteric isolation for 1 week
- Respiratory precautions in case of herpangina

CRIMEAN–CONGO HEMORRHAGIC FEVER VIRUS

GROUP Nairovirus

MICROBIOLOGIC CHARACTERISTICS
- Crimean–Congo virus belongs to the *Nairovirus* genus, which belongs to the Bunyaviridae family
- 3 segments of single-stranded, circular RNA
- Enveloped
- Helicoidal symmetry

EPIDEMIOLOGY
- The virus is transmitted to humans by ticks.
- Eastern Europe, Central Asia, the Balkans, the Middle East, and Africa

INFECTIONS
- Hemorrhagic fever (acute hepatitis with jaundice, disseminated intravascular coagulation, thrombocytopenia, bleeding)
- Infections caused by other viruses of the Bunyaviridae family include California encephalitis, Rift Valley fever, hemorrhagic fever with renal syndrome, and hantavirus pulmonary syndrome.

DIAGNOSIS
- Cell culture
- Serology
- Antigen nucleic acid detection
- PCR

TREATMENT
- Symptomatic
- High mortality (30–40%) in cases of severe Crimean–Congo hemorrhagic fever

ALTERNATIVE TREATMENT
- There is no specific antiviral treatment.

PREVENTION
- Strict isolation of affected patients

CRYPTOCOCCUS NEOFORMANS

See Section II, "Cryptococcal Infections"

CRYPTOSPORIDIUM PARVUM

See Section II, "Cryptosporidiosis"

CUNNINGHAMELLA BERTHOLETIAE

GENUS Cunninghamella

SPECIES
- *C. bertholetiae*

MICROBIOLOGIC CHARACTERISTICS
- Filamentous fungus (mold) with nonseptate hyaline hyphae

EPIDEMIOLOGY
- Worldwide, rare infection
- It affects more frequently immunosuppressed people and patients on hemodialysis.

INFECTIONS
- Zygomycosis (mucormycosis)

DIAGNOSIS
- Identification of the fungus in tissue biopsies
- Culture

TREATMENT
- Amphotericin B i.v.

ALTERNATIVE TREATMENT
- There are limited data on the efficacy of azoles (itraconazole).

CURVULARIA SPECIES

GENUS Curvularia

SPECIES
- *C. boedijn*
- *C. geniculata*
- *C. lunata*
- *C. pallescens*
- *C. senegalensis*

MICROBIOLOGIC CHARACTERISTICS
- Dematiaceous, filamentous fungus (mold)
- Yeasts, pseudohyphae, or septate pigmented hyphae *in vivo*

EPIDEMIOLOGY
- Rare cause of infection

INFECTIONS
- Keratitis
- Skin and subcutaneous tissue infection
- Rarely a cause of deep-tissue infection (e.g., pneumonia, endocarditis, osteomyelitis)

DIAGNOSIS
- Tissue biopsy
- Culture

TREATMENT
- Amphotericin B

ALTERNATIVE TREATMENT
- There are limited data on the efficacy of azoles.

CYCLOSPORA CAYETANENSIS

GENUS Cyclospora

SPECIES
- *C. cayatanensis*

MICROBIOLOGIC CHARACTERISTICS
- Protozoon
- Acid-fast organism
- Designated previously as coccidian-like body

EPIDEMIOLOGY
- Found in Nepal, Caribbean, Peru, and in travelers coming from various regions (Turkey, Pakistan, Sri Lanka, India, Morocco, Mexico, Australia, Malaysia)
- Worldwide distribution
- Rare in the US
- There are few reports from other countries but it is probably a pathogen affecting people worldwide.
- If there is no travel history, consider whether the patient is immunocompromised (HIV status). However, keep in mind that immunocompetent patients with cyclosporiasis and with no travel history have been reported.

INFECTIONS
- Prolonged, watery diarrhea; self-limited; with fluorescent microscopy

DIAGNOSIS
- Examination of concentrated stools, Kinyoun stain
- Fresh examination with fluorescent microscopy

TREATMENT
- Trimethoprim–sulfamethoxazole (TMP–SMX; 160–800 mg q12h for 3–5 days in immunocompetent patients and for 7 days in patients with AIDS)
- Second line (or first line if allergy to sulfamethoxazole): Ciprofloxacin (500 mg q12h for 3 days in immunocompetent and 7 days in immunocompromised)
- Consider secondary prophylaxis because recurrences may occur: One TMP–SMX 3 times per week for 4 weeks in immunocompetent and 10 weeks in immunocompromised patients

CYTOMEGALOVIRUS

See Section II, "Cytomegalovirus Infections"

DENGUE VIRUS

See Section II, "Dengue"

DERMATOBIA HOMINIS

See "Myiasis Agents"

DICROCOELIUM DENDRITICUM

GENUS Dicrocoelium

SPECIES
- *D. dendriticum*

MICROBIOLOGIC CHARACTERISTICS
- A trematode helminth

EPIDEMIOLOGY
- Worldwide, rare infection

INFECTIONS
- Ova of *D. dendriticum* are sometimes seen in examination of human stool specimens. However, the parasite rarely causes a symptomatic infection.
- It occasionally causes biliary colic.

DIAGNOSIS
- Parasitologic examination of stools

TREATMENT
- Praziquantel 25 mg/kg p.o. q8h (for 3 doses) for the exceptional patient with symptomatic *D. dendriticum* infection and other possible causes of symptoms are absent

DIENTAMOEBA FRAGILIS

GENUS Dientamoeba

SPECIES
- *D. fragilis*

MICROBIOLOGIC CHARACTERISTICS
- Protozoon
- It should not be confused with *Entamoeba histolytica*, the cause of amebiasis.

EPIDEMIOLOGY
- Worldwide

INFECTIONS
- It usually leads to an asymptomatic infection.
- The organism sometimes causes abdominal pain and/or diarrhea.

DIAGNOSIS
- Direct stool examination and ferrous hematoxylin stain

TREATMENT
- Paromomycin 500 mg q8h for 7 days
- Iodoquinol 650 mg q8h for 20 days

ALTERNATIVE TREATMENT
- Tetracycline for 7–10 days
- Metronidazole for 7 days

DIPHYLLOBOTHRIUM SPECIES

GENUS Diphyllobothrium

SPECIES
- *D. dalliae*
- *D. dendriticum*
- *D. latum*
- *D. pasificum*
- *D. ursi*

MICROBIOLOGIC CHARACTERISTICS
- Cestode helminths

INCUBATION PERIOD
- 3–6 weeks from ingestion to passage of eggs in the stool
- However, symptoms may appear months or years later (with continued infection).

EPIDEMIOLOGY
- The infection is acquired by humans by eating inadequately cooked or raw fish.
- The infection is not transmitted directly from person to person. A cycle of transmission including a first and a second intermediate host is necessary for the development of the worm.
- The first intermediate host is copepods of the genera *Cyclops* and *Diaptomus*.
- Freshwater fish (salmon, perch, pike, turbots) ingest infected copepods and become the second intermediate host.
- Humans and fish-eating mammals can then become infected by eating infected fish.
- Infection by *Diphyllobothrium* species occurs mainly in lake regions, where eating undercooked or raw fish is common. Eskimos in Alaska and Canada are more likely to be infected than are other populations, due to food preparation practices which increase the probability of infection with *Diphyllobothrium* species.

INFECTIONS
- Infection by *Diphyllobothrium* species is usually asymptomatic.
- The parasite occasionally causes diarrhea and/or abdominal discomfort (in massive infection).
- Obstruction of the bile duct or the bowel may be rarely seen.
- A small minority of infected patients develop vitamin B12 deficiency.

DIAGNOSIS
- Macroscopic stool examination (for proglottids) and examination of concentrated stools (for eggs)

TREATMENT
- Praziquantel 10–20 mg/kg in a single dose

ALTERNATIVE TREATMENT
- Niclosamide 2 g in a single dose
- Niclosamide tablets should be chewed completely before swallowing.

PREVENTION
- Avoid eating undercooked or raw fish.

DIPYLIDIUM CANINUM

GENUS Dipylidium

SPECIES
- *D. caninum*

MICROBIOLOGIC CHARACTERISTICS
- Cestode (tapeworm) helminth

EPIDEMIOLOGY
- Adult *D. caninum* worms are found in dogs and cats worldwide.
- Children (usually toddler-aged) occasionally become infected with the parasite.

INFECTIONS
- Infected humans are usually asymptomatic.
- Humans may have seed-like proglottids in the stool or the anal area.
- The parasite may occasionally cause gastrointestinal symptoms such as abdominal discomfort in cases of massive infection.

DIAGNOSIS
- Stool examination for proglottids or eggs

TREATMENT
- Praziquantel 10–20 mg/kg in a single dose

ALTERNATIVE TREATMENT
- Niclosamide 2 g in a single dose

DIROFILARIA SPECIES

GENUS Dirofilaria

SPECIES
- *D. immitis*
- *D. repens*
- *D. tenuis*
- *D. ursi*

MICROBIOLOGIC CHARACTERISTICS
- Nematode helminth

EPIDEMIOLOGY
- *D. immitis* is the dog heartworm (few reported cases of human disease worldwide).
- *D. tenuis,* a raccoon parasite in the US
- *D. repens,* a parasite of dogs and cats (Europe)
- *D. ursi,* a parasite of bears in Canada

INFECTIONS
- *D. immitis* may cause pulmonary or cutaneous disease in humans.
- Other *Dirofilaria* species occasionally may cause cutaneous manifestation in humans.
- Microfilaremia is rare in humans.

DIAGNOSIS
- By the detection of worms in tissue biopsies of excised lesions

TREATMENT
- Surgical removal of the affected areas

DRACUNCULUS MEDINENSIS

GENUS Dracunculus

SPECIES
- *D. medinensis*

MICROBIOLOGIC CHARACTERISTICS
- Nematode helminth

INCUBATION PERIOD
- About a year

EPIDEMIOLOGY
- Infection due to *D. medinensis* is seen in sub-Saharan African countries, the Middle East, and Asia.
- Humans become infected by drinking water from infected step wells and ponds.

INFECTIONS
- Guinea worm (skin vesicle and a subsequent ulcer where the worm emerges)
- Secondary infections due to bacteria are common in skin lesions due to the Guinea worm.

DIAGNOSIS
- Identification of worms in skin lesions (adult worms may protrude from skin lesions)
- Microscopic identification of skin lesions may reveal the presence of larvae of the parasite.

TREATMENT
- Extraction of the worm

ALTERNATIVE TREATMENT
- Thiabendazole 50 mg/kg/d orally (in 2 doses) for 2 days or metronidazole 10 mg/kg (divided in 3 doses) for 1 week to reduce the inflammation of the skin lesions (although the drugs have no effect on the worm)

PREVENTION
- Patients with skin lesions should not enter any source of drinking water.
- Drink potable, safe water.
- Immunization against tetanus reduces the risk of tetanus associated with secondary infection of Guinea worm skin lesions.

EBOLA–MARBURG VIRAL DISEASES

GROUP Filovirus

SPECIES
- Ebola virus
- Marburg virus

MICROBIOLOGIC CHARACTERISTICS
- Single-stranded, RNA virus
- Helicoidal symmetry
- Enveloped

INCUBATION PERIOD
- 2 days to 3 weeks for Ebola virus
- 3–9 days for Marburg virus

EPIDEMIOLOGY
- Fortunately, a rare cause of infections
- Ebola virus outbreaks occurred in Africa.
- Marburg virus cases were reported, rarely, from Africa and Europe.

INFECTIONS
- These viruses cause severe illnesses with high-case fatality rates (specifically, 50–90% for Ebola virus and 30% for Marburg virus).
- Sudden onset of illness manifested by high fever, myalgia, headache, vomiting, diarrhea, pharyngitis, and maculopapular rash

DIAGNOSIS
- Cell culture
- Serology tests

TREATMENT
- Symptomatic

ALTERNATIVE TREATMENT
- There is no specific antiviral treatment.

PREVENTION
- Strict isolation of patients
- No sexual intercourse for 3 months (or until semen is shown to be free of virus)

ECHINOCOCCUS SPECIES

See Section II, "Echinococcosis"

ECHINOSTOMA ILOCANUM

GENUS Echinostoma

SPECIES
- *E. ilocanum*

MICROBIOLOGIC CHARACTERISTICS
- Trematode helminth

EPIDEMIOLOGY
- Philippines, Indonesia, Malaysia, and China

INFECTIONS
- A rare cause of small bowel infection

DIAGNOSIS
- Examination of concentrated stools (parasitologic examination)

TREATMENT
- Praziquantel 25 mg/kg p.o. q8h for 2 days

ECHOVIRUS

GROUP Enterovirus

MICROBIOLOGIC CHARACTERISTICS
- Single-stranded, RNA viruses
- Icosahedral symmetry
- Naked

INCUBATION PERIOD
- Usually a few days (depends on the syndrome caused by the virus)

EPIDEMIOLOGY
- The virus is isolated from stool specimens for a week in cases of gastroenteritis.

INFECTIONS
- Common cause of human infection manifested by different syndromes
- Exanthems and enanthems
- Upper respiratory infection
- Herpangina
- Pleurodynia
- Myopericarditis
- Disseminated infection in the newborn
- Chronic meningoencephalitis in immunosuppressed individuals, particularly those with agammaglobulinemia
- Meningitis and encephalitis, rarely paralysis

DIAGNOSIS
- Cell culture
- Serology tests
- Immunohistochemistry performed on biopsy material
- Reverse transcriptase polymerase chain reaction for the detection of viral genome

TREATMENT
- Symptomatic

ALTERNATIVE TREATMENT
- There is no specific antiviral treatment.

PREVENTION
- Enteric isolation for 7 days decreases the possibility of transmission of the virus to other people.

EDWARDSIELLA TARDA

GENUS Edwardsiella

SPECIES
- E. tarda

MICROBIOLOGIC CHARACTERISTICS
- Aerobic, Gram-negative bacillus

EPIDEMIOLOGY
- Worldwide, rare infection
- Part of the normal bowel flora of animals and snakes

INFECTIONS
- Gastroenteritis
- Bacteremia

DIAGNOSIS
- Culture

TREATMENT
- Fluoroquinolone (intravenous treatment with a quinolone is needed for patients with bacteremia due to this pathogen)

ALTERNATIVE TREATMENT
- Ampicillin, aminoglycosides, or a cephalosporin

EHRLICHIA SPECIES

See Section II, "Ehrlichiosis"

EIKENELLA CORRODENS

GENUS Eikenella

SPECIES
E. corrodens

MICROBIOLOGIC CHARACTERISTICS
- Microaerophilic, Gram-negative bacillus
- Belongs to the HACEK group

EPIDEMIOLOGY
- Worldwide, rare infection

INFECTIONS
- Part of the normal oral flora
- Human bite-wound infection
- Skin infection in intravenous drug users
- Internal jugular vein thrombophlebitis
- Endocarditis
- Lung infection (pneumonia, abscess, empyema), usually polymicrobial in origin

DIAGNOSIS
- Culture

TREATMENT
- Penicillin G or amoxicillin–clavulanate

ALTERNATIVE TREATMENT
- Doxycycline, aminoglycoside, or a second- or third-generation cephalosporin
- Resistant to metronidazole, oxacillin, first-generation cephalosporins, and clindamycin
- These antibiotics should not be used empirically to treat human-bite wound infections.
- Some strains produce beta-lactamases.

EMMONSIA PARVA

GENUS Emmonsia

SPECIES
- E. parva

MICROBIOLOGIC CHARACTERISTICS
- Filamentous fungus (mold)

EPIDEMIOLOGY
- Worldwide, rare infection

INFECTIONS
- Rare cases of osteomyelitis, prosthetic valve endocarditis, rhinitis, sinusitis with extension to the CNS, pneumonia, or dissemination in immunocompromised patients have been reported.

DIAGNOSIS
- Culture
- Identification of the fungus in tissue biopsies

TREATMENT
- Amphotericin B i.v.

ALTERNATIVE TREATMENT
- Surgical intervention is also helpful in most cases (removal of lesions).

ENCEPHALITIS VIRUSES OF THE FLAVIVIRIDAE FAMILY

GROUP Flavivirus

STRAINS
- Arthropod-borne viral encephalitides are classified in 2 categories: Arboviral encephalitides and tick-borne arboviral encephalitides.
- Mosquito-borne arboviral encephalitides are caused by a specific virus in 1 of the following 3 groups: Togaviridae/Alphaviridae (Eastern equine encephalitis virus and Western equine encephalitis virus), Bunyaviridae (La Crosse virus, California encephalitis virus, Jamestown Canyon virus, and Snowshoe hare virus), and Flaviviridae (Japanese encephalitis virus, Kunjin virus, Murray Valley encephalitis virus, St. Louis encephalitis virus, and Rocio encephalitis virus).

MICROBIOLOGIC CHARACTERISTICS
- Single-stranded, positive RNA virus
- Spheric
- Enveloped

INCUBATION PERIOD
- 5–15 days

EPIDEMIOLOGY
- Rare cause of infection

INFECTIONS
- Epidemic outbreaks of encephalitis

DIAGNOSIS
- Cell culture
- Serology tests are helpful
- PCR

TREATMENT
- Symptomatic

ALTERNATIVE TREATMENT
- There is no specific antiviral treatment.

PREVENTION
- Avoid mosquito bites.
- Japanese encephalitis virus vaccine (inactivated) is recommended for travelers who stay for a long time (more than 2 months) in rural areas with endemicity of the virus.

ENDOLIMAX NANA

GENUS Endolimax

SPECIES
- *E. nana*

MICROBIOLOGIC CHARACTERISTICS
- Protozoon

EPIDEMIOLOGY
- Worldwide

INFECTIONS
- *E. nana* is thought to be nonpathogenic.

DIAGNOSIS
- Examination of concentrated stools

TREATMENT
- Not required because of the commensal-type nature of the parasite

ENTAMOEBA HISTOLYTICA

See Section II, "Amebiasis"

ENTAMOEBA SPECIES

GENUS Entamoeba

SPECIES
- *E. coil*
- *E. hartmanni*
- *E. polecki*

MICROBIOLOGIC CHARACTERISTICS
- Protozoon, which should not be confused with *Entamoeba histolytica*, the cause of amebiasis

EPIDEMIOLOGY
- Worldwide

INFECTIONS
- These protozoa do not appear to cause symptoms.
- Some experts support that these protozoa may rarely cause diarrhea.

DIAGNOSIS
- Parasitologic examination of stool specimens

TREATMENT
- No treatment is usually required.

ALTERNATIVE TREATMENT
- Metronidazole 500 mg q8h for 6 days or tinidazole 1 g q12h for 3 days may be given to the occasional patient with *Entamoeba* parasites and a syndrome of diarrhea with no other clear cause.

ENTEROBACTER SPECIES

GENUS Enterobacter

SPECIES
- *E. aerogenes*
- *E. cloacae*
- *E. sakazakii*
- *E. tayorae*
- Others

MICROBIOLOGIC CHARACTERISTICS
- Aerobic, Gram-negative bacillus

INCUBATION PERIOD
- Unknown

EPIDEMIOLOGY
- Part of the normal enteric flora
- Infections due to *Enterobacter* species are caused by strains that have already colonized the patient's bowel flora.
- However, there are also documented reports of nosocomial outbreaks of *Enterobacter* infections, showing that human-to-human transmission or common source (e.g., contaminated intravenous solutions) infections also occur.

INFECTIONS
- Generally, nosocomial infections
- Urinary and pulmonary infections
- Bacteremia associated with catheters
- Contamination of intravenous infusion
- Surgical wound infection
- Neonatal meningitis

DIAGNOSIS
- Culture of the pathogen

TREATMENT
- Carbapenem (imipenem, meropenem)
- Piperacillin–tazobactam
- Fluoroquinolone

ALTERNATIVE TREATMENT
- A third-generation cephalosporin
- Aztreonam
- Aminoglycoside

ENTEROBIUS VERMICULARIS

GENUS Enterobius

SPECIES
- *E. vermicularis*

MICROBIOLOGIC CHARACTERISTICS
- An intestinal nematode (pinworm infection)

INCUBATION PERIOD
- The life cycle of *E. vermicularis* is 2–6 weeks. However, successive reinfections with the parasite are usually needed to cause symptoms.

EPIDEMIOLOGY
- Worldwide

INFECTIONS
- Enterobiasis (pinworm infection, oxyuriasis)

DIAGNOSIS
- Macroscopic examination of the stools
- Finding characteristic eggs on adhesive tape preparations taken from the perianal skin

TREATMENT
- Pyrantel pamoate 11 mg/kg in a single dose (maximum, 1 g)
- Treatment should be repeated after 2 weeks.
- Treatment of the whole family should be considered, especially if more than 1 family member is infected with the parasite.

ALTERNATIVE TREATMENT
- Mebendazole 100 mg p.o. q12h for 3 days
- Albendazole 400 mg in a single dose

PREVENTION
- Good personal hygiene practices

ENTEROCOCCUS SPECIES

GENUS Enterococcus

SPECIES
- *E. avium*
- *E. casseliflavus*
- *E. durans*
- *E. faecalis*
- *E. faecium*
- *E. gallinarum*
- *E. hirae*
- Others

MICROBIOLOGIC CHARACTERISTICS
- Aerobic, Gram-positive coccus

INCUBATION PERIOD
- Usually, infection follows a prolonged period of colonization with *Enterococcus*.

EPIDEMIOLOGY
- Infections due to *Enterococcus* species have become more frequent the last 2 decades.
- *Enterococcus* isolates are the second most common cause of bacteremia after *Staphylococcus* species in many hospitals.

INFECTIONS
- Bacteremia (polymicrobial in some cases)
- Urinary tract infection
- Acute or subacute endocarditis
- Neonatal, intraabdominal, or pelvic infection
- Meningitis
- Pneumonia
- Skin and soft-tissue infections

DIAGNOSIS
- Culture of the pathogen

TREATMENT
- *E. faecalis:* Amoxicillin, ampicillin, or penicillin G
- In endocarditis or other serious infections, ampicillin 12 g or penicillin 20–30 million units/d with gentamicin (if the MIC is <2,000 μg/mL for gentamicin)
- Endocarditis requires 6 weeks of therapy.
- *E. faecium:* Teicoplanin or vancomycin combined with gentamicin (if the MIC is <2000 μg/mL)

ALTERNATIVE TREATMENT
- Imipenem, vancomycin, teicoplanin, or the combination of amoxicillin–clavulanate, ampicillin–sulbactam, or piperacillin–tazobactam
- For cystitis: Ciprofloxacin, trimethoprim–sulfamethoxazole, and nitrofurantoin are frequently active.

ENTEROCYTOZOON BIENEUSI

See "Microsporidia"

ENTEROVIRUS

GROUP Enterovirus

SUBGROUPS
- Enteroviruses and rhinoviruses are the 2 groups of viruses in the family Picornaviridae that cause disease in humans.
- The group of enteroviruses includes polioviruses (serotypes 1–3), coxsackievirus A and B (several serotypes), enterovirus serotypes 68–71, and hepatitis A virus (enterovirus 72).

MICROBIOLOGIC CHARACTERISTICS
- Single-stranded, RNA viruses

INCUBATION PERIOD
- For acute hemorrhagic conjunctivitis, 12–72 hours

EPIDEMIOLOGY
- Worldwide, common infections

INFECTIONS
- Acute hemorrhagic conjunctivitis (serotype 70)
- Meningoencephalitis, skin rash, and a syndrome similar to poliomyelitis (serotype 71)

DIAGNOSIS
- Cell culture
- Serology may be helpful.

TREATMENT
- Symptomatic treatment

ALTERNATIVE TREATMENT
- There is no effective, specific antiviral treatment.

PREVENTION
- No sharing of towels (to avoid transmission of enterovirus); it may cause acute hemorrhagic conjunctivitis.

EPIDERMOPHYTON FLOCCOSUM

GENUS Epidermophyton

SPECIES
- *E. floccosum*

MICROBIOLOGIC CHARACTERISTICS
- Filamentous fungus (mold) with septated hyaline hyphae

EPIDEMIOLOGY
- Common cause of infection worldwide

INFECTIONS
- Infection of skin (dermatomycosis, tinea)
- All types of tinea (cruris, corporis, pedis, inguinal), except capitis

DIAGNOSIS
- Finding the fungus in clinical samples
- Growth in culture

TREATMENT
- Extensive or inflammatory manifestations: Itraconazole 200 mg/d for 2–4 weeks
- Localized, noninflammatory manifestations: Cyclopyroxolomine (1 application q12h)

ALTERNATIVE TREATMENT
- Onychomycosis: Itraconazole 200 mg/d for 3–6 months

EPSTEIN–BARR VIRUS

See Section II, "Infectious Mononucleosis"

ERYSIPELOTHRIX RHUSIOPATHIAE

GENUS Erysipelothrix

SPECIES
- E. rhusiopathiae

MICROBIOLOGIC CHARACTERISTICS
- Aerobic, Gram-positive bacillus

INCUBATION PERIOD
- Unknown

EPIDEMIOLOGY
- Rare cause of infection (worldwide)

INFECTIONS
- Skin infection (erysipeloid)
- It may also cause a diffuse cutaneous eruption accompanied by systemic symptoms (fever, myalgias, arthralgias).
- Occasionally, systemic infection with endocarditis or bacteremia
- Associated with handling fish, crustaceans, animals, or soil

DIAGNOSIS
- Culture

TREATMENT
- Penicillin G for 10 days

ALTERNATIVE TREATMENT
- Cephalosporin, clindamycin, ciprofloxacin, or carbapenem (imipenem, meropenem)

ESCHERICHIA COLI

See Section II, "*Escherichia coli*"

EUBACTERIUM SPECIES

GENUS Eubacterium

SPECIES
- E. lentum
- E. nodatum
- E. timidum
- Others

MICROBIOLOGIC CHARACTERISTICS
- Anaerobic, pleomorphic, Gram-positive bacillus

EPIDEMIOLOGY
- *Eubacterium* species are part of the normal human flora.
- Subsequently, culture of the organism does not necessarily mean infection due to this organism.

INFECTIONS
- Abscesses and other infections at various sites (almost always mixed infections)
- Periodontal disease
- Septic arthritis in patients with colonic lesions (E. lentum)
- Endometritis in women who wear an IUD (E. nodatum)

DIAGNOSIS
- Culture in anaerobic media

TREATMENT
- Penicillin G or a cephamycin
- Metronidazole

ALTERNATIVE TREATMENT
- Imipenem, meropenem, clindamycin, or a ureidopenicillin

EWINGELLA AMERICANA

GENUS Ewingella

SPECIES
- E. americana

MICROBIOLOGIC CHARACTERISTICS
- Aerobic, Gram-negative bacillus
- Belongs to the Enterobacteriaceae group

EPIDEMIOLOGY
- Rarely grown in cultures
- Its clinical significance is unclear.

INFECTIONS
- Bacteremia, wound infection in immunocompromised patients
- Respiratory tract infection rarely

DIAGNOSIS
- Culture

TREATMENT
- There are scarce data for the efficacy of antimicrobial agents against *E. americana*. More so, multidrug resistance has been reported.
- Cefotaxime, piperacillin/tazobactam, or trimethoprim–sulphomethoxazole have been reported to be active against the bacterium.
- In clinical practice, combinations of trimethoprim–sulfamethoxazole or cefotaxime or an antipseudomonal penicillin, plus an aminoglycoside have been used.

EXOPHIALA SPECIES

GENUS Exophiala

SPECIES
- E. dermatitidis
- E. jeanselmei
- E. moniliae
- E. pisciphila
- E. spinifera

MICROBIOLOGIC CHARACTERISTICS
- Dematiaceous, filamentous fungus (mold)
- Yeasts, pseudohyphae, and septate pigmented hyphae *in vivo*

EPIDEMIOLOGY
- Worldwide

INFECTIONS
- Rare cause of infection
- Occasional cases of corneal, subcutaneous, and systemic infection (prosthetic valve endocarditis, arthritis, brain abscess, pneumonia) due to *Exophiala* species have been reported.

DIAGNOSIS
- Culture of the fungus
- Histopathology

TREATMENT
- Amphotericin B, with or without flucytosine

ALTERNATIVE TREATMENT
- Itraconazole

FASCIOLA SPECIES

GENUS Fasciola

SPECIES
- *F. gigantica*
- *F. hepatica*

MICROBIOLOGIC CHARACTERISTICS
- Trematode helminth (about 3 cm long)

EPIDEMIOLOGY
- Worldwide, rare infection
- Humans are an accidental host.
- Natural parasite of sheep, cattle, and other animal worldwide
- Human disease has been reported in sheep- and/or cattle-raising areas.

INFECTIONS
- The parasites cause fascioliasis, a liver and biliary tree disease.
- Infection outside the liver and the biliary tree may be seen rarely, especially with *F. gigantica*.

DIAGNOSIS
- Similar to *Clonorchis sinensis*
- Serology
- PCR to identify *Fasciola* species

TREATMENT
- There is no satisfactory antiparasitic drug for this infection.
- Bithionol 30–50 mg/kg on alternate days for 10–14 doses has moderate results.
- Endoscopic removal of the parasite through ERCP (endoscopic retrograde cholangiopancreatography) if obstructive cholangiitis occurs
- Triclabendazole is a *veterinary* product that has occasionally been used in humans as a single 10 mg/kg dose. This product is not FDA approved for use in humans.

ALTERNATIVE TREATMENT
- Praziquantel

FASCIOLOPSIS BUSKI

GENUS Fasciolopsis

SPECIES
- *F. buski*

MICROBIOLOGIC CHARACTERISTICS
- Trematode helminth (about 7 cm long)

EPIDEMIOLOGY
- Rural Southeast Asia and India

INFECTIONS
- *F. buski* causes fasciolopsiasis, a disease manifested by gastrointestinal symptoms such as diarrhea, constipation, vomiting, and anorexia. In rare cases, acute intestinal obstruction is caused by the parasites.

DIAGNOSIS
- Parasitologic stool examination

TREATMENT
- Praziquantel 25 mg/kg p.o. q8h for 1 day

ALTERNATIVE TREATMENT
Niclosamide 2 g in a single dose

FLAVIMONAS ORYZIHABITANS

GENUS Flavimonas

SPECIES
- *F. oryzihabitans*

MICROBIOLOGIC CHARACTERISTICS
- Aerobic, Gram-negative bacillus

EPIDEMIOLOGY
- Rare cause of infection

INFECTIONS
- Bacteremia, frequently polymicrobial and associated with intravascular lines
- Peritonitis in patients undergoing peritoneal dialysis
- CNS shunt infection
- Prosthetic joint infection
- Prosthetic valve endocarditis
- Meningitis
- Wound infection

DIAGNOSIS
- Culture

TREATMENT
- An antipseudomonal beta-lactam
- Carbapenem (imipenem, meropenem)

ALTERNATIVE TREATMENT
- Ciprofloxacin, aminoglycoside

FLAVOBACTERIUM SPECIES

GENUS Flavobacterium

SPECIES
- *F. indologenes*
- *F. meningosepticum*
- *F. odoratum*
- Others

MICROBIOLOGIC CHARACTERISTICS
- Aerobic, Gram-negative bacillus
- The taxonomy of these bacteria has not been settled.

INFECTIONS
- Meningitis and bacteremia (*F. meningosepticum,* especially in newborns)
- Endocarditis, particularly on prosthetic valve
- Few reports of nosocomial outbreaks of bacteremia due to *Flavobacterium* associated with contaminated solutions
- Wound infection

DIAGNOSIS
- Culture

TREATMENT
- Ciprofloxacin

ALTERNATIVE TREATMENT
- There are reports of successful use of vancomycin to treat meningitis due to *Flavobacterium* in neonates. This is interesting, because *Flavobacterium* is the only Gram-negative organism for which vancomycin seems to be effective.

FONSECAEA SPECIES

See "Chromoblastomycosis Agents"

FRANCISELLA TULARENSIS

See Section II, "Tularemia"

FOREST DISEASE VIRUS, KYASANUR

GENUS Flavivirus

SPECIES
- N/A

MICROBIOLOGIC CHARACTERISTICS
- Single-stranded, positive RNA virus
- Spheric
- Enveloped

EPIDEMIOLOGY
- Found in several parts of India, China, Southeast Asia, Saudi Arabia

INCUBATION PERIOD
- 3–8 days

INFECTIONS
- Hemorrhagic fever with renal syndrome

DIAGNOSIS
- Cell culture and serology
- PCR

TREATMENT
- Symptomatic

FUSARIUM SPECIES

GENUS Fusarium

SPECIES
- *F. moniliforme*
- *F. oxysporum*
- *F. solani*
- Others

MICROBIOLOGIC CHARACTERISTICS
- Filamentous fungus (mold), with septate hyphae

EPIDEMIOLOGY
- Worldwide infection

INFECTIONS
- Localized infection of skin and subcutaneous tissue
- Keratitis
- Endophthalmitis
- Osteomyelitis and arthritis following trauma or surgery
- Peritonitis in peritoneal dialysis
- Disseminated infections (similar to disseminated aspergillosis, but with higher incidence of cutaneous lesions and fungemia)
- Catheter-associated infections in neutropenic patients and in patients with major burns

DIAGNOSIS
- Identification of the fungus in tissue biopsies
- Culture of the fungus

TREATMENT
- There are limited data on the efficacy of antifungal agents in patients with *Fusarium* infections.
- Amphotericin B i.v. (1.0–1.5 mg/kg/d), with or without flucytosine

ALTERNATIVE TREATMENT
- Surgical removal of operable lesions may be necessary in difficult-to-manage patients with *Fusarium* infections when using only antifungal agents.

FUSOBACTERIUM SPECIES

GENUS Fusobacterium

SPECIES
- *F. alocis*
- *F. mortiferum*
- *F. necrophorum*
- *F. nucleatum*
- *F. periodonticum*
- *F. sulci*
- *F. ulcerans*
- *F. varium*
- Others

MICROBIOLOGIC CHARACTERISTICS
- Anaerobic, Gram-negative bacillus

INCUBATION PERIOD
- Infections are usually endogenous (i.e., from the patient's microbial flora).

EPIDEMIOLOGY
- *Fusobacterium* species are found frequently as part of the normal human oral and bowel flora.

INFECTIONS
- Cervicofacial, pleuropulmonary, abdominal, or pelvis infection (abscesses, usually polymicrobial)
- Soft-tissue infections
- Wound infections (surgical or bite wound)
- Postangina sepsis
- Jugular vein thrombophlebitis and abscesses in the lungs, bones, and CNS
- Endocarditis

DIAGNOSIS
- Anaerobic culture

TREATMENT
- Metronidazole
- Penicillin G

ALTERNATIVE TREATMENT
- Clindamycin
- Cefotetan or cefoxitin
- Carbapenem (imipenem, meropenem)
- Chloramphenicol

GARDNERELLA VAGINALIS

GENUS Gardnerella

SPECIES
- *G. vaginalis*

MICROBIOLOGIC CHARACTERISTICS
- Aerobic, Gram-negative bacillus

EPIDEMIOLOGY
- Worldwide

INFECTIONS
- *G. vaginalis* has been implicated in the pathogenesis of bacterial vaginosis.
- Postpartum endometritis
- Urinary infection in pregnant women
- Bacteremia

DIAGNOSIS
- Culture in specific media
- Clue cells on vaginal smears are diagnostic of bacterial vaginosis.

TREATMENT
- Metronidazole is highly effective for the treatment of vaginosis, although *G. vaginalis* is relatively resistant *in vitro*.
- Metronidazole or clindamycin as a topical application

ALTERNATIVE TREATMENT
- Amoxicillin–clavulanate
- Clindamycin
- In systemic or urinary infection, ampicillin or amoxicillin should be used.

GEMELLA SPECIES

GENUS Gemella

SPECIES
- *G. haemolysans*
- *G. morbillorum*

MICROBIOLOGIC CHARACTERISTICS
- Gram-positive coccus
- Gemella strains are sometimes confused with *viridans* streptococci.

EPIDEMIOLOGY
- Worldwide, rare cause of infection

INFECTIONS
- Endocarditis
- Bacteremia
- *Gemella* strains have been also isolated, rarely, from patients with pneumonia, urinary tract infection, wound infection, abscesses, total knee arthroplasty-related infection, and arteriovenous shunt infection.

DIAGNOSIS
- Culture

TREATMENT
- Penicillin G

ALTERNATIVE TREATMENT
- Vancomycin
- Macrolide

GEOTRICHUM CANDIDUM

GENUS Geotrichum

SPECIES
- *G. candidum*

MICROBIOLOGIC CHARACTERISTICS
- Filamentous fungus (mold), with septate hyphae
- *In vivo*, septate hyaline hyphae with arthroconidia

EPIDEMIOLOGY
- Rare, worldwide infection

INFECTIONS
- Disseminated disease in neutropenics

DIAGNOSIS
- Finding the fungus in tissue biopsies
- Culture of the fungus

TREATMENT
- There are few data about the efficacy of antifungal agents against this fungus.
- Amphotericin B (i.v.) has been used with moderate results.

GIARDIA LAMBLIA

See Section II, "Giardiasis"

GNATHOSTOMA SPINIGERUM

GENUS Gnathostoma

SPECIES
- *G. spinigerum*

MICROBIOLOGIC CHARACTERISTICS
- Most reported cases are from Thailand.
- Nematode helminth of dogs and cats

EPIDEMIOLOGY
- Japan, China, and other Southeast Asian countries
- People and animals are infected with ingestion of undercooked fish or poultry.

INFECTIONS
- The parasites migrate through several tissues of humans or animals, causing gnathostomiasis (transient pruritic, erythematous edema with eosinophilia).
- The brain may be affected, too (focal cerebral lesions and eosinophilic pleocytosis of the CSF are common in patients with gnathostomiasis).

DIAGNOSIS
- Extraction and identification of the parasite

TREATMENT
- The effectiveness of antihelminthic agents is unclear. However, they are commonly used.
- Albendazole 400 mg q12h for 14 days may be given.

ALTERNATIVE TREATMENT
- Successful treatment of ocular lesions has been reported with mebendazole 200 mg q3h for 6 days.

HAEMOPHILUS DUCREYI

GENUS Haemophilus

SPECIES
- *H. ducreyi*

MICROBIOLOGIC CHARACTERISTICS
- Aerobic, Gram-negative coccobacillus

INCUBATION PERIOD
- Usually 3–5 days (sometimes up to 2 weeks)

EPIDEMIOLOGY
- More common in tropical and subtropical climates
- Outbreaks of infections due to *H. ducreyi* have occurred in the US, mainly in inner-city residents and migrant farm workers.
- Men are more likely to develop this infection.

INFECTIONS
- Chancroid (genital ulcer with inguinal adenopathy)

DIAGNOSIS
- Culture in special medium

TREATMENT
- Ceftriaxone 250 mg i.m. (single dose)
- Azithromycin 1 g (single dose)
- Ciprofloxacin 500 mg p.o. q12h for 3 days

ALTERNATIVE TREATMENT
- Erythromycin 0.5 g p.o. q6h for 7 days
- Trimethoprim–sulfamethoxazole (320 and 1600 mg/d, respectively) for 7 days
- Ofloxacin
- Inguinal adenopathy that is fluctuant and larger than 5 cm in diameter should be drained by needle aspiration.

PREVENTION
- Safe-sex practices

HAEMOPHILUS INFLUENZAE

GENUS Haemophilus

SPECIES
- *H. influenzae*

MICROBIOLOGIC CHARACTERISTICS
- Aerobic, Gram-negative coccobacillus

INCUBATION PERIOD
- The incubation period for meningitis due to *H. influenzae* is unknown; however, most data support an incubation period of 2–4 days.

EPIDEMIOLOGY
- Worldwide
- Vaccination programs against *H. influenzae* have led to a dramatic decrease of infections due to this pathogen.

INFECTIONS
- In children, epiglottitis, meningitis, cellulitis, and arthritis are caused by encapsulated strains (serotype b) and are often associated with bacteremia.
- Nonencapsulated strains cause otitis, sinusitis, exacerbations of chronic bronchitis, pneumonia, and, less often, bacteremia; it is seen more frequently in adults.
- In splenectomized patients, it may cause a severe sepsis with a fulminant course.
- Epididymitis
- Orchitis

DIAGNOSIS
- Antigen detection techniques (coagglutination, counterimmunoelectrophoresis, latex) in secretions or body fluids

TREATMENT
- Amoxicillin–clavulanate or a second- or third-generation cephalosporin

ALTERNATIVE TREATMENT
- Trimethoprim–sulfamethoxazole, fluoroquinolones, azithromycin, aztreonam, or carbapenem (imipenem or meropenem)

PREVENTION
- There are several protein–polysaccharide vaccines against *H. influenzae* type B that have been proved effective in children older than 2 months.
- Rifampin and ciprofloxacin have been used as protective measures for close household contacts of patients with *H. influenza* meningitis.

HAEMOPHILUS SPECIES

GENUS Haemophilus

SPECIES
- *H. aegyptius*
- *H. aphrophilus*
- *H. haemolyticus*
- *H. parahaemolyticus*
- *H. parainfluenzae*
- *H. paraphrophilus*
- *H. segnis*

MICROBIOLOGIC CHARACTERISTICS
- Aerobic, Gram-negative coccobacillus

EPIDEMIOLOGY
- Worldwide infections

INFECTIONS
- Bacteremia
- Upper respiratory infection
- Epiglottitis
- Pneumonia exacerbation of chronic bronchitis
- Soft-tissue infection
- Endocarditis
- Meningitis
- Brain abscess
- Urinary tract infection
- Conjunctivitis, sepsis with purpuric manifestations (*H. aegyptius*)

DIAGNOSIS
- Culture

TREATMENT
- Ampicillin (combined with an aminoglycoside in case of endocarditis or sepsis)

ALTERNATIVE TREATMENT
- Third-generation cephalosporin or carbapenem (imipenem or meropenem)

HAFNIA ALVEI

GENUS Hafnia

SPECIES
- *H. alvei*

MICROBIOLOGIC CHARACTERISTICS
- Aerobic, Gram-negative bacillus

INCUBATION PERIOD
- Usually an endogenous infection (*H. alvei* may be a part of the normal human bowel flora)
- In cases of infection associated with contaminated intravenous fluids, symptoms usually start within 1–2 days.

EPIDEMIOLOGY
- The incidence of infections due to *H. alvei* has increased during the past 2 decades (usually nosocomial infections).

INFECTIONS
- Generally nosocomial infections
- Urinary tract infections
- Pneumonia
- Bacteremia associated with intravenous catheters

DIAGNOSIS
- Culture

TREATMENT
- Third-generation cephalosporin
- Aztreonam
- The combination of beta-lactam agent (with antipseudomonal action) with an aminoglycoside is frequently done in severe infections due to Gram-negative bacilli, including *H. alvei*.

ALTERNATIVE TREATMENT
- Carbapenem (imipenem or meropenem)
- Ureidopenicillins
- Ciprofloxacin
- Aminoglycoside

HANSENULA SPECIES

GENUS Hansenula

SPECIES
- *H. anomala*
- *H. polymorpha*

MICROBIOLOGIC CHARACTERISTICS
- Yeast

EPIDEMIOLOGY
- Culture
- Identification of the fungus in clinical biopsy specimens

INFECTIONS
- Fungemia
- Endocarditis
- Meningitis
- Mediastinal lymphadenitis (usually in immunocompromised patients)

DIAGNOSIS
- Rare infection

TREATMENT
- Amphotericin B i.v., with or without flucytosine

HANTAAN VIRUS

GROUP Hantavirus

SPECIES
- Several (see below)

MICROBIOLOGIC CHARACTERISTICS
- 3 circular segments of single-stranded, negative RNA virus
- Helicoidal symmetry
- Enveloped

EPIDEMIOLOGY
- Rare viral infections

INFECTIONS
- Sin nombre virus, Muerto Canyon virus (in southwestern US)
- Fever and pulmonary disease with respiratory failure
- May be associated with hemorrhagic manifestations and renal failure
- In Far East, epidemic hemorrhagic fever, hemorrhagic fever with renal syndrome
- The genus *Hantavirus* includes several species (Seoul, Belgrade, Puumala, Prospect Hill) that are the agents of less severe hemorrhagic fever with renal syndrome.

DIAGNOSIS
- Celt culture serology

TREATMENT
- Ribavirin, 33 mg/kg i.v. initially, followed by 16 mg/kg for 4 days, followed by 8 mg/kg q8h for 6 more days, has been used in China.
- This regimen has been disappointing in early trials in the US.

PREVENTION
- Strict isolation during the entire illness

HELICOBACTER SPECIES

See Section II, "*Helicobacter pylori* Infection"

HENDERSONULA TORULOIDEA

GENUS Hendersonula

SPECIES
- *H. toruloidea*

MICROBIOLOGIC CHARACTERISTICS
- Filamentous fungus (mold) with septate hyphae

INCUBATION PERIOD
- Unknown

EPIDEMIOLOGY
- Worldwide

INFECTIONS
- Similar to tinea (dermatomycosis), affecting the hands, feet, and nails
- Traumatic wound infections
- Sinusitis in diabetics

DIAGNOSIS
- Detection of the fungus in specimens of affected tissue
- Culture of the fungus

TREATMENT
- There are limited reported data for the optimal treatment of this fungal infection.
- Surgical removal of the affected nail may be necessary to eradicate the infection in cases of onychomycosis.
- Amphotericin B should be given in cases of severe, invasive disease.

HEPATITIS VIRUSES

See Section II, "Hepatitis"

HERPES SIMPLEX VIRUS TYPE 1 AND 2

See Section II, "Herpes Simplex Virus Infections"

HUMAN HERPESVIRUS TYPE 6

GROUP Herpesvirus

SPECIES
- N/A

MICROBIOLOGIC CHARACTERISTICS
- Double-stranded DNA virus
- Icosahedral symmetry
- Enveloped

INCUBATION PERIOD
- The mean incubation period, based on experimental infection, is estimated to be approximately 9–10 days.

EPIDEMIOLOGY
- Worldwide

INFECTIONS
- Roseola infantum or exanthem subitum (a febrile infection with or without a rash after defervescence)
- Interstitial pneumonitis
- Mononucleosis-like syndrome in adults with primary infection
- Bone marrow suppression, encephalitis, pneumonia, hepatitis, and exanthem, in bone marrow transplant recipients and immunocompromised patients
- Spontaneous abortion in primary infection during the first trimester of pregnancy

DIAGNOSIS
- Cell culture and serology

TREATMENT
- Symptomatic

HUMAN HERPESVIRUS TYPE 8

GROUP Herpesvirus

SPECIES
- N/A

MICROBIOLOGIC CHARACTERISTICS
- Double-stranded DNA virus

INCUBATION PERIOD
- Unknown

INFECTIONS
- The virus is associated with Kaposi's sarcoma.

DIAGNOSIS
- Cell culture and serology

TREATMENT
- Foscarnet

ALTERNATIVE TREATMENT
- Symptomatic treatment only

HERPES ZOSTER VIRUS

See Section II, "Herpes Zoster"

HETEROPHYES HETEROPHYES

GENUS Heterophyes

SPECIES
- H. heterophyes

MICROBIOLOGIC CHARACTERISTICS
- Nematode helminth
- Small size (2 mm in length)

INCUBATION PERIOD
- Unknown

EPIDEMIOLOGY
- Egypt (Nile delta), Israel, Russia, Japan, Southeast Asia
- Infection is acquired by the consumption of undercooked or salted fish.

INFECTIONS
- Heterophyiasis (frequently asymptomatic, but patients sometimes complain of dyspepsia, mucous diarrhea, and abdominal pain)

DIAGNOSIS
- Parasitologic examination of stools (identification 30 × 15-μm eggs)

TREATMENT
- Praziquantel 25 mg/kg p.o. q8h for 1 day
- No treatment is necessary for asymptomatic patients.

PREVENTION
- Avoid consumption of undercooked fish.

HYMENOLEPSIS SPECIES

GENUS Hymenolepsis

SPECIES
- H. diminuta
- H. nana

MICROBIOLOGIC CHARACTERISTICS
- Very small tapeworms
- H. nana is the only human tapeworm without an obligatory intermediate host.
- H. diminuta is a rat tapeworm (with accidental infection in humans).

INCUBATION PERIOD
- The development of mature worms of H. nana takes about 2 weeks. However, the time to symptoms is variable and depends on the number of worms in the person's bowel.

EPIDEMIOLOGY
- A worldwide infection
- More common in warm than in cold climates
- The most common tapeworm infection in the US
- Infection is usually acquired by ingestion of eggs via contaminated foods or water or directly from fecally contaminated fingers (person-to-person transmission or autoinfection).

INFECTIONS
- Light infection (small number of worms) usually causes no symptoms.
- Heavy infection may cause dyspepsia, abdominal discomfort, and/or diarrhea.

DIAGNOSIS
- Examination of concentrated stools (eggs)

TREATMENT
- Praziquantel 25 mg/kg in a single dose

ALTERNATIVE TREATMENT
- Niclosamide 2 g in a single dose is also effective.

PREVENTION
- Protect food and water from contamination with human and rodent feces.

HYPODERMA SPECIES

See "Myiasis Agents"

INFLUENZA A, B, AND C VIRUS

See Section II, "Influenza"

ISOSPORA BELLI

GENUS Isospora

SPECIES
- I. belli

MICROBIOLOGIC CHARACTERISTICS
- A protozoon

INCUBATION PERIOD
- Unknown

EPIDEMIOLOGY
- Worldwide

INFECTIONS
- Isosporiasis (diarrhea, malabsorption, eosinophilia), particularly in patients with AIDS

DIAGNOSIS
- Examination of concentrated stools (parasitologic examination)
- Kinyoun stain

TREATMENT
- 2 tablets of trimethoprim–sulfamethoxazole (160 mg and 800 mg, respectively) q6h for 10 days, followed by same dose q12h for 3 weeks

ALTERNATIVE TREATMENT
- Pyrimethamine 75 mg/d p.o. and folinic acid 10 mg/d for 2 weeks.
- Doxycycline combined with nitrofurantoin

JUNIN VIRUS (ARGENTINE HEMORRHAGIC FEVER)

See "Arenaviral Hemorrhagic Fevers in South America"

KINGELLA SPECIES

GENUS Kingella

SPECIES
- K. denitrificans
- K. kingae

MICROBIOLOGIC CHARACTERISTICS
- Aerobic, Gram-negative coccobacillus
- Facultative, anaerobic bacterium
- The organism belongs to the HACEK group of bacteria.

INCUBATION PERIOD
- Unknown

EPIDEMIOLOGY
- Usually an endogenous infection (Kingella species may be a part of the normal human flora)

INFECTIONS
- Endocarditis
- Arthritis and osteomyelitis
- Bacteremia (more frequently in children)
- Suttonella indologenes, a bacterium previously called Kingella indologenes, has been associated with eye infections.

DIAGNOSIS
- Culture

TREATMENT
- Penicillin G combined with an aminoglycoside

KLEBSIELLA GRANULOMATIS

GENUS Klebsiella

SPECIES
K. granulomatis (formerly *Calymmatobacterium*)

MICROBIOLOGIC CHARACTERISTICS
- Aerobic, pleomorphic, Gram-negative coccobacillus

INCUBATION PERIOD
- Unknown (probably between 1 and 12 weeks)

EPIDEMIOLOGY
- A sexually transmitted infection
- Rare in industrialized countries
- Cluster outbreaks occasionally occur in the US.
- Endemic in tropical and subtropical areas

INFECTIONS
- Granuloma inguinale (donovanosis): Chronic and progressively destructive disease of the genitalia, inguinal area, and anal area

DIAGNOSIS
- Histologic examination
- A Wright or Giemsa stain of a smear of affected areas reveals the presence of intracytoplasmic, rod-shaped inclusions known as Donovan bodies.
- Culture is difficult and unreliable.

TREATMENT
- Doxycycline 100 mg q12h orally for at least 3 weeks

ALTERNATIVE TREATMENT
- Azithromycin 1 g p.o. once per week
- Ciprofloxacin 750 mg p.o. twice a day
- Erythromycin base 500 mg p.o. q.i.d.
- Trimethoprim–sulfamethoxazole: 1 double-strength tablet twice daily
- Treatment is given for at least 3 weeks and until all lesions have completely healed

PREVENTION
- Safe-sex practice

KLEBSIELLA SPECIES

GENUS Klebsiella

SPECIES
- *K. oxytoca*
- *K. pneumoniae*

MICROBIOLOGIC CHARACTERISTICS
- Aerobic, Gram-negative bacillus

INCUBATION PERIOD
- Usually an endogenous infection (from strains that are part of the normal human flora)

EPIDEMIOLOGY
- Worldwide

INFECTIONS
- Pneumonia, urinary infection, bacteremia
- Atrophic rhinitis
- Rhinoscleroma

DIAGNOSIS
- Culture

TREATMENT
- Consider local epidemiological data regarding potential resistance (i.e. extended spectrum beta-lactamase production)
- Third-generation cephalosporin
- Aztreonam

ALTERNATIVE TREATMENT
- Ciprofloxacin
- Carbapenem (imipenem or meropenem)
- Amoxicillin–clavulanate
- Piperacillin–tazobactam
- Aminoglycoside

KLUYVERA SPECIES

GENUS Kluyvera

SPECIES
- *K. ascorbata*
- *K. cryorencens*

MICROBIOLOGIC CHARACTERISTICS
- Aerobic, Gram-negative bacillus

INCUBATION PERIOD
- Usually an endogenous infection

EPIDEMIOLOGY
- Rare cause of infection
- Worldwide distribution

INFECTIONS
- Bacteremia
- Soft-tissue infection
- Urinary infection
- Pneumonia in immunosuppressed persons

DIAGNOSIS
- Culture

TREATMENT
- There are limited data on *in vitro* susceptibility of *Kluyvera* species to antimicrobial agents.
- Third-generation cephalosporins, antipseudomonal agents, fluoroquinolones, and aminoglycosides are usually effective. There is documented resistance to ampicillin, first- and second-generation cephalosporins.

ALTERNATIVE TREATMENT
- Chloramphenicol

KURTHIA SPECIES

GENUS Kurthia

SPECIES
- *K. gibsonii*
- *K. sibirica*
- *K. zopfii*

MICROBIOLOGIC CHARACTERISTICS
- Aerobic, Gram-positive bacillus

INCUBATION PERIOD
- Unknown

EPIDEMIOLOGY
- Rare cause of infections
- Worldwide distribution
- Intravenous drug users are at higher risk for developing infections due to aerobic, Gram-positive bacilli, including *Kurthia* species.

INFECTIONS
- Endocarditis
- Bacteremia

DIAGNOSIS
- Culture

TREATMENT
- Penicillin G associated with an aminoglycoside (in case of endocarditis)

ALTERNATIVE TREATMENT
- Trimethoprim–sulfamethoxazole
- Chloramphenicol
- Erythromycin

LACTOBACILLUS SPECIES

GENUS Lactobacillus

SPECIES
- *L. acidophilus*
- *L. casei*
- *L. plantarum*
- *L. rhamnosus*
- *L. salivarius*
- Others

MICROBIOLOGIC CHARACTERISTICS
- Gram-positive bacillus
- Microaerophilic

INCUBATION PERIOD
- Usually an endogenous infection

EPIDEMIOLOGY
- *Lactobacillus* strains are part of the normal human vaginal, oral, and bowel flora.
- *Lactobacillus* strains also are found in a variety of food products.
- Changes of the hormonal environment of the vagina lead to changes of the number of lactobacilli locally, which is implicated in the pathogenesis of urinary tract infections (these conditions may permit the overgrowth of other bacterial species).

INFECTIONS
- Endocarditis
- Neonatal meningitis
- Amnionitis
- Bacteremia (especially in neutropenic patients)
- Mediastinitis

DIAGNOSIS
- Culture

TREATMENT
- Penicillin G
- Clindamycin

ALTERNATIVE TREATMENT
- Amoxicillin

LASSA VIRUS

GROUP Arenavirus

SPECIES
- N/A

MICROBIOLOGIC CHARACTERISTICS
- 2 single-stranded, circular RNA segments
- Helicoidal symmetry
- Enveloped

EPIDEMIOLOGY
- Found in West Africa
- Exposure to feces of mouse host (*Mastomys natalensis*)

INFECTIONS
- Lassa fever (hemorrhagic fever)

DIAGNOSIS
- Cell culture and serology

TREATMENT
- Ribavirin

PREVENTION
- Strict isolation for the duration of illness

LECLERCIA ADECARBOXYLATA

GENUS Leclercia

SPECIES
- *L. adecarboxylata*

MICROBIOLOGIC CHARACTERISTICS
- Aerobic, Gram-negative bacillus

INCUBATION PERIOD
- Unknown

EPIDEMIOLOGY
- Worldwide, rare cause of infection

INFECTIONS
- Bacteremia
- Respiratory tract infections
- May be a component of polymicrobial infections such as abscesses

DIAGNOSIS
- Culture

TREATMENT
- Fluoroquinolone

ALTERNATIVE TREATMENT
- Trimethoprim–sulfamethoxazole
- A combination of a beta-lactam agent with an inhibitor of beta-lactamase

LEGIONELLA SPECIES

See "Legionellosis"

LEISHMANIA SPECIES COMPLEX

See Section II, "Leishmaniasis"

LEPTOMYXID SPECIES

GENUS Leptomyxid

SPECIES
- Now referred to as *Balamuthia mandrillaris*

MICROBIOLOGIC CHARACTERISTICS
- Other free-living amoebae of clinical significance include *Naegleria* and *Acanthamoeba*.

INCUBATION PERIOD
- Unknown

EPIDEMIOLOGY
- Worldwide
- Rare cause of infection

INFECTIONS
- Meningoencephalitis
- Most patients are diagnosed postmortem.

DIAGNOSIS
- CSF evaluation
- Direct immunofluorescence and immunoblot to distinguish various strains

TREATMENT
- There is no known effective treatment.

LEPTOSPIRA SPECIES

See Section II, "Leptospirosis"

LEUCONOSTOC SPECIES

GENUS Leuconostoc

SPECIES
- *L. citreum*
- *L. lactis*
- *L. mesenteroides*
- *L. paramesenteroides*
- Others

MICROBIOLOGIC CHARACTERISTICS
- Anaerobic, Gram-positive coccus
- *Leuconostoc* species are sometimes confused with *Enterococcus* species or *viridans group* streptococci.
- The growth of *Leuconostoc* species may represent contamination, but should always be taken seriously in blood cultures for risk of endovascular infection such as endocarditis.

INCUBATION PERIOD
- Unknown

EPIDEMIOLOGY
- Worldwide distribution

INFECTIONS
- The clinical significance of *Leuconostoc* species has not been clarified.
- There are a few reports of bacteremia in newborns and immunocompromised patients.
- Rare cause of endocarditis

DIAGNOSIS
- Culture

TREATMENT
- Penicillin G or ampicillin (high intravenous doses are recommended for severe cases)

ALTERNATIVE TREATMENT
- First-generation cephalosporin
- Clindamycin
- Imipenem
- *Leuconostoc* species are resistant to vancomycin.

LINGUATULA SERRATA

GENUS Linguatula

SPECIES
- *L. serrate*

MICROBIOLOGIC CHARACTERISTICS
- Pentastome helminth (tongue worm)

INCUBATION PERIOD
- Unknown

EPIDEMIOLOGY
- More frequent in the Middle East and Africa
- Parasite of reptiles, birds, and mammals

INFECTIONS
- Immature (nymphal) stages of this parasite sometimes lodge in the human nasopharynx, causing obstruction and irritation. This condition is known as "halzoun and marrara".

DIAGNOSIS
- Histologic examination of biopsy

TREATMENT
- Surgical removal

LISTERIA MONOCYTOGENES

See Section II, "Listeriosis"

LOA LOA

GENUS Loa

SPECIES
- *L. loa*

MICROBIOLOGIC CHARACTERISTICS
- Filarial nematode

INCUBATION PERIOD
- Microfilariae may appear in the peripheral blood roughly 4 months after infection with Loa loa.
- Symptoms may appear as early as 4 months after infection; however, these typically appear after several years.

EPIDEMIOLOGY
- A common infection in Central and West Africa
- Up to 13 million people are infected.
- Loa loa is transmitted to humans by the bite of an infected deer fly.

INFECTIONS
- Most people are asymptomatic.
- Chronic disease (loiasis) manifested by transient swelling of potentially any part of the body (skin, subcutaneous, and deeper tissues). Pruritus and localized pain are common symptoms. These manifestations are from the migration of the adult worm to different parts of the body and are referred to as "Calabar" swellings. Adult worms may also migrate across the eye under the conjunctiva.

DIAGNOSIS
- Finding microfilariae in peripheral blood smear (diurnal blood sample)
- Extracting microfilariae from subcutaneous tissue
- Visualizing worms under the conjunctiva
- Serology

TREATMENT
- Diethylcarbamazine (DEC) is the most effective agent. It kills microfilariae. The drug also may kill adult worms, leading to complete cure in roughly 50% after a single course.
- Hypersensitivity reactions during DEC treatment in patients with a heavy burden of infection may be life threatening.
- Treatment with DEC should be done under careful supervision, especially in cases with severe microfilaremia (>2000/mL of blood), due to the risk of severe meningoencephalitis.

ALTERNATIVE TREATMENT
- Ivermectin
- Albendazole

LYMPHOCYTIC CHORIOMENINGITIS VIRUS

GROUP Arenavirus

SPECIES
- N/A

MICROBIOLOGIC CHARACTERISTICS
- 2 single-stranded, circular RNA segments
- Helicoidal symmetry
- Enveloped

EPIDEMIOLOGY
- Rare cause of infection
- Rodent vector

INFECTIONS
- Fever, adenitis, skin rash, meningoencephalitis with significant lymphocytic pleocytosis

DIAGNOSIS
- Cell culture
- Serology

TREATMENT
- Symptomatic

LYMPHOTROPIC T-CELL HUMAN VIRUS

GROUP Human T-lymphocyte viruses (HTLV-1 and HTLV-2)

SPECIES
- N/A

MICROBIOLOGIC CHARACTERISTICS
- Single stranded, positive RNA; retroviruses
- Enveloped

INCUBATION PERIOD
- Unknown

EPIDEMIOLOGY
- The geographic distribution of these viruses (HTLV-1 and HTLV-2) is not well known, but it is likely that they are found worldwide.
- High seropositivity rates of HTLV-1 have been found in the islands of southeastern Japan and the Caribbean basin.
- Antibodies against HTLV-2 are found in a considerable proportion of intravenous drug users in several countries.

INFECTIONS
- Adult T-cell leukemia and tropical spastic paraparesis
- No disease has been causally associated with HTLV-2 (the virus was initially isolated from 2 patients with hairy-cell leukemia).

DIAGNOSIS
- Cell culture
- Serology
- Antigen detection

TREATMENT
- Symptomatic
- There are limited data about the efficacy of antiviral agents against HTLV-1 or HTLV-2.

PREVENTION
- Methods of prevention are similar to those for HIV.

MACHUPO VIRUS (BOLIVIAN HEMORRHAGIC FEVER)

See "Arenaviral Hemorrhagic Fevers in South America"

MADURELLA SPECIES

GENUS Madurella

SPECIES
- *M. grisea*
- *M. mycetomatis*

MICROBIOLOGIC CHARACTERISTICS
Filamentous fungus (mold), with septate hyaline hyphae

INCUBATION PERIOD
- Months

EPIDEMIOLOGY
- *Madurella* fungi are widespread in nature, found often in soil.
- Symptomatic infection due to these organisms is rare.
- Most cases occur in tropical and subtropical areas (including Northern Africa, Southern Asia, and Central America).

INFECTIONS
- Infection with *Madurella* may lead to local chronic inflammation with formation of sinus tracts.
- Lesions usually appear on the foot or tibia.
- Subcutaneous nodules
- Osteomyelitis

DIAGNOSIS
- Isolation of fungus in cultures from affected tissues
- Granules visible without microscopy are frequently seen in purulent discharge.

TREATMENT
- Ketoconazole

ALTERNATIVE TREATMENT
- Itraconazole
- Surgical removal of lesions

PREVENTION
- Avoiding puncture wounds in endemic areas.

MALASSEZIA SPECIES

GENUS Malassezia

SPECIES
- *M. furfur*
- *M. pachydermatis*
- *M. sympodialis*

MICROBIOLOGIC CHARACTERISTICS
- Lipophilic yeasts
- Supplementation of culture media with lipids help *Malassezia* grow.
- *M. furfur* was previously known as *Pityrosporum orbiculare* or *P. ovale*.

INCUBATION PERIOD
- Unknown

EPIDEMIOLOGY
- Worldwide distribution
- Patients with Cushing syndrome or on total parenteral nutrition are at risk of developing infection.

INFECTIONS
- Pityriasis versicolor (previously called tinea versicolor)
- *M. furfur* may also cause systemic infection in patients (especially immunocompromised patients and neonates) receiving intravenous fluids with high lipid content (e.g., total parenteral nutrition).
- Patients with continuous ambulatory peritoneal dialysis catheters may develop peritonitis due to *M. furfur*.
- A few cases of pneumonia have also been reported.
- *M. pachydermatis* has been reported to cause systemic infection in low-birth-weight children receiving lipid emulsions via a central venous catheter.
- The role of *M. sympodialis* as a cause of a human disease is unclear.

DIAGNOSIS
- Blood culture: The laboratory will often be able to grow the organism in a lipid-rich environment.

TREATMENT
- Pityriasis versicolor is managed with local or systemic azole treatment.
- Itraconazole 200 mg/d by mouth for 7 days usually suffices. A shorter regimen (400 mg itraconazole given once) may be enough for a considerable proportion of patients.
- Some cases of pityriasis versicolor are self-limited.
- Systemic infections due to *Malassezia* require intravenous treatment with azoles (and removal of the central catheters).

ALTERNATIVE TREATMENT
- Selenium sulfur used topically (1 daily application of selenium sulfur 2.5% for half an hour for 2 weeks) is also effective for pityriasis versicolor.

MANSONELLA SPECIES

GENUS Mansonella

SPECIES
- *M. ozzardi*
- *M. perstans*
- *M. streptocerca*

MICROBIOLOGIC CHARACTERISTICS
- Filarial nematode

INCUBATION PERIOD
- Unknown

EPIDEMIOLOGY
- *M. ozzardi* infections occur in Central and South America and in the West Indies.
- *M. perstans* infections occur in West Africa and northeastern South America. It is likely that the organism has a wider geographic distribution than is estimated.
- *M. streptocerca* infections occur in West and Central Africa.

INFECTIONS
- Hypopigmented pruritic dermatitis
- Thought to be milder compared to other filarial infections.

DIAGNOSIS
- Histopathology of skin biopsy
- Finding of microfilariae in affected tissues
- Serology

TREATMENT
- Diethylcarbamazine 50 mg on the first day, 100 mg on the second and third days, followed by 50 mg q8h for 3 weeks

ALTERNATIVE TREATMENT
- Possibly a role for doxycycline

MARBURG VIRUS

See "Filoviruses"

MEASLES VIRUS

See Section II, "Measles"

METAGONIMUS YOKOGAWAI

GENUS Metagonimus

SPECIES
- *M. yokogawai*

MICROBIOLOGIC CHARACTERISTICS
- Trematode helminth

INCUBATION PERIOD
- *Unknown*

EPIDEMIOLOGY
- Rare cause of symptomatic human infection
- Cases of *M. yokogawai* infection have been reported from several areas of the world, including Russia, the Middle East (Israel, Egypt), India, Indonesia, Philippians, China, Japan, and Taiwan.

INFECTIONS
- *M. yokogawai* infection is usually asymptomatic.
- The parasite sometimes leads to gastrointestinal symptoms, including diarrhea, abdominal discomfort, and dyspepsia.

DIAGNOSIS
- Microscopic examination of stool specimens

TREATMENT
- Praziquantel 25 mg/kg p.o. q8h for 1 day (3 doses)

METHYLOBACTERIUM SPECIES

GENUS Methylobacterium

SPECIES
- *M. extorquens*
- *M. mesophilicum*
- Others

MICROBIOLOGIC CHARACTERISTICS
- Aerobic, Gram-negative bacillus
- Previously named *Protomonas* spp.

INCUBATION PERIOD
- Unknown

EPIDEMIOLOGY
- Very rare cause of infection.
- Reports of infections due to these Gram-negative bacilli, which produce pink-pigmented colonies, have increased recently.

INFECTIONS
- Bacteremia
- *Methylobacterium* species may cause infections in immunosuppressed individuals (as opportunistic pathogens).
- Peritonitis (in patients undergoing peritoneal dialysis)

DIAGNOSIS
- Culture

TREATMENT
- Trimethoprim–sulfamethoxazole

ALTERNATIVE TREATMENT
- Ciprofloxacin
- Aminoglycoside

MICROSPORIDIA

GENERA/SPECIES
- The phylum Microspora includes over 100 genera and about 1000 species. Among them, species of certain or possible clinical significance are the following:
- *Enterocytozoon bieneusi*
- *Enterocytozoon cuniculi*
- *Enterocytozoon hellem*
- *Nosema connori*
- *Nosema corneum*
- *Nosema ocularum*
- *Pleistophora species*
- *Septata intestinalis*

MICROBIOLOGIC CHARACTERISTICS
- Microsporidia comprises a group of obligate intracellular, spore-forming protozoa.
- Microsporidia may be reclassified as fungi.

EPIDEMIOLOGY
- Possible routes of transmission include fecal–oral route and the urine–oral routes.
- There is limited understanding about the epidemiology, pathogenesis, and optimal management of infections due to microsporidia.

INFECTIONS
- Microsporidiosis may lead to watery and nonbloody diarrhea. Infection may also lead to biliary tree disease and pulmonary, renal, CNS, and cornea infections. Many immunocompetent individuals may be asymptomatic. Immunocompromised hosts will often have severe diarrheal symptoms.

DIAGNOSIS
- Histologic examination of affected tissue or stool, using light (and electron) microscopy

TREATMENT
- Albendazole

ALTERNATIVE TREATMENT
- Fumagillin preparations (topical treatment) appear to be effective in patients with conjunctival and/or corneal microsporidiosis.

MICROSPORUM SPECIES

GENUS Microsporum

SPECIES
- *M. audouinii*
- *M. canis*
- Others

MICROBIOLOGIC CHARACTERISTICS
- Filamentous fungus (mold)

INCUBATION PERIOD
- Unknown

EPIDEMIOLOGY
- Worldwide infection

INFECTIONS
- All forms of tinea infection (fungal infection of the head, face, trunk, extremities, inguinal areas, interdigital areas, and nails)

DIAGNOSIS
- Identification of the fungus in scrapings of lesions

TREATMENT
- Topical terbinafine twice a day for 2–4 weeks
- Prolonged treatment is needed (2–6 months) for onychomycosis.

ALTERNATIVE TREATMENT
- Itraconazole

MOBILUNCUS SPECIES

GENUS Mobiluncus

SPECIES
- *M. curticei*
- *M. mulieris*

MICROBIOLOGIC CHARACTERISTICS
- Anaerobic, curved, motile, bacillus
- It may be Gram-negative (it is sometimes a Gram-variable organism).

INCUBATION PERIOD
- Unknown

EPIDEMIOLOGY
- *Mobiluncus* strains have been isolated from the vagina in over 50% of women with bacterial vaginosis, and in about 5% of women with no evidence for bacterial vaginosis.

INFECTIONS
- Other bacteria (mainly *Gardnerella vaginalis*) are also frequently isolated from the vaginal fluid of women with bacterial vaginosis.

DIAGNOSIS
- Culture (anaerobic)
- Direct immunofluorescence of vaginal fluid

TREATMENT
- Penicillin

ALTERNATIVE TREATMENT
- Amoxicillin–clavulanate
- Metronidazole is the drug of choice for bacterial vaginosis, regardless of the presence or absence of *Mobiluncus* in vaginal fluid.

MOLLUSCUM CONTAGIOSUM VIRUS

FAMILY Poxviridae

GENUS Molluscipoxvirus

MICROBIOLOGIC CHARACTERISTICS
- Double-stranded DNA virus
- Complex symmetry

INCUBATION PERIOD
- The incubation period varies between 2 and 7 weeks but may be as long as 6 months.

EPIDEMIOLOGY
- Worldwide
- It is spread by direct skin-to-skin contact (including sexual contact and by fomites).
- Humans are the only source of the virus.

INFECTIONS
- Typically few (usually 2–20) papular, waxy, discrete skin lesions with central umbilication
- In patients with AIDS or other causes of immunodeficiency, lesions tend to be larger and more numerous, often affecting extensive areas of skin.

DIAGNOSIS
- Typically a clinical diagnosis; however, may be confused with *Cryptococcus* or *Histoplasma* infection.
- Can also be diagnosed with electron microscopy

TREATMENT
- Lesions are usually self-limited and will regress in 2–4 months in immunocompetent hosts.
- Removal of lesions via cryotherapy or curettage is recommended because of the possibility of autoinoculation and to prevent transmission to others.
- Reconstitution of the immune system will aid recovery in immunocompromised hosts, such as antiretroviral therapy in patients with AIDS.

ALTERNATIVE TREATMENT
- Topical application of several agents, including cantharidin (0.7% in collodion) or peeling agents (e.g., salicylic acid preparations), is also helpful.
- Liquid nitrogen for destruction of lesions can also be successful.

PREVENTION
- In cases of outbreaks, restriction of direct body contact and avoidance of sharing of fomites (such as towels) is recommended.

MORAXELLA (BRANHAMELLA) SPECIES

GENUS Moraxella (Branhamella)

SPECIES
- *M. altantae*
- *M. catarrhalis*
- *M. lacunata*
- *M. nonliquefaciens*
- *M. osloensis*
- *M. phenylpyruvica*

MICROBIOLOGIC CHARACTERISTICS
- Aerobic, Gram-negative coccobacillus

INCUBATION PERIOD
- Unknown

EPIDEMIOLOGY
- *M. catarrhalis* is a common human pathogen.
- *Moraxella* species are part of the normal oral flora of humans and animals.

INFECTIONS
- *Moraxella* species may cause ear and upper and lower respiratory tract infections, including otitis media, sinusitis, laryngitis, acute bronchitis, pneumonia, and bronchopneumonia.
- Neonatal conjunctivitis (usually due to *M. catarrhalis*), blepharoconjunctivitis (due to several *Moraxella* species, usually *M. lacunata*)
- Bacteremia
- Endocarditis
- Arthritis

DIAGNOSIS
- Culture

TREATMENT
- Amoxicillin–clavulanate

ALTERNATIVE TREATMENT
- A macrolide antibiotic
- Fluoroquinolones
- A second-generation cephalosporin
- Trimethoprim–sulfamethoxazole
- *M. catarrhalis* strains frequently produce beta-lactamases.

MORGANELLA MORGANII

GENUS Morganella

SPECIES
- *M. morganii*

MICROBIOLOGIC CHARACTERISTICS
- Aerobic, Gram-negative bacillus

INCUBATION PERIOD
- Unknown

EPIDEMIOLOGY
- Worldwide

INFECTIONS
- Usually nosocomial infections: Urinary, pulmonary, sepsis, also found in snake mouths and may infect bite wounds.

DIAGNOSIS
- Culture

TREATMENT
- Carbapenem (imipenem, meropenem)
- Ciprofloxacin

ALTERNATIVE TREATMENT
- A third-generation cephalosporin, but increasing resistance.
- Aztreonam
- Ofloxacin
- Piperacillin–tazobactam
- Aminoglycoside

MUCOR SPECIES

See Section II, "Mucormycosis"

MUERTO CANYON VIRUS

See "Hantaan Virus"

MULTICEPS MULTICEPS

GENUS Multiceps

SPECIES
- *M. multiceps*

MICROBIOLOGIC CHARACTERISTICS
- Cestode helminth

INCUBATION PERIOD
- Unknown

EPIDEMIOLOGY
- *M. multiceps* is a parasite of dogs.
- Humans acquire infection via ingestion of eggs in dog feces.
- Worldwide distribution

INFECTIONS
- A rare cause of human infection
- Scattered cases of cenurosis (a disease that causes cysts in the CNS) have been reported.

DIAGNOSIS
- Histopathology of removed affected tissues may reveal the parasite.

TREATMENT
- Surgical removal of the cysts, if possible

ALTERNATIVE TREATMENT
- Praziquantel at high doses (>50 mg/kg) may also help.

MUMPS VIRUS

See Section II, "Mumps"

MYCOBACTERIUM, ATYPICAL

See "Atypical Mycobacterial Infections"

MYCOBACTERIUM BOVIS

GENUS Mycobacterium

SPECIES
- *M. bovis*

MICROBIOLOGIC CHARACTERISTICS
- Aerobic, acid-fast bacillus

EPIDEMIOLOGY
- Generally acquired by ingestion of contaminated unpasteurized milk but also via aerosolized respiratory droplets.

INFECTIONS
- *M. bovis* may cause lymphadenitis, pulmonary infection, and gastrointestinal tract infection.

DIAGNOSIS
- Culture

TREATMENT
- INH plus rifampin and either ethambutol or streptomycin
- Some strains have primary resistance to pyrazinamide.
- Most infections require 9 or more months of therapy.

MYCOBACTERIUM LEPRAE

See Section II, "Leprosy"

MYCOBACTERIUM TUBERCULOSIS

See Section II, "Tuberculosis"

MYCOPLASMA SPECIES

GENUS Mycoplasma

SPECIES
- *M. buccale*
- *M. faucium*
- *M. felis*
- *M. genitalium*
- *M. hominis*
- *M. laidlawii*
- *M. lipophilum*
- *M. oculi*
- *M. orale*
- *M. penetrans*
- *M. pirum*
- *M. pneumoniae*
- *M. primatum*
- *M. salivarium*
- *M. spermatophilum*
- *M. urealyticum*

MICROBIOLOGIC CHARACTERISTICS
- Aerobic coccoid bacteria of small size
- *Mycoplasma* species do not have a cell wall.

INCUBATION PERIOD
- *M. pneumoniae* causes clinical syndromes with an incubation period of 6–32 days.

EPIDEMIOLOGY
- Worldwide distribution for all *Mycoplasma* species
- *Mycoplasma* species are frequently commensal organisms, which may be isolated from several human sites. *M. pneumoniae* has a predilection for the oral cavity and the respiratory tract, while *M. hominis* is usually isolated from the genitourinary tract.
- Respiratory tract infection (including pneumonia due to *M. pneumoniae*) is common, especially between the ages of 10 and 40 years.
- Infections due to *M. pneumoniae* may occur in a sporadic, endemic, or even epidemic form.
- Transmission of *M. pneumoniae* occurs, most likely, mainly by droplet inhalation.
- Infection occurs year round.

INFECTIONS

- *M. pneumoniae* is a common cause of upper and lower respiratory tract infections, including pneumonia, bronchitis, tracheobronchitis, pharyngitis, sinusitis, and myringitis.
- *M. pneumoniae* also may cause (rarely) hemolytic anemia, pericarditis, myocarditis, meningoencephalitis, erythema multiforme, and hepatitis.
- *M. fermentans* has been associated with pneumonia, encephalitis, hepatitis, myopericarditis, sepsis, and diarrhea.
- *M. hominis* has been isolated from the endometrium and/or fallopian tubes of about 10% of women with salpingitis. However, an etiologic role cannot be established with certainty in these women, as several microorganisms are often present.
- *M. genitalium* has obtained increasing attention during the past decade as a cause of genitourinary tract infections, including urethritis and pelvic inflammatory disease.
- There are some data that support the role of *Mycoplasma* species in infertility.

DIAGNOSIS

- Culture
- Serology
- Detection of cryoagglutinins for *M. pneumoniae*
- PCR on respiratory samples for *M. pneumoniae*

TREATMENT

- Doxycycline 100 mg p.o. q12h for 7–14 days

ALTERNATIVE TREATMENT

- A macrolide or a fluoroquinolone for *M. pneumoniae* infections
- A fluoroquinolone for other *Mycoplasma* species

PREVENTION

- Avoidance of crowded living and sleeping quarters may decrease the possibility of *M. pneumoniae* infections.
- Safe sexual activity (use of condoms) may decrease the possibility of transmission of *Mycoplasma* species that are part of the urethral and vaginal flora.

MYIASIS AGENTS

GENERA

- Several genera of dipterous flies may cause myiasis. Among them are the following:
- *Calliphora*
- *Chrysomyia*
- *Cochliomyia*
- *Cordylobia*
- *Dermatobia*
- *Gasterophilus*
- *Lucilia*
- *Phormia*
- *Sarcophaga*
- *Wohlfahrtia*

SPECIES

- There are several species in each genus of flies capable of causing myiasis.

MICROBIOLOGIC CHARACTERISTICS

- Flying larvae (arthropods)

EPIDEMIOLOGY

- Tropical and subtropical climates

INFECTIONS

- Myiasis
- Larvae invade skin and subcutaneous tissue and cause local inflammation.

DIAGNOSIS

- Identification of larvae in the affected area

TREATMENT

- 1 usually successful technique is occlusion of the orifice with Vaseline (or other petroleum jelly). Often pork fat is used in endemic countries. The larva's oxygen supply is reduced and larvae will often spontaneously emerge from the skin. Larvae can be gently removed with tweezers. Larvae should not be forcibly removed.

ALTERNATIVE TREATMENT

- Surgical removal of the larvae may be necessary if the previous technique is not successful.

NAEGLERIA FOWLERI

GENUS Naegleria

SPECIES

- *N. fowleri*

MICROBIOLOGIC CHARACTERISTICS

- Free-living amoeba

INCUBATION PERIOD

- 1–3 days

EPIDEMIOLOGY

- Worldwide (temperate regions) in soil, fresh water, brackish water

INFECTIONS

- Rapidly progressing and fulminant meningoencephalitis

DIAGNOSIS

- Fresh examination of CSF and Giemsa or Wright stain
- Culture in special medium

TREATMENT

- An effective treatment is not known.
- Intrathecal and intravenous amphotericin B (1 mg/kg), and miconazole in combination with i.v. or p.o. rifampin, may be tried.

NANOPHYETUS SALMINCOLA

GENUS Nanophyetus

SPECIES

- *N. salmincola*

MICROBIOLOGIC CHARACTERISTICS

- Trematode helminth

INCUBATION PERIOD

- Unknown

EPIDEMIOLOGY

- *N. salmincola* infections in humans have been reported from the northwestern US.

INFECTIONS

- Infection of the gastrointestinal tract, presenting with various nonspecific gastrointestinal symptoms

DIAGNOSIS

- Parasitologic examination of stool specimens (for identification of eggs of the parasite, 64–97 μm long × 43–55 μm wide)

TREATMENT

- Praziquantel 60 mg/kg/d in 3 doses for 1 day

PREVENTION

- Avoidance of eating raw, incompletely cooked, or smoked salmon.

NECATOR AMERICANUS

GENUS Necator

SPECIES
- N. americanus

MICROBIOLOGIC CHARACTERISTICS
- Nematode helminth

EPIDEMIOLOGY
- Common infection in tropical and subtropical regions of the Americas

INFECTIONS
- May be asymptomatic, anemia, diarrhea, abdominal cramping, or anorexia. Patients may have a localized area of pruritis at the site of initial infection and intermittent cough or shortness of breath as the larvae are entering the respiratory tract.

DIAGNOSIS
- Microscopy of stools sample for ova.

TREATMENT
- Mebendazole 100 mg p.o. q12h for 3 days
- Patients with anemia due to a large number of parasites should receive a second cycle of treatment 1–2 weeks after the first cycle.

ALTERNATIVE TREATMENT
- Albendazole 400 mg p.o. in a single dose
- In children, pyrantel pamoate for 3 days may be used.

NEISSERIA GONORRHOEAE

See Section I, "Urethral Discharge/Urethritis"

NEISSERIA MENINGITIDIS

See Section II, "Meningitis, Acute"

NEISSERIA SPECIES

GENUS Neisseria

SPECIES
- N. canis
- N. cinerea
- N. elongata
- N. flavescens
- N. gonorrhoeae
- N. lactamica
- N. meningitidis
- N. mucosa
- N. polysaccharea
- N. sicca
- N. subflava
- N. weaveri

MICROBIOLOGIC CHARACTERISTICS
- Aerobic, Gram-negative cocci

INCUBATION PERIOD
- The incubation period for gonorrhea (caused by N. gonorrhoeae) is usually 2–7 days; occasionally, a longer incubation period may be observed.
- The incubation period of meningitis due to N. meningitidis is usually 3–4 days; occasionally, a shorter (2 days) or longer (5–10 days) incubation period may be observed.
- The incubation period of infections due to other Neisseria species is unknown.

EPIDEMIOLOGY
- Common cause of human infections
- N. gonorrhoeae is usually sexually transmitted.
- N. gonorrhoeae also may be transmitted from mother to neonate and cause neonatal conjunctivitis.
- Other Neisseria species are transmitted, usually, by air droplets.

INFECTIONS
- Meningitis
- Endocarditis
- Bacteremia
- Dog-bite wound infection (N. weaveri)
- N. gonorrhoeae may cause several syndromes, including urethritis, epididymitis, prostatitis, cervicitis, pelvic inflammatory disease, proctitis, pharyngitis, perihepatitis (Fitz-Hugh–Curtis syndrome). A systemic infection can be manifested by monoarthritis, tenosynovitis, and a pustular rash.
- N. meningitidis may cause meningitis, bacteremia, lower and upper respiratory tract infections, conjunctivitis, and a systemic syndrome manifested by rash, fever, and arthritis.

DIAGNOSIS
- Blood culture
- Thayer Martin culture media should be used for synovial, cervical, urethral, rectal, or skin specimens

TREATMENT
- Third-generation cephalosporin
- Please see corresponding chapters for details on treatment of urethritis, pelvic inflammatory disease, cervicitis, and meningitis.

ALTERNATIVE TREATMENT
- Spectinomycin for penicillin allergic patients.

NOCARDIA SPECIES

See Section II, "Nocardiosis"

NORWALK VIRUS

See "Caliciviruses and Calici-like Viruses"

NOSEMA SPECIES

See "Microsporidia"

OCHROBACTRUM ANTHROPI

GENUS Ochrobactrum

SPECIES
- O. anthropi

MICROBIOLOGIC CHARACTERISTICS
- Aerobic, Gram-negative bacillus

INCUBATION PERIOD
- Unknown

EPIDEMIOLOGY
- Rare cause of human infection
- This microorganism has been isolated from various environmental sources and human specimens.

INFECTIONS
- Central venous catheter-related bacteremia is the main infection caused by O. anthropi.
- Peritonitis and septic arthritis has been reported

DIAGNOSIS
- Culture

TREATMENT
- Trimethoprim–sulfamethoxazole

ALTERNATIVE TREATMENT
- Imipenem
- Aminoglycosides
- Fluoroquinolone

OERSKOVIA SPECIES

GENUS Oerskovia

SPECIES
- *O. turbata*
- *O. xanthineolytica*

MICROBIOLOGIC CHARACTERISTICS
- Aerobic (facultatively anaerobic), Gram-positive bacillus
- Branching filamentous bacteria, which fragment into pleomorphic rods
- Catalase-positive microorganism
- Some experts believe that this genus should be combined with the genus *Cellulomonas*.

INCUBATION PERIOD
- Unknown

EPIDEMIOLOGY
- Infections due to *Oerskovia* species were underestimated until recently because of problems related to microbiologic recognition of the pathogen.
- Sources of isolation of *Oerskovia* species include CSF, blood, heart tissue, ascitic fluid, and urine.
- Infection is frequently associated with a foreign body.
- Bacteremia (especially in patients with central venous catheters)
- Endocarditis
- Endophthalmitis
- Meningitis
- Peritonitis
- Urinary tract infection

INFECTIONS
- Line-associated sepsis
- Prosthetic valve endocarditis

DIAGNOSIS
- Culture

TREATMENT
- There are very limited data for the efficacy of antimicrobial agents.
- Removal of a foreign body (e.g., central venous catheter)
- Ampicillin or penicillin has been successfully used.

ALTERNATIVE TREATMENT
- Third-generation cephalosporin, vancomycin, aminoglycoside, imipenem, or trimethoprim–sulfamethoxazole

OLIGELLA SPECIES

GENUS Oligella

SPECIES
- *O. ureolytica*
- *O. urethralis*

MICROBIOLOGIC CHARACTERISTICS
- Anaerobic, Gram-negative coccobacillus

INCUBATION PERIOD
- Unknown

EPIDEMIOLOGY
- Most isolates of *Oligella* have been found in urine specimens.

INFECTIONS
- Rare cause of urinary tract infection

DIAGNOSIS
- Culture

TREATMENT
- There are very limited available data for the *in vitro* susceptibility of *Oligella* species to various antimicrobial agents.
- Penicillin may be effective.

ALTERNATIVE TREATMENT
- Cephalosporin

OMSK VIRUS (HEMORRHAGIC FEVER)

See "Hantaan Virus"

ONCHOCERCA VOLVULUS

GENUS Onchocerca

SPECIES
- *O. volvulus*

MICROBIOLOGIC CHARACTERISTICS
- Filarial (nematode) worm

INCUBATION PERIOD
- The incubation period from larval inoculation to microfilariae in the skin is approximately 6–12 months.

EPIDEMIOLOGY
- Sub-Saharan Africa, southwestern Saudi Arabia, Yemen, Central and South America
- Infection is transmitted to humans only by the bite of infected black flies of the genus *Simulium*.

INFECTIONS
- *O. volvulus* causes onchocerciasis, a chronic, nonfatal disease manifested by subcutaneous nodules.
- Microfilariae may reach the eye and cause visual abnormalities and even blindness (river blindness).

DIAGNOSIS
- Microscopic examination of fresh skin biopsy incubated in water or saline may show the presence of microfilariae.
- Slit lamp examination
- Serology is nonspecific and will cross react with other filarial infections.
- Detection of adult worms in excised nodules

TREATMENT
- Ivermectin
- Retreatment every 6 months to 1 year is recommended.
- Caution in using ivermectin in those co-infected with Loa loa.

ALTERNATIVE TREATMENT
- Suramin: Treatment with suramin should be done under close medical supervision, due to possible nephrotoxicity and other adverse effects.
- Diethylcarbamazine should not be used, due to the possible, severe adverse effects, which are observed in patients with heavy burden of infection.

PREVENTION
- Avoiding bug bites in endemic areas.

OPISTHORCHIS SPECIES

GENUS Opisthorchis

SPECIES
- *O. felineus*
- *O. viverrini*

MICROBIOLOGIC CHARACTERISTICS
- Trematode helminth

INCUBATION PERIOD
- 10–30 days after consumption of contaminated fish.

EPIDEMIOLOGY
- About 2 million people in the countries of the former Soviet Union are infected with *O. felineus*.
- High rates of infections due to *O. viverrini* are found in Thailand, especially in the northern part of the country.

INFECTIONS
- Opisthorchiasis is manifested by obstructive jaundice and cholangitis.
- Opisthorchiasis is considered to be a risk factor for cholangiocarcinoma (as is thought for clonorchiasis, which is caused by *Clonorchis sinensis*).
- Chronic symptoms of dyspepsia, fatigue, and vague abdominal pain may occur as well.

DIAGNOSIS
- Parasitologic examination of stools
- Serology may be helpful but is not specific

TREATMENT
- Praziquantel 25 mg/kg every 8 hours for 1 day

PREVENTION
- Cook or freeze freshwater fish.

ORF VIRUS

GROUP Parapoxvirus (family Poxviridae)

SPECIES
- N/A

MICROBIOLOGIC CHARACTERISTICS
- Double-stranded DNA virus

INCUBATION PERIOD
- Usually 3–6 days

EPIDEMIOLOGY
- Worldwide infections
- Infection is usually transmitted to humans by direct contact with infected animals (usually sheep or goats; rarely deer or reindeer).
- A common infection in persons who are at risk because of their professions (shepherds, abattoir workers, and veterinarians in areas producing sheep and goats, such as New Zealand).

INFECTIONS
- Small, painless nodule(s), usually localized in the hands
- A lesion is usually solitary.
- Lesions may become pustular when secondary bacterial infection occurs.

DIAGNOSIS
- Direct identification of the virus under electron microscopy (ovoid parapoxvirus are seen in affected tissues)
- Serology tests
- Growth of virus in cell cultures of ovine, bovine, or primate origin

TREATMENT
- Usually a self-limited infection

ALTERNATIVE TREATMENT
- There is no specific antiviral treatment.

PREVENTION
- Good personal hygiene of persons exposed to the virus
- General cleanliness of animal-housing areas

PAECILOMYCES SPECIES

GENUS Paecilomyces

SPECIES
- *P. javanicus*
- *P. litacinus*
- *P. marquandii*
- *P. variotii*

MICROBIOLOGIC CHARACTERISTICS
- Filamentous fungus (mold)
- It resembles *Penicillium* species in morphology.

INCUBATION PERIOD
- Unknown

EPIDEMIOLOGY
- Worldwide distribution
- Rare cause of human infection

INFECTIONS
- *Paecilomyces* isolates were usually considered contaminants. However, recent data support the idea that the fungus has a pathogenetic potential and may lead to infection of several sites.
- Keratitis
- Endophthalmitis
- Sinusitis
- Fungemia
- Respiratory tract infection
- Skin and subcutaneous tissue infection
- Endocarditis

DIAGNOSIS
- Culture
- Tissue biopsy (histopathology)

TREATMENT
- Amphotericin B i.v.
- Voriconazole

ALTERNATIVE TREATMENT
- Flucytosine may be added to treatment with amphotericin B.
- Surgical management may be necessary in cases of endophthalmitis, sinusitis, or endocarditis.

PANTOEA AGGLOMERANS

GENUS Pantoea

SPECIES
- *P. agglomerans*

MICROBIOLOGIC CHARACTERISTICS
- Aerobic, Gram-negative bacillus
- Formerly called *Enterobacter agglomerans*

INCUBATION PERIOD
- Unknown

EPIDEMIOLOGY
- Rare, worldwide infection

INFECTIONS
- *P. agglomerans* is usually a cause of nosocomial infections.
- Urinary tract infection
- Bacteremia (related to central venous catheter or not)
- Pneumonia
- A rare cause of meningitis in neonates
- Liver abscess

DIAGNOSIS
- Culture

TREATMENT
- Third-generation cephalosporin

ALTERNATIVE TREATMENT
- Ciprofloxacin
- Carbapenem (imipenem or meropenem)
- Aminoglycoside
- Aztreonam

PAPILLOMAVIRUS

See Section II, "Warts" and "Cervicitis"

PARACOCCIDIOIDES BRASILIENSIS

GENUS Paracoccidioides

SPECIES
- *P. brasiliensis*

MICROBIOLOGIC CHARACTERISTICS
- Dimorphic fungus

INCUBATION PERIOD
- The incubation period is highly variable, ranging from 1 month to many years.

EPIDEMIOLOGY

P. brasiliensis is endemic in tropical and subtropical areas of South and Central America.

Farmers and workers in construction are at risk of infection due to exposure to contaminated soil.

INFECTIONS
- *P. brasiliensis* causes paracoccidioidomycosis (also called South American blastomycosis).
- Paracoccidioidomycosis is a potentially fatal infection that usually affects the lungs (pneumonia) and the oral, nasal, and gastrointestinal tract mucosa (ulcerative lesions); lymphadenopathy is common.
- The infection may affect any organ.
- Adrenal glands are commonly affected.
- Bone marrow involvement is common in the acute form of the infection.

DIAGNOSIS
- Serologic tests
- Identification of the organism in biopsies, sputum, or aspirates from affected tissue (e.g., ascites, lymph nodes).

TREATMENT
- Itraconazole or ketoconazole are preferred for mild-to-moderate infection. They should be given for a prolonged period (at least 6 months).
- In cases of severe infection or CNS involvement, amphotericin B is the drug of choice.

ALTERNATIVE TREATMENT
- Sulfadiazine 4–6 g/d for several months and then 2–3 g/d for 3–5 years
- Voriconazole

PARAGONIMUS SPECIES

GENUS Paragonimus

SPECIES
- *P. africanus*
- *P. kellicotti*
- *P. mexicanus (P. peruvianus)*
- *P. skrjabini*
- *P. uterobilateralis*
- *P. westermani*

MICROBIOLOGIC CHARACTERISTICS
- Trematode helminth

INCUBATION PERIOD
- The interval between infection and symptoms is several months.

EPIDEMIOLOGY
- Infection is transmitted to humans after consuming infected crabs or crayfish.
- *P. africanus* and *P. uterobilateralis* are endemic in Africa (especially in Central Africa).
- *P. mexicanus* is endemic in the Americas.
- *P. westermani* and *P. skrjabini* are endemic in Asia.
- *P. kellicotti* has been found in the US and Canada.

INFECTIONS
- Most infections are asymptomatic.
- Lungs are usually involved in paragonimiasis.
- Clinical features include cough, pleuritic chest pain, and hemoptysis.
- Diffuse or segmental infiltrates, cavities, ring cysts, nodules, and/or pleural effusions may be seen in lung imaging (chest x-rays or CT scan).
- Extrapulmonary manifestations of paragonimiasis are also seen frequently. The infection may affect any organ.

DIAGNOSIS
- Eggs of *Paragonimus* species may be found in sputum specimens.
- Eggs of the parasite also may be found in stool specimens.
- Serologic tests are available.
- Chest x-ray abnormalities due to paragonimiasis may be mistakenly attributed to tuberculosis.

TREATMENT
- Praziquantel 25 mg/kg p.o. q8h for 3 days

ALTERNATIVE TREATMENT
- Bithionol 15–25 mg/kg q12h (alternate days) for 10–14 doses
- Steroids may be beneficial in cases of CNS involvement.

PREVENTION
- Thorough cooking of crustacea

PARAINFLUENZA VIRUS

GROUP/TYPES Paramyxovirus (types 1–4)

SPECIES
- N/A

MICROBIOLOGIC CHARACTERISTICS
- Single-stranded, RNA virus (large)
- Helicoidal symmetry
- Enveloped virus

INCUBATION PERIOD
- From 2 to 6 days

EPIDEMIOLOGY
- Worldwide infection
- Parainfluenza virus infections may present in an epidemic or sporadic fashion.

INFECTIONS
- Major cause of laryngotracheobronchitis (croup)
- Frequent cause of other upper respiratory tract infections
- Rare cause of pneumonia and bronchiolitis
- Immunosuppressed individuals may develop severe parainfluenza viral infections.

DIAGNOSIS
- Serology tests
- Antigen detection assays
- Viral cultures
- PCR is recommended in immunocompromised hosts

TREATMENT
- In mild infections, only symptomatic treatment suffices.
- Racemic epinephrine aerosol reduces airway obstruction in patients with severe laryngotracheobronchitis (croup).
- Intubation may be necessary in patients with severe croup.

PREVENTION
- Handwashing is emphasized in an effort to reduce nosocomial transmission rates of parainfluenza infections.

PARVOVIRUS B-19

See Section II, "Parvovirus Infections"

PASTEURELLA SPECIES

GENUS Pasteurella

SPECIES
- *P. aerogenes*
- *P. canis*
- *P. gallinarum*
- *P. haemolytica*
- *P. multocida*
- *P. pneumotropica*
- Others

MICROBIOLOGIC CHARACTERISTICS
- Aerobic, Gram-negative bacillus

INCUBATION PERIOD
- Usually less than 24 hours

EPIDEMIOLOGY
- Part of the normal oropharyngeal flora of many animals, including 70–90% of cats and 20–50% of dogs
- Transmission usually occurs to humans from animal bites.
- Respiratory spread from animals to humans also occurs.
- Human-to-human transmission has not been documented.

INFECTIONS
- Cellulitis at the site of a scratch or bite of a cat, dog, or other animal
- Regional lymphadenopathy is common.
- Septic arthritis, tenosynovitis, or osteomyelitis may occur locally at the site of the animal scratch or bite.
- *Pasteurella* species also may cause infection of other sites, including respiratory tract infections, meningitis, peritonitis, urinary tract infection, appendicitis, hepatic abscess, and ocular infections (conjunctivitis, keratitis, and endophthalmitis).

DIAGNOSIS
- Culture

TREATMENT
- Penicillin G or amoxicillin–clavulanic acid for 7–10 days in cases of cellulitis.
- The duration of treatment should be at least 14 days in invasive infection.

ALTERNATIVE TREATMENT
- Doxycycline
- Third-generation cephalosporin
- Ofloxacin
- Trimethoprim–sulfamethoxazole

PREVENTION
- Avoid animal bites and scratches.
- Promptly clean, irrigate, and debride (if needed) areas of animal bites and scratches.
- Antibiotic prophylaxis may be given after an animal bite, but data to support its use are lacking.

PEDICULUS AND PHTHIRUS SPECIES (LICE)

GENERA Pediculus/Phthirus

SPECIES
- *Pediculus humanus capitis*
- *Pediculus humanus corporis*
- *Phthirus pubis*

MICROBIOLOGIC CHARACTERISTICS
- Lice

INCUBATION PERIOD
- The life cycles of *Pediculus* and *Phthirus* species are composed of 3 stages: Eggs, nymphs, and adults. Under optimal temperature conditions, the eggs hatch in 7–10 days, and the nymphal stage lasts about 7–13 days.
- The egg-to-egg cycle lasts about 3 weeks.

EPIDEMIOLOGY
- Worldwide distribution
- More common in populations with poor personal hygiene

INFECTIONS
- *Pediculus humanus capitis* causes head lice and is found on the hair, eyelashes, and eyebrows.
- *Pediculus humanus corporis* causes body lice.
- *Phthirus pubis* (crab lice) causes infestation on the pubic hair. In cases of heavy infestation, *P. pubis* may be found on the facial hair, axillae, and body surfaces.
- Both *Pediculus* and *Phthirus* species may cause severe itching.
- Local lymphadenitis may be caused from secondary bacterial infection.

DIAGNOSIS
- Visual inspection of the organism.

TREATMENT
- Head and pubic lice: 1% pyrethrin cream rinse or 1% gamma benzene hexachloride lotion. Retreatment may be necessary 7–10 days after the first treatment (if eggs of the parasite survive).
- Body lice: Clothing and bedding should be washed with the hot-water cycle of an automatic washing machine or dusted with pediculicides.

PREVENTION
- Regular inspection of children (by direct examination)
- Effective, prompt treatment of patients with lice
- Avoidance of physical contact with infected individuals

PEDIOCOCCUS SPECIES

GENUS Pediococcus

SPECIES
- *P. acidilactici*
- *P. pentosaceus*

MICROBIOLOGIC CHARACTERISTICS
- Aerobic, Gram-positive coccus
- May be confused with *Leuconostoc* species

INCUBATION PERIOD
- Unknown

EPIDEMIOLOGY
- Worldwide

INFECTIONS
- Isolates of *Pediococcus* have been traditionally considered contaminants.
- However, recent data support the pathogenic role of *Pediococcus* species, especially in immunosuppressed patients.
- Bacteremia
- Respiratory tract infections

DIAGNOSIS
- Culture

TREATMENT
- Penicillin G
- Ampicillin
- Daptomycin

ALTERNATIVE TREATMENT
- Aminoglycoside
- Imipenem

PENICILLIUM SPECIES

GENUS Penicillium

SPECIES
- *P. chrysogenum*
- *P. commune*
- *P. marneffei*
- Others

MICROBIOLOGIC CHARACTERISTICS
- Filamentous fungus (mold), with septate hyaline hyphae

INCUBATION PERIOD
- Unknown

EPIDEMIOLOGY
- *P. marneffei* is a common cause of infection in the East Asia.

INFECTIONS
- It has been traditionally considered a contaminant.
- More recent data support a pathogenic role for *Penicillium* species.
- *P. marneffei* usually causes disseminated infection in immunosuppressed patients.
- *Penicillium* species also may cause infection in several organs, including the heart valves (endocarditis), the cornea (keratitis), external ear (otitis externa), and the respiratory and urinary tract systems.
- *P. marneffei* has caused significant morbidity in untreated HIV-infected patients of South East Asia

DIAGNOSIS
- Culture
- Tissue biopsy

TREATMENT
- Amphotericin B i.v. is the recommended agent for severe *Penicillium* infections.

ALTERNATIVE TREATMENT
- Itraconazole in a high dose (at least 400 mg/d) is also effective.

PEPTOCOCCUS NIGER

GENUS Peptococcus

SPECIES
- *P. niger*

MICROBIOLOGIC CHARACTERISTICS
- Anaerobic, Gram-positive coccus
- Usually an endogenous infection: *P. niger* is part of the normal human bowel flora.

EPIDEMIOLOGY
- A frequent isolate in mixed infections (due to anaerobic and aerobic bacteria)
- Worldwide

INFECTIONS
- *P. niger* is isolated from patients with polymicrobial infections, such as intraabdominal, pelvic, brain, and lung abscesses.
- It also may cause bacteremia of unclear etiology.

DIAGNOSIS
- Culture under anaerobic conditions.

TREATMENT
- Penicillin G

ALTERNATIVE TREATMENT
- Clindamycin
- Cephamycin
- Carbapenem (imipenem or meropenem)
- Vancomycin
- Piperacillin–tazobactam

PEPTOSTREPTOCOCCUS SPECIES

GENUS Peptostreptococcus

SPECIES
- *P. anaerobius*
- *P. asaccharolyticus*
- *P. magnus*
- *P. prevotii*
- Others

MICROBIOLOGIC CHARACTERISTICS
- Anaerobic, Gram-positive coccus

INCUBATION PERIOD
- Usually a cause of endogenous infection

EPIDEMIOLOGY
- Part of the normal human mouth, vaginal, and bowel flora
- Worldwide distribution

INFECTIONS
- The pathogen is sometimes isolated from specimens of patients with polymicrobial infections, such as intraabdominal, pelvic, lung, and brain abscess.
- Rare cause of endocarditis
- Bacteremia
- Skin and soft tissue infection
- Surgical wound infections
- Septic arthritis

DIAGNOSIS
- Culture under anaerobic conditions.

TREATMENT
- Penicillin G

ALTERNATIVE TREATMENT
- Clindamycin
- Cephamycin
- Carbapenem (imipenem or meropenem)
- Vancomycin

PHIALOPHORA SPECIES

See "Chromoblastomycosis Agents"

PHTHIRUS PUBIS

See "*Pediculus* and *Phthirus* Species (Lice)"

PIEDRAIA HORTAE

GENUS Piedraia

SPECIES
- P. hortae

MICROBIOLOGIC CHARACTERISTICS
- A fungus
- Hyphae are closely septate, dark, and thick walled.

INCUBATION PERIOD
- Unknown

EPIDEMIOLOGY
- Mainly seen in tropical countries

INFECTIONS
- P. hortae causes black piedra, an infection seen most commonly in the tropics.
- Black piedra is manifested by small, gritty, dark nodules along the hair shafts.
- Black piedra should be differentiated from white piedra, which is manifested by soft, pasty nodules on the hair shafts and is caused by Trichosporon beigelii.

DIAGNOSIS
- Visualization fungus on hair shaft with microscopy and fungal stains.
- Culture

TREATMENT
- Shaving of the affected area

ALTERNATIVE TREATMENT
- Terbinafine

PLASMODIUM SPECIES

See Section II, "Malaria"

PLEISTOPHORA SPECIES

See "Microsporidia"

PLESIOMONAS SHIGELLOIDES

GENUS Plesiomonas

SPECIES
- P. shigelloides

MICROBIOLOGIC CHARACTERISTICS
- Aerobic, Gram-negative bacillus

INCUBATION PERIOD
- The exact incubation period is unclear. Evidence from patients with traveler's diarrhea supports a short incubation period (a few days).

EPIDEMIOLOGY
- Ubiquitous freshwater and soil inhabitant

INFECTIONS
- P. shigelloides may cause diarrhea ranging from mild self-limited disease to severe, bloody diarrhea associated with fever, malaise, and white blood cells in stool specimens.
- The pathogen also may rarely cause bacteremia, skin and subcutaneous tissue infection, septic arthritis, osteomyelitis, cholecystitis, endophthalmitis, and meningitis, especially in neonates.
- P. Shigelloides is an major cause of traveler's diarrhea

DIAGNOSIS
- Culture

TREATMENT
- Fluids and electrolytes
- Fluoroquinolone

ALTERNATIVE TREATMENT
- Chloramphenicol
- Trimethoprim–sulfamethoxazole
- Carbapenems
- Aminoglycosides

PNEUMOCYSTIS CARINII

See Section II, "Pneumocystis carinii"

POLIOMYELITIS VIRUS

See Section II, "Poliomyelitis"

POLYOMAVIRUSES

See Section II, "Progressive Multifocal Encephalopathy"

PORPHYROMONAS SPECIES

GENUS Porphyromonas

SPECIES
- P. asaccharolytica
- P. endodontalis
- P. gingivalis
- P. salivosa

MICROBIOLOGIC CHARACTERISTICS
- Anaerobic, Gram-negative bacillus
- Porphyromonas species were classified previously in the genus Bacteroides.

INCUBATION PERIOD
- Usually an endogenous infection

EPIDEMIOLOGY
- Porphyromonas species are part of the normal human flora of the mouth, bowel, and vagina.

INFECTIONS
- Porphyromonas species are isolated in many polymicrobial aerobic and anaerobic infections, such as intraabdominal, pelvic, brain, and lung abscesses, as well as empyema.
- Porphyromonas species are often an etiology of periodontal and oropharyngeal infections.
- Rare cause of bacteremia
- It may be associated with infections due to human bites.
- Skin and subcutaneous tissue infections, including diabetic foot infections

DIAGNOSIS
- Culture under anaerobic conditions

TREATMENT
- Clindamycin or metronidazole

ALTERNATIVE TREATMENT
- Penicillin
- Amoxicillin
- Ticarcillin–clavulanate
- Piperacillin–tazobactam
- Chloramphenicol
- Carbapenem (imipenem or meropenem)

PREVOTELLA SPECIES

GENUS Prevotella

SPECIES
- P. bivia
- P. buccae
- P. buccalis
- P. corporis
- P. denticola
- P. disiens
- P. heparinolytica
- P. intermedia
- P. loescheii
- P. melaninogenica
- P. nigrescens
- P. oralis
- P. oulorum
- P. pallens
- Others

MICROBIOLOGIC CHARACTERISTICS
- Anaerobic, Gram-negative bacillus
- Prevotella species were classified previously in the Bacteroides genus.

INCUBATION PERIOD
- Usually an endogenous infection

EPIDEMIOLOGY
- Prevotella species are part of the normal human flora (oral, bowel, and vagina).

INFECTIONS
- Lung, intraabdominal, brain abscess
- Dental infections
- Pelvic infections (mainly P. disiens and P. bivia)
- Human bite infections
- Skin and subcutaneous tissue infection including diabetic foot infections
- Surgical wound infections

DIAGNOSIS
- Culture under anaerobic conditions.

TREATMENT
- Clindamycin or metronidazole

ALTERNATIVE TREATMENT
- Amoxicillin
- Ampicillin–sulbactam
- Piperacillin–tazobactam
- Ticarcillin–clavulanate
- Chloramphenicol
- Cefoxitin
- Cefotetan
- Carbapenem (imipenem or meropenem)

PRIONS

GENUS N/A

SPECIES
- N/A

MICROBIOLOGIC CHARACTERISTICS
- Prions are thought to be proteinaceous material and are often referred to as proteinaceous infectious particles
- Although they lack nucleic acid, it seems that they possess severe infectious capabilities.

INCUBATION PERIOD
- The incubation period is unknown, but likely quite long in most cases (often several years to decades).
- Cases of a variant of Creutzfeldt–Jakob disease have recently caused considerable concern in Europe.

INFECTIONS
- Kuru
- Creutzfeldt–Jakob disease (sporadic and familial, including the variant possibly related to the agent of bovine spongiform encephalopathy [BSE]) and Gerstmann–Straussler syndrome
- Insomnia secondary to thalamic destruction
- Slow encephalopathy with a very prolonged incubation, scant inflammatory reaction and spongiform changes, with progressive neuro-deterioration and death

DIAGNOSIS
- Direct visualization of the infectious proteinaceous particles using electron microscopy
- CSF with 14-3-3 protein
- Characteristic EEG findings

TREATMENT
- There is no effective treatment.

PROPIONIBACTERIUM PROPIONICUS

See Section II, "Actinomycosis"

PROPIONIBACTERIUM SPECIES

GENUS Propionibacterium

SPECIES
- P. ances
- Others

MICROBIOLOGIC CHARACTERISTICS
- Anaerobic, Gram-positive bacillus

INCUBATION PERIOD
- Unknown (usually an endogenous infection from the patient's flora)

EPIDEMIOLOGY
- Propionibacterium species are part of the normal human flora (mainly skin).

INFECTIONS
- Acne
- Infection related to prosthetic material, including arthroplasty materials (common in shoulder), CSF shunts, endocarditis in the context of prosthetic material, and brain abscesses. Also meningitis after neurosurgical procedures
- Bacteremia

DIAGNOSIS
- Culture (anaerobic)

TREATMENT
- Tetracycline or a macrolide

ALTERNATIVE TREATMENT
- Trimethoprim–sulfamethoxazole
- Vancomycin
- The pathogen is resistant to metronidazole.

PREVENTION
- Good antiseptic technique during surgery.

PROTEUS SPECIES

GENUS Proteus

SPECIES
- P. mirabilis
- P. myxofaciens
- P. penneri
- P. vulgaris

MICROBIOLOGIC CHARACTERISTICS
- Aerobic, Gram-negative bacillus

INCUBATION PERIOD
- Usually an endogenous infection

EPIDEMIOLOGY
- Worldwide distribution
- Part of the normal human bowel flora
- Common cause of infection

INFECTIONS
- Proteus species are a common cause of urinary tract infection, especially in patients with nephrolithiasis.
- The pathogen is also frequently isolated in polymicrobial abscesses.
- Bacteremia

DIAGNOSIS
- Culture

TREATMENT
- Amoxicillin–clavulanate
- Fluoroquinolone

ALTERNATIVE TREATMENT
- Second- or third-generation cephalosporins
- Aztreonam
- Carbapenem (meropenem or imipenem)
- Ureidopenicillins
- Trimethoprim–sulfamethoxazole
- Aminoglycoside

PROTOMONAS SPECIES

See "Methylobacterium species"

PROTOTHECA SPECIES

GENUS Prototheca

SPECIES
- P. stagnora
- P. wickerhamii
- P. zopfii

MICROBIOLOGIC CHARACTERISTICS
- Prototheca species are unicellular, achloric algae that grow in a fungus medium as yeast.
- It reproduces by endosporulation.

EPIDEMIOLOGY
- Prototheca organisms are ubiquitous in nature and commonly found in sewage and soil.

INFECTIONS
- Several cases of Prototheca infections have been reported from around the world.
- The best-described clinical syndrome caused by Prototheca species is a skin and soft-tissue infection manifested by a single, painless, plaque or papulonodular lesion that ulcerates sometimes.
- A few cases of olecranon bursitis have also been reported.
- Rare cause of other infections, such as peritonitis in patients on continuous ambulatory peritoneal dialysis and meningitis in patients with AIDS.
- Algaemia has been reported in immunocompromised hosts.

DIAGNOSIS
- Culture
- Finding the pathogen in pathology specimens of lesions

TREATMENT
- Amphotericin B

ALTERNATIVE TREATMENT
- Ketoconazole or itraconazole
- Posaconazole
- Voriconazole

PROVIDENCIA SPECIES

GENUS Providencia

SPECIES
- *P. alcalifaciens*
- *P. rettgeri*
- *P. rustigianii*
- *P. stuartii*
- Others

MICROBIOLOGIC CHARACTERISTICS
- Aerobic, Gram-negative bacillus

INCUBATION PERIOD
- Usually an endogenous infection

INFECTIONS
- *Providencia* species may cause infection in several sites, including the urinary tract, intraabdominal infection, central venous catheter-related infections, and bacteremia.
- The pathogen has been recognized as an important cause of nosocomial infections.

DIAGNOSIS
- Culture

TREATMENT
- Carbapenem (meropenem, imipenem); if suspected, extended spectrum beta-lactamase
- Ciprofloxacin

ALTERNATIVE TREATMENT
- Third-generation cephalosporin
- Aztreonam
- Ofloxacin
- Piperacillin–tazobactam
- Aminoglycoside

PSEUDALLESCHERIA BOYDII

GENUS Pseudallescheria

SPECIES
- *P. boydii*

MICROBIOLOGIC CHARACTERISTICS
- Filamentous fungus (mold), with septate hyaline hyphae
- Fungal aggregates (granules) *in vivo* (mycetoma)
- Septate hyaline hyphae in hyalohyphomycosis
- Also termed *Scedosporium apiospermum*

INCUBATION PERIOD
- Unknown

EPIDEMIOLOGY
- Worldwide distribution
- Mycetomas are seen more commonly in the tropics.

INFECTIONS
- *P. boydii* has been recognized recently as an important opportunistic pathogen, causing a variety of infections.
- The fungus is a cause of mycetoma, manifested by a slowly growing, tumor-like skin and subcutaneous tissue lesions. Mycetoma lesions may drain granular pus through sinuses.
- Mycetomas may be caused by a variety of fungal species, as well as *Nocardia* and *Actinomyces* spp.
- Mycetoma lesions usually appear on the feet and hands. However, they may occur on any exposed part of the body.
- Manifestations of *P. boydii* infections in sites other than the skin are similar to those of *Aspergillus* (clinical manifestations, histopathology findings, and appearance of hyphae).

- *P. boydii* also may cause the following:
  – Osteomyelitis
  – Brain abscess
  – Meningitis
  – Eye infections
  – Pneumonia
  – Sinusitis
  – Endocarditis
  – Fungal balls in various sites
  – Disseminated infection

DIAGNOSIS
- The granules of pus drained through mycetoma lesions contain fungal elements of various shapes.
- Culture
- Identification of the fungus in tissue biopsy specimens

TREATMENT
- There are limited published data for the treatment of *P. boydii* infections
- Amphotericin B does not seem to be effective for this fungus.
- Azoles: High doses of itraconazole, miconazole, or ketoconazole are recommended.

PSEUDOMONAS AERUGINOSA

See Section II, *"Pseudomonas Infections/Melioidosis/Glanders"*

PSEUDOMONAS LUTEOLA

GENUS Pseudomonas

SPECIES
- *P. luteola* (formerly *Chryseomonas luteola*)

MICROBIOLOGIC CHARACTERISTICS
- Gram-negative bacillus

EPIDEMIOLOGY
- Worldwide, rare infection

INFECTIONS
- Septicemia, sometimes polymicrobial and in association with central venous catheters
- Wound infection
- Peritonitis in patients with peritoneal dialysis
- Prosthetic valve endocarditis
- Meningitis

DIAGNOSIS
- Culture

TREATMENT
- Ceftazidime

ALTERNATIVE TREATMENT
- Ureidopenicillins
- An aminoglycoside
- Imipenem, meropenem
- Ciprofloxacin

PSYCHROBACTER IMMOBILIS

GENUS Psychrobacter

SPECIES
- P. immobilis

MICROBIOLOGIC CHARACTERISTICS
- Gram-negative coccobacillus
- The classification of pathogens, which may belong to the genus *Psychrobacter* or similar genera, is incomplete.

INCUBATION PERIOD
- Unknown

EPIDEMIOLOGY
- *P. immobilis* has been isolated from food, found in colder environments.

INFECTIONS
- Isolated from blood, urine, and wound specimens
- There are only a few reports of disease due to *P. immobilis*.

DIAGNOSIS
- Culture

TREATMENT
- There are not enough published data to make recommendations.
- Selection of antimicrobial agents should be based on *in vitro* susceptibility results.

RABIES VIRUS

See Section II, "Rabies"

RESPIRATORY SYNCYTIAL VIRUS

See Section II, "Respiratory Syncytial Virus (RSV) Infection"

RHINOCLADIELLA AQUASPERA

See "Chromomycosis Agents"

RHINOSPORIDIUM SEEBERI

GENUS Rhinosporidium

SPECIES
- R. seeberi

MICROBIOLOGIC CHARACTERISTICS
- Sporangia containing sporangiospores (biopsy material)
- Large, round sporangia
- Mature sporangia may contain both immature and mature spores.

EPIDEMIOLOGY
- Worldwide distribution (rare infection), but most commonly isolated from Sri Lanka, India, Africa, and South America.

INFECTIONS
- Rhinosporidiosis, which is manifested by chronic, usually painless nasal or conjunctival lesions that resemble polyps.

DIAGNOSIS
- Finding sporangia in tissue biopsies

TREATMENT
- Surgical resection of the nasal or conjunctival polyps
- Lesions may recur after surgical management.

ALTERNATIVE TREATMENT
- The efficacy of antifungal treatment is unknown.

RHINOVIRUS

GROUP Rhinovirus

SPECIES
- N/A

MICROBIOLOGIC CHARACTERISTICS
- Single-stranded, positive RNA virus
- There are more than 100 recognized serotypes of rhinovirus.

INCUBATION PERIOD
- Usually 2–3 days (range, 12 hours to 5 days)

EPIDEMIOLOGY
- Worldwide distribution

INFECTIONS
- Common cold

DIAGNOSIS
- Cell culture
- Usually no diagnostic investigations are warranted.

TREATMENT
- Symptomatic

PREVENTION
- Frequent hand washing
- Covering the mouth and nose when coughing and sneezing
- Sanitary disposal of nasal and oral secretions

RHIZOBIUM RADIOBACTER

GENUS Rhizobium

SPECIES
- R. radiobacter (formerly Agrobacterium radiobacter)

MICROBIOLOGIC CHARACTERISTICS
- Aerobic, Gram-negative bacillus

INFECTIONS
- Present in soil and plants worldwide
- Plant pathogens; rare cause of human infection.
- Catheter-associated sepsis or bacteremia
- Peritonitis in patients receiving ambulatory peritoneal dialysis
- Urinary tract infection in patients with nephrostomy tubes
- Prosthetic valve endocarditis

DIAGNOSIS
- Culture

TREATMENT
- Trimethoprim–sulfamethoxazole
- Chloramphenicol

ALTERNATIVE TREATMENT
- Gentamicin (most isolates are resistant to tobramycin)
- Ciprofloxacin

RHIZOMUCOR SPECIES

See Section II, "Mucormycosis"

RHIZOPUS SPECIES

See Section II, "Mucormycosis"

RHODOCOCCUS SPECIES

GENUS Rhodococcus

SPECIES
- R. aurantiacus
- R. bronchialis
- R. equi (the most clinically relevant species)
- R. erythropolis
- R. luteus
- R. rhodochrous
- R. rubropertinctus

MICROBIOLOGIC CHARACTERISTICS
- Aerobic, Gram-positive coccobacillus
- It may be acid-fast stain-positive.
- Intracellular pathogen

EPIDEMIOLOGY
- Worldwide, rare infection

INFECTIONS
- R. equi has been isolated more frequently during the past 2 decades. It is often an opportunistic infection in immunocompromised hosts.
- R. equi is mainly implicated in pulmonary infections.
- However, the pathogen has been isolated from clinical specimens of patients with a variety of infections, including the following:
  - Brain abscess
  - Osteomyelitis
  - Prostatic abscess
  - Bacteremia
  - Lymphadenitis
  - Endophthalmitis
  - Intraabdominal infections
- Pneumonia due to R. equi may take an acute, subacute, or chronic course. It may resemble tuberculosis, nocardiosis, and actinomycosis, as it can present with cavitation or as a solitary pulmonary nodule.
- Isolation of R. equi from a clinical specimen should prompt investigations for impaired cellular immunity, such as HIV infection.
- Rhodococcus species other than R. equi are usually associated with surgical infections.

DIAGNOSIS
- Culture of the pathogen

TREATMENT
- Vancomycin
- Erythromycin
- Ciprofloxacin
- Imipenem
- Treatment is typically several weeks in duration.

ALTERNATIVE TREATMENT
- Azithromycin

RHODOTORULA SPECIES

GENUS Rhodotorula

SPECIES
- R. glutinis
- R. rubra

MICROBIOLOGIC CHARACTERISTICS
- Yeast
- Rapid growth (mature in 4 days)
- In culture, budding cells (round or oval) and few rudimentary pseudohyphae are seen.

INCUBATION PERIOD
- Unknown

EPIDEMIOLOGY
- Worldwide

INFECTIONS
- Rhodotorula species are usually contaminants of cultures.
- Rhodotorula species play pathogenic role in immunocompromised hosts.
- Rhodotorula species may cause several infections, including fungemia, especially in patients with central venous catheters, peritonitis in patients with peritoneal dialysis, and endocarditis.

DIAGNOSIS
- Culture
- Histopathology

TREATMENT
- Amphotericin B with or without flucytosine

RICKETTSIA SPECIES

GENUS Rickettsia

SPECIES
- R. akari
- R. australis
- R. conorii
- R. mooseri
- R. orientalis
- R. prowazekii
- R. rickettsii
- R. sibirica
- R. tsutsugamushi
- R. typhi

MICROBIOLOGIC CHARACTERISTICS
- Small, intracellular coccobacillus

INCUBATION PERIOD
- Depends on the specific Rickettsia species
- It is 3–14 days for R. rickettsii, the cause of Rocky Mountain spotted fever.
- Incubation period for other Rickettsia species:
  - R. conori: Usually 5–7 days
  - R. sibirica: 2–7 days
  - R. australis: Usually 7–10 days

EPIDEMIOLOGY
- Common cause of human infections

INFECTIONS
- Rickettsia species cause several infections, with various manifestations.
- R. rickettsii: Rocky mountain spotted fever (see dedicated chapter).
- R. conorii: Boutonneuse fever (Mediterranean spotted fever, India tick typhus, African tick typhus), which is manifested frequently by fever, a primary lesion at the site of a tick bite, which ulcerates and has a black center, regional lymphadenopathy (not always present), and, later, a generalized maculopapular erythematous rash.
- R. australis: Queensland tick typhus (similar manifestations with R. conorii).
- R. sibirica: North Asian tick fever (similar manifestations with R. conorii).
- R. akari: Rickettsialpox (transmitted to humans by mite bites and manifested with disseminated vesicular skin rash generally not involving the soles and palms, fever, and lymphadenopathy).
- R. prowazekii: Louse-borne typhus, classic typhus fever.
- R. typhi (R. mooseri): Flea-borne typhus, endemic typhus fever.
- R. tsutsugamushi (R. orientalis): Scrub typhus.

DIAGNOSIS
- Serology

TREATMENT
- Doxycycline 100 mg p.o. q12h for 7 days

ALTERNATIVE TREATMENT
- Chloramphenicol

PREVENTION
- Avoiding tick and other insect bites

ROTAVIRUS, HUMAN

GROUP Rotavirus

SPECIES
- N/A

MICROBIOLOGIC CHARACTERISTICS
- RNA virus that belongs to the Reoviridae family

INCUBATION PERIOD
- The incubation period is usually from 1 to 3 days.

EPIDEMIOLOGY
- Worldwide distribution
- Clinically apparent infections appear in infants and young children.

INFECTIONS
- Rotavirus causes gastroenteritis, which may be sporadic or seasonal and is manifested by fever, vomiting, and watery nonbloody diarrhea.
- The infection may lead to severe dehydration, especially in infants and young children.

DIAGNOSIS
- Rotavirus antigen detection in stool specimens
- Direct visualization of the virus with electron microscopy

TREATMENT
- Symptomatic

ALTERNATIVE TREATMENT
- There is no specific antiviral treatment.

PREVENTION
- Hand hygiene
- Gloves

ROTHIA DENTOCARIOSA

GENUS Rothia

SPECIES
- *R. dentocariosa*

MICROBIOLOGIC CHARACTERISTICS
- Aerobic, pleomorphic, Gram-positive bacillus

INCUBATION PERIOD
- Unknown

EPIDEMIOLOGY
- Worldwide

INFECTIONS
- Endocarditis
- It is implicated in the pathogenesis of dental caries.
- Periodontal disease and abscesses

DIAGNOSIS
- Culture

TREATMENT
- Penicillin with aminoglycosides in endocarditis

ALTERNATIVE TREATMENT
- Cephalosporin
- Erythromycin
- Aminoglycosides

RUBELLA VIRUS

See Section II, "Rubella (German Measles)"

SACCHAROMYCES CEREVISIAE

GENUS Saccharomyces

SPECIES
- *S. cerevisiae*

MICROBIOLOGIC CHARACTERISTICS
- Yeast
- Rapid growth

INCUBATION PERIOD
- Unknown

EPIDEMIOLOGY
- Worldwide distribution

INFECTIONS
- *S. cerevisiae* traditionally has been considered a nonpathogenic fungal organism.
- However, recent data support its pathogenicity, especially in immunocompromised patients, including those with advanced HIV infection.
- *S. cerevisiae* may cause fungemia in patients with central venous catheters, peritonitis in patients on chronic ambulatory peritoneal dialysis, septic arthritis, respiratory tract infection, and vaginitis.

DIAGNOSIS
- Culture

TREATMENT
- Amphotericin B i.v. for systemic infections
- Topical azole treatment for patients with vaginitis

SAKSENAEA VASIFORMIS

GENUS Saksenaea

SPECIES
- S. vasiformis

MICROBIOLOGIC CHARACTERISTICS
- Filamentous fungus (mold), with nonseptate hyaline hyphae

INCUBATION PERIOD
- Unknown

EPIDEMIOLOGY
- The usual method of transmission is via traumatic inoculation.
- Immunocompetent individuals may be infected after inoculation.

INFECTIONS
- A cause of zygomycosis manifested by rhinocerebral, cutaneous, subcutaneous, bone, and lung lesions.

DIAGNOSIS
- Culture
- Histopathology

TREATMENT
- Amphotericin B i.v. is the recommended treatment.

ALTERNATIVE TREATMENT
- Posaconazole

SALMONELLA SPECIES

See Section II, "Typhoid Fever"

SARCOCYSTIS SPECIES

GENUS Sarcocystis

SPECIES
- *S. bovihominis*
- *S. suihominis*

MICROBIOLOGIC CHARACTERISTICS
- A protozoon with characteristics similar to those of *Isospora belli*

INCUBATION PERIOD
- Unclear

EPIDEMIOLOGY
- Worldwide distribution
- Most cases are reported from Southeast Asia.

INFECTIONS
- Muscular sarcocystosis: Typically asymptomatic, however, may present with myalgias and muscle swelling.
- Mild intestinal disease.

DIAGNOSIS
- Parasitologic examination of stool specimens.
- Muscle biopsy (often an incidental finding).

TREATMENT
- Not usually necessary for gastrointestinal infection.
- Metronidazole has been used in myositis.

SARCOPTES SCABIEI

See Section II, "Scabies"

SCEDOSPORIUM PROLIFICANS

GENUS Scedosporium

SPECIES
- *S. prolificans*

MICROBIOLOGIC CHARACTERISTICS
- Filamentous fungus (mold) with septate hyaline hyphae
- Formerly called *Scedosporium inflatum*
- Growth is inhibited by cycloheximide

INCUBATION PERIOD
- Unknown

EPIDEMIOLOGY
- Worldwide distribution

INFECTIONS
- It may cause invasive infection (usually arthritis and/or osteomyelitis, but it may affect various organs such as lungs and pleura).
- Asymptomatic colonization may occur.

DIAGNOSIS
- Culture
- Histopathology

TREATMENT
- Amphotericin B

ALTERNATIVE TREATMENT
- Azoles

SCHISTOSOMA SPECIES

See Section II, "Schistosomiasis"

SCOPULARIOPSIS SPECIES

GENUS Scopulariopsis

SPECIES
- *S. brevicaulis*
- *S. brumptii*
- Others

MICROBIOLOGIC CHARACTERISTICS
- Filamentous fungus (mold)

INCUBATION PERIOD
- Unknown

EPIDEMIOLOGY
- Worldwide distribution

INFECTIONS
- Onychomycosis
- Locally invasive disease (otitis externa) and disseminated disease in neutropenic patients.
- Cutaneous lesions in patients with advanced HIV infection.
- Keratitis
- Pulmonary infection
- Rare cause of endocarditis
- Invasive infections found in immunocompromised hosts.

TREATMENT
- Chemical nail removal with 40% urea for patients with onychomycosis

ALTERNATIVE TREATMENT
- Surgical removal of the affected nail(s).
- There are limited data about the efficacy antifungal agents.
- Amphotericin B i.v. for invasive infections.

SEPTATA INTESTINALIS

See "Microsporidia"

SERRATIA SPECIES

GENUS Serratia

SPECIES
- *S. ficaria*
- *S. fonticola*
- *S. grimesii*
- *S. liquefaciens*
- *S. marcescens* (most clinically relevant species)
- *S. odorifera*
- *S. plymuthica*
- *S. rubidaea*
- Others

MICROBIOLOGIC CHARACTERISTICS
- Aerobic, Gram-negative bacillus

INCUBATION PERIOD
- Usually a nosocomial infection.

EPIDEMIOLOGY
- Worldwide distribution
- Risk factors for infection include hospitalization with invasive procedures or intravenous drug use.

INFECTIONS
- *Serratia* species have been isolated more frequently during the past 2 decades.
- A common cause of nosocomial infection of various sites (bacteremia, urinary tract infections, respiratory tract infections, intraabdominal infections)

DIAGNOSIS
- Culture

TREATMENT
- Based on sensitivity data
- Ciprofloxacin or other fluoroquinolones often susceptible.

ALTERNATIVE TREATMENT
- Third-generation cephalosporin
- Carbapenem (imipenem, meropenem)
- Aztreonam
- Ureidopenicillins
- Aminoglycosides
- Ofloxacin
- Trimethoprim–sulfamethoxazole

SHIGELLA SPECIES

See Section II, "Shigellosis"

SMALLPOX VIRUS

GROUP Orthopoxvirus

SPECIES
- N/A

MICROBIOLOGIC CHARACTERISTICS
- A DNA virus

INCUBATION PERIOD
- About 12 days

EPIDEMIOLOGY
- Smallpox (variola) has been eradicated. The last reported case of smallpox was in October 1977 in Somalia.
- Smallpox virus is held under tight security in select research laboratories.

INFECTIONS
- Smallpox
- Papular eruption evolving into vesicles. Diffuse eruption occurs; however, a heavy burden of lesions is present on the face and distal extremities. Lesions are all at the same stage of development.

DIAGNOSIS
- Clinical features
- Cell culture
- Electron microscopy of clinical samples
- Serology

TREATMENT
- Possibly cidofovir
- Vaccination

PREVENTION
- Smallpox vaccine: Typically for military personnel who may be exposed to biologic warfare agents.

SPHINGOBACTERIUM SPECIES

GENUS Sphingobacterium

SPECIES
- *S. multivorum*
- *S. spiritivorum*
- Others

MICROBIOLOGIC CHARACTERISTICS
- Aerobic, Gram-negative bacillus

INCUBATION PERIOD
- Unknown

EPIDEMIOLOGY
- Rare cause of infections (worldwide)
- *Sphingobacterium* species usually cause nosocomial infections.

INFECTIONS
- Peritonitis
- Bacteremia
- Skin and soft-tissue infections
- Respiratory tract infections
- Urinary tract infections

DIAGNOSIS
- Culture

TREATMENT
- Ampicillin

ALTERNATIVE TREATMENT
- Trimethoprim–sulfamethoxazole
- Fluoroquinolones
- Third-generation cephalosporins
- Carbapenems

SPIRILLUM MINUS (MINOR)

GENUS Spirillum

SPECIES
- *S. minus* (*minor*)

MICROBIOLOGIC CHARACTERISTICS
- Aerobic, Gram-negative bacillus

INCUBATION PERIOD
- 2 days to 3 weeks.

EPIDEMIOLOGY
- Worldwide distribution (rare in the US)
- More common in Asia, especially in Japan

INFECTIONS
- Rat-bite fever (Sodoku).
- Relapsing fevers, polyarthritis, maculopapular rash, myalgias, arthralgias.
- The case fatality rate for untreated cases is about 10%.

DIAGNOSIS
- The microbiology laboratory has to culture *Spirillum* on special media and should be notified prior to obtaining a sample.
- Requires 2–3 weeks to culture.
- No serology available.
- PCR techniques under development for commercial use.

TREATMENT
- Penicillin

ALTERNATIVE TREATMENT
- Doxycycline
- Ampicillin
- Azithromycin
- Streptomycin

SPIROMETRA SPECIES

GENUS Spirometra
SPECIES
- *S. spargana*
- *S. mansonoides*

MICROBIOLOGIC CHARACTERISTICS
- A cestode helminth
- The developmental stage found in humans is the larval cyst.
- The source of transmission to human is cysts from infected copepods, frogs, and snakes.

EPIDEMIOLOGY
- Most cases have been reported from Southeast Asia and Africa.

INFECTIONS
- Sparganosis (localized inflammatory edema)

DIAGNOSIS
- Parasitologic examination of biopsy specimen.

TREATMENT
- Surgery

SPOROBOLOMYCES SPECIES

GENUS Sporobolomyces

SPECIES
- *S. holsaticus*
- *S. roseus*
- *S. salmonicolor*

MICROBIOLOGIC CHARACTERISTICS
- Yeast

INCUBATION PERIOD
- Unknown

EPIDEMIOLOGY
- Most commonly isolated from environmental sources

INFECTIONS
- Rare cause of infections in humans (usually mycetoma)
- It may cause systemic infection in immunocompromised patients, including those with advanced HIV infection.

DIAGNOSIS
- Culture

TREATMENT
- Amphotericin B for systemic infection

SPOROTHRIX SCHENCKII

See Section II, "Sporotrichosis"

STAPHYLOCOCCUS SPECIES

GENUS Staphylococcus

SPECIES
- S. aureus
- S. capitis
- S. cohnii
- S. epidermidis
- S. galinarum
- S. haemolyticus
- S. hominis
- S. intermedius
- S. lugdunensis
- S. warneri
- S. xylosus
- Others

MICROBIOLOGIC CHARACTERISTICS
- Aerobic, Gram-positive coccus
- Staphylococcus species are classified into 2 main categories:
  - Coagulase-positive (mainly S. aureus)
  - Coagulase-negative (most Staphylococcus species, including S. epidermidis)

INCUBATION PERIOD
- The incubation period for staphylococcal infections is highly variable.

EPIDEMIOLOGY
- Worldwide distribution

INFECTIONS
- Staphylococcus species are a common cause of human infections of practically all body sites.
- Among all Staphylococcus species, S. aureus and S. epidermidis are the most common isolates from clinical specimens.
- The incidence of staphylococcal infections has increased considerably recently, partly because of the frequent use of central venous catheters.
- S. aureus tends to cause abscesses.
- Staphylococcus species are a common cause of endocarditis.

DIAGNOSIS
- Culture

TREATMENT
- Antistaphylococcal penicillins (e.g., oxacillin, nafcillin, or cloxacillin) are the best drugs for Staphylococcus species sensitive to methicillin.
- A significant proportion of coagulase-negative Staphylococcus species and S. aureus strains are resistant to methicillin.
- A glycopeptide (vancomycin or teicoplanin) may be needed to treat infections due to these strains.
- Often, doxycycline, clindamycin, or trimethoprim–sulfamethoxazole will be effective against coagulase-negative Staphylococcus and methicillin-resistant Staphylococcus aureus.

STENOTROPHOMONAS SPECIES

GENUS Stenotrophomonas

SPECIES
- S. africana
- S. maltophilia

MICROBIOLOGIC CHARACTERISTICS
- Aerobic, Gram-negative bacillus

INCUBATION PERIOD
- Unclear

EPIDEMIOLOGY
- Worldwide distribution
- Hydrophilic bacteria often found in secretions
- An important cause of nosocomial infections is found especially in patients who have received a prolonged course of antibiotics, long stays in the ICU, or are intubated.

INFECTIONS
- Bacteremia
- Pneumonia, particularly ventilator-associated pneumonia
- Skin and soft-tissue infections
- Urinary tract infection

DIAGNOSIS
- Culture

TREATMENT
- Trimethoprim–sulfamethoxazole

ALTERNATIVE TREATMENT
- Ceftazidime
- Ciprofloxacin
- Minocycline
- Piperacillin–tazobactam
- Ticarcillin and aztreonam–clavulanate
- Many S. maltophilia strains are resistant to carbapenems and aztreonam.

STOMATOCOCCUS MUCILAGINOSUS

GENUS Stomatococcus

SPECIES
- S. mucilaginosus

MICROBIOLOGIC CHARACTERISTICS
- Aerobic, Gram-positive coccus

EPIDEMIOLOGY
- Worldwide, rare infection

INFECTIONS
- Bacteremia associated with central venous catheters
- Oral mucositis in patients with neutropenia, especially those receiving antibiotics for intestinal decontamination
- Endocarditis
- Meningitis

DIAGNOSIS
- Culture

TREATMENT
- Vancomycin
- Carbapenems

ALTERNATIVE TREATMENT
- Penicillin G
- Macrolide

STREPTOBACILLUS MONILIFORMIS

GENUS Streptobacillus

SPECIES
- S. moniliformis

MICROBIOLOGIC CHARACTERISTICS
- Aerobic, pleomorphic, Gram-negative bacillus

INCUBATION PERIOD
- 3–10 days, sometimes longer

EPIDEMIOLOGY
- Worldwide distribution
- Rare cause of infection in North America and Europe
- Most patients with infection report a rat bite.

INFECTIONS
- Rat-bite fever (Haverhill fever or streptobacillosis). It is manifested by fever, headache, and malaise, followed by a maculopapular rash.
- Untreated patients with streptobacillosis may develop endocarditis, pericarditis, tenosynovitis, and abscesses in several organs, including the brain.

DIAGNOSIS
- Culture in specific medium.

TREATMENT
- Penicillin

ALTERNATIVE TREATMENT
- Doxycycline
- Azithromycin

STREPTOCOCCUS AGALACTIAE (GROUP B)

GENUS Streptococcus

SPECIES
- *S. agalactiae* (group B)

MICROBIOLOGIC CHARACTERISTICS
- Aerobic, Gram-positive coccus

INCUBATION PERIOD
- The incubation period of early-onset neonatal disease is less than 6 days.

EPIDEMIOLOGY
- Worldwide distribution

INFECTIONS
- Sepsis and meningitis in the newborn
- Urinary and genital tract infection (endometritis) in pregnant women
- Recent data support the increasing significance of *S. agalactiae* infections in men and nonpregnant women.

DIAGNOSIS
- Culture
- Antigen detection techniques in body fluids (including CSF)

TREATMENT
- Penicillin G or ampicillin

ALTERNATIVE TREATMENT
- Macrolide antibiotic

STREPTOCOCCUS PNEUMONIAE

See Section II, "Pneumonia"

STREPTOCOCCUS PYOGENES (GROUP A β-HEMOLYTIC STREPTOCOCCUS)

GENUS Streptococcus

SPECIES
- *S. pyogenes*

MICROBIOLOGIC CHARACTERISTICS
- Aerobic, Gram-positive coccus

INCUBATION PERIOD
- The incubation period of streptococcal pharyngitis is 2–5 days.
- For impetigo, a 7- to 10-day period between the acquisition of the pathogen on healthy skin and development of lesions

EPIDEMIOLOGY
- Worldwide distribution

INFECTIONS
- Tonsillitis, scarlet fever, otitis, sinusitis, pneumonia
- Skin and soft-tissue infections (impetigo, erysipelas, cellulitis, others)
- Bacteremia
- Necrotizing fasciitis and toxic shock syndrome (TSS)
- Late nonsuppurative (immune-mediated) complications include rheumatic fever, erythema nodosum, and glomerulonephritis.

DIAGNOSIS
- Culture
- Serology

TREATMENT
- Penicillin G.
- Amoxicillin
- Clindamycin

ALTERNATIVE TREATMENT
- Macrolide antibiotics

STRONGYLOIDES SPECIES

See Section II, "Strongyloidiasis"

TAENIA SAGINATA

GENUS Taenia

SPECIES
- *T. saginata*

MICROBIOLOGIC CHARACTERISTICS
- A tapeworm

INCUBATION PERIOD
- Eggs appear in the stool 10–14 weeks after infection with *T. saginata*.

EPIDEMIOLOGY
- Worldwide
- More frequent in populations where insufficiently cooked beef is consumed

INFECTIONS
- Beef tapeworm infection, which is usually asymptomatic. It may cause mild gastrointestinal symptoms like dyspepsia, nausea

DIAGNOSIS
- Parasitologic examination of the stool

TREATMENT
- Praziquantel

ALTERNATIVE TREATMENT
- Niclosamide

PREVENTION
- Thorough cooking of beef

TAENIA SOLIUM

See Section II, "Cysticercosis"

TOXOCARA SPECIES

GENUS Toxocara

SPECIES
- *T. canis*
- *T. catis*

MICROBIOLOGIC CHARACTERISTICS
- Nematode helminth

INCUBATION PERIOD
- Weeks to months
- Manifestation from eye infection may appear several years (2–10) after infection.

EPIDEMIOLOGY
- Worldwide distribution
- Ingestion of soil contaminated with dog (*T. canis*) or cat (*T. catis*) feces containing eggs.
- Young children are at risk for infection

INFECTIONS
- Visceral larva migrans: Typically mild infection, but may have fever, malaise, hepatomegaly, cough, and wheezing.
- The eosinophil count may increase significantly (up to 80,000/mm^3 of blood) in patients with heavy infection.
- *Ocular larva migrans* refers to eye infection by *Toxocara* species.

DIAGNOSIS
- Clinical presentation
- ELISA
- Microscopic visualization of larvae in tissue biopsy (rarely indicated)

TREATMENT
- Usually no treatment necessary.
- Albendazole in heavy infections.

ALTERNATIVE TREATMENT
- Ophthalmology evaluation for eye involvement

TOXOPLASMA GONDII

See Section II, "Toxoplasmosis"

TREPONEMA CARATEUM

GENUS Treponema

SPECIES
- *T. carateum*

MICROBIOLOGIC CHARACTERISTICS
- A spirochete

INCUBATION PERIOD
- Usually 2–3 weeks

EPIDEMIOLOGY
- Tropical areas of South America

INFECTIONS
- Pinta: A plaque-like cutaneous infection, typically involving the dorsum of the foot and legs.
- Regional lymph node enlargement
- Lesions get pigmented with age.

DIAGNOSIS
- Nontreponemal and treponemal serologic tests (rapid plasma regain, venereal disease research laboratory, treponema pallidum particle agglutination)
- Dark-field examination of samples taken from the lesions

TREATMENT
- Benzyl penicillin

ALTERNATIVE TREATMENT
- Tetracycline or chloramphenicol

TREPONEMA PALLIDUM

See Section II, "Syphilis"

TRICHINELLA SPIRALIS

GENUS Trichinella

SPECIES
- *T. spiralis*

MICROBIOLOGIC CHARACTERISTICS
- Nematode helminth (round worm)

INCUBATION PERIOD
- Gastrointestinal symptoms may appear within a few days after infection.
- Systemic symptoms appear 5–45 days after infection.

EPIDEMIOLOGY
- Worldwide
- Variable incidence, depending partially on practices of preparing and eating pork or wild animal meat (e.g., bear, fox, boar)

INFECTIONS
- *T. spiralis* causes an infection with variable severity, depending on the number of ingested larvae and the susceptibility of the host.
- Asymptomatic infection is common.
- Diffuse myalgias, weakness, accompanied by edema of the upper eyelids
- Gastrointestinal symptoms, including mild diarrhea, may precede the ocular manifestations.
- Other sites, including the heart and the CNS, may be affected in trichinellosis.

DIAGNOSIS
- Serology
- Muscle biopsy
- Marked eosinophilia may be found in *Trichinella* infections.

TREATMENT
- Mebendazole or albendazole early in infection

ALTERNATIVE TREATMENT
- Steroids may be necessary with CNS or cardiac manifestations

PREVENTION
- Properly cook all fresh pork and pork products and meat from wild animals.

TRICHOMONAS VAGINALIS

See Section II, "Trichomonas Vaginalis"

TRICHOPHYTON SPECIES

See Section II, "Superficial Skin and Soft-Tissue Infections"

TRICHOSPORON BEIGELII

GENUS Trichosporon

SPECIES
- *T. beigelii*

MICROBIOLOGIC CHARACTERISTICS
- Yeast capable of developing arthroconidia, hyphae, blastoconidia, and pseudohyphae

INCUBATION PERIOD
- Unknown

EPIDEMIOLOGY
- Found in soil, more common in tropical regions but also in temperate zones

INFECTIONS
- White piedra (superficial infection manifested by small yellow concretions on the hair shafts)
- The fungus may also cause a systemic infection in immunocompromised patients, including transplant recipients and patients with advanced HIV infection.

DIAGNOSIS
- Culture
- A false-positive latex agglutination test for *Cryptococcus* antigen may occur in systemic *T. beigelii* infections.
- Histopathology specimens

TREATMENT
- Shaving hair in the affected region followed by topical azole therapy.
- Systemic infections should be managed with systemic antifungal agents. Data are lacking; however, amphotericin B and voriconazole are likely helpful.

TRICHOSTRONGYLUS SPECIES

GENUS Trichostrongylus

SPECIES
- *T. orientalis*
- *T. colubriformis*

MICROBIOLOGIC CHARACTERISTICS
- Nematode

INCUBATION PERIOD
- Unclear

EPIDEMIOLOGY
- Worldwide distribution
- More commonly found in rural areas where herbivorous animals are raised

INFECTIONS
- Usually an asymptomatic infection
- It may occasionally cause mild gastrointestinal symptoms (e.g., dyspepsia) and anemia.

DIAGNOSIS
- Parasitologic examination of stool
- *Trichostrongylus* eggs resemble hookworm eggs, but *Trichostrongylus* eggs are usually larger.

TREATMENT
- Mebendazole

ALTERNATIVE TREATMENT
- Albendazole 400 mg p.o. in a single dose

TRICHURIS TRICHIURA

GENUS Trichuris

SPECIES
- *T. trichiura*

MICROBIOLOGIC CHARACTERISTICS
- Nematode helminth

INCUBATION PERIOD
- Symptoms may appear a few weeks after infection.

EPIDEMIOLOGY
- Worldwide distribution
- More common in regions with moist and warm soil

INFECTIONS
- Trichuriasis is usually an asymptomatic infection of the large bowel.
- Heavy infections (large number of *T. trichiura* in the large bowel) may cause diarrhea, with mucoid and bloody stools.
- Heavy infection with *T. trichiura* in children may be complicated by rectal prolapse, anemia, hypoproteinemia, and growth retardation.

DIAGNOSIS
- Parasitologic examination of stools (detection of eggs)
- Colonoscopy may reveal worms attached to the large bowel wall.

TREATMENT
- Mebendazole

ALTERNATIVE TREATMENT
- Albendazole

PREVENTION
- Good hygienic practices, clean water facilities for bathing, cooking, toileting.

TROPHERYMA WHIPPELII

GENUS Tropheryma

SPECIES
- *T. whippelii*

MICROBIOLOGIC CHARACTERISTICS
- Intracellular, Gram-positive bacillus

INCUBATION PERIOD
- Unknown

EPIDEMIOLOGY
- Probably worldwide distribution

INFECTIONS
- Whipple disease (a syndrome manifested by migratory arthralgias, diarrhea, malabsorption, fever, neurologic disorder, and lymphadenopathy)

DIAGNOSIS
- Histologic examination of intestinal biopsy or lymph node
- PCR

TREATMENT
- Trimethoprim–sulfamethoxazole

ALTERNATIVE TREATMENT
- Penicillin V
- Chloramphenicol
- Tetracycline

TRYPANOSOMA SPECIES

See Section II, "Trypanosomiasis: African (Sleeping Sickness) and American (Chagas)"

TUNGA PENETRANS

GENUS Tunga

SPECIES
- *T. penetrans*

MICROBIOLOGIC CHARACTERISTICS
- Hematophagous flea

INCUBATION PERIOD
- Unknown

EPIDEMIOLOGY
- Mainly found in developing countries of Africa, South and Central America, and the Far East

INFECTIONS
- Tungiasis is manifested by painful nodules, usually on the feet. The lesions may be confused with those caused by myiasis. Tungiasis is caused by invasion of the skin by the mature female flea, *T. penetrans*.

DIAGNOSIS
- Finding and examination of the flea in lesions

TREATMENT
- Surgical excision of the lesions.
- Often topical antibiotics may be required.
- Oral antibiotics for bacterial superinfection after surgical excision

UREAPLASMA UREALYTICUM

GENUS Ureaplasma

SPECIES
- *U. urealyticum*
- *Ureaplasma parvum*

MICROBIOLOGIC CHARACTERISTICS
- Small bacterium
- No cell wall

INCUBATION PERIOD
- The incubation period of nongonococcal urethritis (a common infection that is caused, in some patients, by *U. urealyticum*) after sexual transmission is 10–20 days.

EPIDEMIOLOGY
- Common cause of infections worldwide

INFECTIONS
- Urethritis
- Chorioamnionitis
- Disseminated infection in the newborn

DIAGNOSIS
- Culture on special media
- Serology tests
- PCR

TREATMENT
- Macrolide antibiotic for 7–14 days

ALTERNATIVE TREATMENT
- Doxycycline
- Ofloxacin
- Ciprofloxacin should not be used, because a large proportion (up to 50%) of *U. urealyticum* strains are resistant to this antibiotic.

VARICELLA ZOSTER VIRUS

See Section II, "Chickenpox (Varicella)" and "Herpes Zoster"

VEILLONELLA PARVULA

GENUS Veillonella

SPECIES
- *V. parvula*

MICROBIOLOGIC CHARACTERISTICS
- Anaerobic, Gram-negative coccus

INCUBATION PERIOD
- Unknown

EPIDEMIOLOGY
- Worldwide
- Part of the normal oropharyngeal flora

INFECTIONS
- It may contribute to mixed infection of the female genital tract.
- A probable cause of oral infections

DIAGNOSIS
- Culture (anaerobic conditions)
- Culture requires prolonged incubation for growth of *V. parvula*.

TREATMENT
- Clindamycin

ALTERNATIVE TREATMENT
- Penicillin G
- Metronidazole

VIBRIO CHOLERAE

See Section II, "Cholera"

VIBRIO SPECIES

GENUS Vibrio

SPECIES
- *V. alginolyticus*
- *V. cholerae* non-0:1
- *V. cincinnatiensis*
- *V. damselae*
- *V. fluvialis*
- *V. furnissii*
- *V. hollisae*
- *V. metschnikovii*
- *V. mimicus*
- *V. parahaemolyticus*
- *V. vulnificus*

MICROBIOLOGIC CHARACTERISTICS
- Aerobic, Gram-negative bacillus

INCUBATION PERIOD
- The incubation period of enteritis due to most *Vibrio* species is 24 hours, with a range of 5–92 hours.

EPIDEMIOLOGY
- Ubiquitous in sea water
- Highest risk associated with consumption of raw clams, mussels, and oysters

INFECTIONS
- Gastroenteritis
- Wound infection and secondary sepsis
- Necrotizing skin infection and severe sepsis (mainly *V. vulnificus*)

DIAGNOSIS
- Culture

TREATMENT
- Doxycycline
- Minocycline and cefotaxime are synergistic and can be used in serious infections.
- Supportive measures (fluid and electrolytes) are necessary for patients with gastroenteritis.

ALTERNATIVE TREATMENT
- Fluoroquinolone, aminoglycoside, chloramphenicol, third-generation cephalosporin, carbapenem

WEEKSELLA SPECIES

GENUS Weeksella

SPECIES
- *W. virosa*
- *W. zoohelcum*

MICROBIOLOGIC CHARACTERISTICS
- Aerobic, Gram-negative bacillus

EPIDEMIOLOGY
- Unclear

INFECTIONS
- Rare cause of infections
- Animal bite wound infection (*W. zoohelcum*)
- Urinary infection (*W. virosa*)
- Peritonitis in patients with peritoneal dialysis (*W. virosa*)

DIAGNOSIS
- Culture

TREATMENT
- There are limited data about the antimicrobial susceptibility of *Weeksella* species.
- Penicillin

ALTERNATIVE TREATMENT
- Ciprofloxacin
- Trimethoprim–sulfamethoxazole
- Tetracycline
- Aminoglycoside

PREVENTION
- N/A

WOHLFAHRTIA MAGNIFICA

See "Myiasis Agents"

WUCHERERIA BANCROFTI

See Section II, "Filariasis"

YELLOW FEVER VIRUS

See Section II, "Yellow Fever"

YERSINIA PESTIS

See Section II, "Plague"

YERSINIA SPECIES

See Section II, "*Yersinia enterocolitica* Infections"

Drugs and Vaccines

Matthew E. Falagas
Eleftherios Mylonakis

Petros M. Karsaliakos
Petros I. Rafailidis
Paschalis I. Vergidis

Table 1a. Adverse Reactions to Antimicrobial Agents

Reaction	Common for	Infrequent for
Hypersensitivity-allergic		
Anaphylaxis	Penicillin G	Cephalosporins, imipenem
Fever	—	All agents
SLE-like reactions	Isoniazid	Griseofulvin, nitrofurantoin
Cutaneous reactions	Sulfonamides, penicillins	All agents
Histamine reactions	Vancomycin	—
Phototoxicity	Tetracyclines	Quinolones, chloroquine, primaquine, griseofulvin
Hematopoietic		
Pancytopenia	—	Chloramphenicol
Neutropenia	Sulfonamides, trimethoprim, pyrimethamine, zidovudine	Penicillins, cephalosporins, dapsone
Hemolytic anemia (G6PD-associated)	Sulfonamides, nitrofurans, chloramphenicol, sulfones, nalidixic acid, primaquine	—
Immune hemolysis	Penicillins, cephalosporins, isoniazid, rifampin	—
Sideroblastic anemia	Isoniazid	—
Thrombocytopenia	Sulfonamides, penicillins, cephalosporins, rifampin, trimethoprim, pyrimethamine, linezolid	Vancomycin, teicoplanin
Platelet dysfunction	Carbenicillin, ticarcillin, moxalactam	Extended-spectrum penicillins
Hypoprothrombinemia	Moxalactam, cefoperazone, cefamandole	Cefotetan, ceftriaxone, cefmetazole
Gastrointestinal		
Nausea, emesis, abdominal pain	Erythromycin	Almost any agent, including oral penicillins, quinolones, metronidazole, clindamycin, nystatin, tetracyclines, TMP-SMX, ketoconazole, tigecycline
Diarrhea	Ampicillin-sulbactam, amoxicillin-clavulanate, cefixime, cefoperazone, ceftriaxone	Any agent
Pseudomembranous enterocolitis (*Clostridium difficile*)	Almost any agent, more commonly ampicillin, TMP-SMX, cefoxitin, clindamycin	Quinolones (ciprofloxacin)
Malabsorption	Neomycin	Other aminoglycosides
Hepatic		
Transaminase level increase	Penicillins, particularly oxacillin, aztreonam	Azoles
Cholestatic jaundice	Oleandomycin, erythromycin estolate, nitrofurans, sulfonamides	—
Hepatitis	Isoniazid, nitrofurantoin, trovafloxacin	Rifampin, sulfonamides, ketoconazole

Table 1a. Adverse Reactions to Antimicrobial Agents (continued)

Reaction	Common for	Infrequent for
Pulmonary		
Histamine release	Polymyxin by aerosol	—
Interstitial infiltrates	Nitrofurantoin	—
Cardiovascular		
Arrhythmias	Amphotericin B, miconazole	Penicillin G
Hypotension	Pentamidine, emetine	—
Metabolic		
Hypokalemia	Carbenicillin, amphotericin B	—
Hypogonadal effects	Ketoconazole	—
Hyperglycemia	Nalidixic acid	—
Pancreatitis	Pentamidine, nitrofurantoin, TMP-SMX	—
Diabetes	Pentamidine	—
Hypomagnesemia	Amphotericin B, aminoglycosides	—
Renal		
Hypersensitivity nephritis	Sulfonamides	—
Interstitial nephritis	All beta-lactams	—
Tubular toxocity	Aminoglycosides, polymyxins	Vancomycin, teicoplanin
Distal tubular acidosis	Amphotericin B, tetracyclines	—
Crystal deposition	Fluoroquinolones, acyclovir	—
Neurologic		
Peripheral neuropathy	Nitrofurans, metronidazole, polymyxins, griseofulvin, cycloserine, isoniazid, linezolid	Tetracyclines
Muscular blockade	Polymyxins, aminoglycosides, capreomycin	Clindamycin, lincomycin
Central nervous excitation	—	Fluoroquinolones
Seizures	Penicillin, imipenem, cycloserine	Amantadine, isoniazid, metronidazole, fluoroquinolones, thiabendazole
Ophthalmic		
Opthalmic disturbances	Ethambutol	Isoniazid, chloramphenicol, quinolones, chloroquine
Ototoxicity		
Deafness	Aminoglycosides, vancomycin	Erythromycin
Vestibulotoxicity	Aminoglycosides, minocycline	—

Abbreviations: SLE, systemic lupus erythematosus; G6PD, glucose-6-phosphate dehydrogenase; TMP-SMX, trimethoprim-sulfamethoxazole.

Table 1b. Reported Percentage Frequency of Selected Adverse Effects after Oral Administration of Antibacterial Drugs in Different Studies

Drug	No. of patients	Percentage with					Other Adverse Effects
		Nausea	Vomiting	Diarrhea	Rash	Therapy stopped	
Cephalosporins							
Cephalexin	116	4.0	10	6.0	1.0	NP	"Serum sickness"
	305	2.3	0.7	1.3	1.0	1.3	0.02–0.5%
Cefaclor	245	4.5	0.4	5.7	0.4	—	
	129	NP	NP	3.0	2.0	—	
	435	1.0	1.0	2.0	1.0	—	
	374	2.4	0.5	3.7	1.3	—	
	NP	NP	NP	1.0	1.5	2.4	
Cefuroxime axetil	84	5.0	1.0	8.0	0	—	
	NP	2.4	2.0	3.5	0.6	—	
Cefixime	134	NP	NP	16	3.0	—	
	NP	7.0	NP	16	<2.0	3.8	
Cefprozil	2,383	2.3	0.7	1.2	0.7	2.0	
	NP	3.5	1.0	2.9	0.9	2.0	
Cefpodoxime	762	1.0	NP	4.0	NP	2.0	
Proxetil	3,650	—	2.0	—	NP	NP	
	1,468	1.0	0.2	4.6	0.5	2.3	
Loracarbef	4,506	1.9	1.4	4.1	1.2	1.5	
Ceftibuten	1,870	1.0	2.0	4.0	<1.0	—	
Penicillins							
Penicillin V	630	3.3	1.3	3.7	0.6	2.5	
	199	0	0	5.0	0	—	
	918	NP	NP	NP	1.2–3.0	—	
	NP	NP	NP	NP	2.5–4.2	—	
Ampicillin	1,775	NP	NP	NP	5.2	—	
	2,998	NP	NP	—	5.2	—	
Amoxicillin	574	1.7	0.5	4.5	1.6	1.9	
	1,225	NP	NP	NP	3.9–6.4	—	
Amoxicillin-clavulanate	129	NP	1.6	8.5	0.8	—	
	267	NP	2.0	22.0	1.0	1.0	
	110	5.0	2.0	18.0	4.0	—	
	306	NP	9.2	24.0	NP	—	
	NP	3.0	1.0	9.0	3.0	2.0–3.0	

Table 1b. Reported Percentage Frequency of Selected Adverse Effects after Oral Administration of Antibacterial Drugs in Different Studies (continued)

Drug	No. of patients	Percentage with					Other Adverse Effects
		Nausea	Vomiting	Diarrhea	Rash	Therapy stopped	
Lincosamide							
Clindamycin	52	NP	NP	31.0	21.0	31.0	CDT antibiotic associated diarrhea in 0.01–18% of treated patients
Macrolides							
Erythromycin base	128	2.0	3.0	2.0	0	NP	Rare idiosyncratic hepatitis
	147	NP	NP	NP	NP	0.4–0.6	
Enteric coated	441	5.5	2.9	5.3	0.6	4.9	
	112	—	27.0	—	0	19.0	
	21	—	52.0	—	0	14.0	
Azithromycin	3,995	2.6	0.8	3.6	0.2	0.7	
	229	2.6	NP	5.2	NP	NP	
	NP	3.0	<1.0	5.0	<1.0	0.7	
Clarithromycin	3,768	3.8	NP	3.0	NP	NP	
	NP	3.0	NP	3.0	0	4.0	
Fluoroquinolones							
Ciprofloxacin	4,287	—	2.3	1.5	0.8	1.2	Symptoms referable to CNS (i.e., headache, agitation, dizziness, and sleep disturbances in 1–4%)
	2,799	5.2	2.0	2.3	1.1	3.5	
Ofloxacin	3,184	—	5.4	—	NP	—	In high dose, headache, tremor disorientation
	15,641	—	0.9	0.4	0.3	1.5	
	NP	3.0	1.3	1.0	NP	4.0	
Lomefloxacin	2,869	3.7	<1.0	1.4	1.0	2.6	
Temafloxacin	2,602	5.6	1.1	2.8	1.5	4.1	
TMP-SMX	1,066	—	—	—	—	2.4–4.7	
	47	—	18.0	—	2.0	2.0	
	47	11.0	NP	0	6.0	11.0	
	196	8.2	—	0	5.0	4.0	
	180	—	4.0	—	2.0	3.9	
	129	—	7.0	—	7.0	NP	
	216	9.3	NP	NP	NP	5.1	

Abbreviations: NP, not provided; CNS, central nervous system; CDT, *Clostridium difficile* toxin; TMP-SMX, trimethoprim-sulfamethoxazole.
Source: Modified from Gilbert DN. Aspects of the safety profile of oral antibacterial agents. *Infect Dis Clin Pract* 1995;4[Suppl 2]:S103–S112.

Table 1c. Selected Drug–Drug Interactions Involving an Oral Antibacterial Agent

Antibacterial Agent (A)	Other Drug (B)	Effect	Significance/Certainty
Erythromycin (includes azithromycin and clarithromycin)	Carbamazepine	↑ Levels[a] of B	Avoid combination
	Corticosteroids	↑ Levels[a] of B	Awareness
	Digoxin	↑ Levels[a] of B	Awareness
	Theophylline	↑ Levels[a] of B	Dosage adjustment
	Terfenadine or astemizole	↑ Levels[a] of B	Avoid risk of serious cardiovascular adverse drug reactions
Fluoroquinolones			
All agents	Cimetidine	↑ Levels[a] of A	Awareness
	Multivalent cations (i.e., aluminum, chromium, iron, magnesium, zinc)	↓ Absorption of A	Awareness
Ciprofloxacin	Theophylline	↑ Levels[a] of B	Dosage adjustment
	Caffeine	↑ Levels[a] of B	Awareness
	Oral anticoagulants	↑ Prothrombin time	Monitor prothrombin time
Ofloxacin	Oral anticoagulants	↑ Prothrombin time	Monitor prothrombin time
Tetracyclines (includes doxycycline)	Multivalent cations (i.e., aluminum, bismuth, iron, magnesium, and others)	↓ Absorption of A	Awareness
	Digoxin	↑ Levels[a] of B	Awareness
	Phenytoin	↓ Serum half-life of A	Awareness
Trimethoprim-sulfamethoxazole	Phenytoin	↑ Levels[a] of B	Dosage adjustment
	Oral anticoagulants	↑ Prothrombin time	Monitor prothrombin time
	Sulfonylureas	↑ Effects of B	Monitor blood glucose

[a]Serum levels.
Source: From Gilbert DN. Aspects of the safety profile of oral antibacterial agents. *Infect Dis Clin Pract* 1995;4[Suppl 2]:S103–S112.

Table 2a. Antimicrobial Dosing Regimens in Renal Failure

GENERAL PRINCIPLES
The initial dose is not modified in renal failure. Adjustments in subsequent doses for renally excreted drugs may be accomplished by the following:
- Usual maintenance dose at extended intervals, usually 3 half-lives (extended interval method)
- Reduced doses at the usual intervals (dose reduction method)
- A combination of each

Adjustments in dose are usually based on creatinine clearance that may be estimated by the Cockroft–Gault equation that corrects for 3 critical variables: Age, weight, and gender (Nephron 1976;16:31)

$$\text{Male: } \frac{\text{weight (kg)} \times (140 \text{ minus age in years})}{72 \times \text{serum creatinine (mg/dL)}}$$

Female: above value $\times$ 0.85

Pitfalls and notations with calculations follow.
- Elderly patient: Serum creatinine may be deceptively low (with danger of overdosing) due to reduced muscle mass.
- Pregnancy, ascites, and other causes of volume expansion: GFR may be increased (with danger of underdosing) in the third trimester of pregnancy and in patients with normal renal function who receive massive parenteral fluids.
- Obese patients: Use lean body weight.
- Renal failure: Formulas assume stable renal function; for patients with anuria or oliguria assume creatinine clearance of 5–8 mL/min.

AMINOGLYCOSIDE DOSING

Guidelines of the Johns Hopkins Hospital Clinical Pharmacology Department

Agent	Loading Dose Regardless of Renal Function (mg/kg)	Subsequent Doses (before level measurements) CCr > 70 mL/min	Subsequent Doses (before level measurements) CCr < 70 mL/min	Therapeutic Levels 1 Hour after Start of Infusion over 20–30 Minutes (μg/mL)
Gentamicin[a]	2.0	1.7–2.0 mg/kg/8 h	0.03 CCr = mg/kg/8 h	5–10
Tobramycin[a]	2.0	1.7–2.0 mg/kg/8 h	0.03 CCr = mg/kg/8 h	5–10
Netilmicin[a]	2.2	2.0–2.2 mg/kg/8 h	0.03 CCr = mg/kg/8 h	5–10
Amikacin	7.5	7.5–8.0 mg/kg/8 h	0.12 CCr = mg/kg/8 h	20–40
Kanamycin	7.5	7.5–8.0 mg/kg/8 h	0.12 CCr = mg/kg/8 h	20–40

Initial dose: Gentamicin, tobramycin, netilmicin 1.5–2.0 mg/kg; amikacin, kanamycin 5.0–7.5 mg/kg.
Maintenance dose: Usual daily dose creatinine clearance/100. CCr, creatinine clearance.
[a] Doses should be written in multiples of 5 mg; doses of amikacin and kanamycin should be written in multiples of 25 mg. For obese patients use calculated lean body weight plus 40% of excess adipose tissue. For patients who are oliguric or anuric, use CCr of 5–8 mL/min. Seriously ill patients with sepsis often need higher loading doses to achieve rapid therapeutic levels despite third spacing, for example, 3 mg/kg for gentamicin and tobramycin.
Mayo clinic guidelines follow Van Scoy RE, Wilson WR. *Mayo Clin Proc* 1987;62:1142.

ONCE-DAILY AMINOGLYCOSIDES
Rationale
Efficacy.
High serum levels achieve concentration-dependent killing properties; the post-antibiotic effect (PAE) refers to continued bacterial growth suppression when the serum concentration is below the minimum inhibitory concentration (MIC). The PAE usually lasts 2–4 hours. The implication is that therapeutic levels are readily achieved and the antibiotic continues to suppress bacteria at concentrations below the MIC. Meta-analysis of 17 studies showed that clinical outcome is comparable with once-daily aminoglycosides and standard treatment with multiple daily doses.

(continued)

Table 2a. Antimicrobial Dosing Regimens in Renal Failure (continued)

Toxicity.
- Renal: Longer dosing intervals are associated with reduced renal cortical accumulation and a trend toward reduced nephrotoxicity.
- Ototoxicity: This side effect is related to perilymph accumulation of aminoglycoside rather than to concentration. Meta-analysis of 17 reports showed a 33% reduction in ototoxicity.

Clinical Trials

A review of 24 published trials involving once-daily aminoglycoside compared with standard multiple dosing treatment showed the following.

	Once-Daily Dosing	Multiple Dosing
Favorable outcome		
Clinical	1,041/1,163 (90%)	929/1,097 (84%)
Bacteriologic	636/718 (89%)	557/668 (83%)
Toxicity		
Nephrotoxicity	73/1,617 (5%)	86/1,564 (6%)
Ototoxicity	28/674 (4%)	34/636 (5%)

Contraindications

Patients receiving aminoglycosides for synergy with β-lactam agents versus enterococcus (enterococcal endocarditis) should receive standard multiple daily-dosing regimens. There is limited experience with once-daily aminoglycosides in selected clinical settings, such that some authorities consider them relative contraindications in the following settings: Neutropenic patients, critically ill or septic patients, pregnant patients, renal failure, elderly and pediatric patients, infections involving gram-positive bacteria, endocarditis, or burn patients.

Monitoring

Some authorities suggest monitoring pre-dose levels (18 hours) that should show gentamicin or tobramycin levels <0.5 μg/mL and amikacin levels <4–5 μg/mL; higher levels should lead to dose reduction.

Regimen

- Standard dose: Gentamicin and tobramycin 5–6 mg/kg/d (some use a range of 4–7 mg/kg); amikacin and streptomycin 15–20 mg/kg/d
- Dose adjustment based on trough levels; gentamicin and tobramycin ≤0.5 μg/mL; amikacin <5 μg/mL.
- Dose adjustment is based on renal function.

| | Creatinine clearance (mL/min) | | | |
Agent	>80	60–80	40–60	30–40
Gentamicin or tobramycin (mg/kg/d)	5	4	3.5	2.5
Amikacin (mg/kg/d)	15	12	7.5	4.0

Dose may be based on anatomic site of infection: High dose for pneumonia; low dose for urinary tract infection.

Hartford Hospital Regimen

| Creatinine Clearance (mL/min) | Aminoglycoside Dosage | |
	Gentamicin or Tobramycin	Amikacin
>60	7 mg/kg[a] q24h	15 mg/kg q24h
40–59	7 mg/kg q36h	15 mg/kg q36h
20–39	7 mg/kg q48h	15 mg/kg q48h

Experience with 2,184 patients: Mean dose, 450 mg; mean peak serum level, 26 μg/mL (gentamicin, tobramycin); frequency of nephrotoxicity (creatinine increase of 0.5 mg/dL above baseline), 1.2%; nephrotoxicity with >6 days of therapy, 2.0%; nephrotoxicity with >13 days of therapy, 3.3%; ototoxicity, 0.2%.
[a] Obese patients >20% above ideal body weight: Ideal weight +0.4 (actual weight–ideal weight); aminoglycoside was delivered over 60 min in 50-mL increments.
Source: Adapted from Nicolau DP, Freeman CD, Belliveau PP, Nightingale CH, Ross JW, Quintiliani R. Experience with a once-daily aminoglycoside program administered to 2,184 adult patients. *Antimicrob Agents Chemother* 1995;39:650.

Table 2b. Drug Therapy Dosing Guidelines

Drug	Major Excretory Route	Half-life (hr) Normal	Half-life (hr) Anuria	Usual regimen Oral	Usual regimen Parenteral	Maintenance regimen renal failure glomerular filtration rate (mL/min) 50–80	10–50	<10
Acyclovir	Renal	2.0–2.5	20	200 mg 3–5 times/d 400 mg b.i.d 800 mg 5 times/d —	— — — 5–10 mg/kg q8h	Usual Usual 800 mg q8h Usual	Usual Usual 800 mg q8h 5–12 mg/kg q12–24h	200 mg q12h 200 mg q12h 800 mg q12h 2.5–6.0 mg/kg q24h
Albendazole	Hepatic	8	8	400–800 mg b.i.d	—	Usual	Usual	Usual
Amantadine	Renal	15–20	170	100 mg b.i.d	—	100–150 mg per day	100–200 mg 2–3 times/wk	100–200 mg QWK
Amikacin	Renal	2	30	—	7.5 mg/kg q12h	12 mg/kg q24h (60–80 CCr) 7.5 mg/kg q24h (40–60 CCr)	7.5 mg/kg q48–72h	7.5 mg/kg q24h (40–60 CCr) 4 mg/kg q24h (30–40 CCr)
Amoxicillin	Renal	1	15–20	250–500 mg q8h	—	0.25–0.5 g q12h	0.25–0.5 g q12–24h	0.25–0.5 g q12–24h
Amoxicillin-clavulanic acid	Renal	1	8–16	250–500 mg q8h	—	Usual	0.25–0.5 g q12h	0.25–0.5 g q24–36h
Amphotericin B	Hepatic	15 d	15 d	—	0.3–1.4 mg/kg/d	Usual	Usual	Usual
Amphotericin B lipid complex	Hepatic	8 d	8 d	—	5 mg/kg	Usual	Usual	Usual
Ampicillin	Renal	1	8–12	0.25–0.5 g q6h	1–3 g q4–6h	Usual	0.5 g q8h 1–2 g IV q8h	0.5 g q12h 1–2 g IV q12h
Ampicillin-Sulbactam	Renal	1	8–12	—	1–2 g q6h	1–2 g IV q8h	1–2 g IV q8h	1–2 g IV q12h
Atovaquone	Gut	70	70	750 mg b.i.d suspension	—	Usual	Usual	Unknown
Azithromycin	Hepatic	68	68	250 mg/d	—	Usual	use caution	—
Aztreonam	Renal	1.7–2.0	6–9	—	1–2 g q6h	1–2 g q8–12h	1–2 g q12–18h	1–2 g q24h
Bacampicillin	Renal	1	8–12	0.4–0.8 g q12h	1 g per day (IM)	Usual	Usual	0.4–0.8 q 24h
Capreomycin	Renal	4–6	50–100	—	—	—	—	Avoid
Carbenicillin	Renal	1	13–16	0.5–1.0 g q6h	—	Usual	Usual	Usual
Cefaclor	Renal	0.75	2.8	0.25–0.5 g q8h	—	Usual	Usual	0.5 g q36h
Cefadroxil	Renal	1.4	20–25	0.5–1.0 g q12–24h	—	Usual	0.5 g q12–24h	0.5–0.75 g q12h
Cefamandole	Renal	0.5–2.1	10	—	0.5–2.0 g q4–8h	0.5–2.0 g q6h	0.5–1.0 g q8–12h	0.25–0.75 g q18–24h
Cefazolin	Renal	1.8	18–36	—	0.5–2.0 g q8h	0.5–1.5 q8h	0.5–1.0 g q24h	250–500 mg q24h
Cefepime	Renal	2	13	—	0.5–2.0 g q12h	0.5–2.0 g q24h	300 mg/d	200 mg/d
Cefixime	Renal	3–4	12	200 mg q12h	—	Usual	1–2 g q18–24h	1–2 g q48h
Cefmetazole	Renal	1.2	—	—	2 g q6–12h	1–2 g q12h	4–8 mg/kg q24h	4 mg/kg q3–5d
Cefonicid	Renal	4–5	50–60	—	0.5–2.0 g q24h	8–25 mg/kg q24h	Usual	Usual
Cefoperazone	Gut	1.9–2.5	2.0–2.5	—	1–2 g q6–12h	Usual	Usual	0.5–1.0 g q48–72h
Ceforanide	Renal	3	20–40	—	0.5–1.0 g q12h	Usual	0.5–1.0 g q24h	1–2 g q6–12h
Cefotaxime	Renal	1.1	3	—	1–2 g q4–8h	Usual	1–2 g q24h	1–2 g q12h
Cefotetan	Renal	3–4	12–30	—	1–2 g q12h	Usual	1–2 g q8–12h	1–2 g q48h
Cefoxitin	Renal	0.7	13–22	—	1–2 g q6–8h	1–2 g q8–12h	1–2 g q12–24h	0.5–1.0 g q12–48h
Cefpodoxime	Renal	2.4	10	200–400 mg q12h	—	200–400 mg q24h	200–400 mg 3 times/wk	200–400 mg/wk
Cefprozil	Renal	1.3	5–6	0.25–0.5 g q12h	—	Usual	0.25–0.5 g q24h	0.25 g q12–24h

(continued)

Table 2b. Drug Therapy Dosing Guidelines (continued)

Drug	Major Excretory Route	Half-life (hr) Normal	Half-life (hr) Anuria	Usual regimen Oral	Usual regimen Parenteral	Maintenance regimen renal failure glomerular filtration rate (mL/min) 50–80	10–50	<10
Ceftazidime	Renal	0.9–1.7	15–25	—	1–2 g q8–12h	Usual	1 g q12–24h	0.5 g q24–48h
Ceftibuten	Renal	2.4	22	400 mg/d	—	Usual	200 mg/d	100 mg/d
Ceftizoxime	Renal	1.4–1.8	25–35	—	1–3 g q6–8h	0.5–1.5 g q8h	0.25–1.0 g q12h	0.25–0.5 g q24h
Ceftriaxone	Renal and Gut	6–9	12–15	—	0.5–1.0 g q12–24h	-Usual	Usual	Usual
Cefuroxime	Renal	1.3–1.7	20	—	0.75–1.5 g q8h	Usual	0.75–1.5 g q8–12h	0.75 g q24h
Cefuroxime axetil	Renal	1.2	20	250 mg q12h	—	Usual	Usual	250 mg q24h
Cephalexin	Renal	0.9	5–30	0.25–1.0 g q6h	—	Usual	0.25–1.0 g q8–12h	0.25–1.0 g q24–48h
Cephalothin	Renal	0.5–0.9	3–8	—	0.5–2.0 g q4–8h	0.5–2.0 g q6h	1.0–1.5 g q6h	0.5 g q8h
Cephapirin	Renal	0.6–0.9	2.4	—	0.5–2.0 g q4–6h	Usual	0.5–2.0 g q8h	0.5–2.0 g q12h
Cephradine	Renal	0.7–2.0	8–15	0.25–1.0 g q6h	0.25–1.0 g q6h	0.5–2.0 g q6h	0.5 g q6h	0.25 g q12h
Chloramphenicol	Hepatic	2.5	3–7	0.25–0.75 g q6h	—	Usual	Usual	Usual
Chloroquine	Renal and metabolized	48–120	—	300–600 mg PO per day	—	Usual	Usual	150–300 mg PO per day
Cidofovir	Renal	17–65	↑	—	5 mg/kg qwk for 2 wk (induction); 5 mg/kg qwk for 22 wk (maintenance)	Usual	Dosage titrated to creatinine clearance	Contraindicated
Cinoxacin	Renal	1.5	8.5	0.25–0.5 g q12h	—	0.25 g q8h	0.25 g q12h	0.25 g q24h
Ciprofloxacin	Renal and hepatic metabolism	4	5–10	0.25–0.75 g q12h	—	Usual	0.25–0.5 g q12h	0.25–0.5 g q18h
Clarithromycin	Hepatic and renal metabolism	4	↑	250–500 mg q12h	400 mg q12h	Usual / Usual	0.4 g q18h	0.4 g q24h / 250–500 mg q24h
Clindamycin	Hepatic	2.0–2.5	2.0–3.5	150–300 mg q6h	300–900 mg q6–8h	Usual	Usual	Usual
Clofazimine	Hepatic	8 d	8 d	50 mg per day; 100 mg t.i.d	—	Usual	Usual	Usual
Cloxacillin	Renal	0.5	0.8	0.5–1.0 g q6h	—	Usual	Usual	Usual
Colistin	Renal	3–8	10–20	—	1.5 mg/kg q6–12h	2.5–3.8 mg/kg q24h	1.5–2.5 mg/kg q24–36h	0.6 mg/kg q24h
Cycloserine	Renal	8–12	—	250–500 mg b.i.d	—	Usual	250–500 mg q24h	250 mg q24h
Dapsone	Hepatic metabolism	30	↑	50–100 mg/d	—	Usual	Usual	—
Daptomycin	Renal	7.7–8.3	30.5	—	4–6 mg/kg q24h	Usual	<30 mL/min: Every 48h	Usual
Dicloxacillin	Renal	0.5–0.9	1.0–1.6	0.25–0.5 g q6h	—	Usual	Usual	Usual
D₄T (see Stavudine)								
Dideoxyinosine (ddI, didanosine)	Renal, nonrenal	1.3–1.6	—	200 mg b.i.d	—	Usual	Consider dose reduction; note Mg load—60 mEq/tablet	
Dideoxycytidine (ddC, zalcitabine)	Renal	2	8	0.75 mg t.i.d	—	Usual	0.75 mg b.i.d	0.75 mg
Dirithromycin	Bile	30–44	30–44	500 mg q24h	—	Usual	Usual	Usual
Doripenem	Renal	1	—	—	500 mg q8h	Usual	30–50 mL/min: 250 mg q8h	10–30 mL/min: 250 mg q12h
Doxycycline	Renal and gut	14–25	15–36	100 mg b.i.d	100 mg b.i.d	Usual	Usual	Usual

Drug	Route of elimination	Half-life, normal (h)	Half-life, reduced renal function (h)	Dose for normal renal function	Usual	Half usual dose	Half usual dose
Enoxacin	Renal and hepatic metabolism	3–6	—	200–400 mg b.i.d	Usual		
Ertapenem	Renal	4	—	1 g q24h	Usual	<30 mL/min: 0.5 g q24h	
Erythromycin	Hepatic	1.2–1.6	4–6	0.25–0.5 g q6h; 1 g q6h	Usual	Usual	
Ethambutol	Renal	3–4	8	15–25 mg/kg q24h	15 mg/kg q24h	15 mg/kg q24–36h	15 mg/kg q48h
Ethionamide	Metabolized	4	9	0.5–1.0 g q24h (in 1–3 doses)	Usual	Usual	5 mg/kg q48h
Famciclovir	Renal	2.3	13	125 mg q12h; 500 mg q8h	Usual	125 mg q24h; 500 mg q12–24h	125 mg q48h; 250 mg q48h
Fluconazole	Renal	20–50	100	100–400 mg q24h	Usual	One-half usual dose	25–50 mg q24h
Flucytosine	Renal	3–6	70	37 mg/kg q6h	Usual	37 mg/kg q12–24h	Adjust to keep 2-hr concentration at 50–100 µg/mL
Foscarnet — Induction	Renal	3	8	60 mg/kg q8h	40–50 mg/kg q8h	20–30 mg/kg q8h	Contraindicated (CCr <20 mL/min)
Foscarnet — Maintenance				90 mg/kg/d	60–70 mg/kg per day	50–70 mg/kg per day	Contraindicated (CCr <20 mL/min)
Foscarnet — Maintenance				120 mg/kg/d	80–90 mg/kg per day	60–80 mg/kg per day	Contraindicated (CCr <20 mL/min)
Ganciclovir — Induction	Renal	2.5–3.6	10	5 mg/kg b.i.d	2.5 mg/kg b.i.d	2.5 mg/kg per day	1.25 mg/kg per day
Ganciclovir — Maintenance (half of induction dose)			—	5 mg/kg/d	2.5 mg/kg/d	1.2 mg/kg/d	0.6 mg/kg/d
Ganciclovir (oral)	GI	3–7	10	1,000 mg t.i.d	500 mg t.i.d	500 mg per day	500 mg 3 times/wk
Gentamicin	Renal	2	48	1.7 mg/kg q8h	4 mg/kg q24h (60–80 CCr); 3.5 mg/kg q24h (40–60 CCr)	3.5 mg/kg q24h (40–60 CCr); 2.5 mg/kg q24h (30–40 CCr)	
Griseofulvin	Hepatic metabolism						
Microsize	Same	24	24	0.5–1.0 g q24h	Usual	Usual	Usual
Ultramicrosize		24	24	0.33–0.66 g q24h	Usual	Usual	Usual
Imipenem-cilastatin	Renal	0.8–1.0	3.5	0.5–1.0 g q6h	0.5 g q6–8h	0.5 g q8–12h	0.25–0.5 g q12h
Indinavir	Hepatic metabolism	1.5–2.0	2–10	800 mg tid	Usual	Usual	Usual
Isoniazid	Hepatic	0.5–4.0		300 mg q24h	Usual	Usual	Slow acetylators, half-dose
Itraconazole	Hepatic	20–60	20–60	100–200 mg/d	Usual	Usual	Usual
Ketoconazole	Hepatic metabolism	1–4	1–4	200–400 mg q12–24h	Usual	Usual	Usual
Lamivudine (3TC)	Renal	3–6 h		150 mg b.i.d	Usual	100–150 mg/d	25–50 mg/d
Levofloxacin	Renal	6.3	35	500 mg q24h	Usual	250 mg q24h	250 mg q48h
Linezolid	Nonrenal	6.4	7.1	600 mg q12h	Usual	—	
Lomefloxacin	Renal	8	45	400 mg q24h	Usual	400 mg q24h; then 200 mg q24h	—
Loracarbef	Renal	1	32	200–400 mg q12h	Usual	200–400 mg q24h	200–400 mg q3–5d
Mefloquine	Hepatic	2–4 wk	2–4 wk	250 mg/wk	Usual	Usual	Usual
Meropenem	Renal	1	↑	1 g q8h	Usual	500 mg q12h	500 mg q24h

(continued)

Table 2b. Drug Therapy Dosing Guidelines (continued)

Drug	Major Excretory Route	Half-life (hr) Normal	Half-life (hr) Anuria	Usual regimen Oral	Usual regimen Parenteral	Maintenance 50–80	Maintenance 10–50	Maintenance <10
Methenamine								
Hippurate	Renal	3–6	—	1 g q12h	—	Usual	Avoid	Avoid
Mandelate	Renal	3–6	—	1 g q6h	—	Usual	Avoid	Avoid
Metronidazole	Hepatic	6–14	8–15	0.25–0.75 g t.i.d	0.5 g q6h	Usual	Usual	Usual
Mezlocillin	Renal	1	1.5	—	3–4 g q4–6h	Usual	3 g q8h	2 g q8h
Miconazole	Hepatic	0.5–1	0.5–1.0	—	0.4–1.2 g q8h	Usual	Usual	Usual
Minocycline	Hepatic and metabolized	11–26	17–30	100 mg q12h	100 mg q12h	Usual	Usual	Usual or slight decrease
Nafcillin	Hepatic metabolism	0.5	1.2	0.5–1.0 g q6h	0.5–2.0 g q4–6h	Usual	Usual	Usual
Nalidixic acid	Renal and hepatic metabolism	1.5	21	1 g q6h	—	Usual	Usual	Avoid
Nelfinavir	Hepatic metabolism	3.5–5.0	3.5–5.0	750 mg t.i.d	—	Usual	Usual	Usual
Netilmicin	Renal	2.5	35	—	2 mg/kg q8h	0.03 × CCr mg/kg/8 h	0.03 × CCr mg/kg/8 h	0.03 × CCr mg/kg/8 h
Nevirapine	Hepatic	25	1	200 mg b.i.d	—	Usual	Usual	Usual, "with caution"
Nitrofurantoin	Renal	0.3	1	50–100 mg q6–8h	—	Usual	Avoid	Avoid
Norfloxacin	Renal and hepatic metabolism	3.5	8	400 mg b.i.d	—	Usual	400 mg per day	400 mg per day
Nystatin	Not absorbed	—	—	0.4–1.0 million units 3–5 times/d	—	Usual	Usual	Usual
Ofloxacin	Renal	6	40	200–400 mg b.i.d	200–400 mg q12h	Usual	200–400 mg per day / 200–400 mg q24h	100–200 mg per day / 100–200 mg q24h
Oxacillin	Renal	0.5	1	0.5–1.0 g q6h	1–3 g q6h	Usual	Usual	Usual
Penicillin								
Crystalline (G)	Renal	0.5	7–10		1–4 million units q4–6h	Usual	Usual	Half usual dose
Procaine	Renal	24	—		0.6–1.2 million units IM q12h	Usual	Usual	Usual
Benzathine	Renal	Days	—		0.6–1.2 million units IM	Usual	Usual	Usual
V	Renal	0.5–1.0	7–10	0.4–0.8 million units q6h	—	Usual	Usual	Usual
Pentamidine	Nonrenal	6	6–8	—	4 mg/kg q24h	Usual	4 mg/kg q24–36h	4 mg/kg q48h
Piperacillin	Renal	1	3	—	3–4 g q4–6h	Usual	3 g q8h	3 g q12h
Piperacillin + Tazobactam	Renal	1	3	—	3/0.375 g q6h	Usual	2/0.25 g q6g	2/0.25 q 8h
Praziquantel	Hepatic metabolism	0.8–1.5	—	10–25 mg/kg t.i.d	—	Usual	Usual	Usual
Pyrazinamide	Metabolized	10–16	—	15–35 mg/kg/d	—	Usual	Usual	12–20 mg/kg/d
Pyrimethamine	Hepatic metabolism	1.5–5.0 d	—	25–75 mg/d	—	Usual	Usual	Usual
Quinacrine	Renal	5 d	—	100–200 mg q6–8h	—	Usual	—	—
Quinine	Hepatic	4–5	4–5	650 mg t.i.d	7.5–10.0 mg/kg q8h	Usual	Usual	Usual

Drug	Route of elimination	Half-life, normal (h)	Half-life, ESRD (h)	Dose for normal renal function	GFR >50 mL/min	GFR 10–50 mL/min	GFR <10 mL/min
Rifampin	Hepatic	Early 2–5, Late 2	2–5	600 mg/d	Usual	Usual	Usual
Rimantadine	Hepatic	24–30	48–60	100 mg b.i.d	Usual	Usual	100 mg/d
Ritonavir	Hepatic metabolism	3–4	—	600 mg b.i.d	Usual	Usual	Usual
Saquinavir	Hepatic metabolism	1–2	1–2	600 mg t.i.d	Usual	Usual	Usual
Sparfloxacin	Renal	20	↑	200 mg q24h	Usual	200 mg q48h	200 mg q48h
Spectinomycin	Renal	1–3	—	2 g d IM	Usual	Usual	Usual
Stavudine	Renal and hepatic metabolism	1	—	40 mg b.i.d	Usual	20 mg 1–2 times/d	—
Streptomycin	Renal	2–5	100–110	500 mg q12h	15 mg/kg q24–72h	15 mg/kg q72–96h	7.5 mg/kg q72–96h
Sulfadiazine	Renal	8–17	22–34	0.5–1.5 g q4–6h; 30–50 mg/kg q6–8h	Usual; Usual	0.5–1.5 g q8–12h; 30–50 mg/kg q12–18h	0.5–1.5 g q12–24h; 30–50 mg/kg q18–24h
Sulfisoxazole	Renal	3–7	6–12	1–2 g q6h	Usual	1 g q8–12h	1 g q12–24h
Teicoplanin	Renal	6	41	6–12 mg/kg/d	Usual	Half usual dose	One-third usual dose
Tetracycline	Renal	8	50–100	0.5–1.0 g q12h; 0.25–0.5 g q6h	Usual	Use doxycycline	Use doxycycline
Ticarcillin	Renal	1.0–1.5	16	3 g q4h	Usual	2–3 g q6–8h	2 g q12h
Ticarcillin + clavulanic acid	Renal	1.0–1.5	16	3 g q4–6h	Usual	2–3 g q6–8h	2 g q12h
Tigecycline	Biliary and renal	27.1	—	100 mg initially and then 50 mg q12h	Usual	usual	Usual
Tobramycin	Renal	2.5	56	1.7 mg/kg q8h	0.03 × CCr mg/kg/8 h	0.03 × CCr mg/kg/8 h	0.03 × CCr mg/kg/8 h
Trimethoprim	Renal	8–15	24	100 mg q12h	Usual	100 mg q24h	Avoid
Trimethoprim-sulfamethoxazole (TMP-SMX)	Renal	TMP: 8–15; SMX: 7–12	24; SMX: 22–50	3–5 mg/kg q6–12h; 1–2 tablets q12h or 1–2 double-strength tablets q12h	Usual	Half dose	Avoid
Trimetrexate	Metabolized	11	14	45 mg/m2 q24h	Usual	3–5 mg/kg q12–24h	—
Valacyclovir	Renal	2.5–3.3	—	1,000 mg t.i.d; 500 mg b.i.d	Usual; Usual	1 g q12–24h; 500 mg q12–24h	500 mg q 24h
Vancomycin	Renal	6–8	200–250	15 mg/kg q12h; 0.125–0.5 g q6h	1 g q24h	Usual	1 g q5–10d; 0.125 g PO q6h
Zidovudine	Hepatic and renal metabolism	1	3	200 mg t.i.d	Usual	Usual	100 mg q6–8h

Abbreviations: GI, gastrointestinal; CCr, creatinine clearance

Source: Adapted from American Hospital Formulary Service. AHFS Drug Information. Bethesda, Md: American Society of Health System Pharmacists; 1996:37–612.

Table 3. Antimicrobial Dosing Regimens in Severe Liver Disease

Dose Unchanged	Dose Reduced	Avoid
Aminoglycosides	Cephalosporins[a,b]	Ketoconazole
Amphotericin B	Chloramphenicol	Pyrazinamide
Capreomycin	Clindamycin	Sulfonamides
Cephalosporins	Clofazimine	Tetracycline
Cycloserine	Dapsone	
Doxycycline	Erythromycin,[c] other macrolides	
Ethambutol	Isoniazid	
Penicillin	Metronidazole	
Pentamidine	Nitrofurantoin	
Polymyxin	Penicillins (antistaphylococcal)	
Quinolones[d]	Penicillins (antipseudomonal)	
Spectinomycin	Ribavirin	
Trimethoprim	Rifampicin	
	Tigecycline	
Vancomycin	Zidovudine	

Data are not as accurate as in kidney failure.
[a] Cephalothin, cefotaxime, cefoperazone, ceftriaxone, and cefotetan
[b] Dose reduced particularly for coexisting kidney and liver failure
[c] Avoid using estolate salt
[d] Except Pefloxacin

Table 4a. Recommended Adult Immunization Schedule, by Vaccine and Age Group

Vaccine ▼ Age group ▶	19–26 years	27–49 years	50–59 years	60–64 years	≥65 years
Influenza*	1 dose annually				
Tetanus, diphtheria, pertussis (Td/Tdap)*	Substitute 1-time dose of Tdap for Td booster; then boost with Td every 10 years				Td booster every 10 years
Varicella*	2 doses				
Human papillomavirus (HPV)*	3 doses (females)				
Zoster				1 dose	
Measles, mumps, rubella (MMR)*	1 or 2 doses		1 dose		
Pneumococcal (polysaccharide)	1 or 2 doses				1 dose
Meningococcal*	1 or more doses				
Hepatitis A*	2 doses				
Hepatitis B*	3 doses				

*Covered by the Vaccine Injury Compensation Program

For all persons in this category who meet the age requirements and who lack evidence of immunity (e.g., lack documentation of vaccination or have no evidence of previous infection)

Recommended if some other risk factor is present (e.g., based on medical, occupational, lifestyle, or other indications)

No recommendation

Drugs and Vaccines

Table 4b. Vaccines that Might be Indicated for Adults, Based on Medical and Other Indications

INDICATION ► / Vaccine ▼	Pregnancy	Immunocompromising conditions (excluding human immunodeficiency virus [HIV])	HIV infection CD4+ T lymphocyte count <200 cells/µL	HIV infection CD4+ T lymphocyte count ≥200 cells/µL	Diabetes, heart disease, chronic lung disease, chronic alcoholism	Asplenia (including elective splenectomy) and persistent complement component deficiencies	Chronic liver disease	Kidney failure, end-stage renal disease, receipt of hemodialysis	Healthcare personnel
Influenza*	1 dose TIV annually								1 dose TIV or LAIV annually
Tetanus, diphtheria, pertussis (Td/Tdap)*	Td	Substitute 1-time dose of Tdap for Td booster; then boost with Td every 10 years							
Varicella*	Contraindicated			2 doses					
Human papillomavirus (HPV)*		3 doses through age 26 years							
Zoster	Contraindicated			1 dose					
Measles, mumps, rubella*	Contraindicated			1 or 2 doses					
Pneumococcal (polysaccharide)		1 or 2 doses							
Meningococcal*	1 or more doses								
Hepatitis A*	2 doses								
Hepatitis B*	3 doses								

*Covered by the Vaccine Injury Compensation Program

For all persons in this category who meet the age requirements and who lack evidence of immunity (e.g., lack documentation of vaccination or have no evidence of previous infection)

Recommended if some other risk factor is present (e.g., on the basis of medical, occupational, lifestyle, or other indications)

No recommendation

- **Influenza vaccination [Trivalent inactivated influenza vaccine (TIV), Live, attenuated influenza vaccine (LAIV)]**
  - Healthy, nonpregnant adults <50 years without high-risk medical conditions can receive either intranasally administered live, attenuated influenza vaccine (FluMist), or inactivated vaccine.
  - Other persons should receive the inactivated vaccine.
  - Adults >65 years can receive the standard influenza vaccine or the high-dose (Fluzone) influenza vaccine.
- **Tetanus, diphtheria, and acellular pertussis (Td/Tdap) vaccination**
  - Administer a 1-time dose of Tdap to adults <65 years who have not received Tdap previously or for whom vaccine status is unknown to replace 1 of the 10-year Td boosters.
  - Adults >65 years who have not previously received Tdap and who have close contact with an infant aged <12 months also should be vaccinated.
  - Adults with uncertain or incomplete history of completing a 3-dose primary vaccination series with Td-containing vaccines should begin or complete a primary vaccination series.
  - If a woman is pregnant and has received the most recent Td vaccination 10 or more years previously, administer Td during the second or third trimester.
  - If the woman received the most recent Td vaccination <10 years previously, administer Tdap during the immediate postpartum period.
- **Varicella vaccination**
  - All adults without evidence of immunity to varicella should receive 2 doses of single-antigen varicella vaccine.
- **Human papillomavirus (HPV) vaccination**
  - HPV vaccination with either quadrivalent or bivalent vaccine is recommended for females at age 11 or 12 years and catch-up vaccination for females aged 13–26 years.
  - HPV4 may be administered to males aged 9 years through 26 years to reduce their likelihood of genital warts.
  - Ideally, vaccine should be administered before potential exposure to HPV through sexual activity.
  - A complete series consists of 3 doses. The second dose should be administered 1–2 months after the first dose; the third dose should be administered 6 months after the first dose.
- **Herpes zoster vaccination**
  - A single dose is recommended for adults aged >60 years regardless of whether they report a previous episode of herpes zoster.
- **Measles, mumps, rubella (MMR) vaccination**
  - Adults born before 1957 generally are considered immune to measles and mumps.
  - Measles/mumps component: A second dose, administered a minimum of 28 days after the first dose, is recommended for adults who:
    - Have been recently exposed to measles or are in a measles/mumps outbreak setting
    - Are students in postsecondary educational institutions
    - Work in a health-care facility
    - Plan to travel internationally
  - If no evidence of immunity, women who are not pregnant should be vaccinated.

(continued)

Table 4b. Vaccines that Might be Indicated for Adults, Based on Medical and Other Indications (continued)

- **Pneumococcal polysaccharide (PPSV) vaccination**

Vaccinate all persons with the following indications:
- Chronic lung disease (including asthma)
- Chronic cardiovascular diseases
- Diabetes mellitus
- Chronic liver diseases
- Cirrhosis
- Chronic alcoholism
- Functional or anatomic asplenia (if elective splenectomy is planned, vaccinate at least 2 weeks before surgery)
- Immunocompromising conditions (including chronic renal failure or nephrotic syndrome)
- Cochlear implants and cerebrospinal fluid leaks
- Vaccinate as close to HIV diagnosis as possible
- Residents of nursing homes
- Persons who smoke cigarettes

Revaccination with PPSV

1-time revaccination after 5 years is recommended for persons aged 19–64 years with:
- Chronic renal failure or nephrotic syndrome
- Functional or anatomic asplenia
- For persons with immunocompromising conditions

For persons >65 years, 1-time revaccination is recommended if they were vaccinated 5 or more years previously and were aged <65 years at the time of primary vaccination.

- **Meningococcal vaccination**

A 2-dose series of meningococcal conjugate vaccine is recommended for adults with
- Anatomic or functional asplenia
- Persistent complement component deficiencies
- Adults with HIV infection who are vaccinated should also receive a routine 2-dose series

A single dose of meningococcal vaccine is recommended for:
- Unvaccinated first-year college students living in dormitories
- Microbiologists routinely exposed to isolates of *Neisseria meningitidis*
- Military recruits
- Persons who travel to or live in countries in which meningococcal disease is hyperendemic or epidemic

Conjugate quadrivalent vaccine (MCV4) is preferred for adults who are aged 55 years or younger

Polysaccharide vaccine (MPSV4) is preferred for adults aged 56 years or older

Revaccination every 5 years is recommended for adults previously vaccinated who remain at increased risk for infection

- **Hepatitis A vaccination**

Vaccinate persons with any of the following indications and any person seeking protection from Hepatitis A virus (HAV) infection:
- Men who have sex with men
- Persons who use injection drugs
- Persons working with HAV-infected primates or with HAV in a research laboratory setting.
- Persons with chronic liver disease and persons who receive clotting factor concentrates.
- Persons traveling to or working in countries that have high or intermediate endemicity of hepatitis A

Single-antigen vaccine formulations should be administered in a 2-dose schedule at either 0 and 6–12 months (Havrix), or 0 and 6–18 months (Vaqta)

- **Hepatitis B vaccination**

Vaccinate persons with any of the following indications and any person seeking protection from Hepatitis B virus (HBV) infection:
- Sexually active persons not in a long-term, mutually monogamous relationship
- Persons seeking evaluation or treatment for a sexually transmitted disease
- Current or recent injection-drug users
- Men who have sex with men
- Health-care personnel and public-safety workers who are exposed to blood or other potentially infectious body fluids.
- End-stage renal disease, including patients receiving hemodialysis
- Persons with HIV infection
- Persons with chronic liver disease
- Household contacts and sex partners of persons with chronic HBV infection
- Clients and staff members of institutions for persons with developmental disabilities
- International travelers to countries with high or intermediate prevalence of chronic HBV infection

Adapted from Centers for Disease Control and Prevention. Recommended adult immunization schedule–United States, 2011. *MMWR Morb Mortal Wkly Rep* 2011;60(4):1–4.

Table 5a. Recommended Immunization Schedule for Persons Aged 0 Through 6 years

Vaccine ▼ Age ►	Birth	1 month	2 months	4 months	6 months	12 months	15 months	18 months	19–23 months	2–3 years	4–6 years
Hepatitis B	HepB	HepB				HepB					
Rotavirus			RV	RV	RV						
Diphtheria, Tetanus, Pertussis			DTaP	DTaP	DTaP		DTaP				DTaP
Haemophilus influenzae type b			Hib	Hib	Hib	Hib					
Pneumococcal			PCV	PCV	PCV	PCV				PPSV	
Inactivated Poliovirus			IPV	IPV		IPV					IPV
Influenza						Influenza (Yearly)					
Measles, Mumps, Rubella						MMR					MMR
Varicella						Varicella					Varicella
Hepatitis A						HepA (2 doses)				HepA Series	
Meningococcal											MCV4

Range of recommended ages for all children

Range of recommended ages for certain high-risk groups

- **Hepatitis B vaccine (HepB)** (Minimum age: Birth)
  - **At birth:**
    - Administer monovalent HepB to all newborns before hospital discharge.
    - If mother is hepatitis B surface antigen (HBsAg)-positive, administer HepB and 0.5 mL of hepatitis B immune globulin (HBIG) within 12 hours of birth.
  - **Doses following the birth dose:**
    - The second dose should be administered at age 1 or 2 months. Monovalent HepB should be used for doses administered before age 6 weeks.
- **Rotavirus vaccine (RV)** (Minimum age: 6 weeks) [Pentavalent human-bovine reassortant rotavirus vaccine (RotaTeq), Attenuated human rotavirus vaccine (Rotarix)]
  - Administer the first dose at age 6 through 14 weeks (maximum age: 14 weeks 6 days). Vaccination should not be initiated for infants aged 15 weeks 0 days or older.
  - The maximum age for the final dose in the series is 8 months 0 days.
  - If Rotarix is administered at ages 2 and 4 months, a dose at 6 months is not indicated.
- **Diphtheria and tetanus toxoids and acellular pertussis vaccine (DTaP)** (Minimum age: 6 weeks)
  - The fourth dose may be administered as early as age 12 months, provided at least 6 months have elapsed since the third dose.
- ***Haemophilus influenzae* type b conjugate vaccine (Hib)** (Minimum age: 6 weeks) [PRP-outer membrane protein conjugate vaccine (PedvaxHIB), PRP-tetanus toxoid conjugate vaccine (ActHIB, Hiberix)]
  - If PRP-OMP (PedvaxHIB or Comvax [HepB-Hib]) is administered at ages 2 and 4 months, a dose at age 6 months is not indicated.
  - Hiberix should not be used for doses at ages 2, 4, or 6 months for the primary series but can be used as the final dose in children aged 12 months through 4 years.
- **Pneumococcal vaccine** (Minimum age: 6 weeks for pneumococcal conjugate vaccine [PCV]; 2 years for pneumococcal polysaccharide vaccine [PPSV])
  - PCV is recommended for all children aged younger than 5 years. Administer 1 dose of PCV to all healthy children aged 24 through 59 months who are not completely vaccinated for their age.
  - A PCV series begun with 7-valent PCV (PCV7) should be completed with 13-valent PCV (PCV13).
  - A single supplemental dose of PCV13 is recommended for all children aged 14 through 59 months who have received an age-appropriate series of PCV7.
  - A single supplemental dose of PCV13 is recommended for all children aged 60 through 71 months with underlying medical conditions who have received an age-appropriate series of PCV7.
  - The supplemental dose of PCV13 should be administered at least 8 weeks after the previous dose of PCV7.
  - Administer PPSV at least 8 weeks after last dose of PCV to children aged 2 years or older with certain underlying medical conditions, including a cochlear implant.
- **Inactivated poliovirus vaccine (IPV)** (Minimum age: 6 weeks)
  - If 4 or more doses are administered prior to age 4 years, an additional dose should be administered at age 4 through 6 years.
  - The final dose in the series should be administered on or after the fourth birthday and at least 6 months following the previous dose.
- **Influenza vaccine (seasonal)** (Minimum age: 6 months for trivalent inactivated influenza vaccine [TIV]; 2 years for live, attenuated influenza vaccine [LAIV])
  - For healthy children aged 2 years and older, either LAIV or TIV may be used, except LAIV should not be given to children aged 2 through 4 years who have had wheezing in the past 12 months.
  - Administer 2 doses (separated by at least 4 weeks) to children aged 6 months through 8 years who are receiving seasonal influenza vaccine for the first time or who were vaccinated for the first time during the previous influenza season but only received 1 dose.
- **Measles, mumps, and rubella vaccine (MMR)** (Minimum age: 12 months)
  - The second dose may be administered before age 4 years, provided at least 4 weeks have elapsed since the first dose.
- **Varicella vaccine** (Minimum age: 12 months)
  - The second dose may be administered before age 4 years, provided at least 3 months have elapsed since the first dose.
  - For children aged 12 months through 12 years, the recommended minimum interval between doses is 3 months. However, if the second dose was administered at least 4 weeks after the first dose, it can be accepted as valid.
- **Hepatitis A vaccine (HepA)** (Minimum age: 12 months)
  - Administer 2 doses at least 6 months apart.
  - HepA is recommended for children aged older than 23 months who live in areas where vaccination programs target older children, who are at increased risk for infection, or for whom immunity against hepatitis A is desired.
- **Meningococcal conjugate vaccine, quadrivalent (MCV4)** (Minimum age: 2 years)
  - Administer 2 doses of MCV4 at least 8 weeks apart to children aged 2–10 years with persistent complement component deficiency and anatomic or functional asplenia, and 1 dose every 5 years thereafter.
  - Persons with HIV infection who are vaccinated with MCV4 should receive 2 doses at least 8 weeks apart.
  - Administer 1 dose of MCV4 to children aged 2 through 10 years who travel to countries with highly endemic or epidemic disease and during outbreaks caused by a vaccine serogroup.
  - Administer MCV4 to children at continued risk for meningococcal disease who were previously vaccinated with MCV4 or meningococcal polysaccharide vaccine after 3 years if the first dose was administered at age 2–6 years.

Table 5b. Recommended Immunization Schedule for Persons Aged 7 Through 18 years

Vaccine ▼ Age ►	7–10 years	11–12 years	13–18 years	
Tetanus, Diphtheria, Pertussis		**Tdap**	**Tdap**	Range of recommended ages for all children
Human Papillomavirus		**HPV (3 doses)(females)**	**HPV Series**	
Meningococcal	**MCV4**	**MCV4**	**MCV4**	
Influenza	**Influenza (Yearly)**			Range of recommended ages for catch-up immunization
Pneumococcal	**Pneumococcal**			
Hepatitis A	**HepA Series**			
Hepatitis B	**Hep B Series**			
Inactivated Poliovirus	**IPV Series**			Range of recommended ages for certain high-risk groups
Measles, Mumps, Rubella	**MMR Series**			
Varicella	**Varicella Series**			

- **Tetanus and diphtheria toxoids and acellular pertussis vaccine (TDaP)** (Minimum age: 10 years for Boostrix and 11 years for Adacel)
  - Persons aged 11–18 years who have not received Tdap should receive a dose followed by Td booster doses every 10 years thereafter.
  - Persons aged 7–10 years who are not fully immunized against pertussis should receive a single dose of Tdap.
  - Tdap can be administered regardless of the interval since the last tetanus and diphtheria toxoid-containing vaccine.
- **Human papillomavirus vaccine (HPV)** (Minimum age: 9 years)
  - Quadrivalent HPV vaccine (HPV4) or bivalent HPV vaccine (HPV2) is recommended in females.
  - HPV4 may be administered in a 3-dose series to males aged 9–18 years to reduce their likelihood of genital warts.
  - Administer the second dose 1 to 2 months after the first dose and the third dose 6 months after the first dose.
- **Meningococcal conjugate vaccine, quadrivalent (MCV4)** (Minimum age: 2 years)
  - Administer MCV4 at age 11–12 years with a booster dose at age 16 years.
  - Administer 1 dose at age 13–18 years if not previously vaccinated.
  - Persons who received their first dose at age 13–15 years should receive a booster dose at age 16–18 years.
  - Administer 1 dose to previously unvaccinated college freshmen living in a dormitory.
  - Administer 2 doses at least 8 weeks apart to children aged 2–10 years with persistent complement component deficiency and anatomic or functional asplenia, and 1 dose every 5 years thereafter.
  - Persons with HIV infection who are vaccinated with MCV4 should receive 2 doses at least 8 weeks apart.
  - Administer 1 dose of MCV4 to children aged 2–10 years who travel to countries with highly endemic or epidemic disease and during outbreaks caused by a vaccine serogroup.
  - Administer MCV4 to children at continued risk for meningococcal disease who were previously vaccinated after 3 years (if first dose administered at age 2–6 years) or after 5 years (if first dose administered at age 7 years or older).
- **Influenza vaccine (seasonal)**
  - For healthy nonpregnant persons aged 7 through 18 years, either live, attenuated influenza vaccine (LAIV) or trivalent inactivated influenza vaccine (TIV) may be used.
- **Pneumococcal vaccines**
  - A single dose of 13-valent conjugate vaccine (PCV13) may be administered to children aged 6 through 18 years who have functional or anatomic asplenia, HIV infection or other immunocompromising condition, cochlear implant or CSF leak.
  - The dose of PCV13 should be administered at least 8 weeks after the previous dose of PCV7.
  - Administer polysaccharide vaccine at least 8 weeks after the last dose of PCV to children aged 2 years or older with certain underlying medical conditions, including a cochlear implant. A single revaccination should be administered after 5 years to children with functional or anatomic asplenia or an immunocompromising condition.
- **Hepatitis A vaccine (HepA)**
  - Administer 2 doses at least 6 months apart.
  - HepA is recommended for children aged older than 23 months who live in areas where vaccination programs target older children, or who are at increased risk for infection, or for whom immunity against hepatitis A is desired.
- **Hepatitis B vaccine (HepB)**
  - Administer the 3-dose series to those not previously vaccinated.
  - A 2-dose series (separated by at least 4 months) of adult formulation Recombivax HB is licensed for children aged 11 through 15 years.
- **Inactivated poliovirus vaccine (IPV)**
  - The final dose in the series should be administered on or after the fourth birthday and at least 6 months following the previous dose.
  - If both oral poliovirus vaccine (OPV) and IPV were administered as part of a series, a total of 4 doses should be administered, regardless of the child's current age.
- **Measles, mumps, and rubella vaccine (MMR)**
  - The minimum interval between the 2 doses of MMR is 4 weeks.
- **Varicella vaccine**
  - For persons aged 7 through 18 years without evidence of immunity, administer 2 doses if not previously vaccinated or the second dose if only 1 dose has been administered.
  - For persons aged 7 through 12 years, the recommended minimum interval between doses is 3 months. However, if the second dose was administered at least 4 weeks after the first dose, it can be accepted as valid.
  - For persons aged 13 years and older, the minimum interval between doses is 4 weeks.

(Adapted from Centers for Disease Control. Recommended immunization schedules for persons aged 0 through 18 years–United States, 2011. *MMWR Morb Mortal Wkly Rep.* 2011;60(5):1–4.)

Table 6. Vaccines Available for Use in Adults

Vaccine	Type	Route and Usual Regimen
Anthrax	Avirulent nonencapsulated strain	0.5 mL IM at 0, 1, 6, 12, and 18 months followed by annual boosters
Bacille Calmette-Guerin (BCG)	Live attenuated strain of *Mycobacterium bovis*	Percutaneous (0.2–0.3 mL)
Cholera	Killed *Vibrio cholerae* O1 bacteria and recombinant cholera toxin B subunit. Provides protection for enterotoxigenic *E. coli*.	2 doses PO at intervals of more than 1 week
Diphtheria (Td) (combined with tetanus or tetanus and pertussis)	Diphtheria toxoid. Td contains the same amount of tetanus toxoid as DT but a reduced dose of diphtheria toxoid	0.5 mL IM
Haemophilus influenzae b	Polysaccharide conjugated to protein	0.5 mL IM once
Hepatitis A	Inactivated virus	1.0 mL IM (deltoid muscle) Booster given in 6–12 months
Hepatitis B	Inactivated viral antigen (surface antigen)	1.0 mL IM 3 times at 0, 1, and 6 months
Human papilloma virus	Inactive HPV proteins. Quadrivalent (types 6, 11, 16, 18) Bivalent (types 16, 18)	0.5 mL IM at 0, 2, and 6 months
Influenza	Inactivated vaccine (trivalent)	0.5 mL IM once annually
	Live attenuated vaccine	0.2 mL intranasally
Japanese B encephalitis	Inactivated JE virus	Ixiaro: 0.5 mL IM on days 0, 28 Je-Vax: 1 mL SC on days 0, 7, 30
Measles (combined with mumps, rubella)	Live attenuated virus (all 3 serotypes)	No longer licensed in the US
Meningococcal	Live attenuated virus vaccine	0.5 mL SC in outer aspect of upper arm
	Capsular polysaccharides of serotypes A/C/Y/W-135	0.5 mL SC once
	Conjugated vaccine (serotypes A/C/Y/W-135)	0.5 mL SC once
Mumps (combined with measles, rubella)	Live attenuated virus vaccine	0.5 mL SC in outer aspect of upper arm
Pertussis (combined with diphtheria and tetanus)	Acellular vaccine (purified components of the bacteria and detoxified toxin)	0.5 mL IM
	Whole-cell vaccine	No longer available in the US
Plague	Inactivated bacteria	1.0 mL IM, then 0.2 mL at 1, 6 months (not available in US)
Pneumococcal	Polysaccharide vaccine (23 pneumococcal types)	0.5 mL IM or SC
	Conjugate vaccine (7-valent, 13-valent)	Recommended only in children
Poliovirus	Inactivated virus (all 3 serotypes)	0.5 mL SC once (completely vaccinated, at risk for exposure)
	Live attenuated	Oral (no longer available in US)
Rabies	Inactivated virus	1.0 mL IM on days 0, 7, 21, 28
Rubella (combined with measles, mumps)	Live attenuated virus vaccine	0.5 mL SC in outer aspect of upper arm
Tetanus (combined diphtheria, pertussis)	Tetanus toxoid	0.5 mL IM
Typhoid	Vi capsular polysaccharide vaccine	0.5 mL IM once
	Live attenuated vaccine (Ty21a strain)	1 capsule every other day (total of 4 capsules)
Varicella	Live attenuated virus	0.5 mL SC 2 times, separated by 4–8 weeks
Yellow fever	Live virus (17D strain)	0.5 mL SC once
Zoster vaccine	Live attenuated virus (Oka-Merch strain). Lower potency than varicella vaccine	0.65 mL IM once

Table 7a. Summary of Recommendations on Immunization in the Immunocompromised Host

Vaccine	HIV Infection	Organ Transplantation	Asplenia	Renal Failure, Alcoholism, Alcoholic Cirrhosis
Haemophilus influenzae b	Recommended	Recommended	Recommended	Use if indicated
Hepatitis A	Recommended	Recommended	Recommended	Recommended
Hepatitis B	Recommended	Recommended	Recommended	Recommended
Human papilloma virus	Consider in the recommended age range	Recommended	Recommended	Recommended
Influenza (inactivated)	Recommended (Live vaccine contraindicated)	Recommended (Live vaccine contraindicated)	Recommended	Recommended
Measles, mumps, rubella	Consider in patients with CD4 $>200/mm^3$	Contraindicated	Use if indicated	Use if indicated
Meningococcal	Use if indicated	Use if indicated	Recommended	Use if indicated
Pneumococcal	Recommended	Recommended	Recommended	Recommended
Tetanus, diphtheria (Td)	Recommended	Recommended	Recommended	Recommended
Pertussis (TdaP)	Recommended	Recommended	Recommended	Recommended
Varicella	Consider in patients with CD4 $>200/mm^3$	Contraindicated	Use if indicated	Use if indicated
Zoster	Consider in patients with CD4 $>200/mm^3$	Contraindicated	Use if indicated	Use if indicated

Sources: Recommendations of the Advisory Committee on Immunization Practices (ACIP): Use of vaccines and immune globulins in persons with altered immunocompetence. *MMWR Recomm Rep.* 1993;42(RR-4):1–18.
Danzinger-Isakov L, Kumar D. AST Infectious Diseases Community of Practice. Guidelines for vaccination of solid organ transplant candidates and recipients. *Am J Transplant* 2009;9 (Suppl 4):S258–62.
Aberg JA, Kaplan JE, Libman H et al. Primary care guidelines for the management of persons infected with HIV. *Clin Infect Dis* 2009;49(5):651–81.

Table 7b. Summary of Recommendations on Nonroutine Immunization of Immunocompromised Persons

Vaccine	HIV/AIDS, Organ Transplantation, Severe Immunosuppression[a]	Asplenia, Renal Failure, Alcoholism, and Alcoholic Cirrhosis
Live vaccines		
BCG	Contraindicated	Use if indicated
Oral polio	Contraindicated	Use if indicated
Vaccinia	Contraindicated	Use if indicated
Typhoid, Ty21a	Contraindicated	Use if indicated
Yellow fever[b]	Contraindicated	Use if indicated
Killed or inactivated vaccines		
Anthrax	Use if indicated	Use if indicated
Inactivated cholera	Use if indicated	Use if indicated
Inactivated polio	Use if indicated	Use if indicated
Japanese encephalitis	Use if indicated	Use if indicated
Plague	Use if indicated	Use if indicated
Typhoid, inactivated	Use if indicated	Use if indicated
Rabies	Use if indicated	Use if indicated

[a] Severe immunosuppression can be the result of congenital immunodeficiency, HIV infection, leukemia, lymphoma, aplastic anemia, generalized malignancy, or therapy with alkylating agents, antimetabolites, radiation, large amounts of corticosteroids, or TNF-alpha blockers.
[b] Yellow fever vaccine should be considered for patients when exposure to yellow fever cannot be avoided.

Table 8a. Characteristics, Activity, and Adverse Effects of Immunoglobulins

Pooled Human Immunoglobulin	Hyperimmune-Specific Human Immunoglobulin	Animal (Equine) Immunoglobulin or Antitoxin
	Characteristics	
Obtained from pooled human plasma Contains IgG for several common infections in the population	Obtained from immune persons. High concentration of specific IgG Half-life = 25 days	Obtained from animals immunized with toxoids (inactivated diphtheria or botulinum toxoids)
Half-life = 25 days Prevention of Hepatitis A Measles Poliomyelitis if given early after exposure	**Activity** Prevention of Hepatitis B Varicella zoster virus (VZV) Rabies, Tetanus	**Half-life = 7 days** Treatment relatively effective for Diphtheria Botulism
Little protection against Hepatitis B Congenital rubella (when given to pregnant women with rubella)	**Effectiveness unclear and _not_ recommended for** Whooping cough Mumps	
Local symptoms	**Adverse Effects** Local symptoms	May cause anaphylaxis (perform intradermic testing before administration)
May be used in pregnancy Use only IM; intravenous injection may cause anaphylaxis because it contains IgG aggregates of high molecular weight[a]	May be used in pregnancy Rarely causes anaphylaxis	Fever Serum sickness

Intravenous immunoglobulin may cause headache, abdominal pain, lumbar pain, nausea and vomiting, chills, fever, and myalgias, which may be alleviated by decreasing the infusion rate and administering aspirin or corticosteroids. In patients with IgA deficiency, a severe anaphylactic reaction may be seen. A preparation with low IgA content should be used (Gammagard).

[a] Human immunoglobulin preparations without anticomplement activity are available and may be given at high doses intravenously. They are indicated in patients with hypogammaglobulinemia, prevention of VZV and cytomegalovirus infections, Kawasaki disease, idiopathic thrombocytopenic purpura, and treatment of chronic parvovirus B19 infection in patients with immunosuppression. Other indications are prophylactically given after bone marrow transplantation, in children with AIDS and recurrent bacterial infections, and in patients with Guillain-Barre syndrome.

Human immunoglobulin has been tested and is negative for HBs antigen and for antibodies against Hepatitis C and HIV 1 and 2.

Live virus vaccines should be administered 3 weeks before or 3 months after the injection of pooled human immunoglobulin. The exception is yellow fever vaccine since the immunoglobulin does not contain yellow fever antibodies.

Pooled human immunoglobulin is considered for individuals who have been in close contact with confirmed Hepatitis A and are prone to severe disease. It is also indicated for adults and children with immunodeficiency who have been exposed to measles: the administration should be implemented the first 72 hours after exposure. Protection against developing congenital rubella is minimal.

Hepatitis B – specific immunoglobulin should be administered in individuals who were exposed to a potential viral transmission and to prevent the vertical transmission from seropositive mother to the neonate. Rabies – specific immunoglobulin should be coadministered with the vaccine in different sites of injection.

Table 8b. Use of Vaccines and Immunoglobulins

Disease	Indication	Vaccine	Immunoglobulin
Botulism	Patient with botulism	Not available	Horse antitoxin
CMV disease	Transplant recipient, especially bone marrow and liver transplant; seronegative for CMV	Not available	CMV IG *Dose:* 0.15–1.0 g/kg/wk *Efficacy:* Decreases frequency and severity of disease
Cholera	Travel to area where vaccination is required Person >6 years	*Action:* Killed whole-cell-recombinant B subunit vaccine. *Dose:* 2 doses orally 7–42 days Apart *Efficacy:* 85–90% Booster: every 2 years	Not available
Diphtheria	Age >6 months	*Action:* Diphtheria and tetanus toxoids and acellular pertussis vaccine	—
	Unimmunized persons	*Dose:* 5 doses IM at 2, 4, 6, and 12 months and 4 through 6 years.	
	Immunized persons	*Dose Booster:* Every 10 years (95% efficacy) *Efficacy:* Prevents toxic effects but does not prevent infection	—
	Patient with diphtheria	N/A	Horse antitoxin
Japanese encephalitis	Travel to endemic area (Southeast Asia and China) Persons >3 years for JE-VAX (Biken)	*Action:* Killed virus *Dose:* 3 doses SC at days 0, 7, and 30 Efficacy: 2 doses 80%, 3 doses 99%. Booster: Every 3years	Not available
Yellow fever	Travel to endemic area (equatorial Africa and South America)	*Action:* Live attenuated virus *Dose:* Single dose 0.5 mL SC Contraindicated in patients with egg protein allergy and pregnant women except exposure is unavoidable *Efficacy:* 10-year protection Must be given at least 10 days prior to the entry to the specific country to meet official requirements. YF vaccine-associated neurotropic disease in 5/1,000,000 doses. YF vaccine-associated viscerotropic disease in 1/55,000 doses for people >60 years	Not available
Typhoid fever	Travel to endemic area; natural disasters (floods, earthquakes)	*Action:* Live attenuated bacterial *Vaccine suspension (Vivotif). Live attenuated vaccine capsule. Injectable typhoid polysaccharide vaccine.* *Dose:* 3 doses of suspension taken orally on days 0, 1, 4. 4 capsules administered on alternative days; avoid antibiotics for at least 1 week Typhim Vi vaccine single 0.5-mL (25-μg) dose IM Booster recommended every 3 years *Efficacy:* Effectiveness of all typhoid vaccines is approximately 65%	Not available
Influenza	Adults >age 65 years	*Action:* Killed whole or fractionated virus or surface antigens	Not available
	Health care workers, especially those caring for high-risk persons High-risk persons: Military, police headquarters Patients with chronic lung, heart, liver, kidney disease, diabetes, immunosuppression, or HIV Children 6 months to 18 years on chronic aspirin therapy	*Dose:* Administer annually in a single 0.5-mL dose IM in the deltoid muscle in fall; intramuscular; contraindicated in patients with egg protein allergy. In children younger than the age of 13 years, must use fractionated virus vaccine *Efficacy:* 75% for 6 months in the young, but less in the elderly	

(continued)

Table 8b. Use of Vaccines and Immunoglobulins (continued)

Disease	Indication	Vaccine	Immunoglobulin
Hepatitis A	Susceptible persons older than the age of 2 years traveling to, living in, or relocating to an area of high endemic risk Military personnel Ethnic and geographic populations that experience cyclic hepatitis A epidemics, such as native peoples of Alaska and the Americas Persons engaging in high-risk sexual activity Users of illicit injectable drugs Residents of a community experiencing outbreak of hepatitis A Persons with possible occupational exposure to hepatitis A virus, such as primate handlers and laboratory workers Children and adults in contact with a person with hepatitis A	Two vaccines available: Havrix and VAQTA *Havrix for Adults:* *Dose:* single dose IM of 1440 EL.U. in 1 mL. Booster dose is recommended any time between 6 and 12 months after initiation of the primary course. *Havrix for Children 2–18 years:* *Dose:* 2 doses containing 360 EL.U., each in 0.5 mL IM 1 month apart *VAQTA for Adults:* *Dose:* Single dose IM of 50 U of hepatitis A virus antigen in 1 mL. Booster dose of 1 mL is recommended 6 months after the initial vaccination. *VAQTA for Children 2–17 yr:* *Dose:* Single dose IM of 25 U of hepatitis A virus antigen in 0.5 mL. Booster dose of 0.5 mL is recommended 6–18 months after the initial vaccination.	Pooled human IG 0.02 mL/kg IM for stays <3 months; for longer stays, 0.06 mL/kg/5 m; concurrent administration with vaccine at a different site for late initiation Pooled human IG 0.02 mL/kg IM within first 14 days after exposure
Hepatitis B	Unimmunized persons	*Action:* HBsAg *Dose, Adult:* 3 doses of 1 mL (20 μg) IM in the deltoid at 0, 1, and 6 months *Dose, Children:* 0.5 mL (10 μg) The vaccine should be administered to all newborns before hospital discharge. Do not restart series, no matter how long since previous dose. *Dose, Elderly and Immunosuppressed:* 2 mL, (40 μg) The vaccination with 3-dose series can be implemented at any age. *Efficacy:* 95% *Rapid schedule for travelers:* 2 doses at 2-week interval has >80% protection.	—
	Newborn of HBsAg-positive mother	First dose of 0.5 mL at birth (10 μg) IM at different site from IG, then at 1 and 6 months	Specific IG, 0.5 mL IM within 12 hours of birth
	Accidental exposure (percutaneous, mucosal, sexual)	Immunize the week after administration of IG	Specific IG, 0.06 mL/kg IM within 48 hours after exposure. Obtain serum for HBsAg. If negative, give a second dose of specific IG 1 month later.
Haemophilus influenza type b	Children < 5 years Children >5 years and adults: No efficacy data available. Good immunogenicity in persons with Sickle cell disease, Leukemia, HIV, and splenectomy	Action: Conjugate vaccine Dose, Routine: Children 2 months, 4 months, 6 months, and 12 months. Minimum age 6 weeks. If PRP-OMP is administered at ages 2 and 4 months, a dose at age 6 months is not indicated. For immunogenicity in persons over 5 years, 1 dose is enough.	

(continued)

Table 8b. Use of Vaccines and Immunoglobulins (continued)

Disease	Indication	Vaccine	Immunoglobulin
Pneumococcal	Children >6 weeks for PCV and >2 years for PPSV High Risk children: Sickle cell disease; anatomic or functional asplenia; chronic cardiac, pulmonary, or renal disease; diabetes; cerebrospinal fluid leaks; HIV infection; immunosuppression; diseases associated with immunosuppressive and/or radiation therapy; or who have or will have a cochlear implant. Adults and children older than age of 2 years with chronic lung disease, chronic heart disease, chronic liver disease, chronic kidney disease, diabetes, nephrotic syndrome, and immunosuppression, including asplenia (anatomic or functional), myeloma, immunosuppressive treatment, transplant, CSF fistulas, HIV Adults age >65 years	*Action:* Conjugate 13 serotypes (PCV13). Pneumococcal polysaccharide (PPSV) 23 serotypes. *Dose, Routine:* Children 2 months, 4 months, 6 months, and 12–15 months with PCV13 IM. A single dose to unvaccinated children of 24 months–59 months. PCV13 is not given routinely to children >5 years old. For high-risk children >2 years, give a single dose of PPSV IM at least 8 weeks after PCV last dose. For adults 1 dose of PPSV IM or SC. *Dose, High-Risk:* Consider booster in 4–5 years after "routine" dose; may be administered with flu shot (different sites) *Dose, Transplant:* Administer 2 weeks prior to transplant. *Efficacy:* 70%; lower in patients with immunosuppression or under the age of 2 years	Not available
Meningococcal	Outbreak Complement deficiency Asplenia (anatomic or functional) Travelers visiting endemic areas Contact with meningococcus caused by serogroups included in the vaccine	*Action:* Polysaccharide of serotypes A, C, Y, and W135. Quadrivalent conjugate A, C, Y and W135 *Dose:* Single dose 0.5 mL IM or SC *Efficacy: Polysaccharide* 90%, Conjugate >97% after 28 days of injection; confers no protection against serogroup B Booster: Every 3 years if risk exposure continues	Not available
Mumps	Unimmunized persons	*Action:* Live attenuated virus *Dose:* 0.5 mL SC; contraindicated in persons with egg protein allergy *Efficacy:* 95%	—
Plague	Exposure in an endemic area	*Action:* Killed bacilli *Dose:* Three 1-mL doses SC at 0, 1, and 4 months *Booster Dose:* At 6 months if exposure continues	Not available
Poliomyelitis	Unimmunized persons under age 18 years Unimmunized persons over age 18 years traveling to endemic area Immunosuppressed person Immunized persons over age 18 years traveling to an endemic area	*Action:* Live attenuated virus (Sabin) *Dose:* Orally *Action:* Killed virus (Salk) *Dose:* 3 doses of 0.5 mL SC at 0, 1, and 12 months *Booster Dose:* Live attenuated vaccine (Sabin)	—
Rabies[a]	Exposure to animals in areas where disease is endemic Animal bite or contact of a wound or the mucosae with saliva of an animal suspected of being rabid in an endemic area[a] (Unimmunized persons) Immunized persons	*Action:* Killed virus *Dose:* 3 doses of 1 mL IM in deltoid area at 0, 7, and 28 days *Day 0:* 2 doses of 1 mL *Day 7:* 1 dose of 1 mL *Day 28:* 1 dose of 1 mL *Booster Dose:* Every 2–3 years *Dose:* 2 doses of 1 mL each IM at 0 and 3 days	— HRIG (specific human IG) 20 IU/kg; Half IM and half around wound Not needed if Ab response is good

(continued)

Table 8b. Use of Vaccines and Immunoglobulins (continued)

Disease	Indication	Vaccine	Immunoglobulin
Rotavirus	Children >6 weeks	*Action:* Live attenuated viruses *Dose:* 2 doses at 2 and 4 months Orally. *Efficacy:* 90% after first dose	—
Rubella	Unimmunized persons	*Action:* Attenuated virus *Dose:* 0.5 mL SC *Efficacy:* 95% *Adverse Effects:* May cause arthralgias, adenopathy, and fever	
Measles	Unimmunized persons	*Action:* Attenuated virus *Dose:* 0.5 mL SC; second dose given >1 month later	0.25 mL/kg IM up to 15 mL (healthy host) 0.5 mL/kg up to 15 mL (immunocompromised host)
	Susceptible contacts, in particular, children, pregnant women, and immunocompromised patients	—	IG
Tetanus	Unimmunized persons	*Action:* Inactivated toxin *Dose:* 3 doses of 0.5 mL IM at 2, 4, 6, and 15 months and 4 years *Booster Dose:* Every 10 years	—
	Immunized persons Wound (prophylaxis) Tetanus (treatment)	—	Specific IG 3,000 IU IM
Pertussis	Unimmunized, <age 7 years	*Action:* Acellular vaccine (aP) *Dose:* 8 formulations available	—
Varicella (chickenpox)	Children >age 12 months	*Action:* Live attenuated virus *Children >12 months and <12 years:* *Dose:* Single dose 0.5 mL SC *Adults and children age >13 years* *Dose:* 0.5 mL SC initial dose; 0.5 mL Sc 4–8 weeks later	—
	Susceptible, immunocompetent adults Health care workers Household contacts of immunosuppressed persons living or working in high-risk areas (schools and day care centers) Young adults in military or colleges Nonpregnant women and those of childbearing potential International travelers		
	Immunocompromised or newborn contact	—	VZIG (specific IG) 125 U/10 kg IM up to 625 U
Tuberculosis	PPD-negative patients exposed to known TB who cannot be followed (immigrants, the noncompliant) Persons living in an area of high prevalence of resistant tuberculosis *Avoid* in HIV-infected patients and, possibly, in all immunosuppressed hosts	*Action:* Bacillus Calmette-Guérin *Dose:* single dose SC *Efficacy:* 60–80% *Adverse Effects:* May cause ulcer at vaccination site and local adenopathy	—

Abbreviations: CMV, cytomegalovirus; IG, immunoglobulin.

[a] If the animal is captured, treatment may be delayed until the disease is confirmed with immunofluorescence testing of brain tissue. Immunized animals that exhibit normal behavior may be kept under continued observation for 10 days before the decision is made to kill them.

Table 9a. Prophylaxis of Endocarditis

Prophylaxis is recommended	Prophylaxis is not recommended

• Patients with a prosthetic valve or a prosthetic material used for cardiac valve repair.[a]
• Patients with previous IE.[a]
• Patients with congenital heart disease:
  – Cyanotic congenital heart disease without surgical repair, or with residual defects, palliative shunts, or conduits.
  – Congenital heart disease with complete repair with prosthetic material whether placed by surgery or by percutaneous technique, up to 6 months after the procedure.
  – When a residual defect persists at the site of implantation of a prosthetic material or device by cardiac surgery or percutaneous technique.[a]
	Other forms of valvular or congenital heart disease.

DENTAL PROCEDURES In high-risk patients requiring manipulation of the gingival or periapical region of the teeth or perforation of the oral mucosa.	Local anesthetic injections in noninfectious tissue, removal of sutures, dental x-rays, placement or adjustment of removable prosthodontic or orthodontic appliances or braces. Following the shedding of deciduous teeth or trauma to the lips and oral mucosa.
RESPIRATORY PROCEDURES Invasive respiratory tract infections in high-risk patients for treating an established infection (e.g., abscess drainage)	Respiratory tract procedures including bronchoscopy or laryngoscopy, transnasal, or endotracheal intubation under no infection.
GASTROINTESTINAL OR UROGENITAL PROCEDURES In case of an established infection that implicates the procedure	Gastroscopy, colonoscopy, cystoscopy, or transesophageal echocardiography
SKIN AND SOFT TISSUE	Not recommended for ANY procedure

[a] High risk patients.

Table 9b. Prophylactic Regimens for Dental, Respiratory Tract, or Esophageal Procedures

Situation	Agent	Regimen[a]
Dental procedures in high-risk patients	Amoxicillin	*Adults:* 2 g PO *Children:* 50 mg/kg PO 1 hour before procedure
Cannot take oral medication	Ampicillin	*Adults:* 2 g IM or IV *Children:* 50 mg/kg IM or IV Within 30 minutes before procedure
Allergic to penicillin	Clindamycin	*Adults:* 600 mg PO or IV *Children:* 20 mg/kg PO 1 hour before procedure
	Cephalexin[b]	*Adults:* 2 g IV *Children:* 50 mg/kg IV 1 hour before procedure
	Cefazolin[b] or ceftriaxone[b]	*Adults:* 1g IV *Children:* 50 mg/kg IV 1 hour before procedure
Allergic to penicillin and cannot take oral medications	Clindamycin	*Adults:* 600 mg IV *Children:* 20 mg/kg IV Within 30 minutes before procedure
	Cefazolin[b]	*Adults:* 1 g IM or IV *Children:* 25 mg/kg IM or IV Within 30 minutes before procedure

[a] The total children's dose should not exceed the adult dose.
[b] Cephalosporins should not be used in individuals with immediate-type hypersensitivity reactions (urticaria, angioedema, or anaphylaxis) to penicillins.

Table 9c. Prophylactic Regimens for Respiratory, Dermatological or Musculoskeletal, and Genitourinary, Gastrointestinal Procedures Implicating an Infection in High-Risk Patients

Situation	Agents[a]
Respiratory tract	Anti-staphylococcal penicillin or a cephalosporin.
	Consider vancomycin if β-lactam antibiotics are not tolerated or if there is high suspicion of MRSA infection.
Gastrointestinal or genitourinary procedures	Consider coverage against enterococci with ampicillin, amoxicillin, or vancomycin. In case of suspicion of resistant enterococcus strain, ask for a specialist advice.
Dermatological or musculoskeletal procedures	Anti-staphylococcal penicillin or a cephalosporin against staphylococci and β-hemolytic streptococci.
	Consider vancomycin or clindamycin in cases with no tolerability of β-lactams.
	Vancomycin should be given in cases of MRSA suspicion.
Body piercing and tattooing	Case reports of Infectious endocarditis after these procedures are increasing.
	More data are needed to assess the implementation or not of the antimicrobial prophylaxis.

Table 10. Trade Names of Antimicrobial Agents

Trade Name	Generic Name	Trade Name	Generic Name	Trade Name	Generic Name
Abelcet	Amphotericin (B-lipid complex)	Cefzil	Cefprozil	Furantoin	Nitrofurantoin
Abreva	dosoconasol	Ceptaz	Ceftazidime	Furoxone	Furazolidone
A-cillin	Amoxicillin	Chero-Trisulfa V	Trisulfapyrimidine	Fuzeon	Enfuvirtide
AK-chlor	Chloramphenicol	Chloromycetin	Chloramphenicol	G-Mycin	Gentamicin
Achromycin	Tetracycline	Cinobac	Cinoxacin	Gantanol	Sulfamethoxazole
Aerosporin	Polymyxin B	Cipro	Ciprofloxacin	Gantrisin	Sulfisoxazole
Aftate	Tolnaftate	Cipro XR	Ciprofloxacin	Garamycin	Gentamicin
Ala-Tet	Tetracycline	Claforan	Cefotaxime	Geocillin	Carbenicillin indanyl Sodium
Agenerase	Amprenavir	Cleocin	Clindamycin		
Albamycin	Novobiocin	Cloxapen	Cloxacillin	Germanin	Suramin
Albenza	Albendazole	Cofatrim	Trimethoprim-sulfamethoxazole	Grifulvin	Griseofulvin
Alferon N	Interferon alfa-n3			Grisactin	Griseofulvin
Aldara	Imiquimod	Coly-Mycin M	Colistimethate	Gulfasin	Sulfisoxazole
Alinia	Nitazoxanide	Combivir	Zidovudine+3TC	Halfan	Halofantrine
AmBisome	Amphotericin B-liposomal	Cancidas	Caspofungin	Hepsera	Adefovir
Amcap	Ampicillin	Condylox	Podophyllotoxin	Herplex	Idoxuridine
Amficot	Ampicillin	Copegus	Ribavirin	Hetrazan	Diethylcarbamazepine
Amikin	Amikacin	Cotrim	Trimethoprim-sulfamethoxazole	Hiprex	Methenamine Hippurate
Amoxil	Amoxicillin				
Amphotec	Amphotericin lipid complex	Crixivan	Indinavir	HIVID	Zalcitabine
Amplin	Ampicillin	Cubicin	Daptomycin	Humatin	Paromomycin
Ancef	Cefazolin	Cytovene	Ganciclovir	Ilosone	Erythromycin estolate
Ancobon	Flucytosine	D-Amp	Ampicillin		
Anspor	Cephradine	Daraprim	Pyrimethamine	Ilotycin	Erythromycin
Antepar	Piperazine	Declomycin	Demeclocycline	Intelence	Etravirine
Antiminth	Pyrantel pamoate	Denavir	Penciclovir	Intron A	Interferon-alfa-2b
Aoraciain B	Penicillin G	Dendrid	Idoxuridine	Isentress	Raltegravir
Aptivus	Tipranavir	Diflucan	Fluconazole	Invirase	Saquinavir
Aralen	Chloroquine	Doribax	Doripenem	Invanz	Ertapenem
Arsobal	Melarsoprol	Doryx	Doxycycline	Jenamicin	Gentamicin
Artabax	Retapamulin	Doxy-caps	Doxycycline	Kaletra	Lopinavir/rectonavir
Atabrine	Quinacrine	Doxy-D	Doxycycline	Kantrex	Kanamycin
Atripla	Efavirenz/Emtricitabine/Tenofovir	Duricef	Cefadroxil	Keflex	Cephalexin
		Dycill	Dicloxacillin	Keflin	Cephalothin
Augmentin	Clavulanic acid plus amoxicillin	DynaPak	Dirithromycin	Keftab	Cephalexin
Augmentin ES-600		Dynapen	Dicloxacillin	Kefurox	Cefuroxime
Augmentin XR		Ecalta	Anidulafugin	Kefzol	Cefazolin
Azactam	Aztreonam	E-mycin	Erythromycin	Ketek	Telithromycin
Avelox	Moxifloxacin	EES	Erythromycin Ethylsuccinate	Kwell	Lindane
Azulfidine	Sulfasalazine			Lamisil	Terbinafine
Bactrim	Trimethoprim-sulfamethoxazole	Elimite	Permethrin	Lampit	Nifurtimox
		Emtet-500	Tetracycline	Lamprene	Clofazimine
Bactroban	Mupirocin	Emtriva	Emtricitabine	Lanacillin	Penicillin V
Baraclude	Entecavir	Epivir	Lamivudine	Lariam	Mefloquine
Beepen-VK	Penicillin V	Epzicom	Abacavir + Lamivudine	Ledercillin VK	Penicillin V
Biaxin	Clarithromycin	Erothricin	Erythromycin	Levaquin	Levofloxacin
Biaxin XL	Clarithromycin	ERYC	Erythromycin	Lexiva	Fosamprenavir
Bicillin	Benzathine Penicillin G	Ery-Tab	Erythromycin	Lice-Enz	Pyrethrins
		Erythrocot	Erythromycin	Lincocin	Lincomycin
Biltricide	Praziquantel	Eryzole	Erythromycin Sulfisoxazole	Lincorex	Lincomycin
Bio-cef	cephalexin			Lorabid	Loracarbef
Bitin	Bithionol	Factive	Gemifloxacin	Lotrimin	Clotrimazole
Brodspec	Tetracycline	Famvir	Famciclovir	Lyphocin	Vancomycin
Cancidas	caspofugin	Fansidar	Pyrimethamine plus Sulfadoxine	Macrobid	Nitrofurantoin
C-Lexin	Cephalexin			Macrodantin	Nitrofurantoin
Capastat	Capreomycin	Fasigyn	Tinidazole	Malarone	Atovaquone/proguanil
Caropen-VK	Penicillin V	Femstat	Metronidazole	Mandelamine	Methenamine mandelate
Ceclor	Cefaclor	Flagyl	Metronidazole		
Ceclor CD	Cefaclor	Floxin	Ofloxacin	Mandol	Cefamandole
Cedax	Ceftibutin	Flumadine	Rimantadine	Marcillin	Ampicillin
Cefadyl	Cephapirin	Fortaz	Ceftazidime	Maxaquin	Lomefloxacin
Cefanex	Cephalexin	Fortovase	Saquinavir	Maxipime	Cefepime
Cefizox	Ceftizoxime	Foscavir	Foscarnet	Mectizan	Ivermectin
Cefobid	Cefoperazone	Fulvicin	Griseofulvin	Mefoxin	Cefoxitin
Cefotan	Cefotetan	Fungizone	Amphotericin B	Mepron	Atovaquone
Ceftin	Cefuroxime axetil	Furacin	Nitrofurazone	Merrem	Meropenem
		Furadantin	Nitrofurantoin	Metric	Metronidazole
		Furamide	Diloxanide furoate	Metro-IV	Metronidazole

(continued)

499

Table 10. Trade Names of Antimicrobial Agents (continued)

Trade Name	Generic Name	Trade Name	Generic Name	Trade Name	Generic Name
Mezlin	Mezlocillin	Proloprim	Trimethoprim	Tavanic	Levofloxacin
Minocin	Minocycline	Pronto	Pyrethrins	Ticar	Ticarcillin
Mintezol	Thiabendazole	Prostaphlin	Oxacillin	Tindamax	Tinidazole
Monocid	Cefonicid	Protostat	Metronidazole	Tobrex	Tobramycin
Monodox	Doxycycline	Pyopen	Carbenicillin	Trecator SC	Ethionamide
Monurol	Fosfomycin	Rebetron	Ribavirin+Interferon	Triazole	Trimethoprim-
Monistat	Miconazole	Rebetol	Ribavirin		sulfamethoxazole
Myambutol	Ethambutol	Relenza	Zanamivir	Trimox	Amoxicillin
Mycamin	micafungin	Rescriptor	Delavirdine	Trimpex	Trimethoprim
Mycelex	Clotrimazole	Retrovir	Zidovudine	Trisulfam	Trimethoprim
Mycobutin	Rifabutin	Reyataz	Atazanivir		Sulfamethoxazole
Mycostatin	Nystatin	RID	Pyrethrins	Trizivir	AZT and 3TC and ABC
MyE	Erythromycin	Rifadin	Rifampin	Trobicin	Spectinomycin
Nafcil	Nafcillin	Rifamate	Rifampin-INH	Truvada	Emtricitabine+Tenofovir
Nallpen	Nafcillin	Rifater	Rifampin, INH,	Truxcillin	Penicillin G
Natacyn	Natamycin		pyrazinamide	Tygacil	Tygecycline
Nebcin	Tobramycin	Rimactane	Rifampin	Tyzeka	Telbivudine
NebuPent	Pentamidine	Robicillin VK	Penicillin V	Ultracef	Cefadroxil
	aerosol	Robimycin	Erythromycin	Unasyn	Ampicillin-sulbactam
NegGram	Nalidixic acid	Robitet	Tetracycline	Unipen	Nafcillin
Netromycin	Netilmicin	Rocephin	Ceftriaxone	Urex	Methenamine hippurate
Neutrexin	Trimetrexate	Rochagan	Benzimidazole	Uri-Tet	Oxytetracycline
Niclocide	Niclosamide	Roferon-A	Interferon-alpha-2a	Uroplus	Trimethoprim-
Nilstat	Nystatin	Rovamycine	Spiramycin		sulfamethoxazole
Nix	Permethrin	Selzentry	Maraviroc	V-Cillin	Penicillin V
Nizoral	Ketoconazole	Seromycin	Cycloserine	Valcyte	Valganciclovir
Noroxin	Norfloxacin	Silvadene	Silver sulfadiazine	Valtrex	Valacyclovir
Nor-Tet	Tetracycline	Soxa	Sulfisoxazole	Vancocin	Vancomycin
Norvir	Ritonavir	Spectracef	cefditoren	Vancoled	Vancomycin
Noxafil	Posaconazole	Spectrobid	Bacampicillin	Vansil	Oxamniquine
Nydrazid	INH	Sporanox	Itraconazole	Vantin	Cefpodoxime proxetil
Nystex	Nystatin	Staphcillin	Methicillin	Veetids	Penicillin V
Omnicef	Cefdinir	Storz-G	Gentamicin	Velosef	Cephradine
Omnipen	Ampicillin	Stoxil	Idoxuridine	Vermox	Mebendazole
Ornidyl	Eflornithine	Stromectol	Ivermectin	Vfend	Voriconazole
Ovide	Malathion	Sulfamar	Trimethoprim-	Vibramycin	Doxycycline
Paludrine	Proguanil		sulfamethoxazole	Vibra-Tabs	Doxycycline
Panmycin	Tetracycline	Sulfamethoprim	Trimethoprim-	Videx	Didanosine
PAS	Aminosalicylic acid		sulfamethoxazole	Vira-A	Vidarabine
Pathocil	Dicloxacillin	Sulfamylon	Mefenide	Viracept	Nelfinavir
Pediamycin	Erythromycin	Sulfimycin	Erythromycin	Viramune	Nevirapine
	Ethylsuccinate		sulfisoxazole	Virazole	Ribavirin
Pediazole	Erythro/sulfizoxazole	Sumycin	Tetracycline	Viread	Tenofovir
Peflacine	Pefloxacin	Suprax	Cefixime	Viroptic	Trifluridine
Pegasys	Peginterferon alfa 2a	Suspen	Penicillin V	Vistide	Cidofovir
Pen-G	Penicillin G	Sustiva	Efavirenz	Wesmycin	Tetracycline
Pen-V	Penicillin V	Symadine	Amantadine	Win-cillin	Penicillin V
Pen-VK	Penicillin V	Symmetrel	Amantadine	Wintrocin	Erythromycin
Penetrex	Enoxacin	Synagis	Palivizumab	Wyamycin S	Erythromycin
Pentam 300	Pentamidine	Synercid	Quinupristin-dalfopristin	Wycillin	Penicillin G
	isethionate	TAO	Troleandomycin	Wymox	Amoxicillin
Pentids	Penicillin G	Tamiflu	Oseltamivir	Xifaxan	Rifaximin
Pentostam	Sodium	Tazicef	Ceftazidime	Yodoxin	Iodoquinol
	stibogluconate	Tazidime	Ceftazidime	Zagam	Sparfloxacin
Permapen	Penicillin G	Teebactin	Aminosalicylic acid	Zartan	Cephalexin
	benzathine	Tegopen	Cloxacillin	Zefazone	Cefmetazole
Pipracil	Piperacillin	Teline	Tetracycline	Zevtera	Ceftobiprole
Plaquenil	Hydroxychloroquine	Tequin	Gatifloxacin	Zinacef	Cefuroxime
	sulfate	Terramycin	Oxytetracycline	Ziagen	Abacavir
Polycillin	Ampicillin	Tetracap	Tetracycline	Zentel	Albendazole
Polymox	Amoxicillin	Tetracon	Tetracycline	Zerit	Stavudine (d4T)
Povan	Pyrvinium pamoate	Tetralan	Tetracycline	Zithromax	Azithromycin
Prezista	Darunavir	Tetram	Tetracycline	Zmax	Azithromycin ER
Priftin	Rifapentine	Tiberal	Ornidazole	Zolicef	Cefazolin
Primaxin	Imipenem plus	Ticar	Ticarcillin	Zosyn	Piperacillin-
	Cilastatin	Timentin	Clavulanic acid plus		tazobactam
Primachine	Primaquine		ticarcillin	Zovirax	Acyclovir
Principen	Ampicillin	Tinactin	Tolnaftate	Zyvox	Linezolid

Table 11. Prevention of Travel-Related Illness

PRETRAVEL ASSESSMENT
The following information should be obtained from travelers to assess their medical needs and potential risks, to provide itinerary-specific advice, immunizations, and prophylactic medications:
- Date of departure
- Itinerary
- Types of accommodations
- Medical history
- Vaccination history
- Current medications
- Allergies
- For women: Are they pregnant or planning to conceive within the next 3 months?

TRAVEL MEDICAL KIT
Following are suggestions for a traveler's personal medical kit. The contents should be tailored to the type of trip, duration of travel, and potential risk of travel-related illness.
- Summary of medical history and drug allergies
- ABO blood and Rh-factor types
- List of current medications (including both trade and generic names)
- Names and telephone numbers of the traveler's usual physician and emergency contacts
- Current immunization record (ideally, the International Certificate of Vaccination)
- Medical insurance information
- Prescription medications (should have enough to last the whole trip plus a week, in case of unexpected delays)
- Antibiotics and/or antimotility drugs (such as a fluoroquinolone and loperamide) for the self-treatment of traveler's diarrhea or azithromycin for travelers to SE Asia.
- Malaria pills
- Epinephrine for injection and an antihistamine (if the traveler has a history of severe, life-threatening allergic reactions)
- An antibiotic such as erythromycin (if the individual is prone to frequent respiratory tract infections)
- Analgesics (acetaminophen, aspirin, or ibuprofen)
- Antifungal vaginal cream or suppository (for women who have frequent episodes of vaginitis or who may be taking antibiotics en route)
- Topical antibacterial cream for minor cuts or abrasions
- Band-Aids, 2 × 2 or 4 × 4 sterile gauze pads, adhesive tape
- Thermometer
- Elastic bandage (i.e., Ace wrap) for minor sprains
- Venom-extractor pump
- An extra pair of eyeglasses (if corrective lenses are used)
- Insect repellent with DEET up to 40%. For children advice a pediatrician.
- Insecticide
- Menstrual supplies
- Sunscreen (with sun protective factor >15)
- Spare toilet paper
- Water disinfection device or tablets for water treatment

NONINFECTIOUS HAZARDS OF TRAVEL
Jet Lag
Symptoms
- Daytime sleepiness
- Insomnia
- Difficulty concentrating
- Slowed reflexes
- Indigestion
- Hunger at odd hours
- Irritability

Tips to Prevent Jet Lag
- Avoid alcohol during flights (but drink plenty of water or juices to prevent dehydration).
- 3 days before departure, attempt to maintain the time schedule you will experience during the trip.
- Adjust the sleep pattern at home for a few days before departure.
- Exercise daily in the new setting during sunlight hours.
- Consider using a short-acting benzodiazepine at bedtime.

(continued)

Table 11. Prevention of Travel-Related Illness (continued)

Approaches That May Help Reduce Effects of Jet Lag
- Phototherapy (makes use of bright lights to reset the circadian clock)
- Argonne National Laboratory Jet Lag Diet (alternately feasting and fasting before departure)
- Melatonin (5 mg PO per day for 3 days before departure and 3 days after arrival at destination). This hormonal preparation may be available in pharmacies and health food stores, but quality may vary because it is not an FDA-regulated preparation.

Motion Sickness
- Motion sickness usually manifested by nausea, which may be accompanied by loss of color, sweating, and vomiting.
- Preventive treatments include oral antihistamines, such as dimenhydrinate, meclizine, or terfenadine, and scopolamine patches. All measures are most effective if started before the onset of motion sickness.

Road Safety
- Driving in many developing countries can be dangerous because of poor road and automobile conditions, a lack of traffic regulations, and unsafe driving practices of vehicle operators. If a traveler plans to drive, he or she should learn the local rules of the road and be sure to bring a car seat for any infants or toddlers.

Altitude Sickness
- Acute mountain sickness (AMS) can occur at any altitude above 5,000 ft (1,600 m) but is more likely to occur at altitudes above 12,000 ft (3,600 m).
- Risk factors for AMS include rapid ascent (more than 2,000 ft in a 24-hour period) and a history of AMS.
- Symptoms of AMS include headache, loss of appetite, nausea, vomiting, insomnia, fatigue, and shortness of breath, especially with exertion.
- More severe forms of disease include high-altitude pulmonary edema (characterized by severe dyspnea, cough productive of frothy sputum, and cyanosis) and high-altitude cerebral edema (manifested by severe headache, drowsiness, ataxia, impaired judgment, erratic behavior, and loss of consciousness that may progress to coma).

Altitude Sickness Prevention
- Gradually ascending to higher altitude (600 m/d)
- Resting 1 day for every 900-m increase in altitude
- Avoiding overexertion
- Drinking plenty of fluids
- Consuming multiple small meals instead of a few large meals
- Consuming a high-carbohydrate diet
- Avoiding alcoholic beverages and smoking

Drugs Used for Prevention of Acute Mountain Sickness
- Acetazolamide 125–250 mg PO b.i.d or t.i.d should be started on the day of ascent and continued until peak altitude is reached. It is also useful for the treatment of mild AMS.
- Dexamethasone 4 mg PO q6h: This is generally not recommended, due to its potential to cause side effects such as hyperglycemia and dpsychosis, which may be especially dangerous at higher altitudes.
- Nifedipine, 20–30 mg (slow-release) PO t.i.d

Sexually Transmitted Diseases
- High-risk groups include migrant laborers, younger travelers, long-distance truckers, seafarers, military personnel, and expatriates.
- High-risk travelers should be educated about the risks of HIV and other sexually transmitted diseases, regardless of destination.
- High-risk travelers should be advised to carry condoms and to avoid having unprotected sex, especially with prostitutes or casual acquaintances.
- High-risk travelers should receive the hepatitis B vaccine.

PREVENTION OF MALARIA
- Avoid exposure to mosquitoes by wearing clothing that covers the arms and legs when outside.
- Stay indoors in a screened area during the hours between dusk and dawn.
- Sleep under mosquito netting (ideally, permethrin-impregnated) in a screened room or in a closed, air-conditioned room.
- Apply a non-aerosol mosquito repellent to exposed skin when outdoors. Repellents that contain DEET are best. DEET concentrations >35% may be toxic and should be avoided.
- Consider impregnating clothes with permethrin.
- At dusk, spray the sleeping area with an insect repellent containing pyrethroids, after securing screens and closing windows and doors.
- Depending on the region of travel and time of year, prophylactic medications should be prescribed (Table 11, on page 503).

Table 11. Prevention of Travel-Related Illness (continued)

- The choice of prophylaxis depends on the traveler's itinerary, previous tolerance of antimalarials, and concomitant medications.
- Chloroquine-sensitive strains of *Plasmodium falciparum* exist in Central America, Mexico, Haiti, the Dominican Republic, and the Middle East (Figure 1 on page 505).
- Consider impregnating clothes with permethrin.
- At dusk, spray the sleeping area with an insect repellent containing pyrethroids, after securing screens and closing windows and doors.
- Depending on the region of travel and time of year, prophylactic medications should be prescribed (Table A).
- The choice of prophylaxis depends on the traveler's itinerary, previous tolerance of antimalarials, and concomitant medications.
- Chloroquine-sensitive strains of *Plasmodium falciparum* exist in Central America, Mexico, Haiti, the Dominican Republic, and the Middle East (Figure 1 on page 05).
- Chloroquine-resistant strains have been reported in all other malarious regions.
- Mefloquine-resistant strains of *P. falciparum* have been reported in rural areas of Thailand along the Myanmar and Cambodian borders and in Papua New Guinea.
- Atovaquone-proguanil (Malarone) is the drug of choice for these areas. Gastrointestinal irritation is the most prominent complication.
- Doxycycline is an alternative prophylactic agent for these areas.

IMMUNIZATIONS
Routine Childhood Vaccines
- Guidelines for immunizations in travelers are reviewed in Table B, on page 504.
- All travelers who have not completed a primary series or who have not had a booster during the past 10 years should receive a booster.
- Travelers who will be visiting countries where poliomyelitis remains endemic should receive a single booster of the polio vaccine. Because of the rare risk of vaccine-associated poliomyelitis, the enhanced inactivated polio vaccine (eIPV) should be used, unless the traveler can verify previous immunization with the live attenuated oral vaccine (OPV).
- All adult travelers born after 1956 should have received at least 2 doses of the live attenuated MMR vaccine.
- Hepatitis B vaccination should be considered for travelers who plan to spend prolonged periods abroad (i.e., 6 months), health care workers not previously vaccinated, and short-term travelers who may engage in high-risk sexual activity.
- Varicella immunization should be considered for nonimmune travelers, especially if they plan to have extensive contact with local populations.

Vector-borne Disease
- Yellow fever, a mosquito-borne viral infection, is found in certain parts of sub-Saharan Africa and South America (Figure 2 on page 507). Although yellow fever is rare in travelers, the risk of 1:280 in epidemic areas and 1:4,200 in endemic areas for Africa and 1:2,800 and 1: 42,000 to South America respectively underline the importance of vaccination for this disease. Yellow fever vaccine is required for all travelers for entry into some countries (e.g., Liberia). Some countries require travelers who have recently been in a yellow fever zone to provide documentation of vaccination (International Certificate of Vaccination).
- Japanese encephalitis is a mosquito-borne viral encephalitis common in many parts of Asia. Peak transmission generally occurs during the summer and autumn in regions with temperate climates. The vaccine should be considered for expatriates and travelers who will be spending 30 days in rural areas during seasons of peak transmission. Personal protection measures, as described for malaria prevention, should be followed.
- Tick-borne encephalitis is a form of viral encephalitis transmitted by the tick, *Ixodes ricinus*, in Scandinavia, Western and Central Europe, and many former Soviet Union countries. Peak transmission occurs from April to August. A closely related disease, Russian spring–summer encephalitis, is transmitted by *Ixodes persulcatus* ticks in eastern Russia, Korea, and China. Travelers who visit forested areas or consume unpasteurized dairy products should be advised. Effective vaccines are available in Europe but not in the US.

Food- And Water-Borne Disease
- Proof of cholera vaccination is no longer officially required for entry into any country. Because cholera is rare in travelers and because the vaccine is not very effective (only about 50% protective for *Vibrio cholerae* 01), it is rarely recommended. Travelers who will be staying in highly endemic areas with poor access to clean water, sanitary facilities, and medical care or who have compromised gastric defenses (achlorhydria, antacid therapy, or status post-gastrectomy) should be considered for vaccination.
- Hepatitis A is hyperendemic in all developing countries and is the most common vaccine-preventable disease in returning travelers in whom it is responsible for significant morbidity and productive time lost from work. Young children tend to have mild to asymptomatic infections. The risk of severe infection with jaundice increases with age. For travelers, the risk of hepatitis A acquisition increases with the length of stay. At highest risk are travelers who visit rural areas, hike in back country, and consume food and beverages or have close contact with locals in settings with poor sanitation. Immigrants from developing countries frequently are immune; if time permits, serologic testing for hepatitis A antibody should be performed, because vaccination may be unnecessary. Immunoglobulin provides short-term protection from hepatitis A (85% effective). It should be considered for short-term travelers and can be administered in combination with the hepatitis A vaccines if immediate travel to a developing country is planned. For individuals who travel frequently to endemic areas or who will be at high risk, there are two highly effective, inactivated-virus vaccines for hepatitis A licensed in the US: Havrix and Vaqta. Both provide 95–100% protection. Vaccines will develop a protective immune response in 2–4 weeks.
- Travelers who will be spending several weeks in endemic areas, eating or drinking in the setting of poor sanitation, or visiting rural areas should be considered for typhoid vaccination. Countries with especially high rates of typhoid fever include India, Nepal, Pakistan, and Peru. 3 vaccines are available for the prevention of typhoid fever, and they vary in terms of side effects. Ty21a is a live, attenuated, oral typhoid vaccine administered as 4 capsules; is must be stored in a refrigerator and must be taken on an empty stomach. A newer, purified, capsular polysaccharide vaccine consists of a single infection and can be used in young children who cannot swallow capsules. The original typhoid vaccine (composed of phenol-inactivated *Salmonella typhi*) is rarely used because it has many side effects. All 3 vaccines have similar protective efficacy (ranging from 50–80%) but have never been evaluated prospectively in travelers or in comparative clinical trials.

(continued)

Table 11. Prevention of Travel-Related Illness (continued)

Additional Immunization

- Influenza vaccine should be considered for travelers to tropical countries at any time of the year, or to the Southern Hemisphere from April to September. The most recently released, available vaccine should be used.
- Meningococcal vaccination should be considered for travelers to countries known to have epidemic meningococcal disease caused by a vaccine-preventable serogroup (A, C, W-135, Y). High-risk countries include sub-Saharan countries in savanna areas from Mali to Ethiopia, Kenya, Rwanda, Burundi, Tanzania, India, and Nepal. Travelers to Saudi Arabia during the hajj also should be immunized.
- Dogs are an important reservoir of rabies in less-developed areas of the world. Preexposure vaccination is recommended for persons who will be living in or spending prolonged periods (30 days) in areas of the world where rabies is endemic. In addition, vaccination should be considered for short-term travelers involved in activities that place them at high risk of exposure, such as spelunking, hunting, trekking, and veterinary work. Travelers should be advised that, if bitten or scratched by a potentially rabid animal, they must clean the wound with soap and water and receive postexposure prophylaxis.

SPECIAL SITUATIONS

Immunocompromised Travelers

- Because morbidity and, potentially, mortality from many enteric infections may be increased in immunocompromised travelers, they should be advised to adhere strictly to food and water precautions. Attention to personal protection measures also must be emphasized, because certain vector-borne diseases may be more severe or more difficult to treat in certain immunocompromised groups (e.g., patients with HIV and visceral leishmaniasis). Certain countries have imposed restrictions on the entry of HIV-seropositive travelers and may even require HIV testing for certain risk groups before entry.
- All live attenuated vaccines should be avoided in immunocompromised subjects (although HIV-seropositive persons may receive the MMR vaccine). HIV-seropositive or other immunocompromised travelers should be given a letter of waiver for the yellow fever vaccine if they are traveling to regions where yellow fever is endemic or proof of vaccination is required. (Vaccination can be considered for asymptomatic HIV-seropositive patients with CD4 cell counts of 200 if the risk of yellow fever exposure is high). Inactivated vaccines should be considered for immunocompromised travelers as indicated by itinerary. However, the response to immunization may be impaired, depending on the degree of immune impairment. If time permits, post-vaccination serologic testing should be performed to verify a response to vaccination.

Pregnant Travelers

- The pregnant traveler should be sure that proper prenatal and obstetric medical care will be available at her destinations and that her health insurance will provide coverage there for her and her child. Vigorous exercise, high altitude (generally 1,500 m), and high-risk adventure travel should be avoided.
- Flying after week 35 of pregnancy is not advised, and may be prohibited by many airlines. During the flight, pregnant travelers should frequently move about the cabin to prevent deep venous thrombosis but should avoid being traumatized.
- Chloroquine and proguanil are considered safe for use during pregnancy. Mefloquine may be considered for use after the first trimester. Doxycycline should be avoided because it may lead to staining of fetal bones and teeth. Atuone-proguanil is a category C drug.
- Pregnant travelers should adhere strictly to food and water precautions. Prophylactic drug therapy should generally be avoided. The antimotility agents, loperamide and diphenoxylate are not known to be teratogenic and have been used safely in pregnancy. Fluoroquinolones and doxycycline should be avoided. Trimethoprim–sulfamethoxazole may be used safely for the treatment of traveler's diarrhea in the second trimester only.
- Live attenuated vaccines are generally contraindicated in pregnancy and during the 3 months before conception. Yellow fever and oral polio vaccines may be administered if the risk of exposure is high. Inactivated vaccines are probably safe.

SCHISTOSOMIASIS

- This infection is endemic in many areas of Latin America, the Caribbean, Africa, and Asia. Wading or swimming in freshwater bodies in rural areas where the appropriates nail host exists places travelers at risk for the acquisition of schistosomiasis. Swimming and wading in freshwater bodies in rural areas of endemic countries, therefore, should be avoided. Swimming in adequately chlorinated swimming pools or in salt water is unlikely to lead to schistosomiasis.

Table A. Malaria Chemoprophylaxis Regimes

Drug	Adults	Children	Adverse Effects	Contraindications and Warnings
Chloroquine[a]	300 mg base/wk	5 mg base/kg/wk (maximum 300 mg)	Nausea, headache, pruritus, dizziness, blurred vision	May exacerbate psoriasis; may impede antibody response to intradermal rabies vaccine
Mefloquine[a]	250 mg (1 tablet)/wk	<3 months or 5 kg: no data 5–9 kg; 1/8 tablet/wk 10–19 kg: 1/4 tablet/wk 20–30 kg: 1/2 tablet/wk 31–34 kg: 3/4 tablet/wk >45 kg: 1 tablet/wk	Nausea, dizziness, insomnia, rash, nightmares; rarely, seizures, psychosis, hallucinations, mood changes	Known hypersensitivity to mefloquine, history of seizures or severe psychiatric disorders, cardiac conduction abnormalities, concomitant use of β-blockers for arrhythmias
Doxycycline[b]	100 mg daily	Contraindicated if age <8 yr ≥8 yr: 2 mg/kg/d up to adult dose	Photosensitivity, nausea, vomiting, vaginal yeast infections	Pregnancy, children <8 yr
Chloroquine + proguanil[c]	300 mg base/wk + 200 mg daily	5 mg base/kg/wk to maximum of 300 mg <2 yr: 1/4 adult dose 2–6 yr: 1/2 adult dose 7–10 yr: 3/4 adult dose 10 yr: 200 mg daily	Proguanil may cause nausea, vomiting, mouth ulcers, hair loss	
Atovaquone-proguanil[d]	250 mg atovaquone + 100 mg proguanil	5–8 kg 1/2 pediatric tablet 8–10 kg 3/4 pediatric tablet 10–20 kg 1 pediatric tablet 20–30 kg 2 pediatric tablets 30–40 kg 3 pediatric tablets 40 kg 1 adult tablet	Nausea, vomiting, abdominal pain, diarrhea, hepatitis, seizures, rash	Pregnancy

[a] Should be started 2 weeks before entering malarious area, then each week during travel, and for 4 weeks after exiting the malarious region.
[b] Should be started 2 days before entering malarious area, continued daily during travel, and for 4 weeks after exiting the malarious region.
[c] Proguanil is not licensed for use in the US but is available in Canada and most West European countries.
[d] Should be started 2 days before entering malarious area, continued daily during travel, and for 1 week after exiting the malarious region. Taken with fat meal.
Source: From Gorbach SL. 1999 *Guidelines for infectious diseases in primary care* and Keystone S. J. 2008 *Travel Medicine*

Table B. Immunizations for Travel

Vaccine	Primary Series[a]	Booster	Adverse Effects	Contraindications and Precautions
Routine vaccines				
Tetanus/diphtheria	Adults and children >7 yr: 3 doses (0.5 mL IM or SC) at 0, 4–8 wk, 6–12 mo	Every 10 yr	Pain or erythema at injection site, fever; rarely, anaphylaxis	History of neurologic or severe hypersensitivity reaction to the vaccine
Polio[b]	Adults: eIPV preferable. 3 doses (0.5 mL SC) at 0, 4–8 wk, 6–12 mo	Single dose once as an adult if traveling to endemic areas	Pain or erythema at injection site	Concurrent moderate-to-severe illness; history of anaphylactic reaction to the vaccine or to neomycin, polymyxin B, or streptomycin
Measles, mumps, rubella[b]	Adults born in or after 1957 should have received 2 doses (0.5 mL Sc) of MMR 1+ mo apart		Injection site discomfort, fever, lymphadenopathy, arthralgias; rarely, transient arthritis (especially in women)	Concurrent moderate-to-severe illness; history of anaphylactic reaction to the vaccine or to eggs; pregnancy; should not be given to immunocompromised persons, except those with HIV
Hepatitis B	Adults >20 yr: 3 doses (1.0 mL IM) at 0, 4, and 24 wk Children 11–19 yr: 3 doses (0.5 mL IM) at 0, 4, and 24 wk	Need for boosters has not yet been determined; nonresponders should receive 3 additional doses	Injection site discomfort, fatigue, fever, headache, nausea	Concurrent moderate-to-severe illness; history of anaphylactic reaction to the vaccine, thimerosal, or yeast
Varicella	Adults and adolescents ≥13 yr: 2 doses (0.5 mL SC) at 0 and 4–8 wk	Not currently recommended	Redness, swelling, or pain at the injection site; fever, varicella-like rash (may be local or generalized)	Concurrent moderate-to-severe illness; adolescents undergoing aspirin therapy; history of anaphylactic reaction to the vaccine, gelatin, or neomycin; pregnancy; should not be given to immunocompromised individuals
Vector-borne diseases				
Yellow fever[b]	>9 mo of age: 0.5 mL SC	1 dose every 10 yr	Injection site discomfort, headaches, low-grade fevers, myalgias; rarely, hypersensitivity reactions	History of anaphylactic reaction to the vaccine or to eggs; avoid in children <4 mo of age, pregnancy, immunocompromised individuals
Japanese B encephalitis	>3 yr: 3 doses (1.0 mL SC), at 0,7, 14–28 d 1–3 yr: 3 doses (1.0 mL SC) at 0, 7, 14–28 d	Single dose of 1.0 mL SC for all age groups at ≥3 yr	Local reactions, fever, headaches, myalgias; less commonly, hypersensitivity reactions (may be delayed as long as 1 week after immunization)[c]	History of anaphylactic reaction to the vaccine; pregnancy; increased risk of allergic reactions in persons with a history of urticaria

Table B. Immunizations for Travel (continued)

Vaccine	Primary Series[a]	Booster	Adverse Effects	Contraindications and Precautions
Food- and water-borne diseases				
Cholera	Given as 2 doses, IM or SC ≥1 wk apart 6 mo–4 yr: 0.2 mL 5–10 yr: 0.3 mL ≥10 yr: 0.5 mL	Single dose every 6 mo	Pain, swelling, and redness at injection site; fever, fatigue, headache	Concurrent moderate-to-severe illness; history of anaphylactic reaction to the vaccine; should be administered ≥3 wk apart from yellow fever vaccine
Hepatitis A	Immunoglobulin: 2–5 mL IM shortly before travel	Immunoglobulin: Must be repeated every 4 mo	Immunoglobulin: Injection site discomfort	Concurrent moderate-to-severe illness; history of anaphylactic reaction to the vaccine
	Havrix or Vaqta: >18 yr—1.0 mL IM 2–18 yr—0.5 mL IM; both given ≥2 wk before travel	Havrix or Vaqta: >18 yr—1.0 mL IM at 6–12 mo; 2–18 yr—0.5 mL IM at 6–12 mo	Harvix or Vaqta: injection site pain, fatigue, fever, headache	
Typhoid fever	Ty21a (oral vaccine) ≥6 yr: 4 capsules on days 1, 3, 5, and 7 Purified Vi polysaccharide vaccine ≥2 yr: 1 dose (0.5 mL IM)	Ty21a: Repeat full series every 5 yr Vi: Every 2 yr	Ty21a: Nausea, abdominal cramps; rarely, vomiting, fever, rash, headache Vi: Local pain, fever, headache	Concurrent moderate-to-severe illness, history of anaphylactic reaction to either vaccine; Ty21a: avoid in immunocompromised patients, pregnancy, children <6 yr, and during antibiotic use

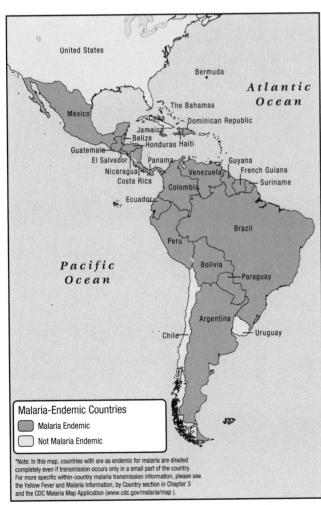

Malaria-Endemic Countries
- Malaria Endemic
- Not Malaria Endemic

*Note: In this map, countries with are as endemic for malaria are shaded completely even if transmission occurs only in a small part of the country. For more specific within-country malaria transmission information, please see the Yellow Fever and Malaria Information, by Country section in Chapter 3 and the CDC Malaria Map Application (www.cdc.gov/malaria/map).

FIGURE 1. Distribution of malaria and chloroquine-resistant *Plasmodium falciparum*. From Centers for Disease Control and Prevention. CDC Health Information for International Travel 2012. New York: Oxford University Press; 2012. (*continued*)

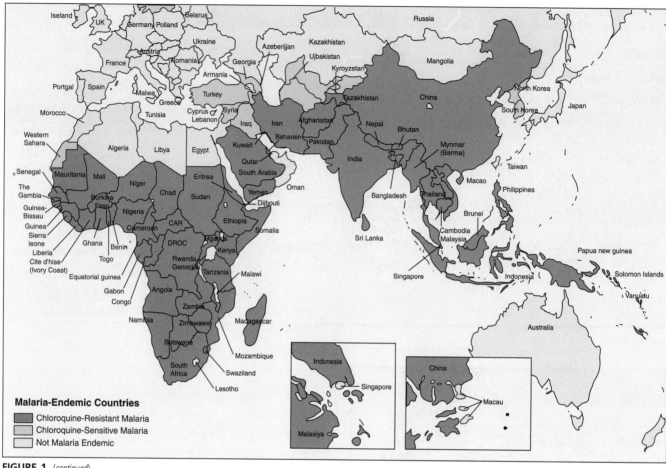

FIGURE 1. (*continued*)

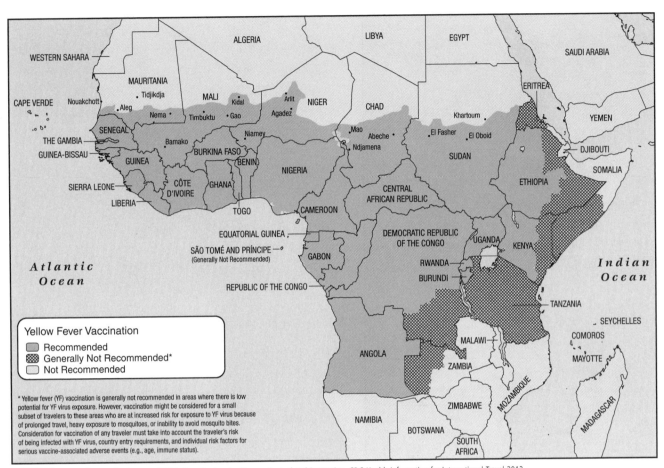

FIGURE 2. Yellow fever endemic zones (2009). From Centers for Disease Control and Prevention. CDC Health Information for International Travel 2012. New York: Oxford University Press; 2012. (*continued*)

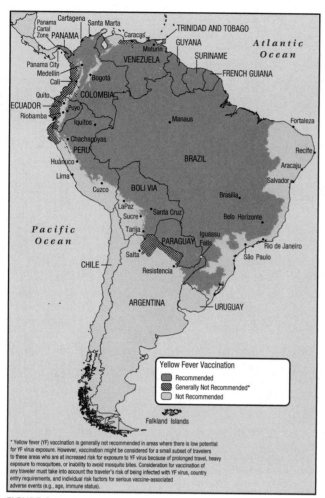

* Yellow fever (YF) vaccination is generally not recommended in areas where there is low potential for YF virus exposure. However, vaccination might be considered for a small subset of travelers to these areas who are at increased risk for exposure to YF virus because of prolonged travel, heavy exposure to mosquitoes, or inability to avoid mosquito bites. Consideration for vaccination of any traveler must take into account the traveler's risk of being infected with YF virus, country entry requirements, and individual risk factors for serious vaccine-associated adverse events (e.g., age, immune status).

FIGURE 2. (*continued*)

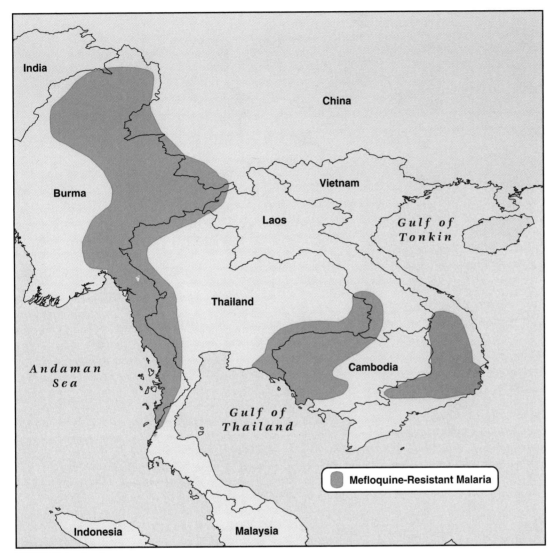

FIGURE 2. (*continued*)

INDEX